# CRITICAL CARE
# ECHOCARDIOGRAPHY
## *REVIEW*
# 1200+
## QUESTIONS AND ANSWERS

# CRITICAL CARE ECHOCARDIOGRAPHY

## *REVIEW*

### 1200+ QUESTIONS AND ANSWERS

## EDITORS

**Marvin G. Chang, MD, PhD**
Director, Perioperative Transthoracic Echocardiography (Point of Care Ultrasound)
Assistant Program Director, Critical Care Fellowship
Assistant Professor, Harvard Medical School
Division of Critical Care and Cardiac Anesthesia
Department of Anesthesia, Critical Care and Pain Medicine
Massachusetts General Hospital
Boston, Massachusetts

**Abraham Sonny, MD, FASE**
Assistant Professor, Harvard Medical School
Division of Critical Care and Cardiac Anesthesia
Department of Anesthesia, Critical Care, and Pain Medicine
Massachusetts General Hospital
Boston, Massachusetts

**David M. Dudzinski, MD, FASE**
Director, Cardiac Intensive Care Unit
Cardiac Ultrasound Laboratory, Division of Cardiology
Assistant Professor, Harvard Medical School
Department of Medicine and Heart Center
Massachusetts General Hospital
Boston, Massachusetts

**Sheri M. Berg, MD**
Medical Director, Post-Anesthesia Care Units
Director of Anesthesia, ECT Service
Director of Anesthesia, MGH Ketamine Clinic
Assistant Professor, Harvard Medical School
Division of Critical Care
Department of Anesthesia, Critical Care and Pain Medicine
Massachusetts General Hospital
Boston, Massachusetts

**Christopher R. Tainter, MD, RDMS**
Program Director, Critical Care Fellowship
Associate Clinical Professor
Division of Critical Care
Department of Anesthesiology
University of California San Diego School of Medicine
La Jolla, California

**Ryan J. Horvath, MD, PhD**
Instructor, Harvard Medical School
Division of Critical Care and Cardiac Anesthesia
Department of Anesthesia, Critical Care and Pain Medicine
Massachusetts General Hospital
Boston, Massachusetts

**Edward A. Bittner, MD, PhD, MSEd, FCCM**
Associate Director, Surgical Intensive Care Unit
Program Director, Critical Care Fellowship
Associate Professor, Harvard Medical School
Division of Critical Care
Department of Anesthesia, Critical Care and Pain Medicine
Massachusetts General Hospital
Boston, Massachusetts

. Wolters Kluwer

Philadelphia • Baltimore • New York • London
Buenos Aires • Hong Kong • Sydney • Tokyo

*Senior Acquisitions Editor:* Keith Donnellan
*Senior Development Editor:* Ashley Fischer
*Editorial Coordinator:* Ann Francis
*Marketing Manager:* Kirstin Watrud
*Senior Production Project Manager:* Alicia Jackson
*Manager, Graphic Arts & Design:* Stephen Druding
*Senior Manufacturing Coordinator:* Beth Welsh
*Prepress Vendor:* S4Carlisle Publishing Services

9 8 7 6 5 4 3 2 1

Printed in Mexico

**Library of Congress Cataloging-in-Publication Data**
ISBN-13: 978-1-9751-4413-5
ISBN-10: 1-9751-4413-9
Library of Congress Control Number: 2021913874

Cataloging in Publication data available on request from publisher.

shop.lww.com

# DEDICATION

To our families, colleagues, and trainees who inspired us to create this resource

# PREFACE

Critical care ultrasound is an invaluable bedside tool for diagnosis and facilitating treatment of patients in a wide number of clinical settings including the intensive care unit, emergency department, operating room, postanesthesia care unit, hospital ward, and prehospital setting. With the introduction of the Examination of Special Competence in Critical Care Echocardiography (CCEeXAM) by the National Board of Echocardiography in 2019, there is now a defined pathway for critical care physicians to obtain formal certification in critical care echocardiography. While there are a number of excellent resources available for critical care echocardiography in a variety of formats and media, there is no stand-alone comprehensive question and answer resource available to facilitate learning and review for all practitioners. This book was designed to fill this educational gap by providing a comprehensive question and answer resource designed for practitioners preparing for the CCEeXAM as well as those interested in expanding their knowledge of critical care ultrasound through a self-paced, iterative, and active learning process. We were inspired by our trainees and faculty colleagues who were seeking such a resource that would cover the major areas of critical care ultrasonography. The chapters in this book are authored by leaders in their field including cardiology, cardiac critical care, medical and surgical critical care, emergency medicine, hospital medicine, and anesthesiology as well as echocardiography and ultrasound imaging. In addition to critical care echocardiography, this book covers all aspects of critical care ultrasonography including heart, lung, vascular, and abdominal imaging as well as applications in airway management, ventilator weaning, extracorporeal support device insertion, and real-time procedural guidance. Our hope is that this book will provide readers, in diverse practice settings, with both the qualitative and quantitative assessment skills to pass the written CCEeXAM, the confidence to better integrate ultrasonography into their clinical practice, and ultimately to improve the care of their patients. We are thankful and grateful for the hard work of our contributors and editors from diverse clinical backgrounds and leaders in critical care ultrasound to provide our trainees and colleagues worldwide with the best available question and answer resource on critical care ultrasound, and hope to improve on this resource in future editions.

# ASSOCIATE EDITORS

**John C. Klick, MD, FCCP, FASE, FCCM**
Associate Professor
Department of Anesthesiology
University of Vermont Larner College of
    Medicine
Cardiothoracic Anesthesiologist and
    Intensivist
University of Vermont Medical Center
Burlington, Vermont

**Thomas Carver, MD, FACS**
Medical Director, Surgical Intensive Care Unit
Program Director, Surgical Critical Care
    Fellowship
Associate Professor
Division of Trauma and Critical Care
Department of Surgery
Medical College of Wisconsin
Milwaukee, Wisconsin

**Jan Kasal, MD, FASE**
Co-Director, Critical Care Ultrasound
    Training Program
Associate Professor
Division of Critical Care
Department of Anesthesiology
Washington University School of
    Medicine
St. Louis, Missouri

**Michael J. Lanspa, MD, FASE, FCCM**
Adjunct Associate Professor
Department of Medicine
University of Utah School of Medicine
Salt Lake City, Utah
Director
Critical Care Echocardiography Service
Intermountain Medical Center
Murray, Utah

# CONTRIBUTORS

**Suresh "Mitu" Agarwal, MD, FACS, FCCM**
Professor and Division Chief
Trauma, Acute and Critical Care Surgery
Department of Surgery
Duke University Health System
Durham, North Carolina

**Katherine Albutt, MD, MPH**
Surgical Critical Care Fellow, Harvard
    Medical School
Division of Trauma, Emergency Surgery
    and Surgical Critical Care
Department of Surgery
Massachusetts General Hospital
Boston, Massachusetts

**Fawaz Alenezi, MD, MSc**
Assistant Professor of Medicine
Division of Cardiology
Department of Internal Medicine
Duke University Medical Center
Durham, North Carolina

**Osaid Alser, MD, MSc (Oxon)**
Postdoctoral Research Fellow, Harvard
    Medical School
Division of Trauma, Emergency Surgery
    and Surgical Critical Care
Massachusetts General Hospital
Boston, Massachusetts

**Lovkesh Arora, MBBS, MD**
Clinical Associate Professor
Department of Anesthesia
University of Iowa Hospitals and
    Clinics
Iowa City, Iowa

**Aranya Bagchi, MBBS**
Assistant Professor, Harvard Medical
    School
Staff Intensivist
Department of Anesthesia, Critical Care
    and Pain Medicine
Massachusetts General Hospital
Boston, Massachusetts

**Jina Bai, PA-C**
Instructor in Hospital Medicine
Weill Cornell Medicine
Internal Medicine
New York Presbyterian
New York, New York

**Brittany K. Bankhead-Kendall, MD, MS**
Assistant Professor
Department of Surgery
Texas Tech University Health Sciences
    Center
Lubbock, Texas

**William Beaubien-Souligny, MD, PhD**
Assistant Professor
Staff Nephrologist—Researcher
Department of Medicine
Université de Montréal
Centre Hospitalier de l'Université de
    Montréal
Montreal, Quebec, Canada

**Ali H. Bedair, MD**
Clinical Fellow, Adult Cardiothoracic
    Anesthesiology
Department of Anesthesiology
Vanderbilt University School of
    Medicine
Vanderbilt University Medical Center
Nashville, Tennessee

**Samuel Bernard, MD**
Cardiac Ultrasound Laboratory
Harvard Medical School
Massachusetts General Hospital
Boston, Massachusetts

**Philippe B. Bertrand, MD, PhD**
Staff Cardiologist/Echocardiography
Department of Cardiology
Ziekenhuis Oost-Limburg
Genk, Belgium
Hasselt University
Hasselt, Belgium

**Charles Lessard Brassard, MD, FRCPC**
Department of Anesthesiology and
    Intensive Care Medicine
Université Laval
Department of Anesthesiology
Institut universitaire de cardiologie et de
    pneumologie de Québec (IUCPQ)
Quebec City, Quebec, Canada

**Yuriy S. Bronshteyn, MD, FASE**
Assistant Professor
Intensivist, Anesthesiologist
Department of Anesthesiology
Duke University School of Medicine
Department of Anesthesiology
Duke University Health System
Durham, North Carolina

**Casey D. Bryant, MD**
Assistant Professor
Department of Anesthesiology—
    Section on Critical Care
Department of Emergency Medicine
Wake Forest University School of Medicine
Winston-Salem, North Carolina

**Nibras Bughrara, MD, FCCM, FASA**
Chief, Anesthesia Critical Care Division
Director, Critical Care Echocardiography
    Program
Medical Director, MSICU
Associate Professor
Departments of Anesthesiology and
    Surgery
Albany Medical College
Department of Anesthesiology
Albany Medical Center
Albany, New York

**Arielle Butterly, MD**
Director, Cardiovascular
    Critical Care
Department of Anesthesia and
    Critical Care
Maine Medical Center
Portland, Maine

**Stephanie Cha, MD**
Assistant Professor
Department of Anesthesiology and Critical
    Care
Johns Hopkins University School of
    Medicine
Baltimore, Maryland

**Andrew N. Chalupka, MD, MBA**
Assistant Professor of Anesthesiology
Senior Associate Consultant
Department of Anesthesiology and
    Perioperative Medicine
Mayo Clinic College of Medicine
Department of Anesthesiology and
    Perioperative Medicine
Mayo Clinic
Rochester, Minnesota

**Lydia Chang, MD, FCCP**
Clinical Associate Professor
Division of Pulmonary and Critical
    Care Medicine
University of North Carolina School
    of Medicine
Chapel Hill, North Carolina

**Chuan-Jay Jeffrey Chen, MD**
Resident Physician, Harvard Medical
    School
Harvard Affiliated Emergency Medicine
    Residency
Department of Emergency Medicine
Brigham and Women's Hospital
Massachusetts General Hospital
Boston, Massachusetts

**Vinca W. Chow, MD**
Assistant Professor of Anesthesiology,
    Geisel School of Medicine at
    Darthmouth
Department of Anesthesiology
Geisel School of Medicine at
    Dartmouth
Hanover, New Hampshire
Physician Anesthesiologist
Department of Anesthesiology
Dartmouth-Hitchcock Medical Center
Lebanon, New Hampshire

**Gian Alfonso Cibinel, MD**
Consultant in Emergency Medicine and
    Strategic Planning
Department of Emergency Medicine
"E. Agnelli" General Hospital
Pinerolo, Turin, Italy

**Jacob Clark, MD**
Assistant Clinical Professor
Department of Anesthesia
Tufts University School of Medicine
Boston, Massachusetts
Clinical Anesthesiologist
Department of Anesthesia
Southcoast Health
St. Luke's Hospital
New Bedford, Massachusetts

**Christopher Collins, MD**
Fellow
Division of Anesthesia Critical
    Care
Department of Anesthesia
Duke University Medical Center
Durham, North Carolina

**Daniel S. Cormican, MD, FCCP**
Anesthesiologist and Intensivist
Anesthesiology Institute
Allegheny Health Network
Pittsburgh, Pennsylvania

**Etienne J. Couture, MD, FRCPC**
Clinical Instructor
Department of Anesthesiology and
    Intensive Care
Université Laval
Anesthesiologist and Intensivist
Department of Anesthesiology and Intensive
    Care Medicine
Department of Medicine
Institut universitaire de cardiologie et
    de pneumologie de Québec
    (IUCPQ)
Quebec City, Quebec, Canada

**Morgan J. Crigger, MD**
Resident
Department of Surgery
University of Arizona School of
    Medicine—Phoenix
Resident
Department of Surgery
Banner University Medical Center—
    Phoenix
Phoenix, Arizona

**Talal Dahhan, MD, MMEL, FACP, FCCP**
Assistant Professor of Medicine
Division of Pulmonary, Allergy
    and Critical Care Medicine
Department of Medicine
Duke University School of
    Medicine
Durham, North Carolina

**Adam A. Dalia, MD, MBA, FASE**
Assistant Professor, Harvard Medical
    School
Department of Anesthesia, Critical Care
    and Pain Medicine
Director of Perioperative Echocardiography
Division of Cardiac Anesthesiology
Massachusetts General Hospital
Boston, Massachusetts

**Robert Deegan, MB, ChB, BAO, PhD, FFARCSI**
Professor
Division of Cardiothoracic Anesthesiology
Department of Anesthesiology
Vanderbilt University School of Medicine
Vanderbilt University Medical Center
Nashville, Tennessee

**Andre Y. Denault, MD, PhD, FRCPC, FASE, ABIM-CCM, FCCS**
Professor
Critical Care Division, Department of
    Anesthesia
Université de Montréal
Point-of Care Ultrasound Fellowship
    Program Director
Critical Care Division, Department of
    Anesthesia
Institut de Cardiologie de Montréal
Montreal, Quebec, Canada

**Lev Deriy, MD**
Associate Professor
Department of Anesthesiology and
    Critical Care
University of New Mexico School
    of Medicine
Albuquerque, New Mexico

**Rasesh Desai, MD**
Assistant Professor
Department of Anesthesiology
Duke University School of Medicine
Duke University Medical Center
Durham, North Carolina

**Ranjit Deshpande, MD, FCCM**
Assistant Professor of Anesthesiology
Director of Transplant Anesthesiology
Director Ultrasound Education

Yale School of Medicine
Yale University Medical Center
New Haven, Connecticut

**David M. Dudzinski, MD, FASE**
Director, Cardiac Intensive Care Unit
Cardiac Ultrasound Laboratory, Division of
    Cardiology
Assistant Professor, Harvard Medial School
Department of Medicine and Heart Center
Massachusetts General Hospital
Boston, Massachusetts

**Susan Eagle, MD**
Professor
Division of Cardiothoracic
    Anesthesiology
Department of Anesthesiology
Vanderbilt University School of Medicine
Vanderbilt University Medical Center
Nashville, Tennessee

**Sarah Ellis, MD**
Assistant Professor
Department of Anesthesiology
McGovern Medical School at UTHealth
Houston, Texas

**Allison C. Ferreira, MD**
Assistant Clinical Professor
Critical Care Division
Department of Emergency
    Medicine
David Geffen School of Medicine
    at UCLA
Los Angeles, California

**Natalie Ferrero, MD**
Assistant Professor
Department of Anesthesiology
Emory University School of Medicine
Atlanta, Georgia

**Vikram Fielding-Singh, MD, JD**
Clinical Assistant Professor
Department of Anesthesiology,
    Perioperative and Pain Medicine
Stanford University School
    of Medicine
Stanford, California

**Karim Fikry, MD**
Assistant Professor
Department of Anesthesia
Tufts University School of Medicine
Boston, Massachusetts
Division Director, Anesthesia Critical
    Care
Department of Anesthesia, Critical Care
    and Pain Medicine
Lahey Hospital and Medical Center
Burlington, Massachusetts

**Babar Fiza, MD**
Assistant Professor, Program Director,
    Anesthesiology Critical Care Medicine
    Fellowship
Department of Anesthesiology
Emory University School of Medicine
Atlanta, Georgia

**Molly Flannagan, MD**
Assistant Professor
Department of Anesthesiology
Uniformed Services University of Health
    Sciences
Bethesda, Maryland
Cardiovascular and Critical Care
    Anesthesiologist
Department of Anesthesiology
Brooke Army Medical Center
Fort Sam Houston, Texas

**Rachel C. Frank, MD**
Fellow, Cardiovascular Medicine
Department of Medicine
Massachusetts General Hospital
Boston, Massachusetts

**John P. Gaillard, MD**
Associate Professor
Department of Anesthesiology—Section on
    Critical Care
Department of Emergency Medicine
Department of Internal Medicine—Section
    of Pulmonary, Critical Care, Allergy and
    Immunologic Diseases
Wake Forest University School of Medicine
Wake Forest Baptist Health
Winston Salem, North Carolina

**Elaine Y. Gee, MD**
Assistant Professor
Department of Medicine
Weill Cornell Medicine
Assistant Attending Physician
Department of Medicine
New York-Presbyterian Hospital/Weill
    Cornell Medical Center
New York, New York

**Lyle Gerety, MD**
Division Chief, Critical Care Medicine
Division of Critical Care Medicine
Department of Anesthesiology
University of Vermont Larner College of
    Medicine
University of Vermont Medical Center
Burlington, Vermont

**Neal S. Gerstein, MD, FASE**
Professor of Anesthesiology
Department of Anesthesiology and Critical
    Care Medicine
University of New Mexico School of
    Medicine
Albuquerque, New Mexico

**Mariya Geube, MD, FASE**
Assistant Professor of Anesthesiology
Department of Cardiothoracic Anesthesiology
Cleveland Clinic Lerner College of Medicine
Cleveland, Ohio

**Alberto Goffi, MD**
Assistant Professor
Interdepartmental Division of Critical Care
    Medicine
University of Toronto
Intensivist, Critical Care Medicine
Unity Health Toronto—St. Michael's Hospital
Toronto, Ontario, Canada

**Timothy P. Goldhardt II, MD**
Assistant Professor
Department of Anesthesia
West Virginia University School of Medicine
Cardiothoracic Anesthesiologist
Department of Anesthesia
Ruby Memorial Hospital
Morgantown, West Virginia

**Ellyn Gray, MD**
Anesthesia Resident
Department of Anesthesia
University of Iowa Carver College of
    Medicine
Iowa City, Iowa

**Dusan Hanidziar, MD, PhD**
Anesthesiologist and Intensivist
Instructor in Anesthesia
Department of Anesthesia, Critical Care
    and Pain Medicine
Boston, Massachusetts

**Ahmed Al Hazmi, MBBS**
Emergency Ultrasound Fellow
Department of Emergency Medicine
University of Maryland Medical
    Center
Baltimore, Maryland

**Megan Henley Hicks, MD**
Assistant Professor
Department of Anesthesiology
Wake Forest University School of
    Medicine
Wake Forest Baptist Health
Winston-Salem, North Carolina

**Maxwell A. Hockstein, MD**
Assistant Professor
Department of Emergency Medicine
Georgetown University School of Medicine
Assistant Professor
Department of Critical Care Medicine
Washington Hospital Center
Washington, District of Columbia

**McKenzie M. Hollon, MD, FASE**
Associate Professor of Anesthesiology
Emory University School of Medicine
Director of Perioperative Echocardiography
Department of Anesthesiology
Grady Memorial Hospital
Atlanta, Georgia

**Pamela Y. F. Hsu, MD**
Assistant Professor
Division of Cardiology

Department of Internal Medicine
University of New Mexico School of
    Medicine
Assistant Professor
Division of Cardiology
Department of Internal Medicine
University of New Mexico Hospital
Albuquerque, New Mexico

**Craig S. Jabaley, MD**
Associate Professor
Department of Anesthesiology
Emory University School of Medicine
Critical Care Medicine Division Chief
Department of Anesthesiology
Emory University Hospital
Atlanta, Georgia

**Jonathan T. Jaffe, MD**
Former Critical Care Fellow
Department of Anesthesiology
Wake Forest Baptist Health
Winston-Salem, North Carolina
Intensivist
Department of Critical Care
Houston Methodist Sugar Land Hospital
Sugar Land, Texas

**Todd A. Jaffe, MD**
Clinical Fellow in Emergency Medicine
Department of Emergency Medicine
Harvard Medical School
Resident Physician
Department of Emergency Medicine
Massachusetts General Hospital
Boston, Massachusetts

**Sana Na Javeed, MD**
Faculty
Department of Anesthesiology
NYU Langone
New York, New York

**Christina Anne Jelly, MD, MS**
Assistant Professor of Anesthesiology
Department of Anesthesiology
Vanderbilt University School of Medicine
Vanderbilt University Medical Center
Nashville, Tennessee

**Shawn Jia, MD**
Assistant Professor
Department of Anesthesiology
University of North Carolina School
of Medicine
Chapel Hill, North Carolina

**Zeid Kalarikkal, MD**
Division of Critical Care Medicine
Department of Anesthesiology
University of Nebraska Medical Center
Omaha, Nebraska

**Jan Kasal, MD**
Co-Director, Critical Care Ultrasound
Training Program
Associate Professor
Division of Critical Care
Department of Anesthesiology
Washington University School of
Medicine
St. Louis, Missouri

**George Kasotakis, MD, MPH, FACS, FCCM**
Assistant Professor of Surgery
Division of Trauma and Critical Care
Surgery
Department of Surgery
Duke University School of Medicine
Durham, North Carolina

**Sung Kim, MD**
Fellow, Adult Cardiothoracic
Anesthesiology
Department of Anesthesiology
University of Iowa Carver College of
Medicine
Iowa City, Iowa

**John C. Klick, MD, FCCP, FASE, FCCM**
Associate Professor
Department of Anesthesiology
University of Vermont Larner College
of Medicine
Cardiothoracic Anesthesiologist and
Intensivist
University of Vermont Medical Center
Burlington, Vermont

**Michael Nasr Boles Kot, MD**
Staff Anesthesiologist and Intensivist
Anesthesia Department
Anesthesiology Institute
Cleveland Clinic
Cleveland, Ohio

**Gunter Michael Krauthamer, MD, MA**
Instructor in Emergency Medicine
Geisel School of Medicine at Dartmouth
Lebanon, New Hampshire
Staff Physician
Department of Emergency Medicine
Gifford Medical Center
Randolph, Vermont

**Michael J. Lanspa, MD, MS**
Adjunct Associate Professor
Department of Medicine
University of Utah School of Medicine
Salt Lake City, Utah
Director
Critical Care Echocardiography Service
Intermountain Medical Center
Murray, Utah

**William S. Lao, MD**
Fellow
Division of Surgical Critical Care
Department of Surgery
Duke University School of Medicine
Duke University Medical Center
Durham, North Carolina

**Jarone Lee, MD, MPH, FCCM**
Associate Professor, Harvard Medial School
Departments of Emergency Medicine and
Surgery
Director, Surgical Critical Care
Department of Surgery
Massachusetts General Hospital
Boston, Massachusetts

**Ryan Lefevre, MD**
Assistant Professor
Department of Anesthesiology
Vanderbilt University School of Medicine
Vanderbilt University Medical Center
Nashville, Tennessee

**Tara Ann Lenk, DO**
Anesthesiologist
Boulder Valley Anesthesiology
Boulder, Colorado

**Benjamin S. Levin, MS, MD**
Critical Care Anesthesiologist
Department of Anesthesia and
    Critical Care
Maine Medical Center
Portland, Maine

**Frederick Wilhelm Lombard, MBChB, FANZCA**
Associate Professor
Division of Cardiothoracic Anesthesiology
Department of Anesthesiology
Vanderbilt University School of Medicine
Vanderbilt University Medical Center
Nashville, Tennessee

**Shu Y. Lu, MD**
Clinical Instructor, Harvard Medical School
Division of Cardiac Anesthesia
Department of Anesthesia, Critical Care
    and Pain Medicine
Massachusetts General Hospital
Boston, Massachusetts

**David Luu, MD**
Critical Care Fellow
Department of Anesthesiology
Duke University
Durham, North Carolina
Anesthesiologist Intensivist
Department of Surgery
Baylor University Medical Center
Dallas, Texas

**Jeffrey T. Lyvers, MD**
Staff Physician
Departments of Anesthesiology and
    Critical Care Medicine
Aurora St. Luke's Medical Center
Milwaukee, Wisconsin

**Layne Alan Madden, MD**
Critical Care Fellow
Department of Anesthesiology
Emory University School of Medicine
Atlanta, Georgia

Physician
Departments of Emergency Medicine and
    Critical Care Medicine
Roper St. Francis Healthcare
Charleston, South Carolina

**Negmeldeen Mamoun, MD, PhD**
Assistant Professor
Department of Anesthesiology
Duke University School of
    Medicine
Cardiothoracic Anesthesiologist
Department of Anesthesiology
Duke University Medical Center
Durham, North Carolina

**Hassan Mashbari, MD, MBBS**
Clinical Fellow, Harvard Medical
    School
Division of Trauma, Acute Care Surgery
    and Surgical Critical Care
Massachusetts General Hospital
Boston, Massachusetts

**Sharon L. McCartney, MD, FASE**
Assistant Professor
Department of Anesthesiology
Duke University School of Medicine
Duke University Medical Center
Durham, North Carolina

**Stephen M. McHugh, MD**
Assistant Professor
Department of Anesthesiology and
    Perioperative Medicine
University of Pittsburgh School of
    Medicine
Faculty Anesthesiologist
Department of Anesthesiology and
    Perioperative Medicine
University of Pittsburgh Medical Center
Pittsburgh, Pennsylvania

**Duncan J. McLean, MBChB**
Assistant Professor
University of North Carolina School of
    Medicine
Critical Care Anesthesiologist
UNC Hospitals
Chapel Hill, North Carolina

**Emily Methangkool, MD, MPH**
Associate Clinical Professor
Department of Anesthesiology and
    Perioperative Medicine
Vice Chair, Quality and Patient Safety
Department of Anesthesiology and
    Perioperative Medicine
David Geffen School of Medicine at UCLA
Los Angeles, California

**Gregory Mints, MD, FACP**
Assistant Professor
Department of Medicine
Weill Cornell Medicine
Attending Physician
Department of Medicine
New York Presbyterian Hospital
New York, New York

**John T. Moeller, MD, MS, MHA**
Assistant Professor of Emergency Medicine
Geisel School of Medicine at Dartmouth
Hanover, New Hampshire
Department of Emergency Medicine
Dartmouth Hitchcock Medical Center
Lebanon, New Hampshire

**Matthew Mueller, DO, MPH**
Fellow in Emergency Medicine and
    Anesthesia Critical Care Medicine
Division of Critical Care
Department of Anesthesiology
University of California San Diego School
    of Medicine
La Jolla, California

**William P. Mulvoy III, MD, MPH, MBA**
Assistant Professor
Department of Anesthesiology, Division of
    Critical Care Medicine
Emory University School of Medicine
Department of Anesthesiology
Emory University Hospital
Atlanta, Georgia

**Emily E. Naoum, MD**
Instructor in Anesthesia, Harvard Medical
    School
Department of Anesthesia, Critical Care
    and Pain Medicine
Massachusetts General Hospital
Boston, Massachusetts

**Rohan K. Panchamia, MD**
Assistant Professor of Clinical
    Anesthesiology
Department of Anesthesiology
Weill Cornell Medicine
Assistant Attending Anesthesiologist
Department of Anesthesiology
New York-Presbyterian Hospital
New York, New York

**Christopher N. Parkhurst, MD, PhD**
Instructor of Medicine
Division of Pulmonary and Critical Care
    Medicine
Weill Cornell Medicine
New York-Presbyterian Hospital
New York, New York

**Bhavik P. Patel, MD**
Internal Medicine Resident
Division of General Internal Medicine
Department of Medicine
Duke University School of Medicine
Durham, North Carolina

**Deepa M. Patel, MD**
Assistant Professor
Department of Emergency Medicine
Division of Critical Care, Department
    of Anesthesiology
Emory University School of Medicine
Attending Physician
Department of Emergency Medicine
Division of Critical Care, Department
    of Anesthesiology
Emory University Hospital
Atlanta, Georgia

**Sammy Pedram, MD**
Associate Professor
Division of Pulmonary and Critical Care
    Medicine
Department of Internal Medicine
Virginia Commonwealth University School
    of Medicine
VCU Medical Center
Richmond, Virginia

**Paolo Persona, MD, PhD**
Attending Physician
Institute of Anesthesia and
    Intensive Care
University Hospital of Padua
Padua, Italy

**Alejandro Pino, MD**
Pulmonary and Critical Care Fellow
Division of Pulmonary and Critical Care
    Medicine
Duke University School of Medicine
Durham, North Carolina

**Amit Prabhakar, MD, MS**
Assistant Professor
Department of Anesthesiology
Emory University School of Medicine
Atlanta, Georgia

**Aliaksei Pustavoitau, MD, MHS, FCCM**
Associate Professor
Department of Anesthesiology and Critical
    Care Medicine
Johns Hopkins University School of
    Medicine
Baltimore, Maryland

**Venkatakrishna Rajajee, MD**
Clinical Professor
Departments of Neurosurgery and
    Neurology
University of Michigan Medical School
Medical Director, Neurocritical Care
Michigan Medicine
Ann Arbor, Michigan

**Mohammad R. Rasouli, MD**
Clinical Assistant Professor
Department of Anesthesiology,
    Perioperative and Pain Medicine
Stanford Unversity School of Medicine
Stanford, California

**Matthew D. Read, MD**
Assistant Professor
Department of Anesthesiology
Uniformed Services University of Health
    Sciences

Bethesda, Maryland
Cardiovascular and Critical Care
    Anesthesiologist
Department of Anesthesiology
Brooke Army Medical Center

**J. Mauricio Del Rio, MD, FASE**
CT Surgical Critical Care Physician
Department of Critical Care Medicine
Advent Health Orlando/Florida Hospital
Orlando, Florida

**S. Michael Roberts, DO, FASE**
Assistant Professor
Department of Anesthesiology and
    Perioperative Medicine
Penn State Health Hershey Medical
    Center
Hershey, Pennsylvania

**Radwan Safa, MD, PhD**
Assistant Professor
Departments of Anesthesiology and Sur-
    gery
Albany Medical College
Albany, New York

**Aarti Sarwal, MD, FNCS, FAAN, FCCM**
Professor
Department of Neurology
Wake Forest University School of Medicine
Medical Director/Section Chief
Department of Neurocritical Care
Wake Forest Baptist Health
Winston Salem, North Carolina

**William J. Sauer, MD**
Assistant Professor
Department of Anesthesia
Tufts University School of Medicine
Maine Medical Center
Portland, Maine

**Raghu Seethala, MD**
Division of Emergency Critical Care
    Medicine
Department of Emergency Medicine
Brigham and Women's Hospital
Boston, Massachusetts

**Vicki Sein, MD**
Clinical Instructor
Department of Surgery
The University of Arizona College of
  Medicine—Phoenix
Phoenix, Arizona
Surgeon, Trauma and Critical Care
Banner Thunderbird Medical Center
Glendale, Arizona

**Michael Self, MD**
Fellow
Department of Emergency Medicine
Division of Critical Care, Department
  of Anesthesiology
University of California San Diego School
  of Medicine
La Jolla, California

**Samir Sethi, MD**
Fellow, Cardiac and Critical Care
  Anesthesiology
Department of Anesthesiology
Weill Cornell Medicine
New York, New York

**Archit Sharma, MD, MBA**
Clinical Assistant Professor
Divisions of Cardiothoracic Anesthesiology
Department of Anesthesia, Divisions of
  Solid Organ Transplant and Critical Care
Fellowship Director, Critical Care
  Fellowship
University of Iowa Carver College of Med-
  icine
Iowa City, Iowa

**Matthew Sigakis, MD**
Clinical Assistant Professor
Department of Anesthesiology
University of Michigan Medical School
Ann Arbor, Michigan

**Martin Ingi Sigurdsson, MD, PhD**
Professor of Anesthesiology and Critical
  Care Medicine
Faculty of Medicine
University of Iceland
Chief Physician

Department of Anesthesiology and
  Critical Care
Landspitali—The University Hospital of
  Iceland
Reykjavik, Iceland

**Bryan Simmons, MD**
Staff Anesthesiologist, Intensivist
Departments of Critical Care and
  Anesthesia
Aurora St. Luke's Medical Center
Milwaukee, Wisconsin

**Cameron Smyres, MD**
Clinical Faculty
Department of Emergency Medicine
University of California San Diego School
  of Medicine
La Jolla, California
Clinical Faculty
Department of Emergency Medicine
UC San Diego Medical Center
San Diego, California

**Brian Starr, MD**
Professor of Anesthesiology
Department of Anesthesiology
University of New Mexico School of
  Medicine
University of New Mexico Health Sciences
  Center
Albuquerque, New Mexico

**Genevieve Staudt, MD**
Assistant Professor
Division of Pediatric Cardiac Anesthesiology
Department of Anesthesiology
Vanderbilt University School of
  Medicine
Vanderbilt University Medical Center
Nashville, Tennessee

**Kevin M. Swiatek, DO**
Fellow
Division of Pulmonary and Critical Care
  Medicine
Department of Internal Medicine
Virginia Commonwealth University
Richmond, Virginia

**Christopher R. Tainter, MD, RDMS**
Program Director, Critical Care
    Fellowship
Associate Clinical Professor
Division of Critical Care
Department of Anesthesiology
University of California San Diego School
    of Medicine
La Jolla, California

**Shaun L. Thompson, MD**
Assistant Professor
Department of Anesthesiology
University of Nebraska College of Medicine
Nebraska Medicine
Omaha, Nebraska

**Eli L. Torgeson, MD**
Anesthesiologist
Albuquerque, New Mexico

**Justin G. Vaughan, MD**
Fellow
Division of Surgical Critical Care
Department of Surgery
Duke University Medical Center
Durham, North Carolina

**Carlos E. Vazquez, MD**
Cardiology Chief Fellow
Cardiology Division, Department
    of Internal Medicine
University of New Mexico School of
    Medicine
Cardiology Chief Fellow
Cardiology Division, Department
    of Internal Medicine
University of New Mexico Hospital
Albuquerque, New Mexico

**Chakradhar Venkata, MD**
Clinical Associate Professor, Pulmonary
    and Critical Care Medicine
Saint Louis University School of
    Medicine
Staff Physician
Critical Care Medicine
Mercy Hospital
St Louis, Missouri

**Ranjani Venkataramani, MD, FRCA**
Clinical Assistant Professor
Department of Anesthesiology and
    Critical Care Medicine
University of New Mexico School of
    Medicine
Albuquerque, New Mexico

**Nathan H. Waldron, MD, MHS**
Anesthesiologist/Intensivist
Department of Anesthesiology
UCHealth
Colorado Springs, Colorado

**Trent Lee Wei, MD**
Resident Physician
Department of Medicine
Duke University School of Medicine
Resident Physician
Department of Medicine
Duke University Hospital
Durham, North Carolina

**Meredith L. Whitacre, MD**
Assistant Professor
Department of Anesthesiology
Duke University School of Medicine
Duke University Hospital
Durham, North Carolina

**Tanping Wong, MD**
Associate Professor
Department of Medicine
Weill Cornell Medicine
New York, New York

**Amanda Xi, MD**
Staff Anesthesiologist/Intensivist
Department of Anesthesia, Critical Care,
    and Pain Medicine
Massachusetts General Hospital
Boston, Massachusetts

**Andrew T. Young, MD**
Assistant Clinical Professor
Department of Anesthesiology &
    Perioperative Medicine
David Geffen School of Medicine at UCLA
Ronald Reagan UCLA Medical Center
Los Angeles, California

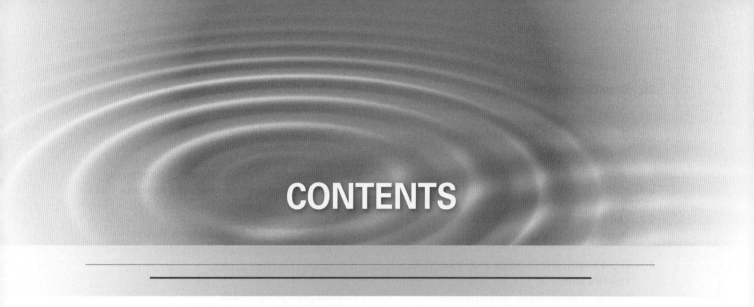

# CONTENTS

# 1 | BASIC ULTRASOUND WAVE PROPERTIES

Michael J. Lanspa

---

**1.** Which of the following will increase the speed of sound transmitting through a medium?

**A.** Increasing the frequency of the sound
**B.** Increasing the density of the medium
**C.** Increasing the stiffness of the medium
**D.** Increasing the wavelength of the sound

---

**2.** Which of the following is true regarding sound?

**A.** Sound is a transverse wave.
**B.** Sound is a longitudinal wave.
**C.** Sound waves transfer mass, not energy, from place to place.
**D.** Sound waves propagate at a constant velocity in a vacuum.

---

**3.** Which of the following remains constant with increasing depth?

**A.** Frequency
**B.** Power
**C.** Amplitude
**D.** Intensity

---

**4.** You perform a chest ultrasound on a patient with a pneumothorax. What is true regarding the ultrasound beam as it travels from soft tissue to air?

**A.** The velocity increases
**B.** The pulse duration increases
**C.** The wavelength decreases
**D.** The frequency decreases

---

**5.** What is the wavelength of a 5 MHz ultrasound traveling through soft tissue?

**A.** 3.25 mm
**B.** 0.308 mm
**C.** 0.154 mm
**D.** 0.616 mm

6. The probe sends out a sound wave and records an echo 0.1 ms later. How deep is the structure that reflected an echo, assuming the medium is soft tissue?

   A. 1.54 cm
   B. 3.08 cm
   C. 7.7 cm
   D. 15.4 cm

7. What is true about the pulse repetition period (PRP) in ultrasound?

   A. The sonographer can change the PRP by increasing the pulse duration.
   B. As the PRP increases, the imaging depth increases.
   C. The PRP is the inverse of the sound frequency.
   D. The sonographer cannot change the PRP.

8. Which of the following is true regarding acoustic impedance and attenuation (**Figure 1.1**)?

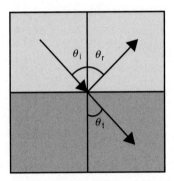

**Figure 1.1** Ultrasound refraction and reflection.

   A. When moving from a low-impedance to a high-impedance medium, the angle of incidence ($\theta_i$) in a non-orthogonal ultrasound beam is less than the angle of transmission ($\theta_t$).
   B. As the speed of sound increases, acoustic impedance decreases.
   C. In a fixed propagation distance, attenuation increases with higher frequency sound.
   D. Acoustic impedance is higher in lower density medium.

9. What is the theoretical shortest PRP when the maximum imaging depth is 5 cm?

   A. 65 μs
   B. 77 μs
   C. 130 μs
   D. 308 μs

10. What is the maximal theoretical frame rate of a B-mode ultrasound image using single line acquisition? The image has 128 lines, with a depth of 15 cm.

   A. 20 Hz
   B. 40 Hz
   C. 60 Hz
   D. 80 Hz

# Chapter 1 ▪ Answers

**1.** Correct Answer: C. Increasing the stiffness of the medium

*Rationale:* The propagation speed is determined by the medium. The speed of sound increases with lower density and higher stiffness media. All sound, regardless of the frequency, travel at the same speed through any specific medium. This means that sound with a frequency of 5 MHz and sound with a frequency of 3 MHz travel at the same propagation speed if they are traveling through the same medium. Increasing the wavelength will decrease the frequency of sound, but since the speed of sound is determined by the medium, it will not affect the propagation speed.

### Selected References
1. Edelman SK. *Understanding Ultrasound Physics.* 4th ed. E.S.P. Ultrasound; 2000.
2. Ziskin MC. Fundamental physics of ultrasound and its propagation in tissue. *Radiographics.* 1993;13:705-709.

**2.** Correct Answer: B. Sound is a longitudinal wave.

*Rationale:* Sound waves are mechanical, longitudinal waves. In longitudinal waves, the particles move along the same axis as the direction of propagation (**Figure 1.2**).

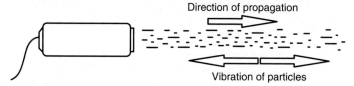

**Figure 1.2** Longitudinal wave.

In transverse waves (e.g., ocean waves), the particles move in a perpendicular direction (orthogonal) to the direction of the wave (**Figure 1.3**).

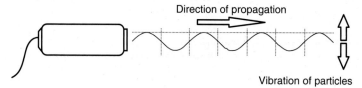

**Figure 1.3** Transverse wave.

Traditionally speaking, sound waves transfer vibration energy, not matter or mass, although a new theoretical study suggests ordinary sound waves carry a small amount of negative mass in Newtonian conditions. Lastly, sound must travel through a medium. Sound cannot propagate in a vacuum.

### Selected References
1. Edelman SK. *Understanding Ultrasound Physics.* 4th ed. E.S.P. Ultrasound; 2000.
2. Nicolis A, Penco R. Mutual interactions of phonons, rotons, and gravity. *Phys Rev B.* 2018;97:134516.
3. Ziskin MC. Fundamental physics of ultrasound and its propagation in tissue. Radiographics. 1993;13:705-709.

**3.** Correct Answer: A. Frequency

*Rationale:* Frequency, pulse duration, period, and axial resolution do not change with depth. If the medium is homogeneous, velocity and wavelength do not change either, although they can change when traveling from one medium to another. Amplitude (defined by the maximum variation of a sound wave from its mean) attenuates (decreases) with depth. Power is the amount of energy transfer, measured in Watts. Power is proportional to the square of the amplitude. Therefore, power will decrease with depth because the amplitude decreases. Intensity is the power divided by the cross-sectional area of the beam. As the beam diameter increases (past the focal point) and the power decreases with depth, both cause the intensity to decrease as well.

Selected References
1. Edelman SK. *Understanding Ultrasound Physics.* 4th ed. E.S.P. Ultrasound; 2000.
2. Ziskin MC. Fundamental physics of ultrasound and its propagation in tissue. *Radiographics.* 1993;13:705-709.

**4.** Correct Answer: C. The wavelength decreases

*Rationale:* The velocity of sound through soft tissue is 1540 m/s, while it is 330 m/s in air, thus the velocity will decrease when traveling from soft tissue to air. Frequency and pulse duration remain unchanged with change in medium. Wavelength will decrease proportional to the decrease in velocity (speed = wavelength × frequency), making option C the correct choice. Although not mentioned, the acoustic impedance of air is much higher than soft tissue, which would result in an increase in amplitude and power as the ultrasound travels from soft tissue to air.

Selected References
1. Edelman SK. *Understanding Ultrasound Physics.* 4th ed. E.S.P. Ultrasound; 2000.
2. Ziskin MC. Fundamental physics of ultrasound and its propagation in tissue. *Radiographics.* 1993;13:705-709.

**5.** Correct Answer: B. 0.308 mm

*Rationale:* Wavelength multiplied by frequency equals velocity. The velocity of sound in soft tissue is 1540 m/s (1.54 mm/µs). One can calculate the wavelength in mm by taking 1.54 mm/µs and dividing by frequency in MHz. 1.54/5 = 0.308 mm.

Selected References
1. Edelman SK. *Understanding Ultrasound Physics.* 4th ed. E.S.P. Ultrasound; 2000.
2. Ziskin MC. Fundamental physics of ultrasound and its propagation in tissue. *Radiographics.* 1993;13:705-709.

**6.** Correct Answer: C. 7.7 cm

*Rationale/Critique:* Ultrasound calculates the depth of an object by measuring the time it takes the signal to return to the transducer and assumes the wave velocity is 1540 m/s. The distance of a reflector is the time in flight divided by 2 (to account for travel toward and back from the reflector), multiplied by velocity.

$$\text{Depth (cm)} = \frac{\text{Time in flight (ms)}}{2} \times 1540 \text{ m/s} \times \left(\frac{100 \text{ cm}}{1 \text{ m}}\right)\left(\frac{1 \text{ s}}{1000 \text{ ms}}\right)$$

The above equation yields an answer of 7.7 cm for 0.1 ms. The other choices are incorrect.
An abbreviated method to calculate the distance for sound traveling through soft tissue is to simply multiply the time in flight by 77 cm/ms (1540/2 m/s). 77 cm/ms × 0.1 ms = 7.7 cm.

Selected References
1. Edelman SK. *Understanding Ultrasound Physics.* 4th ed. E.S.P. Ultrasound; 2000.
2. Ziskin MC. Fundamental physics of ultrasound and its propagation in tissue. *Radiographics.* 1993;13:705-709.

**7.** Correct Answer: B. As the PRP increases, the imaging depth increases.

*Rationale:* The PRP is the amount of time from the start of one pulse to the start of another pulse. It includes both the pulse duration and the "listening time." The PRP can be adjusted by the sonographer and is adjusted for depth of view. Deeper imaging is associated with longer PRP (**Figure 1.4B**). The sonographer can adjust the listening time, not the pulse duration. Typically, the listening time is hundreds of times longer than the pulse duration. The pulse repetition frequency (PRF) is the number of pulses created by the system in 1 s and is the inverse of PRP (shallow image [**Figure 1.4.A**] is associated with higher PRF). The sound frequency is not related to the PRF, and therefore is not related to the PRP.

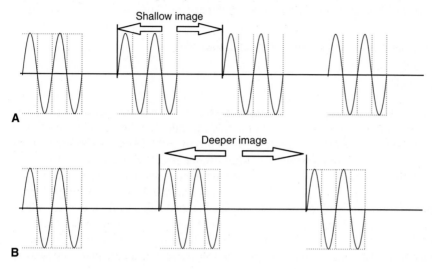

**Figure 1.4** Pulse repetition period demonstrating longer "listening time" with increased depth. A. Shallow image. B. Deeper image.

### Selected References
1. Edelman SK. *Understanding Ultrasound Physics*. 4th ed. E.S.P. Ultrasound; 2000.
2. Terslev L, Diamantopoulos AP, Møller Døhn U, Schmidt WA, Torp-Pedersen S. Settings and artefacts relevant for Doppler ultrasound in large vessel vasculitis. *Arthritis Res Ther.* 2017;19:167.
3. Ziskin MC. Fundamental physics of ultrasound and its propagation in tissue. *Radiographics.* 1993;13:705-709.

**8.** Correct Answer: C. In a fixed propagation distance, attenuation increases with higher frequency sound.

*Rationale:* Attenuation is the decrease of amplitude and intensity of ultrasound waves as they travel through tissue. Attenuation is generally proportional to the square of the frequency of the wave. Attenuation affects higher frequency ultrasound waves more than lower frequency waves. Attenuation is the reason that lower frequency transducers are selected for deeper areas of interest, albeit at the expense of lower spatial resolution. The attenuation coefficient is a representation of a medium's intrinsic property to attenuate sound waves at a given frequency. For example, both aerated lung and cortical bone have very high attenuation coefficients (>20), while blood has an extremely low attenuation coefficient (0.18). When a non-orthogonal beam encounters a boundary between different media with different acoustic impedances, the transmission angle ($\theta_t$) is different than the incident angle ($\theta_i$). If the acoustic impedance of the second media is higher (refraction), the transmission angle will be smaller, so answer A is incorrect. The transmission angle ($\theta_t$) is larger than the incident angle ($\theta_i$) if the acoustic impedance of the second media is lower (also refraction). If the acoustic impedances of the media are significantly different, there will be little transmission, and nearly complete reflection, with reflection angle ($\theta_r$) always equal to the incident angle ($\theta_i$). Acoustic impedance is a physical property of the medium and is proportional to the product of the density of the medium and the propagation velocity through the medium, so answer B is incorrect. The propagation velocity is related to the stiffness and the density of the medium, therefore density has the strongest effect on impedance, and answer D is incorrect.

### Selected Reference
1. Edelman SK. *Understanding Ultrasound Physics*. 4th ed. E.S.P. Ultrasound; 2000.

**9.** Correct Answer: A. 65 μs

*Rationale:* The time needed to travel to the bottom of an image and back is the PRP. Only after the PRP has elapsed can an ultrasound transmit another pulse.

$$\text{Time (}\mu\text{s)} = \frac{2 \times \text{Depth (cm)}}{1540 \text{ m/s}}\left(\frac{1 \text{ m}}{100 \text{ cm}}\right)\left(\frac{1{,}000{,}000 \text{ }\mu\text{s}}{1 \text{ s}}\right)$$

One simple rule of thumb is to recognize that it takes 13 μs for sound to travel 2 cm (1 cm round trip).
Therefore, PRP is the imaging depth of the reflector multiplied by 13 μs/cm (5 cm × 13 μs/cm = 65 μs).

Selected Reference
1. Edelman SK. *Understanding Ultrasound Physics.* 4th ed. E.S.P. Ultrasound; 2000.

**10.** Correct Answer: B. 40 Hz

*Rationale:* There are two methods to reach this answer. One is to calculate the time of flight for each line (see **Answer 1.9**) and then multiply by 128 lines. This will calculate the period for each frame. The frame rate is the inverse of this period. We can use the 13 μs/cm "rule" (**Answer 1.9**) to say it must take 195 μs to travel 15 cm and back. Multiplying by 128 lines/frame results in 24.96 ms or 0.02496 s/frame. The inverse of this results in 40 Hz, or 40 frames/second. In practice, the actual frame rate may be lower, although multiple line acquisition (MLA) may improve the frame rate. In MLA imaging, a signal is sent from a wide transmit beam, and multiple receiver crystals (beams) will acquire the image, allowing for an increased number of lines for a given period. While MLA improves temporal resolution, the lateral resolution is worse, as the wider transmit beam has a smaller transmit aperture. The decreased focus results in lower penetration. Additionally, the multiple beams increase side lobe artifact and increase angle discrepancy between transmit and receive beams.
The other method to calculate the frame rate is to determine the PRF.

$$\text{PRF (Hz)} = \frac{154{,}000 \text{ cm/s}}{2 \times \text{imaging depth (cm)}} = \frac{77{,}000 \text{ cm/s}}{\text{imaging depth (cm)}}$$

This equation is derived from taking the speed of sound (154,000 cm/s) and dividing it by twice the imaging depth. The PRF is the amount of time it takes for one scan. Therefore, the frame rate is the PRF divided by the number of lines (77,000 cm/s/15 cm)/128 lines/frame = 40 frames/second.

Selected Reference
1. Edelman SK. *Understanding Ultrasound Physics.* 4th ed. E.S.P. Ultrasound; 2000.

# 2 | PULSED-WAVE VS. CONTINUOUS-WAVE DOPPLER

Chakradhar Venkata and Jan Kasal

1. A 25-year-old woman is admitted in septic shock from a suspected urinary source. After a 30 mL/kg intravenous (IV) fluid bolus, her HR is 110 bpm and BP is 100/55 mm Hg. A point-of-care echocardiogram is performed to measure the velocity-time integral (VTI) at the left ventricular outflow tract (LVOT) to predict fluid responsiveness. Which of the following statements is *most* accurate with regard to this mode of spectral Doppler (**Figure 2.1**)?

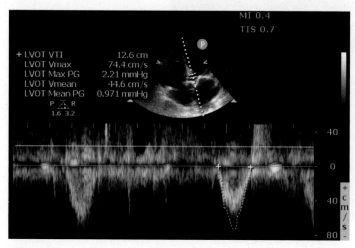

**Figure 2.1**

A. Ultrasound waves are transmitted and received continuously.
B. The sampling rate of the ultrasound transducer is at least half the frequency of blood flow.
C. Range specificity is affected by the physical length of the pulse.
D. The duty factor for this mode is 1.

2. Which of the following is an advantage of continuous-wave Doppler (CWD) over pulsed-wave Doppler (PWD)?

A. Ability to distinguish the location of the acoustic signal
B. Ability to measure high velocities across a stenotic valve
C. Ability to measure low-velocity, high-amplitude signals of the myocardium
D. Ability to measure VTI to calculate stroke volume

3. Decreasing the wall filter cutoff frequency may be necessary for the evaluation of which of the following velocities?

   A. Aortic stenosis jet velocity
   B. Pulmonary venous flow
   C. Mitral regurgitation
   D. Velocity-time integral

4. The axial resolution of PWD is *most* affected by which of the following?

   A. The spatial pulse length (SPL)
   B. The velocity of the ultrasound wave in the medium
   C. The ultrasound beam width
   D. The pulse repetition period (PRP)

5. An 86-year-old man with congestive heart failure and aortic stenosis is admitted to the intensive care unit (ICU) for dyspnea. The following Doppler tracing was recorded in the apical five-chamber view (**Figure 2.2**).

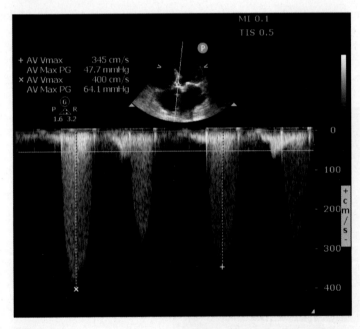

**Figure 2.2**

Which of the following statements is the *most* accurate with regard to this spectral Doppler mode?
A. It is measuring the blood velocity at the level of the aortic valve.
B. It is measuring the blood velocity at the level of the LVOT.
C. It is measuring the velocity signals from the entire length of the ultrasound beam.
D. This spectral Doppler mode is prone to signal aliasing.

6. A 77-year-old man was admitted to the ICU for dyspnea. A point-of-care echocardiography examination was performed to narrow the differential diagnoses for his dyspnea. Which of the following statements is *most* accurate in describing the Doppler mode shown in **Figure 2.3**?

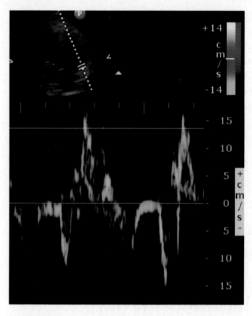

**Figure 2.3**

A. It uses continuous-wave ultrasound
B. It detects high-amplitude, low velocities from tissues
C. It detects low-amplitude, high velocities from blood cells
D. It has poor temporal resolution

7. **Figure 2.4** was obtained while measuring the VTI of the LVOT with pulsed-wave spectral Doppler.

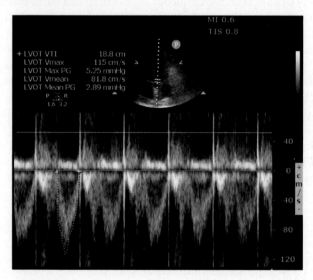

**Figure 2.4**

Which of the following is the *most likely* reason for the spectral window seen in the Doppler envelope?
A. There is laminar blood flow at the LVOT.
B. There is turbulent blood flow at the LVOT.
C. The ultrasound machine transmit power is high.
D. The ultrasound machine gain is high.

# Chapter 2 ▪ Answers

---

**1.** Correct Answer: C. Range specificity is affected by the physical length of the pulse

*Rationale:* Spectral Doppler echocardiography is used to quantify cardiovascular hemodynamics and blood flow characteristics, including velocities and direction. Spectral Doppler includes pulsed-wave Doppler (PWD) and continuous-wave Doppler (CWD) modes, as well as color flow Doppler, which is a type of PWD. Figure 2.1 shows the PWD tracing of the VTI at the LVOT.

In this mode, ultrasound waves are transmitted intermittently in pulses, and the returning waves are "listened to" during the time between the transmitted pulses (**Figure 2.5**).

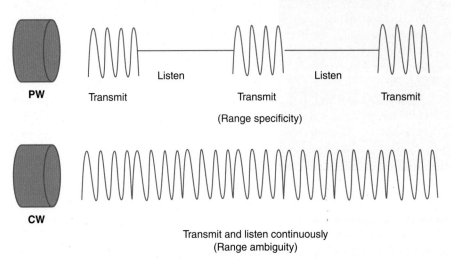

**Figure 2.5**

The advantage of PWD is range specificity, that is, it allows calculation of blood velocities from a specific location by isolating and measuring short bursts of reflected frequency signals from that particular location. The ability of PWD to detect acoustic signals from a specific location of interest (range specificity) is affected by the physical length of the pulse (ie, spatial pulse length). A shorter SPL produces better axial resolution (the ability to detect two points as separate), and a longer SPL will lead to loss of range specificity. Among the answer choices, choice C represents the principle of PWD; hence, it is the correct choice.

The sampling rate (frequency) of the ultrasound transducer should be at least twice as fast as the frequency of the signal being measured; hence, choice B is incorrect.

The duty factor is the percentage of time the transducer is actively transmitting ultrasound signals. It is calculated as the pulse duration (PD) divided by the pulse repetition period (PRP). PD is the time from the start of a pulse to the end of that pulse, that is, the time that the pulse is "on." The time between initiation of transmit events is the PRP. For PWD, the duty factor should be <1; hence, choice D is incorrect. **Figure 2.6** depicts pulsed-wave parameters as a function of time and distance.

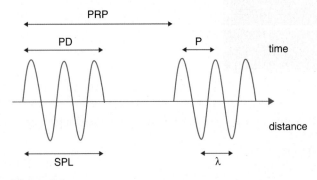

**Figure 2.6**

In contrast to PWD, CWD transmits and receives ultrasound waves continuously. Due to simultaneous transmission and receiving of ultrasound signals, CWD cannot distinguish the origin of the echo, hence it has no range specificity. Figure 2.1 used PWD, hence choice A is incorrect. As CWD is continuously sending and receiving pulses, the duty factor for CWD is 1.

**Selected References**
1. Miele FR. *Essentials of Ultrasound Physics*. Pegasus Lectures; 2008 (Chapters 4 and 7).
2. Otto CM, Schwaegler RG, Freeman RV. *Echocardiography Review Guide*. 3rd ed. Chapter 1. Elsevier; 2016.

**2.** Correct Answer: B. Ability to measure high velocities across a stenotic valve

*Rationale:* CWD uses two ultrasound crystals to emit and receive ultrasound signals continuously. This principle allows CWD to detect very high-velocity shifts. However, CWD cannot distinguish the location of the acoustic reflection. Every single velocity along the Doppler line of interrogation is recorded, producing the Doppler envelope. As the blood velocities across a stenotic valve are higher, CWD is employed to measure peak velocities and to calculate pressure gradients.

In contrast, the advantage of PWD is its ability to interrogate the acoustic signal from a specific location. This principle allows the user to place the sample volume at a specific point of interest and measure the frequency shifts from only that location. PWD is used in the measurement of myocardial tissue velocities (tissue Doppler imaging [TDI]) for diastolic function assessment and to measure the blood flow velocity at the LVOT. Tracing the outer edge of the Doppler envelope measured at the LVOT via PWD gives the VTI to calculate the left ventricular stroke volume. Although VTI can often be measured with CWD, it does not confer any advantage for this application.

**Selected Reference**
1. Boyd AC, Schiller NB, Thomas L. Principles of transthoracic echocardiographic evaluation. *Nat Rev Cardiol*. 2015;12:426-440.

**3.** Correct Answer: B. Pulmonary venous flow

*Rationale:* Wall filters in spectral Doppler are used to suppress low velocities around the baseline. They eliminate the low-velocity, high-amplitude signals arising from the body tissues (eg, myocardium movement, arterial wall motion) and allow higher frequency signals originating from the blood to pass through. This will improve the signal "clutter." However, certain situations require adjustment of wall filter settings. Venous flows require the ability to detect low-frequency Doppler shifts; hence, wall filters may need to be set to a lower cutoff frequency to register these changes. Low-frequency Doppler shifts, such as those arising from the pulmonary vein into the left atrium, may be eliminated when the wall filters are set too high. Aortic stenosis, mitral regurgitation, and tricuspid regurgitation jet velocities are typically high-frequency velocities, hence lowering of wall filter cutoff frequency is not needed.

**Selected Reference**
1. Miele FR. *Essentials of Ultrasound Physics*. Chapter 4 and Chapter 7. Pegasus Lectures; 2008.

**4.** Correct Answer: A. The spatial pulse length (SPL)

*Rationale:* Axial resolution is the ability of the ultrasound wave to distinguish two points as separate in the direction parallel to the ultrasound beam. Wavelength is an important parameter that affects axial resolution. Shorter wavelengths can discriminate two points close to each other as separate in space, hence resulting in better axial resolution. Recall from the pulsed-wave properties diagram (Figure 2.6) that SPL is the physical distance the ultrasound pulse occupies in the medium.

It is the product of wavelength ($\lambda$) and the number of waves in the pulse. A shorter pulse length will be able to differentiate the structures located at neighboring depths more accurately, hence there is better axial resolution. Axial resolution is equal to half of the SPL because of the roundtrip effect (axial resolution = SPL/2). To understand the roundtrip effect, imagine two structures A and B that are separated by a distance "*x*." The acoustic signals reflected from structure A and structure B are separated by twice the actual distance (2*x*) by which these two structures are separated because a wave traveling between them must travel "there and back." Because of this, the physical length of the pulse (ie, SPL) can be almost twice as long as the distance between two structures, but still results in two distinct echoes. If the SPL becomes longer than twice the separation distance, the reflecting echoes from both structures cannot be distinguished, resulting in being interpreted as one structure instead of two distinct structures (i.e., loss of axial resolution).

PRP is the time between transmitting a pulse and receiving a pulse (Figure 2.6), hence it is related to the ability to detect changes in time, that is, temporal resolution, not axial resolution.

Ultrasound beam width is related to lateral resolution, that is, the ability to resolve structures located perpendicular to the direction of the ultrasound beam. A narrow beam width gives better lateral resolution.

The velocity of the ultrasound wave (the speed of the sound wave in a medium) is constant for a given medium and does not affect the axial resolution. The propagation velocity is determined by the stiffness and density of the medium. The propagation velocity in soft tissue is assumed to be 1540 m/sec.

### Selected Reference
1. Edelman SK. *Ultrasound Physics and Instrumentation*. Chapter 1. ESP Inc; 2002.

---

**5.** Correct Answer: C. It is measuring the velocity signals from the entire length of the ultrasound beam

*Rationale:* The spectral Doppler tracing in Figure 2.2 is a CWD tracing. This can be identified by several clues in the image presented here: the velocity scale measuring up to 400 cm/sec, the typical spectral Doppler envelope where the velocities from the entire length of Doppler beam interrogation are recorded (rather than a "hollow" envelope), and the rhomboid- or diamond-shaped sign on the Doppler interrogation line instead of a sample volume gate. Moreover, the question stem states that the patient has aortic stenosis, which would suggest a high-velocity flow through the aortic valve that would not be measured appropriately with PWD.

CWD cannot distinguish the location of the reflected signal. Every velocity along the Doppler line of interrogation is recorded, producing the complete Doppler envelope. As the blood velocities across the stenotic valve are higher, CWD is employed to measure peak velocities and to calculate the pressure gradients.

Signal aliasing occurs with PWD modes (PWD, color Doppler) when measuring high velocities. With aliasing, the Doppler signal "wraps around" the baseline from the top of the display to the bottom of the spectrum display (**Figure 2.7**). This is due to the intermittent Doppler sampling rate (i.e., pulse repetition frequency, PRF) being too low in comparison to the measured Doppler shift. The main advantage of CWD over PWD is its ability to detect very high-velocity shifts, as it is not affected by signal aliasing.

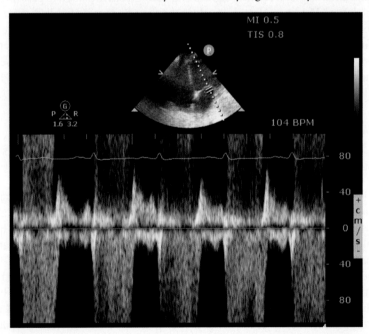

**Figure 2.7**

### Selected References
1. Boyd AC, Schiller NB, Thomas L. Principles of transthoracic echocardiographic evaluation. *Nat Rev Cardiol*. 2015;12:426-440.
2. Harris P, Kuppurao L. Quantitative Doppler echocardiography. *BJA Educ*. 2016;16(2):46-52.

**6.** Correct Answer: B. It detects high-amplitude, low velocities from tissues

*Rationale:* The question requires an understanding of various Doppler techniques that are commonly used in critical care echocardiography. Figure 2.3 is obtained by tissue Doppler imaging (TDI). This technique measures the velocity of myocardial tissue movement at a specific site and is used in the assessment of left ventricular diastolic function. In the heart, both blood and myocardial contraction cause frequency shifts that can be detected by Doppler imaging. As the velocity of small red blood cells (RBCs) is higher than tissue velocity, reflections cause high-frequency, low-amplitude signals that are detected by conventional Doppler techniques. TDI is designed to detect low-velocity but high-amplitude signals arising from myocardial movement, and this is done by the use of contrasting filters that omit high velocities of low-amplitude scattering structures such as RBCs. The cardiac cycle is represented by three distinct waveforms in TDI, as depicted in **Figure 2.8**: systolic myocardial velocity (S) that is above the baseline as the annulus descends toward the apex, an early diastolic myocardial relaxation velocity (e') below the baseline as the annulus ascends away from the apex, followed by a late diastolic velocity (a') associated with atrial contraction.

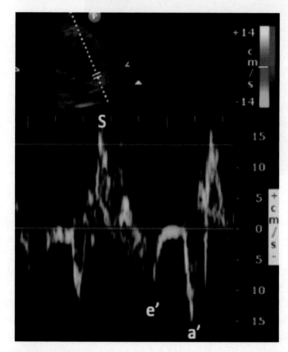

**Figure 2.8**

TDI uses a pulsed-wave ultrasound mode, so choice A is incorrect. The sample volume is placed at the lateral mitral annulus to obtain the spectral contour of myocardial motion. As the TDI measures the longitudinal component of myocardial contraction at the specific area of interest, it has a very high temporal resolution (hence choice D is incorrect).

Selected References
1. Ho CY, Solomon SD. A clinician's guide to tissue Doppler imaging. *Circulation.* 2006;113:e396-e398.
2. Kadappu KK, Thomas L. Tissue Doppler imaging in echocardiography. *Heart Lung Circ.* 2015;24:224-233.

**7.** Correct Answer: A. There is laminar blood flow at the LVOT

*Rationale:* Spectral Doppler measures the velocity of flow over time. Although spectral Doppler does not directly measure the flow, flow characteristics can be determined by the spectral Doppler signal. In the spectral Doppler tracing shown in Figure 2.4, a lucency is seen in the middle of the PWD envelope. This signal-free zone below the narrow bands of accelerating and decelerating velocities of RBCs in systole is called a spectral window (**Figure 2.9**). The presence of a spectral window implies laminar (as opposed to turbulent) flow.

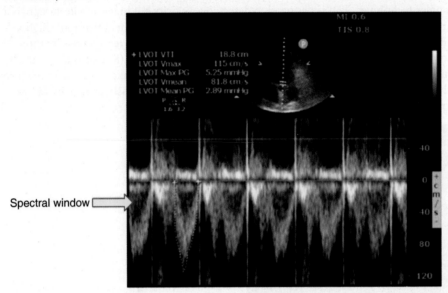

**Figure 2.9**

Interrogation of the VTI provides a flow length that can be multiplied by a cross-sectional area to obtain volumetric flow. Obtaining a good Doppler profile with the presence of a spectral window indicates that the sample volume is placed appropriately in the cylindrical part of the LVOT. The optimal LVOT VTI signal should be narrow with a rapid upstroke and an end-systolic click terminating the flow signal. The sample volume should be 5 mm proximal to the aortic valve and in the center of LVOT.

Although the presence of a spectral window implies laminar flow, its absence does not necessarily imply turbulent blood flow at the sample gate. Loss of the spectral window may happen from various causes, including a large sample volume, larger angle of insonation, or sampling from a shallow imaging depth. Increasing the signal strength either by using a high transmit power or by increasing the receiver gain can also diminish or abolish the spectral window (hence, choices C and D are incorrect). The spectral window is usually seen only with PWD.

### Selected References

1. Miele FR. *Essentials of Ultrasound Physics*, Chapter 4 and Chapter 7. Pegasus Lectures; 2008.
2. Mitchell C, Rahko PS, Blauwet LA, et al. Guidelines for performing a comprehensive transthoracic echocardiographic examination in adults: recommendations from the American Society of Echocardiography. *J Am Soc Echocardiogr.* 2019;32(1):1-64.

# 3 | ULTRASOUND PROPAGATION THROUGH TISSUE

Molly Flannagan

1. Which of the following is the *most* significant cause of ultrasound attenuation in diagnostic ultrasonography?

    A. Thermal absorption
    B. Specular reflection
    C. Scattering
    D. Diffuse reflection

2. What nonthermal effect of ultrasound is *most* responsible for the ability of shock wave lithotripsy to treat nephrolithiasis?

    A. Ionizing radiation
    B. Acoustic radiation force
    C. Acoustic streaming
    D. Cavitation

3. Which ultrasound wave array is correctly matched with the field of view or beam structure it produces?

    A. Linear sequential array—ultrasound waves exiting transducer at 90°, but splay out as they move away from the transducer resulting in a fan-shaped field of view
    B. Curvilinear sequential array—radially increasing rings which create a long focal ultrasound beam
    C. Phased array—pulsed beams emanating from a single point of origin
    D. Annular array—parallel arranged breams created in sequence resulting in a rectangular field of view

4. The acoustic impedance of various tissues affects the reflection and transmission of an ultrasound beam as it travels through tissues. Which tissue has the lowest acoustic impedance?

    A. Air
    B. Fat
    C. Skin
    D. Bone

5. While performing a right upper extremity ultrasound to find intravenous (IV) access, the practitioner notes a hypoechoic area on the screen deep to the location of the radius. The image appears this way because of which type of ultrasound artifact (**e-Figure 3.1**)?

   **A.** Refraction
   **B.** Shadowing
   **C.** Enhancement
   **D.** Reverberation

# Chapter 3 ▪ Answers

1. Correct Answer: A. Thermal absorption

   *Rationale:* Ultrasound attenuation is the decrease in amplitude and intensity of ultrasound waves as they travel through tissue, which occurs as a result of the interaction of the sound waves with the tissue. It is predominantly affected by three factors: thermal absorption, reflection, and scattering. Of these three, thermal absorption is the most significant cause of attenuation.

   Thermal absorption is the conversion of ultrasound wave energy into heat as a beam travels through and interacts with tissue boundaries. It occurs in a predictable fashion, and the amount of heat generation can be calculated by using characteristics including wave frequency, ultrasound pressure, tissue density, and the speed of sound. This is the principle behind thermal cellular destruction in ultrasound ablation of lesions such as malignancies.

   Specular and diffuse reflection cause attenuation of an ultrasound beam because only a portion of the transmitted wave bounces off the tissue interface and returns to the ultrasound transducer. The point of reflection can be smooth, as in specular reflection, and cause the sound wave to be reflected in a singular direction. In contrast, diffuse reflection results when a structure has an uneven surface and ultrasound waves are reflected back at various angles, resulting in a more unpredictable surface pattern. Regardless of the pattern, both specular and diffuse reflection partially contribute to ultrasound wave attenuation. (See **Figure 3.1**.)

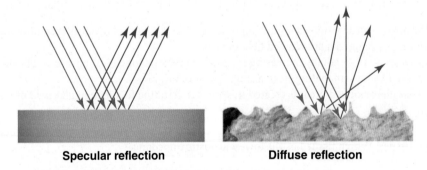

   **Specular reflection**          **Diffuse reflection**

   **Figure 3.1** Specular vs. diffuse reflection.

   The cumulative effect of these phenomena is diminished, returning echoes and poorer image intensity of deeper structures. One way to compensate for this effect is by altering the transmission frequency. High-frequency ultrasound waves generate images with higher axial resolution, but because of the increased number of points of interaction with the tissue, these waves are subject to more attenuation. Low-frequency waves, while providing lower resolution, can visualize deeper structures because they undergo less attenuation. Time gain compensation (TGC) is another method to compensate for attenuation, by progressively increasing the signal gain for later returning echoes, making deeper structures appear more bright on the resulting display. (See **Figure 3.2**.)

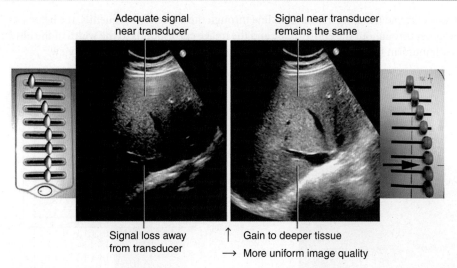

Adequate signal near transducer

Signal near transducer remains the same

Signal loss away from transducer

↑ Gain to deeper tissue

→ More uniform image quality

**Figure 3.2** Abdominal imaging with attenuation and B with gain added.

### Selected Reference
1. O'Brien, W. Ultrasound—Biophysics mechanisms. *Prog Biophys Mol Biol.* 2007;93(1-3):212-255.

## 2. Correct Answer: D. Cavitation

*Rationale:* As ultrasound waves propagate, they produce both thermal and nonthermal effects on the surrounding tissues. The safety profile of ultrasound, with its lack of ionizing radiation, has allowed for its use both diagnostically and therapeutically. Thermal effects are exploited in high-intensity focused ultrasound (HIFU) by focusing ultrasound waves to selected areas causing a predictable degree of tissue heating, resulting in coagulation necrosis and cell death. Clinical applicability of this technology has been used in catheter-based ablation of both benign and malignant lesions.

The nonthermal effects of ultrasound energy include acoustic radiation force, acoustic streaming, and cavitation. Acoustic radiation force and acoustic streaming refer to the transfer of momentum from an ultrasound wave onto an external medium such as tissue- or fluid-filled structures, causing observable displacement of the tissues adjacent to the ultrasound wave. The degree of displacement is dependent upon the intrinsic stiffness of the surrounding tissue, thus the viscoelastic properties of a given tissue can be calculated noninvasively with ultrasonography.

Cavitation is the process by which fluctuations in pressure cause the formation of gas bubbles often from existing gas nuclei within the tissue. Continuous exposure to ultrasound waves causes the microbubbles to grow to a maximal size, then collapse on itself to create a shock wave. This mechanism is the principle behind which ultrasound lithotripsy of kidney stones is achieved.

### Selected References
1. American Institute of Ultrasound in Medicine, Official Statement, ALARA principle; 2014.
2. Izadifar Z, Babyn P, Chapman D. Mechanical and biological effects of ultrasound: a review of present knowledge. *Ultrasound Med Biol.* 2017 Jun;43(6):1085-1104.

## 3. Correct Answer: C. Phased array—pulsed beams emanating from a single point of origin

*Rationale:* An ultrasound wave array refers to both the activation and organization of the piezoelectric crystals within the actual ultrasound transducer. Depending on the position and function of each of the crystals, the resulting ultrasound image on the screen will vary. Ultrasound arrays are broadly grouped into three functional categories—sequential, phased, and annular.

In sequential arrays, multiple crystals are aligned side by side and fire in sequence. A single scan line will run from one crystal, reflect off the tissue, and return back to the probe. The resulting images are built from numerous ultrasound scan lines next to each other, running in straight lines the length of the tissue and then returning to the receiver. Sequential arrays can be linear or curvilinear, depending on the organization of the piezoelectric crystals within the transducer footplate. In linear sequential arrays (**Figure 3.3**), also known as switched arrays, crystals are parallel to one another and produce waves 90°

from the transducer head traveling in a straight line through the tissue. Consequently, the beams stay parallel to one another throughout the entire tissue and the image corresponds to the width of the ultrasound transducer with uniform beam density throughout. This creates a rectangular field of view.

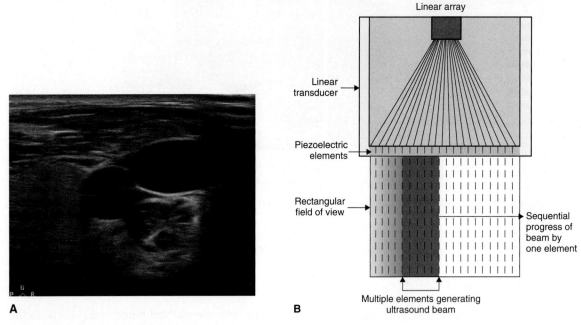

**Figure 3.3** Linear sequential array.

Curvilinear sequential arrays (**Figure 3.4**) have the crystals aligned along a curved transducer head. The beams are again emitted at a 90° angle from the transducer head, traveling in straight lines through the tissue. But because of the initial positioning of the crystals in the head, the beams diverge from one another as they move away from the transducer, resulting in decreased beam density farther from the probe head. While curvilinear probes allow for a wider field of view, they sacrifice resolution at increasing depths.

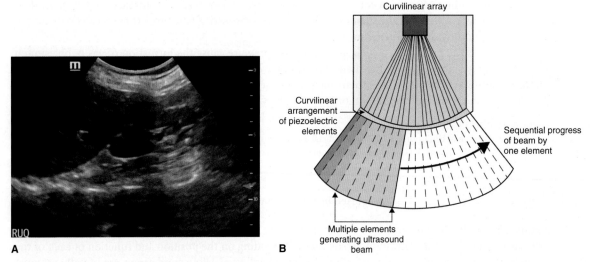

**Figure 3.4** Curvilinear sequential array.

Phased arrays (**Figure 3.5**) have crystals tightly aligned together, but instead of emitting sequential perpendicular waves, the crystals are activated in pulses at various angles. There are fewer crystals in the transducer, but since they are activated in an oscillating fashion, each crystal can create multiple nonparallel ultrasound scan lines per image. Sound waves are generated from a single point on the transducer and then fan out as they move through the tissue. With each pulse from a single piezoelectric crystal, the resulting ultrasound wave is steered in a slightly different degree. This generates a sector- or wedge-shaped image with a narrow field of view closer to the probe and a wider field of view farther away. The receiver is then able to spatially sort the returning waves based upon time to return and wave amplitude, allowing for image construction with the interrogation of areas from multiple angles. Phased array probes are useful for evaluation of areas with small footplate contact, but a large underlying area of interest, such as cardiac ultrasonography between intervening rib spaces.

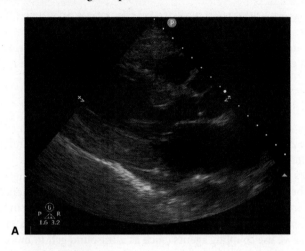

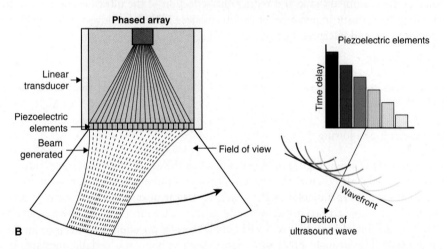

**Figure 3.5** Phased array.

Annular arrays (**Figure 3.6**) are constructed from piezoelectric crystals cut into rings with larger diameter crystals on the outer edge and smaller diameter crystals internally. Each ring has a different acoustic property and will produce different frequency waves, resulting in various depths of natural focus. This creates a long focal zone within the ultrasound beam. This type of array is used predominantly in ophthalmologic evaluations.

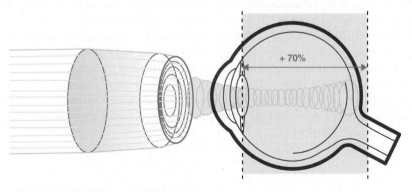

**Figure 3.6** Diagram of annular array.

Selected References

1. Markowitz J. Probe selection, machine controls, and equipment. In: Carmody KA, Moore CL, Feller-Kopman D, eds. *Handbook of Critical Care and Emergency Ultrasound*. McGraw-Hill Education; 2011:25-39.
2. Whittingham R, Martin K. Transducers and beam-forming. In: Hoskins P, Martin K, Thrush A, eds. *Diagnostic Ultrasound: Physics and Equipment*. Cambridge University Press; 2010:23-46.

**4.** Correct Answer: A. Air

*Rationale:* Acoustic impedance is a physical property of a tissue that describes the amount of resistance an ultrasound beam encounters as it moves through the tissue. Impedance is proportional to the density of the material:

$$Z = \rho \times c$$

where impedance is $Z$ (kg/(m²s)), $\rho$ is the density of the tissue (kg/m³), and $c$ is the speed of the sound wave in the tissue (m/s).

Each tissue has its own impedance, which is a characteristic of the tissue medium and it is the difference in impedance between two tissues at an interface that generates the reflecting echoes. For example, while air has a low acoustic impedance (0.00042 kg/(m²s)), the difference in the impedance between air and the underlying examined tissue results in a reflecting echo that limits visibility of deeper tissues. It is for this reason that we use coupling agents (such as ultrasound gel) to more closely match the acoustic impedance of the examined tissue and reduce the reflection of the ultrasound beam off the soft tissue. Understanding the acoustic impedances of various tissues (**Table 3.1**) allows the operator to better understand, troubleshoot, and interpret the resulting image.

Selected References

1. Azhari H. *Basics of Biomedical Ultrasound for Engineers*. John Wiley & Sons, Inc; 2010.
2. Bakhru RN, Schweickert WD. Intensive care ultrasound: I. Physics, equipment, and image quality. *Ann Am Thorac Soc*. 2013;10(5):54-548.

**5.** Correct Answer: B. Shadowing

*Rationale:* Refraction (*arrow,* **Figure 3.7A**) occurs when the assumption that ultrasound waves travel in a straight line is violated. When a transmitted ultrasound pulse reaches a curved surface, it may strike the interface at a non-perpendicular angle, which bends the ultrasound wave away in an oblique angle, resulting in a hypoechoic artifact posterior to the surface. This effect is also known as an edge artifact.

Acoustic shadowing (*arrow,* **Figure 3.7B**) appears as a hypoechoic area deep to an area of strongly attenuating tissue. This strongly attenuating tissue (such as bone or a metallic implant) has either high reflective or absorptive properties that result in limited transmission of ultrasound waves into the tissues deep to the structure. As a result, the underlying tissue appears hypoechoic and obscures evaluation of structures deep to the attenuating tissue.

Acoustic enhancement (*arrow,* **Figure 3.7C**) occurs as a result of **decreased** attenuation of the ultrasound wave as it passes through an overlying area tissue with low impedance (e.g., water). The resulting reflections deep to the low-attenuating structure appears brighter than the adjacent tissue. This increased echogenicity of the deeper tissues is not because that section of tissue is inherently more reflective, but because the intensity of the ultrasound beam in that area is increased compared to the flanking areas.

Reverberation (*arrow,* **Figure 3.7D**) occurs when a single emitted ultrasound wave is reflected multiple times between either a strongly reflective object and the transducer (e.g., A-lines on lung ultrasound) or two strongly reflecting objects (e.g., B-lines on lung ultrasound). This causes a single emitted ultrasound beam to be received multiple times by the ultrasound transducer as the wave bounces back and forth between these two objects. The resulting ultrasound image will show a series of bright bands running parallel to the ultrasound main axis, separated by the same distance as the two reflectors. This artifact can be minimized by angling the ultrasound transducer so as to remove the oscillation between the two strong parallel reflectors.

**Table 3.1 Density, Speed of Sound, and Acoustic Impedance of Common Tissues**

| | Density (g/cm$^3$) | Speed of Sound (m/s) | Acoustic Impedance [kg/(sec m$^2$)] $\times$ 10$^6$ |
|---|---|---|---|
| Air | 0.0013 | 330 | 0.0004 |
| Water | 1 | 1480 | 1.48 |
| Blood | 1.055 | 1575 | 1.66 |
| Fat | 0.95 | 1450 | 1.38 |
| Skin | 1.15 | 1730 | 1.99 |
| Skeletal muscle (varies) | 1.065 | 1575-1590 | 1.68-1.69 |
| Bone (varies) | 1.9 | 2800-4080 | 5.32-7.75 |

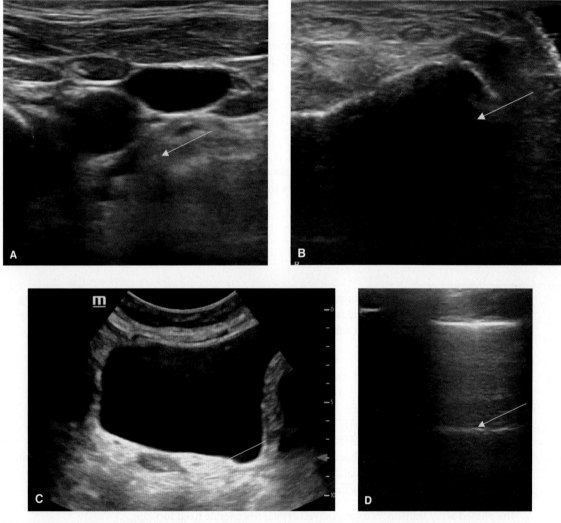

**Figure 3.7** A, Refraction. B, Shadowing. C, Enhancement. D, Reverberation.

### Selected References

1. Baad M, Lu ZF, Reiser I, Paushter D. Clinical significance of US artifacts. *RadioGraphics*. 2017;37(5):1408-1423.
2. Prabhu SJ, Kanal K, Bhargava P, Vaidya S, Dighe MK. Ultrasound artifacts: classification, applied physics with illustrations, and imaging appearance. *Ultrasound Q*. 2014;30(2):145-157.

# 4 | ULTRASOUND TRANSDUCER AND SYSTEM

Christopher R. Tainter, Cameron Smyres, Michael Self, and Raghu Seethala

1. A 37-year-old woman who is 34 weeks pregnant presents with acute shortness of breath. In order to evaluate for cardiogenic causes of her symptoms, which of the following transducers would be most appropriate?

   A. 1 to 2 MHz
   B. 2 to 5 MHz
   C. 5 to 12 MHz
   D. 12 to 15 MHz

2. You want to get the best quality image of a deep structure while performing echocardiography with a phased array transducer. Which transducer crystal will have the best lateral resolution in the Fraunhofer zone?

   A. 10-mm-thick crystal
   B. 8-mm-thick crystal
   C. 6-mm-thick crystal
   D. 4-mm-thick crystal

3. A 65-year-old man with long-standing hypertension is being evaluated for severe chest pain radiating to his back. Point-of-care ultrasound is being used to identify the descending aorta in a long-axis view. Which of the following transducers will provide the best resolution of the descending aorta?

   A. 4 MHz, 4 mm crystal diameter
   B. 7.5 MHz, 8 mm crystal diameter
   C. 4 MHz, 8 mm crystal diameter
   D. 7.5 MHz, 4 mm crystal diameter

4. A 28-year-old man is admitted to the intensive care unit (ICU) in cardiogenic shock from myocarditis. You prepare to perform transthoracic echocardiography to assess his response to resuscitation. The ultrasound machine is equipped with a linear sequential transducer and a phased array transducer. Which of the following options best describes how the phased array transducer differs from the linear transducer?

   A. The phased array transducer uses a curved crystal to generate fixed focusing.
   B. The phased array transducer uses delays in electronic impulses to electronically steer and focus the ultrasound beam.
   C. The phased array transducer uses piezoelectric crystals arranged in a curve to provide a natural sector image.
   D. The phased array transducer uses an external lens to generate adjustable focusing.

5. A 40-year-old man with a history of intravenous drug use presents with fever and difficulty breathing. You suspect endocarditis and use bedside echocardiography to assess for valve vegetations by visualizing the mitral valve in an apical four-chamber view, but are unable to identify the fine details of the valve. Changing which of the following will magnify the image and improve spatial resolution?

    **A.** Increasing zoom
    **B.** Decreasing depth
    **C.** Increasing gain
    **D.** Changing to a higher frequency probe

6. A 56-year-old woman with a history of chronic obstructive pulmonary disease (COPD) and congestive heart failure (CHF) is being evaluated with point-of-care ultrasound for shortness of breath. A parasternal long-axis view is being attempted. The images obtained (**Figure 4.1**) are dark and the structures are not clear (**Figure 4.1A**). An adjustment is made and **Figure 4.1B** is achieved.

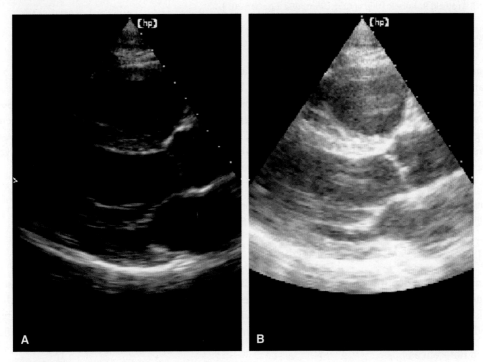

**Figure 4.1**

Which of the following occurred with this adjustment?
**A.** The strength of the transmitted ultrasound wave is increased.
**B.** Correction for beam attenuation is occurring.
**C.** The received signal is amplified.
**D.** The focal zone is adjusted to improve resolution.

7. By switching from a 10 MHz transducer to a 5 MHz transducer, which of the following will occur?

    **A.** There will be more aliasing with pulsed-wave Doppler.
    **B.** There will be improved lateral resolution.
    **C.** There will be increased penetration of the ultrasound waves.
    **D.** More energy will be absorbed by the patient's tissues.

# Chapter 4 ▪ Answers

### 1. Correct Answer: B. 2 to 5 MHz

*Rationale:* In order to evaluate cardiogenic causes of her symptoms, a transthoracic echo would be the most appropriate first step. This would most commonly be performed with a phased array probe, with a frequency of about 2 to 5 MHz. A 1 to 2 MHz probe is more likely to be used for deeper structures, with less movement, like a curvilinear probe used for abdominal imaging, although commonly these probes also have a wider range, like 2 to 5 MHz. A higher frequency probe, like 5 to 12 MHz, would be used to image more superficial structures, for example, vasculature with a linear array probe. A 12 to 15 MHz probe is not likely to be used for clinical imaging.

##### Selected Reference
1. Soni NJ, Arntfield R, Kory P. *Point of Care Ultrasound*. Elsevier; 2019.

### 2. Correct Answer: D. 4-mm-thick crystal

*Rationale:* A 4-mm-thick crystal will have the best lateral resolution. The Fraunhofer zone, or far zone, is the area deep to the focal zone where ultrasound beams diverge. Divergence describes the spread of the ultrasound beam and is determined by the transducer diameter and ultrasound frequency. Sound beams with more divergence spread over a larger area, decreasing lateral resolution. Higher frequencies and larger transducer diameters decrease divergence, improving lateral resolution. Ultrasound frequency is inversely proportional to the piezoelectric crystal thickness. Therefore, the 4-mm-crystal will have the highest frequency, least divergence, and best lateral resolution in the Fraunhofer zone.

##### Selected References
1. Edelman SK. *Ultrasound Physics and Instrumentation*. Education for the Sonographic Professional; 2011.
2. Hoskins P, Martin K, Thrush A. *Diagnostic Ultrasound: Physics and Equipment*. Cambridge University Press; 2019.

### 3. Correct Answer: B. 7.5 MHz, 8 mm crystal diameter

*Rationale:* The focal depth is the area with the best lateral image resolution and depends on ultrasound frequency and the diameter of the active element. Less divergence produces a narrower beam in the far field, also improving lateral resolution. Transducers with a larger active element and higher frequency will have a deeper focal length and less divergence, and therefore improved lateral resolution in the far field.

##### Selected References
1. Edelman SK. *Ultrasound Physics and Instrumentation*. Education for the Sonographic Professional; 2011.
2. Hoskins P, Martin K, Thrush A. *Diagnostic Ultrasound: Physics and Equipment*. Cambridge University Press; 2019.

### 4. Correct Answer: B. The phased array transducer uses delays in electronic impulses to electronically steer and focus the ultrasound beam.

*Rationale:* Phased array probes are designed with the unique ability of electronic focusing and steering. They are composed of an array of hundreds of individual crystal elements. Electronic signals from the ultrasound machine excite the elements, creating a sound pulse, but with variable time delays of approximately 10 ns between each element. These time delays are called phasing and act as an electronic lens that "steers" and focuses the beam. Linear sequential arrays are linear arrangements of piezoelectric elements that sequentially fire. Linear sequential arrays use either a curved crystal (option A) or an external lens to generate fixed focusing (option D). A convex or curved array (e.g., curvilinear probe) uses piezoelectric crystal elements arranged in a curve to provide a natural sector image (option C).

##### Selected References
1. Aldrich JE. Basic physics of ultrasound imaging. *Crit Care Med*. 2007;35(5 suppl):S131-S137.
2. Hoskins P, Martin K, Thrush A. *Diagnostic Ultrasound: Physics and Equipment*. Cambridge University Press; 2019.

**5.** Correct Answer: B. Decreasing depth

*Rationale:* Decreasing the depth will bring the image closer to the focal zone and the transducer, decreasing attenuation and increasing the size of the image without decreasing spatial resolution. Increasing the zoom will magnify the image display, but will not affect spatial resolution. Increasing gain will increase the brightness of the received image, but does not change the resolution, nor magnify the image. Increasing the frequency may improve lateral resolution of a nearby structure, but will not magnify the image.

Selected References
1. Edelman SK. *Ultrasound Physics and Instrumentation*. Education for the Sonographic Professional; 2011.
2. Hoskins P, Martin K, Thrush A. *Diagnostic Ultrasound: Physics and Equipment*. Cambridge University Press; 2019.

**6.** Correct Answer: C. The received signal is amplified.

*Rationale:* The "dark" image (Figure 4.1A) was optimized by increasing the overall gain. This amplifies the received signal to enhance areas of reflected waves, but may also enhance artifacts. It does not affect the strength of the transmitted wave. Time gain compensation (TGC) increases the gain relative to the depth (increased depth = increased time for the wave to travel) to compensate for beam attenuation. However, in Figure 4.1B, we can see increased brightness *throughout* the image, so we know that the overall gain has increased. An adjustment of the focal zone will improve resolution in the area of the focal zone only, but again we see that the entire image has been adjusted.

Selected Reference
1. Noble V, Nelson B, Sutingco N. *Emergency and Critical Care Ultrasound*. Cambridge University Press; 2007.

**7.** Correct Answer: C. There will be increased penetration of the ultrasound waves.

*Rationale:* Decreasing the frequency of the transmitted ultrasound wave will have several effects. It will increase the Nyquist limit, decreasing the amount of aliasing. There will be decreased lateral resolution. Because there is less attenuation, the waves will more effectively penetrate deeper tissues, and less energy will be absorbed in the tissues.

Selected Reference
1. Soni NJ, Arntfield R, Kory P. *Point of Care Ultrasound*. Elsevier; 2019.

# 5 | ULTRASOUND MODES

Christopher R. Tainter, Michael Self, and Cameron Smyres

1. Which of the following ultrasound modes is used to create **Figure 5.1**?

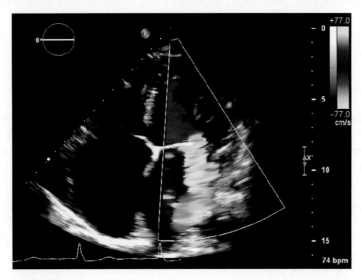

Figure 5.1

A. B-mode
B. Color Doppler
C. Pulsed-wave Doppler
D. All of the above

2. A 38-year-old woman with a history of heavy vaginal bleeding and recent hysterectomy presents with tachycardia, hypotension, and respiratory distress. While performing a point-of-care cardiac ultrasound, you notice she has significant right ventricular dilatation. To evaluate her right ventricular function you assess her "tricuspid annular plane systolic excursion" (TAPSE). What ultrasound mode is the most accurate in measuring the change in distance of the tricuspid annulus along a single ultrasound crystal?

A. B-mode
B. M-mode
C. A-mode
D. C-mode

3. A 67-year-old man presents after a syncopal episode while walking. On examination, a systolic murmur is noted, with a prominent S4. You use ultrasound to assess the flow across the aortic valve, and the pressure gradient between the left ventricle and the aorta to determine the severity of the abnormality. Which imaging mode is the most appropriate for this scenario?

    **A.** Color flow Doppler
    **B.** Color power Doppler
    **C.** Continuous-wave Doppler
    **D.** Pulsed-wave Doppler

4. Which of the following will decrease the artifact seen in **Figure 5.2**?

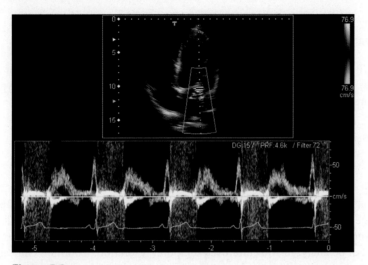

**Figure 5.2**

    **A.** Decreasing the pulse rate frequency (PRF)
    **B.** Reducing the image depth
    **C.** Selecting a higher frequency transducer
    **D.** Increasing the gain

5. While using the linear probe to assist in the placement of an intravascular catheter, you place the machine in color Doppler mode and obtain **Figure 5.3**.

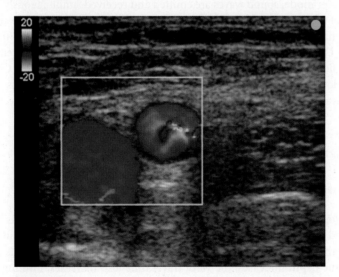

**Figure 5.3**

6. Which of the following associations is correct?

   **A.** Blue: blood flow coming toward the transducer
   **B.** Red: received signal with shorter wavelengths
   **C.** Blue: venous blood flow
   **D.** Red: higher velocity blood flow

# Chapter 5 ▪ Answers

**1.** Correct Answer: D. All of the above

*Rationale:* Figure 5.1 shows a B-mode (brightness mode, or 2-D) background, with overlying color flow Doppler. Color flow Doppler applies a color scale to pulsed-wave Doppler signals, thus it is a type of pulsed-wave Doppler; therefore all three imaging modes are used to create Figure 5.1.

Selected Reference
1. Soni NJ, Arntfield R, Kory P. *Point of Care Ultrasound.* Elsevier; 2019.

**2.** Correct Answer: B. M-mode

*Rationale:* "M-mode," which stands for motion mode, assesses images within a 2-D mode. After applying a cursor along a single line within the 2-D image, the movement of tissues along that single line is analyzed over time. Any movement of structures, including the changes in cavity sizes and movements of structures along that line, can be analyzed with improved temporal resolution. Common clinical applications include changes in the size of cardiac chambers, movement of cardiac valve leaflets throughout the cardiac cycle, changes in the diameter of the inferior vena cava during respiration, and the presence or absence of pleural sliding in assessing for possible pneumothorax.

Selected Reference
1. Ng A, Justiaan S. Resolution in ultrasound imaging. *Contin Educ Anaesth Crit Care Pain.* 2011 Oct;11(5):186-192. doi: 10.1093/bjaceaccp/mkr030.

**3.** Correct Answer: C. Continuous-wave Doppler

*Rationale:* In continuous-wave Doppler mode, sound waves are emitted and received simultaneously and continuously along the entire path of the ultrasound beam. As there is no pulsed cycle, it avoids the aliasing effect of pulsed-wave Doppler imaging and can accurately measure high-velocity blood flow without a Nyquist limit. Both pulsed-wave Doppler and color-flow Doppler are limited by this aliasing effect, making them less effective for high-flow states, like evaluating stenotic or regurgitant valvular flow. Color power Doppler is more sensitive to low velocity than color Doppler, but is limited in that it analyzes only the amplitude of returning sound waves and does not provide any information regarding the direction of flow.

Selected Reference
1. Maus T, Nhieu S, Herway ST, eds. *Essential Echocardiography.* Springer; 2016

**4.** Correct Answer: B. Reducing the image depth

*Rationale:* Although pulsed-wave Doppler allows measurement of velocity at a precise location, it is limited by the aliasing effect. As pulsed waves are transmitted into tissues, the transducer must await the returning wave before emitting further pulses. The PRF is the rate at which the transducer emits and receives these pulsed cycles. As tissue depth increases, the wave travel time also increases, limiting the maximum PRF. When the pulse transmission rate becomes too long relative to the velocity of blood flow, the direction and velocity of blood flow become ambiguous and "aliasing" occurs. The maximum wave frequency that can be measured before aliasing occurs is known as the "Nyquist limit" and is equal to one-half of the PRF. The Nyquist limit can be increased by increasing the PRF, reducing the image depth, or using a lower frequency transducer. Switching to continuous-wave Doppler also eliminates aliasing, because there is no pulse repetition, although it is unable to localize the position of the measurement along its path.

Selected Reference

1. Soni NJ, Arntfield R, Kory P. *Point of Care Ultrasound*. Elsevier; 2019.

**5.** Correct Answer: B. Red: received signal with shorter wavelengths

*Rationale:* The Doppler shift is the change in frequency of sound waves reflected from a moving reflector and is proportional to the relative velocity between the reflector and the ultrasound transducer. Blood flowing in the direction toward the transducer causes the returning ultrasound wavelength to decrease and have higher frequency. Reflection from blood flowing away from the transducer causes the returning ultrasound waves to increase in wavelength and have a lower frequency. In color flow Doppler mode, the direction and magnitude of these velocities are color-coded, as indicated by the legend at the top of the screen. In this case (Figure 5.3), red and yellow indicate flow toward the probe with decreasing wavelength (higher frequency), and dark blue and light blue indicate flow away from the probe with increasing wavelength (lower frequency).

Selected Reference

1. Soni NJ, Arntfield R, Kory P. *Point of Care Ultrasound*. Elsevier; 2019.

# 6 | LONGITUDINAL, LATERAL, AND TEMPORAL RESOLUTION

Michael J. Lanspa

1. Which of the following changes will improve the axial (longitudinal) resolution of an ultrasound image?

   A. Decrease the image sector depth
   B. Narrow the image sector width
   C. Use a higher frequency probe
   D. Change the imaging from fundamental to harmonic (tissue harmonic imaging [THI])

2. Which of the following statements is *most* true regarding lateral resolution?

   A. Lateral resolution is best at the focus.
   B. Lateral resolution worsens with a smaller beam diameter.
   C. Lateral resolution worsens as scan line density increases.
   D. Lateral resolution is typically better than axial resolution.

3. Which of the following will increase temporal resolution?

   A. Changing from B-mode to color flow Doppler imaging
   B. Increasing the frequency from 3 MHz to 5 MHz
   C. Increasing the scan line density
   D. Increasing the pulse repetition frequency

4. Which of the following statements is true regarding resolution and color Doppler imaging?

   A. Temporal resolution will increase with smaller Doppler packet size.
   B. Color Doppler has better axial resolution than B-mode imaging.
   C. Color Doppler has better lateral resolution than B-mode imaging.
   D. Axial resolution varies with depth in color imaging.

5. Which ultrasound probe offers the best axial resolution?

   A. 5 MHz, 4 cycles/pulse, 0.8 μs pulse duration
   B. 5 MHz, 2 cycles/pulse, 0.4 μs pulse duration
   C. 2 MHz, 4 cycles/pulse, 2 μs pulse duration
   D. 2 MHz, 2 cycles/pulse, 1 μs pulse duration

# Chapter 6 ▪ Answers

**1.** Correct Answer: C. Use a higher frequency probe

*Rationale:* Axial resolution (also called longitudinal, range, radial, or depth resolution) is the ability to resolve two structures that are close to each other along the beam's main axis. Axial resolution is determined by the frequency and spatial pulse. Axial resolution improves with higher frequency sound, which has a shorter wavelength. Axial resolution may also improve with fewer cycles per pulse (short pulse length or short pulse duration). The frequency of the transducer is determined by the thickness of the piezoelectric crystals and the damping material behind them, which shortens the pulses of sound waves emitted. Changing these settings requires changing the probe; neither frequency nor pulse duration can be adjusted by the sonographer. Changing sector depth or width may improve temporal resolution, but not axial resolution. Axial resolution is identical throughout an image. While harmonic imaging may improve black-white border definition and reduce some artifacts, it will decrease axial resolution due to its narrowed bandwidth.

### Selected References
1. Anvari A, Forsberg F, Samir AE. A primer on the physical principles of tissue harmonic imaging. *Radiographics*. 2015;25:1955-1964.
2. Edelman SK. *Understanding Ultrasound Physics*. 4th ed. E.S.P. Ultrasound; 2000.
3. Kremkau FW. *Diagnostic Ultrasound: Principles and Instruments*. WB Saunders Company; 2005.

**2.** Correct Answer: A. Lateral resolution is best at the focus.

*Rationale:* Lateral resolution (also called angular, transverse, or azimuthal resolution) is the minimum distance between two reflectors that can be distinguished when they are located perpendicular to the ultrasound beam (**Figure 6.1**). The ultrasound beam width determines the lateral resolution, and a narrower beam produces improved lateral resolution (**Figure 6.2**). Unlike axial resolution, which is uniform throughout the image, the lateral resolution varies with depth, because the ultrasound beam width changes with depth. The lateral resolution is the smallest (best) at the focus, or one near zone length from the transducer (focal depth) because the sound beam is narrowest at that point (Figure 6.1). *Option B* is incorrect, as the lateral resolution is equal to the beam diameter, meaning it improves with smaller diameter beams. *Option C* is incorrect because the lateral resolution is improved by increasing the number of scan lines per image, although increasing the scan line density may worsen the temporal resolution (frame rate). Axial resolution is usually much better than lateral resolution, because spatial pulse length, which determines axial resolution, is typically much smaller than the ultrasound beam width, which determines lateral resolution.

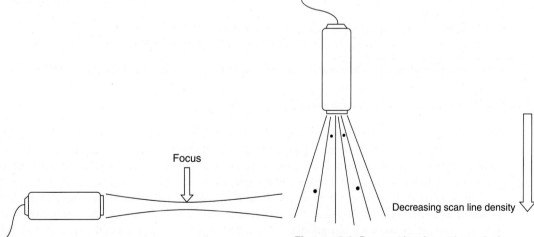

**Figures 6.1** Diagram of lateral resolution.

**Figures 6.2** Decreasing lateral resolution with decreasing line density.

### Selected References
1. Edelman SK. *Understanding Ultrasound Physics*. 4th ed. E.S.P. Ultrasound; 2000.
2. Ng A, Swanevelder J. Resolution in ultrasound imaging. *Contin Educ Anaesth Crit Care Pain*. 2011;11(5):186-192.

**3.** Correct Answer: D. Increasing the pulse repetition frequency

*Rationale:* Temporal resolution depends only on the frame rate (the number of images per second). The frame rate is determined by two factors: the imaging depth and the number of pulses per frame. Shallower image depth and fewer pulses will increase the frame rate and lead to improved temporal resolution. The frame rate is calculated as 77,000 cm/s divided by the pulses/frame and sector depth in centimeters. Pulse repetition frequency (the reciprocal of the pulse repetition period) is the number of pulses created by the system in 1 s. It is inversely related to imaging depth, which can be changed by the sonographer. Decreasing the imaging depth will increase the pulse repetition frequency and will also improve temporal resolution because less time will be required for waves to return to the transducer. Changing from B-mode to color imaging will decrease the frame rate. Any sort of Doppler imaging requires multiple ultrasound pulses to accurately determine velocities. The frame rate in color imaging depends on several factors, including the width and depth of the color box. The wider the box, the more scan lines are required, and the longer it will take to acquire the data to produce the image. Increasing the transducer frequency is not something adjustable by the sonographer, unless the probe is exchanged for a higher frequency probe, and this alone will not change the frame rate (although a different probe may use a different sector type). Increasing the scan line density will result in more scan lines and more pulses per frame, which will decrease the frame rate. Additionally, although not a choice, increasing the image sector width would increase the number of pulses per frame and decrease temporal resolution, while narrowing the sector width would increase temporal resolution.

### Selected References
1. Edelman SK. *Understanding Ultrasound Physics.* 4th ed. E.S.P. Ultrasound; 2000.
2. Kruskal JB, Newman PA, Sammons LG, Kane RA. Optimizing Doppler and color flow US: application to hepatic sonography. *Radiographics.* 2004;24(3):657-675.
3. Ng A, Swanevelder J. Resolution in ultrasound imaging. *Contin Educ Anaesth Crit Care Pain.* 2011;11(5):186-192.

**4.** Correct Answer: A. Temporal resolution will increase with smaller Doppler packet size.

*Rationale:* When performing Doppler imaging, multiple ultrasound pulses are needed to measure velocities. These multiple pulses are called a packet. A packet is the number of pulses per line. A smaller packet size means fewer pulses per line, which will improve temporal resolution (frame rate). Neither axial nor lateral resolution is improved in color Doppler compared to B-mode. Furthermore, color Doppler usually has worse lateral resolution than B-mode. To maintain adequate temporal resolution in color Doppler, the B-mode image is often compromised by reducing the number of focal zones to one or two and by reducing the scan line density, which lowers the lateral resolution. Axial resolution does not vary with depth, regardless of imaging mode.

### Selected References
1. Edelman SK. *Understanding Ultrasound Physics.* 4th ed. E.S.P. Ultrasound; 2000.
2. Kruskal JB, Newman PA, Sammons LG, Kane RA. Optimizing Doppler and color flow US: application to hepatic sonography. *Radiographics.* 2004;24(3):657-675.
3. Ng A, Swanevelder J. Resolution in ultrasound imaging. *Contin Educ Anaesth Crit Care Pain.* 2011;11(5):186-192.

**5.** Correct Answer: B. 5 MHz, 2 cycles/pulse, 0.4 μs pulse duration

*Rationale:* Axial (longitudinal) resolution is calculated by dividing the spatial pulse length by 2. The spatial pulse length is calculated by multiplying the wavelength with the number of cycles per pulse. If the number of cycles per pulse was not provided, one could calculate it by dividing the pulse duration by the period or multiplying the pulse duration by the frequency. For A, the pulse has four cycles (5,000,000 Hz × 0.0000008 s). Wavelength is 1540 m/s divided by 5 MHz = 0.31 mm. The spatial pulse length = 4 cycles/pulse × 0.31 mm = 1.23 mm. The axial resolution = one-half of 1.23 mm = 0.62 mm. For B, the pulse has two cycles and a wavelength of 0.31 mm, which gives a resolution of 0.31 mm. C has a pulse of four cycles and a wavelength of 0.77 mm, yielding an axial resolution of 1.54 mm. D has a pulse of two cycles and a wavelength of 0.77 mm, yielding an axial resolution of 0.77. Of these choices, B has the best (smallest) axial resolution. When given a choice between numerical values, the best axial resolution will be the highest frequency and the fewest cycles per pulse, which will result in the shortest pulse duration. If pulse duration is provided, one can calculate the axial resolution by multiplying pulse duration by 770 m/s (one-half of the speed of sound in soft tissue).

Spatial pulse length = Wavelength $\times$ Cycles / pulse

$$\frac{Cycles}{pulse} = \frac{Pulse\ duration}{Period} = Pulse\ duration\ (s) \times Frequency(Hz)$$

$$Axial\ resolution = \frac{Spatial\ pulse\ length}{2}$$

$$Axial\ resolution = \frac{Cycles\ /\ pulse \times 1540\ m\ /\ s}{2 \times Frequency(Hz)}$$

$$Axial\ resolution = \frac{Pulse\ duration\ \times 1540\ m\ /\ s}{2}$$

Selected References

1. Edelman SK. *Understanding Ultrasound Physics*. 4th ed. E.S.P. Ultrasound; 2000.
2. Ng A, Swanevelder J. Resolution in ultrasound imaging. *Contin Educ Anaesth Crit Care Pain.* 2011;11(5):186-192.

# 7 | DOPPLER EFFECT AND PRINCIPLES

Jan Kasal and Chakradhar Venkata

1. Please select the parameters that best match **Figure 7.1**.

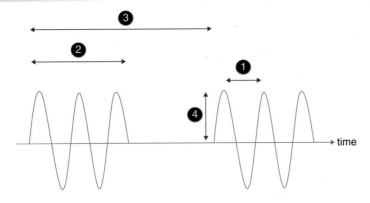

**Figure 7.1**

**A.** 1—pulse duration, 2—period, 3—pulse repetition period (PRP), 4—amplitude
**B.** 1—wavelength, 2—pulse duration, 3—pulse repetition frequency (PRF), 4—amplitude
**C.** 1—period, 2—pulse duration, 3—PRP, 4—amplitude
**D.** 1—frequency, 2—period, 3—spatial pulse length (SPL), 4—amplitude

2. The following Doppler tracing was recorded from an apical four-chamber view in a patient receiving mechanical ventilation, with a mean airway pressure of 28 cmH$_2$O, and positive end-expiratory pressure (PEEP) of 16 cmH$_2$O (**Figure 7.2**). Which of the following statements is *most* accurate?

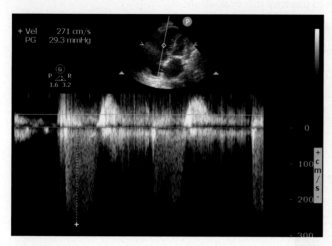

**Figure 7.2**

   **A.** Small deviations in cursor angle may cause a large underestimation in maximal velocity
   **B.** Lowering the lateral resolution underestimates the maximal recorded velocity
   **C.** Increasing the signal-to-noise ratio (SNR) will overestimate the maximal recorded velocity
   **D.** Manipulation of the time gain compensation will improve the estimation of the correct velocity

3. If the frequency of the probe is 2 MHz and the returned signal frequency coming back toward the probe is 2.05 MHz, the Doppler shift ($\Delta f$) is:

   **A.** −50 kHz
   **B.** 50 kHz
   **C.** −50 Hz
   **D.** 50 Hz

4. While examining the left ventricular outflow tract (LVOT) velocity, there is no pulsed-wave (PW) Doppler signal obtained. Which of the following is the *most likely* reason for the inadequate signal?

   **A.** The difference in direction between the ultrasound beam and blood flow
   **B.** High volumetric blood flow
   **C.** Wall filters set too low
   **D.** Dynamic LVOT obstruction

5. A 75-year-old man is admitted with septic shock. After a 30 mL/kg lactated Ringer's bolus, he remains hypotensive. In an attempt to assess for preload responsiveness by measuring breath-to-breath variability in stroke volume, a Doppler waveform is obtained through the LVOT (**Figure 7.3**). Which of the following would be *most* effective to improve this evaluation?

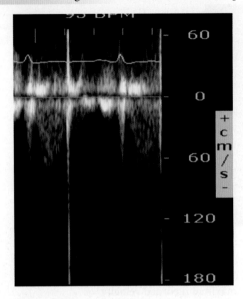

**Figure 7.3**

A. Increase the Doppler velocity scale
B. Measure the LVOT cross-sectional area
C. Increase the sweep speed
D. Move the sample volume to a different location

6. The following image is obtained from an apical long-axis (three-chamber) view, with a Doppler tracing through the LVOT (**Figure 7.4**). There are two Doppler flow patterns present, LVOT velocity-time integral (VTI), and a second signal. Which of the following would *most* effectively optimize the second Doppler flow signal?

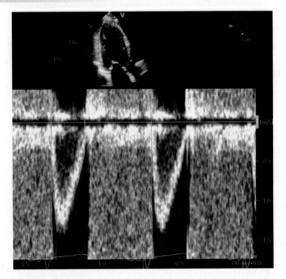

**Figure 7.4**

A. Decrease PRF
B. Increase depth
C. Decrease baseline
D. Change to continuous-wave (CW) mode

7. What would be the maximum detectable Doppler shift, using PW Doppler, if the PRP is 0.125 ms?

    A. 0.125 kHz
    B. 2 kHz
    C. 4 kHz
    D. 8 kHz

8. Which of the following modes does *not* have a Nyquist limit?

    A. Color Doppler
    B. Tissue Doppler
    C. CW Doppler
    D. PW Doppler

9. The following Doppler pattern was obtained during a transthoracic echo examination of an intensive care unit (ICU) patient with heart failure (**Figure 7.5A** and **B**). Which flow does this waveform *most likely* represent?

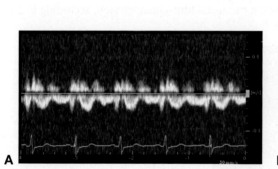

**Figure 7.5**

    A. Right ventricular outflow tract (RVOT)
    B. Pulmonary veins
    C. Hepatic vein (HV)
    D. Descending aorta

10. The following Doppler pattern was obtained in an ICU patient while evaluating for preload responsiveness. **Figure 7.6** shows a suboptimal result. What was the most likely change made in order to optimize the image from Figure 7.6 to **Figure 7.7**?

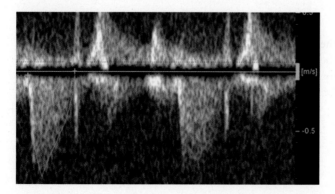

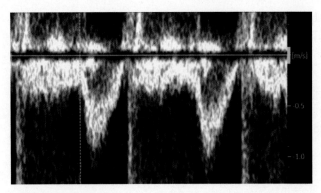

**Figures 7.6 and 7.7**

A. The sample volume was changed from 20 to 3 mm
B. A fluid bolus was given to eliminate the degree of LVOT obstruction
C. The mode was changed to CW to reduce aliasing
D. The sample volume was positioned closer to the aortic valve

11. The following PW Doppler waveforms were obtained from mitral valve inflow during the examination of an ICU patient with respiratory failure secondary to pulmonary edema. **Figure 7.8** shows the initial waveform. After correcting the technique, an optimal waveform was obtained (**Figure 7.9**). What is the correct position of PW Doppler sample volume in the apical four-chamber view, according to American Society of Echocardiography (ASE) guidelines?

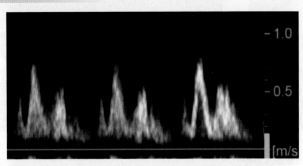

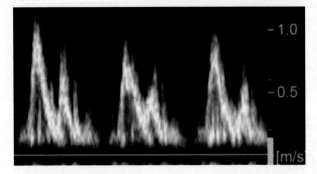

**Figures 7.8 and 7.9**

A. At the mitral leaflet tips, toward the lateral wall of the left ventricle (LV)
B. At the mitral leaflet tips, toward the medial wall of the LV
C. In the center of the long axis of the LV, 10 mm above the mitral leaflet tips
D. In the center of the long axis of the LV, 5 mm below the mitral leaflet tips

12. A 60-year-old man is intubated and placed on mechanical ventilation for severe acute respiratory distress syndrome (ARDS) secondary to COVID-19 pneumonia. He is paralyzed for ongoing ventilator dyssynchrony, and his oxygenation improves. The following Doppler waveform is obtained through his LVOT (**Figure 7.10**). This pattern is *most* consistent with which of the following?

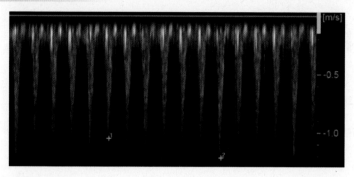

**Figure 7.10**

A. Pulsus alternans
B. Pulsus paradoxus
C. Reverse pulsus paradoxus
D. Annulus reversus or annulus paradoxus

13. A 75-year-old man is admitted to the ICU after he is intubated for acute pulmonary edema secondary to mitral regurgitation related to endocarditis. He is on a stable rate of norepinephrine infusion. The following color flow Doppler (CFD) images are obtained. The change of which variable most likely caused the difference from **Figure 7.11** to **Figure 7.12**?

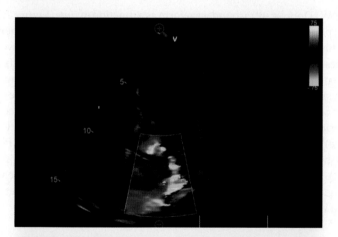

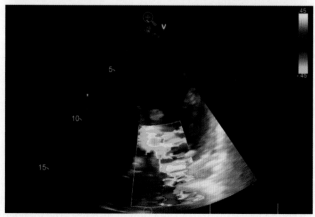

**Figures 7.11 and 7.12**

A. Color Doppler velocity scale
B. Depth and sector size
C. Systolic blood pressure
D. Zoom

# Chapter 7 ▪ Answers

**1.** Correct Answer: C. 1—period, 2—pulse duration, 3—PRP, 4—amplitude

*Rationale:* Several parameters can describe ultrasound waves, which can be viewed as a function of time or a function of distance.

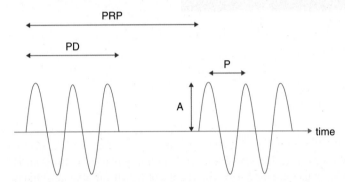

**Figure 7.13**

When visualizing the pulsed-wave (PW) Doppler ultrasound waveform as a function of *time* (**Figure 7.13**), it can be described by the following parameters: (1) is the duration of one wave and is called the **period (P)** (expressed in units of time). Its inverse is called the **frequency (f)** (expressed in Hz). In other words, the frequency is the number of cycles in one second. (2) is the **pulse duration (PD)**, which consists of a discrete pulse of ultrasound energy emitted by the ultrasound probe. Note that in the PW Doppler mode, the PD is limited (the probe sends a signal) and followed by a period of listening without any pulse sent. In CW Doppler, the pulses are sent continuously, without interruption while the probe simultaneously listens. (3) is the pulse repetition period **(PRP)** and describes the duration between the cycles (1 PRP in PW = emitting time + listening time). The inverse of PRP is called the pulse repetition frequency **(PRF)**. PRF limits the maximum Doppler shift (and thus velocity) that the PW Doppler can measure without aliasing (the Nyquist limit = PRF/2). (4) is the **amplitude (A)** and describes the difference between the maximum and the mean value of the acoustic signal. The amplitude contributes to acoustic power and intensity. Higher power is associated with the risk of bioeffects.

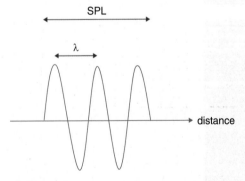

**Figure 7.14**

When visualizing the ultrasound waveform as a function of *distance* (**Figure 7.14**), the **wavelength (λ)** is the spatial distance between individual sound waves, expressed as a unit of distance. The total length of the wave emitted during a PW Doppler pulse is called the spatial pulse length **(SPL)**, and it determines the axial resolution (PW can distinguish between two points along the path of the wave only when the distance between them is more than half of the SPL). One clue for helping to eliminate incorrect answer choices is to pay attention to the units; options offering distance-based parameters (wavelength, SPL) will not be correct here because the x-axis in the diagram is time.

### Selected References
1. Miele FR. *Essentials of Ultrasound Physics*. Pegasus Lectures; 2008:chapter 4.
2. Oh JK, Kane GC, Seward JB, Tajik AJ. *The Echo Manual*. 4th ed. Wolters Kluwer; 2019:chapter 27.

---

**2.** Correct Answer: A. Small deviations in cursor angle may cause a large underestimation in maximal velocity

*Rationale:* Figure 7.2 shows the continuous-wave (CW) Doppler waveform of tricuspid valve regurgitation in a patient with acute cor pulmonale secondary to ARDS, who is on a significant amount of positive pressure. The objective is to correctly measure the velocity of the blood flow of the tricuspid regurgitation jet using CW Doppler and then apply the modified Bernoulli equation to calculate the pressure gradient. The correct measurement of velocity is essential for an accurate estimate of the gradient between the right atrium and the right ventricle (RV), which can be used to estimate the pulmonary artery systolic pressure.

It is important to understand which variables are susceptible to errors in the examination technique. These will lead to inaccurate velocity and pressure calculations, according to the Doppler equation (7.1):

$$\Delta f = (2 f_0 \times v \times \cos \theta)/c \qquad (7.1)$$

where $v$ = velocity of interest, $\Delta f$ = change in frequency between the emitted and received waves, $f_0$ = frequency of the transmitted wave, $\cos \theta$ = incident angle between the blood flow and ultrasound beam (angle of insonation), and $c$ = speed of the ultrasound wave. Because the magnitude of the Doppler shift is proportional to the cosine of the angle of insonation, relatively small deviations in the angle of insonation can result in significant underestimation of flow velocity, so there should be a concerted effort to align the ultrasound beam parallel to the blood flow to obtain the most accurate velocity measurement (choice A is correct). An angle exceeding 20° generally results in an unacceptable underestimation of the velocity. No Doppler shift at all occurs at a completely perpendicular angle (90° or 270°).

Lowering the lateral resolution and time gain compensation is related to properties of a two-dimensional (2D) image, not spectral Doppler velocities (choices B and D are incorrect). With an increased SNR, the correct velocity (the signal) will be more easily differentiated from noise (an incorrect, usually falsely high velocity). The result would be a reduced, not increased, velocity measurement (choice C is incorrect).

### Selected References
1. Miele FR. *Essentials of Ultrasound Physics*. Pegasus Lectures; 2008:chapter 4.
2. Oh JK, Kane GC, Seward JB, Tajik AJ. *The Echo Manual*. 4th ed. Wolters Kluwer; 2019:chapter 27.

---

**3.** Correct Answer: B. 50 kHz

*Rationale:* The Doppler shift describes the difference between the frequency transmitted and received after reflection from a moving reflector ($\Delta f = f_{received} - f_{transmitted}$). In this case, 2.05 − 2 = 0.05 MHz, or 50 kHz. It is important to pay attention to the correct units (MHz = 1000 kHz = 1,000,000 Hz). The positive shift means the object is moving toward the probe (returned frequency increased), while a negative shift implies the object is moving away from the probe (returned frequency decreased).

### Selected References
1. Miele FR. *Essentials of Ultrasound Physics*. Pegasus Lectures; 2008:chapter 4.
2. Oh JK, Kane GC, Seward JB, Tajik AJ. *The Echo Manual*. 4th ed. Wolters Kluwer; 2019:chapter 27.

---

**4.** Correct Answer: A. The difference in direction between the ultrasound beam and blood flow

*Rationale:* Recall the effect of the angle of insonation ($\theta$) in the Doppler equation: $\Delta f = (2 f_0 \times v \times \cos \theta)/c$. An angle of insonation less than 20° (in other words, as parallel as possible) from blood flow direction will result in cosine close to 1 and therefore will not significantly underestimate the measured Doppler shift, and will not reduce Doppler signal substantially. As the angle of insonation approaches 90° (perpendicular), cosine approaches 0 and significantly reduces or eliminates the Doppler shift (choice A is correct).

High volumetric blood flow will result in an increased, not reduced, Doppler signal (choice B is incorrect). Wall filters allow higher frequency signals (blood flow) to pass through while eliminating the low-frequency signals (tissue). Wall filters set too high could eliminate all signals, both low and high frequency, while wall filters set too low could allow lower frequency signals to pass through and increase, not decrease or eliminate, Doppler signal (choice C is incorrect). Dynamic LV tract obstruction increases the velocity of flow and alters the Doppler envelope causing a distinct shape of the Doppler waveform ("dagger shaped"), but does not eliminate the Doppler signal (choice D is incorrect).

### Selected References
1. Miele FR. *Essentials of Ultrasound Physics*. Pegasus Lectures; 2008:chapter 4.
2. Oh JK, Kane GC, Seward JB, Tajik AJ. *The Echo Manual*. 4th ed. Wolters Kluwer; 2019:chapter 4.

**5.** Correct Answer: **D. Move the sample volume to a different location**

*Rationale:* The velocity scale is not optimal. The Doppler signal in Figure 7.3 appears too small due to an excessively large scale. Because of the small Doppler envelope, it would be difficult to trace the VTI contour correctly. Decreasing, not increasing, the Doppler velocity scale would increase the size of VTI contour and would allow more accurate tracing of the VTI (**Figure 7.15**) (choice A is incorrect).

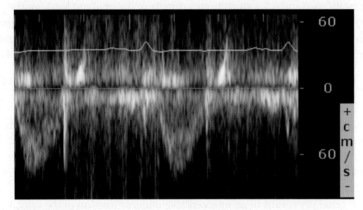

**Figure 7.15**

It is not necessary to measure the LVOT area to compare stroke volume changes in this case, because it will not change with the respiratory cycle. The stroke volume is directly proportional to the VTI ($VTI_{LVOT} \times Area_{LVOT}$) (choice B is incorrect).

Changing the sweep speed will change the number of Doppler tracings on the screen. The number of Doppler tracings (two in this case) is not sufficient to make conclusions about the breath-to-breath variability of stroke volume. Decreasing, not increasing, the sweep speed from 100 mm/s (Figure 7.15) to 35 mm/s (**Figure 7.16**) allows for more waveforms with the LVOT VTI spectral Doppler signal (Figure 7.16) (choice C is incorrect).

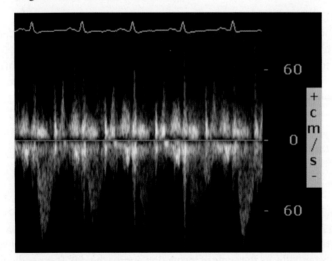

**Figure 7.16**

The Doppler VTI signal through the LVOT in Figure 7.3 is not optimal. An optimal LVOT VTI signal should be narrow, with a central "clearing," reflecting laminar flow. The signal in Figure 7.3 shows spectral broadening. This is consistent with measuring multiple different velocities, raising the suspicion of measuring turbulent, nonlaminar, flow. Additional positioning of the sample volume (ideally 5 mm proximal to the aortic valve in the center of the LVOT) might optimize the Doppler signal (choice D is correct).

### Selected References

1. Miele FR. *Essentials of Ultrasound Physics.* Pegasus Lectures; 2008:chapter 4.
2. Slama M, Masson H, Teboul JL, et al. *Respiratory variations of aortic VTI: a new index of hypovolemia and fluid responsiveness. Am J Physiol Heart Circ Physiol.* 2002;283(4):H1729-H1733.

---

**6.** Correct Answer: D. Change to CW mode

*Rationale:* The image in Figure 7.4 shows a well-defined PW Doppler waveform during systole, directed away from the probe (below the baseline). The second waveform is a diastolic signal both above and below the baseline, caused by aortic regurgitation (AR), which should be directed toward the probe (above the baseline). Aliasing creates this "confusion" of the direction of flow if the velocity measured exceeds the capability of PW Doppler to measure it correctly, resulting in the signal "wrapping around" the baseline (appearing both above and below the line). The maximum measurable velocity is limited by the Nyquist limit ($f_{max}$), which is the frequency equal to one-half of the PRF ($f_{max} = $ PRF/2). Once the detected Doppler shift exceeds half of the PRF, aliasing will occur.

Decreasing PRF would decrease the maximum velocity that PW can measure, and it would increase the likelihood of aliasing (choice A is incorrect).

Increasing the depth means there would be more time needed between transmitting the pulses. The time between transmits is called the PRP. Since PRP = 1/PRF, higher PRP = lower PRF = increased aliasing ($f_{max} = $ PRF/2) (choice B is incorrect).

Changing the baseline on the screen to a higher or lower position **while still in PW Doppler** will move the aliasing flow up or down on the screen, but it would not change the degree of the aliasing (choice C is incorrect).

The best solution would be to use CW Doppler. CW Doppler is not subject to aliasing and will allow the correct examination of high-velocity flows, such as those through stenotic or regurgitant lesions. The limitation of CW is range ambiguity (inability to localize where along the line of interrogation the measurement is occurring), which is not a concern here, since AR would be the highest diastolic flow velocity along the entire tract of ultrasound beam (choice D is correct).

### Selected References

1. Miele FR. *Essentials of Ultrasound Physics.* Pegasus Lectures; 2008:chapter 4.
2. Oh JK, Kane GC, Seward JB, Tajik AJ. *The Echo Manual.* 4th ed. Wolters Kluwer; 2019:chapter 27.

---

**7.** Correct Answer: C. 4 kHz

*Rationale:* According to the Nyquist limit, the maximum detectable shift in PW mode equals one-half of the PRF ($f_{max} = $ PRF/2). PRF is the inverse of PRP (PRF = 1/PRP). If PRP = 0.125 ms, then PRF = 1/0.125 ms = 8 kHz. The maximum detectable shift (Nyquist limit) will be half the PRF = 8 kHz/2 = 4 kHz.

### Selected Reference

1. Miele FR. *Essentials of Ultrasound Physics.* Pegasus Lectures; 2008:chapter 4.

---

**8.** Correct Answer: C. CW Doppler

*Rationale:* PW Doppler (whether measuring blood flow or tissue velocity) is subject to aliasing and therefore has a Nyquist limit. Color Doppler is based on PW Doppler and is also subject to aliasing. CW Doppler is not subject to aliasing and therefore does not have a Nyquist limit.

### Selected References

1. Miele FR. *Essentials of Ultrasound Physics.* Pegasus Lectures; 2008:chapter 4.
2. Oh JK, Kane GC, Seward JB, Tajik AJ. *The Echo Manual.* 4th ed. Wolters Kluwer; 2019:chapter 4.

---

**9.** Correct Answer: C. Hepatic vein (HV)

*Rationale:* Figure 7.5A shows an example of a PW Doppler waveform with relatively slow velocities, with two peaks oriented away from the probe (in systole and diastole) and smaller peaks oriented toward the probe. This is most consistent with flow through the HV. HV flow (Figure 7.5B) is measured from the subcostal view using PW Doppler. The HV waveform morphology displays the flow from the HV into the inferior vena cava (IVC) during systole (S), systolic flow reversal (Sr), the flow into IVC during the first part of diastole (D), and diastolic flow reversal in the HV caused by atrial contraction (Dr). The flow away from the probe (S, D) will be displayed below the baseline and flow toward the probe (Sr, Dr) above the baseline. HV Doppler is useful to assess right atrial (RA) pressure, the severity of tricuspid regurgitation, RV dysfunction, and myopathy versus constrictive pericarditis (CP).

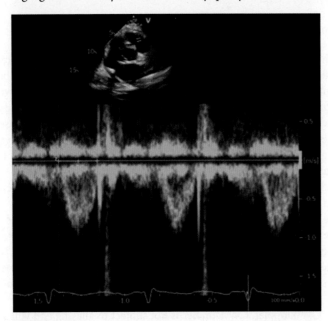

**Figure 7.17**

RVOT flow (**Figure 7.17**) is measured from the parasternal short-axis view and sometimes from the subcostal view using PW Doppler. It is characterized by a symmetric shape with a closing click, similar to the LVOT waveform. RVOT Doppler is useful to assess RV stroke volume and pulmonary hypertension, where its acceleration time shortens and its configuration becomes W-shaped.

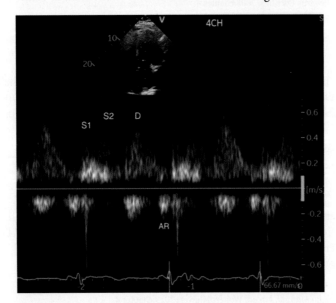

**Figure 7.18**

Pulmonary venous (PV) flow (**Figure 7.18**) is measured using PW Doppler from the apical four-chamber view and is often challenging to obtain due to limited visualization of the left atrium. A typical PV Doppler pattern demonstrates the systolic (S1, S2), diastolic (D), and atrial reversal (AR) flow velocities and is useful for estimating left atrial pressure (LAP).

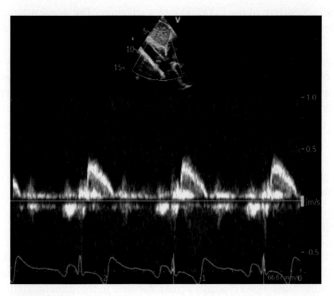

**Figure 7.19**

Descending thoracic aortic flow (**Figure 7.19**) is measured with PW Doppler using the suprasternal notch view. CW Doppler may be used to evaluate for the presence of flow-limiting obstructions. Severe AR results in a marked diastolic flow reversal. Aortic diastolic flow reversal is also present in sinus of Valsalva rupture and decreased aortic compliance in the elderly. Coarctation produces a characteristic pattern obtained by CW Doppler.

### Selected References

1. DeBacker D, Cholley BP, Slama M, Vieillard-Baron A, Vignon P. *Hemodynamic Monitoring Using Echocardiography in the Critically Ill*. Springer; 2011:chapter 16.
2. Mitchell C, Rahko PS, Blauwet LA, et al. Guidelines for performing a comprehensive transthoracic echocardiographic examination in adults: recommendations from the American Society of Echocardiography. *J Am Soc Echocardiogr*. 2019;32(1):1-64.
3. Oh JK, Kane GC, Seward JB, Tajik AJ. *The Echo Manual*. 4th ed. Wolters Kluwer 2019:chapter 4.

**10.** Correct Answer: A. The sample volume was changed from 20 to 3 mm

*Rationale:* The optimal LVOT VTI signal should be narrow with a rapid upstroke and an end-systolic click terminating the flow signal. The sample volume should be 5 mm proximal to the aortic valve and in the center of LVOT. Figure 7.6 shows spectral broadening; in other words, the signal is not narrow (*white arrow*, **Figure 7.20**).

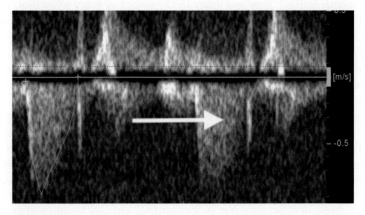

**Figure 7.20**

Decreasing the size of the sample volume gate will demonstrate the correct spectral window (Figure 7.7), indicating that laminar flow is present (choice A is correct).

LVOT obstruction results in a distinct pattern of the LVOT Doppler envelope. The signal may appear asymmetric ("dagger-shaped" envelope), different from the symmetric shape shown in Figures 7.6 and 7.7 (choice B is incorrect).

Changing the mode to CW would result in a wider spectral signal. CW cannot distinguish the location of the flow (range ambiguity) and would capture all velocities measured along the line of the ultrasound beam, resulting in a "filled in" envelope, rather than the "hollow" envelope desired (choice C is incorrect). Positioning the sample volume closer to the aortic valve would result in capturing higher velocities and would increase the risk of aliasing if using PW mode, but it would likely not eliminate spectral broadening (choice D is incorrect).

### Selected Reference

1. Mitchell C, Rahko PS, Blauwet LA, et al. Guidelines for performing a comprehensive transthoracic echocardiographic examination in adults: recommendations from the American Society of Echocardiography. *J Am Soc Echocardiogr*. 2019;32(1):1-64.

---

**11.** Correct Answer: A. At the mitral leaflet tips, toward the lateral wall of the left ventricle (LV)

*Rationale:* Doppler examination of the LV inflow forms the basis of the evaluation for the presence and grade of diastolic dysfunction. The correct placement of the PW Doppler sample volume should be at the mitral leaflet tips toward the lateral wall as blood flows typically across the valve in this direction (choice A is correct). Figure 7.9 shows the characteristic tracing.

It is essential to obtain an optimal Doppler tracing because the incorrect placement of the PW Doppler sample volume will result in an inaccurate estimation of early (E) and atrial (A) velocities, an inaccurate E/A ratio, an inaccurate E/e′ ratio, and an erroneous conclusion about diastolic function. Figure 7.8 shows an example of a suboptimal waveform, with lower velocities and a suboptimal waveform contour. Placing the sample volume erroneously toward the medial wall (choice B), far in the LV (choice C), or toward the left atrium (choice D) would result in a suboptimal tracing like this.

### Selected Reference

1. Mitchell C, Rahko PS, Blauwet LA, et al. (2019). Guidelines for performing a comprehensive transthoracic echocardiographic examination in adults: recommendations from the American Society of Echocardiography. *J Am Soc Echocardiogr*. 2019;32(1):1-64.

---

**12.** Correct Answer: C. Reverse pulsus paradoxus

*Rationale:* Figure 7.10 shows multiple PW Doppler waveforms, compressed in time due to slower sweep speed, with varying peak velocities. There is no respirometer tracing shown, but assuming there is no patient motion and cardiac translation movement, the variability in LVOT flow is most likely caused by changes in ventricular preload (and consequently, stroke volume) due to the intermittent changes in intrathoracic pressure with mechanical ventilation. Several distinct Doppler patterns of the LVOT may appear in ICU patients, and it is useful to be able to distinguish them.

*Pulsus alternans* will result in alternating higher and lower LVOT velocities every other beat, representing variable ventricular filling and stroke volume. It is associated with severe LV dysfunction (choice A is incorrect).

*Pulsus paradoxus* applies to a spontaneously breathing patient. During breathing, LVOT velocities decrease during inspiration and increase during expiration. Exaggerated pulsus paradoxus may be seen in several conditions, including cardiac tamponade. This patient is passively breathing on positive pressure mechanical ventilation (choice B is incorrect).

*Reverse pulsus paradoxus*, on the other hand, can be seen in mechanically ventilated patients. During inspiration, a positive pressure breath will increase pressure within the thoracic cavity and alveolar vessels. During this phase, blood flows from lung vasculature into the LV (LV preload increases and LV afterload decreases) for the duration of several heartbeats while blood flow into the RV decreases (RV preload decreases and RV afterload increases). During expiration, the previously decreased flow from RV is now passed on to the LV (LV preload decreases), which will reduce the flow through the LVOT. The net result is an increase in LVOT velocities on inspiration (i.e., during positive pressure breath) and decrease in LVOT velocities on expiration, sometimes called reverse pulsus paradoxus (*blue crosses*, Figure 7.10). The increased variability between inspiratory and expiratory LVOT velocities becomes clinically relevant during evaluation for preload responsiveness (choice C is correct).

Clinical use of Doppler includes measuring not only blood velocity but also tissue velocity. "*Annulus paradoxus*" describes a phenomenon seen in constrictive pericarditis (CP). In this situation, because tissue velocity (e′) is relatively normal or even increased, the ratio between early diastolic blood velocity mitral inflow (E) and tissue velocity (e′), the E/e′ ratio, is inversely proportional to the left atrial pressure (LAP) and by inference to the pulmonary capillary wedge pressure (PCWP). This "paradoxical" E/e′ and LAP relationship contrasts with myocardial disease where E/e′ is proportional LAP. Also, in CP, the septal e′ usually exceeds the lateral mitral e′ velocity, the opposite of a normal situation (typically, septal e′ < lateral e′). This "*annulus reversus*" is observed in about 80% of patients with constriction. Since there is no information about tissue Doppler, choice D is incorrect.

**Selected References**
1. DeBacker D, Cholley BP, Slama M, Vieillard-Baron A, Vignon P. *Hemodynamic Monitoring Using Echocardiography in the Critically Ill.* Springer; 2011:chapter 4.
2. Oh JK, Kane GC, Seward JB, Tajik AJ. *The Echo Manual.* 4th ed. Wolters Kluwer 2019:chapter 4

**13.** Correct Answer: A. Color Doppler velocity scale

*Rationale:* CFD is a PW Doppler technique that uses a series of multiple sample volumes, along with a series of scan lines, depicted in a region of interest (ROI). Figures 7.11 and 7.12 demonstrate the color Doppler examination of the mitral valve from the apical four-chamber view. There is mitral valve regurgitation, with a turbulent regurgitant flow depicted as a multicolor mosaic. Compared to Figure 7.11, Figure 7.12 shows significantly more regurgitant flow. The change may be related to an interval increase in the amount of the regurgitation, but also may be caused by different echocardiographic techniques without any actual change of the regurgitation itself.

The color Doppler velocity scale setting appears as a numeric value (usually in centimeters per second) seen on the color map (right upper corner in Figures 7.11 and 7.12). This numeric value represents the range of mean velocities that can be displayed. Setting the scale to high-velocity ranges demonstrates some color-flow data without aliasing. This recommendation is particularly true for laminar flow through normal valves and blood vessels. As a default, the color-flow scale (Nyquist limit) should be between 50 and 70 cm/s in each direction for all routine color Doppler interrogation. Such a setting is particularly important for the display of turbulent regurgitant valve jets. The size of the displayed regurgitant jet is affected by several variables, one being the Nyquist limit, in that the same regurgitant volume appears considerably larger at a lower color scale compared with a higher scale. In this case, the velocity scale has been decreased from 75 cm/s in Figure 7.11 to 45 cm/s in Figure 7.12, and is the most likely reason for the perceived increase of the size of regurgitation flow on the CDI (choice A is correct).

The depth and sector size will influence the appearance of the color Doppler. Before initiating CFD, the 2D sector size should be adjusted to the lowest depth and width necessary to accurately depict the anatomic ROI. This will help optimize the color frame rate. The lower the depth and width, the higher the frame rate, and in return, the higher the frequency, the PRF, and Nyquist limit. The color box ROI should be sized to include all of the flow information being evaluated. Setting the ROI as narrow and shallow as possible allows maximum frame rate and velocity scale, thus yielding the best temporal and flow velocity resolution. In this case, the depth, width, and size of the ROI have not appreciably changed (choice B is incorrect).

An increase of the systolic blood pressure would increase the LV afterload and could increase the amount of mitral regurgitation. However, this is less likely as the patient is in ICU without any recent hemodynamic changes indicated by the stable vasopressor rate. In addition, there is also other relevant information (change of color Doppler velocity scale on image) (choice C is incorrect).

The zoom function will magnify the structures of interest on the screen but would not have any effect on anything else. The pixels displaying the regurgitation would appear larger, but within the context of all structures also appearing larger (choice D is incorrect).

**Selected Reference**
1. Mitchell C, Rahko PS, Blauwet LA, et al. (2019). Guidelines for performing a comprehensive transthoracic echocardiographic examination in adults: recommendations from the American Society of Echocardiography. *J Am Soc Echocardiogr.* 2019;32(1):1-64.

# 8 | PHYSICS OF ULTRASOUND BIOEFFECTS

William P. Mulvoy III

1. A higher mechanical index (MI) increases the likelihood that cavitation will occur. A higher MI is *most* likely to occur in which of the following tissues?

   A. Lung
   B. Heart
   C. Adipose tissue
   D. Bone

2. Thermal bioeffects are directly responsible for the temperature elevation in the surrounding tissues caused by absorption and scattering of the ultrasound beam. Which intensity description is associated with thermal bioeffects on the surrounding tissues?

   A. Spatial peak, temporal peak
   B. Spatial peak, temporal average
   C. Spatial peak, pulse average
   D. Spatial peak, pulse peak

3. The biologic effects of ultrasound are directly proportional to the intensity of the ultrasound beam. Which of the following imaging modalities produces the *highest* energy output?

   A. Color Doppler
   B. Continuous-wave Doppler
   C. M-mode
   D. Pulsed-wave Doppler

4. Bubbles that tend to oscillate without bursting when exposed to acoustic waves demonstrate which type of cavitation?

   A. Transient cavitation
   B. Normal cavitation
   C. Inertial cavitation
   D. Stable cavitation

5. Which of the following factors have the *most* impact on the thermal effects on surrounding tissue?

   A. Rarefaction and frequency
   B. Exposure time and temperature
   C. Rarefaction and compression
   D. Amplification and compression

# Chapter 8 ▪ Answers

**1.** Correct Answer: A. Lung

*Rationale:* Microbubbles get bigger during the rarefactions caused by ultrasound waves. When the bubbles expand, it causes a shearing effect and the bubbles may burst, creating cavitation. The MI gives the operator information about the magnitude of energy administered to the patient's tissues during an ultrasound evaluation. The MI is a direct measure of acoustic power per unit time, thus as the number for MI increases, the acoustic power delivered to the surrounding tissues also increases, and cavitation becomes more likely. The organs most sensitive to cavitation are those that are air-filled, such as the lung or the intestine. Thus, the correct answer is the lung, as the other three answers do not have air, which directly relates to the potential for cavitation to occur. MI is a unitless number defined as the peak negative pressure divided by the square root of the frequency of the ultrasound wave:

MI = Peak Rarefaction (Negative) Pressure (MPa)/$\sqrt{}$ frequency (MHz)

The Food and Drug Administration (FDA) considers 1.9 the maximum allowable MI for diagnostic imaging to prevent the biologic effects of cavitation.

### Selected References
1. Apfel RE, Holland CK. Gauging the likelihood of cavitation from short pulse, low duty cycle diagnostic ultrasound. *Ultrasound Med Biol.* 1991;17:179.
2. Şen T, Tüfekçioğlu O, Koza Y. Mechanical index. *Anatol J Cardiol.* 2015;15(4):334-336.

**2.** Correct Answer: B. Spatial peak, temporal average (SPTA)

*Rationale:* SPTA is directly related to tissue heating. SPTA limits are 100 mW/cm$^2$ for unfocused ultrasound and 1 W/cm$^2$ for focused ultrasound. The current FDA output limits for diagnostic ultrasound are an SPTA intensity of less than 720 mW/cm$^2$. The output depends on the power, pulse repetition frequency, and the scanner operation mode (i.e., M-mode, pulsed-wave, or continuous-wave Doppler). The SPTA is the highest intensity measured at any point in the ultrasound beam averaged over the pulse repetition period, which directly relates to the biothermal effects on the surrounding tissues. The maximum allowable increase in tissue temperature approved by the FDA is 2 °C. Temperature elevation in fetal soft tissue is potentially more harmful than adult tissue, and this has been determined safe at this level. An elevation of 4 °C for 5 minutes or more will cause thermal bioeffects to the surrounding tissue and fetus, as this has been well documented in laboratory studies.

### Selected Reference
1. Nelson TR, Fowlkes JB, Abramowicz JS, Church CC. Ultrasound biosafety considerations for the practicing sonographer and sonologist. *J Ultrasound Med.* 2009;28(2):139-150.

**3.** Correct Answer: D. Pulsed-wave Doppler

*Rationale:* Examination exposure time produces the greatest bioeffect on tissues and therefore lengthy examinations should be avoided whenever possible. The lowest output intensity is with grayscale imaging, while the highest output is used with pulsed-wave Doppler signals. When comparing different Doppler output intensities, pulsed-wave Doppler spends about 8% to 10% of the time transmitting compared to grayscale imaging, which transmits only 1% to 2% of the time. This four- to fivefold increase in transmission time directly results in an intensity that is 5-10 times higher, with potentially more bioeffects. Also, the beam is held in a relatively constant position at the point of interest (sampling volume), which may induce a further increase in temporal average intensity. Hence, the intensity of pulsed-wave Doppler is greater than continuous-wave Doppler or color Doppler. Color Doppler is essentially small multiple pulsed-wave Dopplers, which has all the advantages of depth acuity but lacks the ability to measure very high velocities. Even though color Doppler is multiple small pulsed-wave Dopplers, it is still of lower energy when directly compared to pulsed-wave Doppler.

Selected References
1. American Institute of Ultrasound in Medicine Consensus report on potential bioeffects of diagnostic ultrasound: executive summary. *J Diagn Med Sonogr*. 2011;27(1):3-13.
2. Edelman SK. *Understanding Ultrasound Physics*. ESP; 2012.

**4.** Correct Answer: D. Stable cavitation

*Rationale:* Stable cavitation is defined as bubbles that oscillate and do not burst when exposed to small amplitude acoustic waves. Normal cavitation, inertial cavitation, and transient cavitation are all synonyms of one another. These are defined as bubbles that expand during rarefactions (negative pressure changes) causing bubbles to expand and burst. Transient cavitation, inertial cavitation, and normal cavitation cause highly localized, violent effects of enormous pressure waves and significant changes in localized temperature due to friction caused by these microscopic effects.

Selected Reference
1. Edelman SK. *Understanding Ultrasound Physics*. ESP; 2012.

**5.** Correct Answer: B. Exposure time and temperature

*Rationale:* Time and temperature elevation by direct tissue absorption results in thermal bioeffects and potential tissue damage to the surrounding tissues. The bone-tissue interface has the highest absorbent potential of all tissues, and therefore will also be subject to thermal effects more quickly. Thermal effects on tissues are directly related to the length of time exposed to ultrasound energy, as well as the increase in temperature of the surrounding tissue. The FDA states that less than a 2 °C increase in local tissue temperature is unlikely to produce tissue damage. Therefore, to minimize thermal bioeffects, the operator should attempt to reduce exposure time to ultrasound energy, which will minimize the local tissue temperature rise.

Selected References
1. Edelman, S. K. (2012). *Understanding Ultrasound Physics*. Woodlands, TX: ESP.
2. Nelson TR, Fowlkes JB, Abramowicz JS, Church CC. Ultrasound biosafety considerations for the practicing sonographer and sonologist. *J Ultrasound Med*. 2009;28(2):139-150.
3. Shankar H, Pagel PS. Potential adverse ultrasound-related biological effects. *Anesthesiology*. 2011;115(5):1109-1124.

# 9 | PATIENT AND ULTRASOUND MACHINE POSITIONING, PROBE SELECTION AND ORIENTATION, PROPER ULTRASOUND CARE

Aarti Sarwal

1. A 45-year-old man is undergoing fluid resuscitation and vasopressor administration for suspected septic shock. He is intubated and placed on mechanical ventilation. To mitigate the risk of pulmonary edema, you decide to assess for volume responsiveness with a passive leg raise (PLR) before giving more fluids. Which of the following describes this maneuver *most* accurately?

   A. Move the patient from a supine position to a supine position with the legs raised at 30° to 45°, avoiding femoral vein compression
   B. Move the patient from a reverse Trendelenburg position to Trendelenburg position
   C. Move the patient from a semi-recumbent (semi-Fowler's) position to a supine position with the legs raised at 30° to 45°, avoiding femoral vein compression
   D. Move the patient from a semi-recumbent (semi-Fowler's) position to a Trendelenburg position

2. A 75-year-old man with elevated body mass index (BMI) is being admitted to the intensive care unit (ICU) for undifferentiated shock. In order to assess for the etiology, a point-of-care echocardiogram is performed, but with suboptimal images obtained due to his body habitus. Which of the following maneuvers may help improve visualization of the heart from a parasternal or apical window?

   A. Place the patient in a left lateral decubitus position
   B. Place the patient in a right lateral decubitus position
   C. Place the patient in a reverse Trendelenburg position
   D. Place the patient in a Trendelenburg position

3. You are called to evaluate a patient with acute hypoxemia. You elicit a history of recent rib fractures and perform a point-of-care ultrasound examination to evaluate for pneumothorax. Which of the following statements is *most* correct regarding proper probe selection for this examination?

   A. A high-frequency linear array transducer is optimal for the appreciation of the pleural line for diagnosing pneumothorax.
   B. A low-frequency phased array transducer (cardiac probe) is optimal, as its flat and smaller footprint is better suited for imaging in between the ribs and provides better penetration.
   C. Either linear array or phased array transducers can be used to assess for pneumothorax with reliable accuracy.
   D. Ultrasound is not a suitable modality for accurately ruling out pneumothorax.

4. Which of the following statements is *most* accurate with regard to the routine cleaning of the ultrasound machine after use in clinical care?

   A. Ultrasound machines and probes must undergo high-level disinfection between all patient uses with vendor- and institution-approved products.
   B. Ultrasound probes should undergo regularly scheduled disinfection through hospital infection prevention facilities, but the machine can be cleaned only for removal of visible soiling each time in between patient use.
   C. If there is no visible soiling or blood contact, the system (including probes and machine) can be cleaned with wipes between all uses.
   D. For surface use of ultrasound, the machine and probes can be cleaned and disinfected with vendor- and institution-approved products with low-level disinfection in between all patient use, but guidelines for high-level disinfection must be followed for any indications where the system came in contact with blood, body fluids, or mucosal membranes.

5. You are using the cardiology preset to perform a brief, four-view point-of-care assessment of the heart. Which of the following pairings of the echocardiography views are correct for the position of the index marker?

   A. *Parasternal long-axis view:* index marker toward patient's right shoulder; parasternal short-axis view: index marker toward patient's left shoulder; apical four-chamber view: index marker toward patient's left elbow; subcostal view: index marker toward patient's left elbow
   B. *Parasternal long-axis view:* index marker toward patient's left shoulder; parasternal short-axis view: index marker toward patient's right shoulder; apical four-chamber view: index marker toward patient's right elbow; subcostal view: index marker toward patient's right elbow
   C. *Parasternal long-axis view:* index marker toward patient's right shoulder; parasternal short-axis view: index marker toward patient's left shoulder; apical four-chamber view: index marker toward patient's right elbow; subcostal view: index marker toward patient's right elbow
   D. *Parasternal long-axis view:* index marker toward patient's left shoulder; parasternal short-axis view: index marker toward patient's right shoulder; apical four-chamber view: index marker toward patient's left elbow; subcostal view: index marker toward patient's left elbow

# Chapter 9 ■ Answers

1. Correct Answer: C. Move the patient from a semi-recumbent (semi-Fowler's) position to a supine position with the legs raised at 30° to 45°, avoiding femoral vein compression

   *Rationale:* The PLR test is a test for volume responsiveness where the reservoir of venous blood is returned into the central circulation quickly and a hemodynamic response is measured. An increase in cardiac output (CO) or stroke volume (SV) or decrease in inferior vena cava variation denotes volume responsiveness. The PLR is best performed by mobilizing the patient from a semi-recumbent position to a supine position (patient's torso horizontal) with their legs elevated 30° to 45°, and not by manually raising the legs. This avoids compression of the femoral vein, which may reduce the venous return to the heart. Approximately 300 mL of intravascular volume is shifted during a PLR when performed properly. The CO or SV should be assessed 1 minute after the PLR, because at this time the effect seems the highest.

### Selected Reference

1. Orde S, Slama M, Hilton A, Yastrebov K, McLean A. Pearls and pitfalls in comprehensive critical care echocardiography. *Crit Care*. 2017;21:279. doi:10.1186/s13054-017-1866-z.

**2.** Correct Answer A. Place the patient in a left lateral decubitus position

*Rationale:* The parasternal window is located on the left side of the sternum. The apical window is located below the left nipple, where one can feel the apical impulse. Either of the views can be facilitated by turning the patient to their left side, which repositions the content of mediastinum toward the left and anterior, displacing the lung tissue, and facilitating insonation. In addition, raising the patient's left arm above their head (if possible) can widen the rib spaces, further improving visualization. A sustained breath-hold may help lower the diaphragm, improving subcostal visualization (although this usually creates more lung interference and impairs imaging in the parasternal and apical windows).

### Selected Reference

1. Mitchell C, Rahko PS, Blauwet LA, et al. Guidelines for performing a comprehensive transthoracic echocardiographic examination in adults: recommendations from the American Society of Echocardiography. *J Am Soc Echocardiogr*. 2019;32(1):1-64. doi:10.1016/j.echo.2018.06.004.

**3.** Correct Answer: C. Either linear array or phased array transducers can be used to assess for pneumothorax with reliable accuracy.

*Rationale:* Linear or phased array probes can be used to assess for pneumothorax. Comparative performance of the three most common probe types (linear, phased array, and curvilinear) has been tested and showed no difference in the diagnostic performance of the three transducers. Experienced observers perceived the best image quality and needed the least amount of time when they judged the linear array transducer clips (**Figure 9.1**).

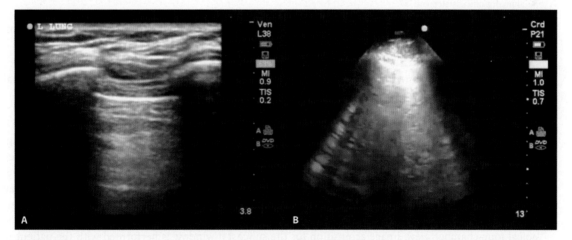

**Figure 9.1** A. Linear array probe used at 3.8 cm depth to visualize the lung between the two ribs. B. Insonation of the lung and ribs but utilizing the low-frequency or phased array probe at 13 cm depth.

### Selected References

1. Ketelaars R, Gülpinar E, Roes T, Kuut M, van Geffen GJ. Which ultrasound transducer type is best for diagnosing pneumothorax?. *Crit Ultrasound J*. 2018;10(1):27. Published 2018 Oct 22. doi:10.1186/s13089-018-0109-0.
2. Husain LF, Hagopian L, Wayman D, Baker WE, Carmody KA. Sonographic diagnosis of pneumothorax. *J Emerg Trauma Shock*. 2012;5(1):76-81. doi:10.4103/0974-2700.93116.

**4.** Correct Answer: D. For surface use of ultrasound, the machine and probes can be cleaned and disinfected with vendor- and institution-approved products with low-level disinfection in between all patient use, but guidelines for high-level disinfection must be followed for any indications where the system came in contact with blood, body fluids, or mucosal membranes.

*Rationale:* Ultrasound system transducers and machines in contact with blood, mucous membranes, or any body fluids (including interventional procedures, injections, tissue sampling, etc.) require high-level disinfection, even if used with protective covers. Institutional guidelines created by an Infection Prevention team for the hospital or clinical center must be integrated with a list of vendor-approved products for that level of disinfection based on clinical indications of ultrasound use.

1. **Cleaning** is the removal of visible soil (e.g., organic and inorganic material) from objects and surfaces and normally is accomplished manually or mechanically using water with soap or enzymatic products. Thorough cleaning is essential before high-level disinfection and sterilization because inorganic and organic material that remains on the surfaces of instruments interfere with the effectiveness of these processes.
2. **Disinfection** describes a process that eliminates many or all pathogenic microorganisms, except bacterial spores.
   - **Low-Level Disinfection**—Destruction of most bacteria, some viruses, and some fungi. Low-level disinfection will not necessarily inactivate *Mycobacterium tuberculosis* or bacterial spores.
   - **Mid-Level Disinfection**—Inactivation of *M. tuberculosis*, bacteria, most viruses, most fungi, and some bacterial spores.
   - **High-Level Disinfection**—Destruction/removal of all microorganisms except bacterial spores.
3. **Sterilization** describes a process that destroys or eliminates all forms of microbial life and is carried out in health care facilities by physical or chemical methods. Steam under pressure, dry heat, ethylene oxide (EtO) gas, hydrogen peroxide gas plasma, and liquid chemicals are the principal sterilizing agents used in health care facilities. When chemicals are used to destroy all forms of microbiologic life, they can be called chemical sterilants. These same germicides used for shorter exposure periods also can be part of the disinfection process (i.e., high-level disinfection).

### Selected References

1. American Institute of Ultrasound in Medicine. Guidelines for Cleaning and Preparing External- and Internal-Use Ultrasound Transducers and Equipment Between Patients as well as Safe Handling and Use of Ultrasound Coupling Gel. 2021. https://www.aium.org/officialstatements/57.
2. Nyhsen CM, Humphreys H, Koerner RJ, et al. Infection prevention and control in ultrasound—best practice recommendations from the European Society of Radiology Ultrasound Working Group. *Insights Imaging.* 2017;8(6):523-535. doi:10.1007/s13244-017-0580-3.

**5.** Correct Answer: A. *Parasternal long-axis view:* index marker toward patient's right shoulder; parasternal short-axis view: index marker toward patient's left shoulder; apical four-chamber view: index marker toward patient's left elbow; subcostal view: index marker toward patient's left elbow

*Rationale:* The parasternal long-axis view is located on the left side of the sternum and will provide imaging planes of the long axis of the heart with the index marker pointed toward the patient's right shoulder. The initial parasternal short-axis view is located in the same location as the parasternal long-axis view, but the index marker is pointed toward the patient's left shoulder. This view provides images of the heart in an axial plane. The apical window is located below the left breast tissue, where one can feel the apical impulse. In the apical window, the index marker is initially placed in the 4 to 5 o'clock position to demonstrate the apical four-chamber view. Image acquisition for the subcostal window is performed with the patient in the supine position to obtain a four-chamber view with the index marker directed toward the patient's left side at the 3 o'clock position.

### Selected Reference

1. Mitchell C, Rahko PS, Blauwet LA, et al. Guidelines for performing a comprehensive transthoracic echocardiographic examination in adults: recommendations from the American Society of Echocardiography. *J Am Soc Echocardiogr.* 2019;32(1):1-64. doi:10.1016/j.echo.2018.06.004

# 10 | OPTIMIZING PROBE POSITION AND KNOBOLOGY FOR IMAGE ACQUISITION

Lydia Chang

1. Which of the following best describes the *tilt* motion used to optimize image acquisition?

    **A.** The transducer remains in the same position and angle against the chest wall while the orientation marker is adjusted in a clockwise or counterclockwise motion.
    **B.** The transducer is moved across the chest wall to a new position.
    **C.** The transducer remains in the same position on the chest wall and the same long-axis orientation to the heart while angled to obtain different imaging planes.
    **D.** The transducer remains in the same position on the chest wall and long-axis imaging plane while adjusted toward or away from the orientation marker.

2. Which of the following motions should be used to optimize the parasternal long-axis view shown in **Figure 10.1**?

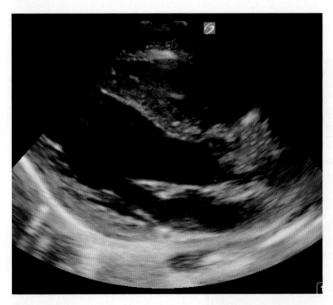

**Figure 10.1**

    **A.** The transducer should be rocked toward the orientation marker and slightly rotated.
    **B.** The transducer should be tilted to obtain a more anterior imaging plane.
    **C.** The transducer should be rotated clockwise by 90°.
    **D.** The transducer should be angled toward the apex.

3. Which motion should be used to acquire the parasternal short-axis from the parasternal long-axis view?

    **A.** The transducer should be angled medially.
    **B.** The transducer should be rotated 90° without any angulation or tilting.
    **C.** The transducer should be tilted anteriorly.
    **D.** The transducer should be rocked away from the orientation marker.

4. Following acquisition and optimization of **Figure 10.2**, which of the following motions should be performed to acquire the right ventricular (RV) outflow tract view?

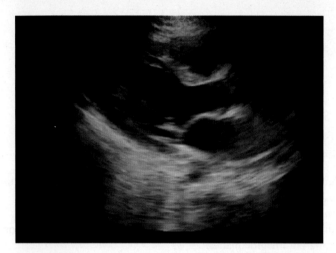

**Figure 10.2**

    **A.** The transducer should be tilted inferiorly to the right hip.
    **B.** The transducer should be rotated clockwise and tilted anteriorly.
    **C.** The transducer should be tilted superiorly.
    **D.** The transducer should be rocked away from the orientation marker.

5. What motion is performed in order to obtain **Figure 10.3** from the parasternal long-axis view?

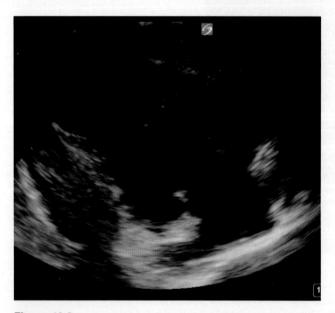

**Figure 10.3**

**A.** The transducer is tilted inferiorly to the right hip.
**B.** The transducer is rotated counterclockwise 90°.
**C.** The transducer is tilted superiorly.
**D.** The transducer is rocked away from the orientation maker.

6. Which of the following motions should be performed to move from the view in **Figure 10.4A** and **10.4B**?

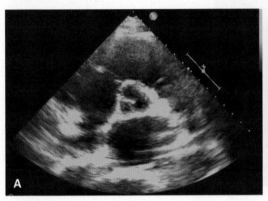 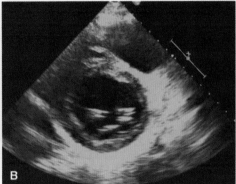

**Figure 10.4**

**A.** Tilting
**B.** Rocking
**C.** Sliding
**D.** Angulation

7. **Figure 10.5** was obtained on a patient erroneously suggesting a hyperdynamic and underfilled left ventricle.

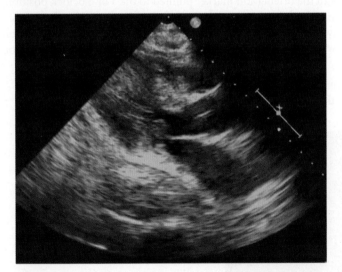

**Figure 10.5**

In addition to slight rotation, how would you maneuver the probe to better view the left ventricle in the long axis?
**A.** Tilt and slightly rotate to capture the left ventricle at its widest dimension.
**B.** Rock away from the orientation marker on the screen and angle toward the apex.
**C.** Slide closer to the sternum to better view the ascending aorta.
**D.** Rotate 90° clockwise.

8. **Figure 10.6** was obtained on a patient, erroneously suggesting that the patient has septal flattening of the left ventricle.

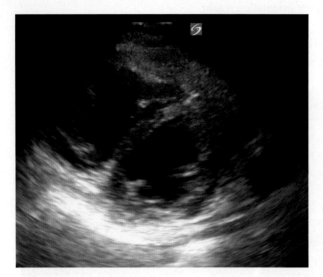

**Figure 10.6**

What likely occurred?
A. Over- or underrotation of the transducer
B. Placement of the transducer too close to the sternum
C. Placement of the transducer too far from the sternum
D. Tilting of the transducer too superiorly

9. A good starting transducer position to obtain the apical four-chamber view is:

A. Inferolaterally to the left nipple with the orientation marker pointed to the 3 or 4 o'clock position
B. Inferolaterally to the left nipple with the orientation marker pointed to the 6 or 7 o'clock position
C. Inferomedially to the left nipple with the orientation marker pointed to the 3 or 4 o'clock position
D. Inferomedially to the left nipple with the orientation marker pointed to the 6 or 7 o'clock position

10. How would you adjust the transducer from the standard apical four-chamber view shown in **Figure 10.7** to optimize the view of the right ventricle?

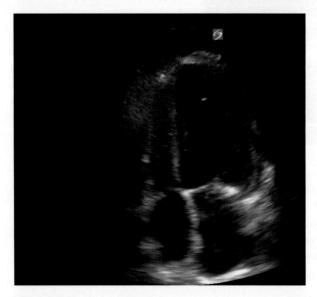

**Figure 10.7**

    **A.** Rotate the probe counterclockwise.
    **B.** Tilt the probe anteriorly.
    **C.** Rock the probe toward the orientation marker.
    **D.** Slide the probe down another intercostal space.

11. In order to evaluate flow across the left ventricular (LV) outflow tract, how should you adjust the transducer from the apical four-chamber view?

    **A.** Tilt the transducer tail up to obtain a more posterior imaging plane.
    **B.** Tilt the transducer tail down to obtain a more anterior imaging plane.
    **C.** Rotate the probe clockwise.
    **D.** Rotate the probe counterclockwise.

12. From the apical four-chamber view, how would you position the transducer to obtain the following view shown in **Figure 10.8**?

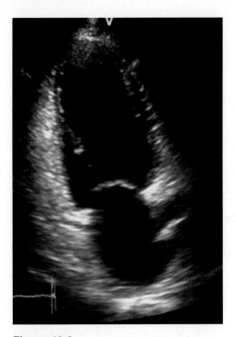

**Figure 10.8**

    **A.** Tilt the transducer posteriorly.
    **B.** Tilt the transducer anteriorly.
    **C.** Rotate the probe clockwise 60°.
    **D.** Rotate the probe counterclockwise 60°.

13. How should the transducer be adjusted in order to view the coronary sinus from the apical four-chamber view?

    **A.** Tilt the transducer tail up to obtain a more posterior imaging plane.
    **B.** Tilt the transducer tail down to obtain a more anterior imaging plane.
    **C.** Rock the transducer toward the orientation marker.
    **D.** Rock the transducer away from the orientation marker.

**14.** How should the transducer be adjusted from the apical two-chamber view to obtain the view shown in **Figure 10.9?**

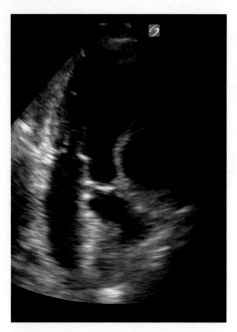

**Figure 10.9**

**A.** Rotate the transducer 60° counterclockwise.
**B.** Tilt the transducer posteriorly.
**C.** Rock the transducer toward the orientation marker.
**D.** Rock the transducer away from the orientation marker.

**15.** Which of the following probe adjustments should be performed to optimize **Figure 10.10?**

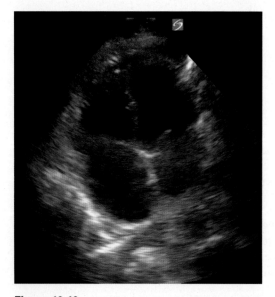

**Figure 10.10**

**A.** The probe should be rotated clockwise by 60°.
**B.** The probe should be rotated slightly counterclockwise.
**C.** The probe position should be adjusted by sliding it more inferiorly and/or laterally.
**D.** The probe should be adjusted by tilting it to acquire a more posterior imaging plane.

**16.** Any of the following adjustments can improve temporal resolution of cardiac ultrasound imaging *except*:

    **A.** Increasing the frame rate
    **B.** Decreasing image depth
    **C.** Decreasing the sector size
    **D.** Increasing the time-gain compensation

**17.** Which of the following statements regarding optimal gain adjustment in cardiac ultrasound is true?

    **A.** Gain should be adjusted so that the blood-endocardial tissue borders are well delineated.
    **B.** Gain should be adjusted to maximize frame rate.
    **C.** Gain should be adjusted in order to maximize harmonic frequency.
    **D.** Gain should be adjusted to reduce biological effects of ultrasound waves.

**18.** Which of the following statements regarding optimization of the dynamic range in cardiac imaging is true?

    **A.** A high dynamic range setting yields an image that is very high contrast.
    **B.** The dynamic range setting should be adjusted so that the compacted and noncompacted myocardium can be distinguished from each other.
    **C.** Increasing dynamic range may be beneficial for studies with poor image quality.
    **D.** Dynamic range can be optimized by increasing the gain.

**19.** How would you optimize **Figure 10.11**?

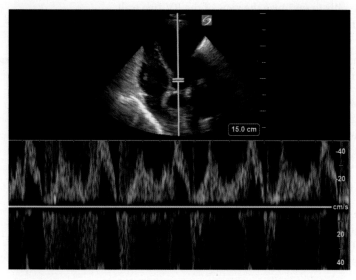

**Figure 10.11**

    **A.** Magnify the region of interest.
    **B.** Adjust the sector size.
    **C.** Increase the velocity scale.
    **D.** Decrease the dynamic range.

20. How would you optimize **Figure 10.12** in order to measure the tricuspid annular systolic planar excursion (TAPSE)?

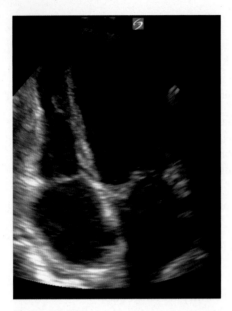

**Figure 10.12**

A. Rotate the transducer to maximize the RV area.
B. Rock the transducer to swing the RV free wall toward the middle of the sector.
C. Tilt the transducer inferolaterally to optimize the view of the RV free wall.
D. Slide the transducer interiorly to view the RV apex.

21. How would you adjust the transducer from the standard position when trying to obtain a parasternal long-axis view in a patient with severe chronic obstructive pulmonary disease?

A. Slide the transducer to a lower ribspace and rotate it in a more cephalocaudal position.
B. Slide the transducer to a higher ribspace and rotate it in a more cephalocaudal position.
C. Slide the transducer to a low ribspace and rotate it in a more transverse position.
D. Slide the transducer to a higher ribspace and rotate it in a more transverse position.

22. Standard methods to optimize the subcostal four-chamber view include all of the following *except*:

A. Having the patient perform a breath-hold
B. Firmer pressure may be required when the view is obscured by bowel gas
C. Repositioning of the patient in the left lateral decubitus position
D. Having the patient bend their knees to relax their abdominal musculature

23. Which of the following adjustments will best optimize color flow Doppler examination of tricuspid valve regurgitation?

A. Minimization of the Doppler angle
B. Changing to subcostal four-chamber view
C. Increase the depth
D. Widen the scan sector

# Chapter 10 ▪ Answers

1. **Correct Answer: C.** The transducer remains in the same position on the chest wall and the same long-axis orientation to the heart while angled to obtain different imaging planes.

   *Rationale:* When *tilting* the probe to optimize acquisition, the transducer remains in the same footprint and long-axis orientation and is moved perpendicular to the axis of the imaging plane to obtain different imaging planes (**Answer C**) (**e-Figure 10.1**). When *rotating* the probe, the transducer remains in the same footprint and angle against the chest, while it is adjusted by rotating clockwise or counterclockwise (**Answer A**). When *rocking* the probe to optimize image acquisition, the transducer remains in the same position against the chest wall and long-axis imaging plane, while the agle of the probe is adjusted parallel to the imaging plane, toward or away from the orientation marker (**Answer D**). Sliding the probe refers to moving the transducer over the patient's skin to a new position (**Answer B**).

   ### Selected References
   1. Mitchell C, Rahko PS, Blauwet LA, et al. Guidelines for performing a comprehensive transthoracic echocardiographic in adults: recommendations from the American Society of Echocardiography. *J Am Soc Echocardiogr.* 2019;32(1):1-64.
   2. Zimmerman JM, Coker BJ. The nuts and bolts of performing Focused Cardiovascular Ultrasound (FoCUS). *Anesth Analg.* 2017 Mar;124(3):753-760. doi: 10.1213/ANE.0000000000001861. PMID: 28207445.

2. **Correct Answer: A.** The transducer should be rocked toward the orientation marker and slightly rotated.

   *Rationale:* The ultrasound beam in an optimized parasternal long-axis view should be perpendicular to the left ventricle such that the left ventricle lies horizontal in the view. The plane should bisect the mitral and aortic valves. Figure 10.1 is both off-angle and off-plane. Rocking the probe toward the orientation marker would angle the left ventricle more perpendicularly to the ultrasound beam and slight rotation would get the aortic valve into plane. Tilting the probe more anteriorly would result in the RV outflow view. Rotation by 90° would result in the parasternal short-axis view. Angling toward the apex would further move the LV cavity away from the horizontal position in the view.

   ### Selected References
   1. Baston CM, Moore C, Krebs EA, Dean AJ, Panebianco N. *Pocket Guide to POCUS: Point of Care Tips for Point of Care Ultrasound.* McGraw Hill; 2018.
   2. Levitov AB, Mayo PH, Slonim AD. *Critical Care Ultrasonography.* McGraw Hill; 2014.
   3. Mitchell C, Rahko PS, Blauwet LA, et al. Guidelines for performing a comprehensive transthoracic echocardiographic in adults: recommendations from the American Society of Echocardiography. *J Am Soc Echocardiogr.* 2019;32(1):1-64.

3. **Correct Answer: B.** The transducer should be rotated 90° without any angulation or tilting.

   *Rationale:* To obtain the parasternal short-axis view from the parasternal long-axis view, the transducer should be rotated 90° clockwise without angulation or tilting. This results in good cross-sectional views of the heart.

   ### Selected References
   1. Baston CM, Moore C, Krebs EA, Dean AJ, Panebianco N. *Pocket Guide to POCUS: Point of Care Tips for Point of Care Ultrasound.* McGraw Hill; 2018.
   2. Levitov AB, Mayo PH, Slonim AD. *Critical Care Ultrasonography.* McGraw Hill; 2014.
   3. Mitchell C, Rahko PS, Blauwet LA, et al. Guidelines for performing a comprehensive transthoracic echocardiographic in adults: recommendations from the American Society of Echocardiography. *J Am Soc Echocardiogr.* 2019;32(1):1-64.

4. **Correct Answer: B.** The transducer should be rotated clockwise and tilted anteriorly.

   *Rationale:* To obtain the parasternal RV outflow view from the standard parasternal long-axis view, the transducer should be rotated slightly clockwise and the probe tilted slightly anteriorly toward the base of the heart. This view should allow visualization of the RV outflow tract, two leaflets of the pulmonic valve, and the pulmonary artery. In some instances, the bifurcation of the pulmonary artery can be viewed.

### Selected Reference
1. Mitchell C, Rahko PS, Blauwet LA, et al. Guidelines for performing a comprehensive transthoracic echocardiographic in adults: recommendations from the American Society of Echocardiography. *J Am Soc Echocardiogr.* 2019;32(1):1-64.

---

**5. Correct Answer: A. The transducer is tilted inferiorly to the right hip.**

*Rationale:* The RV inflow view is obtained from the standard parasternal long-axis view by tilting the probe inferiorly to the rip hip. This view displays only the right ventricle, right atrium, and tricuspid valve. The left ventricle should not be visualized. Two leaflets, the anterior and septal (or posterior) leaflets, of the tricuspid valves are displayed.

### Selected References
1. Levitov AB, Mayo PH, Slonim AD. *Critical Care Ultrasonography.* McGraw Hill; 2014.
2. Mitchell C, Rahko PS, Blauwet LA, et al. Guidelines for performing a comprehensive transthoracic echocardiographic in adults: recommendations from the American Society of Echocardiography. *J Am Soc Echocardiogr.* 2019;32(1):1-64.

---

**6. Correct Answer: A. Tilting**

*Rationale:* The parasternal short-axis view is obtained by rotating 90° clockwise from the parasternal long-axis view. From there, the various levels (or cross sections) of the parasternal short-axis view can be obtained by tilting superiorly and inferiorly. The superior-most view is the level of the great vessels, followed by the level of aortic valve, then the mitral valve, the mid-ventricular tomographic plane, and finally the apex. The mid-ventricular view is particularly important in evaluating global LV function and regional wall motion.

### Selected References
1. Baston CM, Moore C, Krebs EA, Dean AJ, Panebianco N. *Pocket Guide to POCUS: Point of Care Tips for Point of Care Ultrasound.* McGraw Hill; 2018.
2. Levitov AB, Mayo PH, Slonim AD. *Critical Care Ultrasonography.* McGraw Hill; 2014.
3. Mitchell C, Rahko PS, Blauwet LA, et al. Guidelines for performing a comprehensive transthoracic echocardiographic in adults: recommendations from the American Society of Echocardiography. *J Am Soc Echocardiogr.* 2019;32(1):1-64.

---

**7. Correct Answer: A. Tilt and slightly rotate to capture the left ventricle at its widest dimension.**

*Rationale:* The transducer is off-axis and not positioned to identify the LV cavity in its widest dimension, thus end-systolic effacement of the LV cavity appears to be occurring. As Figure 10.5 already includes the long-axis view of the aortic valve and the mitral valve, tilting and slightly rotating the probe to capture the left ventricle at its widest point would probably be the combination of motions most likely to best capture an optimal long-axis view.

Rocking and angling toward the apex would result in further angulation of the left ventricle away from the ultrasound beam. Sliding the probe toward the sternum would move the probe away from the key region of interest, which is the left ventricle. Rotation of the probe by 90° would result in a view of the parasternal short axis at the level of the aortic valve.

### Selected References
1. Levitov AB, Mayo PH, Slonim AD. *Critical Care Ultrasonography.* McGraw Hill; 2014.
2. Mitchell C, Rahko PS, Blauwet LA, et al. Guidelines for performing a comprehensive transthoracic echocardiographic in adults: recommendations from the American Society of Echocardiography. *J Am Soc Echocardiogr.* 2019;32(1):1-64.

---

**8. Correct Answer: A. Over- or underrotation of the transducer**

*Rationale:* The transducer is overrotated in the parasternal short-axis view, resulting in a nonperpendicular tomographic plane. This results in a more elliptical appearance of the left ventricle that could be erroneously interpreted as septal flattening.

### Selected References
1. Levitov AB, Mayo PH, Slonim AD. *Critical Care Ultrasonography.* McGraw Hill; 2014.
2. Mitchell C, Rahko PS, Blauwet LA, et al. Guidelines for performing a comprehensive transthoracic echocardiographic in adults: recommendations from the American Society of Echocardiography. *J Am Soc Echocardiogr.* 2019;32(1):1-64.

**9.** Correct Answer: A. Inferolaterally to the left nipple with the orientation marker pointed to the 3 or 4 o'clock position

*Rationale:* The transducer is best positioned at the anatomic apex of the left ventricle with the patient placed in the left lateral decubitus position. The septum should be oriented vertically along the center of the screen and the tomographic plane adjusted so that it bisects the apex and the midpoint of the tricuspid and mitral orifices.

Selected References
1. Levitov AB, Mayo PH, Slonim AD. *Critical Care Ultrasonography*. McGraw Hill; 2014.
2. Mitchell C, Rahko PS, Blauwet LA, et al. Guidelines for performing a comprehensive transthoracic echocardiographic in adults: recommendations from the American Society of Echocardiography. *J Am Soc Echocardiogr.* 2019;32(1):1-64.

**10.** Correct Answer: A. Rotate the probe counterclockwise.

*Rationale:* The transducer should be rotated slightly counterclockwise to obtain the maximal RV size, that is, the RV focused view. The apical four-chamber is a key view in assessing RV to LV size ratio, thus optimal probe positioning and orientation are critical.

Selected Reference
1. Mitchell C, Rahko PS, Blauwet LA, et al. Guidelines for performing a comprehensive transthoracic echocardiographic in adults: recommendations from the American Society of Echocardiography. *J Am Soc Echocardiogr.* 2019;32(1):1-64.

**11.** Correct Answer: B. Tilt the transducer tail down to obtain a more anterior imaging plane.

*Rationale:* The transducer should be tilted to obtain a more anterior imaging plane in order to obtain the apical five-chamber view. Pulsed-wave Doppler can then be placed at the LV outflow tract in order to obtain the optimal measurement of the velocity time integral and estimate stroke volume. Recall that tilting the probe anteriorly means the tail moves posteriorly, as the probe interface is the pivot point. Be mindful of terminology, as both "tilt" and "tail" are used to describe probe manipulation.

Selected Reference
1. Mitchell C, Rahko PS, Blauwet LA, et al. Guidelines for performing a comprehensive transthoracic echocardiographic in adults: recommendations from the American Society of Echocardiography. *J Am Soc Echocardiogr.* 2019;32(1):1-64.

**12.** Correct Answer: D. Rotate the probe counterclockwise 60°.

*Rationale:* The transducer should be rotated 60° counterclockwise from the apical four-chamber view to obtain the apical two-chamber view. This view provides additional detailed evaluation of the mitral valve using continuous-wave and pulsed-wave Doppler. This view, in combination with the apical four-chamber view, allows calculation of stroke volume and ejection fraction using Simpson's method.

Selected Reference
1. Mitchell C, Rahko PS, Blauwet LA, et al. Guidelines for performing a comprehensive transthoracic echocardiographic in adults: recommendations from the American Society of Echocardiography. *J Am Soc Echocardiogr.* 2019;32(1):1-64.

**13.** Correct Answer: A. Tilt the transducer tail up to obtain a more posterior imaging plane.

*Rationale:* The transducer should be tilted to obtain a more posterior imaging plane in order to visualize the coronary sinus.

Selected Reference
1. Mitchell C, Rahko PS, Blauwet LA, et al. Guidelines for performing a comprehensive transthoracic echocardiographic in adults: recommendations from the American Society of Echocardiography. *J Am Soc Echocardiogr.* 2019;32(1):1-64.

**14.** Correct Answer: A. Rotate the transducer 60° counterclockwise.

*Rationale:* The apical three-chamber view is obtained by rotating the transducer 60° counterclockwise from the apical two-chamber view. The apical three-chamber view corresponds to the parasternal long-axis view with the apex oriented to the transducer.

Selected Reference
1. Mitchell C, Rahko PS, Blauwet LA, et al. Guidelines for performing a comprehensive transthoracic echocardiographic in adults: recommendations from the American Society of Echocardiography. *J Am Soc Echocardiogr.* 2019;32(1):1-64.

**15.** Correct Answer: **C. The probe position should be adjusted by sliding it more inferiorly and/or laterally.**

*Rationale:* Figure 10.10 is a foreshortened apical four-chamber view: the atria comprise more than one-third of the total length of the heart from the apex to the base. Additionally, the apex is rounded rather than tapered. This typically occurs when the probe is not situated over the true cardiac apex; the probe should be adjusted by sliding it more inferiorly and/or more laterally.

Selected References
1. Levitov AB, Mayo PH, Slonim AD. *Critical Care Ultrasonography.* McGraw Hill; 2014.
2. Mitchell C, Rahko PS, Blauwet LA, et al. Guidelines for performing a comprehensive transthoracic echocardiographic in adults: recommendations from the American Society of Echocardiography. *J Am Soc Echocardiogr.* 2019;32(1):1-64.

**16.** Correct Answer: **D. Increasing the time-gain compensation**

*Rationale:* Increasing the time-gain compensation amplifies returning echo signals but does not improve temporal resolution. Cardiac ultrasound requires a high frame rate for best temporal resolution especially for rapidly moving structures. Increased sector depth and width increase the amount of time needed to produce images, decreasing frame rate and thus temporal resolution.

Selected Reference
1. Mitchell C, Rahko PS, Blauwet LA, et al. Guidelines for performing a comprehensive transthoracic echocardiographic in adults: recommendations from the American Society of Echocardiography. *J Am Soc Echocardiogr.* 2019;32(1):1-64.

**17.** Correct Answer: **A. Gain should be adjusted so that the blood-endocardial tissue borders are well delineated.**

*Rationale:* The overall gain control simply amplifies the reflected echo signals equally throughout the entire image sector. Various factors including power of the ultrasound signal determine the biological effect of ultrasound. Gain is a postprocessing function, and changing gain only modifies signal processing for visualization on the screen.

Selected Reference
1. Mitchell C, Rahko PS, Blauwet LA, et al. Guidelines for performing a comprehensive transthoracic echocardiographic in adults: recommendations from the American Society of Echocardiography. *J Am Soc Echocardiogr.* 2019;32(1):1-64.

**18.** Correct Answer: **B. The dynamic range setting should be adjusted so that the compacted and noncompacted myocardium can be distinguished from each other.**

*Rationale:* The dynamic range setting adjusts the ratio between the highest and lowest signal amplitudes in the image, changing the grayscale of the image. A setting with low dynamic range actually is very high contrast with fewer shades of gray, whereas a setting with high dynamic range will have more shades of gray.

Selected Reference
1. Mitchell C, Rahko PS, Blauwet LA, et al. Guidelines for performing a comprehensive transthoracic echocardiographic in adults: recommendations from the American Society of Echocardiography. *J Am Soc Echocardiogr.* 2019;32(1):1-64.

**19.** Correct Answer: **C. Increase the velocity scale.**

*Rationale:* The image demonstrates aliasing, which occurs when the flow velocity at the sampled volume exceeds the Nyquist limit. This occurs when the Doppler shift frequency is higher than half of the transmitted pulse repetition frequency (PRF). The PRF is determined by the velocity scale and image depth.

Selected Reference
1. Mitchell C, Rahko PS, Blauwet LA, et al. Guidelines for performing a comprehensive transthoracic echocardiographic in adults: recommendations from the American Society of Echocardiography. *J Am Soc Echocardiogr.* 2019;32(1):1-64.

**20.** Correct Answer: A. Rotate the transducer to maximize the RV area.

*Rationale:* In order to obtain the apical four-chamber RV focused view, the transducer is typically rotated slightly counterclockwise from the apical four-chamber view in order to maximize the visualized RV area and its lateral dimensions. The RV focused view is recommended for measurement of RV area as well as linear dimensions. Other maneuvers could include tilting toward the right ventricle or sliding more medially.

Selected Reference

1. Mitchell C, Rahko PS, Blauwet LA, et al. Guidelines for performing a comprehensive transthoracic echocardiographic in adults: recommendations from the American Society of Echocardiography. *J Am Soc Echocardiogr.* 2019;32(1):1-64.

**21.** Correct Answer: A. Slide the transducer to a lower ribspace and rotate it in a more cephalocaudal position.

*Rationale:* In patients with hyperinflation, the cardiac position is typically lower and tends to be oriented in a more vertical axis. Patients with large abdomens, on the other hand, have hearts positioned higher in the chest cavity and oriented in a more transverse axis.

Selected References

1. Baston CM, Moore C, Krebs EA, Dean AJ, Panebianco N. *Pocket Guide to POCUS: Point of Care Tips for Point of Care Ultrasound.* McGraw Hill; 2018.
2. Mitchell C, Rahko PS, Blauwet LA, et al. Guidelines for performing a comprehensive transthoracic echocardiographic in adults: recommendations from the American Society of Echocardiography. *J Am Soc Echocardiogr.* 2019;32(1):1-64.

**22.** Correct Answer: C. Repositioning of the patient in the left lateral decubitus position

*Rationale:* The subcostal four-chamber view is best acquired in the supine position. Other methods to optimize the image include firm pressure on the abdomen if there is bowel gas obscuration and having the patient bend their knees to loosen their abdominal muscles and also perform respiratory maneuvers to lower the diaphragm and bringing the heart into view. Turning to a left lateral decubitus position may help optimize an apical viewing window, but is unlikely to help with a subcostal one.

Selected References

1. Baston CM, Moore C, Krebs EA, Dean AJ, Panebianco N. *Pocket Guide to POCUS: Point of Care Tips for Point of Care Ultrasound.* McGraw Hill; 2018.
2. Mitchell C, Rahko PS, Blauwet LA, et al. Guidelines for performing a comprehensive transthoracic echocardiographic in adults: recommendations from the American Society of Echocardiography. *J Am Soc Echocardiogr.* 2019;32(1):1-64.

**23.** Correct Answer: A. Minimization of the Doppler angle

*Rationale:* Color flow Doppler examination is optimized by minimizing the Doppler angle as much as possible, so that the ultrasound beam is near parallel to the blood flow being measured. Reduction of sector width and depth also improves examination by increasing the PRF and thus the frame rate. The direction of tricuspid regurgitation is unlikely to align parallel to the probe in the subcostal views.

Selected References

1. Baston CM, Moore C, Krebs EA, Dean AJ, Panebianco N. *Pocket Guide to POCUS: Point of Care Tips for Point of Care Ultrasound.* McGraw Hill; 2018.
2. Mitchell C, Rahko PS, Blauwet LA, et al. Guidelines for performing a comprehensive transthoracic echocardiographic in adults: recommendations from the American Society of Echocardiography. *J Am Soc Echocardiogr.* 2019;32(1):1-64.

# 11 | KNOBOLOGY, PROBE POSITIONING, AND CONCEPTS OF IMAGE ACQUISITION

Aarti Sarwal

1. You are asked to evaluate the movement of the diaphragm with respiration to assess a patient suspected to be in neuromuscular respiratory failure. Using a curvilinear probe on the abdominal preset imaging mode, you insonate the diaphragm on the right substernal space in the mid-clavicular line, pointing the probe superiorly, posteriorly, and laterally. Which of the modes of ultrasound imaging is the *most* useful to assess the vertical excursion of the diaphragm?

   A. A-mode ultrasound
   B. B-mode ultrasound
   C. M-mode ultrasound
   D. Doppler ultrasound

2. A patient undergoes carotid ultrasound imaging to assess for carotid stenosis. Which of the following Doppler ultrasound modalities is demonstrated in **Figure 11.1**?

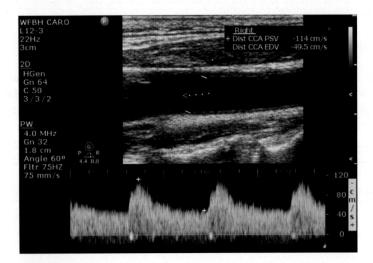

**Figure 11.1**

   A. Power Doppler
   B. Pulsed-wave Doppler
   C. Continuous-wave Doppler
   D. Color flow Doppler

3. During insonation of vascular structures using color flow Doppler, **Figure 11.2** is obtained. Which of the following artifacts is responsible for display of the yellow and aqua blue colors?

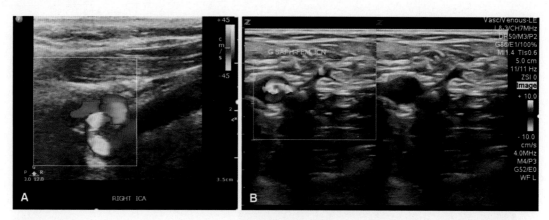

**Figure 11.2**

A. Spontaneous echo contrast ("smoke") produced by an evolving thrombus
B. Aliasing caused by velocities in blood flow higher than color scale specified
C. Twinkling artifact caused by velocities lower than the color scale specified
D. Rainbow artifact caused by turbulent blood flow

4. In an attempt to visualize the left ventricle from the following parasternal long-axis view, which of the following will *most likely* improve the image quality in **Figure 11.3**?

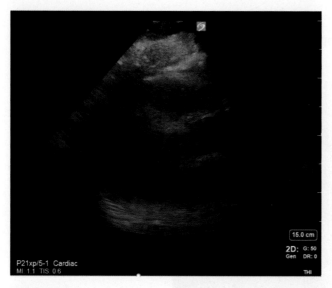

**Figure 11.3**

A. Decrease in depth
B. Increase in gain
C. Decrease in mechanical index
D. Additional transducer gel

5. Which of the following parameters should be adjusted for optimizing the lung base for pleural effusion in **Figure 11.4**?

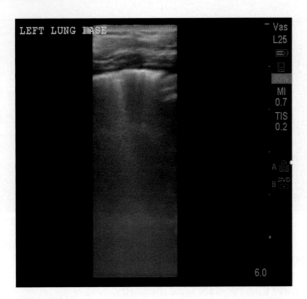

**Figure 11.4**

A. Depth
B. Gain
C. Power
D. Mechanical index

6. **Figure 11.5** shows pulsed-wave Doppler waveforms of a vessel being imaged.

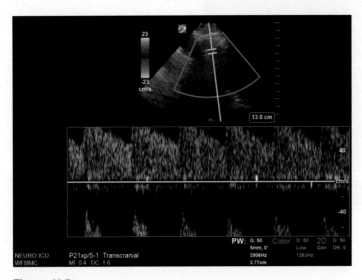

**Figure 11.5**

Which of the following is the *first* step to optimize the spectral waveform pattern for quantitative measurements of peak and end-diastolic velocity (see Figure 11.13A)?
A. Increase the scale
B. Decrease the baseline
C. Decrease the gain of the pulsed-wave Doppler measurement
D. Decrease the depth of the underlying B-mode grayscale image

7. During insonation of the parasternal long-axis view, **Figure 11.6** is obtained.

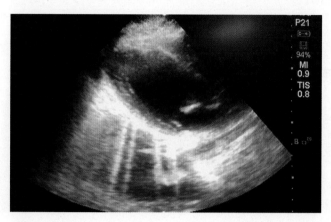

**Figure 11.6**

Which of the following artifacts is present?
A. Pericardial A-lines
B. Acoustic shadowing
C. Reverberation artifact produced by the interventricular septum
D. Mirror artifact produced by the reflective surface of the pericardium

8. A 37-year-old man presents with hypotension after a motor vehicle collision, and a focused assessment with sonography in trauma (FAST) examination is performed. The abdominal preset setting is selected, along with an ultrasound feature called tissue harmonic imaging (THI). Which of the following is *most* correct regarding THI?

A. THI improves visualization of anechoic and hypoechoic structures.
B. THI is useful for depicting cystic lesions and those containing echogenic tissues such as fat, calcium, or air.
C. THI highlights the echoes from the tissues that are composed of the fundamental frequency.
D. THI can be performed in B-mode but not in Doppler mode.

9. Which of the following is the *most* appropriate method to produce images of the liver in the subcostal space, with the probe pointed cranially and posteriorly if the index marker on ultrasound screen is towards left of the screen?

A. A linear high-frequency probe 6-15 MHz with the probe indicator pointed to the right of the patient
B. A linear high-frequency probe 6-15 MHz with the probe indicator pointed to the left of the patient
C. A phased-array low-frequency probe 1 to 3 MHz is used to insonate the liver with the index marker pointed to the right of the patient
D. A phased-array low-frequency probe 1 to 3 MHz with the probe indicator pointed to the left of the patient

10. Which of the following functions describes the ability of an ultrasound machine to adjust this brightness and is marked in **Figure 11.7**?

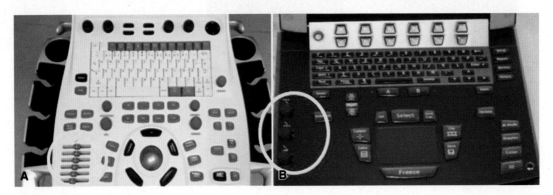

**Figure 11.7**

A. Power
B. Time gain compensation (TGC)
C. Zoom
D. Depth

11. Of the following ultrasound modes, which can be affected by aliasing?

1. M-mode
2. Continuous-wave Doppler
3. Pulsed-wave Doppler
4. Color flow Doppler

A. 1, 2, 3, 4
B. 1, 2, 3
C. 2, 3, 4
D. 3, 4

12. You are evaluating a 25-year-old man for increased intracranial pressure using orbital ultrasound to assess the optic nerve sheath diameter. To perform this ultrasound, which of the following configurations of the preset modes would be *most* appropriate? MI is the Mechanical Index and TI is the Thermal Index.

A. MI 1.0 and TI 0.2
B. MI 0.2 and TI 0.0
C. MI 0.2 and TI 1.0
D. MI 0.5 and TI 0.5

**13.** **Figure 11.8** shows a parasternal long-axis image.

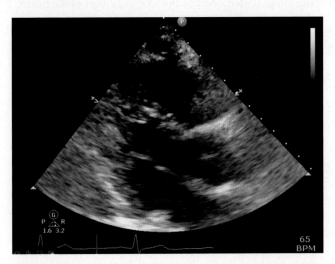

**Figure 11.8**

Which of the following maneuvers would be most useful in optimizing Figure 11.8?
A. Reposition the patient
B. Probe position optimization
C. Increase the gain
D. Change to a curvilinear probe

**14.** A patient is being evaluated for right ventricular strain using the parasternal short-axis view, and **Figure 11.9** is obtained.

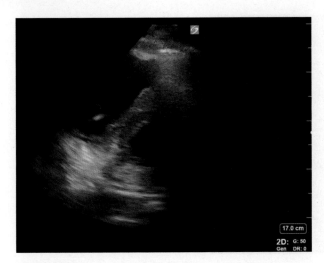

**Figure 11.9**

In an attempt to optimize Figure 11.9, which of the following will be *most* helpful to visualize more of the left ventricle?
A. Increasing the gain of the image to see structures on the right side of the image
B. Reducing the sector width of the image to avoid the lung interfering with imaging
C. Repositioning the probe or patient to allow insonation away from the lung
D. Decreasing the depth of the image

**15.** You are assessing the apical four-chamber view of the heart and encounter a fifth structure in the center of the image. How would you optimize the image to demonstrate the four chambers of the heart?

**A.** Fan the probe further ventrally (anteriorly) to show more anterior portions of the heart
**B.** Fan the probe further dorsally (posteriorly) to show more of the left atrium
**C.** Rotate the probe clockwise
**D.** Rotate the probe counterclockwise

# Chapter 11 ▪ Answers

**1.** Correct Answer: C. M-mode ultrasound

*Rationale:* A-mode ultrasound is the mode used for single-dimensional imaging. A single transducer scans a line through the body with the echoes plotted on screen as a function of depth. Therapeutic ultrasound aimed at a specific tumor or ophthalmologic ultrasound uses A-mode applications when the beam can be directed at a known target. In B-mode ultrasound, a linear array of transducers simultaneously scans a plane through the body that can be viewed as a two-dimensional image, giving a grayscale image of several contiguous beams (similar to several A-mode images placed next to each other). In M-mode (motion mode), a defined line is plotted over time to provide a rapid sequence of B-mode scans only capturing the structures on that line (see **Figure 11.10**). This is the most accurate way to measure movement within a single plane over time, as in diaphragmatic excursion. Doppler ultrasound uses the Doppler effect to measure velocities of structures reflecting ultrasound waves (e.g., tissue movement or blood flow) along the line of insonation.

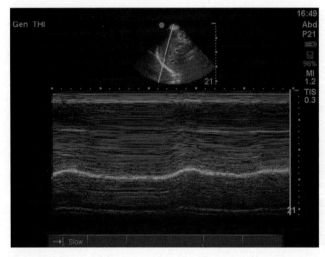

**Figure 11.10**

Selected References

1. Carovac A, Smajlovic F, Junuzovic D. Application of ultrasound in medicine. *Acta Inform Med.* 2011;19(3):168-171. doi:10.5455/aim.2011.19.168-171.
2. Sarwal A, Walker FO, Cartwright MS. Neuromuscular ultrasound for evaluation of the diaphragm. *Muscle Nerve.* 2013;47(3):319-329. doi:10.1002/mus.23671.

**2.** Correct Answer: B. Pulsed-wave Doppler

*Rationale:* Spectral Doppler uses the Doppler principle to convert frequency changes generated by re-flections from moving red blood cells into velocities and displays a "spectrum" of these frequencies as a waveform (at the bottom of the image). Spectral Doppler waveforms can be acquired by pulsed-wave or continuous-wave Doppler depending on sample selection. Continuous-wave Doppler simultaneously transmits and receives sound waves with different receivers and transmitters and samples the entire range of returning frequencies along its beam path. Assessment of velocities along the valves to calculate the valvular gradient utilizes continuous Doppler to ensure capture of all range of velocities encountered. In pulsed-wave Doppler, only the velocities from a user-defined sample within the B-mode image are displayed in the spectral waveforms (the "sampling gate," which is placed within the blood vessel in the image). Most vascular ultrasound utilizes pulsed-wave Doppler waveforms because of its precision and ability to localize the sample site for low-velocity flow. Higher velocity flow (e.g., valvular stenosis or regurgitation) is limited by aliasing and is more appropriate for continuous-wave Doppler. The conven-tional color flow mode utilizes two special colors (red and blue) and indicates the direction of the blood in relation to the probe. In power Doppler (or color power Doppler, CPD) mode, the direction of blood flow is disregarded, and a single color is used, with the gradient reflecting the strength of the Doppler signals. Power Doppler may be useful for lower-flow states, for example, to distinguish between near occlusion or total occlusion in blood vessels like the carotid artery.

Selected References
1. Mitchell C, Rahko PS, Blauwet LA, et al. Guidelines for performing a comprehensive transthoracic echocardiographic exam-ination in adults: recommendations from the American Society of Echocardiography. *J Am Soc Echocardiogr.* 2019;32(1):1-64. doi:10.1016/j.echo.2018.06.004.
2. Oglat AA, Matjafri MZ, Suardi N, Oqlat MA, Abdelrahman MA, Oqlat AA. A review of medical Doppler ultrasonography of blood flow in general and especially in common carotid artery. *J Med Ultrasound.* 2018;26(1):3-13. doi:10.4103/JMU.JMU_11_17.

**3.** Correct Answer: B. Aliasing caused by velocities in blood flow higher than color scale specified

*Rationale:* Aliasing is an artifact produced by attempting to measure velocities exceeding the Nyquist limit. This is a limiting factor for all forms of pulsed-wave Doppler functions, including color flow Dop-pler. When a velocity exceeds the Nyquist limit, the signal may appear to flow in the opposite direction (similar to the "wagon wheel effect" when the frame rate is below the rotational speed of a wagon wheel, and it appears to rotate backward). In color flow Doppler, aliasing can be seen as color signals corre-sponding to the extremes of the color scale (yellow and aqua blue, in this case), in contrast to the red and blue that classically represent directional shifts. M-mode, B-mode, or continuous-wave Doppler do not manifest aliasing.

Selected Reference
1. Kremkau FW. Doppler color imaging. Principles and instrumentation. *Clin Diagn Ultrasound.* 1992;27:7-60.

**4.** Correct Answer: B. Increase in gain

*Rationale:* Increasing gain in this instance will enhance the visualization of the insonated structures and may help optimize the image prior to altering other parameters like depth or changing the probe position and direction. Mechanical and thermal index are preset dependent parameters that can help increase the penetration and output of ultrasound signals. While increasing these may improve imaging in some cases, it would result in more energy transmission to the patient, and adjusting gain would be a more ap-propriate first step. Additional gel would be unlikely to improve the quality of this image, because there appears to be adequate transmission of the ultrasound signal.

Selected Reference
1. Hangiandreou NJ. AAPM/RSNA physics tutorial for residents. Topics in US: B-mode US: basic concepts and new technol-ogy. *Radiographics.* 2003;23(4):1019-1033. doi:10.1148/rg.234035034.

**5.** Correct Answer: A. Depth

*Rationale:* Adjusting the depth to <3 cm will allow a closer look at the pleural space to assess for any possible fluid collections. Given adequate visualization of lung pleura, associated comet tails (B-lines), and diaphragm (left side of Figure 11.4, flush with the pleura), enhancing the gain may not help detect fluid and could obscure anechoic fluid if the gain is too high. Power can be adjusted indirectly by changing imaging modes, but would not help enhance the area of interest in this image. Mechanical index is a dependent parameter and is not adjusted directly, but rather is a consequence of the power delivered.

Selected Reference

1. Patel CJ, Bhatt HB, Parikh SN, Jhaveri BN, Puranik JH. Bedside lung ultrasound in emergency protocol as a diagnostic tool in patients of acute respiratory distress presenting to emergency department. *J Emerg Trauma Shock*. 2018;11(2):125-129. doi:10.4103/JETS.JETS_21_17.

**6.** Correct Answer: B. Decrease the baseline

*Rationale/Critique:* The pulsed-wave Doppler scale is represented on the right lower part of Figure 11.5. Because the measured velocity exceeds the upper limit of the display, "aliasing" appears, as the higher velocities are displayed as negative values at the bottom of the scale. This artifact can be reduced by lowering the baseline or by increasing the scale of the pulsed-wave Doppler spectrum (increasing the pulse rate frequency). Because we are interested in velocity in only one direction, lowering the baseline to focus on the signal "above the line" should be the first step in optimization. The scale can then be adjusted if necessary, but appears to be appropriate for this image after the baseline is adjusted. Adjusting gain on the pulsed-wave Doppler measurement would merely make the waveform appear brighter and not correct the aliasing artifact. Decreasing depth would not affect the Doppler aliasing, but may allow for more accurate measurement.

Selected Reference

1. Oglat AA, Matjafri MZ, Suardi N, Oqlat MA, Abdelrahman MA, Oqlat AA. A review of medical Doppler ultrasonography of blood flow in general and especially in common carotid artery. *J Med Ultrasound*. 2018;26(1):3-13. doi:10.4103/JMU.JMU_11_17.

**7.** Correct Answer: D. Mirror artifact produced by the reflective surface of the pericardium

*Rationale/Critique:* A-lines are the horizontal artifacts arising from and parallel to the pleural line, generated by strong reflections from subpleural air. Because an echodensity is apparent at the bottom of the image, acoustic shadowing does not explain the hypoechoic appearance below the pericardium. **Figure 11.11A** shows B-lines that are reverberation artifacts produced by a thickened serosal surface (e.g., pleura) or interlobular septae, usually in the setting of pulmonary edema. The B-lines here are produced by the excursion of the lung pleura next to the pericardium, not by the septum. The hyperechoic pericardium can serve as a reflector in some cases and produce a mirror image of the heart as seen above it (**Figure 11.11B**).

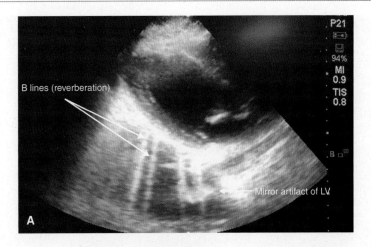

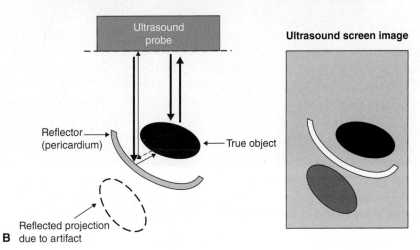

**Figure 11.11**

**Selected Reference**

1. Patel CJ, Bhatt HB, Parikh SN, Jhaveri BN, Puranik JH. Bedside lung ultrasound in emergency protocol as a diagnostic tool in patients of acute respiratory distress presenting to emergency department. *J Emerg Trauma Shock*. 2018;11(2):125-129. doi:10.4103/JETS.JETS_21_17.

**8.** Correct Answer: B. THI is useful for depicting cystic lesions and those containing echogenic tissues such as fat, calcium, or air.

*Rationale/Critique:* An ultrasound wave is altered with time as it traverses tissues with nonlinear motion. THI is a signal processing technique that isolates selected frequencies to reduce image artifacts and improve resolution by improving the signal-to-noise ratio. THI images are obtained by collecting harmonic signals that are tissue-generated and filtering out the fundamental echo signals that are transducer-generated, resulting in crisper images. Harmonic imaging can be performed in B-mode and Doppler modes. THI can be particularly useful for depicting cystic lesions and those containing echogenic tissues such as fat, calcium, or air. THI leads to improved imaging of the liver, gallbladder, pancreas, pelvis, kidneys, and retroperitoneal lymph nodes. Harmonic imaging can involve the injection of contrast agent with the appropriate microbubbles and then scanning the region of interest, but does not mandate the need for contrast (**Figure 11.12**).

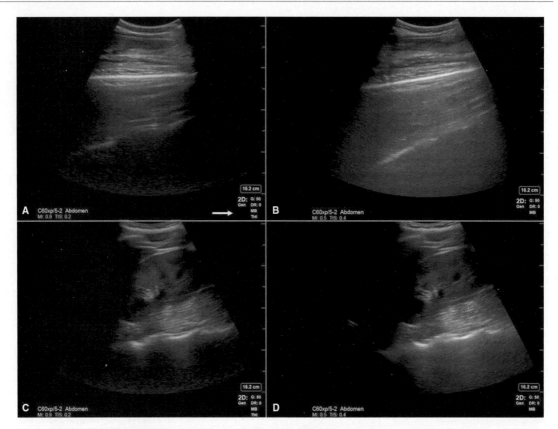

**Figure 11.12** Forearm muscle image on abdominal probe insonation to highlight the image resolution with tissue harmonic imaging (THI; A) and without THI (B). Right flank insonation showing difference in resolution of kidney margins and psoas muscle with THI (C) and without THI (D).

Selected Reference

1. Uppal T. Tissue harmonic imaging. *Australas J Ultrasound Med.* 2010;13(2):29-31. doi:10.1002/j.2205-0140.2010.tb00155.x.

9. Correct Answer: C. A phased-array low-frequency probe 1 to 3 MHz is used to insonate the liver with the index marker pointed to the right of the patient

*Rationale:* For insonation of the liver through the subcostal space, a low-frequency phased-array or curvilinear probe is used with the probe pointed cranially and posteriorly. An abdominal preset function can help optimize images, and the convention is to have the probe indicator directed to the right of the patient, corresponding to the index marker on the left of the screen (**Figure 11.13A**). This creates an anatomically congruent configuration between the probe, patient, and the ultrasound screen (**Figure 11.13B**).

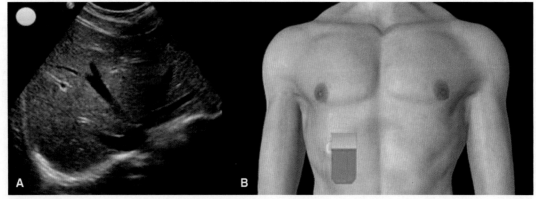

**Figure 11.13**

Selected Reference

1. Luis Enriquez J, Wu TS. An introduction to ultrasound equipment and knobology. *Crit Care Clin.* 2014;30:25-45.

**10.** Correct Answer: B. Time gain compensation (TGC)

*Rationale:* TGC allows adjustment of the gain (or brightness) at a specified depth, as opposed to overall gain, which increases the brightness of the entire image. As an ultrasound wave is attenuated as it travels through tissue, it may be necessary to increase the gain in the area of interest deeper on the image. The top rows of the control allow changing the gain of the field nearest to the probe (near field), and the bottom rows allow changing the gain of the field farthest from the probe (far field). Some machines have controls that allow adjustment of a significant range of depths, like the image on the left. Many point-of-care machines only allow adjustment of two or three bands of depths (near and far gain), as in the image on the right.

Selected Reference

1. Hangiandreou NJ. AAPM/RSNA physics tutorial for residents. Topics in US: B-mode US: basic concepts and new technology. *Radiographics.* 2003;23(4):1019-1033. doi:10.1148/rg.234035034.

**11.** Correct Answer: D. 3, 4

*Rationale:* Aliasing is an artifact produced by sampling a periodic process at a rate much less than the rate at which the process is occurring. Aliasing is a consequence of measuring high velocity with pulsed-wave Doppler modes, which includes color flow Doppler. M-mode, B-mode, and continuous-wave Doppler do not manifest aliasing.

Selected Reference

1. Kremkau FW. Doppler color imaging. Principles and instrumentation. *Clin Diagn Ultrasound.* 1992;27:7-60.

**12.** Correct Answer: B. MI 0.2 and TI 0.0

*Rationale:* The eye is vulnerable to thermal and mechanical damage from excessive ultrasonic energy. TI is the ratio of the total device acoustic power to the power required to increase tissue temperature by 1 °C. According to the European Federation of Societies for Ultrasound in Medicine and Biology (EFSUMB), a diagnostic procedure can be safely undertaken if tissue temperature increases <1.5 °C above physiologic levels. TI is different for soft tissue, bone, and cranial bone, hence specific to these presets on a machine. MI estimates the potential for macro-streaming and cavitation, a process in which ultrasonic vibrations produce tiny gas bubbles, which may also cause tissue damage. The Food and Drug Administration (FDA) and World Federation for Ultrasound in Medicine and Biology have imposed strict TI and MI limits for ocular ultrasound (TI < 1.0, MI < 0.23).

Selected References

1. Duck FA. Hazards, risks and safety of diagnostic ultrasound. *Med Eng Phys.* 2008 Dec;30(10):1338-1348.
2. EFSUMB. European federation of societies for ultrasound in medicine and biology European Committee for medical ultrasound safety bylaw. *Newsletter.* 1998:12.
3. Food and Drug Administration. *Guidance for Industry and FDA Staff Information for Manufacturers Seeking Marketing Clearance of Diagnostic Ultrasound Systems and Transducers.* Maryland; Sept 9, 2008.

**13.** Correct Answer: B. Probe position optimization

*Rationale:* For optimal parasternal long-axis view, the marker on the transducer should point to the right shoulder of the patient. Although this is a good starting point, the probe position needs to be further optimized for each individual patient based on the anatomic position of that patient's heart. **Figure 11.14A** represents a foreshortened left ventricle (i.e., the ultrasound section is *not* through the anatomic long axis of the heart). This can be optimized by rotating the probe. All other options are not useful to optimize a foreshortened image.

For instance, in an obese patient the diaphragm pushed the apex of the heart superiorly, resulting in a more horizontal position of the heart within the mediastinum. In that case the probe needs to be rotated counterclockwise to align with the axis of the heart. On the other hand, the axis of the heart is more vertical in someone with chronic obstructive pulmonary disease (COPD) and emphysema, in whom the probe needs to be rotated clockwise to align with the axis of the heart (**Figure 11.14B**).

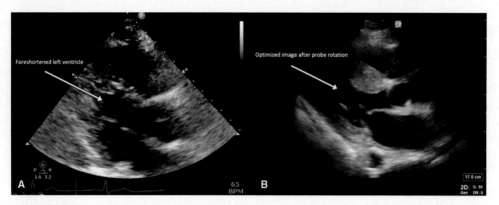

**Figure 11.14**

Selected Reference

1. Mitchell C, Rahko PS, Blauwet LA, et al. Guidelines for performing a comprehensive transthoracic echocardiographic examination in adults: recommendations from the American Society of Echocardiography. *J Am Soc Echocardiogr.* 2019;32(1):1-64. doi:10.1016/j.echo.2018.06.004.

**14.** Correct Answer: **C. Repositioning the probe or patient to allow insonation away from the lung**

*Rationale:* Figure 11.9 shows a parasternal short-axis view of the heart with a straightened septum, showing a "D sign," suggesting elevated right ventricular (RV) pressure. Part of the left ventricle (LV) is obscured by the lung on the right side of the image. Increasing the gain, decreasing the depth or the sector width will not help increase the area of LV visualized. Positioning the probe or the patient to displace the lung laterally may help better visualization of LV.

Selected Reference

1. Mitchell C, Rahko PS, Blauwet LA, et al. Guidelines for performing a comprehensive transthoracic echocardiographic examination in adults: recommendations from the American Society of Echocardiography. *J Am Soc Echocardiogr.* 2019;32(1):1-64. doi:10.1016/j.echo.2018.06.004.

**15.** Correct Answer: **B. Fan the probe further dorsally (posteriorly) to show more of the left atrium**

*Rationale:* The apical four-chamber view demonstrates the two atria and ventricles, and both atrioventricular valves. When the probe is fanned further ventrally from the apical four-chamber view, it images the left ventricular outflow tract and becomes the apical five-chamber view (**Figure 11.15**). To revert to an apical four-chamber view, the probe should be tilted dorsally.

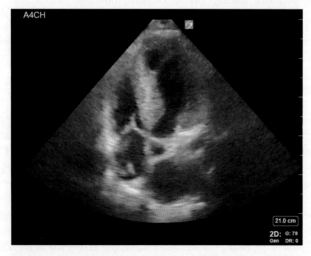

**Figure 11.15** Apical five-chamber view.

Selected Reference

1. Mitchell C, Rahko PS, Blauwet LA, et al. Guidelines for performing a comprehensive transthoracic echocardiographic examination in adults: recommendations from the American Society of Echocardiography. *J Am Soc Echocardiogr.* 2019;32(1):1-64. doi:10.1016/j.echo.2018.06.004.

# 12 | TRANSTHORACIC ECHOCARDIOGRAPHY (TTE) AND TRANSESOPHAGEAL ECHOCARDIOGRAPHY (TEE) VIEWS: TTE VERSUS TEE

Suresh "Mitu" Agarwal, Christopher Collins, Meredith L. Whitacre, Justin G. Vaughan, and William S. Lao

1. A 72-year-old female status post aortic valve replacement 3 years ago is currently being treated for sepsis with concern for endocarditis. Which of the following statements is most appropriate regarding the use of echocardiography?

   A. Due to the anterior location of the aortic valve a transthoracic echocardiography (TTE) will yield more information regarding presence of endocarditis.
   B. TTE is more likely to identify endocarditis involving the mitral valve as compared to the tricuspid valve.
   C. Transesophageal echocardiography (TEE) has a higher sensitivity for detection of endocarditis when evaluating replaced valves as compared to TTE.
   D. Using TTE is a good way to evaluate the extent of perivalvular vegetation.

2. A 31-year-old male presented to the neuro intensive care unit (ICU) following an ischemic stroke. He was initially intubated and sedated at which time a TEE did not reveal the presence of a patent foramen ovale (PFO). Over the course of the next week, he improved and is now following commands with no residual weakness and is ultimately extubated. A PFO is now discovered on TTE with contrast study (**Figure 12.1**).

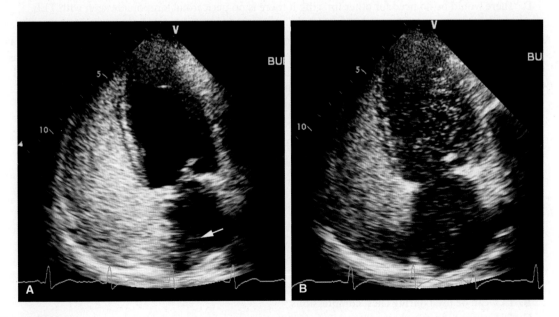

**Figure 12.1**

What is the most likely reason for the new discovery of a PFO?

**A.** TTE with contrast study is better at detecting a PFO as compared to evaluation with TEE.

**B.** A Valsalva breath was performed during the TEE.

**C.** Recognition of the PFO requires a contrast study, and the PFO would have been identified if a contrast had been utilized at the time of TEE.

**D.** The axial resolution of TTE echo is better suited for identifying interatrial anatomy.

3. A 57-year-old female being treated for alcohol withdrawal was admitted to the ICU secondary to hypoxia. On physical examination, she is noted to have jaundice and ascites. Her oxygen saturation is 89% and has not improved with supplemental oxygen via nasal cannula. She is diagnosed with hepatopulmonary syndrome. Would a contrast TEE or contrast TTE be more likely to identify an intrapulmonary shunt and why?

**A.** TTE is more likely to identify an intrapulmonary shunt because the atria are imaged in their entirety.

**B.** TEE is more likely to identify an intrapulmonary shunt as the pulmonary veins are imaged in greater detail.

**C.** TTE is more likely to identify an intrapulmonary shunt because the high sensitivity detection of PFO allows for enhanced differentiation between an interatrial shunt and intrapulmonary shunt.

**D.** TEE is more likely to identify an intrapulmonary shunt because the left atrial appendage (LAA) is better visualized.

4. A 54-year-old male with a history of nonischemic heart failure presents for left ventricular assist device (LVAD) placement. There is concern the patient's right ventricular (RV) function may not be sufficient to meet the output of the LVAD after placement. Which of the following is correct when evaluating RV function?

**A.** TTE and TEE RV s′ values are interchangeable.

**B.** Tricuspid annular plane systolic excursion (TAPSE) by TEE will always be less than TAPSE by TTE.

**C.** RV longitudinal strain by TTE and TEE is similar.

**D.** Optimal RV s′ values with TEE are achieved in the midesophageal four-chamber view.

5. A 51-year-old male on postop day 1 status post a coronary artery bypass grafting (CABG) and mitral valve replacement has become hemodynamically unstable. Due to concern for pericardial tamponade, the plan is to perform a bedside echo. Which of the following is true when comparing TTE and TEE?

**A.** Tamponade is more likely to be seen if TEE is used vs TTE for this patient.

**B.** TEE is considered the gold standard for diagnosing tamponade.

**C.** TTE is better for visualizing pericardial clot in this patient.

**D.** There would be no need for other imaging if there is no pericardial tamponade seen with TEE.

6. A 73-year-old male with a history of uncontrolled hypertension, chronic obstructive pulmonary disease (COPD), 35 pack year smoking, and hyperlipidemia presents to the ICU in hypertensive crisis. He has an elevated creatinine and on examination has an early diastolic murmur heard best at the left sternal border. After becoming unresponsive, he was intubated for airway protection. Given concern for an aortic dissection, which of the following is not an indication for TEE?

**A.** Evaluation of aortic regurgitation

**B.** Evaluation of myocardial wall motion abnormalities

**C.** Evaluation of the abdominal aorta to determine the extent of the dissection

**D.** To determine if there is pericardial effusion

7. A 71-year-old male presented to the Emergency Department with chest pain and shortness of breath. During his examination, he became unresponsive and lost a pulse. While advanced cardiovascular life support (ACLS) is being performed, the code leader requests an echo for evaluation and monitoring. Which of the following is correct pertaining to echo use during a cardiac arrest?

**A.** TEE cannot differentiate pseudo-pulseless electrical activity (PEA) vs PEA.

**B.** TTE can be used during chest compressions.

**C.** TEE cannot identify chest compressions obstructing the left ventricular outflow tract (LVOT).

**D.** TTE has not been shown to lengthen pulse check times.

8. A 67-year-old female is admitted to the ICU for respiratory failure. She was intubated due to acute onset of hypoxia. Upon arrival to the ICU, she was noted to be hypotensive requiring inotropic and vasopressor support. During a TTE, severe mitral regurgitation is identified. When you consider echoing this patient, which of the following is correct when comparing TEE and TTE?

   **A.** TEE provides better 2D imaging of the mitral valve.
   **B.** TTE is better for evaluating pulmonary vein flow.
   **C.** Color flow of the regurgitant jet is better seen with TTE.
   **D.** TTE is useful for localization and determination of pathology that may guide surgical correction.

9. A 68-year-old male with known diastolic dysfunction presents with atrial fibrillation and volume overload. He is admitted to the ICU for respiratory and hemodynamic support. After adequate diuresis and rate control, he still requires hemodynamic support. The decision is made to proceed with cardioversion. Which of the following is correct regarding echo evaluation prior to cardioversion?

   **A.** TTE can evaluate the LAA with higher frequency ultrasound.
   **B.** TEE is better than TTE for capturing different areas of the LAA.
   **C.** LAA velocity >40 cm/s is associated with a higher incidence of cerebrovascular accidents (CVAs).
   **D.** LAA evaluation with TEE is not improved with echo contrast.

10. A 24-year-old male who suffered blunt trauma to the abdomen is intubated in the ICU. He has an intra-abdominal bleed that will require an ex lap. His wife reports that he has some heart condition that she does not know much about. The plan is to perform an echo prior to surgery. Which of the following is true concerning echo?

   **A.** TTE uses a higher frequency probe.
   **B.** The parasternal long axis and midesophageal long axis both look at the inferoseptal and anterolateral portions of the left ventricle.
   **C.** The parasternal short axis and transgastric short axis can visualize the left ventricle with the anterior left ventricle closer to the probe and the inferior left ventricle further from the probe.
   **D.** TEE cannot evaluate the distal ascending aorta due to the left mainstem bronchus.

11. A 78-year-old male with a history of pacemaker placement 5 years ago was found to have bacteremia and sepsis. Infective endocarditis must be ruled out. Which of the following statements is true regarding the use of TTE vs TEE?

   **A.** TTE has been proven to have a greater overall sensitivity when compared to TEE when evaluating for infective endocarditis.
   **B.** TEE provides improved views of the aortic valve and aortic root compared to TTE when evaluating for structural abnormalities.
   **C.** TTE is more accurate than TEE for the diagnosis of pacemaker-associated endocarditis.
   **D.** The costs associated with TEE make it less frequently utilized today in the diagnosis of infective endocarditis.

12. A 48-year-old male status post motor vehicle accident has suffered a sternal fracture with associated retrosternal hematoma and new-onset arrhythmias. Concern for myocardial contusion has been raised. Which of the following statements regarding the use of TTE vs TEE with regard to evaluation of blunt myocardial contusion is correct?

   **A.** TTE has been proven to have a greater overall sensitivity when compared to TEE when evaluating for myocardial contusion.
   **B.** TEE is typically not utilized to evaluate for myocardial contusion in the setting of trauma.
   **C.** TEE has a slightly worse sensitivity compared to TTE for detecting myocardial contusion in the setting of trauma.
   **D.** TEE has been proven to provide a greater sensitivity when evaluating for blunt trauma–associated myocardial contusion.

13. A 58-year-old female just completed transcatheter aortic valve replacement (TAVR) and immediately following the procedure is being evaluated with TEE. A concern for significant paravalvular leak (PVL) is raised based on the results. Which of the following statements regarding the use of TTE vs TEE in the setting of PVL evaluation is correct?

    A. PVL evaluation with TTE has little impact on patient care following TAVR.
    B. Both TTE and TEE have been found to have utility in evaluating PVL following TAVR.
    C. TTE quantification of PVL has no correlation with the results of TEE findings.
    D. Multidetector computed tomography (MDCT) has rendered the use of TTE/TEE obsolete.

14. A 67-year-old male with pancytopenia secondary to chemotherapy treatment for acute myeloid leukemia (AML) has suffered a myocardial infarction. Following resuscitation, he has been transferred to the ICU for further management. His platelet level is 57. The nurse asks you if there are any concerns regarding coagulopathy and thrombocytopenia during TEE. Which of the following statements regarding coagulopathy and TEE are correct?

    A. Any degree of coagulopathy is a contraindication to TEE, and TTE should be performed.
    B. Severe coagulopathy is a relative contraindication to TEE but additional studies are required to more definitively understand the risk.
    C. Platelet counts >100/μL are required prior to performing TEE.
    D. Platelet transfusions should be utilized empirically prior to performing TEE on this patient.

15. A 27-year-old female has been diagnosed with preeclampsia and is having significant hypertension despite extensive medical management. Which of the following statements regarding TEE or TTE in the management of preeclampsia is true?

    A. There is no role for TTE or TEE in the management of preeclampsia.
    B. TEE is the only accepted method of echocardiography in the pregnant patient.
    C. Obstetric anesthesiologists are encouraged to utilize TEE/TTE in the management of preeclampsia.
    D. TEE is preferred over TTE due to the severe limitations in visualization secondary to the body habitus changes of the pregnant patient.

16. A 77-year-old female with severe aortic stenosis is presenting for a TAVR. When using echocardiography to evaluate the aortic valve lesion, which of the following is the best method to measure the LVOT in order to calculate the aortic valve area by continuity equation?

    A. TTE 2D LVOT diameter
    B. TTE 3D LVOT planimetry
    C. TEE 2D LVOT diameter
    D. TEE 3D LVOT planimetry

17. A 32-year-old female presents to the hospital with acute shortness of breath and chest pain. Her past medical history includes type I diabetes, a recent open reduction, internal fixation of a tibial fracture sustained while skiing, and seasonal allergies. Her only medication are oral contraceptive pills. She is currently in visible distress, with significant tachycardia and tachypnea on examination. A bedside electrocardiogram (ECG) demonstrates sinus tachycardia with mild right axis deviation. All other laboratory studies and imaging are pending. Which of the following statements best describes the role of TTE in the workup of this patient?

    A. The presence of left ventricular dysfunction and strain indicates impending cardiovascular collapse and is a commonly visualized sign.
    B. Echocardiography has a high specificity and low sensitivity for pulmonary embolism (PE).
    C. Visualization of an intracardiac thrombus is an indication for urgent embolectomy.
    D. Visualization of RV strain is of little prognostic value.

18. A 76-year-old woman presents for an elective TEE to assess for suspected prosthetic valve dysfunction. Her past medical history is significant for a mechanical mitral valve replacement 20 years ago, hypertension, and rheumatoid arthritis for which she is on chronic steroids. The procedure took noticeably longer due to anatomic challenges but was otherwise uncomplicated and unremarkable. The patient vomited a small amount of gastric succus in the recovery room but remained well enough to be discharged home. She presents 4 days later to the Emergency Department with chest pain, shortness of breath, cough, nausea, and dysphagia. She is hemodynamically stable. CT scan of the chest with intravenous (IV) contrast reveals bibasilar atelectasis with small amount of left-sided pleural effusion, mild mediastinitis, and a dilated stomach. What is the best next step in her management?

   A. Contrast swallow study
   B. Antibiotics followed by discharge home
   C. Insertion of nasogastric (NG) tube for decompression
   D. Upper gastrointestinal (GI) endoscopy

19. A 32-year-old male who recently suffered a series of stroke-like episodes of unclear etiology is undergoing a TEE to rule out a PFO. Which of the following maneuvers is likely to increase the sensitivity of the study and the likelihood of detecting such a defect?

   A. Agitated saline injection
   B. Vagal stimulation maneuvers
   C. Left lateral decubitus positioning
   D. Crystalloid bolus to achieve hypervolemia

20. A 63-year-old female presents to the Emergency Department with severe retrosternal chest pain radiating to the left arm. As part of the workup for suspected acute coronary syndrome (ACS), she undergoes an urgent ECG and bedside TTE. Which of the following statements regarding echocardiography and regional wall motion abnormalities (RWMA) is true?

   A. RWMA is only visualized after at least 1 hour of ischemia and coronary occlusion.
   B. RWMA is a pathognomonic finding of ACS.
   C. There is no role for echocardiography until an ST-elevation myocardial infarction (STEMI) is confirmed on ECG as RWMA are not a sensitive finding for ACS.
   D. RWMA typically occur prior to the onset of ECG changes.

# Chapter 12 ▪ Answers

1. Correct Answer: C. Transesophageal echocardiography (TEE) has a higher sensitivity for detection of endocarditis when evaluating replaced valves as compared to TTE.

*Rationale:* TEE has nearly 100% sensitivity for the detection of endocarditis involving both native and prosthetic valves. Though the sensitivity of TEE is reduced for prosthetic valves, it remains >80% due to the higher frequency ultrasound beam providing better resolution of the cardiac valves. TEE can help determine the extent of vegetations. TTE echo is better for evaluation of the tricuspid valve in comparison to other valves due to its close proximity to the chest wall.

Selected References
1. Biswas A, Yassin MH. Comparison between transthoracic and transesophageal echocardiogram in the diagnosis of endocarditis: a retrospective analysis. *Int J Crit Illn Inj Sci.* 2015;5(2):130-131.
2. Ryan EW, Bolger AF. Transesophageal echocardiography (TEE) in the evaluation of infective endocarditis. *Cardiol Clin.* 2000;18(4):773-787.
3. Sekar P, Johnson JR, Thurn JR, et al. Comparative sensitivity of transthoracic and transesophageal echocardiography in diagnosis of infective endocarditis among veterans with *Staphylococcus aureus* bacteremia. *Open Forum Infect Dis.* 2017;4(2):ofx035.

**2.** Correct Answer: A. TTE with contrast study is better at detecting a PFO as compared to evaluation with TEE.

*Rationale/Critique:* TTE has been shown to be more sensitive ($>80\%$) for PFO detection when utilizing contrast when compared to TEE ($<60\%$) with contrast. TEE usually requires some form of sedation, which can lead to decreased right atrial (RA) pressures as a result of decreased venous return. The decreased RA pressure in comparison to the left atrial pressure may prevent interatrial shunting through a PFO. A Valsalva maneuver helps to generate an increase in RA pressure, which may favor right-to-left shunting through the PFO. However, this may not hold true in patients with markedly elevated left atrial pressure. Axial resolution is improved with higher frequency ultrasound waves. Higher frequency waves do not penetrate tissue as deeply as lower frequency waves because of attenuation. The TEE probe is positioned closer to the interatrial septum, allowing for the use of higher frequencies. See Figure 12.1.

### Selected References

1. Armstrong WF, Ryan T. Left and right atrium, and right ventricle. In: Armstrong WF, Ryan T, eds. *Feigenbaum's Echocardiography*. 8th ed. Wolters Kluwer; 2019:158-193.
2. Thanigaraj S, Valika A, Zajarias A, Lasala JM, Perez JE. Comparison of transthoracic versus transesophageal echocardiography for detection of right-to-left atrial shunting using agitated saline contrast. *Am J Cardiol*. 2005;96(7):1007-1010.
3. Yue L, Zhai YN, Wei LQ. Which technique is better for detection of right-to-left shunt in patients with patent foramen ovale: comparing contrast transthoracic echocardiography with contrast transesophageal echocardiography. *Echocardiography*. 2014;31(9):1050-1055.

**3.** Correct Answer: B. TEE is more likely to identify an intrapulmonary shunt as the pulmonary veins are imaged in greater detail.

*Rationale:* An intrapulmonary shunt is more likely to be identified with a TEE compared to TTE. TTE typically only allows visualization of the pulmonary veins as they empty into the left atrium. On the other hand, portions of the pulmonary veins can be imaged during TEE, allowing visualization of contrast within the veins as a result of intrapulmonary shunt. This can be especially helpful when there is a concomitant interatrial shunt. On TTE, the contrast will be noted within the left atria and make it difficult to determine if contrast is a result of an atrial or an intrapulmonary shunt because of the inability to identify the extent of the pulmonary veins. However, with direct visualization of the pulmonary veins on TEE, the contrast can be seen returning from the lungs.

### Selected References

1. Abushora MY, Bhatia N, Alnabki Z, Shenoy M, Alshaher M, Stoddard MF. Intrapulmonary shunt is a potentially unrecognized cause of ischemic stroke and transient ischemic attack. *J Am Soc Echocardiogr*. 2013;26(7):683-690.
2. Rollan MJ, Munoz AC, Perez T, Bratos JL. Value of contrast echocardiography for the diagnosis of hepatopulmonary syndrome. *Eur J Echocardiogr*. 2007;8(5):408-410.

**4.** Correct Answer: C. RV longitudinal strain by TTE and TEE is similar.

*Rationale:* With TTE the RV s′ value is obtained from the apical four-chamber view. This allows the s′ to be measured at the lateral tricuspid annulus. The tissue movement during systole is toward the ultrasound probe and this provides good alignment for tissue Doppler. Tissue Doppler is angle dependent, and anytime there is an angle between the tissue movement and the ultrasound beam, there will be underestimation of the value. In the TEE midesophageal four-chamber view, the ultrasound beam does not line up well with the movement of the lateral tricuspid annulus. When using another view such as the modified transgastric RV inflow view with TEE, which provides the best ultrasound beam to tissue movement alignment, the inferior portion of the tricuspid valve is being measured. The s′ values in any of the comparisons are not interchangeable. Strain by speckle tracking is angle independent, and RV strain by TTE and TEE is similar. Cardiac magnetic resonance imaging (MRI) is the gold standard for RV measurements.

### Selected References

1. Gebhardt BR, Asher S, Maslow A. The limitations of using transthoracic echocardiographic–derived normative values for grading intraoperative transesophageal echocardiography examinations of the right ventricle: are they really interchangeable? *J Cardiothorac Vasc Anesth*. 2020;34(5):1260-1262.
2. Kurt M, Tanboga IH, Isik T, et al. Comparison of transthoracic and transesophageal 2-dimensional speckle tracking echocardiography. *J Cardiothorac Vasc Anesth*. 2012;26(1):26-31.
3. Roberts SM, Klick J, Fischl A, King TS, Cios TJ. A comparison of transesophageal to transthoracic echocardiographic measures of right ventricular function. *J Cardiothorac Vasc Anesth*. 2020;34(5):1252-1259.

**5.** Correct Answer: A. Tamponade is more likely to be seen if TEE is used vs TTE for this patient.

*Rationale:* Overall, TTE is considered the gold standard for evaluation of tamponade; however, postsurgical changes from an open chest procedure make TTE difficult due to ultrasound beam interference. This can lead to poor differentiation between tissue and hematoma as well as other structures. Patients who have undergone an open cardiac procedure are at risk for pericardial tamponade. In this population, TEE is more sensitive as compared to TTE for identifying pericardial tamponade. The poor windows generated from the postsurgical chest are avoided, with TEE leading to better image acquisition. Unlike typical tamponade, which involves larger portions of the pericardium, postsurgical tamponade can be loculated. If there is concern for pericardial tamponade and echo imaging is inconclusive, then CT imaging would be warranted.

### Selected References
1. Imren Y, Tasoglu I, Oktar GL, et al. The importance of transesophageal echocardiography in diagnosis of pericardial tamponade after cardiac surgery. *J Card Surg.* 2008;23(5):450-453.
2. Kronzon I, Tunick PA, Freedberg RS. Transesophageal echocardiography in pericardial disease and tamponade. *Echocardiography.* 1994;11(5):493-505.

**6.** Correct Answer: C. Evaluation of the abdominal aorta to determine the extent of the dissection

*Rationale:* TEE can evaluate for aortic dissections and the associated findings such as aortic regurgitation, wall motion abnormalities, and pericardial effusion. When a dissection is present, TEE may demonstrate aortic regurgitation, wall motion abnormalities, and pericardial effusion. Due to the close positioning of the esophagus and aorta, TEE can utilize higher frequency imaging for better resolution as compared to TTE. Sensitivity of imaging modalities in aortic dissection: TEE 99%, MRI and CT 95% to 98%. See **Figure 12.2**.

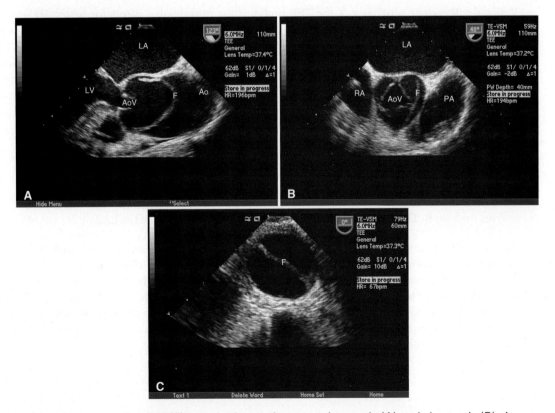

**Figure 12.2** Dissection flap (F) seen in the aortic root on long-axis (A) and short-axis (B) views. (C) The dissection flap extended to the descending thoracic aorta. Ao, aorta; AoV, aortic valve; LA, left atrium; LV, left ventricle; PA, pulmonary artery; RA, right atrium.

Selected References

1. Baliga RR, Nienaber CA, Bossone E, et al. The role of imaging in aortic dissection and related syndromes. *JACC Cardiovasc Imaging*. 2014;7(4):406-424.
2. Banning AP, Masani ND, Ikram S, Fraser AG, Hall RJ. Transoesophageal echocardiography as the sole diagnostic investigation in patients with suspected thoracic aortic dissection. *Br Heart J*. 1994;72(5):461-465.
3. Evangelista A, Flachskampf FA, Erbel R, et al. Echocardiography in aortic diseases: EAE recommendations for clinical practice. *Eur J Echocardiogr*. 2010;11(8):645-658.
4. Garcia-Cortes RS, Rao PK, Quader N. Transesophageal echocardiography. In: Quader N, Makan M, Perez J, eds. *The Washington Manual of Echocardiography*. 2nd ed. Wolters Kluwer; 2017:294-324.
5. Schiller NB, Ren X, Ristow B. Echocardiograpic evaluation of the thoracic and proximal abdominal aorta. In: Manning WJ, Yeon SB, eds. *Uptodate*. Uptodate; Accessed on November 11, 2019.

**7.** Correct Answer: B. TTE can be used during chest compressions.

*Rationale:* Utilizing echo for evaluation of cardiac arrest patients is helpful in identifying reversible causes and may help direct therapy. During pseudo-PEA, echo can help visualize cardiac contraction even if no pulse is palpable as a result of low cardiac output. Absence of contraction is seen with true PEA. TTE has been shown to increase the time during pulse checks beyond 10 sec. This does not decrease TTE utility in this scenario. However, periods of TTE during pulse checks should be monitored to remain less than 10 sec. Many TTE views are not possible and image acquisition can be difficult during chest compressions. However, using the subcostal view can allow for imaging during compressions.

Selected References

1. Long B, Alerhand S, Maliel K, Koyfman A. Echocardiography in cardiac arrest: an emergency medicine review. *Am J Emerg Med*. 2018;36(3):488-493.
2. Price S, Uddin S, Quinn T. Echocardiography in cardiac arrest. *Curr Opin Crit Care*. 2010;16(3):211-215.

**8.** Correct Answer: A. TEE provides better 2D imaging of the mitral valve.

*Rationale:* The close proximity of the TEE probe to the mitral valve allows for better 2D imaging. This makes TEE ideal for localizing specific structural abnormalities that can help guide surgical correction. TEE with color flow can be used in multiple sector angles with better resolution to evaluate the regurgitant jet with more precision as compared to TTE. TTE is better for left atrial dimensions due to the ability to capture the entire atrium. Due to the close positioning of the TEE probe to the left atrium, it generally gets foreshortened. For this same reason TTE is better for measuring maximal mitral regurgitation jet area to left atrial area ratio. Pulmonary vein flow is better evaluated with TEE.

Selected Reference

1. Foster E. Transesophageal echocardiography in the evaluation of mitral valve disease. In: Manning WJ, Gassch WH, eds. *UpToDate*. UpToDate; 2019.

**9.** Correct Answer: B. TEE is better than TTE for capturing different areas of the LAA.

*Rationale:* Due to the close proximity of the esophagus to the LAA, TEE can utilize higher frequency ultrasound to visualize the structure. Different areas of the LAA can be visualized by manipulating the sector angle and probe positioning with TEE. This all contributes to TEE being better able to evaluate the LAA. Echo contrast has been shown to improve imaging of the LAA with TEE. This can be useful when there are obstacles to optimal LAA evaluation such as spontaneous echo contrast and pectinate muscle interference. TEE is considered superior to TTE for LAA evaluation. LAA velocity <40 cm/s indicates an increased risk of stroke. See **Figure 12.3**.

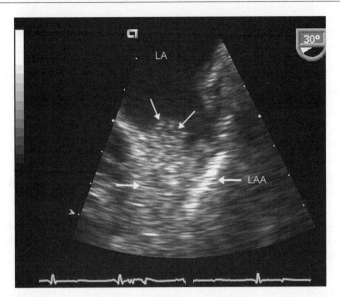

**Figure 12.3** Transesophageal echocardiographic image of the left atrial appendage (LAA) in a patient with rheumatic mitral stenosis and an LAA thrombus. Note the irregular echo density mass filling the LAA (*thin arrows*). The boundary of the wall of the LAA is as noted by the *heavier arrows*. LA, left atrium.

### Selected References

1. Abdelmoneim SS, Mulvagh SL. Techniques to improve left atrial appendage imaging. *J Atr Fibrillation*. 2014;7(1):1059.
2. Beigel R, Wunderlich NC, Ho SY, Arsanjani R, Siegel RJ. The left atrial appendage: anatomy, function, and noninvasive evaluation. *JACC Cardiovasc Imaging*. 2014;7(12):1251-1265.
3. Armstrong WF, Ryan T. Mitral valve disease. In: Feigenbaum H, Armstrong WF, Ryan T, eds. *Feigenbaum's Echocardiography*. 6th ed. Wolters Kluwer; 2004:306-340.
4. Wai SH, Kyu K, Galupo MJ, et al. Assessment of left atrial appendage function by transthoracic pulsed Doppler echocardiography: comparing against transesophageal interrogation and predicting echocardiographic risk factors for stroke. *Echocardiography*. 2017;34(10):1478-1485.

---

**10.** Correct Answer: D. TEE cannot evaluate the distal ascending aorta due to the left mainstem bronchus.

*Rationale:* The left mainstem bronchus blocks imaging of the distal ascending aorta when using TEE due to the anatomic positioning of the bronchus between the probe and distal ascending aorta. TTE evaluation of that area is not affected by the bronchus. Parasternal short axis places the anterior left ventricle closer to the probe and the inferior left ventricle further from the probe. Transgastric short axis places the inferior left ventricle closer to the probe and the anterior left ventricle further from the probe. The parasternal long axis and midesophageal long axis both look at the inferolateral and anteroseptal portions of the left ventricle.

### Selected Reference

1. Shillcutt SK, Bick JS. Echo didactics: a comparison of basic transthoracic and transesophageal echocardiography views in the perioperative setting. *Anesth Analg*. 2013;116(6):1231-1236.

---

**11.** Correct Answer: B. TEE provides improved views of the aortic valve and aortic root compared to TTE when evaluating for structural abnormalities.

*Rationale:* When compared to TTE, TEE is most sensitive for the detection of infective endocarditis. TEE has improved views of the aortic valve and root due to increased frequency that results in improved resolution and better visualization of these structures. TEE should remain the test of choice to rule out infective endocarditis.

### Selected References

1. Lyons K, Bhamidipati K. 4 Comparison of transthoracic and transoesophageal echocardiography in the diagnosis of infective endocarditis—a tertiary centre experience. *Heart*. 2017;103(suppl 6):A3.
2. Sekar P, Johnson JR, Thurn JR, et al. Comparative sensitivity of transthoracic and transesophageal echocardiography in diagnosis of infective endocarditis among veterans with *Staphylococcus aureus* bacteremia. *Open Forum Infect Dis*. 2017;4(2):ofx035.
3. Shively BK, Gurule FT, Roldan CA, Leggett JH, Schiller NB. Diagnostic value of transesophageal compared with transthoracic echocardiography in infective endocarditis. *J Am Coll Cardiol*. 1991;18(2):391-397.

**12.** Correct Answer: D. TEE has been proven to provide a greater sensitivity when evaluating for blunt trauma–associated myocardial contusion.

*Rationale:* When compared to TTE, TEE is most sensitive for the detection of blunt trauma–associated myocardial contusion. TTE may also be further limited due to severe chest trauma.

Selected Reference

1. Karalis DG, Victor MF, Davis GA, et al. The role of echocardiography in blunt chest trauma: a transthoracic and transesophageal echocardiographic study. *J Trauma.* 1994;36(1):53-58.

**13.** Correct Answer: B. Both TTE and TEE have been found to have utility in evaluating PVL following TAVR.

*Rationale:* When evaluating PVL following TAVR, both TEE and TTE remain critical tools for evaluation of the size and significance of the leak. TEE and TTE both allow to quantify the size of the leak better evaluating the risk of mortality following the procedure and need for further surgical intervention.

Selected References

1. Goncalves A, Nyman C, Okada DR, et al. Transthoracic echocardiography to assess aortic regurgitation after TAVR: a comparison with periprocedural transesophageal echocardiography. *Cardiology.* 2017;137(1):1-8.
2. Teeter EG, Dakik C, Cooter M, et al. Assessment of paravalvular leak after transcatheter aortic valve replacement: transesophageal echocardiography compared with transthoracic echocardiography. *J Cardiothorac Vasc Anesth.* 2017;31(4):1278-1284.

**14.** Correct Answer: B. Severe coagulopathy is a relative contraindication to TEE but additional studies are required to more definitively understand the risk.

*Rationale:* TEE use in coagulopathy patients has been understudied. Additional investigations will provide further insight into this area. No specific platelet count or coagulopathy goals are widely accepted in the literature at this time.

Selected Reference

1. Wray TC, Schmid K, Braude D, et al. Safety of transesophageal echocardiography performed by intensivists and emergency physicians in critically ill patients with coagulopathy and thrombocytopenia: a single-center experience. *J Intensive Care Med.* 2021;36(1):123-130. doi:10.1177/0885066619887693.

**15.** Correct Answer: C. Obstetric anesthesiologists are encouraged to utilize TEE/TTE in the management of preeclampsia.

*Rationale:* TTE/TEE use in the management of preeclampsia is widely encouraged in the literature. Additional certifications and training of obstetric anesthesiologists can be expected to become more widespread in the future. TEE is safe during pregnancy. Physiologic periprocedural considerations should be taken into account. This would include: NPO status and gravid uterus, fetal monitoring with administration of sedation, and effects of pregnancy and gravid uterus on respiratory status.

Selected References

1. Dennis AT. Transthoracic echocardiography in women with preeclampsia. *Curr Opin Anaesthesiol.* 2015;28(3):254-260.
2. Regitz-Zagrosek V, Lundqvist CB, Borghi C, et al. ESC Guidelines on the management of cardiovascular diseases during pregnancy: the task force on the management of cardiovascular diseases during pregnancy of the European Society of Cardiology (ESC). *Eur Heart J.* 2011;32(24):3147-3197.

**16.** Correct Answer: D. TEE 3D LVOT planimetry

*Rationale:* Using the LVOT diameter to determine the area of the LVOT makes the assumption that the LVOT is circular. The LVOT is not circular but elliptical in shape. When using 2D planimetry, there is a high likelihood the measurement is from an oblique angle. TEE 3D generally obtains a high-quality dataset that allows for manipulation of the location, cardiac cycle time, and angle at which the LVOT is measured. Using TTE 3D generally yields subpar image quality.

**Selected References**

1. Doddamani S, Grushko MJ, Makaryus AN, et al. Demonstration of left ventricular outflow tract eccentricity by 64-slice multi-detector CT. *Int J Cardiovasc Imaging.* 2009;25:175-181.
2. Gaspar T, Adawi S, Sachner R, et al. Three-dimensional imaging of the left ventricular outflow tract: impact on aortic valve area estimation by the continuity equation. *J Am Soc Echocardiogr.* 2012 Jul;25(7):749-757.
3. Poh KK, Levine RA, Solis J, et al. Assessing aortic valve area in aortic stenosis by continuity equation: a novel approach using real-time three-dimensional echocardiography. *Eur Heart J.* 2008 Oct;29(20):2526-2535.

**17.** Correct Answer: B. Echocardiography has a high specificity and low sensitivity for pulmonary embolism (PE).

*Rationale:* The patient's presentation is suspicious for a PE. She has several risk factors including being a young female, recent surgery, decreased lower extremity mobility, and oral contraceptive use. Echocardiography in the setting of suspected PE is currently not recommended as it cannot directly diagnose the condition and is insensitive, particularly in patients who are hemodynamically stable. When used in this context, it may occasionally be useful to assess for the degree of RV dysfunction and impending hemodynamic collapse. While limited in its use from a diagnostic perspective, the role of echocardiography is more established in prognosticating patients with confirmed PE and RV strain. Echocardiography has a high specificity and low sensitivity for PE, making this modality of imaging favorable in a bedside evaluation workup.

**Selected References**

1. Fields JM, Davis J, Girson L, et al. Transthoracic echocardiography for diagnosing pulmonary embolism: a systematic review and meta-analysis. *J Am Soc Echocardiogr.* 2017;30(7):714.
2. Grifoni S, Olivotto I, Cecchini P, et al. Short-term clinical outcome of patients with acute pulmonary embolism, normal blood pressure, and echocardiographic right ventricular dysfunction. *Circulation.* 2000;101(24):2817-2822.

**18.** Correct Answer: D. Upper gastrointestinal (GI) endoscopy

*Rationale:* Serious complications such as esophageal perforations are overall rare and have been estimated to have an incidence of 1/5000 to 1/10,000. Nevertheless, timely diagnosis of such a complication requires a high index of suspicion as signs and symptoms are generally nonspecific. Urgent upper GI endoscopy is necessary to directly visualize the injury and may simultaneously provide therapy. Though CT scan with oral contrast can be helpful in determining large leaks, a simple upper GI series or contrast swallow study may not be sensitive enough to pick up smaller leaks. Should a perforation be diagnosed, expeditious treatment is required and can range from conservative management, endoscopic stenting, to surgical repair depending on the degree of contamination. Blind insertion of an NG tube is contraindicated in this setting. Though thoracentesis can occasionally yield food particles and bilious fluid if the perforation communicates with the pleural cavity, they have limited role in this scenario.

**Selected References**

1. Herbold T, Chon SH, Grimminger P, et al. Endoscopic treatment of transesophageal echocardiography-induced esophageal perforation. *J Laparoendosc Adv Surg Tech A.* 2018;28(4):422-428.
2. Min JK, Spencer KT, Furlong KT, et al. Clinical features of complications from transesophageal echocardiography: a single-center case series of 10,000 consecutive examinations. *J Am Soc Echocardiogr.* 2005;18(9):925-929.

**19.** Correct Answer: A. Agitated saline injection

*Rationale:* The injection of agitated saline contrast in conjunction with echocardiography is commonly known as a "bubble study" and is a frequently used diagnostic modality for PFOs. The injection of small bubbles into the venous circulation serves as a contrast medium by scattering ultrasound waves and allows for detection of right-to-left shunts. The study can be further enhanced using Valsalva maneuvers to increase right heart pressures. There is no role for vagal stimulation, decubitus positioning, anticoagulation, or hypervolemia in echocardiography for PFOs.

**Selected Reference**

1. Meissner I, Whisnant JP, Khandheria BK, et al. Prevalence of potential risk factors for stroke assessed by transesophageal echocardiography and carotid ultrasonography: the SPARC study. stroke prevention: assessment of risk in a community. *Mayo Clin Proc.* 1999;74(9):862-869.

**20.** Correct Answer: D. RWMA typically occur prior to the onset of ECG changes.

*Rationale:* The role of bedside TTE in the workup of ACS has surged in recent years. Cardiac ischemia from coronary artery occlusion can produce visible RWMA within seconds of severe ischemic changes. These findings, which can be seen prior to the onset of ECG changes, are highly sensitive but relatively nonspecific and must be taken into consideration along with patient symptoms, ECG findings, and laboratory results. Alternate, non-ACS causes of RWMA include prior infarction, previous surgery and implants, baseline cardiomyopathy, and focal myocarditis. Agitated saline (or bubble study) has no role in the diagnosis of ACS.

Selected Reference

1. Hauser AM, Gangadharan V, Ramos RG, Gordon S, Timmis GC. Sequence of mechanical, electrocardiographic and clinical effects of repeated coronary artery occlusion in human beings: echocardiographic observations during coronary angioplasty. *J Am Coll Cardiol.* 1985;5(2 pt 1):183-187.

# 13 | THREE-DIMENSIONAL ECHOCARDIOGRAPHY

Martin Ingi Sigurdsson

1. In which of the following patients might a full volume assessment of the left ventricle ejection fraction (LVEF) via gated acquisition be difficult?

   A. Patient with hypertrophic septal cardiomyopathy
   B. Patient in rate-controlled atrial fibrillation
   C. Patient who is intubated for respiratory distress
   D. Patient with lateral wall dyskinesis

2. Which of the following assessments is greatly improved by using three-dimensional (3D) compared with two-dimensional (2D) echocardiography?

   A. Blood flow in left atrial appendage
   B. Positioning of a ventricular assist device
   C. Assessment of left ventricular dyssynchrony
   D. Location of an aortic insufficiency jet

3. For which of the following assessments does the American Society of Echocardiography (ASE) currently recommend usage of 3D echocardiography?

   A. Tricuspid valve regurgitation
   B. Pulmonary valve stenosis
   C. Aortic valve regurgitation
   D. Mitral valve stenosis

# Chapter 13 ▪ Answers

**1.** Correct Answer: B. Patient in rate-controlled atrial fibrillation

*Rationale:* To improve the resolution during 3D assessment of large structures, such as the left ventricle, gated acquisition stacks together scans of multiple smaller 3D pyramids to generate the image that includes adequate temporal resolution. This is done by electrocardiogram (ECG) gating, and arrythmias such as atrial fibrillation, therefore, render this modality sensitive to stitch artifacts when the image is inaccurately compiled due to the arrhythmia.

Selected Reference
1. Lang RM, Badano LP, Tsang W, et al. EAE/ASE recommendations for image acquisition and display using three-dimensional echocardiography. *Eur Heart J Cardiovasc Imaging.* 2012;13:1-46.

**2.** Correct Answer: C. Assessment of left ventricular dyssynchrony

*Rationale:* Assessment of the left ventricular contraction via 3D echocardiography offers the possibility of assessing the movement of all 17 segments of the left ventricle simultaneously. This allows for a unique assessment of left ventricular dyssynchrony that cannot be replicated with 2D echocardiography.

Selected Reference
1. Lang RM, Badano LP, Tsang W, et al. EAE/ASE recommendations for image acquisition and display using three-dimensional echocardiography. *Eur Heart J Cardiovasc Imaging.* 2012;13:1-46.

**3.** Correct Answer: D. Mitral valve stenosis

*Rationale:* In the 2012 European Association of Echocardiography (EAE)/American Society of Echocardiography (ASE) guidelines describing the current state of evidence for 3D imaging, the society recommends usage of 3D echocardiography for assessment of the mitral valve anatomy, mitral stenosis, and procedural guidance for transcatheter procedures.

Selected Reference
1. Lang RM, Badano LP, Tsang W, et al. EAE/ASE recommendations for image acquisition and display using three-dimensional echocardiography. *Eur Heart J Cardiovasc Imaging.* 2012;13:1-46.

# 14 | PHYSICS OF ARTIFACTS

Karim Fikry and Jacob Clark

1. Which statement below is true regarding side-lobe artifacts?

   A. This artifact is created after ultrasound echoes return from highly reflective objects located within the pathway of the main (central) beam.
   B. All the energy from the ultrasound transducer stays within the main (central) beam.
   C. These artifacts involve the presence of a weakly reflective object that is close to the central ultrasound beam.
   D. With this artifact, an image will appear in the wrong location but at an appropriate distance within the main (central) ultrasound beam.

2. Which of the following is caused by the dark area in the lung ultrasound (**Figure 14.1**)?

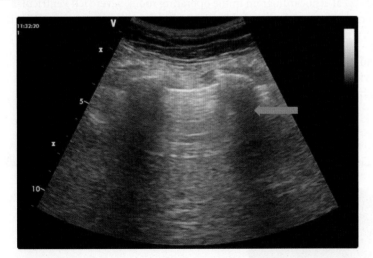

**Figure 14.1**

   A. Shadowing
   B. Lung point
   C. Reverberations
   D. Pulmonary edema

3. Under what circumstances is the artifact in **Figure 14.2** (area indicated by the *arrow*) commonly seen?

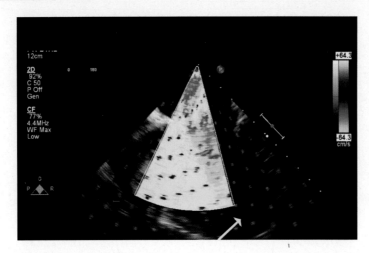

**Figure 14.2**

   **A.** Presence of a pulmonary artery catheter creating multiple side-lobe artifacts
   **B.** Air bubbles seen after cardiopulmonary bypass during cardiac surgery
   **C.** Artifact caused by the use of harmonic imaging
   **D.** Electrocautery artifact

4. Which statement about tissue harmonic imaging is correct?

   **A.** Reverberation artifacts are more common in harmonic imaging.
   **B.** In general, tissue harmonic signals pass through the body wall only once.
   **C.** Harmonics are mainly produced by side-lobe artifacts.
   **D.** Artifacts are less common with fundamental imaging as compared to harmonics.

5. While performing a transesophageal echocardiogram in the operating room, severe left ventricular dysfunction is present and there is a concern for a possible ventricular thrombus at the apex. Which method could help distinguish a true thrombus versus an artifact?

   **A.** Increase the mechanical index
   **B.** Use and optimize a single view
   **C.** Increase the transducer frequency
   **D.** Increase the depth

6. A 73-year-old man presents to the emergency room with shortness of breath and hypotension. A point-of-care lung ultrasound is performed, and an image from the left lung is shown in **Figure 14.3**.

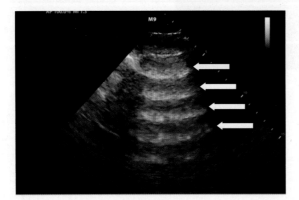

**Figure 14.3**

What do the lines marked by the white arrows indicate?
A. Comet tail artifacts
B. B-lines
C. Reverberation artifacts
D. Bar code sign

7. Which of the following is a true statement about range ambiguity?

A. The pulse repetition frequency (PRF) is not affected by the imaging depth.
B. To help avoid range ambiguity, the PRF is increased when scanning deeper structures.
C. Range ambiguity occurs when the first pulse echoes of deep structures return to the transducer after the second pulse has been emitted.
D. Range ambiguity can result in structures in the image being placed farther from the transducer than their actual location.

8. A reflector is at a depth of 5 cm from the transducer. The resultant image displays it at a depth of 4 cm. What does this most likely mean?

A. Reverberation artifact
B. The speed of sound is lower than 1540 m/s
C. Mirror image artifact
D. The speed of sound is greater than 1540 m/s

9. Which of these interventions would result in worsened "stitching" artifacts during 3D-image acquisition?

A. Pausing respirations in an intubated patient
B. Timing electrocautery with electrocardiogram heart beats
C. Minimizing ultrasound probe movement
D. Performing an electrical cardioversion in a patient with atrial fibrillation to obtain sinus rhythm prior to image acquisition

10. A 60-year-old female is undergoing mitral valve surgery. An intraoperative transesophageal echocardiogram is being performed, and after aortic cannulation, **Figure 14.4** is obtained.

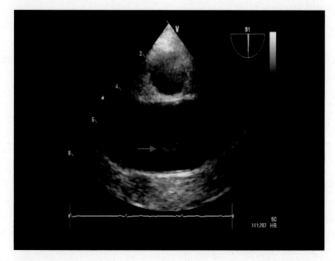

**Figure 14.4**

What type of artifact is occurring depicted by the red arrow?
A. Reverberation artifact
B. Refraction artifact
C. Side-lobe artifact
D. There is no artifact, and an aortic dissection is present

11. An 82-year-old male has a history of aortic stenosis and is now status post aortic valve replacement with new concern of significant aortic regurgitation. When trying to assess the aortic valve in the mid-esophageal long axis of the aortic valve view at 125°, there is significant dropout/shadowing of the regurgitant jet. Which of these methods could be used to improve the assessment of the valve?

   A. Advance the probe and evaluate the valve in a deep transgastric view
   B. Turn down the Nyquist limit of the color Doppler
   C. Turn up the Nyquist limit of the color Doppler
   D. Turn down the overall gain

12. A 45-year-old female patient is admitted to the intensive care unit (ICU) with urosepsis following cystoscopy and stent placement. A right internal jugular central venous line is placed for increasing vasopressor requirement. A transthoracic echocardiography is performed at the bedside. **Figure 14.5** is obtained from the parasternal long axis.

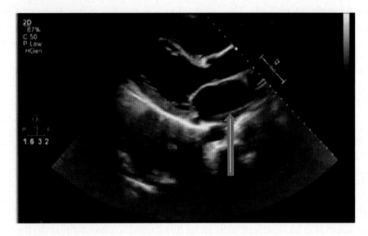

**Figure 14.5**

The arrow in Figure 14.5 is most likely pointing at:
A. Type A aortic dissection
B. Side-lobe artifact
C. Misplaced central line into the carotid artery
D. Reverberation artifact

13. When an ultrasound beam is scanned over a small, point-like reflector, the resultant B-scan image of the reflector is a line. This statement describes what kind of an artifact?

   A. Beam width artifact
   B. Mirror image artifact
   C. Enhancement
   D. Comet-tail artifact

# Chapter 14 ■ Answers

**1.** Correct Answer: **D.** With this artifact, an image will appear in the wrong location but at an appropriate distance within the main (central) ultrasound beam.

*Rationale*: Ultrasound beams leave the transducer and travel in straight lines with most energy concentrated along the main (central) beam. Some energy is also directed adjacent to the central beam, which can also create echoes that the machine could assume originate along the main (central) beam axis. This can make an image appear in the wrong lateral location, but with an appropriate distance from the transducer (side-lobe artifact). In **Figure 14.6A**, a highly reflective structure (solid black ellipse) is interacting with a side-lobe beam (red beam) that is adjacent to the primary beam (yellow), causing a false image artifact (dotted grey ellipse) being depicted in the primary central beam image. An example of a side-lobe artifact (white arrow) can be seen in the ultrasound image (**Figure 14.6B**), where a highly reflective structure (likely the wall of the structure) is causing an artifact to be seen in the lumen of this structure.

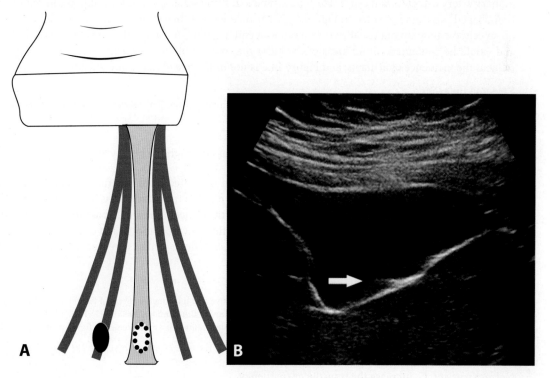

**Figure 14.6**

## Selected References

1. Baad M, Feng Lu Z, Reiser I, Paushter D. Clinical significance of US artifacts. *Radiographics*. 2017;37:1408-1423. doi:10.1148/rg.2017160175
2. Perrino AC, Reeves ST. Chapter 20: Common artifacts and pitfalls of clinical echocardiography. In: Perrino AC Jr, Reeves ST, eds. *A Practical Approach to Transesophageal Echocardiography*. 2nd ed. Lippincott, Williams & Wilkins; 2008:417-434.
3. Quien MM, Saric M. Ultrasound imaging artifacts: how to recognize them and how to avoid them. *Echocardiography*. 2018;35(9):1388-1401.
4. Rubin DN, Yazbek N, Garcia MJ, Stewart WJ, Thomas JD. Qualitative and quantitative effects of harmonic echocardiography imaging on endocardium edge definition and side-lobe artifacts. *J Am Soc Echocardiogr*. 2000;13(11):1012-1018.

**2.** Correct Answer: A. Shadowing

*Rationale:* The dark areas are caused by rib shadowing, as the sound is reflected back to the ultrasound transducer. The lung point occurs at the site of pneumothorax, and it is the point of transition pleural sliding to no sliding in B-mode or from seashore sign to barcode sign in M-mode. Reverberations off the pleural line appear as A-lines, which are horizontal and double the distance of the pleural from the transducer. Pulmonary edema will appear as B-lines, which is not the case in Figure 14.1.

### Selected References
1. Bertrand PB, Levine RA, Isselbacher EM, Vandervoort PM. Fact or artifact in two-dimensional echocardiography: avoiding misdiagnosis and missed diagnosis. *J Am Soc Echocardiogr*. 2016;29(5):381-391.
2. Zagzebski JA. *Essentials of Ultrasound Physics*. 1st ed. Elsevier; 1996.

**3.** Correct Answer: D. Electrocautery artifact

*Rationale:* Artifacts due to electrocautery are very common in the operating room. The artifact produced typically has a geometrically fan-shaped interference pattern, not resembling an anatomic structure. Pulmonary artery catheters can cause side-lobe artifacts in some situations but typically would not have the "fan-shaped" appearance noted in Figure 14.2. Air bubbles post bypass often appear as bright "bubbles" on an echocardiogram but usually are in a random pattern, often display collections in specific locations, and would be contained within areas of the heart that receive blood flow. Harmonic imaging typically reduces the incidence of artifacts, and Figure 14.2 is not indicative of harmonic imaging.

### Selected Reference
1. Quien MM, Saric M. Ultrasound imaging artifacts: how to recognize them and how to avoid them. *Echocardiography*. 2018 Sep;35(9):1388-1401.

**4.** Correct Answer: B. In general, tissue harmonic signals pass through the body wall once.

*Rationale:* In fundamental imaging, the ultrasound beam is emitted from the transducer and first passes through the body wall and a second time during its return to the transducer. Tissue harmonic signals are generated in the body tissue and only travel back to the transducer. The single pass through body tissue by harmonic signals leads to decreased scattering, distortion, reverberations, and other artifacts (including side lobes), although artifacts can still occur at times. Side-lobe artifacts are weaker pulses that rarely produce any harmonics.

### Selected References
1. Rubin DN, Yazbek N, Garcia MJ, Stewart WJ, Thomas JD. Qualitative and quantitative effects of harmonic echocardiography imaging on endocardium edge definition and side-lobe artifacts. *J Am Soc Echocardiogr*. 2000;13(11):1012-1018.
2. Turner SP, Monaghan MJ. Tissue harmonic imaging for standard left ventricular measurements: fundamentally flawed? *Eur J Echocardiogr*. 2006;7(1):9-15.

**5.** Correct Answer: C. Increase the transducer frequency

*Rationale:* Typically, a ventricular thrombus develops in areas of severe wall motion abnormality and may have definable borders. To facilitate diagnosis, they can be further characterized by decreasing the depth, increasing the transducer frequency, and using multiple views (image planes). Contrast agents can also help distinguish thrombus from artifact, but the mechanical index should be decreased in this situation to minimize bubble destruction.

### Selected References
1. Rubin DN, Yazbek N, Garcia MJ, Stewart WJ, Thomas JD. Qualitative and quantitative effects of harmonic echocardiography imaging on endocardium edge definition and side-lobe artifacts. *J Am Soc Echocardiogr*. 2000;13(11):1012-1018.
2. Whalley GA, Gamble GD, Walsh HJ, Sharpe N, Doughty RN. Quantitative evaluation of regional endocardial visualisation with second harmonic imaging and contrast left ventricular opacification in heart failure patients. *Eur J Echocardiogr*. 2005;6(2):134-143.

**6.** Correct Answer: C. Reverberation artifacts

*Rationale:* The lines shown in Figure 14.3 are A-lines, which is a normal finding. A-lines are reverberation artifacts from the pleural line. Reverberation artifacts occur when the echo returning to the transducer is of significant magnitude. It is partially reflected at the transducer surface and redirected toward the interface. The second reflection (reverberation) is interpreted by the transducer as a second interface. Additional reverberations correspond to additional round trips of the sound use between the transducer and the interface. The first echo and the reverberating echoes are all equidistant.

B-lines are longitudinal comet-tail artifacts originating from the pleura. B-lines can indicate interstitial edema. Barcode (stratosphere) sign is present in pneumothorax when the lung is imaged in M-mode.

Selected References
1. Feldman MK, Katyal S, Blackwood MS. US artifacts. *Radiographics.* 2009;29:1179-1189.
2. Scanlan KA. Sonographic artifacts and their origins. *AJR Am J Roentgenol.* 1991;156(6):1267-1272.

**7.** Correct Answer: C. Range ambiguity occurs when first pulse echoes of deep structures return to the transducer after the second pulse has been emitted

*Rationale:* The PRF helps determine the correct imaging of deep structures. As imaging depth increases, the PRF decreases, which helps to limit range ambiguity by allowing the first impulse to return to the transducer before the next impulse is emitted. As an example, if the initial impulse returns from an out-of-image distant structure after the second impulse is emitted, the time delay will be counted from the second impulse (or most recent) and the true object distance will be misregistered. Thus, a range ambiguity artifact in this situation would incorrectly place the distant structure closer to the transducer than its true location in this situation. By increasing the image depth and thus decreasing the PRF appropriately for a particular depth, the "listening time" of the transducer is increased which allows the initial impulse to return to the transducer before sending another impulse too soon.

Selected References
1. Baad M, Lu ZF, Reiser I, Paushter D. Clinical significance of US artifacts. *Radiographics.* 2017;37:1408-1423. doi:10.1148/rg.2017160175
2. Naganuma H, Ishida H, Nagai H, Ogawa M, Ohyama Y. Range-ambiguity artifact in abdominal ultrasound. *J Med Ultrason.* 2019;46(3):317-324.
3. Perrino AC, Reeves ST. Chapter 20: Common artifacts and pitfalls of clinical echocardiography. In: *A Practical Approach to Transesophageal Echocardiography.* 417-434.

**8.** Correct Answer: D. The speed of sound is greater than 1540 m/s

*Rationale:* Ultrasound machines and imaging operate on the assumption that sound travels at a constant speed of 1540 m/s in soft tissues. However, the speed of sound varies according to the type of tissue, for example, sound will travel faster in muscles and slower in fat. If the resulting image is displayed at a smaller depth than what it actually is, this means that the sound waves traveled faster in this tissue and took less time to be reflected back to the transducer. Mirror image and reverberation artifacts will both result in an image of the reflector along with one or multiple reproductions of the same object that are deeper than the original reflector.

Selected References
1. Zagzebski JA. *Essentials of Ultrasound Physics.* 1st ed. Elsevier; 1996.
2. Ziskin MC. Fundamentals physics of ultrasound and its propagation in tissue. *Radiographics* 1993;13:705-709.

**9.** Correct Answer: **B. Timing electrocautery with electrocardiogram heart beats**

*Rationale:* Three-dimensional volume-gated images are created when multiple pyramidal slices/sections obtained over the same number of heartbeats are merged. Most stitching artifacts can be attributed to cardiac patient or probe motion during the image acquisition, so anything that reduces this motion also reduces stitching artifacts. Electrocautery can cause interference and artifacts during image capture. Additionally, irregular heartbeats, like atrial fibrillation, can make the timing of multiple-beat 3D images more challenging to capture appropriately, which can then also cause a stitching artifact when the full image is rendered.

**Selected References**

1. Le HT, Hangiandreou N, Timmerman R, et al. Imaging artifacts in echocardiography. *Anesth Analg.* 2016;122(3):633-646.
2. Faletra FF, Ramamurthi A, Dequarti MC, Leo LA, Moccetti T, Pandian N. Artifacts in three-dimensional transesophageal echocardiography. *J Am Soc Echocardiogr.* 2014;27(5):453-462.

**10.** Correct Answer: **A. Reverberation artifact**

*Rationale:* A reverberation artifact violates the assumption that a pulsed wave returns to the transducer after one reflection. However, sometimes the reflected ultrasound wave can interact with a closer reflector on its way back to the transducer. One portion of the wave makes it back to the transducer as expected/assumed, while the other portion of the wave is reflected back to the original structure. Thus, when that second portion makes its way back to the transducer an artifact (reverberation) image is created that is often twice the distance of the original object and is less "bright" in the final image. Refraction artifacts involve the bending of the ultrasound wave at a structure where the speed of the wave changes depending on the material of the structure, causing an artifact usually to the side of the true image. Side-lobe artifacts occur where side lobes reflect sound from a strong reflector that is outside of the central beam and where the echoes are displayed as if they originated from within the central beam. Figure 14.4 is an artifact, and no continuous dissection flap is appreciated, which could be further confirmed using additional views from alternative imaging planes where the artifact would likely disappear and no flap would be seen.

**Selected References**

1. Lanigan MJ, Chaney MA, Gologorsky E, Chavanon O, Augoustides JG. Case 2–2014: aortic dissection: real or artifact? *J Cardiothorac Vasc Anesth.* 2014;28:398-407.
2. Maltagliati A, Pepi M, Tamborini G, et al. Usefulness of multiplane transesophageal echocardiography in the recognition of artifacts and normal anatomical variants that may mimic left atrial thrombi in patients with atrial fibrillation. *Ital Heart J.* 2003;4:797-802.
3. Pamnani A, Skubas NJ. Imaging artifacts during transesophageal echocardiography. *Anesth Analg.* 2014;118:516-520.

**11.** Correct Answer: **A. Advance the probe and evaluate the valve in a deep transgastric view**

*Rationale:* In a mid-esophageal long axis of the aortic valve view, the highly reflective prosthetic valve induces a "shadowing" artifact to structures in the image plane deep to the valve. This can be overcome by trying other views where the regurgitant jet of interest is closer to the transducer than the highly reflective object, so any shadowing caused by the object does not disrupt the assessment. Adjusting the Nyquist limit can make a regurgitant jet appear more or less severe than it truly is by turning it down and up, respectively; however, this has no effect on shadowing. Adjusting the overall gain brightens and darkens the overall image; however, it will not have a significant impact on the shadowing artifact which is the true cause of the limited regurgitant jet evaluation in the above scenario.

**Selected References**

1. Perrino AC, Reeves ST. Chapter 20: Common artifacts and pitfalls of clinical echocardiography. In: Perrino AC Jr, Reeves ST, eds. *A Practical Approach to Transesophageal Echocardiography.* 2nd ed. Lippincott, Williams & Wilkins; 2008:417-434.
2. Quien MM, Saric M. Ultrasound imaging artifacts: how to recognize them and how to avoid them. *Echocardiography.* 2018;35(9):1388-1401.

**12.** Correct Answer: B. Side-lobe artifact

*Rationale:* Side-lobe artifacts occur when a highly reflective structure is present in the side lobe of the ultrasound beam that is falsely displayed in the center. The white line in **Figure 14.7** (marked by the *arrow*) is a side-lobe artifact, most likely of the pericardium, which is a very bright structure. In order to confirm, other views (especially a parasternal short axis) should be obtained.

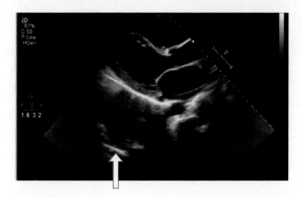

**Figure 14.7**

It is not a Type A aortic dissection, as the left ventricular outlet (LVOT) and ascending aorta in Figure 14.7 appear free in this image. The carotid artery is not visualized in the image in Figure 14.5. Reverberation artifacts appear parallel and equidistant to other bright reflectors. A reverberation artifact of the pericardium is marked by the blue arrow in the image. This is parallel to the pericardium and located at double the distance from the transducer.

Selected References
1. Hedrick W, Hykes D, Starchmen D. *Ultrasound Physics and Instrumentation.* 3rd ed. Mosby; 1995.
2. Zagzebski JA. *Essentials of Ultrasound Physics.* 1st ed. Elsevier; 1996.

**13.** Correct Answer: A. Beam width artifact

*Rationale:* The ultrasound beam changes its width as it leaves the transducer (**Figure 14.8**). The beam gets narrowest at a focal point and then widens again beyond the width of the transducer. Point-like structures, such as calcifications, located in the distal (wide) beam are broadened, appearing as small lines. The length of the line depends on the width of the beam at the location of the imaged structure.

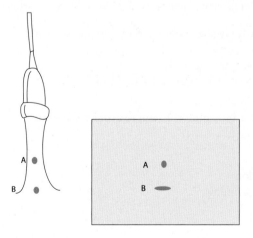

**Figure 14.8**

Selected References
1. Feldman MK, Katyal S, Blackwood MS. US artifacts. *Radiographics.* 2009;29:1179-1189.
2. Quien MM, Saric M. Ultrasound imaging artifacts: how to recognize them and how to avoid them. *Echocardiography.* 2018;35(9):1388-1401.

# 15 | TYPES OF ARTIFACTS

Philippe B. Bertrand, Samuel Bernard, and David M. Dudzinski

1. Which of the following assumptions about ultrasound wave propagation is made when processing the returning ultrasound waves?

   A. Ultrasound propagates in a straight line in the direction of the central ultrasound beam.
   B. The distance of a structure along the scan line is inversely proportional to the travel time of the transmitted wave.
   C. The amplitude of returning ultrasound waves is not affected by tissue characteristics of the reflecting objects.
   D. Structures located outside of the intended path of the beam can generate reflections to the transducer.

2. What statement about reflection and refraction of ultrasound waves is correct?

   A. Ultrasound waves in biologic tissue do not obey Snell's law.
   B. Refraction is determined by differences in acoustic impedance between two tissues.
   C. Reflected waves propagate at lower speed than the incoming (emitted) ultrasound waves.
   D. Along the intended path of the beam, a structure can only reflect the beam once.

3. Which of the following statements regarding reverberation artifacts is correct? Reverberation artifacts:

   A. are typically located at half the distance from the transducer compared to the true structure.
   B. move in opposite direction relative to the true structure.
   C. increase in intensity with increasing distance from the transducer.
   D. are due to the assumption that a given structure will reflect the ultrasound beam only once.

4. Which of the following changes to the ultrasound machine is most useful to avoid reverberation artifacts?

   A. Adjusting the focal zone
   B. Increasing the gain and/or time gain compensation
   C. Moving the transducer to an alternative imaging window
   D. Decreasing the color Doppler gain settings

5. Which of the following favors the finding of an artifact rather than a true structure?

   A. Accelerated or disturbed color Doppler flow
   B. Visualization in multiple imaging views
   C. Lacking well-demarcated borders
   D. Attachments to nearby structures

6. Which of the following statements regarding side lobe artifacts is correct?

   Side lobe artifacts relate to:
   A. the transducer emitting ultrasound energy outside of the central ultrasound beam.
   B. the lateral beam resolution being lower away from the focal zone.
   C. differences in acoustic impedance between two media.
   D. the elevation width of the ultrasound beam.

7. A refraction type artifact will cause a duplicate image of a structure:

   A. at half the distance to the probe than the true structure.
   B. at double the distance from the probe than the true structure.
   C. at a similar distance from the probe than the true structure.
   D. at a distance from the probe equal to the distance between true structure and a wave refractor.

8. A previously healthy person is admitted to the intensive care unit after a motor vehicle accident. A transthoracic echocardiography is performed. The parasternal long-axis image is shown in **Figure 15.1** and ▶ **Video 15.1.** Which of the following statements is correct?

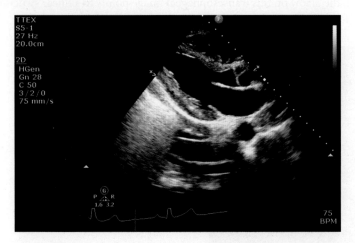

**Figure 15.1**

   A. There are no cardiac abnormalities noted in this image.
   B. There is a loculated left pleural effusion.
   C. There is both pleural and pericardial effusion.
   D. There is evidence of a type B aortic dissection.

9. M-mode echocardiography is most useful in the recognition of which type of artifact?

   A. Reverberation artifact
   B. Side lobe artifact
   C. Refraction artifact
   D. Beam width artifact

**10.** In **Figure 15.2**, the arrow points to a linear structure that corresponds to which of the following?

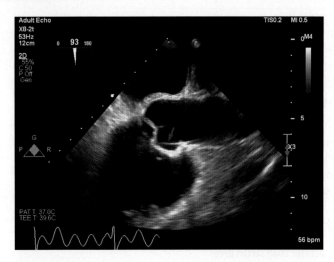

**Figure 15.2**

**A.** Type A aortic dissection
**B.** Side lobe artifact
**C.** Refraction artifact
**D.** Reverberation artifact

**11.** In **Figure 15.3** and ▶ **Video 15.2**, the arrow on this transesophageal image points to a linear structure that corresponds to which of the following?

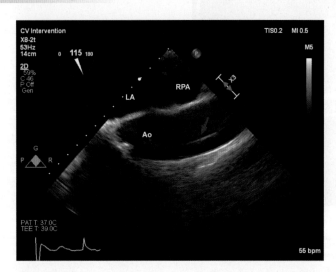

**Figure 15.3** Transesophageal echocardiography image of the ascending aorta (Ao). Notice the right pulmonary artery (RPA) and the left atrium (LA). The arrow points to a linear echodensity in the ascending aorta.

**A.** Type A aortic dissection
**B.** Side lobe artifact
**C.** Refraction artifact
**D.** Reverberation artifact

12. In **Figure 15.4** and ▶ **Video 15.3**, the structure in the left atrium is compatible with:

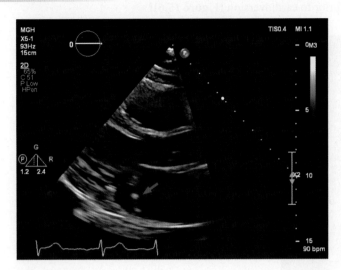

**Figure 15.4**

A. Cor triatriatum
B. Refraction artifact
C. Mirror artifact
D. Reverberation artifact

13. In a patient with recent anterior myocardial infarction, **Figure 15.5 and** ▶ **Video 15.4** show the transthoracic apical two-chamber view of the left ventricle. Which of the following approaches is most appropriate?

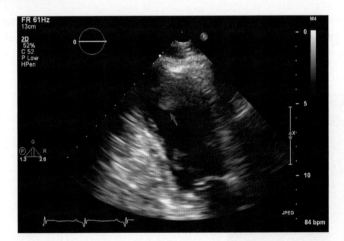

**Figure 15.5**

A. Decrease the transducer frequency
B. Administer ultrasound enhancing agents (UEA, or echo contrast)
C. Increase the ultrasound gain
D. This is near-field clutter, no further approach is needed

**14.** Which type of artifact is the most common mimic of left atrial (LA) appendage clot during transesophageal echocardiography prior to cardioversion (**Figure 15.6**)?

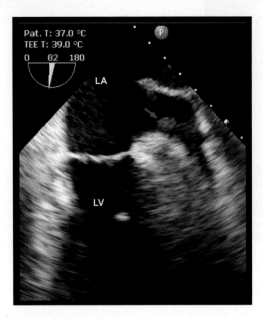

**Figure 15.6**

**A.** Reverberation artifact
**B.** Side lobe artifact
**C.** Mirror artifact
**D.** Refraction artifact

**15.** A patient with a mechanical mitral valve prosthesis is admitted to the intensive care unit with shortness of breath and a systolic murmur. **Figure 15.7** shows the apical four-chamber view in midsystole. (See also ▶ **Video 15.5.**) The color Doppler jet in the left atrium is most compatible with which of the following?

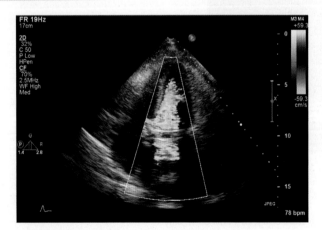

**Figure 15.7**

**A.** Paravalvular mitral regurgitation (MR)
**B.** Valvular MR
**C.** Mirroring of left ventricular outflow tract (LVOT) flow
**D.** Washing jets of the mechanical prosthesis, which is a normal observation

**16.** How would you best describe the findings (**Figure 15.8**, *arrow*) in the left atrium of an asymptomatic patient with a mechanical mitral valve prosthesis?

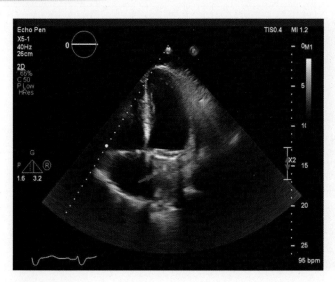

**Figure 15.8**

A. Shadowing
B. Shielding
C. Refraction
D. Attenuation

**17.** A nonmobile structure is intermittently seen in the right atrium without clear attachments (**Figure 15.9**, *arrow*). Given the location, nonmobility, and aspect, this structure most likely represents which of the following?

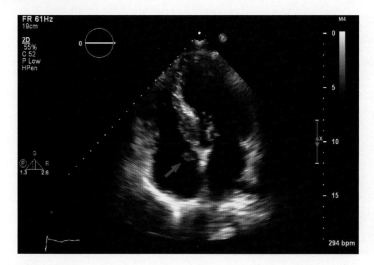

**Figure 15.9**

A. A thrombus
B. A myxoma
C. A prominent/calcified aortic root
D. A reverberation artifact

**18.** Which of the following statements is most accurate regarding the structure in the right atrium (transthoracic parasternal right ventricular inflow view) in **Figure 15.10?**

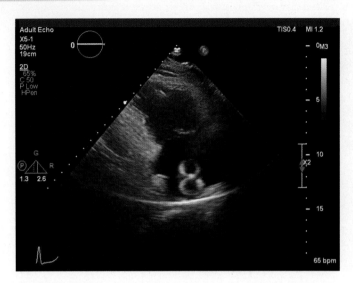

**Figure 15.10**

**A.** There is a central line wire retained in the right atrium.
**B.** There is a percutaneous septal disc occluder in the interatrial septum.
**C.** This is the expected position and appearance of the dual-lumen venovenous (VV) extracorporeal membrane oxygenation (ECMO) cannula.
**D.** The patient has a history of percutaneous tricuspid valve repair.

**19.** During lung ultrasound examination **(Figure 15.11)** a number of artifacts are noted in the scanning field. The presence of this type of artifact:

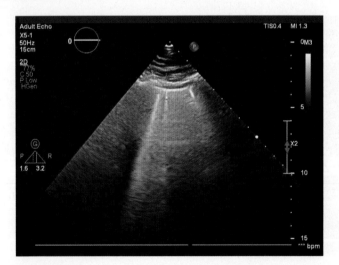

**Figure 15.11**

**A.** renders the examination inconclusive due to shadowing
**B.** can be a diagnostic sign of pneumothorax
**C.** can be a diagnostic sign of lung congestion
**D.** is usually seen in hypovolemia

20. **Figure 15.12** and ▶ **Video 15.6** show the parasternal long-axis image of a patient with an aortic valve bioprosthesis. Name three artifacts (arrows) related to the bioprosthesis that are noted.

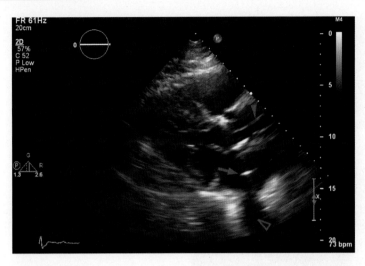

**Figure 15.12**

   **A.** Reverberation—Shadowing—Mirroring
   **B.** Reverberation—Mirroring—Aliasing
   **C.** Reverberation—Refraction—Side Lobe
   **D.** Reverberation—Side Lobe—Shadowing

21. **Figure 15.13** and ▶ **Video 15.7** show a subcostal color Doppler image of the abdominal aorta in an asymptomatic patient. Which mechanism relates to the color Doppler signal that is seen outside of the abdominal aorta?

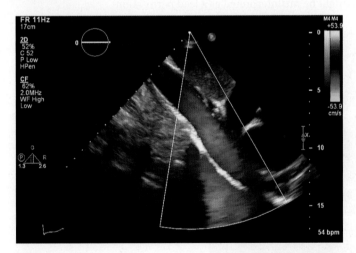

**Figure 15.13**

   **A.** Reflection
   **B.** Refraction
   **C.** Aliasing
   **D.** Presence of ascites

22. Which statement is correct regarding the mean transmitral gradient in a patient with calcific mitral valve disease (**Figure 15.14**)? The mean transmitral gradient is:

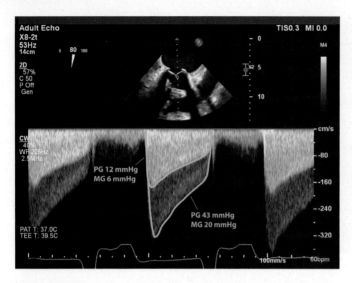

**Figure 15.14**

A. 6 mm Hg
B. 20 mm Hg
C. 13 mm Hg
D. 7.5 mm Hg

23. A patient presents to the emergency department with nonspecific chest pain after a pacemaker implantation. Which type of artifact related to the pacemaker wire is visible in the parasternal short-axis image (**Figure 15.15**, arrow) and might be misinterpreted as a lead perforation?

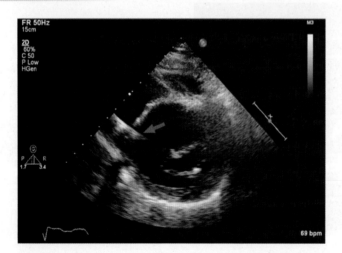

**Figure 15.15**

A. Reverberation
B. Shielding
C. Refraction
D. Side lobe

24. A patient with class IV, stage D heart failure with a reduced ejection fraction (HFrEF) presents to the emergency room with progressive shortness of breath. **Figure 15.16** and ▶ **Video 15.8** show the transthoracic apical four-chamber view of the left ventricle. The color Doppler finding is indicative of which of the following?

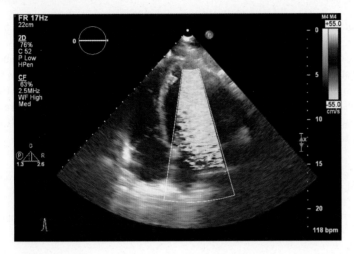

**Figure 15.16**

   **A.** Severe MR
   **B.** Severe aortic insufficiency
   **C.** Artifact related to an implantable cardioverter defibrillator
   **D.** Artifact related to a mechanical assist device

25. A patient in the intensive care unit develops chest pain on day 1 post–major abdominal surgery. A transthoracic echocardiography is performed. The inferolateral myocardial motion in the parasternal short-axis images (**Figure 15.17** and ▶ **Video 15.9**) is most consistent with which of the following?

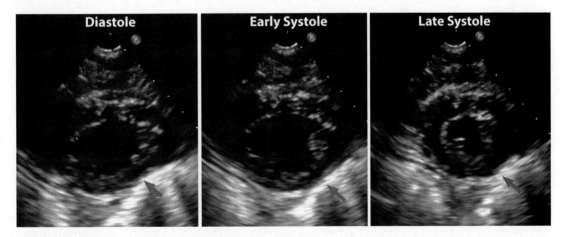

**Figure 15.17**

   **A.** Acute inferolateral wall ischemia
   **B.** Chronic inferolateral wall ischemia with viability
   **C.** Normal inferolateral wall motion
   **D.** Inferolateral wall aneurysm

# Chapter 15 ■ Answers

**1.** Correct Answer: A. Ultrasound propagates in a straight line in the direction of the central ultrasound beam.

*Rationale:* As the transducer emits an ultrasound wave and awaits the returning ultrasound wave to reconstruct an image, certain assumptions are being made with respect to wave propagation: (a) ultrasound propagates in a straight line in the direction of the central beam; (b) a given structure will reflect the beam only once; (c) only structures located within the intended path of the beam will generate reflections back to the transducer; (d) the position of a structure along the scan line is directly proportional to the travel time of the transmitted wave. These assumptions, however, are not always correct, and when they are not, typical ultrasound artifacts may appear. All clinicians who use ultrasonography must be fluent in ultrasound physics and artifacts so as to generate correct image interpretations.

Selected References
1. Bertrand PB, Levine RA, Isselbacher EM, Vandervoort PM. Fact or artifact in two-dimensional echocardiography: avoiding misdiagnosis and missed diagnosis. *J Am Soc Echocardiogr*. 2016;29:381-391. doi:10.1016/j.echo.2016.01.009
2. Weyman AE. *Principles and Practice of Echocardiography*. Lea & Febiger; 1994.
3. Physics and instrumentation. In: Feigenbaum H, Armstrong WF, Ryan T, eds. *Feigenbaum's Echocardiography*. 6th ed. Lippincott Williams & Wilkins; 2005:11-45.

**2.** Correct Answer: B. Refraction is determined by differences in acoustic impedance between two tissues.

*Rationale:* Ultrasound waves traveling through biologic tissue obey the physical laws of reflection and refraction (Snell's law). The boundary of two tissues with different acoustic impedance can act as a specular (mirror-like) reflector if significantly larger than the wavelength of the ultrasound waves. A portion of ultrasound wave energy is reflected with reflection angle equal to the angle of incidence. Another portion will be transmitted with a refraction angle dependent on the magnitude of difference in acoustic impedance between both tissues (**Figure 15.18**).

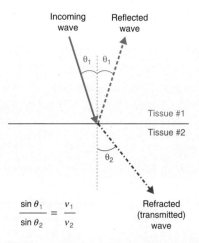

$$\frac{\sin \theta_1}{\sin \theta_2} = \frac{v_1}{v_2}$$

**Figure 15.18** Reflection and refraction of ultrasound waves in biologic tissue. The ultrasound wave propagation velocity (v) in biologic tissues is inversely proportional to the tissue acoustic impedance. The boundary of two tissues with different acoustic impedance can act as a specular (mirror-like) reflector if significantly larger than the wavelength of the ultrasound waves. A portion of ultrasound wave energy will be reflected with reflection angle equal to the angle of incidence. Another portion will be transmitted with a refraction angle dependent on the magnitude of difference in acoustic impedance. The latter is inversely proportional to the wave propagation velocity v.

Selected References
1. Bertrand PB, Levine RA, Isselbacher EM, Vandervoort PM. Fact or artifact in two-dimensional echocardiography: avoiding misdiagnosis and missed diagnosis. *J Am Soc Echocardiogr*. 2016;29:381-391. doi:10.1016/j.echo.2016.01.009.
2. Physics and instrumentation. In: Feigenbaum H, Armstrong WF, Ryan T, eds. *Feigenbaum's Echocardiography*. 6th ed. Lippincott Williams & Wilkins; 2005:11-45.
3. Weyman AE. *Principles and Practice of Echocardiography*. Lea & Febiger; 1994.

**3.** Correct Answer: D. are due to the assumption that a given structure will reflect the ultrasound beam only once.

*Rationale:* A reverberation artifact occurs when a reflected ultrasound wave on its way back to the transducer encounters a reflector in its path that reflects a portion of this returning energy back to the first reflector. A portion of sound energy that was not interrupted by the closer reflector returns to the transducer as expected and the first reflector's structure is mapped accurately. The portion of sound energy that makes a second round trip to the first reflector and back to the transducer will have had a longer travel time. Due to the assumptions of wave propagation (see **Question 15.2**), the transducer interprets this reflected structure as being at a further distance from the transducer and thus maps a structure below the first reflector (at a distance below first reflector equal to the distance between first and second reflector). In clinical practice, the second reflector is often the ultrasound transducer itself—generating an artifact at a distance twice that of the first reflector (**Figure 15.19**). During the cardiac cycle, the motion of the reverberation artifact parallels that of the true structure but with a greater (typically double) amplitude. Multiple reflections between the two reflectors are possible, causing multiple reverberations with gradually diminishing intensity. Indeed, as ultrasound energy decreases with each additional round trip, each reverberation occurs at progressively weaker signal intensity than the true structure (Figure 15.19).

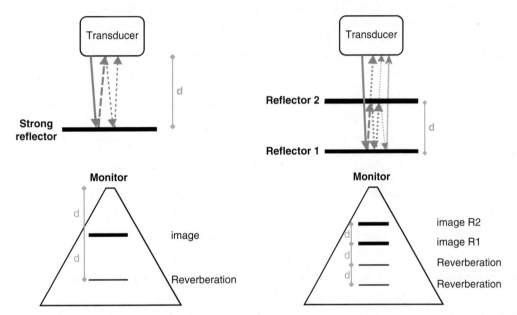

**Figure 15.19** Reverberation artifact. A reverberation artifact occurs when additional reflections occur between a strong reflector and a second reflector. This second reflector can either be the transducer itself (A) leading to a reverberation at twice the distance to the probe, or another strong reflector (B) located closer to the transducer than the first reflector. Reverberations occur at progressively weaker signal intensity than the true structure.

Selected References

1. Bertrand PB, Levine RA, Isselbacher EM, Vandervoort PM. Fact or artifact in two-dimensional echocardiography: avoiding misdiagnosis and missed diagnosis. *J Am Soc Echocardiogr.* 2016;29:381-391. doi:10.1016/j.echo.2016.01.009.
2. Feldman MK, Katyal S, Blackwood MS. US artifacts. *Radiographics.* 2009;29:1179-1189. doi:10.1148/rg.294085199.
3. Kremkau FW, Taylor KJ. Artifacts in ultrasound imaging. *J Ultrasound Med.* 1986;5:227-237. doi:10.7863/jum.1986.5.4.227.

**4.** Correct Answer: C. Moving the transducer to an alternative imaging window

*Rationale:* Decreasing the image gain and using alternative imaging planes to avoid potential reflectors in the near-field are the most common strategies for recognizing and reducing/eliminating reverberation artifacts. Color Doppler (at normal or decreased scale) can be helpful to demonstrate that flow is not affected by the artifactual structure. The basic recognition of reverberation artifacts comes from appreciating structures at a "double distance" (compared to the probe-to-structure difference) exerting parallel motion while not respecting anatomic boundaries.

Selected Reference

1. Bertrand PB, Levine RA, Isselbacher EM, Vandervoort PM. Fact or artifact in two-dimensional echocardiography: avoiding misdiagnosis and missed diagnosis. *J Am Soc Echocardiogr.* 2016;29:381-391. doi:10.1016/j.echo.2016.01.009

**5.** Correct Answer: C. Lacking well-demarcated borders

*Rationale:* One central principle to recall for all forms of artifact is that true structures cannot pass through cardiac or vascular walls and are typically well defined, unlike the indistinct borders of artifacts. True structures are seen in multiple imaging views, whereas artifacts typically cannot be reproduced from alternative probe positions (e.g., a reverberation artifact mimicking a thrombus in the left atrium in parasternal imaging windows cannot be reproduced in apical imaging windows). In addition, unlike true anatomic structures, artifacts will not accelerate or disturb surrounding color Doppler flow in any way. **Table 15.1** summarizes the typical differences between true structures and artifacts, which can aid in the investigation of uncommon echocardiographic findings and offer clues toward a correct interpretation.

**Table 15.1 Clues to the Presence of an Ultrasound Artifact Rather than a True Structure**

|  | **Favors True Structure** | **Favors Artifact** |
|---|---|---|
| **Morphology** | • Distinct edges (unless thrombus) | • Linear<br>• Lacks well-demarcated borders |
| **Motion** | • Independent motion | • Identical to other real structure (parallel or mirror)<br>• Appears to pass through other solid structures |
| **Attachments** | • Attached to other structures | • No clear attachments |
| **Reproducibility** | • Consistently seen in multiple views | • May not be reproduced in other imaging views |
| **Color Doppler flow** | • Affected by real structure | • Not affected by artifact |
| **Others** | • Logical anatomic relationships | • Logical physical explanation for presence of an artifact in that specific location |

Selected Reference

1. Bertrand PB, Levine RA, Isselbacher EM, Vandervoort PM. Fact or artifact in two-dimensional echocardiography: avoiding misdiagnosis and missed diagnosis. *J Am Soc Echocardiogr.* 2016;29:381-391. doi:10.1016/j.echo.2016.01.009

**6.** Correct Answer: A. the transducer emitting ultrasound energy outside of the central ultrasound beam.

*Rationale:* As the ultrasound transducer aims to focus the emitted ultrasound energy within a central ultrasound beam, small amounts of energy inevitably get emitted in other directions as well. These may form so-called "side lobes" of ultrasound energy that propagate off-axis. These small portions of ultrasound energy emitted in "side lobes" are mostly dissipated in the tissue without relevant reflections. However, when this side lobe energy is reflected by a strong reflector (wires, calcifications, pericardium) in its path, these reflections are interpreted by the transducer as originating from the central beam. As the transducer scans the imaging window by sweeping in a radial direction, numerous side lobe artifacts can be generated on both sides of the true reflector. When the true reflector is echodense and wide, these multiple side lobe images can overlap and visually merge, producing a linear arc-like artifact at a radial distance of the transducer (**Figure 15.20**).

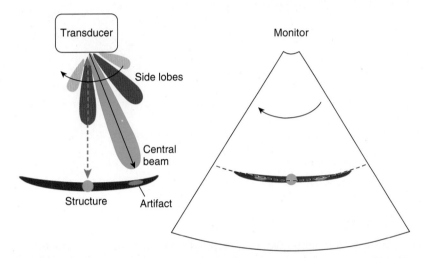

**Figure 15.20** Side lobe artifact. Side lobe energy (red and pink beams) can encounter a strong reflector that is located outside of the central scanning line (blue beam) in which the transducer is actually "looking." Reflections of side lobe energy can only however be interpreted by the machine as if originating from the direction of the scanning line. This results in a linear "arc-like" artifact on both sides of the strong reflector and at a radial distance from the transducer.

### Selected References
1. Feldman MK, Katyal S, Blackwood MS. US artifacts. *Radiographics.* 2009;29:1179-1189. doi:10.1148/rg.294085199
2. Laing FC, Kurtz AB. The importance of ultrasonic side-lobe artifacts. *Radiology.* 1982;145:763-768. doi:10.1148/radiology.145.3.7146410.
3. Lu JY, Zou H, Greenleaf JF. Biomedical ultrasound beam forming. *Ultrasound Med Biol.* 1994;20:403-428. doi:10.1016/0301-5629(94)90097-3.
4. Pamnani A, Skubas NJ. Imaging artifacts during transesophageal echocardiography. *Anesth Analg.* 2014;118:516-520. doi:10.1213/ANE.0000000000000084.

**7.** Correct Answer: C. at a similar distance from the probe than the true structure.

*Rationale:* A refraction artifact, also called a "lens artifact" or "twin artifact," is the false duplication of an object behind a structure that acts as a wave refractor and thus behaves as a lens. Ultrasound waves directed through the "lens" are refracted toward the respective cardiac object and then re-refracted back to the original direction of transmission on the return acoustic path, resulting in a duplicate image of this object along the original direction of the beam, at similar distance from the probe **(Figure 15.21)**. These artifacts mostly occur in subcostal and parasternal imaging planes, with costal cartilage, fascial structures and fat, and pleural and pericardial surfaces acting as the medium inducing refraction of the ultrasound beam. Structures behind an ultrasound lens may not be visible in that plane because the sound beam never reaches them and instead they are "overwritten" by the duplicated image of a nearby structure. Adjusting the probe to avoid the lens or using alternative imaging windows are strategies to avoid the double image and assess the structures that were shadowed.

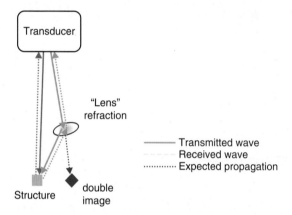

**Figure 15.21** Refraction artifact. Ultrasound waves directed through a "lens" are refracted toward the respective cardiac structure and back, resulting in a duplicate of this object in the initial beam direction at a similar distance from the probe.

### Selected References

1. Buttery B, Davison G. The ghost artifact. *J Ultrasound Med.* 1984;3:49-52. doi:10.7863/jum.1984.3.2.49.
2. Ozeke O, Ozbakir C, Gunel EN. Double mitral valve imaging. *J Am Soc Echocardiogr.* 2010;23:340 e1-e2. doi:10.1016/j.echo.2009.08.017.
3. Spieker LE, Hufschmid U, Oechslin E, Jenni R. Double aortic and pulmonary valves: an artifact generated by ultrasound refraction. *J Am Soc Echocardiogr.* 2004;17:786-787. doi:10.1016/j.echo.2004.04.003.

**8.** Correct Answer: A. There are no cardiac abnormalities noted in this image.

*Rationale:* The echo image shown in Figure 15.1 shows no structural abnormalities. However, there is evidence of a mirror artifact more distal to the posterior pericardium–lung interface **(Figure 15.22)**. A mirror artifact can present below a strong reflective surface that acts much as a mirror, producing a duplicate image behind the mirror of real structures that are located in front (more proximal) of the mirror. In dynamic images, mirrored structures move in the opposite direction from the mirror as do the real structures. The mechanism is similar to that of a reverberation: ultrasound waves hitting a strong reflector are reflected (angle of reflection = angle of incidence) toward objects closer to the transducer than the reflector. These intervening objects reflect the waves back to the strong reflector, which in turn sends them back to the transducer (Figure 15.22). Due to the assumption of wave propagation—that all the returning sound comes from objects in the initial direction of the sound beam—the scanner displays these objects below the strong reflector, at a distance equal to the distance between strong reflector and the true intervening objects. Mirror artifacts can be identified in two-dimensional images as a copy of structures located above a strongly reflective surface.

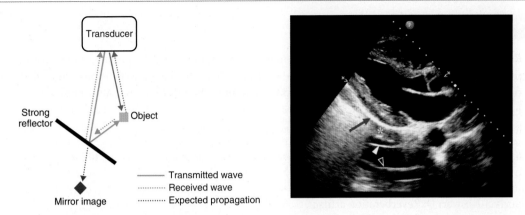

**Figure 15.22** (A) The mechanism underlying mirror artifacts. (B) The parasternal long-axis image of the case presentation shows a mirror artifact below the pericardium–lung interface (red arrow). Notice the mirror image of the posterior myocardial tissue (*), the posterior mitral leaflet (full arrowhead), and the anterior mitral leaflet (empty arrowhead). Comet-tail reverberations below the pericardium due to the strongly reflecting lung interface can be observed as well.

### Selected References

1. Adams MS, Alston TA. Echocardiographic reflections on a pericardium. *Anesth Analg.* 2007;104:506. doi:10.1213/01. ane.0000255056.78259.3c.
2. Bertrand PB, Verhaert D, Vandervoort PM. Mirror artifacts in two-dimensional echocardiography: don't forget objects in the third dimension. *J Am Soc Echocardiogr.* 2015. doi:10.1016/j.echo.2015.07.025.
3. Scanlan KA. Sonographic artifacts and their origins. *AJR Am J Roentgenol.* 1991;156:1267-1272. doi:10.2214/ajr.156.6.2028876.

**9.** Correct Answer: A. Reverberation artifact

*Rationale:* M-mode echocardiography can be particularly useful in determining whether an image finding has independent motion (suggestive of a true structure) versus identical motion that is a copy or mirror of a true structure (suggestive of artifact). This is most relevant in reverberation artifacts, where the artifact and true structures are located on the same scanning line relative to the ultrasound probe. **Figure 15.23** shows an example of a linear structure in the ascending aorta that on M-mode echocardiography shows identical motion compared to the anterior aortic wall and is therefore most likely a reverberation artifact. If the linear structure were a real structure, like a dissection flap, it would be expected to exhibit its own independent motion and not completely mimic the anterior aortic wall. Note also that the long R-R interval in the M-mode tracing reinforces this conclusion because there is again no motion independent of the anterior aortic wall.

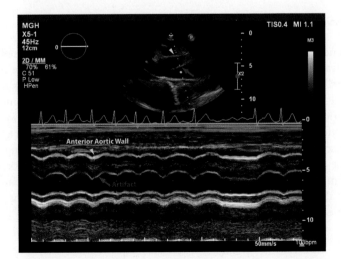

**Figure 15.23** M-mode echocardiography of a linear echo density in the ascending aorta.

**10.** Correct Answer: B. Side lobe artifact

*Rationale:* Figure 15.2 shows a calcified and strongly reflective sinotubular junction, resulting in an arc-like side lobe artifact on both sides of the junction—a finding that can sometimes be misinterpreted as a type A aortic dissection. See also **Answer 15.6** and explanation of the side lobe mechanism in Figure 15.20.

Selected References

1. Laing FC, Kurtz AB. The importance of ultrasonic side-lobe artifacts. *Radiology.* 1982;145:763-768. doi:10.1148/radiology.145.3.7146410.
2. Pamnani A, Skubas NJ. Imaging artifacts during transesophageal echocardiography. *Anesth Analg.* 2014;118:516-520. doi:10.1213/ANE.0000000000000084.

**11.** Correct Answer: D. Reverberation artifact.

*Rationale:* The echodensity in the ascending aorta is linear and lacks well-demarcated borders. Moreover, the motion of this structure (▶ **Video 15.2**) is similar to the posterior aortic wall closer to the probe. As such, this echodensity represents a reverberation artifact, in which ultrasound waves are reflected twice in between the posterior wall of the right pulmonary artery (closest to the echo probe) and the posterior wall of the ascending aorta. See also **Answer 15.3** and explanation of the reverberation mechanisms in Figure 15.19.

M-mode echocardiography could be useful to evaluate the identical motion pattern of the artifact relative to the pulmonary artery and aortic wall. Adequate recognition is essential to avoid misinterpretation of these echo findings as a type A aortic dissection.

Selected Reference

1. Appelbe AF, Walker PG, Yeoh JK, Bonitatibus A, Yoganathan AP, Martin RP. Clinical significance and origin of artifacts in transesophageal echocardiography of the thoracic aorta. *J Am Coll Cardiol.* 1993;21:754-760. doi:10.1016/0735-1097(93)90109-e.

**12.** Correct Answer: B. Refraction artifact

*Rationale:* The visualized structure in the left atrium is a "twin" or duplicate image of the mitral valve at a similar distance to the probe, that is, a refraction artifact. ▶ **Video 15.3** is most helpful to appreciate the duplicate motion of the mitral valve. This artifact occurs due to the presence of a "refractor" in the near field, most commonly rib cartilage. Repositioning the transducer to avoid the refracting tissue is most effective in eliminating the duplicate image.

Selected Reference

1. Ozeke O, Ozbakir C, Gunel EN. Double mitral valve imaging. *J Am Soc Echocardiogr.* 2010;23:340 e1-e2. doi:10.1016/j.echo.2009.08.017.

**13.** Correct Answer: B. Administer ultrasound enhancing agents (UEA, or echo contrast).

*Rationale:* Figure 15.11 shows evidence of "near-field clutter," which is noise in the near field caused by high-amplitude oscillations of the transducer itself. Near-field clutter can cause structures in the near field to be obscured. This is especially relevant for the detection of apical ventricular thrombus as is suspected in this case of a patient with prior anterior myocardial infarction. In contrast to a thrombus, clutter artifact is unaffected by ventricular wall motion and appears to pass through the wall. However, in the presence of clutter, an underlying thrombus cannot be ruled out. When uncertain, one can apply color Doppler and reduce the color scale to demonstrate blood flow through the apex, thus refuting the possible thrombus; alternatively, one can switch to other (parasternal/subcostal) imaging planes or use contrast echocardiography to confirm or refute the presence of an apical thrombus. In this case, contrast echocardiography was performed as the most definitive method, demonstrating an apical thrombus that could have been missed because of near-field clutter (**Figure 15.24**).

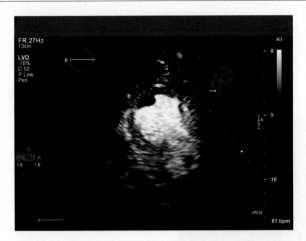

**Figure 15.24** Contrast echocardiography in the same patient demonstrates an apical left ventricular thrombus.

### Selected Reference
1. Garbi M. The general principles of echocardiography. In: Galiuto L, Badano L, Fox K, Sicari R, Zamorano JL, eds. *The EAE Textbook of Echocardiography*. Oxford University Press; 2011:1-13.

---

**14.** Correct Answer: **A. Reverberation artifact**

*Rationale:* The most common artifact mimicking thrombus in the LA appendage is a reverberation artifact due to a double reflection of the warfarin ridge (also known as the ligament of Marshall, a fatty ridge separating the appendage and left superior pulmonary vein). Applying color Doppler or changing the image position is helpful to distinguish this artifact from true structure or thrombus.

### Selected Reference
1. Bertrand PB, Levine RA, Isselbacher EM, Vandervoort PM. Fact or artifact in two-dimensional echocardiography: avoiding misdiagnosis and missed diagnosis. *J Am Soc Echocardiogr*. 2016;29:381-391. doi:10.1016/j.echo.2016.01.009

---

**15.** Correct Answer: **C. Mirroring of left ventricular outflow tract (LVOT) flow.**

*Rationale:* In patients with mechanical mitral valve prostheses, particularly during systole, the prosthesis can act as a mirror deviating ultrasound Doppler waves toward the LVOT and back to the transducer. As such, a mirror image of LVOT flow can occur below the mechanical mitral prosthesis, mimicking MR below the prosthesis (also known as "pseudo-MR"). Clues to pseudo-MR include its pulsed Doppler velocity profile (which is that of LVOT flow) and the absence of a proximal flow convergence region.

### Selected References
1. Linka AZ, Barton M, Attenhofer Jost C, Jenni R. Doppler mirror image artifacts mimicking mitral regurgitation in patients with mechanical bileaflet mitral valve prostheses. *Eur J Echocardiogr*. 2000;1:138-143. doi:10.1053/euje.2000.0024.
2. Rudski LG, Chow CM, Levine RA. Prosthetic mitral regurgitation can be mimicked by Doppler color flow mapping: avoiding misdiagnosis. *J Am Soc Echocardiogr*. 2004;17:829-833. doi:10.1016/j.echo.2004.04.027.

---

**16.** Correct Answer: **B. Shielding**

*Rationale:* There are two phenomena related to mechanical valve prostheses that together almost completely obscure the left atrium in the apical echocardiography windows: "shadowing" and "shielding." Shadowing refers to attenuation of ultrasound due to the prosthesis stent frame, in both biologic and mechanical valves, and presents as a pie-shaped "dropout" below the medial and lateral part of the frame. "Shielding" is more specific for mechanical valve prosthesis and consists of a reverberation-type artifact (similar to "comet tails") below the valve leaflets in systole that similarly obscures all visualization beyond this point. The mechanical prosthesis leaflets thus act as a "shield" for the ultrasound waves. Alternative imaging windows are required to evaluate the left atrium in the presence of a mechanical valve prosthesis and shielding.

**17.** Correct Answer: C. A prominent/calcified aortic root.

*Rationale:* A nonmobile structure in the respective location should raise suspicion of catching part of the aortic root in the imaging plane, which can be evaluated by tilting the transducer out of plane (**Figure 15.25**, arrow).

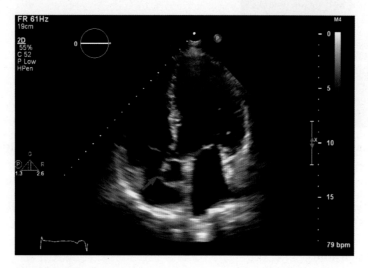

**Figure 15.25**

Remember that the ultrasound beam has a finite width not only in lateral direction but also in the in- and out-of-plane direction. Highly reflective structures that are located in an adjacent imaging plane can sometimes be misinterpreted as structures within the scanning plane (see schematic representation in **Figure 15.26**).

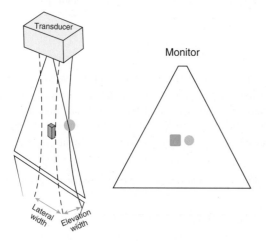

**Figure 15.26** Beam width artifact.

Selected Reference

1. Bertrand PB, Levine RA, Isselbacher EM, Vandervoort PM. Fact or artifact in two-dimensional echocardiography: avoiding misdiagnosis and missed diagnosis. *J Am Soc Echocardiogr.* 2016;29:381-391. doi:10.1016/j.echo.2016.01.009

**18.** Correct Answer: **B. There is a percutaneous septal disc occluder in the interatrial septum.**

*Rationale:* The "figure-of-eight" display in Figure 15.10 is a specific echocardiographic artifact related to interaction of ultrasound waves with the specific morphology of Amplatzer-like percutaneous disc occluders (e.g., the Amplatzer-type LA appendage occluder device, patent foramen ovale (PFO) or atrial septum defect occluders, vascular plugs, and other devices with similar structure). These types of devices have an epitrochoidal mesh configuration, with a characteristic nitinol mesh fiber orientation (**Figure 15.27**). Ultrasound waves interacting with the device are mostly deflected away from the transducer except where the mesh fibers lie orthogonal to the beam direction. Mathematical analysis previously demonstrated that those locations where ultrasound would be reflected back to the probe (horizontal) constitute a "figure-of-eight," explaining the artifact that is frequently seen in apical five-chamber view after LA appendage closure using the Amplatzer Cardiac Plug, but also in off-axis parasternal long-axis views following atrial septal defect (ASD) or PFO closure procedures, as seen in this present example. The reason the figure-of-eight is visualized in the parasternal right ventricular inflow view is because the interatrial septum is just out of plane, and the right atrial aspect of the occluder device is visible when imaging the right ventricle and right atrium.

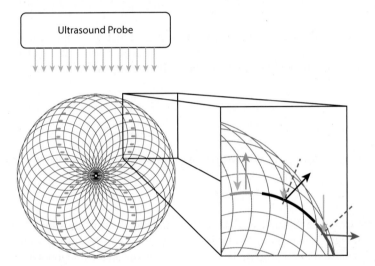

**Figure 15.27** The "figure-of-eight" artifact in the echocardiographic assessment of percutaneous disk occluders.

### Selected References

1. Bertrand PB, Grieten L, De Meester P, et al. Etiology and relevance of the figure-of-eight artifact on echocardiography after percutaneous left atrial appendage closure with the Amplatzer Cardiac Plug. *J Am Soc Echocardiogr.* 2014;27:323-328e1. doi:10.1016/j.echo.2013.11.001.
2. Bertrand PB, Grieten L, Smeets CJ, et al. The figure-of-eight artifact in the echocardiographic assessment of percutaneous disc occluders: impact of imaging depth and device type. *Echocardiography.* 2015;32:557-564. doi:10.1111/echo.12685.
3. de Agustin JA, Rodrigo JL, Marcos-Alberca P, et al. Figure-of-eight artifact after successful percutaneous closure of left atrial appendage. *Int J Cardiol.* 2015;185:101-102. doi:10.1016/j.ijcard.2015.03.100.

**19.** Correct Answer: **C. can be a diagnostic sign of lung congestion.**

*Rationale:* The artifacts seen on this lung ultrasound image are "ring-down" artifacts, also called "B-lines" when presenting in lung ultrasound. A "ring-down" artifact is a series of reverberations below trapp*ed air bubble*s (or similarly, a small amount fluid trapped between air bubbles). Trapped bubbles being struck by ultrasound energy cause an excitation (oscillation) of the bubbles that then results in a persistent series of ultrasound signals emitted back to the transducer. This results in a vertical artifact of closely spaced reverberations that have the appearance of the beam of a flashlight. The finding of B-lines on lung ultrasound is a sign of increased lung water, and therein an artifact can be directly marshaled as a diagnostic sign of pulmonary edema.

Selected Reference

1. Gargani L. Lung ultrasound: a new tool for the cardiologist. *Cardiovasc Ultrasound.* 2011;9:6. doi:10.1186/1476-7120-9-6.

### 20. Correct Answer: D. Reverberation—Side Lobe—Shadowing

*Rationale:* The three most prominent artifacts related to the presence of a biologic aortic valve prosthesis are: (a) a reverberation artifact in the left atrium (*arrow*), related to a double reflection of ultrasound energy in between the stent prostheses; (b) a side lobe artifact in the ascending aorta (*full arrowhead*), due to side lobe energy interacting with one of the bioprosthesis struts, even if the struts are not exactly in plane in this view; and (c) shadowing in the left atrium due to the bioprosthetic stent frame (*hollow arrowhead*).

Selected Reference

1. Bertrand PB, Levine RA, Isselbacher EM, Vandervoort PM. Fact or artifact in two-dimensional echocardiography: avoiding misdiagnosis and missed diagnosis. *J Am Soc Echocardiogr.* 2016;29:381-391. doi:10.1016/j.echo.2016.01.009

### 21. Correct Answer: A. Reflection

*Rationale:* The color Doppler flow outside of the aorta results from a mirror artifact of abdominal aortic flow, likely due to strong reflection at the level of the posterior thoracoabdominal aortic wall (adjacent to lung tissue) acting as a mirror. The mechanism of a mirror artifact is due to **reflection**.

Selected References

1. Adams MS, Alston TA. Echocardiographic reflections on a pericardium. *Anesth Analg.* 2007;104:506. doi:10.1213/01.ane.0000255056.78259.3c.
2. Bertrand PB, Verhaert D, Vandervoort PM. Mirror artifacts in two-dimensional echocardiography: don't forget objects in the third dimension. *J Am Soc Echocardiogr.* 2015. doi:10.1016/j.echo.2015.07.025.
3. Scanlan KA. Sonographic artifacts and their origins. *AJR Am J Roentgenol.* 1991;156:1267-1272. doi:10.2214/ajr.156.6.2028876.

### 22. Correct Answer: A. 6 mm Hg

*Rationale:* The spectral Doppler artifact in this image is a typical example of spectral "ghosting." It is seen with high-gain settings and large signals, which overload system electronics. This results in a signal with double the velocity of the true signal and lower amplitude. It can also be associated with Doppler spectral mirroring. The true signal is the denser signal with the lower velocity. This type of artifact is a common cause of valve gradient misinterpretation and misdiagnosis of valve obstruction. Lowering the Doppler gain is most effective to avoid a spectral ghosting artifact.

Selected Reference

1. Ranjan R, Pressman GS. *Doppler Never Lies. Or Does It?* American College of Cardiology Media File; 2018.

### 23. Correct Answer: D. Side lobe.

*Rationale:* An arc-like artifact at similar distance to the probe is noted on both sides of the pacemaker wire in the right ventricle, hence this is a side lobe artifact. See also **Answer 15.6**, and explanation of the side lobe mechanism in Figure 15.20.

Selected References

1. Laing FC, Kurtz AB. The importance of ultrasonic side-lobe artifacts. *Radiology.* 1982;145:763-768. doi:10.1148/radiology.145.3.7146410.
2. Pamnani A, Skubas NJ. Imaging artifacts during transesophageal echocardiography. *Anesth Analg.* 2014;118:516-520. doi:10.1213/ANE.0000000000000084.

**24.** Correct Answer: D. Artifact related to a mechanical assist device.

*Rationale:* Figure 15.16 depicts a "waterfall" artifact related to the HeartWare (or HVAD) left ventricular assist device. This results from the materials used to construct the device, which causes a large amplitude and long duration of reverberation after insonation. Subsequent pulse interrogations are contaminated, creating a continuous band of color across the designated color box, emanating from the inflow cannula of the ventricular assist device. There is also typically a mosaic color appearance due to the chaotic nature of reverberation and subtle changes in impeller positioning during imaging. This artifact has important implications as it can preclude accurate assessment of the degree of MR or improperly be mistaken for other abnormal lesions. Off-axis views that do not include the inflow cannula can allow for valvular assessment while alleviating this artifact. Of note, the "waterfall" effect is not seen with the HeartMate 2 or HeartMate 3 devices.

### Selected References

1. Lesicka A, Feinman JW, Thiele K, Andrawes MN. Echocardiographic artifact induced by HeartWare left ventricular assist device. *Anesth Analg.* 2015;120:1208-11. doi:10.1213/ANE.0000000000000664
2. Shah NR, Cevik C, Hernandez A, Gregoric ID, Frazier OH, Stainback RF. Transthoracic echocardiography of the HeartWare left ventricular assist device. *J Card Fail.* 2012;18:745-748. doi:10.1016/j.cardfail.2012.06.529.

**25.** Correct Answer: C. Normal inferolateral wall motion

*Rationale:* This case represents apparently abnormal myocardial motion, in which external compression (e.g., related to increased intra-abdominal pressure) causes characteristic diastolic flattening, while the normal systolic contraction causes outward epicardial motion. This motion pattern is consistent with pseudodyskinesis and should not be misinterpreted as a sign of myocardial ischemia.

### Selected Reference

1. Yosefy C, Levine RA, Picard MH, Vaturi M, Handschumacher MD, Isselbacher EM. Pseudodyskinesis of the inferior left ventricular wall: recognizing an echocardiographic mimic of myocardial infarction. *J Am Soc Echocardiogr.* 2007;20:1374-1379. doi:10.1016/j.echo.2007.05.003.

# 16 | ULTRASOUND ARTIFACTS VERSUS PATHOLOGICAL AND NORMAL ANATOMICAL VARIANTS

Sharon L. McCartney and Jeffrey T. Lyvers

1. The artifact in **Figure 16.1** (*arrow*) violates which assumption of ultrasound wave propagation?

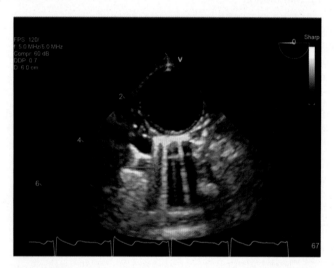

**Figure 16.1**

A. Ultrasound propagates in a straight line in the direction of the central beam
B. A structure will reflect the ultrasound beam only once
C. Only structures located within the intended path of the ultrasound beam will generate reflections back to the transducer
D. The position of the structure along the scan line is proportional to the travel time of the transmitted wave

2. A 65-year-old patient with chronic obstructive pulmonary disease presents with three-vessel coronary artery disease for coronary artery bypass grafting. A transesophageal echocardiogram (ECG) is performed prior to the procedure. Identify the structure in **Figure 16.2** (*arrow*).

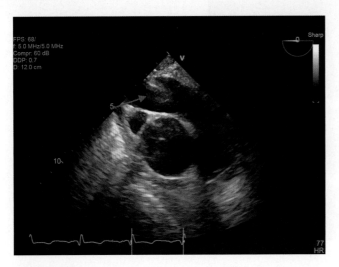

**Figure 16.2**

   A. Pulmonary embolus
   B. Pulmonary artery sarcoma
   C. Near-field artifact
   D. Beam width artifact

3. The imaging artifact in **Figure 16.3** violates which assumption of ultrasound principles?

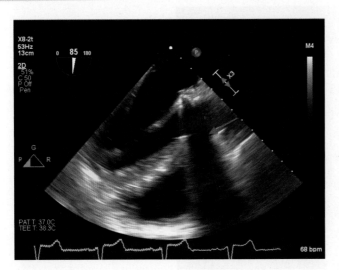

**Figure 16.3**

   A. Echoes return to the transducer after a single reflection
   B. Echoes originate from the main beam
   C. The depth of an object is directly related to the travel time for an ultrasound pulse to return to the transducer
   D. Pulses are propagated uniformly by all tissues

4. A 56-year-old male is undergoing a mitral valve replacement via thoracotomy. What is shown in **Figure 16.4** (*arrow*)?

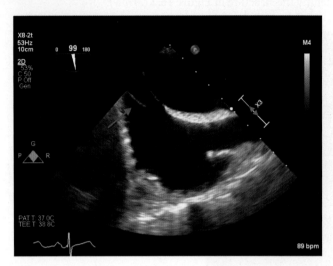

**Figure 16.4**

A. Crista terminalis
B. Side-lobe artifact
C. Chiari network
D. Eustachian valve

5. In **Figure 16.5**, which Doppler artifact is shown?

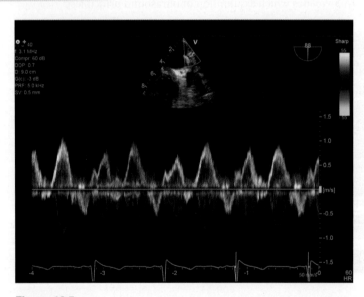

**Figure 16.5**

A. Aliasing
B. Spectral Doppler mirroring
C. Pseudoflow
D. Twinkling

6. The artifact in **Figure 16.6** violates which assumption of ultrasound principles?

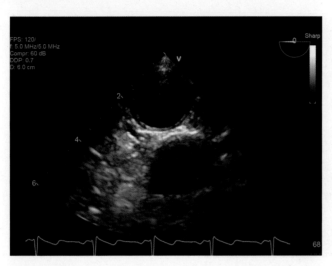

**Figure 16.6**

A. Echoes return to the transducer after a single reflection
B. Pulses travel in a straight line
C. Echoes originate from the main beam
D. Pulses are attenuated uniformly by all tissues

7. A 65-year-old female with a past medical history of osteoporosis and severe mitral regurgitation from P2 prolapse presents for elective mitral valve repair. During her comprehensive preprocedure intraoperative transesophageal echocardiogram (**Figure 16.7**), this is seen in her ascending aorta.

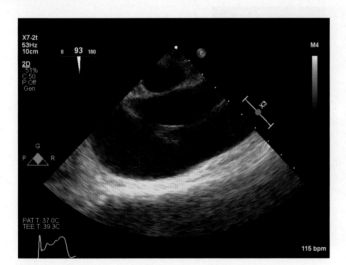

**Figure 16.7**

Which of the following artifacts is it most likely?
A. Ascending aortic dissection
B. Mirror image artifact
C. Side-lobe artifact
D. Beam width artifact

**8.** Which color flow Doppler artifact in **Figure 16.8** is depicted by the *arrow*?

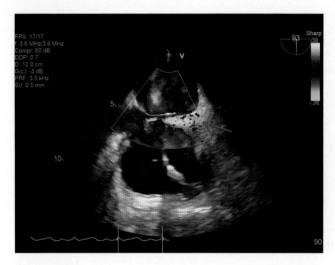

**Figure 16.8**

**A.** Pseudoflow
**B.** Twinkling
**C.** Blooming
**D.** Aliasing

**9.** A 68-year-old female undergoes elective coronary artery bypass grafting. On her comprehensive transesophageal ECG, a mid-esophageal bicaval view is obtained (**Figure 16.9**).

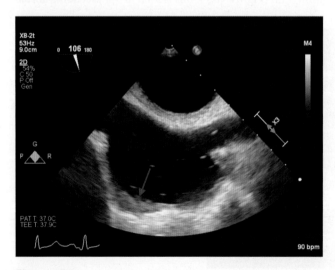

**Figure 16.9**

What is depicted by the *arrow*?
**A.** Nodule of Arantius
**B.** Right atrial myxoma
**C.** Right atrial thrombus
**D.** Right atrial pectinate muscles

**10.** The color flow Doppler artifact represented in **Figure 16.10** is:

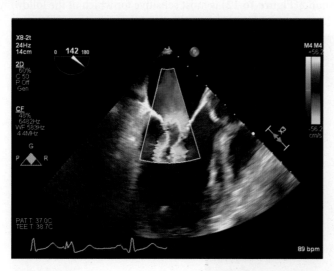

**Figure 16.10**

**A.** Pseudoflow
**B.** Spectral Doppler mirroring
**C.** Aliasing
**D.** Blooming

**11.** A 78-year-old woman presents to the Emergency Department with shortness of breath and acute hypoxemic respiratory failure. Based on the ultrasound artifact in **Figure 16.11**, which of the following is the most likely diagnosis?

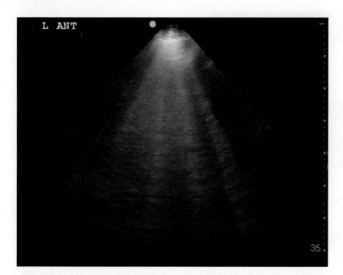

**Figure 16.11**

**A.** Pneumothorax
**B.** Congestive heart failure exacerbation
**C.** COPD exacerbation
**D.** Pneumonia

**12.** A 35-year-old man is being treated for sepsis in the intensive care unit (ICU). The presence of pleural sliding and A-lines on bedside ultrasound (**Figure 16.12**) is most sensitive for which of the following?

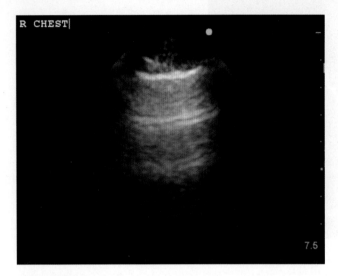

**Figure 16.12**

**A.** Fluid overload
**B.** Pneumonia
**C.** Pulmonary capillary wedge pressure < 18 mm Hg
**D.** Pneumothorax

**13.** During three-dimensional analysis of the mitral valve, the following artifact is observed (**Figure 16.13**).

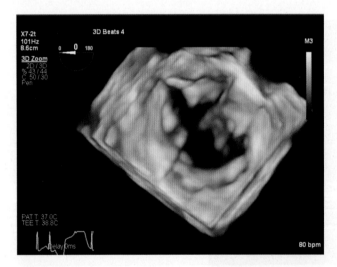

**Figure 16.13**

This finding may result from any of the following EXCEPT?
**A.** Sinus tachycardia
**B.** Positive pressure ventilation
**C.** Electrocautery
**D.** Probe movement

**14.** Which of the following ultrasound artifacts is depicted in **Figure 16.14**?

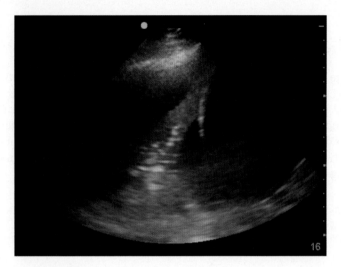

**Figure 16.14**

A. A-lines
B. B-lines
C. Lung point
D. Air bronchogram

**15.** After undergoing an uncomplicated aortic valve replacement, **Figure 16.15** is observed on interrogation of the mitral valve.

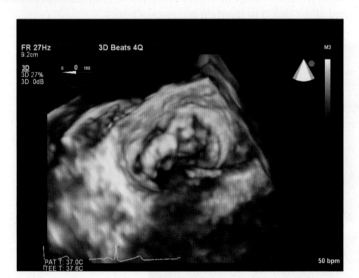

**Figure 16.15**

What is the most likely diagnosis?
A. Retained left ventricular (LV) vent
B. Pacemaker wire
C. Suture material
D. Side-lobe artifact

# Chapter 16 ■ Answers

**1.** Correct Answer: **B. A structure will reflect the ultrasound beam only once**

*Rationale:* Reverberation artifacts are created when the ultrasound beam bounces multiple times between two highly reflective surfaces during the listening phase, before returning to the transducer. This violates the assumption that the ultrasound has returned to the transducer after only a single reflection from the structure. Because the ultrasound beam bounces between two strong reflectors during the listening phase, the reverberation artifact lies distal to the imaged structure and often violates anatomic boundaries. When the distance between the two reflectors is small, the artifact will appear as closely approximated lines (or stepladder), creating a "ring-down" or "comet-tail" artifact.

### Selected References

1. Bertrand PB, Levine RA, Isselbacher EM, Vandervoort PM. Fact or artifact in two-dimensional echocardiography: avoiding misdiagnosis and missed diagnosis. *J Am Soc Echocardiogr.* 2016;29(5):381-391.
2. Le HT, Hangiandreou N, Timmerman R, et al. Imaging artifacts in echocardiography. *Anesth Analg.* 2016;122(3):633-646.

**2.** Correct Answer: **C. Near-field artifact**

*Rationale:* Structures in the near field are sometimes obscured by high-amplitude oscillations by the transducer itself, causing near-field artifacts. These are often seen in structures that are close to the transducer, such as the pulmonary arteries or descending aorta. True pulmonary embolus moves with cardiac motion and will show a lack of color with color flow Doppler. With the addition of color flow Doppler on a near-field artifact, the color will encompass the entire pulmonary artery, without filling defects. In the patient scenario, this patient is coming to the operating room for coronary artery bypass grafting, without evidence of right heart strain or hypoxemia. This helps us to identify from the stem that this is an artifact. Contrast the image in the stem from the image in **Figure 16.16** which is a pulmonary embolus. This image shows a discrete mass and filling defect in the right pulmonary artery.

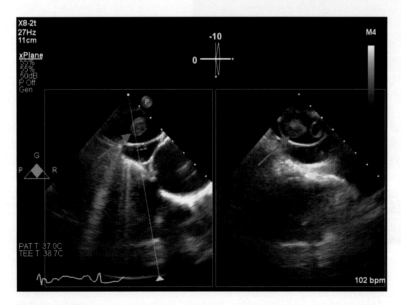

**Figure 16.16**

### Selected Reference

1. Bertrand PB, Levine RA, Isselbacher EM, Vandervoort PM. Fact or artifact in two-dimensional echocardiography: avoiding misdiagnosis and missed diagnosis. *J Am Soc Echocardiogr.* 2016;29(5):381-391.

**3.** Correct Answer: D. Pulses are propagated uniformly by all tissues

*Rationale:* The prosthetic aortic valve in Figure 16.3 acts as a strong reflector preventing ultrasound wave propagation beyond the valve. This creates an artifact called acoustic shadowing. Acoustic shadowing violates the assumption that pulses are propagated uniformly by all tissues. In this case, the prosthetic valve attenuates the pulse distal to the valve.

Selected References

1. Bertrand PB, Levine RA, Isselbacher EM, Vandervoort PM. Fact or artifact in two-dimensional echocardiography: avoiding misdiagnosis and missed diagnosis. *J Am Soc Echocardiogr.* 2016;29(5):381-391.
2. Le HT, Hangiandreou N, Timmerman R, et al. Imaging artifacts in echocardiography. *Anesth Analg.* 2016;122(3):633-646.

**4.** Correct Answer: D. Eustachian valve

*Rationale:* The Eustachian valve is an embryologic remnant that can be seen as a prominent crescent-shaped tissue at the posterior aspect of the inferior vena cava. In fetal life, it directed blood flow across the fossa ovalis. In this view (Figure 16.4), the Eustachian valve separates the inferior vena cava (above) from the coronary sinus (below). A Chiari network is a remnant of the right valve of the sinus venosus and appears as a filamentous structure in the right atrium. The crista terminalis is a ridge of myocardium at the junction of the right atrium and superior vena cava.

Selected Reference

1. Silvestry FE, Cohen MS, Armsby LB, et al. Guidelines for the echocardiographic assessment of atrial septal defect and patent foramen ovale: from the American Society of Echocardiography and Society for Cardiac Angiography and Interventions. *J Am Soc Echocardiogr.* 2015;28(8):910-958.

**5.** Correct Answer: B. Spectral Doppler mirroring

*Rationale:* The duplication of the Doppler spectrum above and below the baseline represents spectral Doppler mirroring. This mirroring is caused by cross-talk, which is erroneous signal transfer when the echo exceeds the operating range of the circuit and results in the appearance of velocities on both sides of the baseline; or by directional ambiguity, which is when the Doppler angle is near 90°. The signal is typically more intense on one side of the baseline compared to the other side. Reducing the Doppler gain in the case of cross-talk will help to resolve the spectral Doppler mirroring, while changing the image such that the Doppler beam intersects close to 0° is helpful in directional ambiguity.

Selected Reference

1. Le HT, Hangiandreou N, Timmerman R, et al. Imaging artifacts in echocardiography. *Anesth Analg.* 2016;122(3):633-646.

**6.** Correct Answer: A. Echoes return to the transducer after a single reflection

*Rationale:* In Figure 16.6, the ultrasound reaches the descending aorta before reaching a strong reflector. The strong reflector then creates a mirror image of the descending aorta inferior to the actual aorta. Mirror images occur because the ultrasound pulse reaches a smooth strong reflector (mirror), which directs the beam to the second reflector (in this case, the descending aorta). The beam then bounces from the target to the mirror-like surface on its return to the probe.

Selected References

1. Bertrand PB, Levine RA, Isselbacher EM, Vandervoort PM. Fact or artifact in two-dimensional echocardiography: avoiding misdiagnosis and missed diagnosis. *J Am Soc Echocardiogr.* 2016;29(5):381-391.
2. Le HT, Hangiandreou N, Timmerman R, et al. Imaging artifacts in echocardiography. *Anesth Analg.* 2016;122(3):633-646.

**7.** Correct Answer: C. Side-lobe artifact

*Rationale:* The main ultrasound beam emits the most energy, while small portions of ultrasound energy emitted in "side-lobes" of the main ultrasound beam are often dissipated in the tissue. However, when this side-lobe energy is reflected by a strong reflector in its path, these reflections are interpreted by the scanner as originating from the central/main ultrasound beam. Numerous side-lobe artifacts can be generated as the transducer scans by sweeping in a radial direction, often merging the side-lobe images, producing a linear arc-like artifact. In the ascending aorta, side-lobe artifacts from highly reflective aortic sinotubular junctions could be mistaken for aortic dissection flaps. Because the patient in the scenario is being imaged for elective mitral repair, without a history of hypertension or connective tissue disorder, and is asymptomatic, Figure 16.7 represents a side-lobe artifact. Imaging in alternative planes and the addition of color flow Doppler can help to distinguish a side-lobe artifact from true pathology.

### Selected References

1. Bertrand PB, Levine RA, Isselbacher EM, Vandervoort PM. Fact or artifact in two-dimensional echocardiography: avoiding misdiagnosis and missed diagnosis. *J Am Soc Echocardiogr*. 2016;29(5):381-391.
2. Le HT, Hangiandreou N, Timmerman R, et al. Imaging artifacts in echocardiography. *Anesth Analg*. 2016;122(3):633-646.

---

**8. Correct Answer: C. Blooming**

*Rationale:* A blooming artifact is seen when soft tissues have red/blue color with color flow Doppler as if they contain true blood flow. This artifact is typically seen with high gain settings. Pseudoflow is seen with motion of fluid other than blood, such as ascites. Twinkling is a mosaic of rapidly changing blue and red patches of color that is seen near strongly reflective surfaces. Aliasing is seen when a velocity reaches the peak velocity of the color scale.

### Selected References

1. Bertrand PB, Levine RA, Isselbacher EM, Vandervoort PM. Fact or artifact in two-dimensional echocardiography: avoiding misdiagnosis and missed diagnosis. *J Am Soc Echocardiogr*. 2016;29(5):381-391.
2. Le HT, Hangiandreou N, Timmerman R, et al. Imaging artifacts in echocardiography. *Anesth Analg*. 2016;122(3):633-646.

---

**9. Correct Answer: D. Right atrial pectinate muscles**

*Rationale:* The right and left atria contain muscle bands known as pectinate muscles that course across the anterior endocardial surfaces and both appendages. Pectinate muscles are more prominent in the right atrium than the left. Pectinate muscles can be differentiated from thrombus or mass by their uniform texture and density. Additionally, pectinate muscles move in synchrony with the cardiac tissues.

### Selected Reference

1. Hahn RT, Abraham T, Adams MS, et al. Guidelines for performing a comprehensive transesophageal echocardiographic examination: recommendations from the American Society of Echocardiography and the Society of Cardiovascular Anesthesiologists. *J Am Soc Echocardiogr*. 2013;26(9):921-964.

---

**10. Correct Answer: C. Aliasing**

*Rationale:* Aliasing occurs in color flow Doppler because the maximum velocity that can be measured with color flow Doppler is limited. The Nyquist limit is reached, at which point, all higher velocities are shown as aliased. In Figure 16.10, aliasing is displayed as patches of light blue adjacent to patches of bright yellow and red, despite the flow going away from the probe in diastole. This is because there is some degree of mitral stenosis and a higher velocity of diastolic blood flow through the mitral valve.

### Selected References

1. Bertrand PB, Levine RA, Isselbacher EM, Vandervoort PM. Fact or artifact in two-dimensional echocardiography: avoiding misdiagnosis and missed diagnosis. *J Am Soc Echocardiogr*. 2016;29(5):381-391.
2. Le HT, Hangiandreou N, Timmerman R, et al. Imaging artifacts in echocardiography. *Anesth Analg*. 2016;122(3):633-646.

---

**11. Correct Answer: B. Congestive heart failure exacerbation**

*Rationale:* The presence of B-lines on lung ultrasound (Figure 16.11) indicates the presence of interstitial edema, the precursor to frank alveolar edema. These comet-tail artifacts fan downward from the surface of the lung and arise from accumulation of fluid in the interlobular septa. This ultrasonographic artifact has been shown to have a sensitivity of 100% and specificity of 92% in the diagnosis of pulmonary edema compared to COPD.

### Selected References

1. Lichtenstein D, Mezière G. A lung ultrasound sign allowing bedside distinction between pulmonary edema and COPD: the comet-tail artifact. *Intensive Care Med*. 1998;24(12):1331-1334.
2. Lichtenstein DA, Mezière GA, Lagoueyte JF, Biderman P, Goldstein I, Gepner A. Lung ultrasound as a bedside tool for predicting pulmonary artery occlusion pressure in the critically ill. *Chest*. 2009;136(4):1014-1020.

**12.** Correct Answer: C. Pulmonary capillary wedge pressure < 18 mm Hg

*Rationale:* A-lines are a reverberation ultrasound artifact seen in normal lungs which appear as repetitive horizontal echoic lines resembling the pleural line. They arise from reflection of the ultrasound beam by subpleural air. A preponderance of A-lines without B-lines on lung ultrasound is a sensitive (85.7%) but not specific (40.0%) finding for PCWP <18 mm Hg. The presence of pleural sliding makes a diagnosis of pneumothorax less likely.

Selected References
1. Lichtenstein DA, Mezière GA, Lagoueyte JF, Biderman P, Goldstein I, Gepner A. Lung ultrasound as a bedside tool for predicting pulmonary artery occlusion pressure in the critically ill. *Chest.* 2009;136(4):1014-1020.
2. Volpicelli G, Skurzak S, Boero E, et al. Lung ultrasound predicts well extravascular lung water but is of limited usefulness in the prediction of wedge pressure. *Anesthesiology.* 2014;121:320-327.

**13.** Correct Answer: A. Sinus tachycardia

*Rationale:* Three-dimensional full-volume images are "stitched" together from multiple ECG-gated sub-volumes to make Figure 16.13. Movement of the probe, movement of the patient, ECG artifact from electrocautery, or changes in cardiac rhythm during image acquisition will lead to geometrical distortion of the final product.

Selected Reference
1. Faletra FF, Ramamurthi A, Dequarti MC, Leo LA, Moccetti T, Pandian N. Artifacts in three-dimensional echocardiography. *J Am Soc Echocardiogr.* 2014;27(5):453-462.

**14.** Correct Answer: D. Air bronchogram

*Rationale:* Air bronchograms may be observed in consolidated lung tissue, indicating the presence of atelectasis or pneumonia. These linear hyperechoic artifacts visualize fluid mixed with air and may be static or dynamic in nature. Static bronchograms are typically associated with resorptive atelectasis, whereas dynamic bronchograms move centrifugally with respiration and are highly specific for the diagnosis of pneumonia.

Selected References
1. Lichtenstein D, Mezière G, Seitz J. The dynamic air bronchogram: a lung ultrasound sign of alveolar consolidation ruling out atelectasis. *Chest.* 2009;135(6):1421-1425.

**15.** Correct Answer: D. Side-lobe artifact

*Rationale:* While iatrogenic origins are always possible and important to rule out, Figure 16.15 is most consistent with a side-lobe artifact. After an uncomplicated procedure, this unexpected curvilinear density appearing on the atrial side of the mitral valve is classic for a side-lobe artifact. While the curvilinear shape of this artifact may resemble a pacemaker wire, the left atrial origin would be incongruent with a pacemaker wire. The artifact does not resemble suture material, which would have a smaller profile. Additionally, after an uncomplicated aortic valve replacement, one would need to question what suture material would be present in the left atrium. Lastly, a retained LV vent would be plausible after an uncomplicated aortic valve replacement (may have been placed due to aortic insufficiency), but the LV vent would be larger in diameter than this artifact and would ideally cross the mitral valve.

Selected References
1. Bertrand PB, Levine RA, Isselbacher EM, Vandervoort PM. Fact or artifact in two-dimensional echocardiography: avoiding misdiagnosis and missed diagnosis. *J Am Soc Echocardiogr.* 2016;29(5):381-391.
2. Le HT, Hangiandreou N, Timmerman R, et al. Imaging artifacts in echocardiography. *Anesth Analg.* 2016;122(3):633-646.

# SECTION IV | QUANTIFICATION AND HEMODYNAMIC CALCULATIONS

# 17 | DOPPLER SHIFT PRINCIPLES

Matthew Sigakis and Venkatakrishna Rajajee

1. For accurate Doppler velocity measurement, the angle of incidence between the direction of motion and the ultrasound beam should be:

   A. 90°
   B. Between 60° and 90°
   C. Between 20° and 60°
   D. Less than 20°

2. The Doppler shift is inversely proportional to:

   A. Red blood cell speed
   B. Frequency of the transducer
   C. Angle between red blood cell flow and ultrasound beam
   D. Speed of sound in the tissue

3. Which of the following statements is *most accurate* regarding the Doppler method shown in **Figure 17.1**?

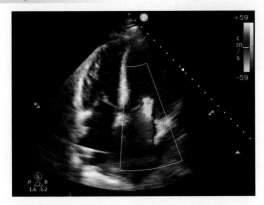

**Figure 17.1**

   A. It is not subject to aliasing
   B. Flow is moving away from the transducer
   C. It is based on the principles of pulsed wave Doppler (PWD)
   D. It reports peak velocities

4. Which statement *best* describes a property of the Doppler method depicted in **Figure 17.2**?

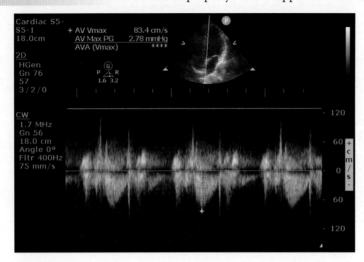

**Figure 17.2**

A. Aliasing will occur at the Nyquist limit
B. It is best applied to low velocities
C. It is limited by range ambiguity
D. One element serves as both the transmitter and the receiver

5. Which statement *best* describes a property of the Doppler method depicted in **Figure 17.3**?

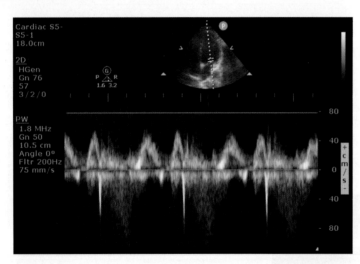

**Figure 17.3**

A. Aliasing occurs at PRP/2 (pulse repetition period)
B. Aliasing occurs at PRF/2 (pulse repetition frequency)
C. Aliasing is reduced by greater depth
D. Aliasing is reduced by using a higher frequency transducer

# Chapter 17 ▪ Answers

---

**1.** Correct Answer: D. Less than 20°

*Rationale:* The magnitude of the Doppler shift depends on the cosine of the angle (Θ, theta) between the direction of motion (i.e., red blood cells in blood) and the ultrasound beam (**Figure 17.4**). The velocity measured is equal to the true velocity multiplied by the cosine of the angle away from parallel.

The greater the angle away from parallel, the greater the measured velocity differs from the true velocity (see **Table 17.1**). To minimize measurement error, the ultrasound beam should be as parallel as possible to the target flow. An angle of less than 20° is recommended because it corresponds to a low level of error, less than 6%.

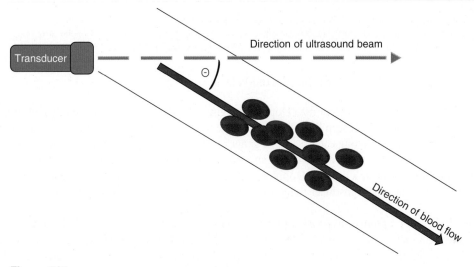

**Figure 17.4**

**Table 17.1**

| Angle (Θ) | Cos (Θ) | Error (%) |
|-----------|---------|-----------|
| 0° | 1 | 0 |
| 10° | 0.985 | 2.5 |
| 20° | 0.940 | 6 |
| 30° | 0.866 | 13 |
| 60° | 0.50 | 50 |
| 90° | 0 | 100 |

Selected References
1. Edelman SK. *Understanding Ultrasound Physics.* 4th ed. E.S.P. Ultrasound; 2012.
2. Mitchell C, Rahko PS, Blauwet LA, et al. Guidelines for performing a comprehensive transthoracic echocardiographic examination in adults: recommendations from the American Society of Echocardiography. *J Am Soc Echocardiogr.* 2019;32(1):1-64.

**2.** Correct Answer: D. Speed of sound in the tissue

*Rationale:*

$$\text{Doppler shift } (f_d) = \frac{2 \times \text{reflector speed } (v) \times \text{incident frequency } (f_O) \times \cos(\theta)}{\text{propagation speed } (c)} \qquad (17.1)$$

The Doppler shift is directly proportional to the reflector speed (flow of red blood cells, $V$), incident frequency (transducer frequency, $f_0$), and cosine of the angle ($\Theta$) between the red blood cell flow and ultrasound beam (Equation 17.1). The Doppler shift is inversely proportional to the propagation speed (speed of sound in the medium, $C$). The equation can be rearranged to solve for blood flow velocity ($V$)—this is the value calculated by the ultrasound machine. The "2" represents a double Doppler shift: the first shift occurs upon the target (red blood cell). The second shift occurs from the reflected ultrasound wave sent back to the ultrasound transducer from the moving red blood cell.

Selected References
1. Edelman SK. *Understanding Ultrasound Physics*. 4th ed. E.S.P. Ultrasound; 2012.
2. Oglat AA, Matjafri MZ, Suardi N, Oqlat MA, Abdelrahman MA, Oqlat AA. A review of medical Doppler ultrasonography of blood flow in general and especially in common carotid artery. *J Med Ultrasound*. 2018;26(1):3-13.

**3.** Correct Answer: C. It is based on the principles of PWD

*Rationale:* Figure 17.1 represents color flow Doppler imaging, also described as 2-D, multigated (multiple scan lines) Doppler. Along each scan line within an image plane, an ultrasound pulse is transmitted, and the reflected waves received along each scan line generate measured Doppler shifts. These shifts (which we interpret as velocities) are coded into colors and superimposed on a 2-D image. Blood flow directed toward the transducer reflects a positive Doppler shift and is color coded in shades of red/orange. Blood flow directed away from the transducer reflects a negative Doppler shift and is color coded in shades of blue.

Color flow Doppler reports *average* (or mean) velocities. It actually uses multiple ultrasound pulses, or "packets," along each scan line to accurately determine blood velocity. There is a trade-off: small packets result in a higher frame rate leading to higher temporal resolution, but result in less accurate velocity measurements. Conversely, large packets require a slower frame rate leading to lower temporal resolution, but result in more accurate velocity measurements. Thus, color low Doppler measures mean velocity to balance temporal resolution and accuracy of velocity measurement.

Color flow Doppler is based on PWD ultrasound principles and therefore is subject to aliasing. Aliasing will occur if the sampling rate (pulse repetition frequency [PRF]) is too low compared to the Doppler shift. Aliasing can be improved by reducing depth (reduces pulse repetition duration and increases PRF), increasing the color scale if previously set lower, adjusting the baseline to allow higher velocities to be displayed, or increasing the angle between flow and beam (at the expense of measurement accuracy).

Selected References
1. Edelman SK. *Understanding Ultrasound Physics*. 4th ed. E.S.P. Ultrasound; 2012..
2. Levitov LB, Mayo PH, Slonim AD. *Critical Care Ultrasonography*. 2nd ed. McGraw-Hill Education/Medical; 2014.

**4.** Correct Answer: C. It is limited by range ambiguity

*Rationale:* Figure 17.2 demonstrates an example of continuous wave Doppler. At least two elements are required for this modality: one element constantly emits the incident ultrasound wave and another element constantly receives the returning signal. Continuous wave Doppler can detect any flow velocity and is particularly useful when measuring high flow velocities. However, it cannot detect where the sample is obtained, called "range ambiguity," because the emitting and receiving signals have large overlap.

Selected References
1. Edelman SK. *Understanding Ultrasound Physics*. 4th ed. E.S.P. Ultrasound; 2012.
2. Levitov LB, Mayo PH, Slonim AD. *Critical Care Ultrasonography*. 2nd ed. McGraw-Hill Education/Medical; 2014.

**5.** Correct Answer: B. Aliasing occurs at PRF/2 (pulse repetition frequency)

*Rationale:* Figure 17.3 demonstrates an example of PWD. Here, echo signals are emitted from the probe, then the transducer must wait until the reflected wave is received before the next incident pulse is emitted. The length of time for each cycle (between emitted and received wave) is pulse repetition period (PRP). And, PRF is 1/PRP.

The Doppler shift measured by the reflected wave is used to calculate the velocity of the reflector (blood cells). However, the upper limit of the Doppler shift that can be displayed is called the Nyquist limit. Nyquist limit is PRF/2 and a higher Doppler shift (due to a faster moving reflector) leads to aliasing and range ambiguity. Aliasing can be reduced (or Nyquist limit can be increased) by decreasing depth of imaging or using a lower frequency probe.

Selected References

1. Edelman SK. *Understanding Ultrasound Physics*. 4th ed. E.S.P. Ultrasound; 2012.
2. Levitov LB, Mayo PH, Slonim AD. *Critical Care Ultrasonography*. 2nd ed. McGraw-Hill Education/Medical; 2014.

Matthew Sigakis and Venkatakrishna Rajajee

1. A 67-year-old woman presents to the intensive care unit (ICU) after a syncopal episode. She is afebrile, heart rate 99 bpm, blood pressure 98/34 mm Hg, and oxygen saturation 96% on room air. Echocardiography is performed, and the results are shown in **Figure 18.1**.

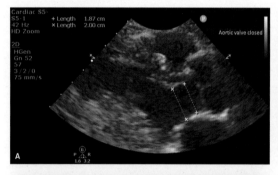
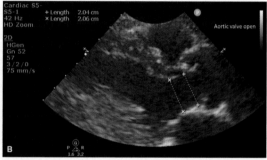
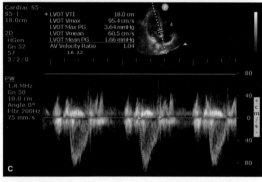
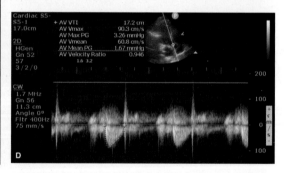

**Figure 18.1**

What is the calculated stroke volume?
A. 59.94 cc
B. 58.80 cc
C. 56.52 cc
D. 57.28 cc

2. Based on Figure 18.1 (noted in **Question 18.1**), calculate the patient's aortic valve area (AVA).

   **A.** 3.33 cm$^2$
   **B.** 3.42 cm$^2$
   **C.** 3.48 cm$^2$
   **D.** 4.02 cm$^2$

3. A 75-year-old man who is being cared for in the ICU develops delirium and, during a period of agitation, pulls out his Swan-Ganz catheter. Instead of replacing the catheter, echocardiography is performed and demonstrates **Figure 18.2**.

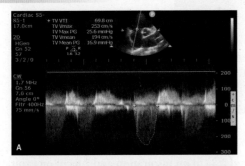

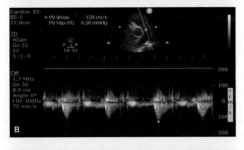

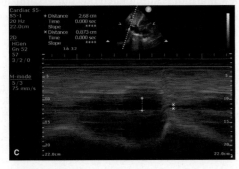

**Figure 18.2**

Calculate the systolic pulmonary artery pressure (SPAP).
   **A.** 33.6 mm Hg
   **B.** 25.6 mm Hg
   **C.** 16.9 mm Hg
   **D.** 24.9 mm Hg

4. If the patient in **Question 18.3** had pulmonary stenosis with a peak pressure gradient of 10 mm Hg, choose the BEST statement:

   **A.** SPAP will be 10 mm Hg higher than right ventricular systolic pressure (RVSP)
   **B.** SPAP will be 10 mm Hg lower than RVSP
   **C.** SPAP = RVSP
   **D.** SPAP cannot be determined

5. A continuous wave Doppler (CWD) flow across the pulmonic valve in the parasternal short-axis view (PSAX) is depicted in **Figure 18.3**.

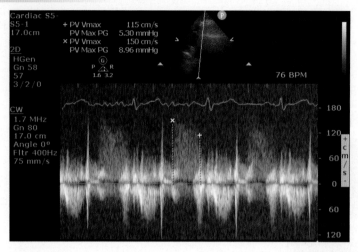

**Figure 18.3**

The inferior vena cava (IVC) is large, with a diameter of 2.8 cm on inspiration and 2.8 cm on expiration. Calculate the diastolic pulmonary artery pressure (DPAP):
   A. 24.00 mm Hg
   B. 22.29 mm Hg
   C. 20.29 mm Hg
   D. 22.00 mm Hg

6. A 78-year-old man presented to the ICU after a percutaneous coronary intervention to the right main, left circumflex, and left anterior descending coronary arteries for ST-elevation myocardial infarction. On ICU day 4, he developed progressive hypotension. A new murmur is auscultated on your examination. Echocardiography is performed and reveals a new ventricular septal defect (VSD) in the mid portion of the interventricular septum. Additional information from the examination is noted in **Table 18.1**.

**Table 18.1 Patient Examination**

| Parasternal Long-Axis View (PLAX) | PSAX: Right Ventricular Outflow Tract (RVOT) | Apical Five-chamber View (A5C): Left Ventricular Outflow Tract (LVOT) |
|---|---|---|
| LVOT diameter: 2.1 cm | $V_{max}$: 93.3 cm/s | $V_{max}$: 96.0 cm/s |
| Aortic valve (AV) diameter: 1.7 cm | | |
| | Maximal instantaneous PG (max-PG): 3.5 mm Hg | Maximal instantaneous PG (max-PG):3.7 mm Hg |
| | Mean PG: 1.8 mm Hg | Mean PG: 1.6 mm Hg |
| | Velocity time integral (VTI): 23.0 cm | VTI: 21.0 cm |
| | Diameter: 2.2 cm | |

PG, peak gradient.

Calculate the shunt fraction.
   A. 1.0
   B. 1.2
   C. 1.4
   D. 1.6

7. A 73-year-old woman with a history of hypertension is admitted to the ICU with acute shortness of breath. She is found to have pulmonary edema and is managed with noninvasive positive pressure ventilation and a diuretic. Echocardiography is performed. The left ventricular (LV) ejection fraction is calculated at 56% using Simpson's method. Her left atrium (LA) is enlarged at 38 mL/m$^2$. The peak tricuspid regurgitant (TR) velocity is measured at 2.95 m/s. There is no significant valvular stenosis or regurgitation. Tissue Doppler imaging assessment of the medial mitral annulus is performed, and the tracing is shown in **Figure 18.4**.

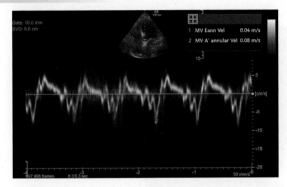

**Figure 18.4**

Based on the information provided, which of the following is the BEST assessment of the patient's LV diastolic function?
A. Normal diastolic function
B. Indeterminate, based on tissue Doppler imaging criteria
C. Indeterminate, based on the presence of normal LV ejection fraction
D. Diastolic dysfunction

8. A 78-year-old man with a history of hypertension, alcohol abuse, coronary artery bypass surgery, and bioprosthetic AV replacement presents with shortness of breath on minimal exertion, chest tightness, and marked pedal edema. On echocardiography, the LV ejection fraction is 62% by Simpson's method and a septal bounce is noted on the apical four-chamber view (A4C). Right ventricular (RV) size and systolic function are normal to subjective assessment. There is no significant valvular stenosis or regurgitation. Mitral inflow velocities reveal an E/A ratio of 1.59. The IVC is seen to be distended at 2.4 cm, and there is only a 10% change in diameter with a sniff. Results of tissue Doppler imaging assessment of the mitral annulus are shown in **Figure 18.5**.

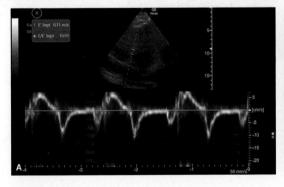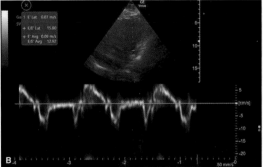

**Figure 18.5**

Based on the information provided, which of the following is *most likely* to be the underlying pathology?
A. Constrictive pericarditis
B. Restrictive cardiomyopathy
C. Mixed constriction restriction
D. RV failure

9. A 68-year-old man with hypertension, diabetes, and chronic kidney disease is admitted to the ICU with suspected pneumonia, requiring intubation and mechanical ventilation. He is on assist control ventilation with an FiO2 of 50% and positive-end expiratory pressure of 12 cm H₂O. A chest X-ray reveals bilateral diffuse airspace opacities. He requires a norepinephrine infusion at 0.5 µg/kg/min. An echocardiogram is performed. LV size and systolic function are normal to subjective assessment. Based solely on the still image from an apical A4C and the results of tissue doppler imaging assessment of the tricuspid annulus (shown in **Figure 18.6**), which of the following is the best assessment of the condition of his right ventricle?

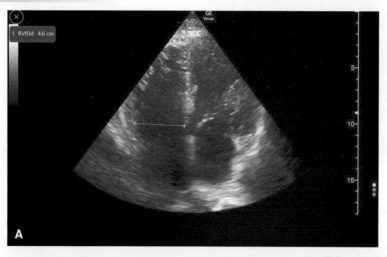

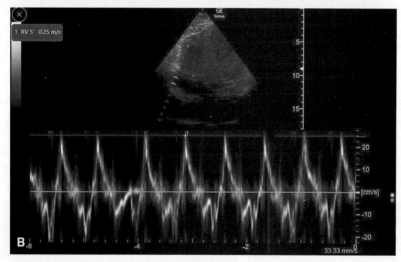

**Figure 18.6**

A. Dilated, decreased systolic function
B. Dilated, normal systolic function
C. Normal size, decreased systolic function
D. Normal size, normal systolic function

**10.** A 54-year-old South Asian woman with no significant past medical history presents with shortness of breath and palpitations. She is in atrial fibrillation. Echocardiography reveals normal LV size and systolic function, an enlarged LA, and a thickened mitral valve with limited excursion. CWD examination of the mitral valve is performed, and the results are shown in **Figure 18.7**.

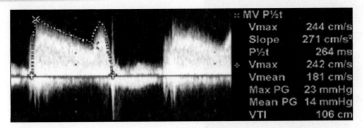

| :: MV P½t | |
|---|---|
| Vmax | 244 cm/s |
| Slope | 271 cm/s² |
| P½t | 264 ms |
| ÷ Vmax | 242 cm/s |
| Vmean | 181 cm/s |
| Max PG | 23 mmHg |
| Mean PG | 14 mmHg |
| VTI | 106 cm |

**Figure 18.7**

What is the estimated mitral valve area (MVA)?
**A.** 0.83 cm²
**B.** 1.00 cm²
**C.** 1.50 cm²
**D.** 2.23 cm²

# Chapter 18 ▪ Answers

**1.** Correct Answer: A. 59.94 cc

*Rationale:* Cardiac output is the product of heart rate and stroke volume. Stroke volume is calculated as the cross-sectional area (CSA) of the LVOT multiplied by the LVOT VTI.

The CSA is calculated as follows: $3.14 \times (D/2)^2 = 0.785 \times D^2$. The LVOT diameter (D) is obtained in the PLAX. It is important to zoom in on the LVOT image to minimize measurement error. The LVOT diameter is measured in mid-systole from inner edge to inner edge at the level of LVOT (within 0.5 to 1 cm of the valve orifice).

$$CSA = 0.785 \times (2.06 \text{ cm})^2 = 3.33 \text{ cm}^2$$

The LVOT VTI is measured with pulsed wave Doppler (PWD), placing the sample volume in the LVOT, which can be obtained in the A5C or apical three-chamber (A3C) view. The PWD sample volume is placed in the center of the LVOT, at the same location where the LVOT diameter was measured (within 0.5 to 1 cm of the valve orifice). The intercept angle should be less than 20° to minimize error in Doppler measurement. The spectral image obtained (PWD velocity curve) should demonstrate a narrow signal, with a rapid upstroke and end-systolic click that terminates the flow signal. The PWD velocity curve is traced to measure the VTI. In the image presented, the LVOT VTI is measured to be 18.0 cm.

Stroke volume = 3.33 cm² × 18.0 cm = 59.94 cc

Incorrect answers:
- *Answer B,* 3.26 cm² × 18.0 cm = 58.80 (AV diameter, valve open, used incorrectly)
- *Answer C,* 3.14 cm² × 18.0 cm = 56.52 (LVOT diameter, valve closed, used incorrectly)
- *Answer D,* 3.33 cm² × 17.2 cm = 57.28 (AV VTI, used incorrectly)

Selected Reference
1. Mitchell C, Rahko PS, Blauwet LA, et al. Guidelines for performing a comprehensive transthoracic echocardiographic examination in adults: recommendations from the American Society of Echocardiography. *J Am Soc Echocardiogr.* 2019;32(1):1-64.

**2.** Correct Answer: C. 3.48 cm$^2$

*Rationale:* The continuity equation is used to solve for the AVA as shown in **Figure 18.8**.

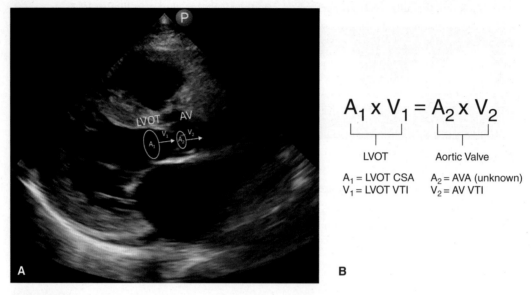

$$A_1 \times V_1 = A_2 \times V_2$$

LVOT      Aortic Valve

$A_1$ = LVOT CSA    $A_2$ = AVA (unknown)
$V_1$ = LVOT VTI     $V_2$ = AV VTI

**Figure 18.8**

The continuity equation represents the concept that all the volume ejected through the LVOT also passes through the AV orifice. The calculation of the continuity equation to determine AVA requires three measurements: the AV VTI by CWD, the LVOT diameter for calculation of the LVOT CSA, and the LVOT VTI by PWD. The equation is rearranged to solve for the unknown, the AVA.

$A1$ = LVOT CSA = 3.33 cm$^2$

$V1$ = LVOT VTI = 18.0 cm

$V2$ = AV VTI = 17.2 cm

$A2$ = (3.33 cm$^2$ × 18.0 cm)/17.2 cm = 3.48 cm$^2$

Selected Reference
1. Mitchell C, Rahko PS, Blauwet LA, et al. Guidelines for performing a comprehensive transthoracic echocardiographic examination in adults: recommendations from the American Society of Echocardiography. *J Am Soc Echocardiogr.* 2019;32(1):1-64.

**3.** Correct Answer: A. 33.6 mm Hg

*Rationale:* SPAP is calculated as the sum of the estimated right atrial pressure (RAP) and the peak pressure gradient measured between the right ventricle and right atrium. In the absence of a gradient across the pulmonic valve or RVOT, the SPAP is considered equal to the RVSP. The peak pressure gradient between the RV and RA is estimated by applying the modified Bernoulli equation ($4V^2$) to the peak velocity obtained by tricuspid regurgitation CWD signal. Therefore, the SPAP = RVSP = 4(V)$^2$ + RAP.

Of note, there may be variation in the measured flow velocity in different views. Ideally, this measurement should be obtained from multiple views including the PLAX (at the aortic valve level) (RV inflow view), PSAX, or A4C. The highest velocity obtained from a good quality signal should be reported for the final calculation.

In this question, the RV-RA peak pressure gradient = 4(2.53 m/s)$^2$ = 25.6 mm Hg.

The RA pressure is measured as the CVP or assumed based on characteristics of the IVC diameter as shown in **Table 18.2.**

**Table 18.2 Characteristics of IVC Diameter**

| Variable | Normal (0-5 mm Hg) [3] | Intermediate (5-10 mm Hg) [8] | | High (15 mm Hg) |
|---|---|---|---|---|
| IVC diameter | ≤2.1 cm | ≤2.1 cm | >2.1 cm | >2.1 cm |
| Collapse with sniff | >50% | >50% | >50% | >50% |
| Secondary indices of elevated RA pressure | | | | • Restrictive filling<br>• Tricuspid E/E' >6<br>• Diastolic flow predominance in hepatic veins (systolic filling fraction <55%) |

In this question, based on the IVC diameter greater than 2.1 cm and 50% collapse with sniff, RAP is estimated as intermediate range, approximately 8 mm Hg.

Therefore, the calculated SPAP = 25.6 + 8 = 33.6.

### Selected Reference

1. Rudski LG, Lai WW, Afilalo J, et al. Guidelines for the echocardiographic assessment of the right heart in adults: a report from the American Society of Echocardiography. *J Am Soc Echocardiogr.* 2010;23:685-713.

---

**4.** Correct Answer: **B. SPAP will be 10 mm Hg lower than RVSP**

*Rationale:* If there is no pulmonic stenosis or RVOT obstruction, then RVSP will be assumed to equal SPAP. In the presence of pulmonic stenosis or RVOT obstruction, RVSP exceeds SPAP because of the gradient of higher to lower pressure over the stenotic region: RVSP = SPAP + ΔP(RV − PA). Thus, SPAP = RVSP − ΔP(RV − PA).

### Selected Reference

1. Rudski LG, Lai WW, Afilalo J, et al. Guidelines for the echocardiographic assessment of the right heart in adults: a report from the American Society of Echocardiography. *J Am Soc Echocardiogr.* 2010;23:685-713.

---

**5.** Correct Answer: **C. 20.29 mm Hg**

*Rationale:* DPAP is calculated from the velocity of the end-diastolic pulmonary regurgitant jet using the modified Bernoulli equation: DPAP = 4 × (end-diastolic pulmonary regurgitant velocity)$^2$ + RAP. The RAP is high based on the explanation above (IVC diameter >2.1 cm and <50% collapsibility) and, therefore, can be estimated at 15 mm Hg.

DPAP = 4 × (1.15)$^2$ + 15 = 20.29

### Selected Reference

1. Rudski LG, Lai WW, Afilalo J, et al. Guidelines for the echocardiographic assessment of the right heart in adults: a report from the American Society of Echocardiography. *J Am Soc Echocardiogr.* 2010;23:685-713.

**6.** Correct Answer: B. 1.2

*Rationale:* The shunt fraction represents the ratio of pulmonary blood flow to systemic blood flow. This ratio informs the clinician about the independence of the two circulations. Although there are normal small anatomic shunts, such as when blood that is supplied to the lungs via the bronchial arteries is returned through the pulmonary veins without passing through the pulmonary capillaries, generally speaking the pulmonary blood flow will approximate the systemic blood flow such that the ratio of flows is close to 1. If the ratio is >1, then there is passage of systemic blood into the pulmonary circulation, resulting in pulmonary flow that is greater than the systemic flow. If the ratio is <1, then there is passage of pulmonary blood flow into the systemic circulation, resulting in systemic flow that is greater than the pulmonic flow. This ratio is used to determine the ratio of the pulmonary to systemic blood flow across an intracardiac shunt, such as an atrial septal defect (ASD), ventricular septal defect (VSD), or patent foramen ovale (PFO). Of note, the calculation below is sensitive to errors in measurement of the diameter, as it is squared. This formula is used when there is a simple left to right shunt.

**Shunt fraction = Qp/Qs**

$Q$ = blood flow

$p$ = pulmonary

$s$ = systemic

$Q_p = \text{RVOT VTI} \times [(\text{RVOT diameter}/2)]^2$

$Q_s = \text{LVOT VTI} \times [(\text{LVOT diameter})/2]^2$

$Q_p = 23.0 \text{ cm} \times [(2.2 \text{ cm}/2)]^2 = 27.83 \text{ cm}^3$

$Q_s = 21.0 \text{ cm} \times [(2.1 \text{ cm})/2]^2 = 23.15 \text{ cm}^3$

**Shunt fraction = Qp/Qs = 1.2**

Selected References
1. Oh J, Seward JB, Tajik AJ. *The Echo Manual*. 3rd ed. Lippincott, Williams & Wilkins; 2007.
2. Sanders SP, Yeager S, Williams RG. Measurement of systemic and pulmonary blood flow and QP/QS ratio using Doppler and two-dimensional echocardiography. *Am J Cardiol*. 1983;51(6):952-956.

**7.** Correct Answer: D. Diastolic dysfunction

*Rationale:* In patients with normal LV ejection fraction, the American Society of Echocardiography's (ASE's) 2016 guidelines for the evaluation of LV diastolic function by echocardiography recommend the use of four variables to identify the presence of diastolic dysfunction, with the following cutoffs: (a) septal e' < 7 cm/s OR lateral e' < 10 cm/s, (b) average E/e' ratio > 14, (c) left atrial (LA) volume index >34 mL/m$^2$, and (c) peak TR velocity >2.8 m/s. The presence of at least three of these four findings identifies the presence of diastolic dysfunction, provided other major pathology, such as valvular insufficiency, is absent. The presence of only two findings suggests indeterminate LV diastolic function, while the presence of only one finding, or none, suggests normal diastolic function. This patient with preserved LV ejection fraction has a dilated LA (volume index 38 mL/m$^2$), elevated peak TR velocity (2.95 m/s), and decreased septal e' (4 cm/s). Diastolic dysfunction is therefore present.

Selected Reference
1. Nagueh SF, Smiseth OA, Appleton CP, et al. Recommendations for the evaluation of left ventricular diastolic function by echocardiography: an update from the American Society of Echocardiography and the European Association of Cardiovascular Imaging. *J Am Soc Echocardiogr*. 2016;29(4):277-314.

**8. Correct Answer: A. Constrictive pericarditis**

*Rationale:* Constrictive pericarditis is characterized by a scarred and inelastic pericardium that limits diastolic filling of the ventricles. Ventricular interdependence is increased, and there is an increase in respiratory variation in ventricular filling. Unlike with tamponade, early diastolic filling is often prominent. This patient does not have evidence of tamponade, valvular dysfunction, or systolic dysfunction of either ventricle. Echocardiographic parameters to differentiate restrictive cardiomyopathy from constrictive pericarditis as a cause of diastolic dysfunction have been proposed and endorsed by the ASE. Common to both conditions is an E/A ratio >0.8 (since early diastolic filling is prominent), a dilated IVC (because limited filling of the right heart in expiration leads to engorgement of the IVC), and the presence of ventricular septal motion abnormality with respiration ("septal bounce"), an otherwise non-specific finding, caused by increased interventricular dependence and reciprocal changes in filling of the left and right heart chambers with respiration. Tissue doppler imaging is critical in distinguishing these two conditions. Tethering of the lateral mitral annulus by the pericardium results in a lateral e' that is lower than the septal e' ("annulus reversus"), which is often increased, to compensate. When the other conditions are satisfied, a mitral septal e' >8 cm/s suggests the presence of constrictive pericarditis, septal e' <6 cm/s suggests a restrictive cardiomyopathy, and septal e' 6-8 cm/s suggests mixed constriction/restriction. When the medial e' is 6-8 cm/s, the presence of annulus reversus suggests constrictive pericarditis is "most likely" present. When hepatic venous end-diastolic flow reversal in expiration is ≥0.8 of forward flow, there is "definite" constriction. This patient has an E/A ratio of 1.59, a dilated IVC, septal bounce, septal e' of 11 cm/s, and annulus reversus (septal e' 11 cm/s > lateral e' 7 cm/s). Constrictive pericarditis is therefore the most likely diagnosis.

### Selected References

1. Klein AL, Abbara S, Agler DA, et al. American Society of Echocardiography clinical recommendations for multimodality cardiovascular imaging of patients with pericardial disease: endorsed by the Society for Cardiovascular Magnetic Resonance and Society of Cardiovascular Computed Tomography. *J Am Soc Echocardiogr.* 2013;26(9):965-1012.e15.
2. Nagueh SF, Smiseth OA, Appleton CP, et al. Recommendations for the evaluation of left ventricular diastolic function by echocardiography: an update from the American Society of Echocardiography and the European Association of Cardiovascular Imaging. *J Am Soc Echocardiogr.* 2016;29(4):277-314.
3. Welch TD, Ling LH, Espinosa RE, et al. Echocardiographic diagnosis of constrictive pericarditis: Mayo Clinic criteria. *Circ Cardiovasc Imaging.* 2014;7(3):526-534. doi:10.1161/CIRCIMAGING.113.001613

**9. Correct Answer: B. Dilated, normal systolic function**

*Rationale:* Moderate-to-severe acute respiratory distress syndrome (ARDS), which is likely present in this case, can result in acute cor pulmonale in 22% to 50% of cases. This finding is associated with increased mortality. Criteria for RV enlargement, as specified by the ASE's 2015 guidelines for cardiac chamber quantification include an RV basal diameter >41 mm, mid-ventricular diameter >35 mm, longitudinal diameter >83 mm, and end-diastolic area >24 cm$^2$ in men (>20 cm$^2$ in women). These guidelines also describe several techniques for the quantification of RV systolic function, including the tricuspid annular peak systolic excursion (abnormal if <17 mm), fractional area change (abnormal if <35%), and tissue Doppler imaging of the tricuspid annulus with measurement of systolic annular velocity (S'). An S' <9.5 cm/s suggests RV systolic dysfunction. Each of these techniques has advantages and limitations. This patient has a basal diameter of 46 mm, suggesting the presence of RV dilatation, while the RV S' is 25 cm/s, suggesting normal RV systolic function. The presence of pulmonary hypertension in ARDS can result in RV dilatation before overt RV systolic dysfunction occurs.

### Selected References

1. Lang RM, Badano LP, Mor-Avi V, et al. Recommendations for cardiac chamber quantification by echocardiography in adults: an update from the American Society of Echocardiography and the European Association of Cardiovascular Imaging. *J Am Soc Echocardiogr.* 2015;28(1):1-39.e14.
2. Zochios V, Parhar K, Tunnicliffe W, Roscoe A, Gao F. The right ventricle in ARDS. *Chest.* 2017;152(1):181-193.

**10.** Correct Answer: A. 0.83 cm$^2$

*Rationale:* This patient has mitral stenosis, possibly of rheumatic etiology, based on the thickened mitral valve with limited excursion, LA enlargement, and presence of atrial fibrillation. She has no other past medical history and is from a region where rheumatic heart disease is more prevalent. While planimetry in the short-axis view is the reference standard for the measurement of MVA, the pressure half-time (PHT or P½T) method can also be used to estimate MVA. The PHT or P½T is defined as the time interval in milliseconds between the maximum mitral gradient in early diastole and the time point where the gradient is half the maximum initial value. The decline in diastolic transmitral flow velocity is inversely proportional to valve area. The deceleration slope of the early mitral inflow velocity (E-wave) obtained using CWD provides the PHT. The PHT can also be calculated as 0.29 × Deceleration time. The MVA in cm$^2$ is then calculated using the empirical formula 220/PHT. Since the PHT (P½T) in this case is 264 ms, the MVA is 220/264 = 0.83 cm$^2$. Mitral stenosis is judged severe when MVA is <1.5 cm$^2$ and very severe when <1 cm$^2$. The PHT is not significantly rate-dependent and can be used in the setting of varying R–R intervals, such as in atrial fibrillation. However, the MVA may be overestimated when the PHT is shortened because of aortic regurgitation, atrial septal defect, or abnormal LV relaxation.

### Selected References

1. Baumgartner H, Hung J, Bermejo J, et al. Echocardiographic assessment of valve stenosis: EAE/ASE recommendations for clinical practice. *J Am Soc Echocardiogr.* 2009;22(1):1-23.
2. Ganesan G. How to assess mitral stenosis by echo—a step-by-step approach. *J Indian Acad Echocardiogr Cardiovasc Imaging.* 2017;1(3):197-205.

# 19 | HEMODYNAMIC CALCULATIONS

Martin Ingi Sigurdsson and Nathan H. Waldron

1. An echocardiographic assessment of left ventricular (LV) output revealed HR 100/min, BP 130/76 mm Hg, and LV outflow tract velocity time integral (LVOT VTI) 10 cm. Following this a bolus of 500 cc of crystalloid was given. Reassessment shows HR 95/min, BP 128/78 mm Hg, and LVOT VTI 12.5 cm. What statement best describes the volume responsiveness of the patient?

   A. The patient is not volume responsive given minimum change in blood pressure.
   B. The patient is considered to be volume responsive based on the change in VTI.
   C. The patient is not volume responsive based on the change in VTI.
   D. Measurement of the LVOT radius is not needed to calculate cardiac output (CO).

2. A patient in mixed cardiogenic and septic shock is assessed by echocardiography. HR is 120/min, mean arterial pressure (MAP) is 70 mm Hg, central venous pressure (CVP) is 10 mm Hg, LVOT diameter is 2.0 cm, and LVOT VTI is 20 cm. What is the patient's systemic vascular resistance (SVR)?

   A. 637 dynes $\times$ sec $\times$ cm$^{-5}$
   B. 742 dynes $\times$ sec $\times$ cm$^{-5}$
   C. 159 dynes $\times$ sec $\times$ cm$^{-5}$
   D. 1152 dynes $\times$ sec $\times$ cm$^{-5}$

3. An adult male patient in mixed cardiogenic and septic shock is assessed by echocardiography. HR is 80 mm Hg, MAP is 50 mm Hg, CVP is 15 mm Hg, LVOT diameter is 2.0 cm, and LVOT VTI is 12 cm. There is no increase in LVOT VTI with a passive leg raise, no valvulopathies are identified, and there are no signs of pericardial tamponade. What is the appropriate next step in his treatment?

   A. Give a 1 L fluid bolus
   B. Initiate esmolol infusion
   C. Initiate norepinephrine infusion
   D. Initiate dobutamine infusion

4. Following the original treatment chosen for the patient in **Question 3**, the patient remains hypotensive. HR is 100, MAP is 55 mm Hg, CVP is 15 mm Hg, LVOT diameter is 2.0 cm, LVOT VTI is 20 cm, and other echocardiographic findings are unchanged. What is the logical next step?

   A. Give 1 L fluid bolus
   B. Initiate esmolol infusion
   C. Initiate norepinephrine infusion
   D. Increase dobutamine infusion

5. A hypotensive patient is evaluated for the etiology of shock. HR is 100/min, MAP is 55 mm Hg, LVOT diameter is 1.8 cm, LVOT VTI is 26 cm, and inferior vena cava (IVC) diameter is 2.4 cm without respiratory variation. What is the most likely etiology of this patient's shock?

   A. Hypovolemic shock
   B. Obstructive shock
   C. Distributive shock
   D. Cardiogenic shock

6. A patient has the following quantification of their intracardiac shunt: LVOT diameter 2.0 cm, LVOT VTI 22 cm, MAP 70 mm Hg, right ventricular outflow tract (RVOT) diameter 2.4 cm, RVOT VTI 24 cm. Which shunt physiology, among the following, could explain this quantification?

   A. Atrial septal defect with left → right shunt
   B. It cannot be determined without HR
   C. Patent foramen ovale with right → left shunt
   D. Ventricular septal defect with right → left shunt

7. **Figure 19.1** shows a continuous VTI assessment over the LVOT in a mechanically ventilated patient in sinus rhythm.

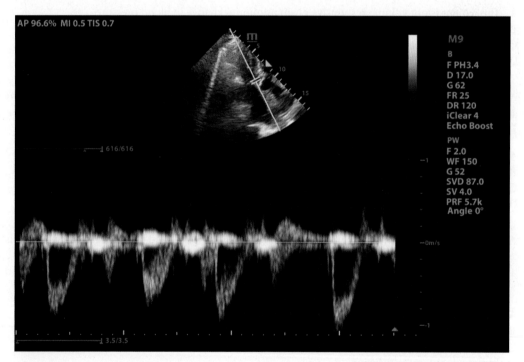

**Figure 19.1**

2D assessment ruled out tamponade and RV failure. What hemodynamic assessment can be made based on the tracing?

A. The patient is likely fluid responsive.
B. Fluid responsiveness cannot be predicted based on the image.
C. The patient has low LV ejection fraction.
D. The patient has a high afterload.

8. **Figure 19.2** shows a continuous Doppler pulse wave assessment of the VTI in the LVOT during a respiratory cycle in a mechanically ventilated patient with a prior history of chronic heart failure admitted currently in septic shock.

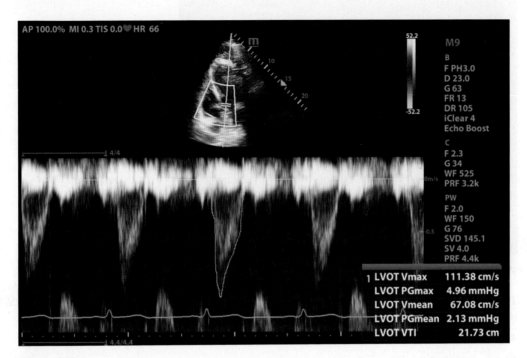

**Figure 19.2**

The patient is in a sinus rhythm. 2D assessment ruled out tamponade and RV failure. Following a fluid bolus of 1000 cc, the $VTI_{LVOT}$ is reassessed and changes by 5% during the respiratory cycle. The patient is still hypotensive and the average $LVOT_{VTI}$ is 21 cm, the LVOT diameter is 2 cm, and the HR is 66/min. What is the next appropriate step?

A. Administer another fluid bolus since the patient is still fluid responsive
B. Administer a diuretic, the patient is now fluid overloaded
C. Initiate an inotrope
D. Initiate a vasopressor

9. A patient with a pulmonary artery (PA) catheter and continuous CO measurement has a measured SVR of 2200 dynes ×sec × cm$^{-5}$, MAP of 80 mm Hg, CVP of 10 mm Hg, LVOT diameter of 2 cm, and LVOT VTI of 10 cm. What is their HR?

A. 75/min
B. 51/min
C. 101/min
D. 81/min

10. **Figure 19.3** is a still from a continuous wave Doppler assessment of the blood flow through a stenotic aortic valve in a critically ill patient.

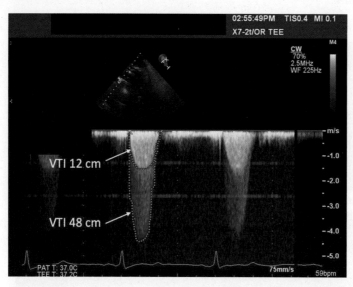

**Figure 19.3**

The LVOT diameter is 2.0 cm and the HR is 80/min, and the patient's body surface area is 1.9 m². What is the cardiac index?

A. 3.00 L/min/m²
B. 1.59 L/min/m²
C. 6.36 L/min/m²
D. 2.54 L/min/m²

11. A patient with known nonischemic cardiomyopathy presents to the intensive care unit (ICU) with hypotension in the setting of a urinary tract infection. A harsh systolic murmur is auscultated. Transthoracic echocardiography is performed and the following values measured from an apical view:

- Aortic valve peak velocity: 2.7 m/s
- Aortic valve peak gradient: 29.2 mm Hg
- LVOT peak velocity: 0.54 m/s
- LVOT peak gradient: 1.2 mm Hg

What is the grade of this patient's aortic stenosis?

A. This patient does not have aortic stenosis.
B. Mild, as the peak velocity is 2.7 m/s
C. Moderate, as the peak gradient is 29.2 mm Hg
D. Severe, as the velocity ratio is 0.2

12. A patient with known nonischemic cardiomyopathy presents to the ICU with hypotension in the setting of a urinary tract infection. A harsh systolic murmur is auscultated. Transthoracic echocardiography is performed and the following values measured from both apical and parasternal views:

- Aortic valve VTI: 116 cm
- LVOT VTI: 16 cm
- LVOT diameter: 3.0 cm
- Aortic valve peak velocity: 3.8 m/s

What is the grade of this patient's aortic stenosis?

**A.** This patient does not have aortic stenosis.
**B.** Moderate, as the peak velocity is 3.8 m/s
**C.** Moderate, as the aortic valve area is 1.3 cm$^2$
**D.** Severe, as the aortic valve area is 0.97cm$^2$

---

**13.** A patient presents to the ICU after elective mitral valve repair with an annuloplasty ring and posterior leaflet resection for fibroelastic deficiency. Shortly after arrival, the patient becomes hypotensive and tachycardic. A transesophageal echocardiography probe is placed. The aortic valve is noted to open without signs of aortic stenosis. Additionally, the following hemodynamic variables are obtained:

- Aortic valve peak velocity: 3.1 m/s
- Mitral regurgitation jet peak velocity: 5.8 m/s
- HR: 116 /min, regular
- LVOT diameter: 2 cm
- Aortic valve diameter: 2.4 cm

What is the cause of this patient's decompensation?

**A.** Residual mitral regurgitation causing flash pulmonary edema
**B.** Aortic dissection
**C.** LVOT obstruction
**D.** Postoperative atrial fibrillation with rapid ventricular response

---

**14.** What is the CO of the patient from **Question 13**?

**A.** 3.68 L/min
**B.** 7.36 L/min
**C.** 5.3 L/min
**D.** Unable to calculate with the numbers provided

---

**15.** A 61-year-old patient with normal LV function and a body surface area of 2.2 m$^2$ undergoes a three-vessel coronary artery bypass grafting procedure. Due to a history of gastric bypass surgery, a transesophageal echocardiography probe is not placed for the procedure. Hemodynamics throughout the procedure are uneventful. Two hours after ICU arrival, plethysmography reads an oxygen saturation of 87%, and initial blood gas reveals a PaO$_2$ of 54 mm Hg. Chest radiography shows a small left pleural effusion, no pneumothorax, and no significant infiltrates. Secretions are scant. Transthoracic echocardiography yields the following values:

- HR: 79/min
- LVOT VTI: 21.2 cm
- LVOT diameter: 2.9 cm
- RVOT VTI: 28.4 cm
- RVOT diameter: 2.1 cm

What is the most likely cause of this patient's hypoxemia?

**A.** Pneumonia
**B.** Right-to-left shunting with a $\dfrac{Qp}{Qs}$ of 0.70
**C.** Left-to-right shunting with a $\dfrac{Qp}{Qs}$ of 1.42
**D.** Right-to-left shunting with a $\dfrac{Qp}{Qs}$ of 0.56

16. A 67-year-old man is admitted to the ICU with septic shock from a presumed urinary source. His past medical history is notable for a long-standing history of cardiac murmur, recent non-ST elevation myocardial infarction (NSTEMI) treated with a drug-eluting stent, 80 pack-year smoking history, moderate chronic obstructive pulmonary disease (COPD), and benign prostatic hypertrophy. A central line is placed due to hypotension and requirement for norepinephrine, and the patient is intubated due to worsening mental status and hypoxemia. Due to persistent hypotension despite increasing doses of norepinephrine, a comprehensive transthoracic echocardiogram is performed, and the following values are obtained:

- LV end-diastolic volume: 127.8 mL
- LV end-systolic volume: 79.6 mL
- Systemic blood pressure: 86/42 mm Hg
- HR: 61/min
- Tricuspid regurgitation peak velocity: 3.9 m/s
- Right atrial pressure (measured from tip of central line): 12 mm Hg
- Pulmonic regurgitation early diastolic velocity: 2.9 m/s
- Pulmonic regurgitation end-diastolic velocity: 1.8 m/s
- Aortic regurgitation end-diastolic velocity: 1.6 m/s

Additionally, the sonographer mentions that the right ventricle is mildly to moderately dysfunctional. What is the estimated RV systolic pressure (RVSP) for this patient?

A. 72.8 mm Hg
B. 27.6 mm Hg
C. Cannot be calculated with the information provided
D. 60.8 mm Hg

17. What is the estimated mean PA pressure for the patient in **Question 16**?

A. 25.0 mm Hg
B. 21.6 mm Hg
C. Cannot be calculated with the information provided
D. 45.6 mm Hg

18. What is the estimated LV end-diastolic pressure (LVEDP) for the patient in **Question 16**?

A. 52.24 mm Hg
B. 42 mm Hg
C. Cannot be calculated with the information provided
D. 31.8 mm Hg

19. What is the estimated LV ejection fraction for the patient in **Question 16**?

A. 60.6%
B. 37.7%
C. Cannot be calculated with the information provided
D. 55%

20. Given the information provided and the hemodynamic calculations performed, what might be a reasonable next step to treat the patient's hypotension in **Question 16**?

A. Administer 1 L balanced crystalloid fluid bolus
B. Initiate a milrinone infusion
C. Initiate an epinephrine infusion
D. Initiate a phenylephrine infusion

# Chapter 19 ▪ Answers

**1.** Correct Answer: B. The patient is considered to be volume responsive based on the change in VTI.

*Rationale:* CO can be quantified using echocardiography by using the equation

$$CO = VTI_{LVOT} \times r^2_{LVOT} \times \pi \times HR$$

where VTI is the velocity time integral of the LVOT, $r$ is the radius of the LVOT, and HR is the heart rate. Since the diameter of the LVOT presumably does not change with a fluid bolus, changes in CO can be assessed by change in HR and the VTI alone. Here, the total change was $\frac{125 \times 95}{100 \times 100} = 1.19$, indicating that the stroke volume increased by 19% with the fluid bolus. This patient would therefore be considered fluid responsive (more than 15% increase in CO).

### Selected References
1. Lamia B, Ochagavia A, Monnet X, Chemla D, Richard C, Teboul JL. Echocardiographic prediction of volume responsiveness in critically ill patients with spontaneously breathing activity. *Intensive Care Med.* 2007 Jul;33(7):1125-1132. doi: 10.1007/s00134-007-0646-7. Epub 2007 May 17. PMID: 17508199.
2. Miller A, Mandeville J. Predicting and measuring fluid responsiveness with echocardiography. *Echo Res Pract.* 2016;3:G1-G12.

**2.** Correct Answer: A. 637 $dynes \times sec \times cm^{-5}$

*Rationale:* CO can be quantified using echocardiography by using the equation

$$CO = VTI_{LVOT} \times r^2_{LVOT} \times \pi \times HR$$

where VTI is the time velocity time integral of the LVOT, $r$ is the radius of the LVOT, and HR is the heart rate. Using the given values, CO=20 cm ×(1 cm)$^2$× $\pi$ × 120 beats/min= 7536 cm$^3$/min= 7.54 L/min

Using Ohm's equation MAP–CVP = CO × SVR and a conversion factor of 80 to convert from peripheral resistance units to the more traditional centimeter-gram-second units (dynes × sec × cm$^{-5}$), we can therefore calculate $SVR = 80 \times \frac{MAP - CVP}{CO} = 80 \times \frac{70 - 10}{7.54} = 637$ dynes × sec × cm$^{-5}$. This patient's SVR is therefore slightly reduced, suggesting that a vasopressor rather than an inotrope would be helpful for management of his shock.

### Selected Reference
1. Miller A, Mandeville J. Predicting and measuring fluid responsiveness with echocardiography. *Echo Res Pract.* 2016;3:G1-G12.

**3.** Correct Answer: D. Initiate dobutamine infusion

*Rationale:* CO can be quantified using echocardiography by using the equation

$$CO = VTI_{LVOT} \times r^2_{LVOT} \times \pi \times HR$$

where VTI is the velocity time integral of the LVOT, $r$ is the radius of the LVOT, and HR is the heart rate. Using the given values, $CO = 12$ cm $\times (1cm)^2 \times \pi \times 80$ beats/min = 3014 cm$^3$/min = 3.0 L/min· The average body surface area of an adult male is 1.9 m$^2$, giving a cardiac index of 1.57 L/min/m$^2$. Using Ohm's equation $MAP - CVP = CO \times SVR$ and a conversion factor of 80 to convert from peripheral resistance units to the more traditional centimeter-gram-second units (dynes × sec × cm$^{-5}$), we can calculate $SVR = 80 \times \frac{MAP - CVP}{CO} = 80 \times \frac{50 - 15}{3.0} = 933$ dynes × sec × cm$^{-5}$. This patient's SVR is therefore normal but the CO is severely reduced, suggesting that an inotrope such as dobutamine would be an appropriate next step in treatment.

### Selected Reference
1. Miller A, Mandeville J. Predicting and measuring fluid responsiveness with echocardiography. *Echo Res Pract.* 2016;3:G1-G12.

**4.** Correct Answer: C. Initiate norepinephrine infusion

*Rationale:* CO can be quantified using echocardiography by using the equation

$$CO = VTI_{LVOT} \times r^2_{LVOT} \times \pi \times HR$$

where VTI is the velocity time integral of the LVOT, $r$ is the radius of the LVOT, and HR is the heart rate. Using the given values, CO = 20 cm $\times$ (1 cm)$^2$ $\times$ $\pi$ $\times$ 100 beats/min = 6280 cm$^3$/min = 6.3 L/min. The average body surface area of an adult male is 1.9 m$^2$, giving a cardiac index of 3.31 L/m$^2$. Using Ohm's equation $MAP - CVP = CO \times SVR$ and a conversion factor of 80 to convert from peripheral resistance units to the more traditional centimeter-gram-second units ($dynes \times sec \times cm^{-5}$), we can calculate $SVR = 80 \times \dfrac{MAP - CVP}{CO} = 80 \times \dfrac{55 - 15}{6.3} = 508$ dynes $\times$ sec $\times$ cm$^{-5}$. This patient's SVR is therefore low but the patient's CO is in the normal range, suggesting that the patient is vasodilated. A vasopressor such as norepinephrine would be an appropriate next step in treatment.

### Selected References

1. Miller A, Mandeville J. Predicting and measuring fluid responsiveness with echocardiography. *Echo Res Pract.* 2016;3:G1-G12.
2. Porter TR, Shillcutt SK, Adams MS, et al. Guidelines for the use of echocardiography as a monitor for therapeutic intervention in adults: a report from the American Society of Echocardiography. *J Am Soc Echocardiogr.* 2015;28:40-56.

**5.** Correct Answer: C. Distributive shock

*Rationale:* CO can be quantified using echocardiography by using the equation

$$CO = VTI_{LVOT} \times r^2_{LVOT} \times \pi \times HR$$

where VTI is the velocity time integral of the LVOT, $r$ is the radius of the LVOT, and HR is the heart rate. Using the given values, CO=26 cm $\times$ (0.9 cm)$^2$ $\times$ $\pi$ $\times$ 100 beats/min = 6612 cm$^3$/min = 6.6 L/min. Given an IVC size of 2.4 cm without a respiratory variation, CVP can be estimated as 15 (10-20) mm Hg. Using Ohm's equation $MAP - CVP = CO \times SVR$ and a conversion factor of 80 to convert from peripheral resistance units to the more traditional centimeter-gram-second units ($dynes \times sec \times cm^{-5}$), we can calculate $SVR = 80 \times \dfrac{MAP - CVP}{CO} = 80 \times \dfrac{55 - 15}{6.6} = 484$ dynes $\times$ sec $\times$ cm$^{-5}$. This patient's right-sided cardiac filling pressure is therefore normal/high, CO is normal/high but SVR is low, suggestive of distributive shock.

### Selected References

1. Miller A, Mandeville J. Predicting and measuring fluid responsiveness with echocardiography. *Echo Res Pract.* 2016;3:G1-G12.
2. Porter TR, Shillcutt SK, Adams MS, et al. Guidelines for the use of echocardiography as a monitor for therapeutic intervention in adults: a report from the American Society of Echocardiography. *J Am Soc Echocardiogr.* 2015;28:40-56.

**6.** Correct Answer: A. Atrial septal defect with left → right shunt

*Rationale:* CO can be quantified using echocardiography by using the equation

$$CO = VTI_{LVOT} \times r^2_{LVOT} \times \pi \times HR$$

This can be done on both the right and left sides of the heart, and if done with the same HR measurements, VTI and radius of LVOT and RVOT can be used to assess intracardiac shunts. Here, both the diameter and VTI of the RVOT are larger than the LVOT, indicating that blood flow through the RVOT is more than the blood flow through the LVOT. This indicates that blood is flowing from the left side of the heart to the right side of the heart prior to the LVOT, making atrial septal defect with left-to-right shunt the most likely answer.

### Selected References

1. Miller A, Mandeville J. Predicting and measuring fluid responsiveness with echocardiography. *Echo Res Pract.* 2016;3:G1-G12.
2. Porter TR, Shillcutt SK, Adams MS, et al. Guidelines for the use of echocardiography as a monitor for therapeutic intervention in adults: a report from the American Society of Echocardiography. *J Am Soc Echocardiogr.* 2015;28:40-56.

**7.** Correct Answer: A. The patient is likely fluid responsive.

*Rationale:* Figure 19.1 shows a continuous VTI assessment of the LVOT during a full respiratory cycle. This reveals that $V_{max}$, the maximum velocity obtained during each contraction, changes by at least 20% during the respiratory cycle (where $V_{max}$ increases during inspiration). This indicates that the patient has a substantial stroke volume variation and is likely fluid responsive.

Selected Reference
1. Miller A, Mandeville J. Predicting and measuring fluid responsiveness with echocardiography. *Echo Res Pract.* 2016;3:G1-G12.

**8.** Correct Answer: D. Initiate a vasopressor

*Rationale:* Figure 19.2 shows a continuous VTI assessment of the LVOT during a full respiratory cycle. This reveals that $V_{max}$, the maximum velocity obtained during each contraction, changes by at least 20% during the respiratory cycle (where $V_{max}$ increases during inspiration). This indicates that the patient has substantial stroke volume variation and is likely fluid responsive. After a fluid bolus the $VTI_{LVOT}$ variability goes down to 5% (VTI and $V_{max}$ can both be used). Therefore the patient is likely no longer fluid responsive. The calculated CO is, $CO = VTI_{LVOT} \times r^2_{LVOT} \times \pi \times HR = 16 \times 1 \times \pi \times 100 = 4.3$ L/min. This is likely an adequate CO, hence a vasopressor is a logical next choice.

Selected Reference
1. Miller A, Mandeville J. Predicting and measuring fluid responsiveness with echocardiography. *Echo Res Pract.* 2016;3:G1-G12.

**9.** Correct Answer: D. 81/min

*Rationale:* Using Ohms equation $MAP - CVP = CO \times SVR$ and a conversion factor of 80 to convert from peripheral resistance units to the more traditional centimeter-gram-second units (dynes $\times$ sec $\times$ cm$^{-5}$), we can calculate $CO = 80 \times \dfrac{MAP - CVP}{SVR} = 80 \times \dfrac{80 - 10}{2200} = 2.54 \dfrac{L}{min} = 2540$ cc/min.

CO (in cc/min) can be quantified using echocardiography by using the equation

$$CO = VTI_{LVOT} \times r^2_{LVOT} \times \pi \times HR$$

where VTI is the velocity time integral of the LVOT, $r$ is the radius of the LVOT, and HR is the heart rate. Using the given numbers $HR = \dfrac{CO}{VTI_{LVOT} \times r^2_{LVOT} \times \pi} = \dfrac{2540}{10 \times 1^2 \times \pi} = 81$/min.

Selected Reference
1. Miller A, Mandeville J. Predicting and measuring fluid responsiveness with echocardiography. *Echo Res Pract.* 2016;3:G1-G12.

**10.** Correct Answer: B. 1.59 L/min/m$^2$

*Rationale:* CO can be quantified using echocardiography by using the equation

$$CO = VTI_{LVOT} \times r^2_{LVOT} \times \pi \times HR$$

Figure 19.3 shows a "double envelope" flow through a stenotic aortic valve, where one pattern (smaller envelope) of dense velocities describes the flow in the LVOT and the second flow pattern (larger envelope) describes the increased velocity flow through the stenotic valve. Therefore the VTI through the LVOT is the smaller envelope and $CO = 12 \times 1^2 \times \pi \times 80 = 3014$ cc/min $= 3.0$ L/min. Given the surface area of 1.9 m$^2$, the cardiac index is $CI = \dfrac{CO}{BSA} = \dfrac{3.0}{1.9} = 1.59$ L/min/m$^2$.

Selected Reference
1. Miller A, Mandeville J. Predicting and measuring fluid responsiveness with echocardiography. *Echo Res Pract.* 2016;3:G1-G12.

**11.** Correct Answer: D. Severe, as the velocity ratio is 0.2

*Rationale:* There are a number of ways to quantify the severity of aortic stenosis, including peak and mean gradients, planimetry, calculation of the aortic valve area using the continuity equation, and utilization of the velocity ratio or dimensionless index. One advantage to the velocity ratio, expressed as $\text{Velocity}^{\text{LVOT}}/\text{Velocity}^{\text{AorticValve}}$, is that it is less variable in terms of grading than the continuity equation. In this case, the velocity ratio is $0.54/2.7 = 0.2$, indicating that this patient has severe aortic stenosis.

Selected Reference
1. Baumgartner H, Hung J, Bermejo J, et al. Recommendations on the echocardiographic assessment of aortic valve stenosis: a focused update from the European Association of Cardiovascular Imaging and the American Society of Echocardiography. *J Am Soc Echocardiogr.* 2017;30(4):372-392.

**12.** Correct Answer: D. Severe, as the aortic valve area is 0.97 cm$^2$

*Rationale:* There are a number of ways to quantify the severity of aortic stenosis, including peak and mean gradients, planimetry, calculation of the aortic valve area using the continuity equation, and utilization of the velocity ratio or dimensionless index. In this case, the necessary data to calculate the aortic valve area via the continuity equation are included. Here, the equation takes advantage of the principle of conservation of mass, whereby $\text{Area}^{\text{Aortic Valve}} \times \text{VTI}^{\text{Aortic Valve}} = \text{Area}^{\text{LVOT}} \times \text{VTI}^{\text{LVOT}}$, which can be rearranged to $\text{Area}^{\text{Aortic Valve}} = \text{Area}^{\text{LVOT}} \times \text{VTI}^{\text{LVOT}}/\text{VTI}^{\text{Aortic Valve}}$. Because area $= \pi \times r^2$ and VTIs are provided, $\text{AVA} = 7.065 \times 16/116 = 0.97$ cm$^2$.

Selected Reference
1. Baumgartner H, Hung J, Bermejo J, et al. Recommendations on the echocardiographic assessment of aortic valve stenosis: a focused update from the European Association of Cardiovascular Imaging and the American Society of Echocardiography. *J Am Soc Echocardiogr.* 2017;30(4):372-392.

**13.** Correct Answer: C. LVOT obstruction

*Rationale:* Sudden decompensation after mitral valve repair should prompt suspicion for LVOT obstruction, often due to redundant anterior mitral leaflet structures causing systolic anterior motion (SAM) of the anterior mitral valve leaflet. In this case, an elevated peak velocity in the LVOT (2.9 m/s) points to LVOT obstruction as the cause of decompensation. Another clue is the regular (sinus) tachycardia, likely a compensatory mechanism for decreased CO in the setting of LVOT obstruction. In this case, the peak gradient across the LVOT is 4 (LVOT peak velocity)$^2$, or 29.4 mm Hg, enough to cause hemodynamically significant obstruction in a hypovolemic patient after cardiac surgery.

**14.** Correct Answer: D. Unable to calculate with the numbers provided

*Rationale:* CO can be quantified using echocardiography by using the equation

$$\text{CO} = \text{VTI}_{\text{LVOT}} \times r^2_{\text{LVOT}} \times \pi \times \text{HR}$$

Common mistakes include using measurements at the level of the aortic valve (not commonly as cylindrical) or forgetting to divide the diameter by 2 in order to arrive at the radius. However, due to the presence of an LVOT obstruction, we are unable to calculate CO.

Selected Reference
1. Baumgartner H, Hung J, Bermejo J, et al. Recommendations on the echocardiographic assessment of aortic valve stenosis: a focused update from the European Association of Cardiovascular Imaging and the American Society of Echocardiography. *J Am Soc Echocardiogr.* 2017;30(4):372-392.

**15.** Correct Answer: B. Right-to-left shunting with a Qp/Qs of 0.70

*Rationale:* CO can be quantified using echocardiography by using the equation

$$\text{CO} = \text{VTI}_{\text{LVOT}} \times r^2_{\text{LVOT}} \times \pi \times \text{HR}$$

This can be done on both the right and left sides of the heart, and if done with the same HR, measurements of VTI and radius of LVOT and RVOT can be used to assess intracardiac shunts. Here the right-sided stroke volume can be calculated as 98.3 mL, whereas the left-sided stroke volume can be calculated as 140.0 mL, indicating markedly higher flow through the left side of the heart. In the setting of hypoxemia and without having previously ruled out an intracardiac shunt, the most likely answer here is right-to-left shunting with the Qp/Qs calculated as 0.70.

### Selected References

1. Miller A, Mandeville J. Predicting and measuring fluid responsiveness with echocardiography. *Echo Res Pract*. 2016;3:G1-G12.
2. Porter TR, Shillcutt SK, Adams MS, et al. Guidelines for the use of echocardiography as a monitor for therapeutic intervention in adults: a report from the American Society of Echocardiography. *J Am Soc Echocardiogr*. 2015;28:40-56.

**16.** Correct Answer: A. 72.8 mm Hg

*Rationale:* **Questions 16-18** are governed by the equation $P_{OC} = 4v^2 + P_{RC}$, where OC stands for originating chamber and RC stands for receiving chamber. Additionally, $v$ in this equation is the velocity of the appropriately timed regurgitant jet. If one can correctly identify the originating and receiving chambers, along with which regurgitant jet velocity to measure—typically the jet between the originating and receiving chambers—then one can estimate a number of intracardiac pressures.

RVSP is the pressure in the originating chamber, where the pressure in the receiving chamber (the right atrium) is known and directly measured. Here, the peak velocity of the tricuspid regurgitation jet is the velocity used in the equation. As such, the rearranged equation ($P_{RC} + 4v^2 = P_{OC}$) becomes $12 + 4$ $(3.9^2) = 72.8$ mm Hg.

**17.** Correct Answer: D. 45.6 mm Hg

*Rationale:* The pressure in question is the originating chamber (the PA) in early diastole—an approximation of the mean PA pressure. The regurgitant jet in question is the peak early diastolic velocity of the pulmonic regurgitation jet—2.9 m/s. An additional assumption of this equation is that the right atrial pressure is equivalent to the right ventricular pressure in early diastole. As such, this equation becomes $PA_m = 4(V_{\text{Peak early diastole PI}})^2 + RAP$, which is equal to 45.6 mm Hg.
*For additional details refer to **Answer 19.16**.*

**18.** Correct Answer: D. 31.8 mm Hg

*Rationale:* Here the pressure in question is the receiving chamber (the left ventricle) where the originating chamber is the aorta, and the regurgitant jet is the end-diastolic velocity of the aortic insufficiency jet. As such, this equation becomes $LVEDP = \text{Diastolic blood pressure} - 4(V_{\text{End-diastolic AI}})^2 = 31.8$ mm Hg.
*For additional details refer to **Answer 19.16**.*

**19.** Correct Answer: B. 37.7%

*Rationale:* Ejection fraction can be calculated as end-diastolic volume – end-systolic volume/end-diastolic volume.

**20.** Correct Answer: C. Initiate an epinephrine infusion

*Rationale:* The patient in **Question 16** has pulmonary hypertension (likely World Health Organization group 3 given long-standing smoking and COPD), right ventricular dysfunction, and aortic insufficiency. They are experiencing no improvement in hemodynamics despite increasing doses of norepinephrine and likely require additional therapy. Given the right ventricular dysfunction and normal right atrial pressure, a crystalloid bolus is not likely to significantly improve hemodynamics and should be given as part of a fluid challenge regimen with pre- and postmeasurements if administered. Milrinone may improve CO but given the preexisting hypotension, it could significantly worsen hemodynamics. Phenylephrine is unlikely to meaningfully impact hemodynamics in a patient receiving escalating doses of norepinephrine. Epinephrine has the benefits of increasing chronotropy—helpful to minimize regurgitant fraction in aortic insufficiency—and improving right ventricular performance.

# 20 | QUANTIFICATION CALCULATIONS

Martin Ingi Sigurdsson and Nathan H. Waldron

1. A patient's left ventricular end systolic volume is 30 mL and end diastolic volume is 72 mL. What is the patient's left ventricular ejection fraction (LVEF)?

   A. 32%
   B. 58%
   C. 42%
   D. 42%

2. **Figure 20.1** shows an M-mode with the focal line through the annular plane and two measurements of the position of the tricuspid annulus in systole and diastole relative to the probe. What is the tricuspid annular plane systolic excursion (TAPSE) measurement and the right ventricular (RV) function based on this measurement?

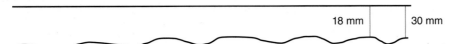

18 mm    30 mm

**Figure 20.1**

   A. TAPSE is 12 mm, RV function is reduced
   B. TAPSE is 18 mm, RV function is normal
   C. TAPSE is 12 mm, RV function is normal
   D. TAPSE is 18 mm, RV function is reduced

3. **Figure 20.2** shows a continuous-wave Doppler assessment through the left ventricular outflow tract (LVOT) and aortic valve. Which of the following statements is correct regarding the aortic valve?

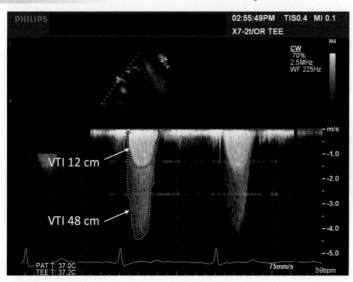

PHILIPS 02:55:49PM TIS0.4 MI 0.1
X7-2t/OR TEE
M4
CW
70%
2.5MHz
WF 225Hz

VTI 12 cm

VTI 48 cm

PAT T: 37.0C
TEE T: 37.2C          75mm/s          59bpm

**Figure 20.2**

A. Maximum gradient over the aortic valve is 16 mm Hg
B. Maximum gradient over the aortic valve is 32 mm Hg
C. Maximum gradient over the aortic valve is 48 mm Hg
D. Maximum gradient over the aortic valve is 64 mm Hg

4. Figure 20.2 shows a continuous-wave Doppler assessment through the LVOT and aortic valve. Which of the following statements is correct regarding the assessment of the aortic valve?

A. Dimensionless index is 0.25, supporting a diagnosis of severe aortic stenosis
B. Dimensionless index is 0.25, supporting a diagnosis of mild aortic stenosis
C. Dimensionless index is 4, supporting a diagnosis of severe aortic stenosis
D. Dimensionless index is 1, supporting a diagnosis of severe aortic stenosis

5. Figure 20.2 shows a continuous-wave Doppler assessment through the LVOT and aortic valve. The LVOT diameter is 2.0 cm. What is the aortic valve area?

A. $0.49 \text{ cm}^2$
B. $0.79 \text{ cm}^2$
C. $0.99 \text{ cm}^2$
D. $3.14 \text{ cm}^2$

6. The following measurements were performed for assessment of aortic valve stenosis: LVOT diameter 2.4 cm, aortic valve annulus (AVA) 2.5 cm, LVOT velocity time integral (VTI) 10 cm, aortic valve VTI 32 cm, and aortic valve max velocity 3.5 m/s. What is the correct statement regarding the aortic valve stenosis assessment?

A. Valve area of $1.41 \text{ cm}^2$ and max velocity of 3.5 m/s support moderate aortic stenosis
B. Valve area of $1.41 \text{ cm}^2$ and max velocity of 3.5 m/s support mild aortic stenosis
C. Valve area of $0.91 \text{ cm}^2$ and max velocity of 3.5 m/s support moderate aortic stenosis
D. Valve area of $2.36 \text{ cm}^2$ and max velocity of 3.5 m/s support mild aortic stenosis

7. **Figure 20.3** shows a continuous-wave Doppler analysis of blood flow through an insufficient aortic valve in diastole (blue triangle). Which statement accurately describes the quantification of aortic regurgitation (AR)?

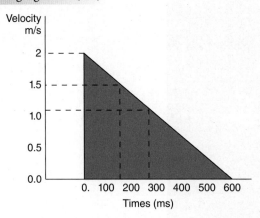

**Figure 20.3**

A. The pressure half-time is 300 ms, supporting moderate AR
B. The pressure half-time is 300 ms, supporting severe AR
C. The pressure half-time is 180 ms, supporting moderate AR
D. The pressure half-time is 180 ms, supporting severe AR

8. **Figure 20.4** shows a continuous-wave Doppler analysis of blood flow through a stenotic mitral valve (blue triangle). Which statement accurately describes the quantification of mitral stenosis?

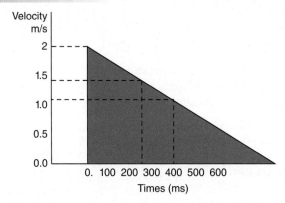

**Figure 20.4**

A. Pressure half-time of 240 ms supports moderate mitral stenosis
B. Pressure half-time of 240 ms supports severe mitral stenosis
C. Pressure half-time of 400 ms supports moderate mitral stenosis
D. Pressure half-time of 400 ms supports severe mitral stenosis

9. The following assessment is performed to quantify pulmonary artery systolic pressure: inferior vena cava (IVC) is 2.4 cm without a respiratory variation, $V_{max}$ of the tricuspid regurgitation jet during systole is 4.8 m/s, and $V_{mean}$ of the tricuspid regurgitation jet during systole is 3 m/s. What is the estimated pulmonary artery systolic pressure?

A. 95 mm Hg
B. 107 mm Hg
C. 36 mm Hg
D. 51 mm Hg

10. The following assessment is performed: central venous pressure (CVP) is 8 mm Hg, velocity of the pulmonary regurgitation jet at end diastole is 2 m/s, and $V_{mean}$ of the tricuspid regurgitation jet during systole is 3 m/s. What is the estimated pulmonary artery diastolic pressure?

   A. 8 mm Hg
   B. 24 mm Hg
   C. 36 mm Hg
   D. 54 mm Hg

11. An 87-year-old patient with severe chronic obstructive pulmonary disease (COPD) and dementia undergoes transcatheter aortic valve implantation. The procedure is uneventful, though the postoperative echocardiogram (**Figure 20.5**) demonstrates the following on short-axis view of the aortic valve during diastole.

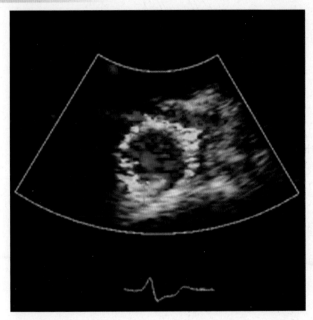

**Figure 20.5**

What is the grade of paravalvular leak (PVL) during this procedure?
A. None
B. Mild
C. Moderate
D. Severe

**12.** A 76-year-old male presents to the intensive care unit (ICU) from the Emergency Department with sudden-onset shortness of breath. A transthoracic echocardiogram is performed, which yields the following values:

LVOT diameter: 23 mm
Mitral annular diameter: 35 mm
VTI LVOT (in systole): 14 cm
VTI mitral valve (in diastole): 19 cm
VTI of mitral regurgitation (MR) jet: 170 cm
What is the stroke volume across the aortic valve?
A. 58 mL
B. 79 mL
C. 183 mL
D. 172 mL

**13.** What is the stroke volume across the mitral valve of the patient in Question 20.12?

A. 58 mL
B. 79 mL
C. 183 mL
D. 172 mL

**14.** What is the regurgitant volume across the mitral valve of the patient in Question 20.12?

A. 11 mL
B. 125 mL
C. 104 mL
D. Cannot be calculated from the information provided

**15.** What is the regurgitant fraction and grade of MR of the patient in Question 20.12?

A. 6%, mild
B. 68%, severe
C. 57%, severe
D. Cannot be calculated from the information provided

**16.** What is the effective regurgitant orifice area (EROA) of the mitrar regurgitation (MR) lesion of the patient in Question 20.12?

A. 0.74 cm$^2$
B. 0.61 cm$^2$
C. 0.58 cm$^2$
D. Cannot be calculated from the information provided

**17.** An 80-year-old female is evaluated for aortic valve stenosis. She has an LVEF of 40% on visual assessment. The mean pressure gradient across the valve is 30 mm Hg. Her LVOT diameter is 1.8 cm$^2$, the peak velocity through the aortic valve is 3 m/s, and the peak velocity through the LVOT is 0.8 m/s. What is the aortic valve area?

A. 0.49 cm$^2$
B. 0.68 cm$^2$
C. 2.71 cm$^2$
D. 3.14 cm$^2$

18. What is the mismatch in the criteria for aortic stenosis for the patient described in Question 20.17?

   A. Severe aortic stenosis by mean gradient, moderate aortic stenosis by aortic valve area
   B. Severe aortic stenosis by peak gradient, moderate aortic stenosis by aortic valve area
   C. Moderate aortic stenosis by mean gradient, severe aortic stenosis by aortic valve area
   D. Moderate aortic stenosis by peak gradient, moderate aortic stenosis by aortic valve area

19. What is the most likely reason for mismatch between the various criteria for aortic stenosis severity for the patient described in Question 20.17?

   A. Small size of the patient resulting in an abnormally small valve area compared to the peak velocity and mean gradient
   B. Small size of the LVOT resulting in an abnormally small valve area compared to the peak velocity and mean gradient
   C. Low ejection fraction, resulting in an incorrect assessment of valve area using the continuity equation
   D. Low ejection fraction, resulting in an abnormally small velocity and gradient compared to the valve area

20. Cardiac output via both right and left heart is performed in a patient with AR. The measurements are: right ventricular outflow tract (RVOT) diameter 2.6 cm, RVOT VTI: 14 cm, LVOT diameter 2.0 cm, LVOT VTI 27 cm. What is the severity of AR?

   A. Mild AR
   B. Moderate AR
   C. Severe AR
   D. Cannot be calculated from the information provided

# Chapter 20 ▪ Answers

1. Correct Answer: B. 58%

*Rationale:* Measurement of LVEF when end systolic (LVESV) and end diastolic (LVEDV) volumes have been measured via 3D echocardiography or Simpson disks by the formula:

$$LVEF = \frac{LVEDV - LVESV}{LVEDV} = \frac{72 - 30}{72} = 58\%$$

Selected Reference
1. Lang RM, Badano LP, Mor-Avi V et al. Recommendations for cardiac chamber quantification by echocardiography in adults: an update from the American Society of Echocardiography and the European Association of Cardiovascular Imaging. *Eur Heart J Cardiovasc Imaging.* 2016;17:412.

2. Correct Answer: A. TAPSE is 12 mm, RV function is reduced

*Rationale:* TAPSE is a measurement of the longitudinal movement of the right ventricle during systole that correlates with overall RV function. This is measured by aligning a M-mode Doppler through the tricuspid annulus and measuring the movement by comparing the position of the annulus in systole and diastole. Here the TAPSE is 30 − 18 = 12 mm. TAPSE values under 16 mm are indicative of reduced RV function.

Selected Reference
1. Lang RM, Badano LP, Mor-Avi V et al. Recommendations for cardiac chamber quantification by echocardiography in adults: an update from the American Society of Echocardiography and the European Association of Cardiovascular Imaging. *Eur Heart J Cardiovasc Imaging.* 2016;17:412.

**3.** Correct Answer: D. Maximum gradient over the aortic valve is 64 mm Hg

*Rationale:* Figure 20.2 shows blood flow through a stenotic aortic valve. The maximum velocity through the stenotic orifice is around 4 m/s, and per the simplified Bernoulli equation this translates to a maximum pressure gradient of $\Delta P = 4v^2 = 4 \times 4^2 = 64 \ mm \ Hg$ over the aortic valve.

Selected Reference
1. Baumgartner H, Hung J, Bermejo J, et al. Recommendations on the echocardiographic assessment of aortic valve stenosis: a focused update from the European Association of Cardiovascular Imaging and the American Society of Echocardiography. *J Am Soc Echocardiogr.* 2017;30:372-392.

**4.** Correct Answer: A. Dimensionless index is 0.25 supporting a diagnosis of severe aortic stenosis

*Rationale:* Figure 20.2 shows blood flow through a stenotic aortic valve. Clearly pictured is a "double envelope" where the smaller envelope describes the blood flow through the LVOT and the larger envelope through the stenotic valve. The ratio of blood flow velocities through the LVOT and the aortic valve is commonly called dimensionless index or velocity ratio and either includes the maximum velocity or the VTI. This ratio ranges from 0 to 1, where a higher ratio indicates a more similar flow velocity through both LVOT and aortic valve, suggesting no marked stenosis. A dimensionless index of 0.25 and less is indicative of severe aortic stenosis.

Selected Reference
1. Baumgartner H, Hung J, Bermejo J, et al. Recommendations on the echocardiographic assessment of aortic valve stenosis: a focused update from the European Association of Cardiovascular Imaging and the American Society of Echocardiography. *J Am Soc Echocardiogr.* 2017;30:372-392.

**5.** Correct Answer: B. 0.79 cm$^2$

*Rationale:* The continuity equation can be used to calculate the aortic valve area given the LVOT diameter as well as a VTI through both the aortic valve and the LVOT. Figure 20.2 shows both integrals, where the smaller and denser envelope represents the LVOT and the larger and less dense envelope represents the aortic valve. Hence, the $AVA = Area_{LVOT} \times \dfrac{VTI_{LVOT}}{VTI_{AV}} = 1^2 \times \pi \times \dfrac{12}{48} = 0.79 \ cm^2$.

Selected Reference
1. Baumgartner H, Hung J, Bermejo J, et al. Recommendations on the echocardiographic assessment of aortic valve stenosis: a focused update from the European Association of Cardiovascular Imaging and the American Society of Echocardiography. *J Am Soc Echocardiogr.* 2017;30:372-392.

**6.** Correct Answer: A. Valve area of 1.41 cm$^2$ and max velocity of 3.5 m/s support moderate aortic stenosis.

*Rationale/Critique:* The continuity equation can be used to calculate the aortic valve area:
$$AVA = Area_{LVOT} \times \dfrac{VTI_{LVOT}}{VTI_{AV}} = 1.2^2 \times \pi \times \dfrac{5}{16} = 1.41 \ cm^2$$

Both this area as well as the max velocity support the assessment of moderate aortic stenosis (see **Table 20.1**).

**Table 20.1 Recommendations for Grading of Aortic Valve Severity by the American Society of Echocardiography (ASE) Guidelines**

|  | Mild | Moderate | Severe |
| --- | --- | --- | --- |
| Peak velocity (m/s) | 2.6-2.9 | 3.0-4.0 | ≥4.0 |
| Mean gradient (mm Hg) | <20 | 20-40 | ≥40 |
| Valve area (cm$^2$) | >1.5 | 1.0-1.5 | <1.0 |
| Velocity ratio (Dimensionless Index) | >0.5 | 0.25-0.50 | <0.25 |

Selected Reference
1. Baumgartner H, Hung J, Bermejo J, et al. Recommendations on the echocardiographic assessment of aortic valve stenosis: a focused update from the European Association of Cardiovascular Imaging and the American Society of Echocardiography. *J Am Soc Echocardiogr.* 2017;30:372-392.

**7.** Correct Answer: D. The pressure half-time is 180 ms supporting severe AR

*Rationale:* Figure 20.3 depicts a continuous-wave Doppler assessment of flow velocity that can be used to quantify pressure half-time. This needs to be converted to pressure to accurately detect the time point (x-axis) where pressure is halved. The peak velocity is 2 m/s, corresponding to a pressure of $P = 4v^2 = 4 \times 2^2 = 16 \, mm \, Hg$ per the simplified Bernoulli equation. Utilizing this equation to calculate the velocity matching 50% of the maximum pressure we find that the corresponding velocity is $v = \sqrt{\dfrac{P}{4}} = \sqrt{\dfrac{8}{4}} = 1.41 \, m/s$. This velocity is reached at approximately 180 ms. Therefore pressure half-time is 180 ms, and this corresponds to severe AR. For AR, pressure half-time of 200-500 ms corresponds to moderate regurgitation and pressure half-time of less than 200 ms corresponds to severe regurgitation.

Selected Reference

1. Zoghbi WA, Adams D, Bonow RO, et al. Recommendations for noninvasive evaluation of native valvular regurgitation: a report from the American Society of Echocardiography developed in collaboration with the Society for Cardiovascular Magnetic Resonance. *J Am Soc Echocardiogr.* 2017;30:303-371.

**8.** Correct Answer: B. Pressure half-time of 240 ms supports severe mitral stenosis.

*Rationale:* Figure 20.4 depicts a continuous-wave Doppler assessment of flow velocity that can be used to quantify pressure half-time. This needs to be converted to pressure to accurately detect the time point (x-axis) where pressure is halved. The peak velocity is 2 m/s, corresponding to a pressure of $P = 4v^2 = 4 \times 2^2 = 16 \, mm \, Hg$ per the simplified Bernoulli equation. Utilizing this equation to calculate the velocity with 50% of the maximum pressure we find that the corresponding velocity is $v = \sqrt{\dfrac{P}{4}} = \sqrt{\dfrac{8}{4}} = 1.41 \, m/s$ This velocity is reached at approximately 240 ms. Therefore, pressure half-time is 240 ms, and this can be converted to estimate effective mitral valve orifice using the equation $MVA = \dfrac{220}{PHT} = \dfrac{220}{240} = 0.91 \, cm^2$, which corresponds to a severely stenotic mitral valve. Quantification of mitral stenosis is shown in **Table 20.2**.

**Table 20.2 Quantification of Mitral Stenosis**

|  | Mild | Moderate | Severe |
| --- | --- | --- | --- |
| Valve area (cm$^2$) | >1.5 | 1.0-1.5 | <1.0 |
| Mean gradient (mm Hg) | <5 | 5-10 | >10 |

Selected Reference

1. Baumgartner H, Hung J, Bermejo J, et al. Echocardiographic assessment of valve stenosis: EAE/ASE recommendations for clinical practice. *J Am Soc Echocardiogr.* 2009;22:1-23; quiz 101-102.

**9.** Correct Answer: B. 107 mm Hg

*Rationale:* The IVC assessment estimates right atrial pressure at 10 to 20 mm Hg, and the $V_{max}$ can be converted to a maximum pressure gradient between the right ventricle and the right atrium of $P = 4v^2 = 4 \times 4.8^2 = 92 \, mm \, Hg$. Thus the peak pulmonary pressure during systole is 15 + 92 = 107 mm Hg.

Selected Reference

1. Zoghbi WA, Adams D, Bonow RO, et al. Recommendations for noninvasive evaluation of native valvular regurgitation: a report from the American Society of Echocardiography developed in collaboration with the Society for Cardiovascular Magnetic Resonance. *J Am Soc Echocardiogr.* 2017;30:303-371.

**10.** Correct Answer: B. 24 mm Hg

*Rationale:* In the presence of pulmonary regurgitation, the pressure gradient during end diastole can be used to quantify diastolic pulmonary pressure, similarly to usage of tricuspid regurgitation to quantify systolic pulmonary pressure. The velocity can be converted to the pressure gradient between the right ventricle and the right atrium (at end diastole), $P = 4v^2 = 4 \times 2^2 = 16 \ mm \ Hg$. Thus, the pulmonary artery diastolic pressure is $8 + 16 = 24$ mm Hg.

Selected Reference

1. Zoghbi WA, Adams D, Bonow RO, et al. Recommendations for noninvasive evaluation of native valvular regurgitation: a report from the American Society of Echocardiography developed in collaboration with the Society for Cardiovascular Magnetic Resonance. *J Am Soc Echocardiogr.* 2017;30:303-371.

**11.** Correct Answer: D. Severe

*Rationale:* In this short-axis view of the aortic valve in diastole, aliasing is depicted outside the valvular ring, indicating a PVL. Though the assessment of PVL after transcatheter aortic valve is complex and multimodal, PVL occupying <10%, 10%-30%, and >30% the circumference of the aortic annulus is typically considered mild, moderate, and severe, respectively, according to Valve Academic Research Consortium (VARC)-2 criteria.

Selected References

1. Geleijnse ML, Di Martino LF, Vletter WB, et al. Limitations and difficulties of echocardiographic short-axis assessment of paravalvular leakage after corevalve transcatheter aortic valve implantation. *Cardiovasc Ultrasound.* 2016 ;14(1):37.
2. Kappetein AP, Head SJ, Généreux P, et al. Updated standardized endpoint definitions for transcatheter aortic valve implantation: the Valve Academic Research Consortium-2 consensus document. *Eur Heart J.* 2012 ;33(19):2403-2418.
3. Zoghbi WA, Asch FM, Bruce C, et al. Guidelines for the evaluation of valvular regurgitation after percutaneous valve repair or replacement. *J Am Soc Echocardiogr.* 2019;32(4):431-475.

**12.** Correct Answer: A. 58 mL

*Rationale:* Quantitative measurements of stroke volume across the LVOT and the mitral valve can be used to grade MR in the absence of other valvular lesions. The following calculations can be used to grade MR in this setting:

$$SV_{LVOT} = CSA_{LVOT} \times VTI_{LVOT} \ = \ \pi \times d^2_{LVOT} \times VTI_{LVOT} \ = \ 58 \ mL$$

$$SV_{mitral} = CSA_{mitral} \times VTI_{mitral} = \pi \times d^2_{mitral} \times VTI_{mitral} \ = \ 183 \ mL$$

$$Regurgitant \ volume = \ SV_{mitral} \ - \ SV_{LVOT} \ = \ 125 \ mL$$

$$Regurgitant \ fraction = Regurgitant \ Volume \ / \ SV_{mitral} \ = \ 68\%$$

$$EROA = Regurgitant \ volume \ / \ VTI_{Regurgitant \ Jet}$$

Selected Reference

1. Zoghbi WA, Adams D, Bonow RO, et al. Recommendations for noninvasive evaluation of native valvular regurgitation: a report from the American Society of Echocardiography developed in collaboration with the Society for Cardiovascular Magnetic Resonance. *J Am Soc Echocardiogr.* 2017;30:303-371.

**13.** Correct Answer: C. 183 mL

See Answer 20.12 for rationale and selected reference.

**14.** Correct Answer: B. 125 mL

See Answer 20.12 for rationale and selected reference.

**15.** Correct Answer: B. 68%

See Answer 20.12 for rationale and selected reference.

**16.** Correct Answer: A. 0.74 cm$^2$

See Answer 20.12 for rationale and selected reference.

**17.** Correct Answer: B. 0.68 cm$^2$

*Rationale:* The simplified continuity equation can be used to calculate the aortic valve area given the LVOT diameter as well as a maximum velocity through the aortic valve and the LVOT. Hence, the

$$AVA = Area_{LVOT} \times \frac{V_{LVOT}}{V_{AV}} = 0.9^2 \times \pi \times \frac{0.8}{3} = 0.68 \ cm^2$$

Selected Reference

1. Baumgartner H, Hung J, Bermejo J, et al. Recommendations on the echocardiographic assessment of aortic valve stenosis: a focused update from the European Association of Cardiovascular Imaging and the American Society of Echocardiography. *J Am Soc Echocardiogr.* 2017;30:372-392.

**18.** Correct Answer: C. Moderate aortic stenosis by mean gradient, severe aortic stenosis by aortic valve area

*Rationale:* $AVA = Area_{LVOT} \times \frac{V_{LVOT}}{V_{AV}} = 0.9^2 \times \pi \times \frac{0.8}{3} = 0.68 \ cm^2$, corresponding to severe aortic stenosis by valve area. However, both the peak velocity (3.0-3.9 m/s) and mean gradient (20-40 mm Hg) are within range for moderate aortic stenosis.

Selected Reference

1. Baumgartner H, Hung J, Bermejo J, et al. Recommendations on the echocardiographic assessment of aortic valve stenosis: a focused update from the European Association of Cardiovascular Imaging and the American Society of Echocardiography. *J Am Soc Echocardiogr.* 2017;30:372-392.

**19.** Correct Answer: C. Low ejection fraction, resulting in an incorrect assessment of valve area using the continuity equation

*Rationale:* This patient represents a classic "low-flow aortic stenosis"—a patient with reduced left ventricular function unable to generate enough pressure with a mean pressure gradient and peak velocity that meets the criteria for severe aortic stenosis, despite a severely reduced aortic valve area. These patients are identified by a mismatch in the severity of peak velocity/mean gradient and an LVEF of 40% or less. Frequently, a dobutamine stress echocardiography is performed to adequately classify the severity of the aortic stenosis in such patients.

Selected Reference

1. Chambers J. Low "gradient", low flow aortic stenosis. *Heart.* 2006;92(4):554-558. doi: 10.1136/hrt.2005.079038 [published Online First: 2006/03/16].

**20.** Correct Answer: A: Mild AR

*Rationale:* Quantitative measurements of stroke volume across the LVOT and RVOT can be used to calculate both regurgitant volume and fraction.

$$SV_{LVOT} = VTI_{LVOT} \times r_{LVOT}^2 \times \pi = 27 \times 1^2 \times \pi = 85 \ mL$$

$$SV_{RVOT} = VTI_{RVOT} \times r_{rVOT}^2 \times \pi = 14 \times 1.3^2 \times \pi = 74 \ mL$$

Regurgitant volume $= SV_{LVOT} - SV_{RVOT} = 85 \ mL - 74 \ mL = 11 \ mL$

Regurgitant fraction $= V_{Regurgitation} - SV_{LVOT} = 11 \frac{mL}{85} mL = 13\%$

This falls under the criteria for mild AR (regurgitant volume <30 mL, regurgitant fraction < 30%). See **Table 20.3**.

**Table 20.3 Criteria for Mild AR**

|  | Mild | Moderate | Severe |
|---|---|---|---|
| Regurgitant volume (mL) | <30 | 30-59 | >59 |
| Regurgitant fraction (%) | <30 | 30-50 | >50 |

### Selected Reference

1. Zoghbi WA, Adams D, Bonow RO, et al. Recommendations for noninvasive evaluation of native valvular regurgitation: a report from the American Society of Echocardiography developed in collaboration with the Society for Cardiovascular Magnetic Resonance. *J Am Soc Echocardiogr*. 2017;30:303-371.

# 21 | QUANTIFICATION OF DIASTOLIC FUNCTION

Shaun L. Thompson and Zeid Kalarikkal

1. A 56-year-old male presents for preoperative evaluation for lung resection. Due to the history of coronary disease, hypertension, and dyspnea on exertion, a transthoracic echocardiogram is ordered. Left ventricular (LV) systolic function is mildly reduced. Which of the following sets of parameters along with an E/A ratio of 1.4 suggests grade II diastolic dysfunction?

   A. E/e′ <14 and left atrial (LA) maximum volume index (VI) <34 mL/m$^2$
   B. Tricuspid regurgitation (TR) jet velocity <2.8 m/s and E/e′ >14
   C. LA maximum VI >34 mL/m$^2$ and TR jet velocity <2.8 m/s
   D. TR jet velocity >2.8 m/s and E/e′ >14

2. A patient presents to the intensive care unit (ICU) in presumed cardiogenic shock. Bedside echocardiography is performed and reveals reduced systolic ejection fraction (EF) of 35%. The intensivist is concerned that there is also diastolic dysfunction and obtains mitral valve inflow velocities shown in **Figure 21.1**.

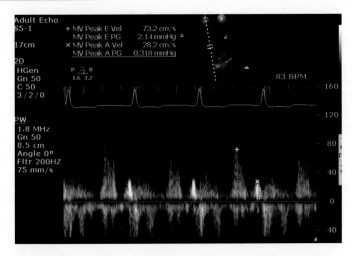

**Figure 21.1** Mitral valve inflow velocities obtained from apical four-chamber view with transthoracic echocardiography.

Based on the information provided, what grade of diastolic dysfunction is present?
   A. Grade I
   B. Grade II
   C. Grade III
   D. None, normal diastolic function is shown in this figure

3. Intraoperative transesophageal echocardiography is requested for a hypotensive patient who is undergoing an anterior approach lumbar laminectomy for spinal stenosis. The patient has no history of heart disease but activity has been limited due to back pain from spinal stenosis. The echo reveals normal systolic function of the left and right ventricles. Mitral inflow velocities show an E/A ratio of 1.2, a TR jet velocity of 1.6 m/s, and an LAVI of 32 mL/m². Tissue Doppler is performed on the lateral aspect of the mitral valve to further investigate diastolic function. Based on **Figure 21.2**, what can be said of this patient's diastolic function?

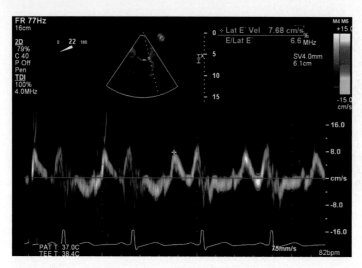

**Figure 21.2** Tissue Doppler velocity of the lateral mitral annulus obtained in four-chamber view with transesophageal echocardiography.

A. Normal
B. Grade I
C. Grade II
D. Grade III

4. A 74-year-old female with a history of congestive heart failure presents to the ICU with new-onset atrial fibrillation. Which of the following findings would be suggestive of elevated LV filling pressure and diastolic dysfunction?

A. Peak acceleration rate of mitral E velocity <1900 cm/s²
B. Mitral deceleration time (DT) of <160 ms
C. E/e′ ratio of <10
D. Isovolumic relaxation time (IVRT) of >70 ms

5. A patient with atrial fibrillation is assessed with echocardiography due to hypotension and concern for hypovolemia and possible septic shock. **Figure 21.3** shows the mitral inflow velocities obtained.

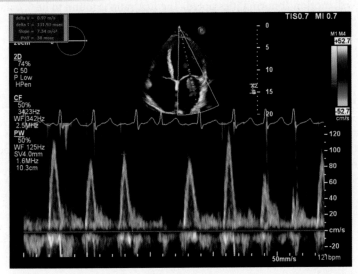

**Figure 21.3** Mitral valve inflow velocities with measurement of mitral deceleration time.

Based on **Figure 21.3**, which of the following is your best assessment of the patient's volume status?
A. Reduced LV end-diastolic pressure
B. Elevated LV end-diastolic pressure
C. Cardiac tamponade
D. LV end-diastolic pressure cannot be measured in atrial fibrillation

6. A patient with new-onset shortness of breath is assessed with transthoracic echocardiography. Due to body habitus, the examination is technically challenging and limited views are obtained. Of the measures to ascertain diastolic function only a TR jet velocity of 3.1 m/s and a lateral e′ velocity of 7 cm/s are able to be reliably obtained. What grade of diastolic dysfunction can be diagnosed based on this data? Assume normal LV systolic function.

A. Grade I
B. Grade II, pseudonormal
C. Grade III, restrictive filling pattern
D. Indeterminate, cannot document

7. A heart transplant recipient undergoes a transthoracic echocardiographic examination on postoperative day 5 to assess heart function. EF is found to be normal and no valvular abnormalities are noted. What type of diastolic function is noted commonly in this patient population?

A. Grade I
B. Grade II, pseudonormal
C. Grade III, restrictive filling pattern
D. Grade IV

8. A patient with coronary disease status post placement of drug-eluting stents 10 months prior undergoes transthoracic echocardiography prior to exploratory laparotomy for resection of colon cancer. Patient's EF is found to be 65% without wall motion abnormalities noted. The E/A ratio is found to be 0.7 and mitral E velocity is 37 cm/s. What grade of diastolic dysfunction is present?

   A. Normal diastolic function is present in this patient
   B. Grade I
   C. Grade II, pseudonormal
   D. Grade III, restrictive filling pattern

9. A patient undergoes transthoracic echocardiography to assess for potential constrictive pericarditis versus restrictive cardiomyopathy. Along with an elevated E/A ratio of 2.5 and medial mitral e′ velocity of 4.6 cm/s, what other echocardiographic parameter is specific for restrictive cardiomyopathy in comparison with constrictive pericarditis?

   A. E/e′ of 12
   B. Mitral DT of 182 ms
   C. IVRT of 46 ms
   D. LAVI of 36 mL/m²

10. A 63-year-old female patient with heart failure with reduced ejection fraction (HFrEF), coronary artery disease, hypertension, and peripheral vascular disease is evaluated in the ICU with transthoracic echocardiography for increased shortness of breath and concern for volume overload following femoral endarterectomy. **Figure 21.4A-C** were captured during the examination.

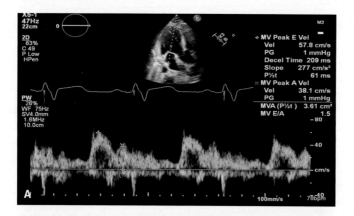

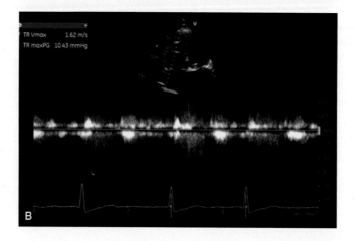

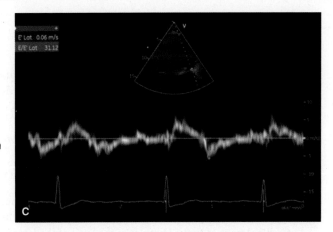

**Figure 21.4** A. Mitral inflow velocity measuring E and A waves in two-chamber view from apical position with transthoracic echocardiography. B. Tricuspid regurgitation jet velocity measured with continuous-wave Doppler. C. Tissue Doppler of lateral mitral annulus measuring e′ velocity.

Based on the information from **Figure 21.4**, what can be determined about the patient's diastolic function?
A. Grade I
B. Grade II
C. Cannot be determined
D. Normal

11. In a patient with normal LVEF, the following parameters are obtained:

- Average E/e′ = 17
- Septal e′ 6 cm/s, Lateral e′ 8 cm/s
- TR velocity 3.4 m/s
- LAVI: not obtained

Based on these results, which of the following answer choices is most appropriate?
A. Normal diastolic function
B. Indeterminate for diastolic dysfunction
C. Diastolic dysfunction present
D. Further information is necessary

12. An 82-year-old male presents to the Emergency Department with shortness of breath. Chest x-ray (CXR) shows bilateral pulmonary infiltrates. He is placed on noninvasive positive pressure ventilation and admitted to the ICU. He has a long-standing history of hypertension as well as known coronary artery disease. His electrocardiogram (ECG) shows evidence of LV hypertrophy and is otherwise unremarkable. You perform a bedside echo and obtain **Figure 21.5**.

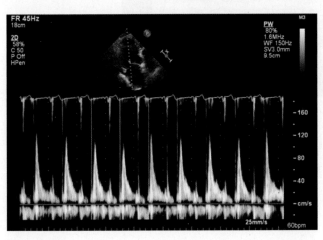

**Figure 21.5**

Additional information available:
- IVRT: 65 ms
- E-wave DT: 130 ms

How would you grade the diastolic function for this patient?
**A.** Normal left atrial pressure (LAP), grade I diastolic dysfunction
**B.** Grade II diastolic dysfunction
**C.** Grade III diastolic dysfunction
**D.** Cannot determine degree of diastolic dysfunction with information available

**13.** In order to obtain peak E and A-wave velocities, which of the following methods should be used?

**A.** Placement of continuous-wave Doppler signal at the level of the mitral valve
**B.** Placement of pulsed-wave Doppler sample gate at the level of the mitral leaflet tips
**C.** Placement of tissue Doppler at the level of the lateral mitral annulus
**D.** Placement of tissue Doppler at the level of the septal mitral annulus

**14.** A 70-year-old female with a history of HFrEF presents to the Emergency Department with 2 days of dyspnea. Bedside ultrasound is shown in **Figure 21.6**.

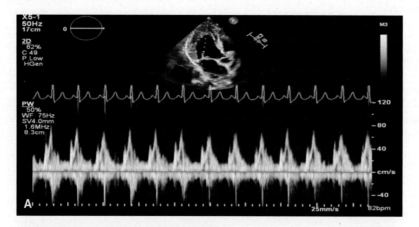

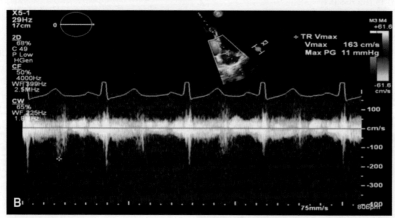

**Figure 21.6**

Additionally, E/e′ is calculated to be 12.

How would you classify the diastolic function for this patient?
**A.** Grade I diastolic dysfunction
**B.** Grade III diastolic dysfunction
**C.** Indeterminate diastolic function
**D.** Normal diastolic function

**15.** A 58-year-old male presents to the hospital with dyspnea. He has a history of hypertension, diabetes, previous myocardial infarction, and ischemic cardiomyopathy. His last performed echo showed an EF of 35%. You repeat a bedside echo and **Figure 21.7** is obtained.

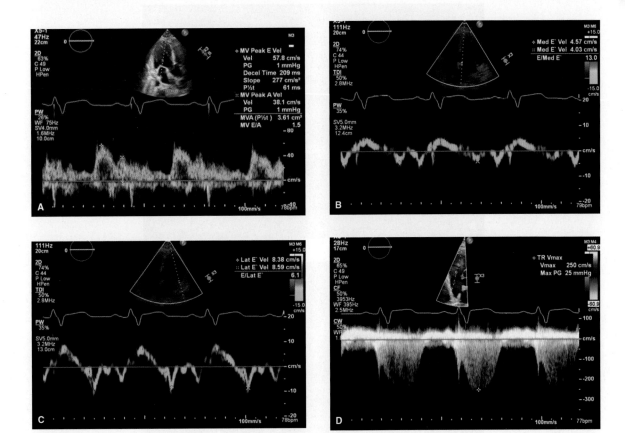

**Figure 21.7**

How would you quantify the diastolic function for this patient?
**A.** Grade I diastolic dysfunction
**B.** Grade II diastolic dysfunction
**C.** Grade III diastolic dysfunction
**D.** Normal diastolic function

**16.** A 78-year-old patient is admitted to the ICU with respiratory failure. He has no known pulmonary disease. **Figure 21.8** is obtained using echocardiography.

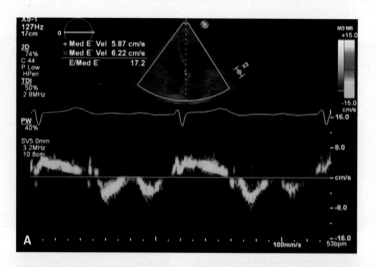

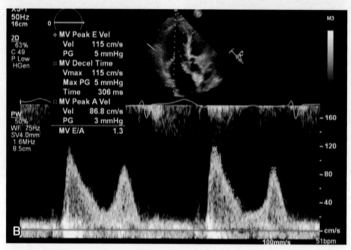

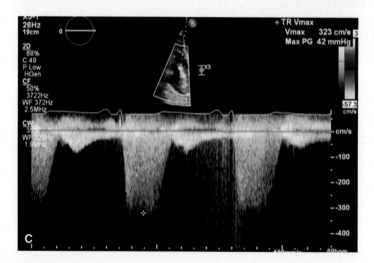

**Figure 21.8**

Based on the information available, which of the following best describes the patient's diastolic function?
A. Grade I diastolic dysfunction
B. Grade II diastolic dysfunction
C. Grade III diastolic dysfunction
D. Normal diastolic function

17. E-wave on mitral valve inflow signal best represents which of the following?

   A. Atrial contraction
   B. Deceleration time
   C. Early rapid filling
   D. Ventricular contraction

18. A 62-year-old woman with a history of hypertension, diabetes, and chronic kidney disease is brought to the ICU from the operating room post–exploratory laparotomy. A Swan-Ganz catheter was placed in the operating room (OR) and central venous pressure (CVP) found to be 10 mm Hg. Bedside echo is performed and reveals the following values:

   - EF: 55%
   - Pulmonary artery systolic pressure (PASP) 74 mm Hg based on CVP of 10 mm Hg
   - LAVI 36 mL/m$^2$
   - Average E/e′ 15

   You diagnose the patient as having diastolic dysfunction. Based on these parameters, what do you expect the peak velocity of the TR jet to be?
   A. 2 m/s
   B. 3 m/s
   C. 4 m/s
   D. 5 m/s

19. An 80-year-old male presents to the Emergency Department with dyspnea. He has a history of coronary artery disease, chronic kidney disease, and peripheral vascular disease. **Figure 21.9** shows a recent echocardiogram.

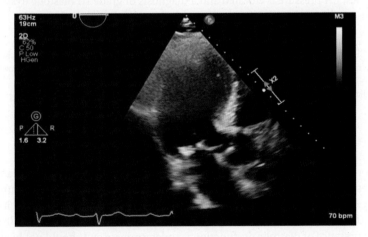

**Figure 21.9**

Given the pathology noted in **Figure 21.9**, what limitation might you face when attempting to classify diastolic function?
A. In patients with an incomplete TR jet, diastolic dysfunction cannot be quantified.
B. In the presence of atrial fibrillation, it is impossible to classify diastolic dysfunction.
C. In the presence of LV hypertrophy, diastolic function cannot be quantified.
D. In the presence of mitral annular calcification (MAC), mitral E and e′ values are unreliable.

**20.** In the presence of increased pulmonary artery pressures, assessment of LV filling pressures can be made using which of the following parameters?

**A.** Diastolic function cannot be assessed
**B.** E/A
**C.** Lateral E/e′
**D.** Pulmonary function tests

# Chapter 21 ▪ Answers

**1.** Correct Answer: **D. TR jet velocity >2.8 m/s and E/e′ >14**

*Rationale:* Based on the 2016 American Society of Echocardiography (ASE) guidelines, grading of diastolic dysfunction in patients with reduced LVEF is dependent on the following variables. First, the E/A ratio will give the first data point to make a determination if there is abnormal diastolic dysfunction. With an E/A ratio of <0.8, grade I diastolic dysfunction can be diagnosed. When the E/A ratio is normal with values >0.8 and <2, then determining between normal and pseudonormal (grade II diastolic dysfunction) takes a few more variables into consideration. The three variables that can be used are the E/e′ ratio (>14), LA maximum VI (>34 mL/m$^2$), and TR jet velocity (>2.8 m/s). If two of three or all three of these variables are positive (at or above values listed), it implies an elevated LA pressure and grade II diastolic dysfunction.

### Selected Reference

1. Nagueh SF, Smiseth OA, Appleton CP, et al. Recommendations for the evaluation of left ventricular diastolic function by echocardiography: an update from the American Society of Echocardiography and the European Association of Cardiovascular Imaging. *J Am Soc Echocardiogr.* 2016;29:277-314.

**2.** Correct Answer: **C. Grade III**

*Rationale:* This patient's E/A ratio is 2.59 (E/A ≥ 2) in the setting of reduced systolic function. Hence, based on the 2016 ASE guidelines, LA pressure is elevated and a diagnosis of grade III diastolic dysfunction or restrictive filling pattern can be made.

### Selected References

1. Nagueh SF, Smiseth OA, Appleton CP, et al. Recommendations for the evaluation of left ventricular diastolic function by echocardiography: an update from the American Society of Echocardiography and the European Association of Cardiovascular Imaging. *J Am Soc Echocardiogr.* 2016;29:277-314.
2. Otto CM. Chapter 7: Ventricular diastolic filling and function. In: Delores Meloni, eds. *Textbook of Clinical Echocardiography.* Elsevier Saunders; 2013. Print.

**3.** Correct Answer: **A. Normal**

*Rationale:* In patients with normal systolic function and without cardiac disease, four criteria can be looked at to determine the presence of diastolic dysfunction. These include E/e′ >14, LA maximum VI of >34 mL/m$^2$, TR jet velocity of >2.8 m/s, and a septal e′ velocity of <7 cm/s or a lateral e′ velocity of <10 cm/s. If less than 50% of these criteria are met, then normal diastolic function is present. If 50% of these criteria are met, then the presence of diastolic dysfunction is indeterminate and should not be documented. If greater than 50% of the criteria are satisfied, then diastolic dysfunction is present. In this patient only one among the four criteria are met (lateral e′ =7.7 cm/s), suggesting normal diastolic function.

### Selected References

1. Andersen OS, Smiseth OA, Dokainish H, et al. Estimating left ventricular filling pressure by echocardiography. *J Am Coll Cardiol.* 2017 Apr 18;69(15):1937-1948.
2. Nagueh SF, Smiseth OA, Appleton CP, et al. Recommendations for the evaluation of left ventricular diastolic function by echocardiography: an update from the American Society of Echocardiography and the European Association of Cardiovascular Imaging. *J Am Soc Echocardiogr.* 2016;29:277-314.

**4. Correct Answer: B. Mitral deceleration time (DT) of <160 ms**

*Rationale:* Atrial fibrillation creates challenges in the diagnosis of diastolic dysfunction due to the fact that many of these patients have preexisting congestive heart failure and enlarged LA. Along with these changes, measurement of E/A ratio can be difficult due to the lack of an A-wave secondary to loss of atrial contraction in atrial fibrillation. There are some parameters that can be measured to ascertain diastolic function in these patients despite these pitfalls. These include a peak acceleration time of mitral E velocity >1900 cm/s$^2$, mitral DT of <160 ms, E/e′ ratio of >11, and IVRT of <65 ms.

Selected References

1. Andersen OS, Smiseth OA, Dokainish H, et al. Estimating left ventricular filling pressure by echocardiography. *J Am Coll Cardiol.* 2017 Apr 18;69(15):1937-1948.
2. Nagueh SF, Smiseth OA, Appleton CP, et al. Recommendations for the evaluation of left ventricular diastolic function by echocardiography: an update from the American Society of Echocardiography and the European Association of Cardiovascular Imaging. *J Am Soc Echocardiogr.* 2016;29:277-314.

**5. Correct Answer: B. Elevated LV end-diastolic pressure**

*Rationale:* Of the listed answers, only the mitral DT of <160 ms (131.9 ms in this question) has been shown to be a reliable indicator of elevated LV filling pressures and diastolic dysfunction in patients with reduced EF and atrial fibrillation. The mitral DT is shown by the delta T in the upper left of the image but can also be calculated using the pressure half-time or PHT. The equation for this is: DT = 38/0.29 = 131 ms. Other parameters that have been shown to be associated with elevated filling pressures in patients with atrial fibrillation include peak acceleration time of mitral E velocity >1900 cm/s$^2$, E/e′ ratio of >11, and IVRT of <65 ms. Variations in mitral inflow velocity cannot be used to identify tamponade physiology in the presence of atrial fibrillation.

Selected References

1. Andersen OS, Smiseth OA, Dokainish H, et al. Estimating left ventricular filling pressure by echocardiography. *J Am Coll Cardiol.* 2017 Apr 18;69(15):1937-1948.
2. Nagueh SF, Smiseth OA, Appleton CP, et al. Recommendations for the evaluation of left ventricular diastolic function by echocardiography: an update from the American Society of Echocardiography and the European Association of Cardiovascular Imaging. *J Am Soc Echocardiogr.* 2016;29:277-314.

**6. Correct Answer: D. Indeterminate, cannot document**

*Rationale:* In a patient with normal LV function, four parameters can be evaluated to assess diastolic function. These include an average E/e′ >14, septal e′ velocity of <7 cm/s or a lateral e′ velocity <10 cm/s, TR jet velocity >2.8 m/s, and LAVI >34 mL/m$^2$. If less than 50% of these criteria are met, then normal diastolic function is present. If 50% of these criteria are met, then the presence of diastolic dysfunction is indeterminate and should not be documented. If greater than 50% of the criteria are satisfied, then diastolic dysfunction is present. In this case, two out of four criteria are met and therefore diastolic function cannot be determined.

Selected References

1. Andersen OS, Smiseth OA, Dokainish H, et al. Estimating left ventricular filling pressure by echocardiography. *J Am Coll Cardiol.* 2017 Apr 18;69(15):1937-1948.
2. Nagueh SF, Smiseth OA, Appleton CP, et al. Recommendations for the evaluation of left ventricular diastolic function by echocardiography: an update from the American Society of Echocardiography and the European Association of Cardiovascular Imaging. *J Am Soc Echocardiogr.* 2016;29:277-314.

**7. Correct Answer: C. Grade III, restrictive filling pattern**

*Rationale:* Patients with heart transplantation pose a special circumstance in regard to evaluating diastolic dysfunction. It is common for patients to have a restrictive filling pattern on echocardiography in the first few weeks following transplantation despite normal EF. Most times, the filling pressures are normal in these patients as the donors are typically young, healthy people at the time of donation. Elevated TR jet velocities can still be a surrogate marker of elevated left-sided filling pressure in this patient population. Diastolic dysfunction findings typically resolve over time with many patients having normal measurements after 1 year following transplant.

Selected Reference

1. Nagueh SF, Smiseth OA, Appleton CP, et al. Recommendations for the evaluation of left ventricular diastolic function by echocardiography: an update from the American Society of Echocardiography and the European Association of Cardiovascular Imaging. *J Am Soc Echocardiogr.* 2016;29:277-314.

---

**8.** Correct Answer: B. Grade I

*Rationale:* In this patient with normal systolic function and myocardial disease, the two parameters noted on the examination of E/A ratio and mitral E velocity are consistent with grade I diastolic dysfunction. Based on most recent guidelines, if values of E/A are less than or equal to 0.8 and E is less than or equal to 50 cm/s, the patient likely has normal LAP with grade I diastolic dysfunction. If the E/A ratio is less than or equal to 0.8 and E is greater than 50 cm/s or the E/A ratio is between 0.9 and 1.9, further information in terms of E/e′, TR velocity, and LAVI is needed to quantify diastolic function more accurately. If the E/A ratio is greater than or equal to 2, then grade III diastolic dysfunction is present along with elevated LAP.

Selected References

1. Andersen OS, Smiseth OA, Dokainish H, et al. Estimating left ventricular filling pressure by echocardiography. *J Am Coll Cardiol.* 2017 Apr 18;69(15):1937-1948.
2. Nagueh SF, Smiseth OA, Appleton CP, et al. Recommendations for the evaluation of left ventricular diastolic function by echocardiography: an update from the American Society of Echocardiography and the European Association of Cardiovascular Imaging. *J Am Soc Echocardiogr.* 2016;29:277-314.

---

**9.** Correct Answer: C. IVRT of 46 ms

*Rationale:* Differentiation between constrictive pericarditis and restrictive cardiomyopathy can be performed utilizing echocardiography, and differences in tissue Doppler velocities, IVRT, DT, and LAVI can be used to differentiate between the two. In the above scenario, the most specific finding to differentiate between constrictive pericarditis and restrictive cardiomyopathy is the drastically shortened IVRT of 46 ms. Other ancillary findings that discern between the two entities are an E/e′ of >15, mitral DT of <160 ms, and an LAVI of >48 mL/m². **Figure 21.10** shows the IVRT in an LV outflow tract measurement with pulse wave. IVRT is normally between 70 and 90 ms.

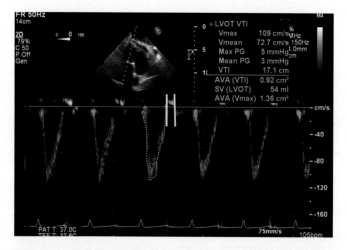

**Figure 21.10** Left ventricular outflow tract (LVOT) Doppler measurement with pulse wave. Isovolumic relaxation time (IVRT) is marked in this image by the yellow lines. Normal values are typically between 70 and 90 ms.

Selected Reference

1. Nagueh SF, Smiseth OA, Appleton CP, et al. Recommendations for the evaluation of left ventricular diastolic function by echocardiography: an update from the American Society of Echocardiography and the European Association of Cardiovascular Imaging. *J Am Soc Echocardiogr.* 2016;29:277-314.

**10.** Correct Answer: **C. Cannot be determined**

*Rationale:* In a patient with heart disease or reduced EF, the determination of diastolic function starts with evaluation of the E/A ratio, which in this case is 1.9. Due to the fact that this patient has underlying cardiac disease, three criteria should be evaluated in order to elucidate if the patient has grade I dysfunction, grade II dysfunction, or not able to determine. These three criteria are an E/e′ >14, TR jet velocity of >2.8 m/s, and an LAVI of >34 mL/m². In this case, we are only presented with two of the three criteria. These two criteria can still be utilized in order to determine the type of diastolic dysfunction. The E/e′ ratio averages between 29 and 31, and the TR jet velocity is 1.6 m/s. Because we have one positive variable (E/e′) and one negative variable (TR jet velocity), the grade of diastolic dysfunction cannot be determined. The lateral mitral annulus e′ velocity is also low in this case at 6 cm/s, suggesting impaired relaxation but this variable is typically utilized in patients with normal EF and without underlying cardiac disease.

Selected References

1. Andersen OS, Smiseth OA, Dokainish H, et al. Estimating left ventricular filling pressure by echocardiography. *J Am Coll Cardiol.* 2017 Apr 18;69(15):1937-1948.
2. Nagueh SF, Smiseth OA, Appleton CP, et al. Recommendations for the evaluation of left ventricular diastolic function by echocardiography: an update from the American Society of Echocardiography and the European Association of Cardiovascular Imaging. *J Am Soc Echocardiogr.* 2016;29:277-314.

**11.** Correct Answer: **C. Diastolic dysfunction present**

*Rationale:* This is a simple application of the algorithm for diagnosis of LV diagnostic dysfunction in subjects with normal LVEF. As per the most recent guidelines, there are four recommended variables:
1. Annular e′ velocity : septal e′ < 7 cm/s or lateral e′ < 10 cm/s
2. Average E/e′ ratio > 14
3. LAVI > 34 mL/m²
4. Peak TR velocity > 2.8 m/s

This patient has three of the four criteria present. Per the guidelines, if <50% of variables are positive this indicates normal diastolic function. If 50% of variables are positive, it is indeterminate for the presence of diastolic dysfunction. If >50% of variables are positive, it is indicative of diastolic dysfunction (Answer C).

Selected Reference

1. Nagueh SF, Smiseth OA, Appleton CP, et al. Recommendations for the evaluation of left ventricular diastolic function by echocardiography: an update from the American Society of Echocardiography and the European Association of Cardiovascular Imaging. *J Am Soc Echocardiogr.* 2016;29:277-314.

**12.** Correct Answer: **C. Grade III diastolic dysfunction**

*Rationale:* Chronic increases in the filling pressure will increase the pressure gradient between the LA and LV. Ultimately, this is represented by a tall E-wave and shortening of the A-wave. This can lead to an observed E/A ratio of >2. In many patients, especially those with a reduced EF, atrial to ventricular flow starts quickly and ends just as quickly as a result of such high filling pressures. This is represented by a shortening of both the DT (normal 140-240 ms) and IVRT (normal 70-100 ms). As shown in the image, an E/A ratio greater than 2 is suggestive of grade III diastolic dysfunction (Answer C).

Selected Reference

1. Nagueh SF, Smiseth OA, Appleton CP, et al. Recommendations for the evaluation of left ventricular diastolic function by echocardiography: an update from the American Society of Echocardiography and the European Association of Cardiovascular Imaging. *J Am Soc Echocardiogr.* 2016;29:277-314.

**13.** Correct Answer: B. Placement of pulsed-wave Doppler sample gate at the level of the mitral leaflet tips

*Rationale:* Optimal acquisition is from the apical view. Pulsed-wave Doppler is then placed with the sample gate between the mitral leaflet tips. Color flow is often used for optimal alignment of the pulsed-wave Doppler. Wall filter and signal gain settings should be set to low for optimal Doppler signal attainment.

Selected Reference

1. Nagueh SF, Smiseth OA, Appleton CP, et al. Recommendations for the evaluation of left ventricular diastolic function by echocardiography: an update from the American Society of Echocardiography and the European Association of Cardiovascular Imaging. *J Am Soc Echocardiogr.* 2016;29:277-314.

**14.** Correct Answer: A. Grade I diastolic dysfunction

*Rationale:* This question tests application of the algorithm for determining grade of LV diastolic dysfunction. Figure 21.6A suggests an E/A ratio of less than 0.8 and an E-wave velocity of <50 cm/s. This would classify the patient as having grade I diastolic dysfunction. Even if you assume the E/A ratio is between 0.8 and 2 or the E-wave velocity is >50 cm/s, the classification would not change. The remainder of the question provides that the E/e′ is less than 14 and the max TR velocity observed is 1.63 m/s. With two of these criteria being negative, this would classify the patient as having grade I diastolic dysfunction.

Selected Reference

1. Nagueh SF, Smiseth OA, Appleton CP, et al. Recommendations for the evaluation of left ventricular diastolic function by echocardiography: an update from the American Society of Echocardiography and the European Association of Cardiovascular Imaging. *J Am Soc Echocardiogr.* 2016;29:277-314.

**15.** Correct Answer: A. Grade I diastolic dysfunction

*Rationale:* Based on the information provided, the patient has an E/A ratio of 1.5. In the presence of a reduced EF, this requires additional information for classification of diastolic dysfunction. The average E/e′ is 9.5 (average of 6.1 and 13) and the max TR jet velocity is displayed as 2.5 m/s. Even without an LAVI, this would classify the patient as having grade I diastolic dysfunction. Note that even in the presence of LA dilation or LAVI of greater than 34, this patient would still only classify as having grade I diastolic dysfunction.

Selected Reference

1. Nagueh SF, Smiseth OA, Appleton CP, et al. Recommendations for the evaluation of left ventricular diastolic function by echocardiography: an update from the American Society of Echocardiography and the European Association of Cardiovascular Imaging. *J Am Soc Echocardiogr.* 2016;29:277.

**16.** Correct Answer: B. Grade II diastolic dysfunction

*Rationale:* This question does not provide you with a lot of information regarding the patient's past medical history of current symptoms besides respiratory failure. It does, however, show an elevated TR jet velocity. In the absence of intrinsic pulmonary disease, this raises the possibility of elevated LV filling pressures. With an E/A ratio of 1.3, the additional criteria being evaluated are TR jet velocity of 3.23 m/s. A medial E/e′ is shown as 17.2. This gives two positive criteria, which regardless of the calculation of an LAVI, classifies the patient as having grade II diastolic dysfunction.

Selected Reference

1. Nagueh SF, Smiseth OA, Appleton CP, et al. Recommendations for the evaluation of left ventricular diastolic function by echocardiography: an update from the American Society of Echocardiography and the European Association of Cardiovascular Imaging. *J Am Soc Echocardiogr.* 2016;29:277-314.

**17.** Correct Answer: C. Early rapid filling

*Rationale:* E-wave on the mitral valve inflow signal represents early rapid filling during diastole (Answer C). The velocity reflects the LA-LV pressure gradient. Atrial contraction is represented by the A-wave on the mitral valve inflow signal.

**Selected Reference**

1. Otto CM. Chapter 7: Ventricular diastolic filling and function. In: Delores Meloni, eds. *Textbook of Clinical Echocardiography*. Elsevier Saunders; 2013. Print.

## 18. Correct Answer: C. 4 m/s

*Rationale:* In the absence of right ventricular outflow tract (RVOT) obstruction, PASP = right ventricular systolic pressure (RVSP) = $4V^2$ (*V* is peak TR jet velocity) + RA. The PASP is given as 74 mm Hg. Knowing the RA pressure is 10 mm Hg, using Bernoulli's equation, the pressure gradient between the RV and RA is calculated as follows:

- $4V^2 = 64$
- $V^2 = 16$
- $V = 4$ m/s

**Selected Reference**

1. Otto CM. Chapter 7: Ventricular diastolic filling and function. In: Delores Meloni, eds. *Textbook of Clinical Echocardiography*. Elsevier Saunders; 2013. Print.

## 19. Correct Answer: D. In the presence of mitral annular calcification (MAC), mitral E and e′ values are unreliable.

*Rationale:* In the presence of MAC, mitral orifice area is decreased. This leads to increased velocities across the mitral valve. Lateral e′ velocities can also be negatively affected due to restriction in movement of the annulus. It is not known if septal e′ velocities can be of any value in these patients. Ultimately this leads to having increased E/e′ velocities but without the ability to separate the contributions from mitral valve calcifications versus diastolic dysfunction.

**Selected Reference**

1. Nagueh SF, Smiseth OA, Appleton CP, et al. Recommendations for the evaluation of left ventricular diastolic function by echocardiography: an update from the American Society of Echocardiography and the European Association of Cardiovascular Imaging. *J Am Soc Echocardiogr*. 2016;29:277-314.

## 20. Correct Answer: C. Lateral E/e′

*Rationale:* In patients with noncardiac pulmonary hypertension (e.g., idiopathic pulmonary hypertension), diastolic function can still be assessed. Lateral E/e′ has been shown to help determine the underlying etiology of increased PA pressures. In the presence of cardiac disease, lateral E/e′ is often > 13. In the presence of pulmonary hypertension due to noncardiac disease, lateral E/e′ is <8. In contrast, the septal e′ (and E/e′) in patients with pulmonary hypertension due to noncardiac disease is increased, likely due to the contribution of RV myocardium to annular velocities measured at the interventricular septum.

**Selected References**

1. Nagueh SF, Smiseth OA, Appleton CP, et al. Recommendations for the evaluation of left ventricular diastolic function by echocardiography: an update from the American Society of Echocardiography and the European Association of Cardiovascular Imaging. *J Am Soc Echocardiogr*. 2016;29:277-314.
2. Ruan Q, Nagueh SF. Clinical application of tissue Doppler imaging in patients with idiopathic pulmonary hypertension. *Chest*. 2007;131(2):395-401, ISSN 0012-3692. doi:10.1378/chest.06-1556.

# 22 | LEFT VENTRICULAR SYSTOLIC FUNCTION

Vikram Fielding-Singh and Emily Methangkool

1. Identify the phase of the cardiac cycle labeled 3 in **Figure 22.1**.

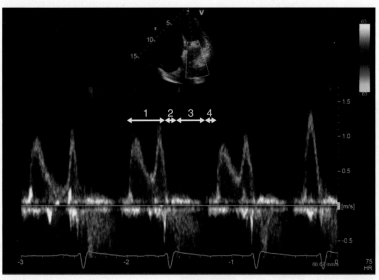

**Figure 22.1**

A. Isovolumic contraction
B. Systolic ejection
C. Isovolumic relaxation
D. Diastolic filling

2. Identify the phase of the cardiac cycle shown in **Figure 22.2**.

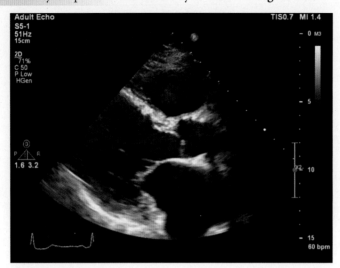

**Figure 22.2**

A. Isovolumic contraction
B. Systolic ejection
C. Isovolumic relaxation
D. Diastolic filling

3. Identify where the left ventricular end-diastolic diameter should be measured in **Figure 22.3**.

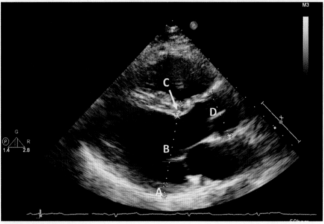

**Figure 22.3**

A. A
B. B
C. C
D. D

4. A patient has the following left ventricular chamber dimensions measured at end diastole with transthoracic echocardiography:

- Posterior wall thickness: 1.4 cm
- Septal wall thickness: 2.0 cm
- End-diastolic diameter: 4.3 cm

How would you describe these left ventricular chamber dimensions?
A. Normal left ventricular geometry
B. Eccentric hypertrophy
C. Concentric hypertrophy
D. Concentric remodeling

5. How would you describe the left ventricular chamber dimensions of the ventricle in Box 4 of **Figure 22.4**?

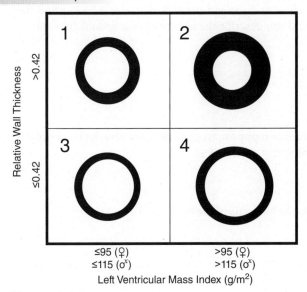

**Figure 22.4**

A. Normal left ventricular geometry
B. Eccentric hypertrophy
C. Concentric hypertrophy
D. Concentric remodeling

6. In the transthoracic apical four-chamber image shown in **Figure 22.5**, which line(s) represent(s) the correct tracing of the left ventricular end-diastolic area from which left ventricular diastolic volume may be calculated?

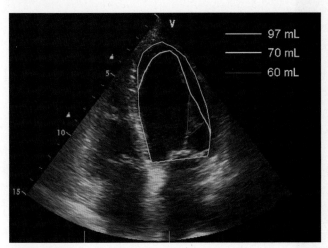

**Figure 22.5**

A. Green
B. Yellow
C. Pink
D. Green and pink

7. A transthoracic echocardiogram shows no significant valvular abnormalities and no left ventricular regional wall motion abnormalities. The left ventricular end-diastolic diameter is 55 mm and the end-systolic diameter is 48 mm. How would you describe the left ventricular systolic function?

   A. Hyperdynamic
   B. Normal
   C. Reduced
   D. Unable to determine

8. When comparing M-mode and 2D echocardiography for assessment of left ventricular systolic function using a parasternal long-axis view, 2D offers what advantages?

   A. Superior temporal resolution
   B. Superior spatial resolution
   C. Avoidance of measurements oblique to the long axis of the ventricle
   D. 2D does not offer any advantages

9. In a patient experiencing a myocardial infarction, which method of assessment of left ventricular systolic function is likely to overestimate the true function?

   A. Qualitative assessment using the apical four-chamber view
   B. Biplane method of disks
   C. Three-dimensional volumetric assessment
   D. Global longitudinal strain

10. Which structure in **Figure 22.6** is most likely to rupture in the setting of myocardial ischemia?

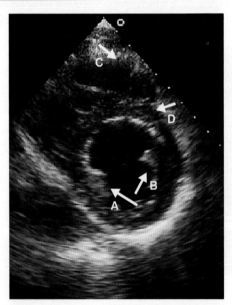

**Figure 22.6**

   A. A
   B. B
   C. C
   D. D

**11.** Using the American Society of Echocardiography's 17-segment model, which transthoracic view allows assessment of the mid-anterior wall?

**A.** Apical four chamber
**B.** Apical two chamber
**C.** Parasternal long axis
**D.** Apical long axis

**12.** A patient in the intensive care unit is experiencing chest pain on postoperative day 2 after a Whipple procedure. The echocardiogram (**Figure 22.7**) shows hypokinesis in the region indicated by the white arrow.

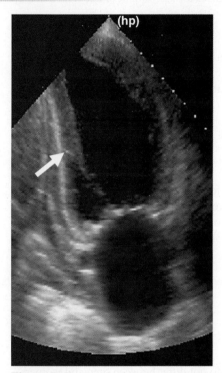

**Figure 22.7**

According to the American Society of Echocardiography's 17-segment model, the name of the wall segment and the coronary blood supply that is likely impaired are:
**A.** Mid-inferior wall; right coronary artery
**B.** Mid-posterior wall; right coronary artery
**C.** Mid-posterior wall; left circumflex artery
**D.** Mid-anterolateral wall; left circumflex artery

**13.** A hypokinetic wall segment might be expected to exhibit what percentage thickening from left ventricular end-diastolic thickness?

**A.** 5%
**B.** 20%
**C.** 35%
**D.** 45%

14. Which of the following methods is currently recommended by the American Society of Echocardiography for quantitative assessment of left ventricular ejection fraction with echocardiography?

    A. Fractional shortening
    B. Fractional area change
    C. Biplane method of disks
    D. Global longitudinal strain

15. Advantages associated with using the biplane method of disks for assessment of left ventricular ejection fraction include:

    A. Avoids foreshortening of the apex
    B. Avoids geometric assumptions compared to linear methods
    C. Avoids endocardial dropout
    D. Visualizes all walls of the ventricle to account for possible shape distortions

16. Which of the following views or measurements is *not* required to calculate a left ventricular ejection fraction using the biplane method of disks in a patient with regional wall motion abnormalities?

    A. Length of the left ventricular long axis from an apical four chamber
    B. Left ventricular end-systolic volume from an apical two chamber
    C. Left ventricular end-systolic volume from an apical four chamber
    D. Left ventricular end-diastolic volume from an apical long axis

17. Reference values for left ventricular systolic function differ between men and women for which category of systolic function?

    A. Normal
    B. Moderately abnormal
    C. Severely abnormal
    D. Reference values for left ventricular systolic function do not differ between men and women

18. Which of the following is least likely to be used for calculation of cardiac output using the Doppler method for hemodynamic assessment?

    A. Diameter of the left ventricular outflow tract
    B. End-systolic and end-diastolic volumes of the left ventricle
    C. Pulsed-wave Doppler–derived velocity-time integral of systolic flow through the left ventricular outflow tract
    D. Heart rate

19. In which of the following clinical conditions would a linear measurement technique such as fractional shortening be most likely to provide an accurate assessment of left ventricular systolic function?

    A. Sepsis with hyperdynamic systolic function
    B. Acute coronary thrombosis of the left circumflex artery
    C. Left bundle branch block
    D. Right ventricular epicardial pacing

20. When using the biplane method of disks to assess left ventricular ejection fraction, the end-diastolic frame is best defined as:

    A. The frame just prior to closure of the mitral valve
    B. The frame when the left ventricular dimensions are largest
    C. The frame just after opening of the aortic valve
    D. The frame corresponding to the T wave in the QRS complex

21. You are called to the bedside to assess a patient who is awaiting mitral valve replacement for severe mitral regurgitation. Using the biplane method of discs, you obtain the following estimates:

    • Left ventricular end-diastolic volume: 100 mL
    • Left ventricular end-systolic volume: 44 mL

    Which among the following statements best describe the predicted ventricular function of this patient after mitral valve replacement?
    A. Normal left ventricular function
    B. Impaired left ventricular function
    C. Impaired right ventricular function
    D. Hyperdynamic left ventricular function

22. You are evaluating a patient preoperatively for coronary artery bypass grafting. The patient is in permanent atrial fibrillation. In order to obtain a left ventricular ejection fraction estimate using biplane method of disks, you should:

    A. Try to capture the largest end-diastolic volume and smallest end-systolic volume that you can and use those values
    B. Wait for a beat that follows a long period of diastole to ensure adequate preload before taking your measurements
    C. Repeat your measurements five times and average the results
    D. Decline to quantitatively measure left ventricular ejection fraction as it cannot be done accurately in atrial fibrillation

23. What left ventricular global longitudinal strain measurement would reassure you that a patient's left ventricular systolic function is likely to be normal?

    A. 30
    B. 0
    C. −10
    D. −30

24. A routine preoperative echocardiogram in a patient waiting for thoracic surgery identified regional left ventricular systolic dysfunction; however, a subsequent cardiac catheterization failed to identify any lesions in the coronary arteries. What are some other potential causes of abnormal wall motion patterns?

    A. Left bundle branch block
    B. Ventricular pacing
    C. Subarachnoid hemorrhage
    D. All of the above

25. You are evaluating a patient suffering from an anterior myocardial infarction. You are interested in calculating a wall motion score index to describe the degree of left ventricular dysfunction. You note akinesia of the mid-anterior wall. For the purposes of calculating a wall motion score index, this wall segment would be assigned a score of:

    A. 1
    B. 2
    C. 3
    D. 4

# Chapter 22 ▪ Answers

**1.** Correct Answer: B. Systolic ejection

*Rationale:* The image depicts the Doppler interrogation of transmitral inflow. This image was taken in the apical four-chamber view, with the sample volume at the coaptation of the mitral valve leaflets. The time period marked 1 indicates the diastolic filling phase, comprised of a large peak due to early diastolic filling (referred to as the E wave) and a smaller peak due to atrial contraction (referred to as the A wave). This is followed by isovolumic contraction (2), systolic ejection (3), and isovolumic relaxation (4).

Selected References
1. Armstrong WF, Ryan T. *Feigenbaum's Echocardiography*. 8th ed. Wolters Kluwer; 2019.

**2.** Correct Answer: A. Isovolumic contraction

*Rationale:* The phase of the cardiac cycle seen in this image is isovolumic contraction. The ventricle is in an isovolumic state because the aortic and mitral valves are closed. The ventricle is in a contractile state (compared to relaxation) because the electrocardiogram (ECG) is at the QRS complex. **Figure 22.8** outlines the relationship between phases of the cardiac cycle and the ECG tracing.

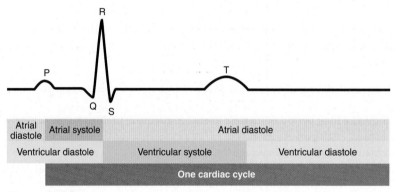

**Figure 22.8**

Selected Reference
1. Sheth PJ, Danton GH, Siegel Y, et al. Cardiac physiology for radiologists: review of relevant physiology for interpretation of cardiac MR imaging and CT. *Radiographics*. 2015;35(5):1335-1351.

**3.** Correct Answer: B.

*Rationale:* Internal linear dimensions of the left ventricle (such as the left ventricular end-diastolic diameter) are typically obtained from the parasternal long-axis view. Electronic calipers are positioned at the interface of the myocardial wall and cavity, with the axis of measurement perpendicular to the long axis of the left ventricle. The measurement is made at or immediately below the level of the mitral valve leaflet tips. Linear measures of left ventricular systolic function use this view. Use of M-mode to obtain internal linear dimensions offers improved spatial and temporal resolution but may not allow measurement perpendicular to the long axis of the left ventricle. Of note, E-point Septal Separation (EPSS) is measured from the parasternal long-axis view at the level of the mitral valve leaflet tips. EPSS measures the distance separating the anterior mitral valve leaflet at maximal excursion during systole and the septal wall, and an EPSS of >7 mm has been shown to be 87% sensitive and 75% specific at identifying reduced EF (<50%). EPSS has limited accuracy when there is significant aortic regurgitation, mitral stenosis, or inferior wall motion abnormalities present.

Answer A is the posterior wall, answer C is the interventricular septum, and answer D is the aortic root. **Figure 22.9** shows examples of EPSS in patients with anterior and inferior myocardial infarction.

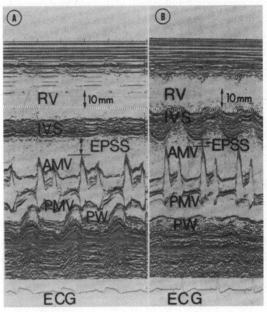

**Figure 22.9**

### Selected References

1. Ahmadpour H, Shah AA, Allen JW, et al. Mitral E point septal separation: a reliable index of left ventricular performance in coronary artery disease. *Am Heart J.* 1983;106(1 Pt 1):21-28.
2. Lang RM, Badano LP, Mor-Avi V, et al. Recommendations for cardiac chamber quantification by echocardiography in adults: an update from the American Society of Echocardiography and the European Association of Cardiovascular Imaging. *J Am Soc Echocardiogr.* 2015;28(1):1-39.e14.

### 4. Correct Answer: C. Concentric hypertrophy

*Rationale/Critique:* Hypertrophy (vs. normal geometry or concentric remodeling) is defined as elevated left ventricular mass, which can be estimated from linear measurements using formulas that you should not be expected to memorize. Practically speaking, knowledge of normal chamber dimensions may be used to diagnose hypertrophy. Normal values for both septal and posterior wall thickness are generally about 0.6 to 0.9 cm. This patient clearly has significant hypertrophy, particularly of the septal wall.

To then characterize the hypertrophy as concentric or eccentric, relative wall thickness may be used. Relative wall thickness is calculated as:

$$(2 \times \text{posterior wall thickness})/\text{end-diastolic diameter}$$

Concentric hypertrophy is defined as a relative wall thickness >0.42 and eccentric hypertrophy is defined as a relative wall thickness ≤0.42. This patient has a relative wall thickness of 0.65, so the hypertrophy is concentric. Note that the relationship between the posterior and septal walls is not used in characterizing hypertrophy as concentric versus eccentric.

### Selected References

1. Armstrong WF, Ryan T. *Feigenbaum's Echocardiography.* 8th ed. Wolters Kluwer; 2019.
2. Lang RM, Badano LP, Mor-Avi V, et al. Recommendations for cardiac chamber quantification by echocardiography in adults: an update from the American Society of Echocardiography and the European Association of Cardiovascular Imaging. *J Am Soc Echocardiogr.* 2015;28(1):1-39.e14.

**5.** Correct Answer: **B. Eccentric hypertrophy**

*Rationale:* Hypertrophy (vs. normal geometry or concentric remodeling) is defined as elevated left ventricular mass. Boxes 2 and 4 show enlarged ventricles with increased left ventricular mass, so Boxes 1 (concentric remodeling) and 3 (normal left ventricular geometry) can be eliminated. To then characterize the hypertrophy as concentric versus eccentric, the relative wall thickness is used. A relative wall thickness >0.42 defines concentric hypertrophy and a relative wall thickness ≤0.42 defines eccentric hypertrophy. Box 4 shows eccentric hypertrophy.

### Selected References

1. Armstrong WF, Ryan T. *Feigenbaum's Echocardiography*. 8th ed. Wolters Kluwer; 2019.
2. Lang RM, Badano LP, Mor-Avi V, et al. Recommendations for cardiac chamber quantification by echocardiography in adults: an update from the American Society of Echocardiography and the European Association of Cardiovascular Imaging. *J Am Soc Echocardiogr.* 2015;28(1):1-39.e14.

**6.** Correct Answer: **A. White**

*Rationale:* An apical four-chamber view is shown in Figure 22.5. Quantification of the left ventricular ejection fraction using a biplane method of discs involves estimating left ventricular end-diastolic volume using an area tracing. The endocardial border should be traced, while papillary muscles (red line) and trabeculations (yellow line) should not be included in the tracing. This method of tracing results in volume estimates that most closely match magnetic resonance imaging (MRI) measurements. For illustrative purposes, another example is provided in **Figure 22.10**. The left panel shows a tracing that does not track the endocardial border for the lateral wall, resulting in an underestimation of left ventricular volume. The right panel shows a corrected tracing that does not involve tracing the borders of either trabeculations or papillary muscles.

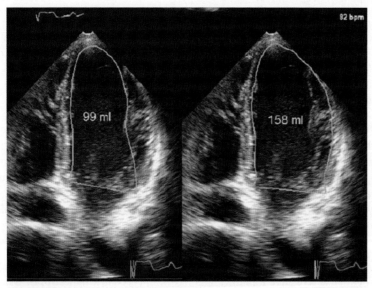

**Figure 22.10**

### Selected Reference

1. Armstrong WF, Ryan T. *Feigenbaum's Echocardiography*. 8th ed. Wolters Kluwer; 2019.

**7.** Correct Answer: **C. Reduced**

*Rationale:* Fractional shortening is defined as:

(Left ventricular end-diastolic diameter − left ventricular end-systolic diameter)/left ventricular end-systolic diameter

The measurements required may be obtained from a parasternal long axis as shown in Figure 22.15 or from an M-mode tracing if the M-mode interrogation beam is perpendicular to the long axis of the left ventricle. Fractional shortening may be a useful way to assess left ventricular systolic function in the absence of regional wall motion abnormalities, conduction abnormalities, and abnormal left ventricular geometry. A fractional shortening ≥25% implies normal left ventricular function. A value <25% implies reduced function. This patient's fractional shortening is 12.7%, suggesting reduced left ventricular systolic function.

Selected References

1. Armstrong WF, Ryan T. *Feigenbaum's Echocardiography*. 8th ed. Wolters Kluwer; 2019.
2. Lang RM, Bierig M, Devereux RB, et al. Recommendations for chamber quantification: a report from the American Society of Echocardiography's Guidelines and Standards Committee and the Chamber Quantification Writing Group, developed in conjunction with the European Association of Echocardiography, a branch of the European Society of Cardiology. *J Am Soc Echocardiogr.* 2005;18(12):1440-1463.

**8.** Correct Answer: C. Avoidance of measurements oblique to the long axis of the ventricle

*Rationale:* M-mode offers superior temporal and spatial resolution compared to 2D echocardiography. However, these advantages are becoming less pronounced as 2D echocardiography has improved. In general, 2D echocardiography on modern echocardiography machines offer sufficient resolution to make linear measurements in different phases of the cardiac cycle. The advantages of M-mode are more pronounced when interrogating rapidly moving objects such as valve leaflets. 2D echocardiography offers the advantage of being able to ensure linear measurements are taken in the correct axis. As illustrated in **Figure 22.11**, the M-mode interrogation beam may not be perpendicular to the left ventricular long axis.

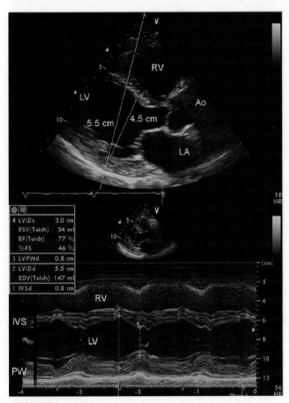

**Figure 22.11**

Selected References

1. Armstrong WF, Ryan T. *Feigenbaum's Echocardiography*. 8th ed. Wolters Kluwer; 2019.
2. Lang RM, Badano LP, Mor-Avi V, et al. Recommendations for cardiac chamber quantification by echocardiography in adults: an update from the American Society of Echocardiography and the European Association of Cardiovascular Imaging. *J Am Soc Echocardiogr.* 2015;28(1):1-39.e14.

**9.** Correct Answer: A. Qualitative assessment using the apical four-chamber view

*Rationale:* Although qualitative assessment of left ventricular systolic function by experienced echocardiographers is felt to be accurate, in the context of a myocardial infarction, a single view may not accurately assess the systolic function. In particular, the apical four-chamber view typically shows the anterolateral and inferoseptal walls. However, severe hypokinesis or akinesis of the inferior or anterior walls (such as a right coronary artery or left anterior descending [LAD] infarct) may not be completely appreciated in this view, leading to an overestimation of left ventricular systolic function. See **Figure 22.12** for additional details.

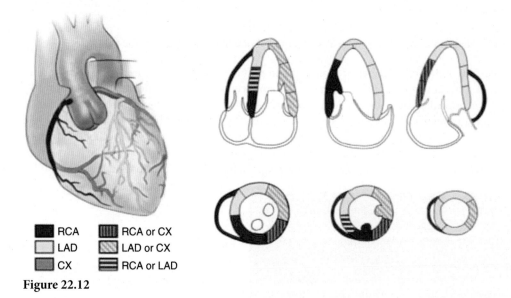

RCA
LAD
CX
RCA or CX
LAD or CX
RCA or LAD

**Figure 22.12**

Selected Reference

1. Lang RM, Badano LP, Mor-Avi V, et al. Recommendations for cardiac chamber quantification by echocardiography in adults: an update from the American Society of Echocardiography and the European Association of Cardiovascular Imaging. *J Am Soc Echocardiogr.* 2015;28(1):1-39.e14.

**10.** Correct Answer: A.

*Rationale:* This is a parasternal short-axis view of the left ventricle. Arrow A points to the posteromedial papillary muscle. Arrow B points to the anterolateral papillary muscle. Arrow C points to the right ventricular free wall, and arrow D points to the interventricular septum.

Although coronary blood supply may vary in individual patients, the anterolateral papillary muscle most commonly draws its blood supply from both the left anterior descending and the left circumflex coronary arteries. In contrast, the posteromedial papillary muscle most commonly draws its blood supply from the right coronary artery. The posteromedial papillary muscle is more likely to rupture in the context of a myocardial infarction because of its single coronary blood supply compared to the dual blood supply of the anterolateral papillary muscle. Rupture of the interventricular spectrum or right ventricular free wall is a rarer event. See **Figure 22.12** for additional details.

Selected Reference

1. Lang RM, Badano LP, Mor-Avi V, et al. Recommendations for cardiac chamber quantification by echocardiography in adults: an update from the American Society of Echocardiography and the European Association of Cardiovascular Imaging. *J Am Soc Echocardiogr.* 2015;28(1):1-39.e14.

## 11. Correct Answer: B. Apical two chamber

*Rationale:* As shown in **Figure 22.13**, the apical two-chamber view typically allows visualization of the mid-anterior wall.

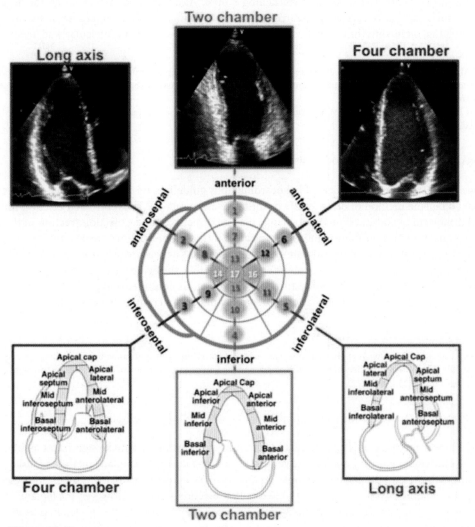

**Figure 22.13**

Selected Reference

1. Lang RM, Badano LP, Mor-Avi V, et al. Recommendations for cardiac chamber quantification by echocardiography in adults: an update from the American Society of Echocardiography and the European Association of Cardiovascular Imaging. *J Am Soc Echocardiogr.* 2015;28(1):1-39.e14.

## 12. Correct Answer: A. Mid-inferior wall; right coronary artery

*Rationale/Critique:* Figure 22.7 is an apical two-chamber view. It is apical because the apex of the left ventricle is at the top of the image. The papillary muscle on the left of the image (as well as the absence of the right ventricle from Figure 22.7) is a clue that it is an apical two chamber. The arrow points to a papillary muscle, which by definition is at a "mid"-level of the ventricle. The papillary muscle in Figure 22.7 is the posteromedial papillary muscle. In the American Society of Echocardiography's 17-segment model (Figure 22.13), there is no posterior wall (answer choices B and C). The wall segment designated by the arrow is the mid-inferior wall, which is supplied by the right coronary artery. The mid-anterolateral wall (answer choice D) is supplied by both the left anterior descending and left circumflex and the arrow does not point to this wall segment in Figure 22.7.

Selected Reference

1. Lang RM, Badano LP, Mor-Avi V, et al. Recommendations for cardiac chamber quantification by echocardiography in adults: an update from the American Society of Echocardiography and the European Association of Cardiovascular Imaging. *J Am Soc Echocardiogr.* 2015;28(1):1-39.e14.

**13.** Correct Answer: B. 20%

*Rationale:* Normal ventricular wall thickening during ventricular systole is commonly defined as an increase in wall thickness of >30% of the end-diastolic thickness. Hypokinesis is defined as reduced thickening during ventricular systole or thickening <30%. Akinesis is defined as absent or negligible thickening such as what occurs with a scarred segment. Dyskinesis is defined as systolic expansion or outward bulging, often with thinning; this can, for example, be seen with a ventricular wall aneurysm.

Selected References
1. Lang RM, Badano LP, Mor-Avi V, et al. Recommendations for cardiac chamber quantification by echocardiography in adults: an update from the American Society of Echocardiography and the European Association of Cardiovascular Imaging. *J Am Soc Echocardiogr.* 2015;28(1):1-39.e14.
2. Mathew JP, Swaminathan M, Ayoub CM. *Clinical Manual and Review of Transesophageal Echocardiography.* 2nd ed. McGraw Hill Medical; 2010.

**14.** Correct Answer: C. Biplane method of disks

*Rationale:* The 2015 American Society of Echocardiography guidelines on cardiac chamber quantification recommend biplane method of disks for 2D quantitative assessment of left ventricular ejection fraction. Fractional shortening and fractional area change may incorrectly estimate ejection fraction in the presence of regional wall motion abnormalities (for instance, if these abnormalities are near the base or apex). Global longitudinal strain does not estimate ejection fraction. As a measure of systolic function, although global longitudinal strain appears to be robust and reproducible, the evidence base for its routine clinical use is far less than 2D ejection fraction estimation. If offered, three-dimensional volumetric assessment would be an acceptable answer choice, as the 2015 guidelines also recommend its use when available and feasible.

Selected Reference
1. Lang RM, Badano LP, Mor-Avi V, et al. Recommendations for cardiac chamber quantification by echocardiography in adults: an update from the American Society of Echocardiography and the European Association of Cardiovascular Imaging. *J Am Soc Echocardiogr.* 2015;28(1):1-39.e14.

**15.** Correct Answer: B. Avoids geometric assumptions compared to linear methods

*Rationale:* Linear methods of left ventricular ejection fraction estimation make significant assumptions about left ventricular geometry, such as the ventricle is bullet-shaped. The biplane method of disks makes significantly fewer assumptions. For example, an aneurysmal segment that is well visualized is incorporated into the volume estimates that are used to calculate ejection fraction. However, the biplane method of disks may have several significant limitations. The apex may be foreshortened, leading to incorrect estimation of ejection fraction. Endocardial dropout remains a significant problem in some patients—echo-contrast administration may assist with endocardial border visualization. Finally, although the biplane method of disks uses two orthogonal views to visualize large parts of the left ventricular wall, subtle regional wall motion abnormalities out of plane from these two views may be missed and not incorporated into the ejection fraction estimate.

Selected Reference
1. Lang RM, Badano LP, Mor-Avi V, et al. Recommendations for cardiac chamber quantification by echocardiography in adults: an update from the American Society of Echocardiography and the European Association of Cardiovascular Imaging. *J Am Soc Echocardiogr.* 2015;28(1):1-39.e14.

**16.** Correct Answer: D. Left ventricular end-diastolic volume from an apical long axis

*Rationale:* The biplane method of disks uses tracings of the endocardial border as well as the length of the left ventricular long axis. The two views used are the apical four chamber and the apical two chamber. The apical long-axis view (also known as the apical three chamber) is not used in the biplane method of disks.

Selected Reference
1. Lang RM, Badano LP, Mor-Avi V, et al. Recommendations for cardiac chamber quantification by echocardiography in adults: an update from the American Society of Echocardiography and the European Association of Cardiovascular Imaging. *J Am Soc Echocardiogr.* 2015;28(1):1-39.e14.

## 17. Correct Answer: A. Normal

*Rationale:* Normal left ventricular ejection fraction for men is 52% to 72%; for women, the reference values are 54% to 74%. Reference values for mildly abnormal function also differ slightly for men and women. For moderately and severely abnormal left ventricular systolic function, the reference values for men and women are the same, with moderately abnormal defined as 30% to 40% and severely abnormal defined as <30%.

### Selected Reference
1. Lang RM, Badano LP, Mor-Avi V, et al. Recommendations for cardiac chamber quantification by echocardiography in adults: an update from the American Society of Echocardiography and the European Association of Cardiovascular Imaging. *J Am Soc Echocardiogr.* 2015;28(1):1-39.e14.

## 18. Correct Answer: B. End-systolic and end-diastolic volumes of the left ventricle

*Rationale/Critique:* To calculate cardiac output, a Doppler spectral profile of flow velocity through the left ventricular outflow tract over time is acquired. The profile is traced, and a time-velocity integral is obtained, which is equivalent to a stroke distance. The diameter of the left ventricular outflow tract is also measured, from which a cross-sectional area is calculated. The time-velocity integral and the cross-sectional area are multiplied, which yields the stroke volume. The stroke volume is then multiplied by the heart rate to obtain the cardiac output. Answer B can be used to calculate cardiac output but does not incorporate any Doppler methods. The equations involved are shown in **Figure 22.14**.

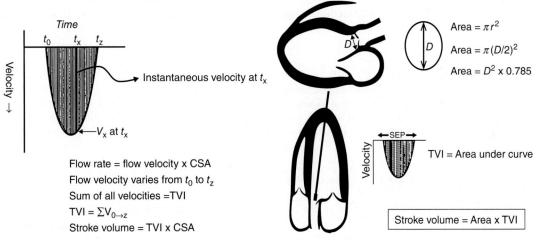

**Figure 22.14**

### Selected Reference
1. Armstrong WF, Ryan T. *Feigenbaum's Echocardiography.* 8th ed. Wolters Kluwer; 2019.

## 19. Correct Answer: A. Sepsis with hyperdynamic systolic function

*Rationale:* Fractional shortening is a linear measurement technique used to estimate left ventricular systolic function:

(Left ventricular end-diastolic diameter − left ventricular end-systolic diameter)/left ventricular end-systolic diameter

A fractional shortening ≥25% implies normal left ventricular function. A value <25% implies reduced function. The measurements are often obtained from a parasternal long-axis view. Fractional shortening may be a useful way to assess left ventricular systolic function in the absence of regional wall motion abnormalities, conduction abnormalities, and abnormal left ventricular geometry. In this question, an acute myocardial infarction (choice B), a left bundle branch block (choice C), and right ventricular pacing (choice D) would all cause regional wall motion abnormalities that may make fractional shortening inaccurate. (See **Figure 22.15** for additional details.)

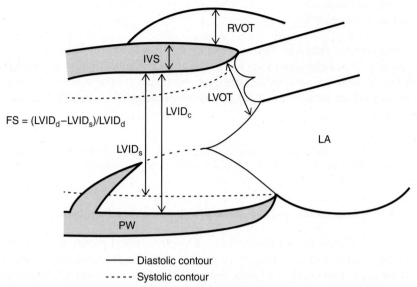

——— Diastolic contour

----- Systolic contour

**Figure 22.15** Schematic of a parasternal long-axis view of the left ventricle depicting linear measurements. By convention, linear measurements of the left ventricle are made at the level of the mitral chordae. From the linear internal dimension of the left ventricle in diastole and systole, fractional shortening can be calculated as noted. When measuring ventricular septal thickness, caution is advised to avoid measuring the most proximal portion of septum, which is frequently an area of isolated hypertrophy and angulation that does not truly represent ventricular wall thickness. FS, fractional shortening; IVS, interventricular septum; LVIDd, left ventricular internal dimension in diastole; LVIDs, left ventricular internal dimension in systole; PW, posterior wall.

Selected References

1. Armstrong WF, Ryan T. *Feigenbaum's Echocardiography.* 8th ed. Wolters Kluwer; 2019.
2. Lang RM, Bierig M, Devereux RB, et al. Recommendations for chamber quantification: a report from the American Society of Echocardiography's Guidelines and Standards Committee and the Chamber Quantification Writing Group, developed in conjunction with the European Association of Echocardiography, a branch of the European Society of Cardiology. *J Am Soc Echocardiogr.* 2005;18(12):1440-1463.

**20.** Correct Answer: B. The frame when the left ventricular dimensions are largest

*Rationale/Critique:* Identification of the correct end-diastolic and end-systolic frames is essential to applying the biplane method of disks. End diastole is defined as the first frame after mitral valve closure or the frame in the cardiac cycle in which the left ventricular dimension or volume measurement is the largest. End systole is defined as the frame after aortic valve closure or the frame in which the left ventricular dimension or volume measurement is smallest. In patients with regular heart rhythms, M-mode measurements of the opening and closing of valves or pulse-wave or continuous-wave Doppler may be used as well.

Regarding the other answer choices, the frame prior to closure of the mitral valve (choice A) would be too early. The frame just after opening of the aortic valve (choice C) is now systole. End diastole is commonly associated with the R wave in the QRS complex (choice D) and use of the ECG by itself without consideration of the 2D image is likely to be less accurate. (See Figure 22.8 for additional details.)

Selected Reference

1. Lang RM, Badano LP, Mor-Avi V, et al. Recommendations for cardiac chamber quantification by echocardiography in adults: an update from the American Society of Echocardiography and the European Association of Cardiovascular Imaging. *J Am Soc Echocardiogr.* 2015;28(1):1-39.e14.

**21.** Correct Answer: B. Impaired left ventricular function

*Rationale:* This question requires calculating an ejection fraction, for which the equation is:

$$\text{Ejection fraction} = (\text{left ventricular end-diastolic volume} - \text{left ventricular end-systolic volume})/\text{left ventricular end-diastolic volume}$$

This patient has an estimated ejection fraction of 56%. In the absence of mitral regurgitation, the correct answer would be normal (A). However, in patients with severe mitral regurgitation, mitral regurgitation may provide a low-impedance pathway for blood during ventricular systole, thus reducing afterload. After correction via mitral valve replacement, the afterload experienced by the left ventricle increases. Recently, this mechanism has been disputed in the literature, particularly if the mitral regurgitation is more in the moderate to severe range.

However, regardless of the mechanism, a preoperative ejection fraction <60% is correlated with reduced left ventricular systolic function and worse outcomes after surgical correction of mitral regurgitation. Hence, options A and D are incorrect. At least based on patient outcomes, adequate preoperative ejection fraction among patients with severe mitral regurgitation who will undergo surgical correction is higher than what is considered normal in other populations. Severe mitral regurgitation increases right heart afterload and when present chronically results in pulmonary hypertension and right ventricular dysfunction. However, surgical correction of mitral regurgitation improves right ventricular afterload and potentially improving right ventricular function. Hence option C is incorrect.

### Selected Reference
1. Carabello BA. A tragedy of modern cardiology: using ejection fraction to gauge left ventricular function in mitral regurgitation. *Heart.* 2017;103(8):570-571.

---

**22.** Correct Answer: C. Repeat your measurements five times and average the results

*Rationale:* Organized left atrial contraction contributes around 15% to 30% of left ventricular diastolic filling. In atrial fibrillation, this contribution is lost, and the filling of the left ventricle can be extremely variable depending on the timing of diastole. For measurements of ventricular systolic function, the 2015 American Society of Echocardiography guidelines on cardiac chamber quantification recommend averaging a minimum of five beats to account for interbeat variability in patients with atrial fibrillation. For patients in normal sinus rhythm, averaging at least three beats is recommended. The committee also added that use of a representative beat is acceptable in the clinical setting, as the previous recommendation may be time consuming. Although "representative beat" was not defined by the committee and is not an available answer choice above, in our practice we look for a beat that qualitatively does not appear to be an outlier in terms of diastolic filling time.

### Selected Reference
1. Lang RM, Badano LP, Mor-Avi V, et al. Recommendations for cardiac chamber quantification by echocardiography in adults: an update from the American Society of Echocardiography and the European Association of Cardiovascular Imaging. *J Am Soc Echocardiogr.* 2015;28(1):1-39.e14.

---

**23.** Correct Answer: D. −30

*Rationale/Critique:* Strain describes deformation of the myocardium, which may occur in the radial, circumferential, or longitudinal directions. Strain is a dimensionless index that describes a change in length, calculated as:

Strain ($\varepsilon$) = (end-systolic length − end-diastolic length)/end-diastolic length

Global **longitudinal** strain has emerged as a relatively robust marker of left ventricular systolic function. However, widespread adoption has been slowed by a significant dependence on image quality and variability between software vendors, limiting reproducibility and comparability among studies.

Based on the strain equation previously mentioned, one can discern that a normal value for global longitudinal strain should be negative, as the end-systolic length of the ventricle should ideally be less than the end-diastolic length. The most commonly cited reference value for normal global longitudinal strain is <−20.

### Selected References
1. Duncan AE, Alfirevic A, Sessler DI, Popovic ZB, Thomas JD. Perioperative assessment of myocardial deformation. *Anesth Analg.* 2014;118(3):525-544.
2. Potter E, Marwick TH. Assessment of left ventricular function by echocardiography: the case for routinely adding global longitudinal strain to ejection fraction. *JACC Cardiovasc Imaging.* 2018;11(2 Pt 1):260-274.

**24.** Correct Answer: **D. All of the above.**

*Rationale/Critique:* Although ischemic disease may be a commonly thought of cause of regional wall motion abnormalities, it is important to be aware of others. Left bundle branch block and ventricular pacing (answer choices A and B) cause regional wall motion abnormalities due to abnormal depolarization of the left ventricle compared to the native conduction system. Patients suffering from subarachnoid hemorrhage or acute stroke may also demonstrate left ventricular regional wall motion abnormalities (answer choice C).

Selected References

1. Armstrong WF, Ryan T. *Feigenbaum's Echocardiography.* 8th ed. Wolters Kluwer; 2019.
2. Choi JY, Cha J, Jung JM, et al. Left ventricular wall motion abnormalities are associated with stroke recurrence. *Neurology.* 2017;88(6):586-594.
3. Medina de Chazal H, Del Buono MG, Keyser-Marcus L, et al. Stress cardiomyopathy diagnosis and treatment: JACC state-of-the-art review. *J Am Coll Cardiol.* 2018;72(16):1955-1971.

**25.** Correct Answer: **C. 3.**

*Rationale:* The wall motion score index is a method of evaluating the degree of ventricular dysfunction. It involves evaluating the wall motion of as many of the 17 segments as can be visualized. Each segment is assigned a numeric score. The scores are then added up and divided by the total number of segments visualized and scored, producing an average wall motion score called the index.

The American Society of Echocardiography's 2015 guidelines on cardiac chamber quantification recommend that each segment be analyzed individually in multiple views. A normal or hyperkinetic segment is given a score of 1; a hypokinetic segment is given a score of 2; an akinetic segment is given a score of 3; and a dyskinetic segment is given a score of 4. Additionally, in the past aneurysmal segments were assigned a score of 5—this is no longer recommended. A normal wall motion score index would be 1.0. The akinetic segment described above would be assigned a score of 3.

Selected Reference

1. Lang RM, Badano LP, Mor-Avi V, et al. Recommendations for cardiac chamber quantification by echocardiography in adults: an update from the American Society of Echocardiography and the European Association of Cardiovascular Imaging. *J Am Soc Echocardiogr.* 2015;28(1):1-39.e14.

# 23 | RIGHT VENTRICULAR FUNCTION AND PULMONARY HYPERTENSION

Etienne J. Couture, Charles Lessard Brassard, and Andre Y. Denault

1. What is the particular finding related to the flattening of interventricular septum (IVS) during cardiac cycle in the situation of right ventricular pressure and/or volume overload?

   A. Flattening of IVS is maximal at end systole for pressure overload and at end diastole for volume overload.
   B. Flattening of IVS is maximal at end diastole for pressure overload and at end systole for volume overload.
   C. Flattening of IVS is maximal at end diastole for both pressure overload and volume overload.
   D. Flattening of IVS is maximal at end systole for both pressure overload and volume overload.

2. The eccentricity index can be used to characterize the left ventricle shape during different parts of the cardiac cycle in order to identify abnormal motion of the IVS in different conditions of right ventricular overload. Which of the following sentences is not appropriate?

   A. Normal eccentricity index is 1 at end systole and 1 at end diastole
   B. Right ventricular volume overload yields an eccentricity index >1 at end diastole
   C. Right ventricular pressure overload yields an eccentricity index >1 at end diastole and end systole
   D. Right ventricular pressure overload yields an eccentricity index <1 at end diastole and end systole

3. Among the following findings, which one should be used to differentiate right ventricle from left ventricle on echocardiography?

   A. Septal attachment of atrioventricular valve is apically displaced in the left ventricle.
   B. Moderator band is a muscle band that generally extends from the anterior papillary muscle to the tricuspid annulus.
   C. The left ventricle wall is thinner than the right ventricle.
   D. There are three papillary muscles in the right ventricle.

4. When measuring the right ventricular dimensions in mid-esophageal four chamber transesophageal echocardiography (TEE), which of the following statements is compatible with right ventricle enlargement?

   A. Right ventricular base diameter of 45 mm
   B. Right ventricular mid-diameter of 31 mm
   C. Right ventricular length of 41 mm
   D. Right ventricular base diameter of 35 mm

5. Using the modified Bernoulli equation, what would be the estimated systolic pulmonary artery pressure (SPAP) from a tricuspid regurgitation (TR) maximal velocity of 2 m/s in a patient with a measured central venous pressure of 12 mm Hg?

   A. 28 mm Hg
   B. 20 mm Hg
   C. 16 mm Hg
   D. 26 mm Hg

6. When calculating the SPAP from the TR peak velocity, which of the following must be taken into consideration?

   A. SPAP can be estimated from TR jet in the presence of pulmonary flow obstruction such as pulmonary stenosis.
   B. TR jet peak velocity has to be squared via Bernoulli equation to convert velocity toward a pressure.
   C. In the presence of severe TR with large non-coaptation area the peak velocity provides a better estimation of the real SPAP.
   D. It is recommended to use parasternal short-axis view to maximize TR peak velocity.

7. Pulmonary regurgitation (PR) continuous-wave Doppler signal can be obtained from a parasternal short-axis view to estimate pulmonary artery pressure. What is the mean pulmonary artery pressure (MPAP) given a PR peak velocity of 3 m/s, PR end-diastolic velocity of 1 m/sec, and right atrial pressure (RAP) of 8 mm Hg?

   A. 36 mm Hg
   B. 44 mm Hg
   C. 12 mm Hg
   D. It is not possible based on the given values

8. Right ventricular systolic function can be assessed by $dP/dt$. Which of the following is a confounder when using it?

   A. Large and eccentric TR
   B. Central regurgitation
   C. Dilated right atrium
   D. Dilated right ventricle

9. Which of the following is not a risk factor for dynamic right ventricular outflow tract (RVOT) obstruction?

   A. Right ventricular hypertrophy
   B. Hypovolemia
   C. Hypervolemia
   D. Inotropic support

10. Right ventricular fractional area change (RVFAC) corresponds to:

   A. A percentage change in the right ventricular volume from end diastole to end systole
   B. Abnormal values if lower than 55%
   C. A global appraisal of right ventricular systolic function
   D. Right ventricular ejection fraction

11. Which of the following applies to linear, two-dimensional measurements of the right ventricle?

   A. Right ventricular dimensions should preferably be visually estimated compared to measured.
   B. Conventional apical four chamber focused on the left ventricle yields the most reliable measurements for right ventricular dimensions.
   C. Adequate right ventricular linear measurements should be taken from an apical four chamber showing the largest possible right ventricular basal diameter while presenting the left ventricular apex in the center of the scanning sector.
   D. Measurements are difficult due to the thinner right ventricular wall compared to the left ventricle.

12. In the presence of pulmonary embolism, McConnell sign refers to which of the following finding?

   A. Moderate-to-severe right ventricular lateral wall hypokinesis with normal or hyperdynamic wall motion of the right ventricular apex
   B. Presence of a right ventricular thrombus
   C. Moderate-to-severe hypokinesis of the right ventricular apex with normal or hyperdynamic right ventricular lateral wall motion
   D. Presence of a thrombus in transit between the right and left atrium

13. Which of the following findings would be diagnostic for a pulmonary embolism?

   A. New enlarged right ventricle
   B. Visualized thrombus in the proximal pulmonary artery
   C. New TR
   D. New PR

14. Which of the following is not a feature of the moderator band?

   A. Muscular trabeculation containing the right bundle branch
   B. It extends from the lower IVS to the anterior papillary muscle
   C. It serves as an anchoring structure for the tricuspid papillary muscle
   D. It is a mobile, net-like structure occasionally seen in the right atrium near the opening of inferior vena cava (IVC) and coronary sinus

15. Which of the following is a sign of severity of TR?

   A. Systolic dominance on hepatic vein flow pulsed-wave Doppler evaluation
   B. Dense and triangular continuous-wave Doppler signal of the tricuspid regurgitant flow
   C. Systolic reversal on hepatic vein flow pulsed-wave Doppler evaluation
   D. TR vena contracta of 4 mm

16. What is not typical with right ventricular blood supply?

   A. The right coronary artery is the primary coronary supply of the right ventricle.
   B. Right ventricular involvement with posterior descending artery occlusion may be limited to a portion of the right ventricular inferior wall.
   C. The left anterior descending artery may supply a portion of the right ventricular apex.
   D. The posterior septal perforators supply the entire septal wall.

17. Which of the following does not result in right ventricular wall thickening?

   A. Chronic obstructive pulmonary disease
   B. Pulmonary arterial hypertension
   C. Pulmonic valve stenosis
   D. Right ventricular arrhythmogenic dysplasia

18. Bedside echocardiography can be useful in the situation of hypoxemia. What particular finding on echo can be seen in a patient with pulmonary hypertension that can explain hypoxemia refractory to high levels of inspired oxygen?

   A. Right ventricular hypertrophy
   B. Severe TR
   C. Patent foramen ovale with right to left shunting
   D. Atrial septal defect with left to right shunting

19. Regarding right ventricular diastolic function evaluation, which of the following is true?

   A. Left atrial filling is more influenced by respiration than right atrial filling.
   B. The left and right ventricular diastolic filling patterns are similar except for lower velocity in the right ventricle.
   C. There is more respiratory variation in diastolic filling in the left ventricle than in the right ventricle.
   D. Right atrial filling is increased during expiration.

20. Variations in hepatic vein flow pattern can be seen with the appearance of right ventricular dysfunction and eventually progress to right ventricular failure. How would the hepatic vein flow systolic-to-diastolic (S/D) ratio be described in situations of end-stage right ventricular diastolic function?

   A. Reversed S and blunted D
   B. S>D
   C. S=D
   D. Blunted S

21. Milrinone is given after a bedside echocardiography examination showing signs of right ventricular dysfunction. Which of the following corresponds to a good response to the proposed therapy?

   A. Increase in right ventricular end-systolic area
   B. Decrease in TR severity
   C. Decrease in systolic lateral tricuspid annulus velocity (S')
   D. Decrease in tricuspid annulus plane systolic excursion (TAPSE)

22. Which of the following corresponds to an echocardiographic sign of tamponade?

   A. Presence of a localized effusion next to the right atrium
   B. Presence of a right ventricular diastolic and right atrial systolic collapse
   C. Presence of reciprocal respiratory change in tricuspid valve inflow pulsed Doppler velocity >15%
   D. Right atrial enlargement

23. Which of the following views is useful to calculate cardiac output from the RVOT?

   A. Parasternal short axis
   B. Parasternal long axis
   C. Apical four chamber
   D. Apical two chamber

24. What should be the estimated value of the RAP based on the following findings: IVC diameter of 3.2 cm with <50% collapsibility with a sniff test?

   A. 0
   B. 3
   C. 8
   D. 15

# Chapter 23 ▪ Answers

**1.** Correct Answer: A. Flattening of IVS is maximal at end systole for pressure overload and at end diastole for volume overload.

*Rationale:* In the situation of right ventricular pressure overload, the IVS is shifted to the left side during the entire cardiac cycle with maximal flattening at the end systole, when pressure in the right ventricle is at its highest level. In the situation of right ventricular volume overload, the IVS is shifted mainly during mid- to end diastole when the right ventricle is being volume loaded. This flattening is reversed during systole-sparing left ventricular deformation at end systole. However, paradoxical systolic septal motion from left to right can be seen.

### Selected References

1. Harjola VP, Mebazaa A, Celutkiene J, et al. Contemporary management of acute right ventricular failure: a statement from the Heart Failure Association and the Working Group on Pulmonary Circulation and Right Ventricular Function of the European Society of Cardiology. *Eur J Heart Fail.* 2016;18(3):226-241.
2. Naeije R, Badagliacca R. The overloaded right heart and ventricular interdependence. *Cardiovasc Res.* 2017;113(12):1474-1485.

**2.** Correct Answer: D. Right ventricular pressure overload yields an eccentricity index <1 at end diastole and end systole

*Rationale:* The eccentricity index has been described as a modality to evaluate IVS motion through the cardiac cycle (**Figure 23.1**).

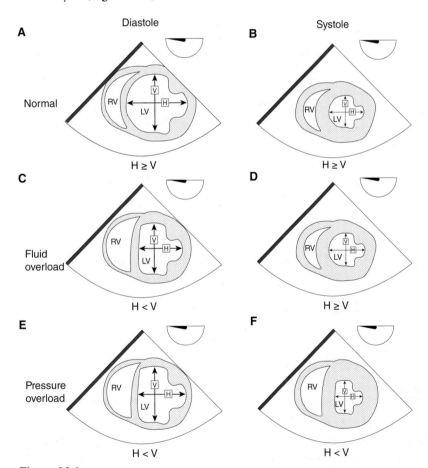

**Figure 23.1**

The eccentricity index is the ratio of the vertical diameter parallel to the IVS over the horizontal diameter perpendicular to the IVS of the left ventricle taken from a transgastric short-axis TEE view or a parasternal short-axis transthoracic echocardiography (TTE) view. The vertical diameter corresponds to the anterior to inferior diameter and the horizontal diameter corresponds to the septal to lateral diameter. These diameters are measured at end diastole and at end systole. Under normal pressure- and volume-loading conditions, the eccentricity index is 1 in order to describe the circular left ventricular geometry as well as the curvature of the IVS. This ratio will increase over 1 during systole and diastole in situations of elevated right ventricular pressure. In situations of volume overload, the ratio will be >1 only during end diastole, where the right ventricle is being overfilled and distended.

### Selected Reference

1. Ryan T, Petrovic O, Dillon JC, Feigenbaum H, Conley MJ, Armstrong WF. An echocardiographic index for separation of right ventricular volume and pressure overload. *J Am Coll Cardiol.* 1985;5(4):918-927.

**3.** Correct Answer: D. There are three papillary muscles in the right ventricle.

*Rationale:* The right ventricle presents anatomic features that allow differentiation from the left ventricle. Among them are apical displacement of the right septal atrioventricular valve leaflet that is also formed by three leaflets, presence of a moderator band in the right ventricle, presence of three papillary muscles, and a frank separation of inflow and outflow. The thickness of the right ventricle is typically less than the left ventricle but can be the same in some pathologic conditions.

### Selected References

1. Haddad F, Hunt SA, Rosenthal DN, Murphy DJ. Right ventricular function in cardiovascular disease, part I: Anatomy, physiology, aging, and functional assessment of the right ventricle. *Circulation.* 2008;117(11):1436-1448.
2. Haddad Fo, Doyle R, Murphy DJ, Hunt SA. Right Ventricular function in cardiovascular disease, Part II. *Circulation.* 2008;117(13):1717-1731.
3. Sanz J, Sánchez-Quintana D, Bossone E, Bogaard HJ, Naeije R. Anatomy, function, and dysfunction of the right ventricle. *J Am Coll Cardiol.* 2019;73(12):1463-1482.

**4.** Correct Answer: A. Right ventricular base diameter of 45 mm

*Rationale:* Right ventricular dimensions should always be measured at end diastole to reflect the largest measurement (**Figure 23.2**).

**A**

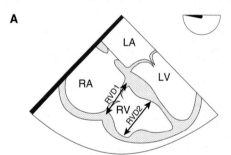

**Normal value for 2D RV chamber size**

| Parameter | Mean ± SD | Normal range |
|---|---|---|
| RVD1 (mm) | 33 ± 4 | 25-41 |
| RVD2 (mm) | 27 ± 4 | 19-35 |
| RV wall thickness (mm) | 3 ± 1 | 1-5 |

**B**

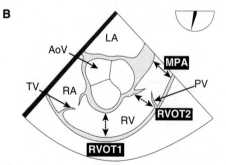

**Normal value for 2D RV chamber size**

| Parameter | Mean ± SD | Normal range |
|---|---|---|
| RVOT1 (mm) | 28 ± 3.5 | 21-35 |
| RVOT2 (mm) | 22 ± 2.5 | 17-27 |
| MPA (mm) | 21 ± 3 | 11-31 |

**Figure 23.2**

Multiple views and alignments should be used in order to get the largest possible diameter. The right ventricular base diameter (RVD1) corresponds to the maximal transverse dimension in the basal one-third of the right ventricular inflow. Values >41 mm correspond to right ventricular dilatation. Mid-cavity right ventricular linear diameter (RVD2) corresponds to the transverse right ventricular diameter in the middle third of right ventricle inflow, approximately halfway between the maximal basal diameter and the apex, at the level of papillary muscles. Values >35 mm correspond to dilatation. Right ventricular length or longitudinal dimension (RVD3) corresponds to the distance between the tricuspid plane and the apex. Values >83 mm refer to dilatation.

Selected References

1. Lang RM, Badano LP, Mor-Avi V, et al. Recommendations for cardiac chamber quantification by echocardiography in adults: an update from the American Society of Echocardiography and the European Association of Cardiovascular Imaging. *J Am Soc Echocardiogr.* 2015;28(1):1-39 e14.
2. Rudski LG, Lai WW, Afilalo J, et al. Guidelines for the echocardiographic assessment of the right heart in adults: a report from the American Society of Echocardiography endorsed by the European Association of Echocardiography, a registered branch of the European Society of Cardiology, and the Canadian Society of Echocardiography. *J Am Soc Echocardiogr.* 2010;23(7):685-713; quiz 86-88.

**5.** Correct Answer: A. 28 mm Hg

*Rationale:* Using the modified Bernoulli equation, $P = 4\,V^2$, where $P$ stands for pressure and $V$ for velocity, the pressure gradient between the right atrium and right ventricle can be calculated. Using continuous-wave Doppler of the TR jet, the difference in pressure between the right ventricle and the right atrium can be calculated with the following modified Bernoulli equation: $P = 4\,(\mathrm{TR_{peak\ velocity}})^2$ where $P$ corresponds to a pressure difference on which the RAP must be added to obtain an estimation of the right ventricular systolic pressure. From the TR, the probability of pulmonary hypertension can be estimated based on the maximal TR jet velocity; $\leq 2.8$ m/s being low probability, 2.9-3.4 m/s being intermediate probability, and $>3.4$ m/s being high probability. MPAP can be estimated from the SPAP using the following formula: MPAP = (0.61 · SPAP) + 2 mm Hg. See **Figure 23.3** for additional details.

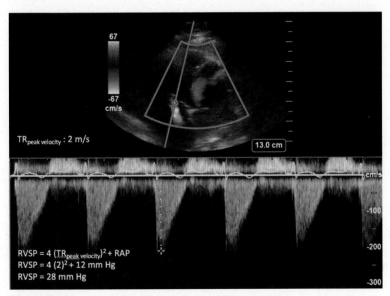

**Figure 23.3**

Selected References

1. Bossone E, D'Andrea A, D'Alto M, et al. Echocardiography in pulmonary arterial hypertension: from diagnosis to prognosis. *J Am Soc Echocardiogr.* 2013;26(1):1-14.
2. Parasuraman S, Walker S, Loudon BL, et al. Assessment of pulmonary artery pressure by echocardiography – a comprehensive review. *Int J Cardiol Heart Vasc.* 2016;12:45-51.

**6.** Correct Answer: B. TR jet peak velocity has to be squared via Bernoulli equation to convert velocity toward a pressure

*Rationale:* Doppler evaluation of TR allows a reliable estimation of pulmonary artery pressure.
The bedside echocardiographer must remember that velocity measurements are angle dependent. Thus, optimal TR jet velocity should be taken after interrogation in multiple, sometimes off-axis views, in order to obtain the best spectral Doppler envelope and maximal velocity as well as the best alignment between regurgitant flow and continuous-flow Doppler interrogation beam.

In the absence of pulmonary flow obstruction or significant pressure gradient between RVOT and pulmonary artery, TR peak velocity squared has a linear positive correlation with SPAP measured by right heart catheterization. In situations of pulmonary valve stenosis or RVOT obstruction, pulmonary artery pressure based on TR peak velocity and the modified Bernoulli equation will estimate the right ventricular systolic pressure but overestimate the pulmonary artery systolic pressure. If this is the case, peak pressure gradient across the pulmonary valve or the RVOT should be subtracted from the measured pulmonary artery systolic pressure.

It is also important to mention that in the presence of severe TR with a large color-flow regurgitant jet due to a large effective regurgitation orifice area (EROA), the TR peak velocity may not reflect the true gradient between the right ventricle and the RAP due to early equalization of right ventricle and RAP.

Selected Reference
1. Bossone E, D'Andrea A, D'Alto M, et al. Echocardiography in pulmonary arterial hypertension: from diagnosis to prognosis. *J Am Soc Echocardiogr*. 2013;26(1):1-14.

**7.** Correct Answer: B. 44 mm Hg

*Rationale:* Evaluation of PR from a parasternal short-axis view allows estimation of both MPAP and diastolic pulmonary artery pressure (DPAP). In this view, color-flow Doppler interrogation of PR will permit estimation of MPAP from peak early diastolic velocity, whereas DPAP will be estimated from end-diastolic velocities. Using the modified Bernoulli equation ($P = 4V^2$), PR peak early diastolic velocity and PR end-diastolic velocity can, respectively, be placed in the equation to find the pressure difference between the pulmonary artery and the right ventricle during diastole. From these values, addition of the RAP will result in MPAP and DPAP, assuming that RAP is equal to right ventricular end-diastolic pressure.

$$MPAP = 4(PR_{peak\ early\ diastolic\ velocity})^2 + RAP$$

$$MPAP = 4\ (3\ m/s)^2 + 8\ mm\ Hg$$

$$MPAP = 44\ mm\ Hg$$

$$DPAP = 4(PR_{end\text{-}diastolic\ velocity})^2 + RAP$$

$$DPAP = 4\ (1\ m/s)^2 + 8\ mm\ Hg$$

$$DPAP = 12\ mm\ Hg$$

Common pitfalls using this technique are misalignment of the PR Doppler signal and presence of constrictive or restrictive physiology that will result in shorter PR signal due to early equalization of pulmonary artery and right ventricular pressure.

MPAP can also be calculated using the SPAP obtained from Bernoulli equation and TR peak velocity and the DPAP obtained from the method previously mentioned using the following equation: $MPAP = 2/3 \cdot DPAP + 1/3 \cdot SPAP$. Lastly, MPAP can also be estimated from velocity-time integral (VTI) obtained from continuous-wave Doppler TR profile tracing. MPAP will thus be obtained by adding RAP to mean pressure obtained from $VTI_{TR}$, which represents mean right ventricular systolic pressure.

Selected References
1. Bossone E, D'Andrea A, D'Alto M, et al. Echocardiography in pulmonary arterial hypertension: from diagnosis to prognosis. *J Am Soc Echocardiogr*. 2013;26(1):1-14.
2. Parasuraman S, Walker S, Loudon BL, et al. Assessment of pulmonary artery pressure by echocardiography – a comprehensive review. *Int J Cardiol Heart Vasc*. 2016;12:45-51.

**8.** Correct Answer: A. Large and eccentric TR

*Rationale:* The right ventricular contractility can be estimated from intraventricular d$P$/d$t$. In order to use d$P$/d$t$ on echocardiography, TR must be present and must be interrogated with continuous Doppler during isovolumetric contraction when there is no significant change in RAP and before pulmonary valve opening. By using a time interval between 0.5 (=1 mm Hg) and 2 (=16 mm Hg) m/s on the Doppler velocity spectrum, the numerator becomes 15 mm Hg (16 mm Hg − 1 mm Hg) using Bernoulli equation. Thus, d$P$/d$t$ = 15 mm Hg/d$t$, where d$t$ represents the time lapse between 0.5 and 2 m/s on the Doppler spectrum. A d$P$/d$t$ value higher that 400 mm Hg/s or a duration of d$t \leq$ 37.5 ms when the velocity goes from 1 to 2 m/s corresponds to normal values, whereas d$P$/d$t$ lower than 400 mm Hg/s (d$t$ >37.5 ms) corresponds to reduced right ventricular systolic function. Finally, eccentric, trivial, or severe TR and presence of regional wall motion abnormality might give wrong estimates of the right ventricular systolic function.

### Selected Reference

1. Rudski LG, Lai WW, Afilalo J, et al. Guidelines for the echocardiographic assessment of the right heart in adults: a report from the American Society of Echocardiography endorsed by the European Association of Echocardiography, a registered branch of the European Society of Cardiology, and the Canadian Society of Echocardiography. *J Am Soc Echocardiogr*. 2010;23(7):685-713; quiz 86-88.

---

**9.** Correct Answer: **C. Hypervolemia**

*Rationale:* Dynamic RVOT obstruction can be seen in up to 4% of patients undergoing cardiac surgery. It is defined by a difference of at least 6 mm Hg between systolic right ventricular pressure and SPAP. Significant RVOT obstruction is defined by a pressure gradient of at least 25 mm Hg. This causes end-systolic obliteration of the RVOT on echocardiography. This condition can be appreciated with the use of M-mode in mid-esophageal right ventricular inflow-outflow view. Management strategies of this condition are similar to left ventricular outflow tract obstruction and include increase in preload, decrease in inotropic support, and decrease in heart rate when possible. Right ventricular dysfunction can be from mechanical compression secondary to mediastinal tumors, blood clots, surgical manipulation, left-sided tension pneumothorax, or any extrinsic condition that reduces the size of the RVOT. The treatment consists of removing the extrinsic cause of obstruction.

### Selected References

1. Denault AY, Chaput M, Couture P, Hébert Y, Haddad F, Tardif J-C. Dynamic right ventricular outflow tract obstruction in cardiac surgery. *J Thorac Cardiovasc Surg*. 2006;132(1):43-49.
2. Raymond M, Gronlykke L, Couture EJ, et al. Perioperative right ventricular pressure monitoring in cardiac surgery. *J Cardiothorac Vasc Anesth*. 2019;33(4):1090-1104.
3. Rochon AG, L'Allier PL, Denault AY. Always consider left ventricular outflow tract obstruction in hemodynamically unstable patients. *Can J Anaesth*. 2009;56(12):962-968.

---

**10.** Correct Answer: **C. A global appraisal of right ventricular systolic function**

*Rationale:* RVFAC is defined as the difference between end-diastolic and end-systolic right ventricular area compared to the end-diastolic right ventricular area (RV end-diastolic area − RV end-systolic right ventricular area)/end-diastolic right ventricular area × 100. RVFAC is obtained by tracing the right ventricular endocardium in diastole and systole from the lateral portion of the tricuspid annulus, along the lateral wall to the apex, and then to the septal portion of the tricuspid annulus, all along the IVS (**Figure 23.4**).

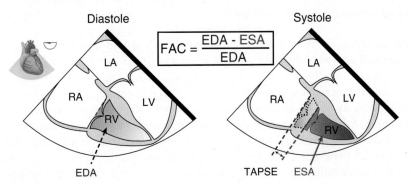

**Figure 23.4**

Right ventricular wall must be traced beneath the trabeculations. The lower reference value for normal right ventricular systolic function for RVFAC is 35%. Some references grade severity of right ventricular dysfunction based on RVFAC according to the following: mild (RVFAC 25%-31%), moderate (RVFAC 18%-24%), and severe (RVFAC < 18%). However, recent iteration of the American Society of Echocardiography does not refer to any such classification. RVFAC provides an estimate of global right ventricular systolic function as it has been shown to correlate with right ventricular ejection fraction by magnetic resonance imaging. It has also been found to be an independent predictor of heart failure, sudden death, stroke, and/or mortality in studies of patients after pulmonary embolism and myocardial infarction.

### Selected References

1. Lang RM, Badano LP, Mor-Avi V, et al. Recommendations for cardiac chamber quantification by echocardiography in adults: an update from the American Society of Echocardiography and the European Association of Cardiovascular Imaging. *J Am Soc Echocardiogr.* 2015;28(1):1-39 e14.
2. Lang RM, Bierig M, Devereux RB, et al. Recommendations for chamber quantification: a report from the American Society of Echocardiography's Guidelines and Standards Committee and the Chamber Quantification Writing Group, developed in conjunction with the European Association of Echocardiography, a branch of the European Society of Cardiology. *J Am Soc Echocardiogr.* 2005;18(12):1440-1463.
3. Rudski LG, Lai WW, Afilalo J, et al. Guidelines for the echocardiographic assessment of the right heart in adults: a report from the American Society of Echocardiography endorsed by the European Association of Echocardiography, a registered branch of the European Society of Cardiology, and the Canadian Society of Echocardiography. *J Am Soc Echocardiogr.* 2010;23(7):685-713; quiz 86-88.

**11.** Correct Answer: C. Adequate right ventricular linear measurements should be taken from an apical four chamber showing the largest possible right ventricular basal diameter while presenting the left ventricular apex in the center of the scanning sector.

*Rationale:* There is a greater interobserver variability when visual assessment of right ventricular chamber size and function is made over direct quantification. The conventional transthoracic apical four-chamber view focused on the left ventricle can induce considerable variability in how the right heart is partitioned. Thus, linear right ventricular dimensions and areas are prone to variations with only minor rotations in transducer position. Right ventricular dimensions are best estimated from an apical four-chamber view dedicated to the right ventricle obtained by lateral or medial transducer rotation. Adequate right ventricular linear measurements should ideally be taken from an apical four chamber showing the largest possible right ventricular basal diameter while presenting the left ventricular apex in the center of the scanning sector. Part of the right ventricular lateral wall might not be well defined due to either its size or its position behind the sternum. Two-dimensional right ventricular measurements are challenging essentially due to its complex geometry and the lack of specific right-sided anatomic landmarks to be used as reference points.

### Selected References

1. Lang RM, Badano LP, Mor-Avi V, et al. Recommendations for cardiac chamber quantification by echocardiography in adults: an update from the American Society of Echocardiography and the European Association of Cardiovascular Imaging. *J Am Soc Echocardiogr.* 2015;28(1):1-39 e14.
2. Ling LF, Obuchowski NA, Rodriguez L, Popovic Z, Kwon D, Marwick TH. Accuracy and interobserver concordance of echocardiographic assessment of right ventricular size and systolic function: a quality control exercise. *J Am Soc Echocardiogr.* 2012;25(7):709-713.

**12.** Correct Answer: A. Moderate-to-severe right ventricular free wall hypokinesis with normal or hyperdynamic wall motion of the right ventricular apex

*Rationale:* The McConnell sign consists of moderate-to-severe basal and mid-lateral hypokinesis with normal or hyperdynamic wall motion of the right ventricular apex in situations where a pulmonary embolism is suspected. This sign is specific for acute right ventricular failure though not only specific to pulmonary embolism. For a diagnosis of pulmonary embolism, this echocardiographic finding yields a sensitivity of 77% and a specificity of 94% in hospitalized patients with RV dysfunction from any cause. The positive predictive value of this finding for the diagnosis of pulmonary embolism is described to be 71% and the negative predictive value of 96% for an overall diagnostic accuracy of 92%. One explanation for this finding is believed to be that in the presence of pulmonary embolism, the left ventricle can become hyperdynamic and create tethering of the right ventricular apex rendering the preserved or hyperdynamic right ventricular apex. Also, in the situation of acute increases in right ventricular afterload, the right ventricle may assume a more spherical shape to equalize regional wall stress when subjected to an abrupt increase in afterload. A more spherical shape with systolic contraction would correspond to a bulging of the mid-right ventricular lateral wall relative to the apex and base. Lastly, increased right ventricular pressures and wall stress can decrease right ventricular coronary artery perfusion pressure and create localized ischemia of right ventricular lateral wall.

### Selected Reference

1. McConnell MV, Solomon SD, Rayan ME, Come PC, Goldhaber SZ, Lee RT. Regional right ventricular dysfunction detected by echocardiography in acute pulmonary embolism. *Am J Cardiol.* 1996;78(4):469-473.

**13.** Correct Answer: B. Visualized thrombus in the proximal pulmonary artery

*Rationale:* Diagnosis of pulmonary embolism can rarely be done by echocardiography. To do so, a thrombus must be seen in the proximal pulmonary artery. The diagnosis of pulmonary embolism can be highly supported without being definitive, by the presence of a clot in the right ventricle. It has been reported in approximately 4% of unselected patients with pulmonary embolism, but their prevalence can reach 18% in patients with pulmonary embolism in the intensive care unit. These findings are associated with high early mortality, especially in patients with right ventricular dysfunction. Nonspecific findings indicating right ventricular strain, present in approximately 30% to 40% of patients with pulmonary embolism, include the presence of an increased right ventricular size, a decreased right ventricular function, TR, and abnormal septal wall motion and regional wall motion abnormalities that spare the right ventricular apex (McConnell's sign). The most useful echocardiographic criteria for right ventricular dysfunction in patients with acute pulmonary embolism include an enlarged hypokinetic right ventricle with McConnell sign, or the 60/60 sign, which is the concomitant decrease in the acceleration time at the RVOT (pulmonary acceleration time) < 60 ms and an RVSP < 60 mm Hg.

Selected Reference

1. Kurnicka K, Lichodziejewska B, Goliszek S, et al. Echocardiographic pattern of acute pulmonary embolism: analysis of 511 consecutive patients. *J Am Soc Echocardiogr.* 2016;29(9):907-913.

**14.** Correct Answer: D. It is a mobile, net-like structure occasionally seen in the right atrium near the opening of IVC and coronary sinus

*Rationale:* The moderator band is a muscular trabeculation containing the right bundle branch. It extends from the lower IVS to the anterior papillary muscle of the right ventricular lateral wall. The moderator band serves as an anchoring structure for the tricuspid papillary muscles. The Chiari network is a mobile, net-like structure in the right atrium near the opening of IVC and coronary sinus occasionally seen during echocardiography imaging.

Selected Reference

1. Sanz J, Sánchez-Quintana D, Bossone E, Bogaard HJ, Naeije R. Anatomy, function, and dysfunction of the right ventricle. *J Am Coll Cardiol.* 2019;73(12):1463-1482.

**15.** Correct Answer: C. Systolic reversal on hepatic vein flow pulsed-wave Doppler evaluation

*Rationale:* TR is severe when the systolic waveform is reversed on hepatic vein flow pulsed-wave Doppler evaluation. Other signs of severity include the presence of a dilated annulus with absence of coaptation or a flail leaflet, a large central jet that occupies >50% of the right atrium area, vena contracta of at least 7 mm, a proximal isovelocity surface area (PISA) of >9 mm using a Nyquist limit of 30-40 mm/s, a dense and triangular-shaped color-wave Doppler jet, and a dilated right ventricle with a preserved function. EROA and regurgitant volume can also be measured and calculated for better evaluation of the severity.

Selected Reference

1. Zoghbi WA, Adams D, Bonow RO, et al. Recommendations for noninvasive evaluation of native valvular regurgitation: a report from the American Society of Echocardiography developed in collaboration with the Society for Cardiovascular Magnetic Resonance. *J Am Soc Echocardiogr.* 2017;30(4):303-371.

**16.** Correct Answer: D. The posterior septal perforators supply the entire septal wall.

*Rationale:* The consequences of an acute myocardial infarction are generally more severe the more proximal the occlusion is. The right ventricle is primarily perfused by acute marginal branches that arise from the right coronary. In the case of right ventricular involvement from a posterior descending artery occlusion, the regional wall motion abnormality might affect right ventricular inferior wall only. The posterior descending artery gives off perpendicular posterior septal perforators that typically supply the posterior third of the ventricular septal wall. In <10% of people, posterolateral branches of the left circumflex artery supply a portion of the posterior right ventricular free wall. The left anterior descending artery may supply a portion of the right ventricular apex, which could be compromised in occlusion of the left anterior descending artery.

Selected Reference

1. Crystal GJ, Pagel PS. Right ventricular perfusion: physiology and clinical implications. *Anesthesiology.* 2018;128(1):202-218.

**17.** Correct Answer: D. Right ventricular arrhythmogenic dysplasia

*Rationale:* Right ventricular free wall hypertrophy is an adaptation to a chronic state of increased afterload. Chronic obstructive pulmonary disease and other respiratory states associated with chronic hypoxemia, pulmonary hypertension due to various etiologies, and pulmonary valve stenosis are among causes of increased right ventricular afterload that produce right ventricular wall hypertrophy. Right ventricular arrhythmogenic dysplasia, myocardial aneurysm after right ventricular myocardial infarction, and Uhl syndrome are all differential diagnoses of right ventricular wall thinning.

### Selected References

1. Lang RM, Bierig M, Devereux RB, et al. Recommendations for chamber quantification: a report from the American Society of Echocardiography's Guidelines and Standards Committee and the Chamber Quantification Writing Group, developed in conjunction with the European Association of Echocardiography, a branch of the European Society of Cardiology. *J Am Soc Echocardiogr.* 2005;18(12):1440-1463.
2. Rudski LG, Lai WW, Afilalo J, et al. Guidelines for the echocardiographic assessment of the right heart in adults: a report from the American Society of Echocardiography endorsed by the European Association of Echocardiography, a registered branch of the European Society of Cardiology, and the Canadian Society of Echocardiography. *J Am Soc Echocardiogr.* 2010;23(7):685-713; quiz 86-88.

**18.** Correct Answer: C. Patent foramen ovale with right to left shunting

*Rationale:* In situations of hypoxemia refractory to high levels of inspired oxygen, the presence of a right to left shunt must be ruled out. Patent foramen ovale can be present in up to 25% of adults. To evaluate shunt, bedside echocardiography can be useful, but interatrial shunt will be better visualized using TEE. Contract enhancing agent or agitated saline can also be used to increase sensitivity.

### Selected References

1. Hara H, Virmani R, Ladich E, et al. Patent foramen ovale: current pathology, pathophysiology, and clinical status. *J Am Coll Cardiol.* 2005;46(9):1768-1776.
2. Silvestry FE, Cohen MS, Armsby LB, et al. Guidelines for the echocardiographic assessment of atrial septal defect and patent foramen ovale: from the American Society of Echocardiography and Society for Cardiac Angiography and Interventions. *J Am Soc Echocardiogr.* 2015;28(8):910-958.

**19.** Correct Answer: B. The left and right ventricular diastolic filling patterns are similar except for lower velocity in the right ventricle.

*Rationale:* The tricuspid valve annulus diameter is larger than the mitral valve diameter, resulting in lower right ventricular inflow velocity. The right ventricle is subject to more respiratory variation in diastolic filling than the left ventricle. The right atrium filling exerts more respiratory variation than the left atrial filling. Right atrial filling patterns are marked by an increase of right atrial inflow during inspiration and a decrease during expiration due to variations in intrathoracic pressure during spontaneous ventilation. Similar to mitral valve inflow, tricuspid valve inflow is characterized by an early diastolic E wave corresponding to right atrial emptying and a late diastolic A wave corresponding to atrial contraction.

Using tissue Doppler analysis, the lateral aspect of the tricuspid annulus can be interrogated. The normal spectral waveform includes a systolic wave (S′) and two diastolic waves (e′ and a′). Normally, the e′ wave is higher than the a′ in a similar fashion to the left ventricle. In a scenario of impaired ventricular relaxation, the E and e′ wave will be decreased and the E/A and e′/a′ will be <1. Transition to a more severe degree of diastolic dysfunction will produce a high E/A ratio (>1.5) due to decreased ventricular compliance and restricted filling. In contrast to the tricuspid E/A ratio, the e′/a′ will remain <1 and continue to decrease as diastolic right ventricular dysfunction progresses.

### Selected References

1. Dahou A, Levin D, Reisman M, Hahn RT. Anatomy and physiology of the tricuspid valve. *JACC Cardiovasc Imaging.* 2019;12(3):458-468.
2. Rudski LG, Lai WW, Afilalo J, et al. Guidelines for the echocardiographic assessment of the right heart in adults: a report from the American Society of Echocardiography endorsed by the European Association of Echocardiography, a registered branch of the European Society of Cardiology, and the Canadian Society of Echocardiography. *J Am Soc Echocardiogr.* 2010;23(7):685-713; quiz 86-88.

**20.** Correct Answer: A. Reversed S and blunted D

*Rationale:* Right ventricular diastolic dysfunction leads to a decrease of the systolic hepatic vein flow velocity and, eventually, a systolic-to-diastolic ratio less than 1 (S/D <1). Progression of right ventricular diastolic dysfunction leads to a blunting of the S wave before it becomes completely reversed, being the reflection of systolic backward flow in the hepatic veins during systole.

Selected Reference

1. Raymond M, Gronlykke L, Couture EJ, et al. Perioperative right ventricular pressure monitoring in cardiac surgery. *J Cardiothorac Vasc Anesth.* 2019;33(4):1090-1104.

**21.** Correct Answer: B. Decrease in TR severity

*Rationale:* Milrinone should increase right ventricular systolic performance. Thus, markers of right ventricular systolic performance should improve. Systolic lateral tricuspid annulus velocity (S') and TAPSE are expected to increase, whereas right ventricular end-systolic area should decrease due to an increase in RVFAC. Due to a decrease in end-systolic right ventricular area, decreased right ventricular afterload, and better right ventricular systolic performance, the severity of TR should decrease.

Selected References

1. Denault AY, Bussières JS, Arellano R, et al. A multicentre randomized-controlled trial of inhaled milrinone in high-risk cardiac surgical patients. *Can J Anesth.* 2016;63(10):1140-1153.
2. Gebhard CE, Rochon A, Cogan J, et al. Acute right ventricular failure in cardiac surgery during cardiopulmonary bypass separation: a retrospective case series of 12 years' experience with intratracheal milrinone administration. *J Cardiothorac Vasc Anesth.* 2019;33(3):651-660.

**22.** Correct Answer: B. Presence of a right ventricular diastolic and right atrial systolic collapse

*Rationale:* Tamponade after cardiac surgery can be seen with moderate-to-severe pericardial effusion that can also be localized. Right atrial systolic and right ventricular diastolic collapse are echocardiographic signs of tamponade. Left atrial and left ventricular collapse can also be seen in very localized tamponade after cardiac surgery. Reciprocal respiratory changes of at least 25% in right and left ventricular filling can be observed using pulse-wave Doppler in the ventricular inflows.

Selected Reference

1. Harjola VP, Mebazaa A, Celutkiene J, et al. Contemporary management of acute right ventricular failure: a statement from the Heart Failure Association and the Working Group on Pulmonary Circulation and Right Ventricular Function of the European Society of Cardiology. *Eur J Heart Fail.* 2016;18(3):226-241.

**23.** Correct Answer: A. Parasternal short axis

*Rationale:* Calculation of right ventricular cardiac output ($CO_{RV}$) from the RVOT is possible with the parasternal short-axis plane. With this view, it is possible to find the diameter of the RVOT ($D_{RVOT}$) and subsequently the area of the RVOT ($Area_{RVOT}$). In fact, $Area_{RVOT}$ can be estimated from the following equation assuming a circular shape: $Area_{RVOT} = \pi \cdot (D_{RVOT}/2)^2$ or its simplified version: $Area_{RVOT} = 0.78 \cdot D_{RVOT}^2$. Pulse-wave Doppler at the same area is used to find the VTI of the RVOT ($VTI_{RVOT}$) during the ejection phase. Estimation of the right ventricular output can thus be made from the following equation: $CO_{RV} = HR \cdot Area_{RVOT} \cdot VTI_{RVOT}$.

Selected Reference

1. Maslow A, Comunale ME, Haering JM, Watkins J. Pulsed wave Doppler measurement of cardiac output from the right ventricular outflow tract. *Anesth Analg.* 1996;83(3):466-471.

**24.** Correct Answer: **D. 15**

*Rationale/Critique:* Specific values of RAP should be reported instead of ranges when estimations of right ventricular or pulmonary artery pressure are made. IVC can be imaged in its long axis after a 90° counterclockwise rotation of the probe from an original subxiphoid view. However, the presence of chest tubes or dressings may prevent access to this view. Imaging through the liver from any lower right intercostal position can provide an adequate acoustic window to the IVC since its distal portion is intrahepatic.

Dynamic interrogation of the IVC allows estimation of the RAP. In spontaneously breathing patients, IVC diameter <2.1 cm and >50% collapsibility with a sniff test suggests low RAP of 3 mm Hg (range 0-5 mm Hg), while IVC diameter >2.1 cm and <50% collapsibility with a sniff test suggests RAP pressure of 15 mm Hg (range 10-20 mm Hg). With intermediate scenarios in which IVC diameter and collapsibility do not fit this classification, a value of 8 mm Hg (range 5-10 mm Hg) may be used. Other surrogates of RAP can also be used to downgrade or upgrade RAP value. In young patients, the IVC may be dilated in the presence of normal pressures. For patients supported by mechanical ventilation, the IVC is commonly dilated and may not collapse due to the constant presence of positive pressure throughout the entire respiratory cycle.

Finally, the IVC size and dynamics change throughout the respiratory cycle can easily be monitored with fluid resuscitation in order to estimate RAP in the absence of direct central venous pressure monitoring. There are several limitations to the use of the IVC. In fact, some patients with right ventricular dysfunction may present with RAP in the range of 25-30 mm Hg. This emphasizes the importance of integrating right heart findings such as right atrial size, ventricular size, and hepatic vein size and not underestimating RAP that might be higher than the prespecified range. Recent studies have shown that estimation of the RAP using both a transverse and a longitudinal view was more precise (**Table 23.1**).

**Table 23.1 Inferior Vena Cava Dynamics**

| Inferior Vena Cava Diameter (cm) | Collapsibility (%) | Estimated Right Atrial Pressure (mm Hg) |
| --- | --- | --- |
| <2.1 | >50 | 3, range 0-5 |
|  | <50 | 8, range 5-10 |
| >2.1 | <50 | 15, range 10-20 |
|  | <50 | 15, range 10-20 |

Selected References

1. Lang RM, Badano LP, Mor-Avi V, et al. Recommendations for cardiac chamber quantification by echocardiography in adults: an update from the American Society of Echocardiography and the European Association of Cardiovascular Imaging. *J Am Soc Echocardiogr.* 2015;28(1):1-39 e14.
2. Seo Y, Iida N, Yamamoto M, Machino-Ohtsuka T, Ishizu T, Aonuma K. Estimation of central venous pressure using the ratio of short to long diameter from cross-sectional images of the inferior vena cava. *J Am Soc Echocardiogr.* 2017;30(5):461-467.
3. Via G, Tavazzi G, Price S. Ten situations where inferior vena cava ultrasound may fail to accurately predict fluid responsiveness: a physiologically based point of view. *Intensive Care Med.* 2016;42(7):1164-1167.

# 24 | AORTIC VALVULAR DISEASE

Ranjani Venkataramani, Michael Nasr Boles Kot, and Mariya Geube

1. While evaluating an elderly patient with hypotension in the emergency room, a bedside point-of-care ultrasound (POCUS) reveals good left and right ventricular systolic function but a heavily calcified aortic valve (AV). What findings suggest severe aortic stenosis (AS) in this scenario?

   A. Color flow Doppler across AV in the AV short-axis (SAX) view showing flow turbulence
   B. Maximal velocity (Vmax) across the AV in the apical five-chamber view >4 m/s
   C. Mean AV gradient >30 mm Hg
   D. Ratio of velocity time integral $(VTI)_{LVOT}$ to $VTI_{AV}$ is 0.5.

2. A 50-year-old male patient with a history of hypertension presented in the emergency room after an episode of unconsciousness at his workplace. His vital signs were blood pressure 76/53 mm Hg, heart rate 98 bpm, respiratory rate 24 breaths/min, and temperature 97.5 F. An urgent transthoracic echocardiography (TTE) as part of his workup reveals **Figure 24.1** and ▶ **Video 24.1**.

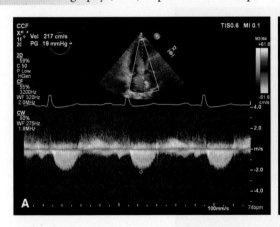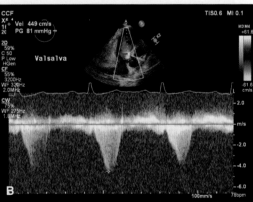

**Figure 24.1** A. Continuous-wave Doppler across left ventricular outflow tract at rest. B. Continuous-wave Doppler across left ventricular outflow tract during Valsalva.

What is the least appropriate next step in the management of his condition?
A. Start epinephrine
B. Start phenylephrine
C. Fluid bolus
D. Esmolol

225

3. A 37-year-old male undergoing an ascending aortic aneurysm repair has a transesophageal echocardiogram (TEE) intraoperatively that reveals **Figure 24.2** and ▶ **Videos 24.2A** and **B**.

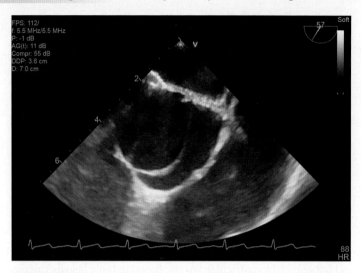

**Figure 24.2**

What other conditions can be associated with this condition?
A. Coronary artery disease
B. Coarctation of aorta
C. Parachute mitral valve
D. All of the above

4. A 60-year-old male with fatigue and dizziness was found to have AS. Calculate AV area (AVA) and assess severity of AS from the images below (**Figures 24.3** and **24.4**), assume left ventricular outflow tract (LVOT) diameter of 2.0 cm.

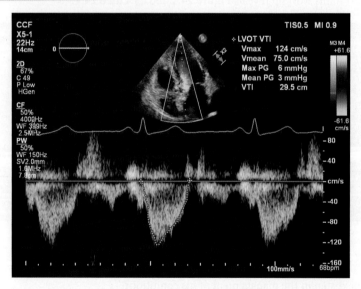

**Figure 24.3** Pulsed-wave Doppler of left ventricular outflow tract.

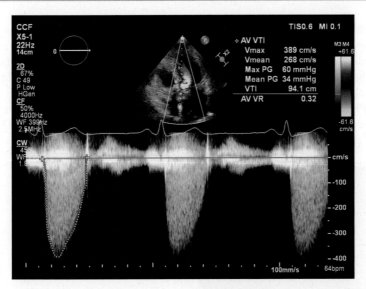

**Figure 24.4** Continuous-wave Doppler of left ventricular outflow tract.

A. 2 cm$^2$ and mild AS
B. 0.98 cm$^2$ and severe AS
C. 0.6 cm$^2$ and severe AS
D. Not enough information to calculate

5. An 82-year-old female is admitted to the intensive care unit (ICU) post–transfemoral aortic valve replacement (TAVR) with the following vital signs: blood pressure 180/110/130 mm Hg, heart rate 62 bpm, and respiratory rate 26 breaths/min. Patient complained of difficulty breathing. Based on **Figure 24.5** and ▶ **Videos 24.3A** and **B**, which of the following should be considered?

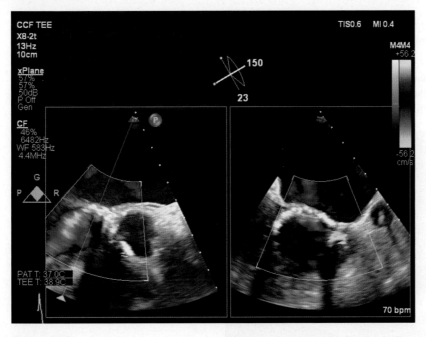

**Figure 24.5**

A. Initiate inotropic support
B. Give 1L crystalloid fluid bolus
C. Consider afterload reduction and discuss the echocardiographic findings with the proceduralist
D. Recommend urgent coronary angiogram

6. A 72-year-old male with a history of poorly controlled hypertension, smoking, and unstable angina underwent percutaneous coronary intervention in the cath lab. The patient had a left anterior descending artery stent and left circumflex artery stent placed. After the procedure, he had an episode of syncope and was found to have a blood pressure of 74/51 mm Hg and heart rate 118 bpm. Bedside TTE revealed normal LV systolic function and absence of regional wall motion abnormalities. TEE was performed and revealed **Figure 24.6** and ▶ **Video 24.4**. Cardiac tamponade is due to rupture of the adventitia or exudate from the adventitia in the ascending aortic hematoma, which is observed in approximately 20% to 36% of cases of type A aortic dissections

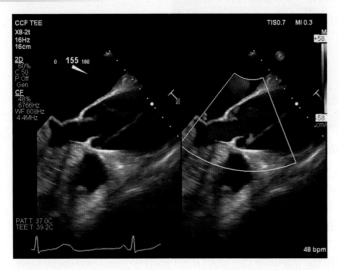

**Figure 24.6** Color compare image of midesophageal long-axis view.

Which complication is *least* likely to be associated with this condition?
A. Myocardial ischemia
B. Tamponade
C. Aortic regurgitation
D. Mitral regurgitation

7. A 52-year-old female on chronic steroids and infliximab (for Crohn disease), with factor V Leiden, presents with worsening shortness of breath with minimal activity, malaise, and cachexia. TEE was performed to further investigate her condition (**Figure 24.7** and ▶ **Videos 24.5A** and **B**).

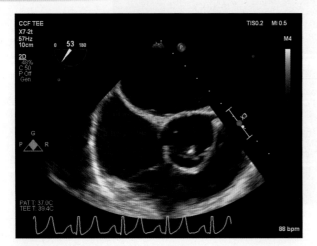

**Figure 24.7** Midesophageal aortic valve short-axis view.

Which of the following is *most* likely?
A. Mobile echogenic mass on the noncoronary cusp
B. Mobile echogenic mass on the right coronary cusp
C. Mobile echogenic mass on the posterior leaflet of the tricuspid valve
D. Mobile echogenic mass on the left coronary cusp

8. A 46-year-old man with a history of previous AV and aortic root replacement is admitted to the emergency room with acute onset of chest pain from his cardiologist's office. A TEE is obtained (**Figure 24.8** and ▶ **Videos 24.6A,B,C**).

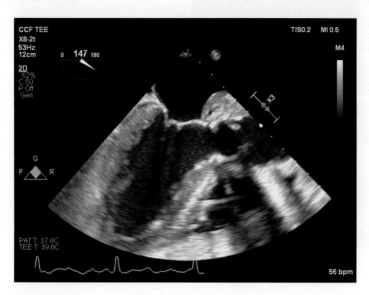

**Figure 24.8**

What is most appropriate next step?
A. Admit to ICU and start nitroprusside
B. Transfuse 2 U red blood cell concentrate
C. Consult cardiac surgery for evaluation
D. Start ceftriaxone and ampicillin for 6 weeks and discharge the patient home

9. A 65-year-old female, body surface area (BSA) 1.6 m², blood pressure 140/70 mm Hg, is admitted to the ICU from the postoperative recovery area after having undergone general anesthesia for a ventral hernia repair. After extubation, the patient had increased work of breathing and increased oxygen requirements. You obtain a formal echo that reveals the following—normal left ventricular ejection fraction (LVEF), LV hypertrophy; AV calcifications, peak and mean AV gradients 35/22 mm Hg, AVA of 0.9 cm² by planimetry; stroke volume index (SVI) 32 mL/m².

Which of the following most likely explains these findings?
A. Low-flow low-gradient (LF-LG) AS
B. Paradoxical LF-LG AS
C. Severe AS, but the transvalvular gradients are low because of poor alignment of the continuous-wave Doppler with the LVOT
D. Mild AS

**10.** A 45-year-old male presents to the hospital for treatment of urosepsis and is found to be hypotensive. The floor nurse requests an ICU evaluation and a bedside ECHO reveals **Figure 24.9** and ▶ **Video 24.7**.

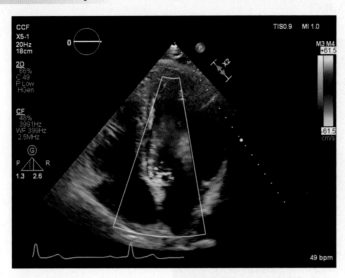

**Figure 24.9**

This pathology when chronic can most likely result in one of the following:
A. Low LV end-diastolic pressure
B. LV dilation
C. Atrial fibrillation
D. High diastolic blood pressure

**11.** A TTE performed in a 70-year-old male who presents with fatigue and light-headedness in the Emergency Department reveals **Figure 24.10**.

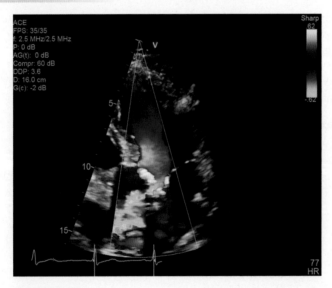

**Figure 24.10**

What is the most likely pathology?
A. Aortic stenosis
B. Aortic aneurysm
C. Mitral stenosis
D. Aortic insufficiency

12. Identify the coronary artery that arises from this coronary sinus in this midesophageal AV SAX view on TEE shown by the *arrow* in **Figure 24.11.**

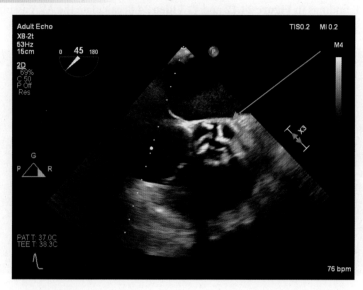

**Figure 24.11**

A. Obtuse marginal artery
B. Left main coronary artery
C. Left anterior descending artery
D. Left circumflex artery

13. Which of the following is least associated with bicuspid aortic valves (BAVs)?

A. Infectious endocarditis
B. Aortic regurgitation
C. Aortic aneurysms
D. Myocardial infarction

14. A 55-year-old male patient has concomitant AV stenosis and LVOT dynamic obstruction due to hypertrophic obstructive cardiomyopathy (HOCM). On 2D echocardiogram, the AV shows severe calcification. What method will most accurately estimate the degree of AS in this patient?

A. Peak/mean AV gradients
B. 3D planimetry
C. Continuity equation using right ventricular outflow tract diameter and VTI
D. Peak velocity through the AV using continuous-wave Doppler >4 m/s

15. A 35-year-old male with past medical history (PMH) of infective endocarditis and known severe tricuspid valve regurgitation was admitted to a community hospital ICU for fever, shortness of breath, and dark color urine. On admission, his vital signs were blood pressure 85/45 mm Hg, heart rate 110 bpm, and respiratory rate 28 breaths/min. In the emergency room he received 30 mL/kg fluid bolus with no improvement in hemodynamics. Bedside TTE was performed with the following findings:

- LVOT VTI 28 cm
- AV VTI 34 cm, LVOT diameter 2.2 cm
- Right ventricular systolic pressure (RVSP) 42 mm Hg

Calculate the cardiac output (CO).
A. 5.8 L/min
B. 8.4 L/min
C. 9.2 L/min
D. 11.7 L/min

**16.** A 69-year-old female presents to the emergency room with intermittent chest pain and shortness of breath with exertion. She has a previous history of a systolic murmur for which she receives medical management. Based on the TTE findings in **Figure 24.12** and ▶ **Video 24.8**, calculate the AVA assuming LVOT diameter is 2.1 cm.

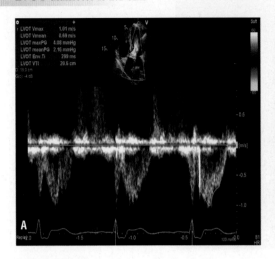 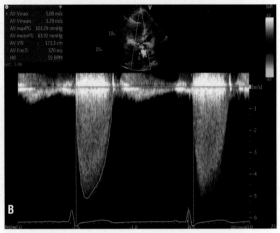

**Figure 24.12**

**A.** 2 cm$^2$

**B.** 0.82 cm$^2$

**C.** 0.41 cm$^2$

**D.** 0.59 cm$^2$

**17.** A 55-year-old female with PMH of diabetes, hypertension, morbid obesity, and sleep apnea complains of acute right upper quadrant abdominal pain, nausea, and vomiting for the last 48 h. She was diagnosed with acute cholecystitis and was taken to surgery for laparoscopic cholecystectomy. After insufflation, she becomes hypotensive and unresponsive to repeated doses of ephedrine and develops cardiac arrest. Cardiopulmonary resuscitation (CPR) was started with recovery of circulatory function. Intraoperative TEE is shown in **Figures 24.13A** and **B**.

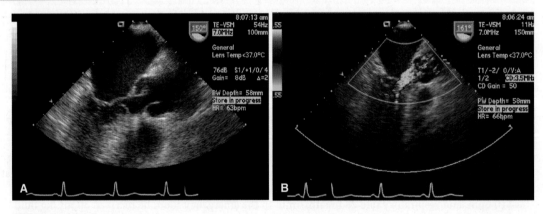

**Figure 24.13**

What is the most likely diagnosis?

**A.** Aortic stenosis

**B.** Hypertrophic obstructive cardiomyopathy

**C.** Membranous subaortic stenosis

**D.** Mitral regurgitation

**18.** A 65-year-old male was admitted to the cardiology ICU for shortness of breath due to acute decompensated heart failure with rapid ventricular response. After administration of metoprolol IV, he converted to SR. On the next day, while the patient was in sinus rhythm, with stable hemodynamics, TTE showed:

- LVEF 35%
- Peak and mean AV gradients 46 and 25 mm Hg accordingly
- AVA 0.9 cm$^2$, SVI 32 mL/m$^2$.

What is your next step of action?
**A.** Patient has severe AS and you should call cardiac surgery to evaluate for AV replacement
**B.** Dobutamine stress echocardiogram
**C.** Discharge patient to follow-up with his cardiologist
**D.** Urgent TAVR

**19.** Review **Figure 24.14** and ▶ **Videos 24.9A** and **B**.

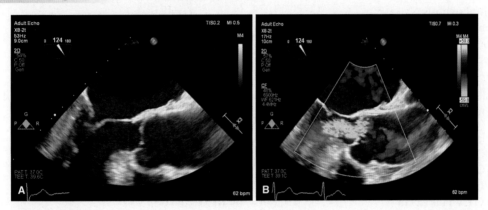

**Figure 24.14**

What is the type of aortic regurgitation according to El Khoury classification?
**A.** Type 1D
**B.** Type 2
**C.** Type 3
**D.** Type 1C

**20.** A 67-year-old female was admitted to the ICU because of shortness of breath after knee surgery replacement. On arrival, her vital signs were as follows: blood pressure 105/45 mm Hg, heart rate 95 bpm, oxygen saturation 85%, and temperature 36.5 °C. Chest X-ray was ordered and showed increased bronchovascular marking, suggestive of interstitial lung edema. She was diagnosed with a heart murmur 7 years ago. TTE and TEE images are shown in **Figures 24.15** and **24.16** respectively and ▶ **Video 24.10**.

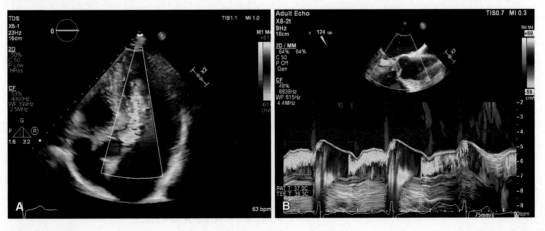

**Figure 24.15**

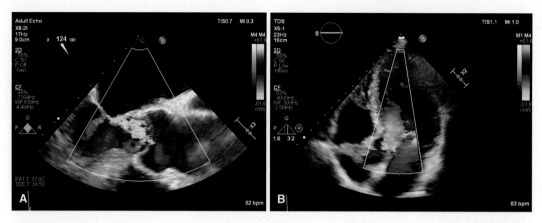

**Figure 24.16**

What is the most likely diagnosis?
A. Mitral stenosis
B. Ventricular septal defect
C. Aortic regurgitation
D. Hypertrophic obstructive cardiomyopathy

21. On follow-up of a 40-year-old male with PMH of Marfan syndrome and BAV, his cardiologist heard a worsening diastolic murmur and so ordered a TTE:

Calculate the effective regurgitant volume of the AV if you know that:
• LVOT diameter is 2.0 cm
• LVOT VTI is 50 cm
• RVOT diameter is 2.4 cm
• RVOT VTI is 22 cm

A. 68 mL
B. 57 mL
C. 43 mL
D. 33 mL

22. A 68-year-old male with PMH of chest pain had a left heart catheterization that demonstrated extensive three-vessel disease. Other history includes type 2 diabetes on oral agents and hyperlipidemia. The patient reports a transient ischemic attack episode a year ago. On the day of the CABG his vitals are temperature 36.9 °C, blood pressure 124/85 mm Hg, and heart rate 68/min. Intraoperative TEE is shown in ▶ **Videos 24.11A** and **B**.

What is your differential diagnosis?
A. Infective endocarditis vegetation
B. Myxoma
C. Lambl's excrescences
D. Left atrial appendage thrombus

23. A patient who has the TEE shown in **Figure 24.17** is at increased risk of all of the following except:

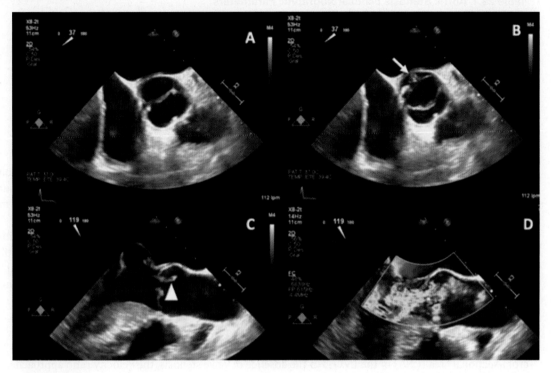

**Figure 24.17**

A. Aortic dissection
B. Coarctation of aorta
C. AV insufficiency
D. Pericarditis

24. An 82-year-old female presents to the cardiology office with complaints of increased shortness of breath and occasional chest pain on exertion and limited physical activity at home. Her cardiologist reports a systolic heart murmur and is concerned about AS. He orders an echocardiogram and subsequent angiography. Which of the following is true regarding AV gradients?

A. Gradients obtained by echo are mean instantaneous gradients
B. Gradients obtained by echo are peak-to-peak gradients
C. Gradients obtained by angiography are peak instantaneous gradients
D. Gradients obtained by echo are peak instantaneous gradients.

# Chapter 24 ▪ Answers

1. Correct Answer: B. Maximal velocity (Vmax) across the AV in the apical five-chamber view >4 m/s

   *Rationale:* The three basic echocardiographic parameters to evaluate the presence of AS include (level 1 recommendation):
   1. Peak velocity across AV using continuous-wave Doppler
   2. Mean transvalvular pressure gradient
   3. AVA by planimetry or continuity

Additional AS echocardiographic parameters can be seen in **Table 24.1**.

**Table 24.1 Aortic Stenosis Echocardiographic Parameters**

|  | **Mild** | **Moderate** | **Severe** |
|---|---|---|---|
| Peak velocity (m/s) | 2.6-2.9 | 3-4 | ≥4 |
| Mean gradient (mm Hg) | <20 | 20-40 | ≥40 |
| AVA (cm²) | >1.5 | 1-1.5 | <1 |
| Indexed AVA (cm²/m²) | >0.85 | 0.65-0.85 | <0.65 |
| Velocity ratio | >0.50 | 0.25-0.50 | <0.25 |

Severe AS is defined by current guidelines as calcified or thickened valve leaflets with reduced systolic opening and antegrade velocity across the valve of >4.0 m/s equivalent to a mean transvalvular pressure gradient of >40 mm Hg. Typically, AVA is <1.0 cm². The guidelines also take into account the BSA of the patient, thus severe AS is defined as AVA <0.65 cm²/m².

Beware of lower velocities (underestimation of the severity of AS) when the Doppler beam is misaligned with the direction of the blood flow. The degree of AS is also underestimated with low stroke volume (SV) (LF-LG AS). The velocity ratio (also referred to as dimensionless index) may be helpful in these circumstances where there is Doppler misalignment and in situations where one may be concerned about LF-LG AS.

Option D refers to the dimensionless index, which is the ratio of subvalvular velocity obtained by pulsed-wave Doppler and the maximum velocity obtained by continuous-wave Doppler across the AV. This dimensionless index expresses the size of the valvular effective orifice area as a proportion of the cross-sectional area (CSA) of the LVOT. In the absence of valve stenosis, the velocity ratio approaches 1, with smaller numbers indicating more severe stenosis. Severe AS is suggested when the velocity ratio is <0.25, corresponding to a valve area 25% of normal.

Selected Reference

1. Baumgartner H, Hung J, Bermejo J, et al. Recommendations on the echocardiographic assessment of aortic valve stenosis: a focused update from the European Association of Cardiovascular Imaging and the American Society of Echocardiography. *J Am Soc Echocardiogr.* 2017;30(4):372-392.

**2.** Correct Answer: **A. Start epinephrine**

*Rationale:* Both fixed lesions such as valvular AS and dynamic LVOT obstruction such as seen in HOCM present with increased LVOT velocities. However, in AS, the orifice remains fixed in systole, whereas in HOCM, the LVOT obstruction is worse in mid- to late systole.

The spectral Doppler waveforms in Figure 24.1A show an elevated LVOT velocity of 2 m/s with a "rounded" velocity profile. Figure 24.1B obtained during a Valsalva maneuver shows a higher velocity of 4 m/s with a "dagger-shaped" velocity profile along with an intracavitary gradient of approximately 80 mm Hg. This increase in velocity across the LVOT with Valsalva occurs in dynamic LVOT obstruction (aka HOCM) due to worsening obstruction with the reduced venous return from the Valsalva maneuver. Dynamic obstruction is made worse with increased inotropy (option A—use of epinephrine), reduced venous return (low preload), and reduced afterload. Hence options B, C, and D (phenylephrine to increase afterload, fluid bolus to maintain preload, and esmolol to reduce inotropy) are appropriate next steps.

Selected References

1. Geske JB, Ommen SR, Gersh BJ. Hypertrophic cardiomyopathy. *JACC Heart Fail.* 2018;6(5):364.
2. Sherrid MV, Wever-Pinzon O, Shah A, Chaudhry FA. Reflections of inflections in hypertrophic cardiomyopathy. *J Am Coll Cardiol.* 2009;54(3):12-219.

**3.** Correct Answer: **B. Coarctation of aorta**

*Rationale:* Figure 24.2 and ▶ **Videos 24.2A** and **B** show a midesophageal aortic valve short axis view (ME AV SAX view) with a BAV. A congenital BAV occurs in approximately 1% to 2% of the general population, making it the most common congenital valvular malformation. Calcification of a congenitally bicuspid valve results in premature onset of AS and represents the most common cause of AS among patients younger than

70 years of age. Commonly associated findings in patients with BAVs include aortic disease, including aortic coarctation, aortic insufficiency, aortic root dilation, ascending/arch aneurysms, and an increased risk of aortic dissection. Coarctation of the aorta can be associated with 20% of BAV or even more.

Notably, BAV is often associated with aortopathy. Type 1 BAV (fusion of right and left coronary cusps) leads to aneurysm of the ascending aorta, while type 2 BAV (fusion of right and noncoronary cusps) leads to arch dilation. Fusion of the non- and left cusp is extremely rare.

### Selected Reference

1. Siu SC, Silversides CK. Bicuspid aortic valve disease. *J Am Coll Cardiol.* 2010;55(25):2789.

---

**4.** Correct Answer: B. 0.98 cm² and severe AS

*Rationale:* The continuity equation is based on the principle of conservation of mass, or "flow in = flow out." In other words, SV through the LVOT must equal SV through the AV.

We can obtain three of the four components of the continuity equation by calculating the SV of the LVOT and measuring the peak AV velocity.

$$SV = VTI \text{ (chamber)} \times CSA \text{ of the chamber}$$

$$SV \text{ (LVOT)} = SV \text{ (AV)}$$

Applying this:

$$\textbf{\textit{AVA}} \times \textbf{\textit{VTI AV}} = \textbf{\textit{CSA LVOT}} \times \textbf{\textit{VTI LVOT}}$$

CSA LVOT = cross-sectional area of LVOT ($\pi r^2$); $r$ is $d/2$ where $d=$ diameter of the LVOT, which is 2.0 cm in this question.

Solving for AVA:

$$AVA = \frac{CSA\ LVOT \times VTI\ LVOT}{VTI\ AV}$$

VTI LVOT is 29.5 cm and the VTI AV is 94.1 cm. Entering these numbers into the equation yields a value of 0.98 cm², which suggests severe AS, as shown in **Table 24.2**.

**Table 24.2 Classification of Aortic Stenosis**

|                                    | Mild      | Moderate  | Severe   |
| ---------------------------------- | --------- | --------- | -------- |
| Peak velocity (m/s)                | 2.6-2.9   | 3-4       | ≥4       |
| Mean gradient (mm Hg)              | <20       | 20-40     | ≥40      |
| Aortic valve area (AVA) (cm²)      | >1.5      | 1-1.5     | <1       |
| Indexed AVA (cm²/m²)               | >0.85     | 0.65-0.85 | <0.65    |
| Velocity ratio                     | >0.50     | 0.25-0.50 | <0.25    |

### Selected Reference

1. Baumgartner H, Hung J, Bermejo J, et al. Recommendations on the echocardiographic assessment of aortic valve stenosis: a focused update from the European Association of Cardiovascular Imaging and the American Society of Echocardiography. *J Am Soc Echocardiogr.* 2017;30(4):372-392.

---

**5.** Correct Answer: C. Consider afterload reduction and discuss the echocardiographic findings with the proceduralist

*Rationale:* Figure 24.5 and ▶ **Videos 24.3A** and **B** demonstrate AV paravalvular leak (PVL). The diagnosis is made based on echocardiographic appearance and quantification, root aortography, and hemodynamics (aortic and LV waveforms). The presence of PVL causes acute aortic regurgitation with increased LV end-diastolic pressure, which may result in pulmonary edema. Giving a fluid bolus would not be recommended. There are certain treatment options if significant postdeployment PVL is noticed on an echocardiographic examination. It can be corrected with repeat dilation of the valve to minimize residual regurgitation or using valve-in-valve technique, in which a second valve is deployed over the first percutaneous valve, or with other percutaneous closure devices. Moderate-to-severe PVL after surgical or transcatheter AV replacement is associated with increased mortality and should be corrected.

Given that patients with at least moderate paravalvular leak (PVL) at 30 days harbor a 2.4-fold increase in 1-year mortality, it is essential to make every effort to avoid more than mild PVL at the time of TAVR. The updated Valve Academic Research Consortium (VARC-2) criteria used in the PARTNER I trial recommended the following with respect to the circumferential extent of PVL in SAX: trace (pinpoint jet), mild (<10% of the valve circumference), moderate (10%-30%), and severe (>30%).

### Selected References

1. Ionescu A, Fraser AG, Butchart EG. Prevalence and clinical significance of incidental paraprosthetic valvar regurgitation: a prospective study using transoesophageal echocardiography. *Heart.* 2003;89(11):1316.
2. Steinvil A, Leshem-Rubinow E, Halkin A, et al. Vascular complications after transcatheter AV implantation and their association with mortality reevaluated by the valve academic research consortium definitions. *Am J Cardiol.* 2015;115(1):100-106.

---

**6.** Correct Answer: **D. Mitral regurgitation**

*Rationale/Critique:* Figure 24.6 and ▶ **Video 24.4** depict an ascending aortic dissection (Stanford type A). The dissected intimal (flap) is visualized to originate near the right sinus of Valsalva (most common origin). If the dissection involves the ostia of the coronary arteries, it may result in myocardial ischemia/infarction. Also, the impingement of the flap during diastole can result in malcoaptation of the AV cusps resulting in aortic regurgitation. In case of rupture, a life-threatening tamponade may occur. This leads to abrupt hemodynamic collapse and requires emergent surgery with institution of cardiopulmonary bypass to establish control of the bleeding and provide cardiopulmonary support.

Complications associated with dissections are aortic regurgitation (50%-70% of the cases), coronary dissections with myocardial ischemia (10%-20%), pleural and pericardial effusions, and global LV dysfunction. TEE midesophageal long-axis view is most helpful to assess the presence and severity of aortic regurgitation in the presence of dissection. LV dysfunction may be secondary to ischemia following coronary dissection and acute aortic regurgitation.

### Selected Reference

1. Patil T, Nierich A. Transesophageal echocardiography evaluation of the thoracic aorta. *Ann Card Anaesth.* 2016;19(5):44-55.

---

**7.** Correct Answer: **B. Mobile echogenic mass on the right coronary cusp**

*Rationale:* Figure 24.7 and ▶ **Videos 24.5A** and **B** TEE images depict a midesophageal AV SAX view. The valve is tricuspid. The leaflet close to the right ventricular outflow tract (6 o' clock position) is the right coronary cusp. The leaflet abutting the interatrial septum is the noncoronary cusp, and the leaflet close to the left atrial appendage is the left coronary cusp.

### Selected Reference

1. Hahn RT, Abraham T, Adams MS, et al. Guidelines for performing a comprehensive transesophageal echocardiographic examination: recommendations from the American Society of Echocardiography and the Society of Cardiovascular Anesthesiologists. *J Am Soc Echocardiogr.* 2013;26(9):921-964.

---

**8.** Correct Answer: **C. Consult cardiac surgery for evaluation**

*Rationale:* The patient has an aortic root abscess, a serious complication of infective endocarditis that is most commonly seen after an aortic valve replacement and aortic root repair. Aortic root abscesses appear as heterogenous hyperechoic lesions and perivalvular thickening. The video shows the presence of a false aneurysm, or pseudoaneurysm, which is a collection of blood that communicates with the aortic lumen as demonstrated by color Doppler flow but is not essentially enclosed by the normal vessel wall; it is contained only by the adventitia or surrounding soft tissue. Pseudoaneurysms can arise from a defect in the aortic wall or a leaking anastomosis after aortic aneurysm repair. The blood flow through the defect of the aortic wall can be observed using Doppler modalities, such as color and pulsed-wave Doppler. Pseudoaneurysms complicate aortic grafting in 1% to 6% of cases. It is an indication for emergent aortic replacement surgery. Uncorrected, it carries 100% mortality from rupture.

### Selected Reference

1. Spencer KT, Kaji E, Drucker D. Transesophageal echocardiographic diagnosis of a mycotic ascending aortic pseudoaneurysm as a source of embolism. *J Am Soc Echocardiogra*. 1998;11(12):1155-1157.

**9.** Correct Answer: **B. Paradoxical LF-LG AS**

*Rationale:* Severe AS is defined by an AVA $\leq 1.0$ cm$^2$ ($<0.65$ cm$^2$/m$^2$) and a mean transvalvular gradient $\geq 40$ mm Hg. Occasionally, there is discordance between AVA $<1$ cm$^2$ and $<0.6$ cm$^2$/m$^2$ (consistent with severe AS) and the mean gradient $<40$ mm Hg (consistent with nonsevere AS) called area-gradient mismatch. Classifying the severity of AS in the presence of area-gradient mismatch is challenging, and they largely fall under two scenarios.

LF-LG AS is found in about 5%-10% of the patients with severe AS and is characterized by area-gradient mismatch, a reduced LVEF ($<50$%), and SVI $<35$ mL/m$^2$. The reduced flow across the AV due to low EF results in insufficient gradient, even in the presence of severe AS. To investigate for the presence of severe AS, further evaluation with dobutamine echocardiography is recommended. Dobutamine administration causes an increase in SV (SVI $>35$) and EF. In patients with truly severe AS (LF-LG AS), echocardiographic measurements obtained at this SV will satisfy all criteria for severe AS and resolve the area-gradient mismatch. If the mean gradient does not increase to $>40$ mm Hg despite a SVI $> 35$, the patient likely does not have severe AS.

Paradoxical LF-LG AS occurs in 5%-15% of patients with AS and it is characterized by area-gradient mismatch, normal LVEF ($>50$%), and SVI $< 35$. This is typically seen in the elderly and women with small/hypertrophied LV cavities resulting in low LV end-diastolic volumes. This low LV end-diastolic volume results in a low SV (despite normal LVEF), creating insufficient gradient across the AV, despite presence of severe AS. These patients are further evaluated either by increasing their SVI with dobutamine administration or by complementary imaging to assess AV calcification with cardiac CT.

### Selected References

1. Baumgartner H, Hung J, Bermejo J, et al. Recommendations on the echocardiographic assessment of aortic valve stenosis: a focused update from the European Association of Cardiovascular Imaging and the American Society of Echocardiography. *J Am Soc Echocardiogr*. 2017;30(4):372-392.
2. Pibarot P, Dumesnil JG. Low-flow, low-gradient aortic stenosis with normal and depressed left ventricular ejection fraction. *J Am Coll Cardiol*. 2012;60:1845-1853.

**10.** Correct Answer: **B. LV dilation**

*Rationale:* Aortic regurgitation can be caused by primary disease of the AV and/or abnormalities of the aortic root and ascending aortic geometry. Degenerative tricuspid and bicuspid aortic regurgitation are the most common etiologies of aortic regurgitation in developed countries. Other causes include congenital variants (BAV), infective endocarditis, aortic dissection, and rheumatic heart disease. This patient had a BAV with severe aortic regurgitation in the setting of systemic infection, which is very suspicious for endocarditis and associated aortic regurgitation.

Infectious endocarditis causes destruction of the leaflets of the AV, and/or invasion into the aortic annulus and the adjacent structures. Thus, it results in acute aortic regurgitation. The physiology is very different from chronic aortic regurgitation developing over time. Acute aortic regurgitation is poorly tolerated, because the ventricle lacks the adaptive mechanisms—LV dilation and eccentric hypertrophy. Thus, there is an abrupt increase in the LV diastolic pressure, which may lead to pulmonary edema and acutely reduced contractility. Chronic aortic regurgitation can lead to significant LV dilation and a reduced EF, which are indications for surgery in the setting of asymptomatic severe aortic regurgitation. In chronic aortic regurgitation, a high LV end-diastolic pressure and high pulse pressure (with low diastolic blood pressure) may be present.

### Selected Reference

1. Baumgartner H, Falk V, Bax JJ, et al. 2017 ESC/EACTS Guidelines for the management of valvular heart disease. *Eur Heart J*. 2017;38(36):2739-2791.

**11.** Correct Answer: A. Aortic stenosis

*Rationale:* Figure 24.10 shows flow turbulence distal from the AV in systole as evidenced by the mosaic-like appearance of the color flow Doppler. This is explained by the increased *blood flow* velocities across the calcified and stenotic AV orifice. As velocities exceed the Nyquist limit, flow turbulence appears on the color flow Doppler image.

Epidemiologic studies have determined that more than one in eight people aged 75 and older have moderate or severe AS due to degeneration of the AV. Symptom onset is a late sign of the disease and usually develops in the seventh to ninth decade, manifested by reduced exercise tolerance. Late symptoms include angina (35%), syncope (15%), and heart failure (50%) and are important predictors of mortality within 2 years of symptom onset.

Selected Reference

1. Nkomo VT, Gardin JM, Skelton TN, et al. Burden of valvular heart diseases: a population-based study. *Lancet.* 2006;368(9540): 1005-1011, https://doi.org/10.1016/S0140-6736 (06)69208-8.

**12.** Correct Answer: B. Left main coronary artery

*Rationale:* The midesophageal SAX TEE view is used to assess the morphology and function of each of the three individual cusps of the AV. The typical "Mercedes Benz" sign during diastole can be obtained by decreasing the omniplane by 90° from the long-axis view of the AV (typically at 40-55°). The right coronary cusp is visualized in the most anterior position and adjacent to the right ventricular cavity. The left coronary cusp is on the right side of the image adjacent to the left atrial appendage; and the noncoronary cusp is located to the left side of the image adjacent to the interatrial septum. The left main coronary artery is usually seen arising at the 1-3 o' clock position adjacent to the left coronary cusp and then bifurcates into the left anterior descending artery and the left circumflex artery, with the latter bifurcating toward the left atrium. The right coronary artery is seen arising from 6 o' clock position toward the right ventricle.

Selected Reference

1. Hahn RT, Abraham T, Adams MS, et al. Guidelines for performing a comprehensive transesophageal echocardiographic examination: recommendations from the American Society of Echocardiography and the Society of Cardiovascular Anesthesiologists. *J Am Soc Echocardiogr.* 2013;26(9):921-964.

**13.** Correct Answer: D. Myocardial infarction

*Rationale:* BAV disease is the most common congenital heart defect, with a prevalence estimated between 0.5% and 2%.

BAV is often associated with other congenital cardiac lesions. The most frequent associated finding is dilation of the proximal ascending aorta secondary to abnormalities of the aortic media. Changes in the aortic media are present independent of whether the valve is functionally normal, stenotic, or incompetent. Complications can include AV stenosis or incompetence, endocarditis, aortic aneurysm formation, and aortic dissection; however, the risk of myocardial infarction is not higher than in the general population.

Selected Reference

1. Siu SC, Silversides CK. Bicuspid aortic valve disease. *J Am Coll Cardiol.* 2010;55(25):2789.

**14.** Correct Answer: B. 3D planimetry

*Rationale:* The peak pressure gradient through the AV is estimated by the Bernoulli formula, which states that $\Delta P = 4(V_2^2 - V_1^2)$. In this equation, $V_2$ is the peak velocity of the blood flow distal from the stenosis, and $V_1$ is the peak velocity proximal from the stenosis (LVOT). Typically, $V_1$ can be ignored, because of the low velocity in the LVOT and the equation can be simplified to $\Delta P = 4V^2$ (simplified Bernoulli equation). This assumption is true only if the proximal velocity ($V_1$) is low. When $V_1$ is above 1.5 m/s (such as in HOCM with increased LVOT velocity), the above-mentioned equation (modified Bernoulli equation) should not be used. Failure to take into account increased proximal velocity (LVOT) will lead to overestimation of the pressure gradient and the degree of AS. For this reason, the most accurate method for estimation of the degree of AS would be 3D planimetry in this patient.

Selected Reference

1. Mathew JP. Aortic valve. In: Mathew JP, Nicoara A, Ayoub CM, Swaminathan M, eds. *Clinical Manual and Review of Transesophageal Echocardiography.* 3rd ed. McGraw-Hill Education; 2018:Chapter 11.

**15.** Correct Answer: D. 11.7 L/min

*Rationale:* The Doppler VTI method for estimating SV and CO is based on the fact that it represents "stroke distance," which is the distance the SV will travel over time, so VTI and CSA will produce SV. It is a quick and easy way to determine CO in urgent situations and also to monitor for fluid responsiveness after fluid challenge. It correlates well with results of thermodilution CO (gold standard) measurements in patients without significant valvular disease.

$$SV = \pi \, \frac{D(LVOT)^2}{2} \times LVOT_{VTI}$$

$$CO = \frac{SV \times HR}{1000}$$

$$SV = 3.14 \times (2.2/2)^2 \times 28 = 106 \text{ mL}$$

$$CO = 106 \times 110 / 1000 = 11.7 \text{ L/min}$$

There are limitations to use VTI for Doppler assessment of the CO. The most common error is due to lack of appropriate alignment of the ultrasound beam with the direction of the flow, which should be less than 20°. The second most common error is due to erroneous measurement of LVOT diameter. The impact of this error can be significant, given the fact that the LVOT radius is squared in the equation. Of note, the pulsed-wave Doppler used to measure VTI and the LVOT diameter should be measured at the same anatomic location.

Fluid responsiveness can be measured using LVOT VTI only with changes >12% indicating responsiveness. This represents a surrogate measure for CO and eliminates the potential error from measuring LVOT diameter. SV can also be calculated from pulmonic valve diameter and VTI, or any other heart structure, where diameter and time velocity interval can be measured.

Selected Reference
1. Miller A, Mandeville J. Predicting and measuring fluid responsiveness with echocardiography. *Echo Res Pract.* 2016;3(2): G1-G12.

**16.** Correct Answer: D. 0.59 cm$^2$

*Rationale:* AVA is calculated using the continuity equation that is based on the concept that the SV ejected through the LVOT passes through the stenotic orifice (aka AVA) and thus SV at valve orifice is equal to the SV at the LVOT:

SV (AV) = SV (LVOT)

Because the amount of flow through any CSA is equal to the CSA multiplied by flow velocity over the ejection period (aka VTI), this equation can be written as:

$AV_{Area} \times AV_{VTI} = LVOT_{Area} \times LVOT_{VTI}$:

$$AV_{Area} = \frac{LVOT_{Area} \times LVOT_{VTI}}{AV_{VTI}}$$

Calculation of the AVA by continuity equation requires three measurements:

1. AS jet velocity by continuous-wave Doppler, obtained from apical five-chamber view or apical three-chamber view.
2. LVOT diameter for calculation of the CSA from parasternal long-axis view.
3. LVOT velocity recorded with pulsed-wave Doppler from apical five-chamber view or apical three-chamber view.

*CSA = 0.785 × d2 or CSA = πr$^2$*

In this example:

VTI LVOT = 20.6 cm, VTI AV = 121.3 cm

CSA LVOT = $3.14 (2.1/2)^2 = 3.46$

AVA = $3.46 \times 20.6/121.3 = 0.59$ cm$^2$

## Selected Reference

1. Baumgartner H, Hung J, Bermejo J, et al. Recommendations on the echocardiographic assessment of aortic valve stenosis: a focused update from the European Association of Cardiovascular Imaging and the American Society of Echocardiography. *J Am Soc Echocardiogr.* 2017;30(4):372-392.

**17.** Correct Answer: **C. Membranous sub-AS**

*Rationale/Critique:* Membranous sub-AS is a rare cause of obstruction of LVOT, which can easily be mistaken for AV stenosis. In sub-AS, there is a fibrinous band or ring just below the AV causing obstruction of the LVOT. This is an example of fixed stenosis—fixed (unchanged) throughout systole, as opposed to HOCM or other causes of systolic anterior motion of the mitral leaflet. Sub-AS is suspected when high gradients are measured in the LVOT in the absence of structural changes of the AV.

As with AS, sub-AS produces a rounded spectral Doppler pattern with a midsystolic peak, as opposed to a dagger-shaped pattern in HOCM, due to late systolic peak of the velocity.

Turbulent flow in the LVOT on color flow Doppler imaging is usually the first clue to the existence of subvalvular obstruction.

## Selected Reference

1. Mathew JP. Aortic valve. In: Mathew JP, Nicoara A, Ayoub CM, Swaminathan M, eds. *Clinical Manual and Review of Transesophageal Echocardiography.* 3rd ed. McGraw-Hill Education; 2018:Chapter 11.

**18.** Correct Answer: **B. Dobutamine stress echocardiogram**

*Rationale/Critique: Low-Flow, Low-Gradient AS* is defined by AVA <1.0 cm$^2$, mean AV pressure gradient <40 mm Hg, and SVI <35 mL/m$^2$. As is obvious from the definition, there is a discordance between the AVA measured by the continuity equation and the mean AV gradient. This condition can be caused by decreased EF in 50% of the cases (heart failure with reduced EF), but also in patients with high degree of diastolic dysfunction or atrial arrhythmias, all of which may decrease the SV. It is recommended that these patients undergo dobutamine stress testing to determine whether the inotropic stimulation will increase their SV. In this setting, if the mean AV gradient increases >40 mm Hg while their SV becomes >35 mL/m$^2$, this means the patient has severe AS. Dobutamine stress test will also demonstrate if contractile or flow reserve is present.

Patients without true severe AS will have an increase in their AVA (>1.0 cm$^2$) and only a small increase in the velocity or gradient (pseudo-severe AS). These patients will not benefit from AV replacement, as their low gradient is due to low SV and diminished valve opening.

*True severe AS* is suggested by >20% increase in SV from baseline or an increase in AS jet velocity ≥4 m/s or a mean gradient ≥40 mm Hg; provided that the valve area does not exceed 1.0 cm$^2$ at any flow rate, these patients benefit from an AV replacement (**Table 24.3**).

**Table 24.3 True severe aortic stenosis versus pseudo-severe aortic stenosis with dobutamine challenge**

| Findings | Fixed Aortic Valve Stenosis | Fixed Aortic Valve Stenosis + Poor Response to Dobutamine | Pseudo-Aortic Valve Stenosis |
|---|---|---|---|
| Baseline AVA | <1.0 cm$^2$ | <1.0 cm$^2$ | <1.0 cm$^2$ |
| Cardiac output during dobutamine | >20%-25% improvement | <20%-25% improvement | >20%-25% improvement |
| AVA during dobutamine | Increase <0.3 cm$^2$ | Increase <0.3 cm$^2$ | Increase >0.3 cm$^2$ |
| Final AVA during dobutamine | <1 cm$^2$ | <1 cm$^2$ | >1 cm$^2$ |
| Benefit from surgery | Yes | Likely | No |

Selected Reference

1. Baumgartner H, Falk V, Bax JJ, et al. 2017 ESC/EACTS Guidelines for the management of valvular heart disease. *Eur Heart J.* 2017;38(36):2739-2791.

**19.** Correct Answer: A. Type 1D

*Rationale/Critique:* The AV regurgitation classification is centered on two components (annulus/aortic root dimension and leaflets), but unlike the mitral valve, the aortic root consists of several components: aortic annulus, sinus of Valsalva, and sinotubular junction.

- **Type 1:** there is normal leaflet motion with functional aortic dilation and/or cusp perforation:
  **Type IA:** due to dilation of sinotubular junction and ascending aorta
  **Type IB:** due to dilation of the sinus of Valsalva and sinotubular junction
  **Type IC:** due to isolated dilation of the aortic annulus
  **Type ID:** due to perforation of leaflet
- **Type II:** due to leaflet prolapse
- **Type III**: due to leaflet restriction

  Patients can have one or more of those pathologies. For example, a patient with type 1C is expected to have a central regurgitant jet; however, if there is evidence of restricted leaflets, the aortic insufficiency jet becomes eccentric. Thus, accurate assessment of leaflet anatomies is essential to delineate different mechanisms for AR.

Selected Reference

1. Boodhawani M, de Kerchove L, Glineur D, et al. Repair-oriented classification of aortic insufficiency: impact on surgical techniques and clinical outcomes. *J Thorac Cardiovasc Surg.* 2009;137(2):286-294.

**20.** Correct Answer: C. Aortic regurgitation

*Rationale/Critique:*

**Table 24.4 Aortic regurgitation severity grading**

|  | **Mild** | **Moderate** | **Severe** |
|---|---|---|---|
| Jet width/LVOT width (%) | <25 | 25-65 | >65 |
| Pressure half-time (ms) | >500 | 500-200 | <200 |
| Diastolic flow reversal in descending aorta | Brief, early diastolic reversal | Intermediate | Prominent holodiastolic reversal |
| Vena contracta width (cm) | <0.3 | 0.3-0.6 | >0.6 |
| Regurgitant volume (mL) | <30 | 30-60 | >60 |
| Regurgitant fraction (%) | <30 | 30-50 | >50 |
| Effective orifice area (cm$^2$) | <0.1 | 0.1-0.3 | >0.3 |

Aortic regurgitation causes increased end-diastolic ventricular volume over time and is the cause of LV volume overload. In certain circumstances, such as in the perioperative period with significant fluid intake, this may cause pulmonary venous congestion and subsequent pulmonary edema. Since the flow turbulence in color flow Doppler is in diastole, it is not HOCM. The septum seems to be intact and the question stem does not suggest the presence of ventricular septal defect, which if new during adulthood, the septal defect is likely an acute and devastating complication of right coronary artery myocardial infarction.

There are some pitfalls in using the echocardiographic parameters for grading aortic insufficiency severity (**Table 24.4**), for example: In patients with elevated LV end-diastolic pressure (eg, ischemia, cardiomyopathy, diastolic dysfunction, chronic aortic regurgitation), the use of pressure half-time may overestimate the true severity of regurgitation because the elevated ventricular pressure will decrease the time required for equalization of pressures between the aorta and the left ventricle. Similarly, decreased systemic vascular resistance (eg, sepsis, post-CPB [cardipulmonary bypass]) results in a steeper deceleration slope.

Holodiastolic flow reversal in abdominal aorta is sensitive and specific for severity of AR.

Vena contracta width is a good measure for severity of aortic regurgitation, it is load-independent and is not affected by changes in afterload or intravascular volume.

**Selected Reference**

1. Zoghbi WA, Adams D, Bonow RO, et al. Recommendations for evaluation of the severity of native valvular regurgitation with two-dimensional and Doppler echocardiography. *J Am Soc Echocardiogr.* 2017;30(4):303-371.

---

**21.** Correct Answer: B. 57 mL

*Rationale:* In the absence of significant valvular regurgitation, the SV through all four valves should be equal. One way to calculate the regurgitant volume through a valve is by the difference between the SV across the regurgitant valve and the SV through a different (reference) valve that does not have significant regurgitation. In the absence of intracardiac shunts and mitral regurgitation, the AV regurgitant volume is the difference between AV SV and pulmonic valve (PV) SV. Mitral valve can also be used as a reference valve (diastolic mitral inflow), as long as there is no significant mitral regurgitation.

Regurgitant volume (AV) = SV (AV) – SV (pulmonic valve).

Since SV = VTI (valve) $\times$ CSA (valve), then:

Regurgitant volume (AV) = (VTI AV $\times$ CSA AV ) – (VTI pulmonic valve $\times$ CSA pulmonic valve)

In the absence of AS and pulmonic stenosis, SV LVOT and RVOT can be used instead of SV of the AV and PV.

In our example:

SV AV = $50 \times 3.14(2/2)^2 = 157$ mL

SV PV = $22 \times 3.14(2.4/2)^2 = 100$ mL

Regurgitant volume across AV = $157 - 100 = 57$ mL, which is equal to moderate-to-severe aortic insufficiency

**Selected Reference**

1. Zoghbi WA, Enriquez-Sarano M, Foster E, et al. Recommendations for evaluation of the severity of native valvular regurgitation with two-dimensional and Doppler echocardiography. *J Am Soc Echocardiogr.* 2003;16(7):777-802.

---

**22.** Correct Answer: C. Lambl's excrescences

*Rationale:* Lambl's excrescences are thin, mobile, filiform structures, often referred to as valvular strands typically occurring at coaptation lines of the left-sided valves. The differential diagnosis for these excrescences includes fibroelastoma, myxoma, thrombus, vegetation, and cardiac neoplasms and metastases.

They have been associated with stroke, but causality has not been proven. TEE remains the gold standard for diagnosis. Asymptomatic Lambl's excrescences are closely monitored, while symptomatic lesions with a history of thromboembolism are managed with antiplatelet drugs or are anticoagulated. Surgery is indicated in case of recurrent thromboembolic episodes occurring while on medications.

**Selected Reference**

1. Ammannaya GKK. Lambl's excrescences: current diagnosis and management. *Cardiol Res.* 2019;10(4):207-212.

---

**23.** Correct Answer: D. Pericarditis

*Rationale:* BAV is the most common congenital cardiac anomaly. It affects 1% to 2% of the general population.

BAV carries a 6% lifetime risk of development of aortic dissection, which is nine times higher than that with trileaflet AV.

Aortic root dilation occurs irrespective of hemodynamics and age and continues after valve repair, suggesting developmental and biochemical defects.

BAV patients may also have patent ductus arteriosus, coarctation of aorta, aneurysm of aorta, dissection, aortic regurgitation, or stenosis. The most common associated lesion is aortic regurgitation; however, the most common indication for surgery is AS.

Selected Reference

1. Verma S, Siu SC. Aortic dilation in patient with BAV. *N Engl J Med.* 2014;370(20):1920-1929.

**24.** Correct Answer: D. Gradients obtained by echo are peak instantaneous gradients.

*Rationale/Critique:* Gradients obtained by continuous-wave Doppler are peak instantaneous gradients. Continuity equation, which takes into account the peak velocities or VTI through the AV are considered gold standard for assessment of AS severity.

Left heart catheterization measurements of AV velocities are peak-to-peak gradients. The peak-to-peak gradient is defined as the difference between peak LV pressure and peak aortic pressure that can be done by pulling a pressure catheter from the left ventricle to the aorta to get the measurement (on a different heartbeat) or by having two catheters—one in the left ventricle and the other in the aorta. Although peak aortic pressure happens milliseconds after peak LV pressure, it is not instantaneous.

Gradients derived by spectral Doppler are peak instantaneous gradients so they are higher than obtained by angiography (**Figure 24.18**).

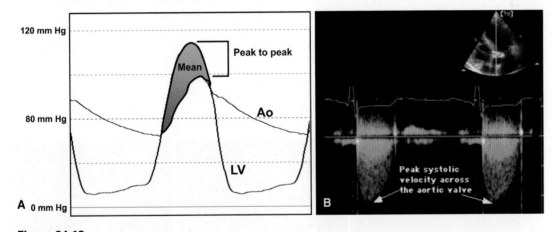

**Figure 24.18**

Selected References

1. Mathew J, Swamiinathan M, Ayoub C. Aortic valve. In: *Clinical and Manual Review of Transesophageal Echo.* 3rd ed. Chapter 11.
2. Yang CS, Jividen K, Kamata T, et al. Discrepancies between direct catheter and echocardiography based values in aortic stenosis. *Catheter Cardiovasc Interv.* 2017;87(3):488-497.

# 25 | MITRAL VALVULAR DISEASE

Gregory Mints

1. A 92-year-old man presents to the emergency room with fatigue, confusion, and shortness of breath. His accompanying friend reports the history of "heart failure" and atrial fibrillation but does not know any details. It is unclear whether he is taking any prescribed medications. His oral intake in the week preceding hospitalization is also questionable. On admission, his vitals are: HR 80 bpm, in atrial fibrillation, BP 120/60 mm Hg, and afebrile. Physical examination reveals 2+ lower extremity edema and elevated jugular venous pressure (JVP). White blood cell (WBC) count is $5 \times 10^9$/L; 20 mg of intravenous furosemide is administered. Six hours after presentation, the patient developed progressive hypoxemia with arterial oxygen saturation reading by pulse oximetry in the 70s. His vitals now are: HR 80 bpm, BP 90/50 mm Hg. He remained afebrile.

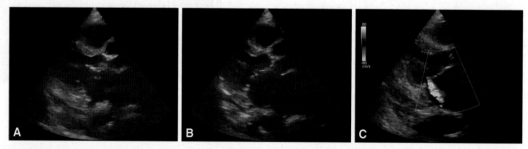

**Figure 25.1** A, Parasternal long-axis (PLAx) diastole. B, PLAx end-systole. C, PLAx with color Doppler.

You determine that this patient has significantly decreased left ventricular (LV) systolic function (**Figure 25.1A-C,** ▶ **Videos 25.1** and **25.2**). Which of the following statements is *most* accurate?

A. Significant left atrial (LA) dilation seen in this clip is virtually pathognomonic for elevated LA pressure.

B. Large LA size and eccentricity of the mitral regurgitation (MR) jet may both lead to overestimation of MR severity.

C. Opening of mitral valve (MV) leaflets in diastole is restricted, which is highly concerning for mitral stenosis (MS). A.fib in the context of MS is likely contributing to the patient's decompensation.

D. The specific type of MR the patient has may be caused by prior inferior wall myocardial infarction (MI).

E. None of the statements above are accurate.

2. An 83-year-old man presents with gradually worsening dyspnea on exertion and lower extremity edema. He is known to have ischemic dilated cardiomyopathy with depressed LV function and atrial fibrillation. He is in obvious congestive heart failure (CHF) by examination, but careful history fails to reveal a trigger for the CHF exacerbation.

On bedside cardiac ultrasound, significant MR is detected (images not shown), which the patient does not recall having been told about previously.

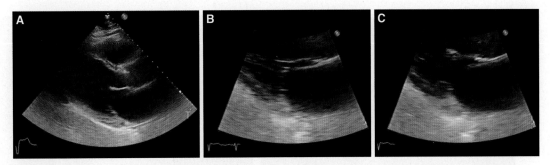

**Figure 25.2** A, Parasternal long-axis (PLAx). Diastole, peak of rapid filling. B and C, PLAx zoomed-in on the mitral valve (MV). (B) End-systole. MV is fully closed. (C) Diastole. MV is fully open.

Based on the available information as well as **Figure 25.2** and ▶ **Videos 25.3, 25.4, 25.5,** which one of the following is most likely concerning the etiology of this patient's MR?
A. Anatomy of the MV is suggestive of acute inferolateral MI.
B. Anatomy of the MV is suggestive of torn chordae tendineae as the etiology of MR.
C. MV anatomy suggests that MR is most likely primary (e.g., rheumatic heart disease [RHD] or endocarditis) and reduced systolic function is likely secondary to the MR.
D. MV anatomy suggests that MR is likely secondary to dilated cardiomyopathy and not its cause.

3. A 92-year-old man presents with shortness of breath. On examination, he has crackles bilaterally, elevated JVP, and a systolic murmur at the apex that radiates to the axilla. He is hemodynamically stable. Lung ultrasound shows bilateral diffuse B-lines in all lung fields, including anteriorly. On bedside cardiac ultrasound, an MR jet is detected, and significant MR is suspected as a contributor to the patient's CHF.

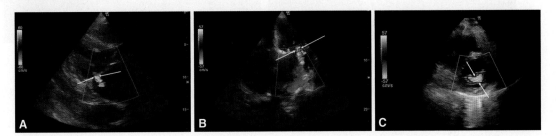

**Figure 25.3** A, Parasternal long-axis (PLAx) view. B, Apical four-chamber view. C, Parasternal short-axis (PSAx) view.

Based on these details as well as **Figure 23.3** and ▶ **Videos 25.6, 25.7, 25.8,** which one of the following is true regarding vena contracta (VC)?
A. Figure 25.3A. VC is properly measured in the parasternal long-axis (PLAx) view.
B. Figure 25.3B. VC is properly measured in A4 view.
C. Either measurement is acceptable, there should not be a difference between the two. If such difference is detected, the technique is at fault.
D. Neither measurement is appropriate. VC is not a useful metric for assessment of MR severity.
E. VC is a valid index of MR severity but neither PLAx nor A4 are appropriate for its measurement, which is best obtained in parasternal short-axis (PSAx) view, as shown in Figure 25.3C.

4. A 40-year-old man presented to a hospital in New York City with 3 weeks of profound dyspnea on exertion, cough with frothy pink sputum, and occasional small amount of blood. He reports that symptoms started suddenly when he was vacationing in Ecuador, where he is originally from. He was hospitalized for a week and had some cardiac procedure performed in Ecuador but is unable to provide any details. He reports not feeling better since then. On presentation, the patient's arterial oxygen saturation by pulse oximetry was 85% while breathing room air. He was tachypneic but was otherwise hemodynamically stable.

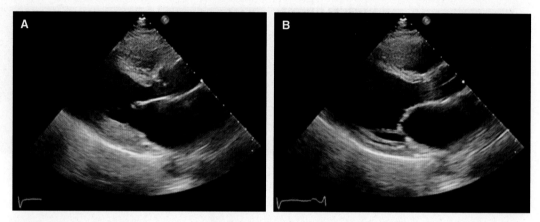

**Figure 25.4** A, Parasternal long-axis (PLAx) in diastole: mitral valve (MV) is open. B, PLAx in systole: MV is closed.

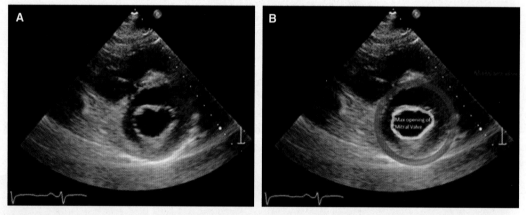

**Figure 25.5** A, Parasternal short-axis (PSAx) in diastole. B, PSAx in diastole, labeled.

Sonographic images demonstrate restriction of the MV opening (**Figures 25.4** and **25.5**, ▶ **Videos 25.9** and **25.10**).

This sonographic appearance of restriction of MV opening is most characteristic of which one of the following?

**A.** Mitral stenosis
**B.** Dilated cardiomyopathy
**C.** Rheumatic MR
**D.** Endocarditis of the MV with MR
**E.** Concomitant significant aortic regurgitation

5. **Figure 25.6A** and **B** shows color Doppler (CD) in PLAx view from a patient with MR.

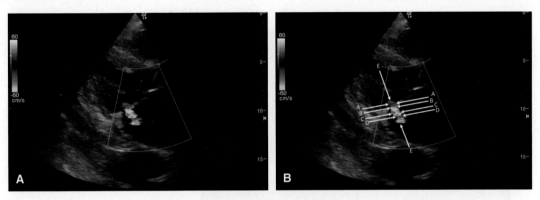

**Figure 25.6** A, Color Doppler (CD) in parasternal long-axis (PLAx) view showing mitral regurgitation (MR). B, CD in PLAx view showing MR, labeled.

Which of the shown measurements in Figure 25.6 and ▶ **Video 25.11** represent VC?
A. A
B. B
C. C
D. D
E. E

6. This 62-year-old man with a history of CHF due to nonischemic cardiomyopathy presents with 3 days of worsening dyspnea on exertion. He has no history of angina, atrial fibrillation, or trauma. His echocardiogram 3 months prior showed trace MR. The patient is mildly tachypneic, but his vitals are otherwise stable.

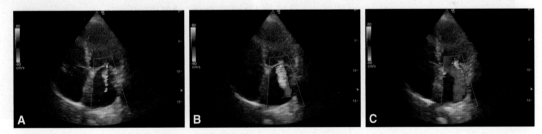

**Figure 25.7** A-C, Color Doppler in apical four-chamber view.

**Figure 25.7A** to C and ▶ **Videos 25.12, 25.13, 25.14** were obtained sequentially from the same patient. The only difference among the recordings is a progressively increasing CD gain from Figure 25.7A to C. What is true regarding this patient's MR?
A. MR is likely minor and is not contributing to this patient's symptoms. Figure 25.7A most accurately represents the degree of MR in this patient, that is, CD is overgained in other images.
B. This is likely a case of acute MR, in which degree of MR by CD may not parallel severity of symptoms.
C. This is a significant MR that is likely contributing to the patient's symptoms. Image in Figure 25.7C is the most representative of the degree of the MR and in other images CD is undergained.
D. The proper gain is shown in Figure 25.7B; MR is likely insignificant.
E. None of the above are true.

7. **Figures 25.8** and **25.9** and ▶ **Video 25.15** were obtained from a 70-year-old man with hypotension, fever, and altered mental status.

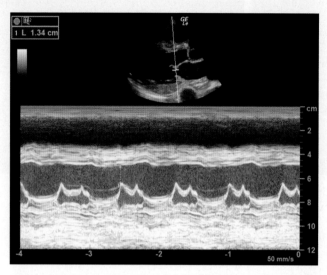

**Figure 25.8** M-mode recording in parasternal long-axis (PLAx) view.

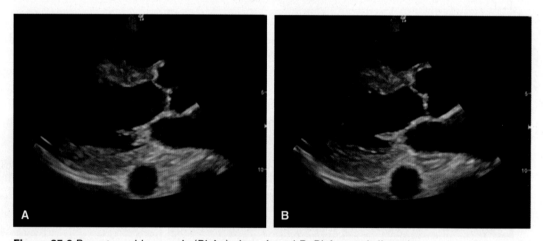

**Figure 25.9** Parasternal long-axis (PLAx) view. A and B, PLAx: end-diastole.

Which of the following is the term used for the distance measured at 1.34 cm?
A. TAPSE (tricuspid annular plane systolic excursion)
B. SAM (systolic anterior motion)
C. S'
D. EPSS or E-point septal separation
E. Pressure half-time of the mitral inflow

8. What is true concerning imaging of MR in the apical two-chamber view?

A. Jet, including VC, may appear broader than in A4C view
B. MR jet may be missed entirely in this view
C. All of the above
D. None of the above

9. A 52-year-old man with an unknown history was brought in by emergency medical services (EMS) after a severe motor vehicle collision (MVC) into the side of a home. On arrival at the Emergency Department (ED), his BP was 90/50 mm Hg, HR 110 bpm, respiratory rate 12 breaths/min, oxygen saturation 95% on 100% non-rebreather mask. His Glasgow coma score (GCS) was 8. The patient was intubated due to labored breathing and inability to control his airway. Extended focused assessment with sonography in trauma (EFAST) examination did not reveal free fluid in the chest, abdomen, pericardium, or pelvis. Lung ultrasound (US) ruled out pneumothorax on both sides of the chest but did reveal significant B-lines in the left upper lung field that correlated with an anteroposterior (AP) chest radiograph. Computed tomography (CT) revealed multifocal airspace consolidations, predominantly in the left upper lobe and right lower lobe, with no evidence of head, chest, or abdominal injury (**Figures 25.10, 25.11, 25.12** and ▶ **Video 25.16**).

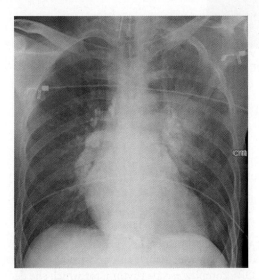

**Figure 25.10** Anteroposterior chest radiograph.

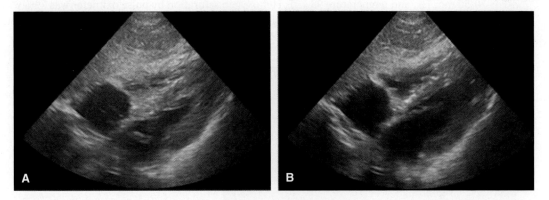

**Figure 25.11** Subcostal four-chamber view. A, Systole. B, Diastole.

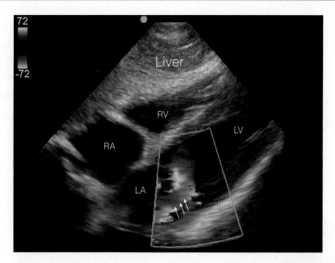

**Figure 25.12** Subcostal four-chamber view. Color Doppler. Systole. LA, left atrium; LV, left ventricle; RA, right atrium; RV, right ventricle.

Which of the following is most likely in this patient?
A. Severe acute MR 2/2 traumatic papillary muscle (PM) rupture
B. Lung contusion, echo is unremarkable
C. Takotsubo cardiomyopathy (TTC) with acute cardiogenic pulmonary edema
D. Aspiration pneumonitis. Echo findings most consistent with normal CD signal from pulmonary veins
E. None of the above

10. A 73-year-old woman presented with progressively worsening shortness of breath over 5 days. Her medical history was significant for poorly controlled hypertension, diabetes, nonobstructive coronary artery disease, and complete heart block with wide QRS complex escape rhythm, for which she declined cardiology referral. The patient collapsed on her way from the hospital's parking lot to the ED, where she was found to be in severe respiratory distress. Her respiratory rate is 28 breaths/min, HR is 52 bpm, BP is 70/50 mm Hg, and temperature 98.1 °F. Her oxygen saturation by pulse oximeter was 79% while breathing room air. Physical examination was significant for bilateral crackles and normal heart sounds with no appreciable murmur. Chest X-ray (CXR) is shown in **Figure 25.13**.

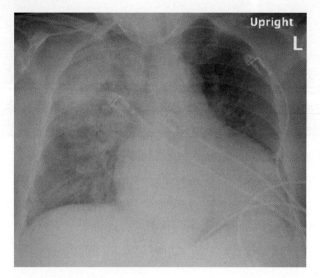

**Figure 25.13** Chest X-ray.

On arrival to the intensive care unit (ICU) the patient developed worsening respiratory failure and was intubated and started on invasive mechanical ventilation.

After an initial hemodynamic improvement, the patient's course rapidly deteriorated, with development of hypotension requiring intravenous norepinephrine and transcutaneous pacing (**Figure 25.14** and ▶ **Videos 25.17, 25.18, 25.19, 25.20**).

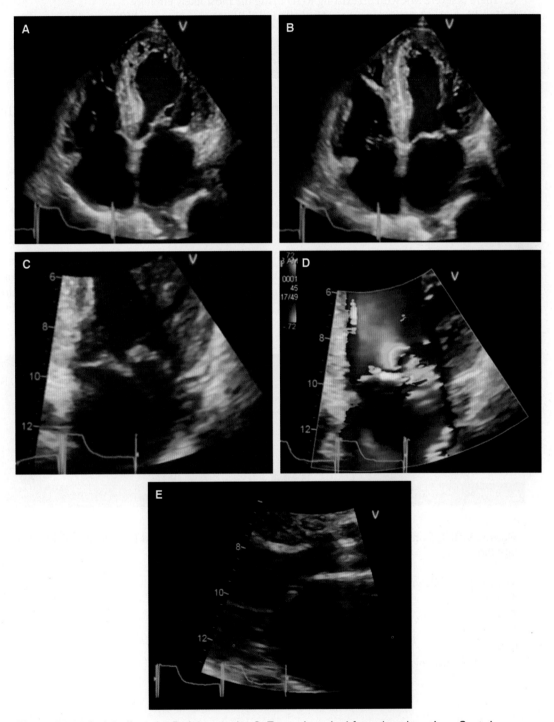

**Figure 25.14** A, A4, diastole. B, A4, systole. C, Zoom-in apical four-chamber view. Systole. D, Zoom-in apical four-chamber view plus color Doppler. Systole. E, Parasternal long-axis view. Zoom-in on mitral valve.

Which of the following statements is the most accurate?

**A.** In this case finding of MR on echo is inconsistent with the rest of the clinical picture and therefore MR is an unlikely contributor to the patient's clinical presentation.

**B.** In this case of acute MR, CD is likely to overestimate the degree of regurgitation. In reality this MR is probably not significant.

**C.** There is severe MR with preexisting RHD being the most likely etiology.

**D.** It is likely that LA enlargement is premorbid in this patient with acute MR.

**E.** None of the above.

11. In which of the following situations would it be most appropriate to use CD jet area (relative to the LA size) for estimation of MR severity?

    **A.** Eccentric posteriorly directed jet of acute MR caused by a flail anterior leaflet secondary to cord rapture in a hemodynamically stable patient

    **B.** Holosystolic regurgitation of chronic central MR in a patient with pulmonary edema who is hemodynamically stable

    **C.** Chronic posteriorly directed MR secondary to prior inferior wall MI with overall preserved LV systolic function and a dilated left atrium

    **D.** Central late systolic MR associated with MV prolapse in a hypotensive patient with septic shock

    **E.** Double jet of MR secondary to MV endocarditis in a hemodynamically stable patient with pulmonary edema

12. **Figure 25.15** is a continuous-wave Doppler (CWD) tracing of mitral inflow obtained from a patient suspected of having MS (Figure 25.15A). (Figure 25.15B shows yellow markings A and B on the velocity scale that corresponds to the yellow markings C and D on the time axis. A marks 71% of Max, and B marks 50% of Max.)

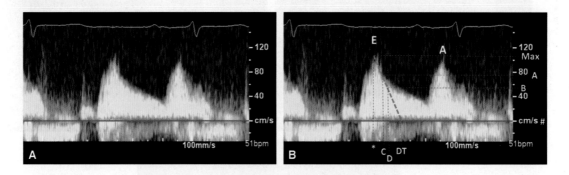

**Figure 25.15** A, Continuous-wave Doppler (CWD) of mitral inflow and B, CWD of mitral inflow, labeled.

Which of the following intervals represents pressure half-time (P½T)?

**A.** A—#

**B.** B—#

**C.** C—*

**D.** D—*

**E.** None of the above

13. The following cases depict three different patients who present with tachycardia, shortness of breath, and pink frothy sputum.

**Case1 (Figure 25.16 and ▶ Videos 25.21, 25.22, 25.23)**

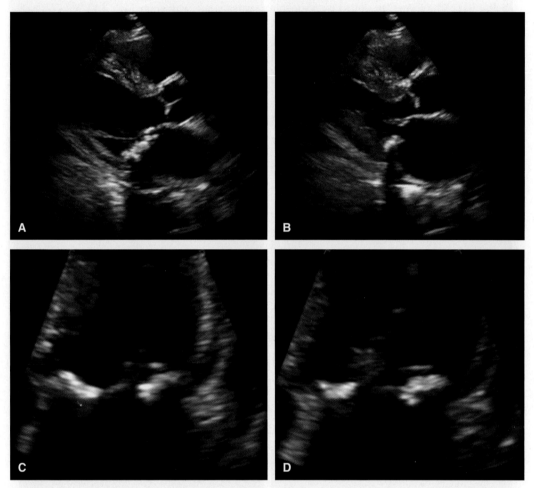

**Figure 25.16** Case 1, Patient 1. A, Parasternal long-axis view. End-systole. Mitral valve (MV) is closed. B, Diastole. MV is open. C, A4, zoomed-in on MV. End-systole. MV is closed. D, A4 zoomed-in on MV. Diastole. MV is open.

**Case 2 (Figure 25.17 and ▶ Videos 25.24, 25.25, 25.26)**

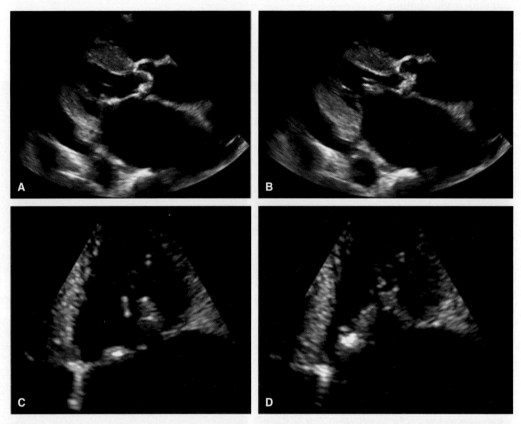

**Figure 25.17** Case 2, Patient 2. A, Parasternal long-axis (PLAx). End-systole. Mitral valve (MV) is closed. B, PLAx. Diastole. MV is open. C, A4, zoomed-in on MV. End-systole. MV is closed. D, A4 zoomed-in on MV. Diastole. MV is open.

**Case 3 (Figure 25.18 and ▶ Videos 25.27, 25.26, 25.27, 25.28, 25.29)**

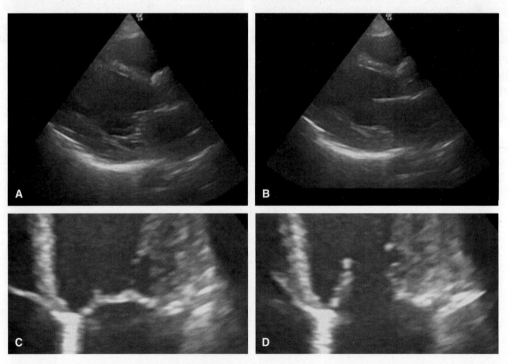

**Figure 25.18** Case 3, Patient 3. A, Parasternal long-axis (PLAx). End-systole. Mitral valve (MV) is closed. B, PLAx. Diastole. MV is open. C, A4, zoomed-in on MV. End-systole. MV is closed. D, A4 zoomed-in on MV. Diastole. MV is open.

Which of these three patients have MS?
A. Case 1
B. Case 2
C. Case 3
D. Cases 1 and 2
E. All of the above

14. "Hockey stick" configuration refers to:

A. Diastolic configuration of the anterior mitral leaflet seen in rheumatic MS
B. Systolic configuration of posterior mitral leaflet seen in severe calcific MS
C. Configuration of apically displaced ("tethered") leaflets of the MV seen in ischemic MR
D. Configuration of the MV in relation to chordae tendineae seen in MS and best visualized in the apical views
E. None of the above

15. All of the following are signs of severe MS *except*:

A. Severely sclerotic and/or calcified valve leaflets
B. Restricted opening of the valve
C. Dilated left ventricle and/or decrease in LV systolic function
D. Dilated left atrium
E. Greater restriction of mobility of posterior (compared to anterior) leaflet of the MV

16. All of the patients in cases 1 to 3 present with fever, hypotension, pulmonary congestion and all have a regurgitant systolic murmur at the apex, radiating to the axilla.

### Case 1 (Figure 25.19 and ▶ Videos 25.30 and 25.31)

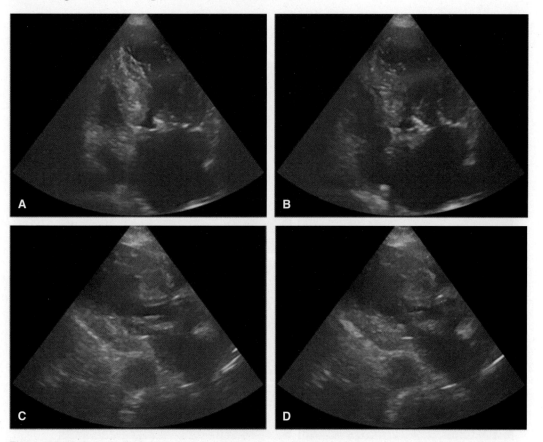

**Figure 25.19** Case 1, Patient 1. A, A4, systole. B, A4, diastole. C, Parasternal long-axis (PLAx), systole. D, PLAx, diastole.

**Case 2 (Figure 25.20 and ▶ Videos 25.32 and 25.33)**

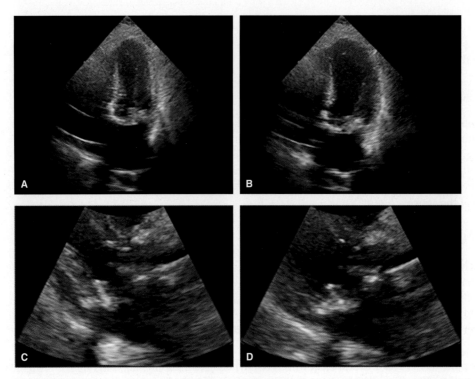

**Figure 25.20** Case 2, Patient 2. A, A4, systole. B, A4, diastole. C, Parasternal long-axis (PLAx) zoomed-in, systole. D, PLAx zoomed-in, diastole.

**Case 3 (Figure 25.21 and ▶ Videos 25.34 and 25.35)**

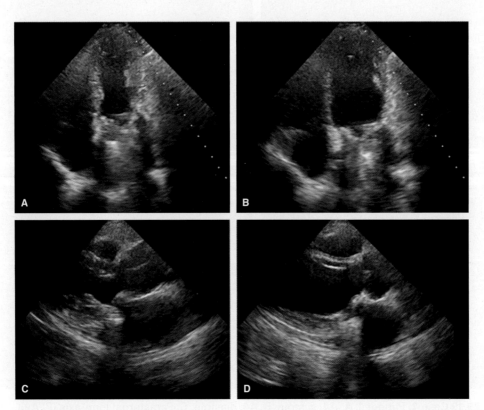

**Figure 25.21** Case 3, Patient 3. A, A4, systole. B, A4, diastole. C, Parasternal long-axis (PLAx), systole. D, PLAx, diastole.

Which of these patients have mitral annular calcification (MAC)?
A. The patient in case 1
B. The patient in case 2
C. The patient in case 3
D. Patients in cases 1 and 2
E. All of the above

17. A 70-year-old man is admitted with shortness of breath, hypoxemia, and hypotension. His JVP is severely elevated and lungs have crackles bilaterally, including in the anterior lung fields. His extremities are cool to touch and he has not made any urine since the day prior.

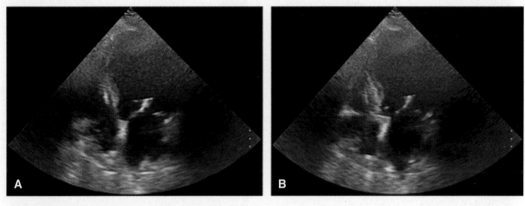

**Figure 25.22** A, A4 diastole. B, A4 systole.

It is evident that the patient has a severely decreased LV systolic function. Based on this sonographic examination (**Figure 25.22** and ▶ **Video 25.36**), what other factors may be contributing to the development of shock in this patient?
A. Severe MS with tachycardia
B. No other contributors can be identified
C. Acute MR secondary to prosthesis failure
D. Acute right ventricular (RV) failure

18. What does **Figure 25.23** and ▶ **Video 25.37** show?

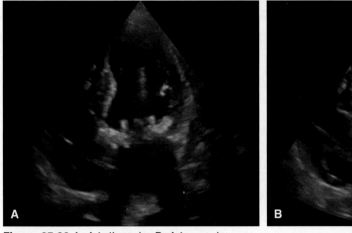

**Figure 25.23** A, A4 diastole. B, A4 systole.

A. Patient has had MV replacement
B. Calcific MS
C. Rheumatic MS
D. Mechanical MV prosthesis
E. None of the above

19. An 82-year-old man with a history of chronic rate-controlled atrial fibrillation (a.fib) and coronary heart disease for which he has received three-vessel coronary bypass some years ago presents with sudden onset of shortness of breath at rest. He is tachypneic at 28 breaths/min, his HR is 83 bpm, arterial BP is 90/50 mm Hg, and oxygen saturation by pulse oximeter is 80% while breathing room air. He denies any chest pain. His electrocardiogram shows a.fib with ventricular rate of 96 bpm and LV hypertrophy by voltage criteria. Physical examination is remarkable for an uncomfortable, orthopneic patient. On lung auscultation, bilateral crackles are heard, including anterior lung fields. Point of maximal cardiac impulse (PMI) is not displaced and there are no murmurs appreciated.

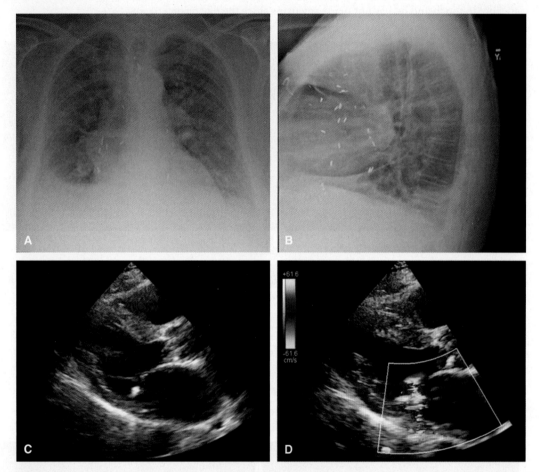

**Figure 25.24** A, Posteroanterior chest X-ray (CXR). B, Lateral CXR. C, Parasternal long-axis (PLAx). Systole. D, PLAx with color Doppler. Systole.

Based on **Figure 25.24** and ▶ **Videos 25.38** and **25.39**, which of the following is most likely?
A. Patient has significant MR secondary to a flail anterior leaflet, which is likely contributing to his presentation.
B. Patient has significant MR secondary to ruptured posterior medial PM, which is likely contributing to his presentation.
C. Patient has significant MR secondary to apical displacement of both PMs and tethered leaflets, which is likely contributing to his presentation.
D. Patient has significant MR secondary to tethered posterior leaflet, likely from a prior inferior wall MI.
E. None of the above.

**20.** Which of the following is *true* of severe *acute* MR? (See also **Figure 25.25**.)

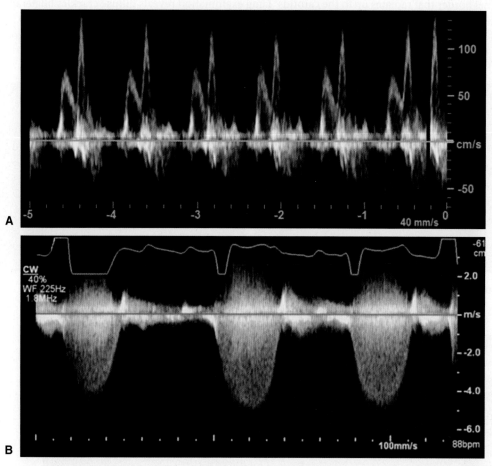

**Figure 25.25** A, Mitral inflow. Pulse-wave Doppler. B, Continuous-wave Doppler of mitral regurgitation.

**A.** LA size correlates well with severity of MR.
**B.** A-wave-dominant pattern of mitral inflow strongly suggests that MR is not severe (see Figure 25.25A).
**C.** Peak velocity of MR by CWD of >4 m/s strongly suggests that MR is severe.
**D.** Characteristic parabolic shape of MR velocity CWD envelope strongly suggests that acute MR is severe (Figure 25.25B).
**E.** None of the above.

**21.** A 79-year-old woman presented with acute hip fracture after a motor vehicle accident (pedestrian struck at a low velocity). There was no loss of consciousness or any other trauma. She has a history of arterial hypertension, but no other known comorbidities. She underwent an uneventful hip repair under general anesthesia on hospital day 2. Postoperatively, in the recovery room, the patient became progressively tachycardic, hypotensive, and hypoxemic. She was thought to be in pulmonary edema from excessive intraoperative fluid administration and was given intravenous furosemide. Her BP continued to drop and she required 50% oxygen supplementation delivered via a face mask to maintain arterial saturation (by pulse oximeter) of 92%. When BP decreased to 80/40 mm Hg, intravenous continuous infusion of dobutamine was started. Urine output was noted to decrease, and the patient now required 100% oxygen supplementation via a non-rebreather mask. CXR was most consistent with bilateral pulmonary edema. On physical examination, there is a loud systolic murmur at the left sternal border that radiates up to the carotids. Lung examination reveals diffuse crackles bilaterally including the anterior lung fields. Cardiac US images are shown. Inferior vena cava (IVC) was 0.5 cm and collapsed completely on inspiration. Lung US showed diffuse B-lines bilaterally in all lung zones. See **Figures 25.26, 25.27, 25.28, 25.29, 25.30** and ▶ **Videos 25.40** to **25.42**.

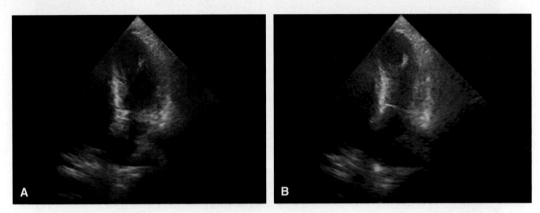

**Figure 25.26** A, A4 end-diastole. B, A4 end-systole.

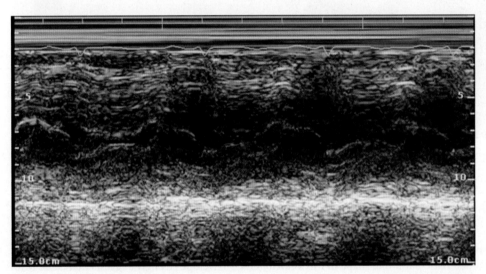

**Figure 25.27** Parasternal long-axis M-mode through the tips of the mitral valve. Note that only the anterior leaflet is well visualized.

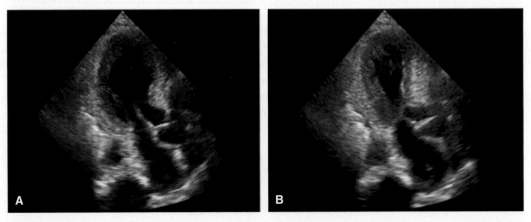

**Figure 25.28** A, Apical three-chamber view (A3). End-diastole. B, Apical three-chamber view (A3). End-systole.

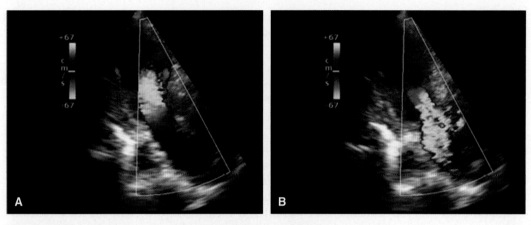

**Figure 25.29** A, A3 color Doppler. Diastole. B, A3 color Doppler. Systole.

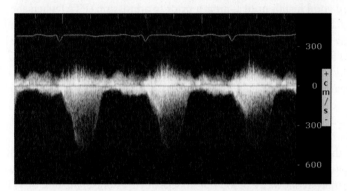

**Figure 25.30** Spectral recording of continuous-wave Doppler through the aortic outflow tract obtained in apical three-chamber view (A3). Peak velocity is 4.5 m/s (peak pressure gradient 81 mm Hg).

Which of the following is correct about this patient?
**A.** Despite low right-sided filling pressure, LA pressure is high and the patient should be aggressively diuresed.
**B.** Intubation is likely to improve hemodynamics and pulmonary edema.
**C.** The patient has significant premorbid MR contributing to her presentation.
**D.** Peripheral vasoconstrictors, such as neosynephrine, should be initiated and inotropes tapered off.
**E.** None of the answer options are correct.

**22.** A 70-year-old man comes in with progressive dyspnea on exertion. He has a history of coronary heart disease and heart failure with reduced ejection fraction (HFrEF). He ran out of his medications 2 weeks prior to the presentation and was not able to refill them. He is hemodynamically stable, has a respiratory rate of 22 breaths/min, and his oxygen saturation by pulse oximeter is 90% while on oxygen supplementation per nasal cannula at 2 L/min.

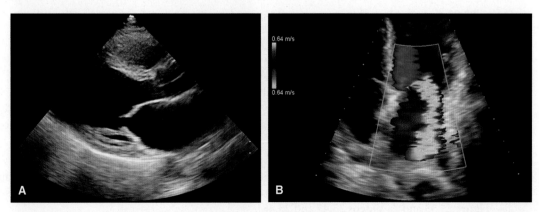

**Figure 25.31** A, Parasternal long-axis. B, Zoomed-in apical four-chamber view with color Doppler. Systole.

Assuming that all the settings have been optimized in **Figure 25.31** and ▶ **Videos 25.43** and **25.44,** which of the following is the most accurate statement about this patient's MR?

A. MR is likely chronic and significant.

B. MR is likely chronic and not significant.

C. Whether this MR is significant or not depends on whether it is acute or chronic, which cannot be determined with any certainty from the provided data.

D. MR is likely acute and significant.

23. A 72-year-old woman is admitted to the ICU with a diagnosis of sepsis and hypoxemia. Her illness started suddenly 2 days prior to admission when she felt generally unwell. The morning before the admission she developed a subjective fever and saw her outpatient provider. In the provider's office she suddenly felt acutely dyspneic. At the time her oxygen saturation by pulse oximetry was 80% while inspiring room air, and her temperature was 101.3 °F. There was no prodrome and she denied any urinary or gastrointestinal symptoms.

The patient was in her usual state of good health until 1-month prior to admission (PTA) when she was in a motor vehicle accident, which, among other things, resulted in a mandibular fracture, as well as diaphragmatic eventration of the bowels requiring multiple abdominal surgeries. Since then she has had very limited oral intake and for the past 3 weeks has been receiving total parenteral nutrition (TPN) at home via a peripherally inserted central venous catheter (PICC).

On physical examination, she appears chronically ill and is in moderate distress. She requires 100% oxygen administered via a non-rebreather mask to maintain oxygen saturation of 91% by pulse oximeter. Her respiratory rate is 24 breaths/min, temperature is 39.2 °C, BP 100/50 mm Hg, and HR 112 bpm. Lung auscultation reveals diffuse bilateral crackles. There is a loud holosystolic murmur best heard at the apex that radiates to the axilla. Laboratory tests are significant for WBC count of 35 × 10⁹/L, serum creatinine of 3.1 mg/dL (from the baseline of 0.8 mg/dL), and venous blood lactate of 4.1 mmol/L. Urinalysis shows 2+ blood but no leukocyte esterase, nitrites, or WBC. Admission CXR shows bilateral infiltrates "concerning for a multifocal pneumonia."

Bedside lung ultrasound shows diffuse B-lines in all lung zones and small bilateral pleural effusions (see **Figure 25.32** and ▶ **Videos 25.45** and **25.46**).

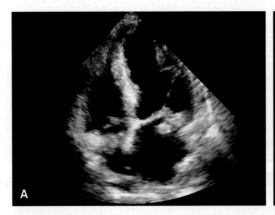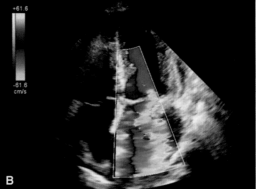

**Figure 25.32** A, Apical four-chamber view. B, Apical four-chamber view with color Doppler in systole.

Which of the following is most accurate?

A. The patient has a flail anterior leaflet of the MV.

B. MR is not significant and is unlikely to contribute to patient's presentation.

C. Urgent CT surgery consultation is indicated.

D. Red CD signal along the interatrial septum is a result of aliasing and indicates very high flow velocity.

E. None of the answer options are accurate.

24. A 72-year-old woman presents with sudden onset of shortness of breath, fever, and pulmonary edema. Bedside lung ultrasound shows diffuse B-lines in all lung zones and small bilateral pleural effusions (see also **Figure 25.33** and ▶ **Videos 25.47** and **25.48**).

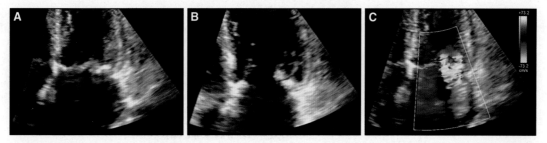

**Figure 25.33.** A, Apical four-chamber view, zoomed-in on the mitral valve. Systole. B, Apical four-chamber view, zoomed-in on the mitral valve. Diastole. C, Apical four-chamber view, zoomed-in on the mitral valve. Color Doppler.

Which of the following is most accurate concerning this patient?
A. This patient has a perforation of an MV leaflet.
B. This patient has a flail anterior mitral leaflet.
C. This patient has an MV clip.
D. In this case, severity of MR is likely overestimated by CD.
E. None of the answer options are accurate.

25. What is a definition of a "flail leaflet"?

A. A leaflet any portion of which is billowing below the plane of the MV (i.e., protrudes in the left atrium) by ≥2 mm in systole
B. A leaflet that has a torn chord seen moving around in the left ventricle during the cardiac cycle
C. A leaflet that fails to close all the way during MV closure and is thus seen above the plane of the MV annulus
D. A prolapsed leaflet with a tip pointing toward the left atrium in systole
E. None of the answer choices above

# Chapter 25 ▪ Answers

1. Correct Answer: D. The specific type of MR the patient has may be caused by prior inferior wall MI.

*Rationale:* This patient has significantly decreased systolic LV function. He also had significant (moderate-severe) MR, despite the CD signature being less than impressive. CHF exacerbation as well as worsening MR (caused by progressively more dilated left ventricle and increasing LV pressures) have likely contributed to his presentation. The MR jet in this case is posteriorly directed. With a structurally normal MV, a posteriorly directed MR jet can be a result of either prolapse of the anterior leaflet or apical tethering of the posterior leaflet. The latter is commonly a sequela of inferior wall infarction. Both leaflets in this case are tethered, but the posterior one more than the anterior one.

Increase in LA size is generally a reflection of chronically elevated LA pressures. However, chronic atrial fibrillation destroys that relationship: significant LA dilation is frequently seen in the absence of elevated LA pressures.

The most basic method of semiquantitatively grading the severity of MR is based on the area of the regurgitant jet relative to the area of the left atrium. Generally, jets occupying >40% of the atrium indicate severe MR, and those which occupy <10% indicate mild, insignificant MR. Eccentric MR jets, however, constitute a special case. When the turbulent jet of MR comes in contact with the atrial wall, kinetic energy is dissipated and CD signal decreases, resulting in visual underestimation of the jet severity (Coanda effect). In general, eccentricity of the jet should upstage its severity, as judged by area of the jet body. Severe dilation of the left atrium may make the jet area appear relatively smaller and thus less significant.

MV leaflets indeed seem not to open all the way in diastole. However, they appear relatively structurally normal. This is not a finding of MS, but rather is most commonly due to dysfunction of the left ventricle. Proximity of the anterior mitral leaflet to the septum during diastole may be used as an indirect index of systolic function. This measure, called EPSS, increases when LV systolic function is poor. In addition, aortic insufficiency (AI), which this patient also happened to have, appears to hit the anterior leaflet of the MV and prevent its full opening in diastole.

### Selected Reference

1. Zoghbi WA, Adams D, Bonow RO, et al. Recommendations for noninvasive evaluation of native valvular regurgitation: a report from the American Society of Echocardiography developed in collaboration with the Society for Cardiovascular Magnetic Resonance. *J Am Soc Echocardiogr.* 2017 Apr;30(4):303-371. doi:10.1016/j.echo.2017.01.007. Epub 2017 Mar 14.

**2.** Correct Answer: D. MV anatomy suggests that MR is likely secondary to dilated cardiomyopathy and not its cause.

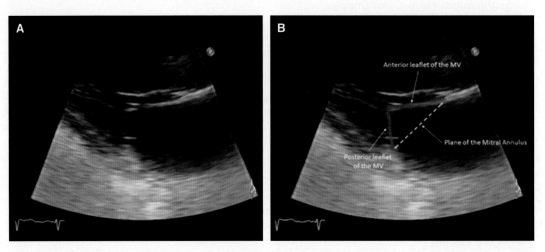

**Figure 25.34** Parasternal long-axis zoomed-in on the mitral valve (MV) in end-systole (A). Leaflets of the MV and the plane of the mitral annulus are labeled (B).

*Rationale:* PLAx view clearly shows that in systole when the MV closes, MV leaflets do not reach the plane of the MV annulus (**Figure 25.34**). This is a result of MV leaflets being tethered by the subvalvular apparatus (PMs and chordae). Tethering of just (or predominantly) the posterior MV leaflet can be seen after an MI, especially after an inferolateral MI, but symmetric tethering is almost invariably secondary to chronic LV dilation and alteration in LV shape with apical and lateral displacement of the PMs. Consequently, MV fails to close in systole, resulting in secondary MR.

### Selected Reference

1. Dudzinski DM, Hung J. Echocardiographic assessment of ischemic mitral regurgitation. *Cardiovasc Ultrasound.* 2014 Nov 21;12:46. doi:10.1186/1476-7120-12-46.

**3.** Correct Answer: A. Figure 25.3A. VC is properly measured in the parasternal long-axis (PLAx) view.

*Rationale:* VC is properly measured in PLAx view, as shown in Figure 25.3A. In the PLAx view, the MR flow is (almost) perpendicular to the insonation beam, while in A4 it is (almost) parallel to it. Because lateral resolution of CD is poor, measurement of VC in A4 will often result in significant overestimation of the width of the jet.

VC width is an established measure of MR severity. It is defined as the narrowest part of the jet on CD and cannot be identified reliably in the transverse PSAx view.

This patient was confirmed to have moderate-severe MR by other echocardiographic measures.

### Selected Reference

1. Zoghbi WA, Adams D, Bonow RO, et al. Recommendations for noninvasive evaluation of native valvular regurgitation: a report from the American Society of Echocardiography developed in collaboration with the Society for Cardiovascular Magnetic Resonance. *J Am Soc Echocardiogr.* 2017 Apr;30(4):303-371. doi:10.1016/j.echo.2017.01.007. Epub 2017 Mar 14.

**4.** Correct Answer: B. Dilated cardiomyopathy.

*Rationale:* The appearance of a small MV relative to the size of the mitral annulus is typical of dilated cardiomyopathy and is also a frequent cause of MR, secondary to the failure of the leaflets to coapt in systole. (See **Figure 25.35** and ▶ **Video 25.49**.)

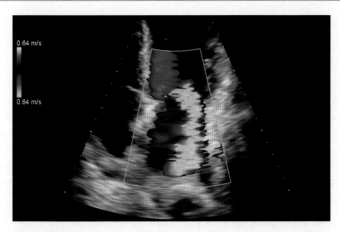

**Figure 25.35** Apical zoomed-in four-chamber view. Color Doppler. Systole.

The appearance of a restricted MV opening is secondary to the leaflets being tethered by the PMs, which are now further away from the MV in dilated cardimyopathy. The restriction is generally uniform without any part of the leaflet affected more than others. Also, a low stroke volume in a patient with dilated cardiomyopathy leads to reduced opening of the mitral leaflets during diastole (due to reduction in diastolic blood flow from the left atrium to the left ventricle). This appearance is commonly misinterpreted by beginner sonographers as MS, which it is not. Presence of rheumatic MV disease is virtually excluded by lack of sclerosis, calcifications, and fusions of the commissures. Endocarditis and AI cannot be excluded, but the appearance of the dilated MV annulus in the presence of decreased LV systolic function is highly characteristic of MV dysfunction secondary to dilated cardiomyopathy. This patient had diabetes with severely decreased LV systolic function. The procedure he had abroad was coronary catheterization.

Selected Reference

1. Zoghbi WA, Adams D, Bonow RO, et al. Recommendations for noninvasive evaluation of native valvular regurgitation: a report from the American Society of Echocardiography developed in collaboration with the Society for Cardiovascular Magnetic Resonance. *J Am Soc Echocardiogr.* 2017 Apr;30(4):303-371. doi:10.1016/j.echo.2017.01.007. Epub 2017 Mar 14.

5. Correct Answer: B. B

*Rationale:* Regurgitant jet is said to have a conversion zone, located above the plane of the valve in the sending chamber (the left ventricle in this case) and a body of the jet, within the receiving chamber (in this case the left atrium). In between the two, just under the valve, the jet narrows. This part of the jet is called VC. VC width correlates with severity of regurgitation.

Selected Reference

1. Zoghbi WA, Adams D, Bonow RO, et al. Recommendations for noninvasive evaluation of native valvular regurgitation: a report from the American Society of Echocardiography developed in collaboration with the Society for Cardiovascular Magnetic Resonance. *J Am Soc Echocardiogr.* 2017 Apr;30(4):303-371. doi:10.1016/j.echo.2017.01.007. Epub 2017 Mar 14.

6. Correct Answer: C. This is a significant MR that is likely contributing to the patient's symptoms. Image in Figure 25.7C is the most representative of the degree of the MR and in other images CD is undergained.

*Rationale:* Changes in Doppler scale and gain significantly affect appearance of MR on CD imaging. The appropriate scale setting depends on prevalent velocities of blood flow. Recognize that:

- Velocities greater than the maximum indicated on the scale will be aliased, that is, appear to be opposite in direction (and therefore color).
- Velocities below the threshold of detection will not be picked up by the instrument at all. A useful estimate is that the detection threshold is approximately 10% of the maximum. Thus, if the scale is set up such that maximum deductible velocity is 60 cm/s (0.6 m/s), the instrument will not pick up any flow slower than 6 cm/s (0.06 m/s). The standard approach to interrogating the MV is to initially set the scale at highest possible value for the preset (60 cm/s in this case).
- Appropriate pulse-wave Doppler and CD scale for most intracardiac structures, including the valves, as well as for arterial structures is 50 to 70 cm/s. Usually your machine's cardiac preset would be correct for most applications. Assessment of venous flows and flow across the septum will require lower scale settings with max of 40 to 50 cm/s.

The standard optimization of color gain is performed as follows:

- The gain is turned all the way up, until color pixelation is seen "bleeding" into the cardiac tissues.
- The gain is then slowly turned down just enough to eliminate this effect.

The gain is *not* excessive in any of the three images shown and therefore the one with the highest gain will reflect the severity of the regurgitation best. The jet in Figure 25.7C occupies >40% of the left atrium and is therefore consistent with severe MR. It is possible that it is still underestimating the degree of MR, but there is no way to upstage MR already assigned the grade of "severe." Therefore, Figure 25.7C is the most accurate. **Remaining** Figures 25.7A and 25.7B are undergained and underestimating the degree of MR.

Acute MR, listed in answer B, is a very important condition that may elude detection by both physical examination and echocardiography. Several typical features of acute MR are worth keeping in mind:

- Left atrium is usually of normal size, as the chamber does not have enough time to accommodate the regurgitant flow of blood.
- Because left atrium has not had enough time to dilate, the pressure within it is high and patients tend to be acutely severely symptomatic and frequently critical.
- Anatomy of acute MR usually falls into one of the four categories:
  1. PM rupture—almost exclusively a result of an acute MI, though it does not tend to occur in the acute setting (tends to occur 3-7 days after the event).
  2. Chordae tendineae rupture, which results in a flail leaflet. This can be degenerative or traumatic.
  3. Perforation of the leaflet from endocarditis.
  4. Tethering of a leaflet (or less commonly, both leaflets) because of acute PM ischemia (but not rupture), acute myocarditis, or TTC.
     - Occasionally, dynamic left ventricular outflow tract (LVOT) obstruction can result in SAM of the anterior leaflet of the MV, causing acute (posteriorly directed) MR. This is most commonly seen in older women (likely a surrogate for smaller body and heart size) with sigmoid interventricular septa who experience acute hypovolemia or peripheral vasodilation, or in the presence of TTC.
     - MR jet of acute MR tends to be eccentric, though central MR can be seen as well.
     - When acute MR is symmetric it is most often due to massive MI, acute myocarditis, or TTC.

Note that this patient's MR is symmetric in appearance, left atrium is dilated, LV systolic function is decreased, and both leaflets appear tethered. This is a typical appearance of MR secondary to dilated cardiomyopathy. The patient is hemodynamically stable and is not in any extremis. He is unlikely to have an acute MR.

Selected Reference

1. Thomas JD. Doppler echocardiographic assessment of valvular regurgitation. *Heart.* 2002 Dec;88(6):651-657. doi:10.1136/heart.88.6.651.

**7.** Correct Answer: D. EPSS or E-point septal separation

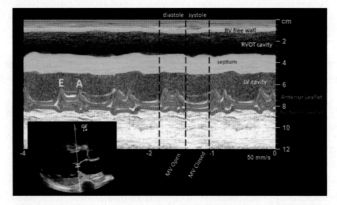

**Figure 35.36** M-mode through the tips of the mitral valve in parasternal long-axis.

*Rationale:* In M-mode displacement is plotted on the Y-axis and time on the X-axis. In **Figure 25.36** the blue line represents the movement of the anterior leaflet and the red line the posterior leaflet over time. The distance between the two increases in diastole when the valve is open and decreases in systole when the valve is closed. The MV opens twice during each cardiac cycle: once during rapid ventricular filling and once during atrial contraction, designated as E and A, respectively. The measured minimal separation between the anterior leaflet of the MV and the septum, which occurs in diastole, specifically during the E-event, is called EPSS. It is an indirect surrogate of the LV systolic function. Values of >7 mm are highly predictive of severely reduced LV systolic function. Note that EPSS is an indirect measure of LV systolic function, a correlate, because the event occurring in diastole may not in principle be a direct reflection of ejection, occurring in systole. As seen in the case images, this patient indeed has severely impaired LV systolic function.

TAPSE is an apicobasal displacement of the tricuspid valve (TV) annulus during systole and is a measure of RV systolic function. S' is the velocity of that (systolic) displacement as captured by tissue Doppler imaging (TDI) and is too a measure of RV contractility. SAM is an abnormal systolic movement of the anterior leaflet of the MV, which would be detected by the same M-mode tracing. Pressure half-time is a measure of rapidity of mitral inflow used for assessment of MS severity and is a spectral Doppler measure.

### Selected Reference

1. McKaigney CJ, Krantz MJ, La Rocque CL, Hurst ND, Buchanan MS, Kendall JL. E-point septal separation: a bedside tool for emergency physician assessment of left ventricular ejection fraction. *Am J Emerg Med*. 2014 Jun;32(6):493-497. doi:10.1016/j.ajem.2014.01.045. Epub 2014 Feb 3.

**8.** Correct Answer: C. All of the above are correct statements.

*Rationale:* The MV has a complex geometric shape, and though in primary MR the regurgitant orifice is roughly circular, it has a more complex shape in secondary MR, which occurs along the coaptation line of the two mitral leaflets. (See **Figure 25.37**.)

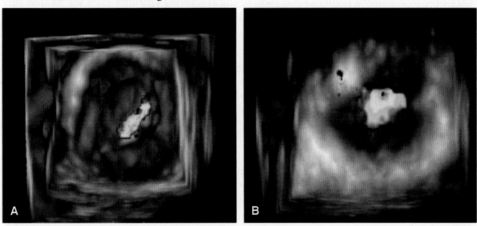

**Figure 35.37** En face color 3D image showing shape of the regurgitant jet. A, Functional mitral regurgitation (MR). B, MR secondary to mitral valve prolapse (MVP).

Consequently, particularly in secondary MR, depending on the tomographic scan plane, the jet of MR may have a different appearance. This is especially striking in the case of the apical two-chamber view, in which the scan plane is parallel to a large segment of the coaptation line between the two leaflets. (See **Figure 25.38**.)

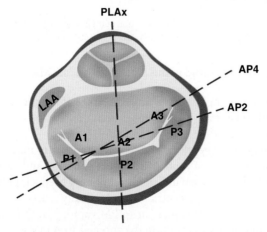

**Figure 35.38** Tomographic planes of standard transthoracic views transecting the mitral valve. PLAx, parasternal long-axis.

In functional MR with its slit-like or oval regurgitant orifice, the jet area will be larger in apical two-chamber view than in apical four-chamber view. (See **Figure 25.39.**)

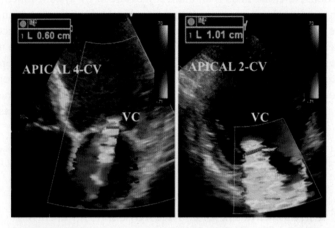

**Figure 35.39** A and B, Vena contracta (VC) width obtained from the apical four-chamber and two-chamber views in a patient with ischemic functional mitral regurgitation.

In primary MR, with a round regurgitant orifice, in the apical two-chamber view the jet may be missed entirely.

**Selected References**
1. Fields A. Mitral valve: echo perspective. Cardioserv. Accessed April 23, 2021. https://www.cardioserv.net/echo-mitral-valve/.
2. Lancellotti P, Tribouilloy C, Hagendorff A, et al. Recommendations for the echocardiographic assessment of native valvular regurgitation: an executive summary from the European Association of Cardiovascular Imaging. *Eur Heart J Cardiovasc Imaging.* 2013 Jul;14(7):611-644. doi:10.1093/ehjci/jet105. Epub 2013 Jun 3.
3. Matsumura Y, Fukuda S, Tran H, et al. Geometry of the proximal isovelocity surface area in mitral regurgitation by 3-dimensional color Doppler echocardiography: difference between functional mitral regurgitation and prolapse regurgitation. *Am Heart J.* 2008 Feb;155(2):231-238. doi:10.1016/j.ahj.2007.09.002. Epub 2007 Oct 25.

**9.** Correct Answer: A. Severe acute MR secondary to traumatic PM rupture

*Rationale:* Torn PM can be seen moving from the left ventricle to the left atrium and back during the cardiac cycle. Even though CD may underestimate the severity of MR in the acute setting, as well as in cases of an eccentric jet, here CD is consistent with severe posteriorly (and superiorly) directed MR. Most cases of unilateral pulmonary edema are right-sided. However, whenever unilateral left-sided pulmonary edema is seen, the cause is very frequently a posteriorly directed MR jet. This can be achieved either by a prolapse of the anterior leaflet or by tethering of the posterior leaflet, with the former being more common in cases of acute MR. Acute MR secondary to blunt chest trauma is more often due to chordae rupture, while acute MR 2 to 5 days after an acute MI is more likely to be secondary to PM rupture.

**Selected Reference**
1. Thomas B, Durant E, Barbant S, Nagdev A. Repeat point-of-care echocardiographic evaluation of traumatic cardiac arrest: a new paradigm for the emergency physician. *Clin Pract Cases Emerg Med.* 2017 May 23;1(3):194-196. doi:10.5811/cpcem.2017.2.33021.

**10.** Correct Answer: D. It is likely that LA enlargement is premorbid in this patient with acute MR.

*Rationale:* Even though measurement of LA AP diameter in PLAx as a single measure of LA size is disarranged, in this case it is obviously and severely dilated at least 4.7 cm (upper limit of normal for women is 3.8 cm).

   Clinical presentation of unilateral right-sided pulmonary edema and hypotension is very much consistent with acute MR. Bilateral pulmonary edema in cases of acute MR is more common and cases of unilateral edema present a significant diagnostic challenge. When unilateral pulmonary edema is present, it is more commonly right-sided and when secondary to acute eccentric MR, it is usually caused by a flail posterior leaflet. Acute flail leaflet may be secondary to chord rupture or to PM rupture. In this case, a chord can be seen flying between the left atrium and the left ventricle in the zoomed-in A4 view. Etiologies of chordae rupture include:

- myxomatous disease. This, by definition, occurs only to people with preexisting chronic MV prolapse
- infective endocarditis
- blunt chest trauma
- RHD
- spontaneous (idiopathic)

Mobility of the MV leaflets does not show signs of fibrosis or calcification and is not restricted, which makes rheumatic MV disease unlikely. (See **Figure 25.40**.)

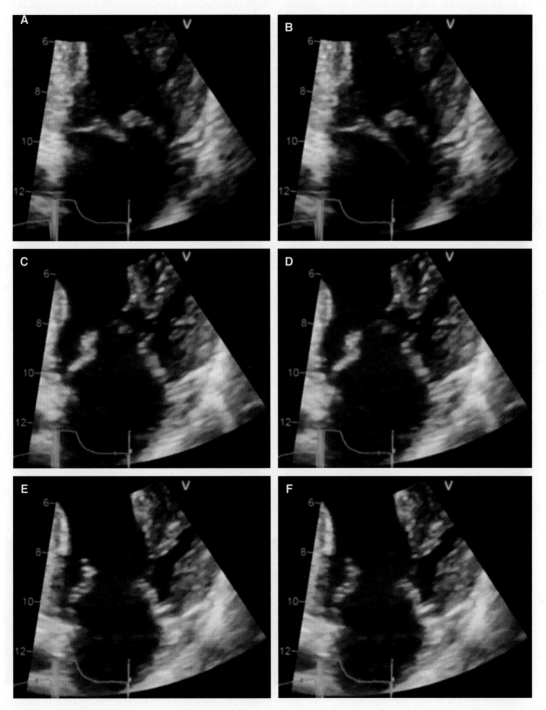

**Figure 25.40.** A, Systole. B, Systole. Torn chordae labeled. C, Early diastole. D, Early diastole, torn chordae labeled. E, Diastole. F, Diastole, torn chordae labeled.

Selected Reference

1. Ravi V, Rodriguez J, Doukky R, Pyslar N. Acute mitral regurgitation: the dreaded masquerader. *CASE (Phila)*. 2018 Jan 3;2(1):12-15. doi:10.1016/j.case.2017.10.002.

**11.** Correct Answer: B. Holosystolic regurgitation of chronic central MR in a patient with pulmonary edema who is hemodynamically stable

*Rationale:* Assumptions behind the use of relative MR jet area are:
- Central (as opposed to eccentric) MR jet.
- A single jet (as opposed to multiple MR jets). Measuring only one of several jets will result in underestimation of the severity of the MR.
- Holosystolic MR. Late systolic regurgitation, which is frequently associated with MV prolapse, is of very short duration and measuring the jet in the frames that contain it will overestimate clinical MR severity.
- MR must be chronic. Velocity of MR jet is, naturally, dependent on the pressure gradient between the left ventricle and left atrium in systole. This will be affected by factors such as systemic hypotension, whether the left atrium had enough time to become dilated, thus accommodating pressure increase, and volume status. In acute MR, measures based on MR jet area will tend to underestimate MR severity.

### Selected References
1. Dudzinski DM, Hung J. Echocardiographic assessment of ischemic mitral regurgitation. *Cardiovasc Ultrasound.* 2014 Nov 21;12:46. doi:10.1186/1476-7120-12-46.
2. Mitral valve disease. In: Armstrong WF, Ryan T, eds. *Feigenbaum's Echocardiography.* 8th ed. Wolters Kluwer; 2019.
3. Zoghbi WA, Adams D, Bonow RO, et al. Recommendations for noninvasive evaluation of native valvular regurgitation: a report from the American Society of Echocardiography developed in collaboration with the Society for Cardiovascular Magnetic Resonance. *J Am Soc Echocardiogr.* 2017 Apr;30(4):303-371. doi:10.1016/j.echo.2017.01.007.

**12.** Correct Answer: E. None of the above

*Rationale:* Both A and B are velocities, not time, so may not be correct.

D marks the time point when velocity has decreased from its peak to half its value. Note that this is *not* pressure half-time. P½T is the time it takes for the *pressure*, not the velocity, to fall to 50% of its value. From modified Bernoulli equation, $\Delta P = 4 \times V^2$, and so $V = \frac{1}{2}\sqrt{\Delta P}$. Consequently,

$$V_{max} = \frac{1}{2}\sqrt{\Delta P_{max}},$$

$$V_{0.5\ max} = \frac{1}{2}\frac{\sqrt{P_{max}}}{\sqrt{2}}, \text{ and}$$

$$\frac{V_{0.5\ max}}{V_{max}} = \frac{\frac{1}{\sqrt{2}}}{1} = \frac{1}{\sqrt{2}} \approx 0.71$$

In English, pressure half-time is achieved at the point where velocity has dropped to 0.71 of its peak value.

Nonetheless, Answer C is wrong because the deceleration slope used to derive these values is incorrect. (See **Figures 25.15** and **25.41**.)

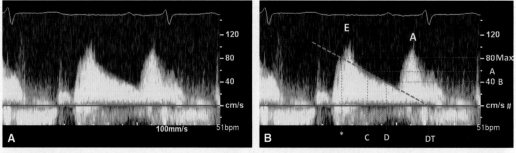

**Figure 25.41.** A, Continuous-wave Doppler (CWD) of mitral inflow and B, CWD of mitral inflow, labeled.

Note that the E-wave has two distinct slopes, the earlier one being much steeper. When such morphology is present, it is the later slope that should be used to obtain pressure half-time and deceleration time, as shown in Figures 25.15 and 25.41. Note also that the $V_{max}$ value used for the calculations is the point of the intersection of the slope with the spectral graph, not the actual maximal velocity of the flow.

Selected Reference

1. Baumgartner H, Hung J, Bermejo J, et al. Echocardiographic assessment of valve stenosis: EAE/ASE recommendations for clinical practice. *J Am Soc Echocardiogr.* 2009 Jan;22(1):1-23.

**13.** Correct Answer: D. Cases 1 and 2 show MS.

*Rationale:* Patients in cases 1 and 2 both have restricted MV opening due to MS. In case 3 the valve itself is normal, but the leaflets are displaced apically (i.e., "tethered") because of dilated cardiomyopathy. As a result, the valve leaflets do not coapt in systole, which results in MR. In diastole, the pressure in the left ventricle is high and the leaflets do not open all the way, but *not* because of any intrinsic valve pathology. Consequently, the anterior leaflet of the MV does not come close to the septum, as it does normally, resulting in increased EPSS—an index correlating with poor LV systolic function. Recognition of significant MS in patients presenting with pulmonary edema is extremely important clinically, as treatment options differ significantly, and a beta-blocker may be indicated. In significant MS of any etiology, posterior leaflet movement tends to be more restricted than that of the anterior leaflet.

The patient in case 1 has significant calcific MS. In MAC, the annulus is affected early and the disease then progresses distally toward the tips of the leaflets. Note that in this case the only mobile part of the anterior leaflet is its tip, while the base of the leaflet is fixed. In the industrialized world, MAC has replaced RHD as the leading cause of MS. (See **Figure 25.42.**)

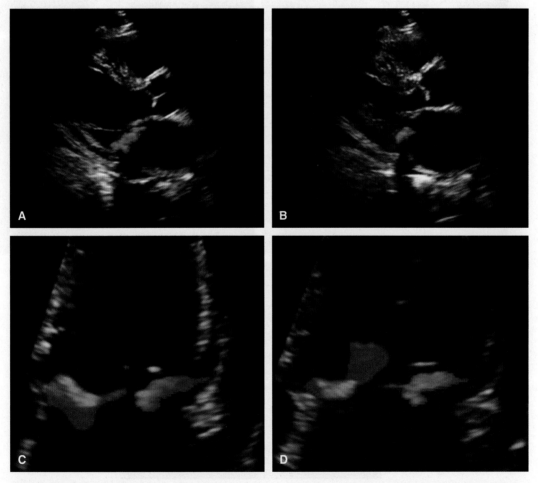

**Figure 25.42** Case 1, Patient 1: significant calcific mitral stenosis. Posterior (blue) and anterior (red) mitral valve (MV) leaflets are labeled. Posterior leaflet is essentially immobile. For the anterior leaflet, note relative sparing of the distal (tip) portion, which is still mobile, and a relatively more severe involvement of the base of the leaflet, which is fixed. Left atrium is dilated and left ventricular systolic function is normal. A, Parasternal long-axis (PLAx). End-systole. MV is closed. B, PLAx. Diastole. MV is open. C, A4, zoomed-in on MV. Systole. MV is closed. D, A4, zoomed-in on MV. Diastole. MV is open.

The patient in case 2 has significant rheumatic MS. In RHD, the leaflets are first affected at their tips, with the rest of the leaflets and the chordae getting involved only later in the course. The leaflet commissures fuse, which prevents the valve from opening fully in diastole. Until the disease involves the entire leaflet, the base of the leaflet tends to retain mobility relative to the more restricted tip. Consequently, when the valve opens in diastole, the base of the leaflet moves into the left ventricle more than the tip does, creating a bend. This configuration of the anterior mitral leaflet has been historically compared to a hockey stick. This is best seen on the PLAx view. Chordae fusion is best seen in apical windows. Note that LV systolic function is normal and there is concomitant significant aortic valve disease (stenosis). (See **Figure 25.43**.)

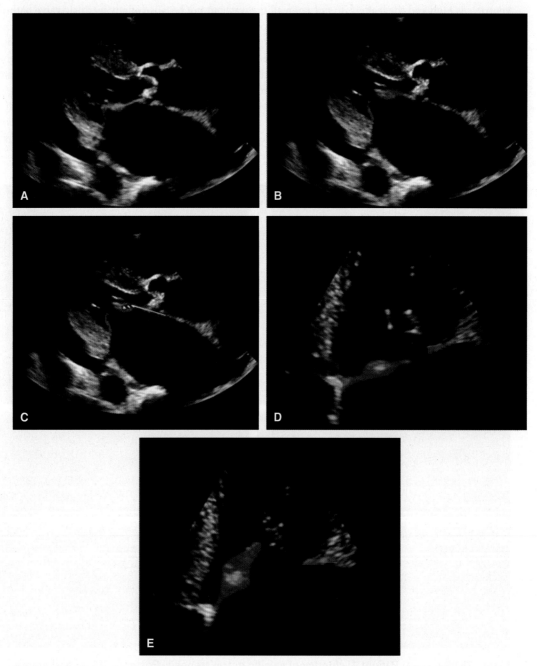

**Figure 25.43** Case 2, Patient 2: significant rheumatic mitral stenosis. Posterior (blue) and anterior (red) mitral valve (MV) leaflets are labeled. Posterior leaflet is essentially immobile. For the anterior leaflet, note relative sparing of the base, which is still mobile, and relatively more severe involvement of the distal (tip) portion of the leaflet, which is fixed. In the parasternal long-axis (PLAx) view this mid-leaflet change in mobility results in diastolic bending of the anterior mitral leaflet and a characteristic "hockey stick" appearance, which in this case can only be intuited.

Chordae thickening and fusion is best appreciated in the apical views. Left atrium is dilated and Left ventricular systolic function is normal. A, PLAx. End-systole. MV is closed. B, PLAx. Diastole. MV is open. C, PLAx. Diastole. MV is open. Hockey stick configuration of the anterior leaflet. D, A4, zoomed-in on MV. Systole. MV is closed. E, A4, zoomed-in on MV. Diastole. MV is open.

The patient in case 3 has a morphologically normal MV. Nonetheless, the appearance of MV in both systole and diastole is abnormal. Note that this patient has dilated left ventricle with poor systolic function. LV dilation displaces both PMs distally and laterally and "tethers" the leaflets. As a result, the cusps come closest to each other (in systole) apically the plane of the MV annulus, which is best seen in the PLAx view. In addition, in diastole, the leaflets do not open all the way, which is thought to reflect a reduced stroke volume, and the minimal distance between the anterior mitral leaflet and the interventricular septum in diastole (EPSS) is increased. EPSS is measured in the PLAx view. This creates an impression of an incomplete valve opening in diastole but must never be mistaken for MS. (See **Figure 25.44**.)

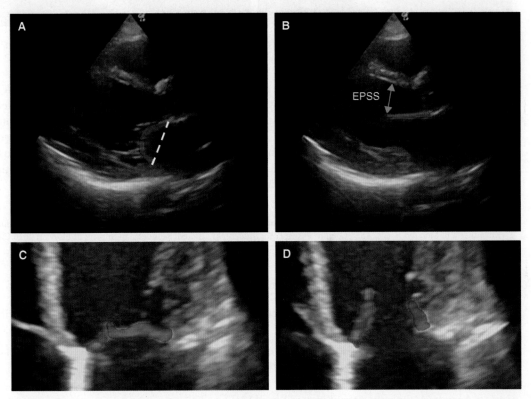

**Figure 25.44** Case 3, Patient 3. A, Parasternal long-axis (PLAx). End-systole. Mitral valve (MV) is closed. B, PLAx. Diastole. MV is open. C, A4, zoomed-in on MV. Systole. MV is closed. D, A4, zoomed-in on MV. Diastole. MV is open. EPSS, E-point septal separation

### Selected Reference

1. Freed BH, Tsang W, Lang RM. Etiologies and mechanisms of mitral valve dysfunction. In: Lang RM, Goldstein SA, Kronzon I, Khandheria B, Mor-Avi V, eds. *ASE's Comprehensive Echocardiography*. 2nd ed. Saunders, an imprint of Elsevier; 2016:Chapter 114. ISBN 9780323260114.

**14.** Correct Answer: A. Diastolic configuration of the anterior mitral leaflet seen in rheumatic MS

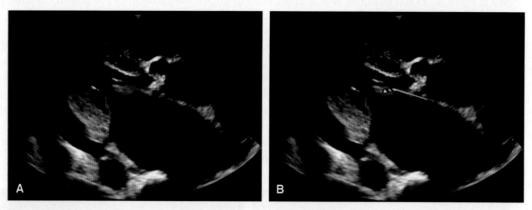

**Figure 25.45** Parasternal long-axis in a patient with significant rheumatic mitral stenosis. Diastole (A). Mitral valve is open (B).

*Rationale:* In **Figure 25.45** and ▶ **Video 25.50**, note the relative sparing of the base of the anterior leaflet, which is still mobile, compared to the relatively more severely affected distal (tip) portion of the leaflet, which is fixed. In PLAx view, this mid-leaflet change in mobility results in diastolic bending of the anterior mitral leaflet and a characteristic "hockey stick" appearance, which in this case is not very pronounced. A similar effect is seen with the posterior leaflet. In calcific MS, the disease process involves the annulus and the base of the leaflets first, and only later spreads to involve the tips of the leaflets. Consequently, tips of the valve remain more, not less, mobile until late in the disease when the entire valve is affected.

Selected Reference

1. Freed BH, Tsang W, Lang RM. Etiologies and mechanisms of mitral valve dysfunction. In: Lang RM, Goldstein SA, Kronzon I, Khandheria B, Mor-Avi V, eds. *ASE's Comprehensive Echocardiography.* 2nd ed. Saunders, an imprint of Elsevier; 2016:Chapter 114. ISBN 9780323260114.

**15.** Correct Answer: C. Dilated left ventricle and/or decrease in LV systolic function

*Rationale:* Typically, severe MS causes neither dilation nor decrease of contractility of the left ventricle.

Selected Reference

1. Saric M, Lang RM, Kronzon I. Rheumatic mitral stenosis. In: Lang RM, Goldstein SA, Kronzon I, Khandheria B, Mor-Avi V. eds. *ASE's Comprehensive Echocardiography.* 2nd ed. Saunders, an imprint of Elsevier; 2016:Chapter 108.

**16.** Correct Answer: A. Only the patient in case 1 has MAC.

*Rationale:* All other patients have prosthetic MVs. Presence of prosthetic valves or the type of the device is not always evident from history, physical examination, and chest radiography.

The patient in case 3 has a mitral mechanical prosthesis. This is evidenced by the "dirty" shadow that the prosthesis casts. "Dirty shadow" is a term used to designate a heterogeneous echo appearance of structures composed of small echogenic bits, such as bowel gas, or in this case, a prosthetic valve, which reflects only part of the insonating ultrasound beam (the rest of the beam permeates the outer layer of the structure or gets scattered). The term stands in contrast to "clean" shadows, cast by larger structures with completely impermeable, fully reflective structures, such as bone or tissue calcifications. (See **Figure 25.46**.)

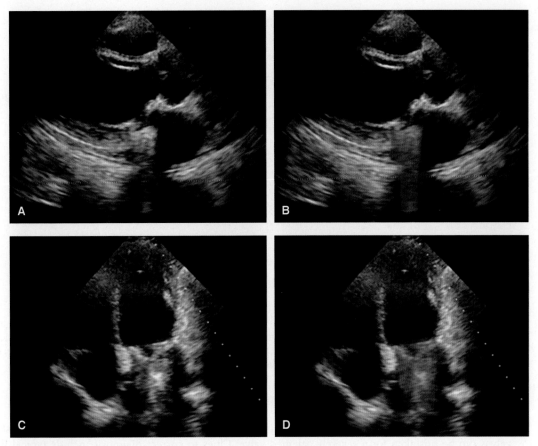

**Figure 25.46** Case 3, Patient 3. A, Parasternal long-axis (PLAx). B, PLAx. Shadow from mechanical mitral valve (MV) prosthesis is shown. C, A4. D, Shadow from mechanical MV prosthesis is shown.

The patient in case 2 has a (stented) biomechanical prosthesis. These create significantly less artifact than mechanical valves do. In the video a three-pronged appearance, characteristic of such valves, is evident. Note that the struts of mechanical valves always point in the direction of the blood flow. See answer to question 18 for additional details.

One useful clue to the prosthetic nature of MVs in cases 2 and 3 is absence of normal chordae, which are removed during surgery. These are usually best seen in apical views and are present in the patient described in case 1.

**17.** Correct Answer: B. No other contributors can be identified.

*Rationale:* No other contributors can be identified based on Figure 25.22. This patient had MV repair with a MitraClip. The apical chamber view shows a typical appearance of the MV after the clip. It is critical to be able to distinguish this from MS. A clip falling off could result in severe acute MR, but in this case, there is no evidence of such an occurrence and the clip is in place. RV function appears to be normal by visual inspection. No other factors are evident. (See also **Figure 25.47.**)

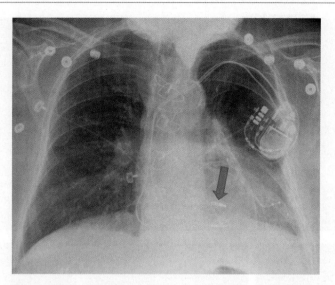

**Figure 25.47** Chest X-ray from the same patient showing mitral clip in situ.

Selected Reference

1. Okada A, Kanzaki H, Amaki M, et al. Successful treatment of mitral regurgitation after transapical transcatheter aortic valve implantation by percutaneous edge-to-edge mitral valve repair (MitraClip®) – the first combination therapy performed in Japan. *Intern Med*. 2018 Apr 15;57(8):1105-1109. doi:10.2169/internalmedicine.9663-17. Epub 2017 Dec 21.

**18.** Correct Answer: A. The patient has had MV replaced (with a bioprosthesis).

This patient's MV has a typical sonographic appearance of a bioprosthesis. Occasionally, bioprosthetic valves can be mistaken for a severely calcified valve. Clues to correct diagnosis include typical three-pronged appearance and absence of chordae, which are removed during valve replacement. Mechanical prosthesis is expected to cast a more pronounced shadow and/or cause a significant artifact deep to it.

Most mitral bioprosthetic valves are of stented construction, which includes three prongs of non-biological material, on which biological tissue (bovine or porcine) is mounted. The biological tissue has very low sonographic signature and may not be visible. The prongs, however, can be readily identified on ultrasound. Unlike mechanical valves, bioprostheses usually cast only limited acoustic shadow. (See **Figure 25.48**.)

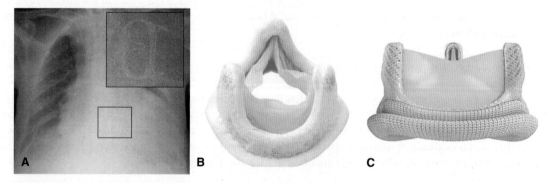

**Figure 25.48** A, Appearance of a stented bioprosthetic valve in mitral position. Note that the prongs of the bioprosthesis always point in the direction of the blood flow. Stented bioprosthesis in the aortic position would have its struts pointing toward the patient's right shoulder. B, Stented porcine bioprosthesis (Medtronic Mosaic). C, Stented pericardial bioprosthesis (Carpentier-Edwards Magna).

Selected References

1. Pibarot P, Dumesnil JG. Prosthetic heart valves: selection of the optimal prosthesis and long-term management. *Circulation*. 2009 Feb 24;119(7):1034-1048. doi:10.1161/CIRCULATIONAHA.108.778886.
2. Zoghbi WA, Chambers JB, Dumesnil JG, et al. Recommendations for evaluation of prosthetic valves with echocardiography and Doppler ultrasound: a report from the American Society of Echocardiography's Guidelines and Standards Committee and

the task force on prosthetic valves, developed in conjunction with the American College of Cardiology Cardiovascular Imaging Committee, Cardiac Imaging Committee of the American Heart Association, the European Association of Echocardiography, a registered branch of the European Society of Cardiology, the Japanese Society of Echocardiography and the Canadian Society of Echocardiography, endorsed by the American College of Cardiology Foundation, American Heart Association, European Association of Echocardiography, a registered branch of the European Society of Cardiology, the Japanese Society of Echocardiography, and Canadian Society of Echocardiography. *J Am Soc Echocardiogr.* 2009 Sep;22(9):975-1014; quiz 1082-4. doi:10.1016/j.echo.2009.07.013. PMID: 19733789.

**19.** Correct Answer: **A. Patient has significant MR secondary to a flail anterior leaflet, which is likely contributing to his presentation.**

*Rationale:* By definition, a leaflet is said to be flail when at any time during the cardiac cycle the tip of the leaflet points toward the left atrium. This usually is a result of a ruptured chordae of a PM. When only a part of the leaflet is flail, the prolapse of the leaflet tissue into the atrium may be difficult to visualize, and care must be taken not to miss it in a patient with an eccentric MR jet. The presence of eccentric MR directed posteriorly may be a result of either a prolapse of the anterior leaflet or tethering of the posterior leaflet, and both possibilities must be investigated. Similarly, anteriorly directed MR jet will result from either prolapse of the posterior MR leaflet or tethering of the anterior leaflet. Apical displacement of both PMs would tend to result in tethering of both leaflets and lack of leaflet coaptation and, usually, a central MR. (See **Figure 25.49.**)

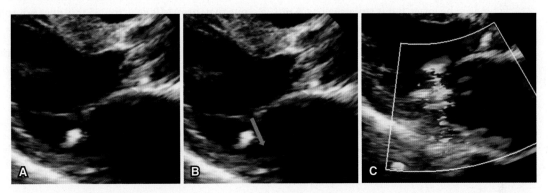

**Figure 25.49** A, Zoomed-in parasternal long-axis (PLAx), systole. Anterior leaflet (red) tip points toward the atrium—that is, is flail. B, Zoomed-in PLAx, systole. Anterior leaflet (red) is flail. Expected direction of the mitral regurgitation jet is indicated with a blue arrow. C, Zoomed-in PLAX with color Doppler. Systole.

Presence of a flail leaflet in a patient with MR of consistent direction strongly correlates with regurgitation being severe.

In this case, there is no evidence of a torn PM and no history suggestive of blunt chest trauma or recent MI. Therefore, a torn chord is the most likely etiology of this patient's acute significant MR. The diagnosis was confirmed by transesophageal echocardiogram (TEE). The patient underwent successful transcatheter bioprosthetic MV replacement.

Selected Reference

1. Oh JK, Park S, Pisralu SV, Nkomo VT. Native valvular heart disease. In: Oh JK, Kane GC, Seward JB, Tajik AJ, Eds. *The Echo Manual.* 4th ed. Wolters Kluwer; 2019:Chapter 13. ISBN 9781496312198.

**20.** Correct Answer: **B. A-wave-dominant pattern of mitral inflow strongly suggests that MR is not severe (see Figure 25.25A).**

*Rationale:* Many other echocardiographic findings have been proposed to identify severe MR. Unfortunately, all of them have limited sensitivity. All these findings are supportive but are not diagnostic.

- **Mitral inflow pattern.** A-wave-dominant mitral inflow pattern (A > E) strongly suggests that MR is not severe.
- **Mitral inflow velocities.** E-wave velocity in severe MR is usually ≥1.2 to 1.5 m/s.
- Characteristic pointed **shape of MR jet** CWD envelope (referred to as a "cutoff sign") suggests that MR is severe; however, normal parabolic shape of the envelope does not rule out severe acute regurgitation. (See also **Figure 24.50.**)

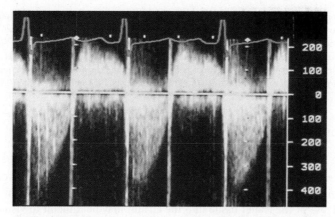

**Figure 25.50** Severe acute mitral regurgitation on continuous-wave Doppler showing a "cutoff" sign.

- **Peak velocity of MR jet** on CWD. As MR severity increases, LA pressure tends to increase as well. In acute MR, LA pressure also tends to be high. As LA pressure increases, the systolic pressure gradient across the regurgitant MV orifice drops, and so does the flow velocity. Characteristically, in chronic severe MR, peak velocity of regurgitant MR jet is <5 m/s. In acute severe MR, transmittal velocity tends to be lower, but is still usually <4 m/s. Despite that, peak MR velocity >5 m/s does not rule out severe regurgitation.

LA dilation is a predictor of MR severity in chronic MR. In acute MR, left atrium is typically normal in size. LA dilation, if present, usually results from other causes. There is no correlation between LA size and regurgitation severity in acute MR.

### Selected References

1. Oh JK, Park S, Pisralu SV, Nkomo VT. Native valvular heart disease. In: Oh JK, Kane GC, Seward JB, Tajik AJ, Eds. *The Echo Manual.* 4th ed. Wolters Kluwer; 2019:Chapter 13. ISBN 9781496312198.
2. Tsang W, Freed BH, Lang RM. Quantification of mitral regurgitation. In: Lang RM, Goldstein SA, Kronzon I, Khandheria B, Mor-Avi V, eds. *ASE's Comprehensive Echocardiography.* 2nd ed. Saunders, an imprint of Elsevier; 2016:Chapter 116. ISBN 9780323260114.

**21.** Correct Answer: **D. Peripheral vasoconstrictors, such as neosynephrine, should be initiated and inotropes tapered off.**

*Rationale:* This patient has TTC, aka transient apical ballooning, likely induced by the stress of trauma and surgery. Cardiogenic shock in TTC can result from acute LV systolic failure itself, but several other mechanisms have been reported. First, TTC may result in LVOT obstruction. It is classically seen in older women with small left ventricles and sigmoid interventricular septa. The postulated mechanism involves compensatory increase in contractility of the base of the left ventricle. The second factor is acute MR. This can develop either as a result of LVOT obstruction or independently of it, in which case symmetric displacement of PMs toward the apex with tethering of both MV leaflets is believed to be responsible. This patient has LVOT obstruction with a high intracavitary pressure gradient. The shape of the CWD spectral Doppler recording is characteristic for LVOT obstruction in that it has a "scooped" proximal limb. This differs significantly from the usual aortic stenosis (AS) envelope, which has a symmetric parabolic shape. As the LVOT gets obstructed, blood flow velocity in LVOT increases. Because of the Bernoulli effect, the pressure within a high-velocity stream drops and a suctioning effect on the walls of the LVOT is created. The posterior wall of the LVOT is formed by the anterior mitral leaflet, which then gets sucked into the LVOT during systole. This abnormal movement is known as SAM and is best seen on M-mode tracing obtained in the PLAx view with the interrogation line through the tips of the mitral leaflets. Systolic displacement of the anterior leaflet creates acute MR, which can be recognized by the presence of a characteristic murmur on examination, and by echo. Acute MR can further contribute to hemodynamic deterioration and pulmonary edema.

    Similar physiology (LVOT obstruction causing acute MR) can be seen in the same group of patients (older women with small hearts and sigmoid interventricular septae) postoperatively even in the absence of TTC. In these cases, relative dehydration, tachycardia, and peripheral vasodilation secondary to anesthetics are likely causative factors. Awareness of this physiology and its recognition are critical, as it has direct management implications. Inotropes and excessive diuresis must be avoided. In the absence of cardiomyopathy, beta-blockers should be considered, along with peripheral vasoconstrictors. Both work by decreasing the gradient across the LVOT and thus ameliorating obstruction and MR.

In this patient, the aortic valve appears structurally normal and the observed LVOT gradient is from dynamic LVOT obstruction, not from the stenotic aortic valve.

Positive pressure ventilation is known to decrease both preload and afterload, both of which are expected to further increase the LVOT gradient and cause progressive hemodynamic deterioration. (See **Figures 25.51** to **25.53**.)

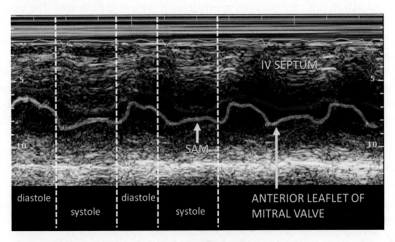

**Figure 25.51** Parasternal long-axis (PLAx) M-mode through the tips of the mitral valve. Anterior leaflet movement is labeled. In systole, the leaflet drifts anteriorly toward the interventricular septum—systolic anterior motion (SAM).

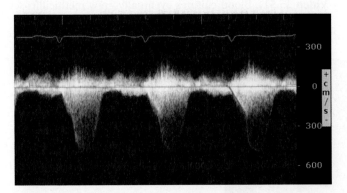

**Figure 25.52** Continuous-wave Doppler spectral Doppler recording through the left ventricular outflow tract (LVOT) obtained in A3 view. Scooped appearance of the ejection envelope, characteristic of (dynamic) LVOT obstruction is highlighted.

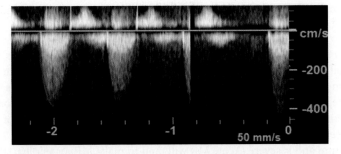

**Figure 25.53** For comparison, "normal" appearance of ejection continuous-wave Doppler envelope recorded through the left ventricular outflow tract in A5 view in a patient with moderate aortic stenosis.

Selected References

1. Baumgartner H, Hung J, Bermejo J, et al. Echocardiographic assessment of valve stenosis: EAE/ASE recommendations for clinical practice. *J Am Soc Echocardiogr.* 2009 Jan;22(1):1-23.
2. Citro R, Lyon AR, Meimoun P, et al. Standard and advanced echocardiography in takotsubo (stress) cardiomyopathy: clinical and prognostic implications. *J Am Soc Echocardiogr.* 2015 Jan;28(1):57-74. doi:10.1016/j.echo.2014.08.020. Epub 2014 Oct 1.

**22.** Correct Answer: **A. MR is likely chronic and significant.**

*Rationale:* The jet area of the MR in this case occupies approximately 40% of the LA area. The suggested cutoff for severe MR is 40%. However, the jet is somewhat eccentric (though not exceedingly so) and some of the energy may be dissipated when the turbulent jet contacts the wall of the left atrium (Coanda effect). Thus, this is at least moderate MR, is likely underestimated, and is probably significant.

All CD-based MR grading schemes assume that MR is chronic. In acute MR, the left atrium does not have enough time to dilate and remains noncompliant with a resultant increase in LA pressure and decrease in transmitral regurgitant pressure gradient in systole. Consequently, in cases of acute MR CD may significantly underestimate the severity of regurgitation. In this case, then, the MR would be significant whether it is chronic or acute.

Given the history of subacute presentation, history of HFrEF, and evidence of LA dilation, the patient most likely has chronic MR secondary to apical displacement of both PMs and leaflet tethering.

Selected Reference

1. Zoghbi WA, Adams D, Bonow RO, et al. Recommendations for noninvasive evaluation of native valvular regurgitation: a report from the American Society of Echocardiography developed in collaboration with the Society for Cardiovascular Magnetic Resonance. *J Am Soc Echocardiogr.* 2017 Apr;30(4):303-371. doi:10.1016/j.echo.2017.01.007. Epub 2017 Mar 14.

**23.** Correct Answer: **C. Urgent CT surgery consultation is indicated.**

*Rationale:* This patient has a vegetation on the posterior leaflet of her MV and severe MR. TEE confirmed the diagnosis (**Figure 25.54** and ▶ **Video 25.51**). Blood cultures eventually grew methicillin-sensitive *Staphylococcus aureus* (MSSA).

Acute heart failure in endocarditis is one of the accepted indications for valve surgery.

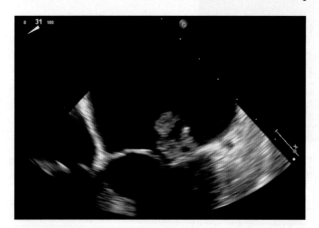

**Figure 25.54** Transesophageal echocardiogram showing a mobile hyperechoic mass on the atrial side of the posterior mitral leaflet.

Diagnosis of MV endocarditis may be difficult in the presence of preexisting valvular disease, such as sclerosis and calcification. A flail leaflet, particularly if a piece of a torn chorda is attached to it, may appear as a hyperechoic density on the leaflet and is certainly in the differential diagnosis. In this case, the density is rather large for the degree of the leaflet prolapse and the appearance in this clinical context must raise a concern for endocarditis. Nonetheless, the leaflet involved in this patient is the posterior one, not the anterior, as offered in choice A.

MR jet occupies the entire atrium and is severe. Acute MR will tend to make MR appear less significant on CD, and so this regurgitation is definitely severe, regardless of acuity, and is likely contributing to the patient's presentation. Aliasing is usually seen proximally in the jet, where blood velocity is at its highest. The red signal shown here is from the blood swirling around the atrium and coming back up toward the transducer.

Selected References

1. Evangelista A, Gonzalez-Alujas MT. Echocardiography in infective endocarditis. *Heart*. 2004 Jun;90(6):614-617. doi:10.1136/hrt.2003.029868.
2. Mügge A, Daniel WG, Frank G, Lichtlen PR. Echocardiography in infective endocarditis: reassessment of prognostic implications of vegetation size determined by the transthoracic and the transesophageal approach. *J Am Coll Cardiol*. 1989 Sep;14(3):631-638. doi:10.1016/0735-1097(89)90104-6.

**24.** Correct Answer: A. This patient has a perforation of an MV leaflet.

*Rationale:* This patient has MV endocarditis. The vegetation is on the atrial side of the posterior mitral leaflet but is not very well visualized (**Figure 25.55**).

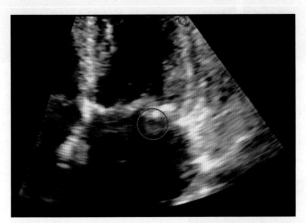

**Figure 25.55** Apical four-chamber view, zoomed-in on the mitral valve. Systole. Vegetation on the atrial side of the posterior leaflet of the mitral valve is marked.

There is a prolapse of the posterior (not anterior) leaflet as well. A flail MV leaflet, especially when torn chordae are present, may be difficult to differentiate from a vegetation.

The most conspicuous feature seen in this clip is the presence of two, not just one, MR jets. With intact MV leaflets, regurgitation, naturally, occurs along the leaflet coaptation line. In certain echocardiographic views (apical two-chamber view of transthoracic echocardiography [TTE]) the tomographic plane transects the coaptation line between the leaflets of the MV twice (see **Answer 8,** Figure 25.38), and a central MR (which results from the gap between the two leaflets in systole) may appear to have two jets. This is usually better appreciated on the equivalent TEE view (**Figure 25.56**). Because apical four-chamber view and PSAx plane (same as apical two-chamber view) transect the coaptation line only once, typical MR with intact MV leaflets should never appear as two separate jets in these views.

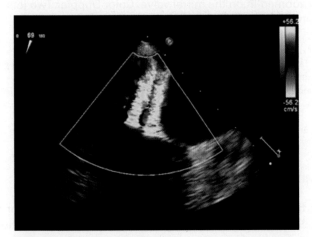

**Figure 25.56** Two-chamber transesophageal echocardiogram view of a single mitral regurgitation jet appearing as two jets.

MV clip effectively separates MV office into two orifices of smaller combined area and frequently results in multiple MR jets (the number of the jets will depend on the imaging plane and number of clips placed). (See **Figure 25.57** and ▶ **Video 25.52**.)

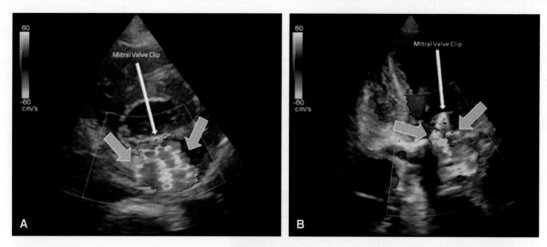

**Figure 25.57** A, Parasternal short-axis view. B, A4 view.

In this case the two jets are present in the A4 view, but there is no evidence of any prosthetic device. This should lead to the conclusion that there are indeed two separate MR jets present: one central and one closer to the posterior valve base. The second jet, remote from the coaptation line, is likely a result of leaflet perforation. (See **Figure 25.58**.)

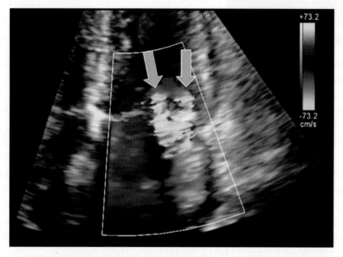

**Figure 25.58** Apical four-chamber view zoomed-in on the mitral valve. Color Doppler. Two jets are indicated with the arrows. The lateral one is secondary to leaflet perforation.

Selected References
1. Cziner DG, Rosenzweig BP, Katz ES, Keller AM, Daniel WG, Kronzon I. Transesophageal versus transthoracic echocardiography for diagnosing mitral valve perforation. *Am J Cardiol.* 1992 Jun 1;69(17):1495-1497. doi:10.1016/0002-9149(92)90911-h.
2. Mügge A, Daniel WG, Frank G, Lichtlen PR. Echocardiography in infective endocarditis: reassessment of prognostic implications of vegetation size determined by the transthoracic and the transesophageal approach. *J Am Coll Cardiol.* 1989 Sep;14(3):631-638. doi:10.1016/0735-1097(89)90104-6.
3. Sidebotham DA, Allen SJ, Gerber IL, Fayers T. Intraoperative transesophageal echocardiography for surgical repair of mitral regurgitation. *J Am Soc Echocardiogr.* 2014 Apr;27(4):345-366. doi:10.1016/j.echo.2014.01.005. Epub 2014 Feb 15.

**25.** Correct Answer: D. A prolapsed leaflet with a tip pointing toward the left atrium in systole

*Rationale:* All flail leaflets are prolapsed, but not all prolapsed leaflets are flail. Flail of a leaflet (or part of a leaflet) is indeed commonly as a result of a torn chord, although PM rupture and extreme chordal elongation without rupture can also be responsible. Unfortunately, chordae are thin structures that are not always seen on the ultrasound and presence of a torn one is not required for the diagnosis. Answer A is a definition of leaflet prolapse. Answer C is a definition of a tethered leaflet.

Selected Reference
1. Oh JK, Park S, Pisralu SV, Nkomo VT. Native valvular heart disease. In: Oh JK, Kane GC, Seward JB, Tajik AJ, Eds. *The Echo Manual.* 4th ed. Wolters Kluwer; 2019:Chapter 13. ISBN 9781496312198.

# 26 | TRICUSPID VALVULAR DISEASE

Babar Fiza, Natalie Ferrero, Amit Prabhakar, and Craig S. Jabaley

**1.** Which of the following *best* describes the three leaflets of the tricuspid valve?

  **A.** Coronary, noncoronary, right coronary
  **B.** Anterior, lateral, posterior
  **C.** Anterior, posterior, septal
  **D.** Anterior, noncoronary, septal

**2.** On an apical four-chamber view of a normal heart, which of the following anatomic features *best* distinguishes the tricuspid valve from the mitral valve?

  **A.** The tricuspid and mitral valves cannot be distinguished on an apical four-chamber view.
  **B.** The insertion of the mitral valve is located closer to the cardiac apex compared to the tricuspid valve.
  **C.** The septal leaflet insertion of the tricuspid valve is located closer to the base compared to the anterior mitral valve.
  **D.** The septal leaflet insertion of the tricuspid valve is located closer to the cardiac apex compared to the septal leaflet insertion of the mitral valve.

**3.** Which of the following echocardiographic features is *most* associated with moderate tricuspid regurgitation (TR)?

  **A.** Vena contracta (VC) width >0.7 cm
  **B.** Dilated right ventricle
  **C.** Systolic blunting of the hepatic vein flow
  **D.** Large central jet >50% of right atrium (RA)

**4.** A 66-year-old woman with a history of rheumatic heart disease presents to the preoperative clinic prior to inguinal hernia repair. Her most recent echocardiographic examination is notable for dilated inferior vena cava (IVC), enlarged RA, and pressure half-time (PHT) of 220 m/s across the tricuspid valve on Doppler interrogation. Based on this information, what is the calculated tricuspid valve area (TVA)?

  **A.** 0.86 cm$^2$
  **B.** 1 cm$^2$
  **C.** 1.15 cm$^2$
  **D.** 1.5 cm$^2$

5. A 76-year-old man presents to the preoperative area prior to scheduled cystoscopy. His most recent echocardiographic examination is notable for an enlarged RA, dilated IVC, mean pressure gradient of 6 mm Hg across the tricuspid valve, and PHT of 200 m/s. His vital signs are notable for a heart rate of 80 bpm and blood pressure of 130/80 mm Hg. These findings *best* describe which of the following?

   A. Nonhemodynamically significant tricuspid stenosis
   B. Hemodynamically significant tricuspid stenosis
   C. Mild physiologic tricuspid stenosis
   D. Normal tricuspid function

6. The *arrow* points to which of the following tricuspid valve leaflets in **Figure 26.1**?

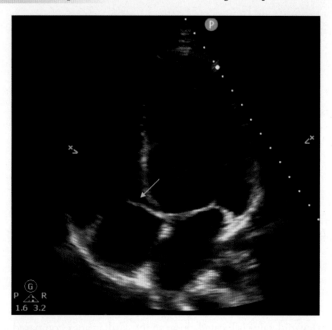

**Figure 26.1**

   A. Anterior
   B. Septal
   C. Posterior
   D. Either septal or posterior

7. A 46-year-old man with a history of intravenous drug use presents to the intensive care unit (ICU) with respiratory failure and circulatory shock. A right internal jugular central venous line is placed, and an echocardiogram is performed by the intensive care team. A parasternal long-axis right ventricular (RV) inflow view of the heart is shown in ▶ **Video 26.1** and a Doppler velocity of TR jet in **Figure 26.2**. Vital signs are as noted in **Table 26.1**.

**Table 26.1 Vital Signs**

| |
| --- |
| Blood pressure 96/40 |
| Heart rate 94 |
| Central venous pressure 10 mm Hg |
| Temperature 38.7 °C |

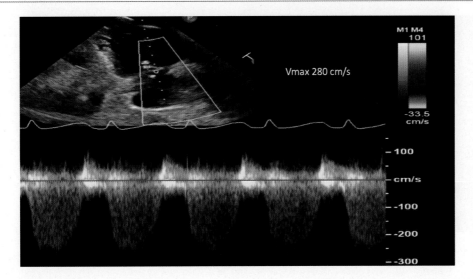

**Figure 26.2**

Based on the hemodynamic data and echocardiographic evaluation, what is the estimated RV systolic pressure (RVSP) in this patient?

A. 41 mm Hg
B. 76 mm Hg
C. 56 mm Hg
D. 96 mm Hg

8. A 60-year-old woman with septic shock due to bacterial pneumonia presents to the ICU. Patient is hypotensive and hypoxemic on arrival to the ICU. A transthoracic echocardiographic (TTE) examination is performed by the intensive care team. Based on the echocardiographic images ( ▶ **Videos 26.2, 26.3, 26.4, 26.5, 26.6, 26.7, Figures 26.3** and **26.4**), what is the estimated RVSP in this patient?

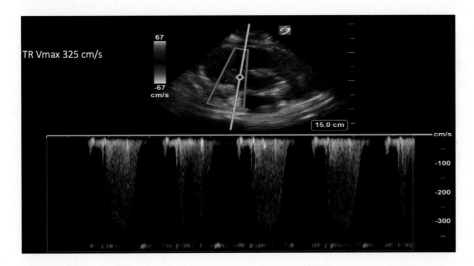

**Figure 26.3**

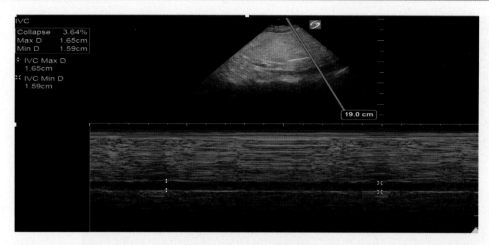

**Figure 26.4**

A. 57 mm Hg
B. 45 mm Hg
C. 50 mm Hg
D. 52 mm Hg

9. A 56-year-old woman with a history of carcinoid syndrome presents to the ICU after an abdominal tumor resection. TTE examination is notable for severe TR and tricuspid regurgitant jet maximum velocity (TR $V_{max}$) of 4 m/s. IVC is >2.1 cm with minimal respiratory variation. Pulmonary stenosis is also noted, and the mean pressure gradient across the pulmonic valve is 15 mm Hg. Based on these findings, what is the pulmonary artery systolic pressure (PASP) in this patient?

A. 79 mm Hg
B. 94 mm Hg
C. 71 mm Hg
D. 64 mm Hg

10. A 31-year-old man presents with complaints of malaise, fevers, and dyspnea. Past medical history is remarkable for a history of intravenous drug abuse. Based on the echocardiographic evaluation (▶ **Videos 26.8, 26.9, 26.10, 26.11**), which of the following is the *most* likely cause of his symptoms?

A. Endocarditis
B. Cardiac fibroma
C. Lambl's excrescence
D. Mesothelioma

11. You are reviewing echocardiogram studies from overnight. You notice that the resident calculated the RVSP based on the TR jet $V_{max}$ at the point identified by the *arrow* in **Figure 26.5**.

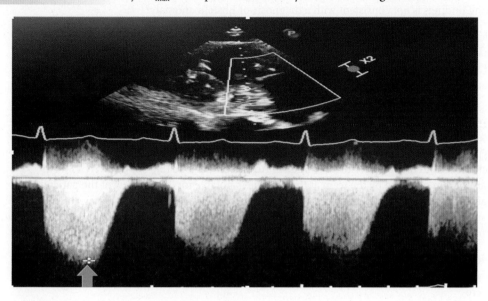

**Figure 26.5**

You conclude that the RVSP calculation in this case is *most* likely:

A. Correct
B. Underestimated
C. Overestimated
D. Not valid as average of acquired jet velocities is needed

12. You notice an abnormal finding while reviewing the RV inflow view (**Figure 26.6** and ▶ **Video 26.12**) from an echocardiogram performed on a patient with septic shock.

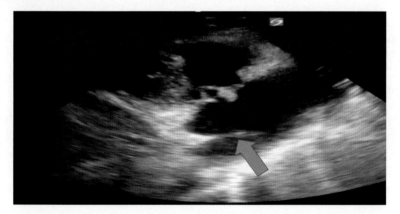

**Figure 26.6**

The structure identified by the *arrow* in Figure 26.6 and **Video 26.12** is *most* likely:

A. Mobile thrombus
B. Eustachian valve (EV)
C. Pores of Kohn
D. Crista terminalis

13. A 34-year-old woman presents with symptoms of fatigue, dyspnea, and palpitations. An echocardiogram is performed, and the patient is diagnosed with Ebstein anomaly. Which of the following findings is *not* consistent with a diagnosis of Ebstein anomaly?

    A. Tricuspid regurgitation
    B. Small RA
    C. RV hypoplasia
    D. An atrialization of the inlet component of the right ventricle

14. A 68-year-old woman with a medical history significant for cervical cancer, deep venous thrombosis, hypertension, and hyperlipidemia presents with a complaint of acute dyspnea. She is hypotensive and hypoxemic on arrival to the Emergency Department and sustains cardiac arrest with return of spontaneous circulation after three rounds of Advanced Cardiac Life Support (ACLS). An echocardiogram obtained by the team at the bedside is notable for TR. Review of the patient's echocardiogram performed 2 months prior did not show any valvular abnormalities. Based on the echocardiographic findings (▶ **Videos 26.13, 26.14, 26.15, 26.16, 26.17**), which of the following *best* describes the severity grade of her TR?

    A. Mild
    B. Moderate
    C. Severe
    D. Unable to determine

15. Which of the following is the *most* likely explanation of the hemodynamic collapse in the patient in **Question 26.14**?

    A. Acute pulmonary embolism (PE)
    B. Acute valvular regurgitation due to infective endocarditis
    C. Left ventricular failure
    D. Pneumonia

# Chapter 26 ▪ Answers

1. Correct Answer: **C. Anterior, posterior, septal**

   *Rationale:* The tricuspid valve consists of three leaflets: anterior, posterior, and septal. The anterior leaflet is the largest leaflet, the posterior leaflet is the smallest, and the septal leaflet is the most medially located and the most immobile.

   Selected Reference
   1. Huttin O, Voilliot D, Mandry D, Venner C, Juillière Y, Selton-Suty C. All you need to know about the tricuspid valve: tricuspid valve imaging and tricuspid regurgitation analysis. *Arc Cardiovasc Dis.* 2016;109:67-80.

2. Correct Answer: **D. The septal leaflet insertion of the tricuspid valve is located closer to the cardiac apex compared to the septal leaflet insertion of the mitral valve.**

   *Rationale:* The septal leaflet of the tricuspid valve is characteristically inserted more apically than the septal insertion of the anterior mitral valve leaflet. This allows for the differentiation of the tricuspid valve from the mitral valve on an apical four-chamber view during two-dimensional TTE.

   Selected Reference
   1. Shah PM, Raney AA. Tricuspid valve disease. *Curr Probl Cardiol.* 2008;33(2):47-84.

**3.** Correct Answer: C. Systolic blunting of the hepatic vein flow

*Rationale/Critique:* Systolic blunting of the hepatic vein is seen in moderate TR.
The following criteria are recommended by the American Society of Echocardiography for grading severe TR:
- Dilated annulus with no valve coaptation or flail leaflet
- Large TR central jet >50% of RA
- Vena contracta (VC) width >0.7 cm
- Proximal isovelocity surface area (PISA) radius >0.9 cm
- Systolic reversal of hepatic vein flow
- Dilated right ventricle with preserved function

Selected Reference
1. Zoghbi WA, Adams D, Bonow RO, et al. Recommendations for noninvasive evaluation of native valvular regurgitation. *J Am Soc Echocardiogr.* 2017;30:303-371.

**4.** Correct Answer: A. 0.86 cm$^2$

*Rationale:* In patients with tricuspid valve stenosis, TVA can be calculated by the PHT method. The TVA is derived using an empirical formula: TVA = 190/PHT. In **Question 26.4**,
- TVA = 190/220 = 0.86 cm$^2$
- PHT is the time required for the pressure gradient across an obstruction to decrease to half of its maximal value.

Thus, the worse the obstruction (e.g., smaller transvalvular orifice), the more time required for the maximal gradient value to decrease. PHT is obtained by tracing the deceleration slope of the E-wave on the Doppler spectral display of the transvalvular flow.

Selected Reference
1. Baumgartner H, Hung J, Bermejo J, et al. Echocardiographic assessment of valve stenosis: EAE/ASE recommendations for clinical practice. *J Am Soc Echocardiogr.* 2009;22:1-23.

**5.** Correct Answer: B. Hemodynamically significant tricuspid stenosis

*Rationale:* Echocardiographic findings that indicate hemodynamically significant tricuspid stenosis include:
- Mean pressure gradient ≥5 mm Hg
- Inflow time-velocity integral >60 cm
- PHT ≥190 ms
- Valve area by continuity equation ≤1 cm$^2$
- Additional supportive findings include enlarged RA and dilated IVC
- Mild TR in the setting of structurally normal tricuspid valve is seen in healthy subjects.

Selected Reference
1. Baumgartner H, Hung J, Bermejo J, et al. Echocardiographic assessment of valve stenosis: EAE/ASE recommendations for clinical practice. *J Am Soc Echocardiogr.* 2009;22:1-23.

**6.** Correct Answer: B. Septal

*Rationale:* Due to the complex anatomy of the tricuspid valve and its retrosternal location, all three leaflets of the valve cannot be visualized simultaneously on 2D TTE. In 2D TTE, the tricuspid valve leaflets can be visualized from the parasternal long (RV inflow), parasternal short at the aortic valve level, apical four-chamber, and the subcostal views. On apical four-chamber view, the anterior and septal leaflets are visible, with the septal leaflet adjacent to the interventricular septum and the anterior leaflet adjacent to the RV free wall (**Figure 26.7**).

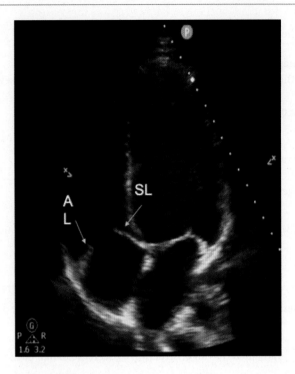

**Figure 26.7**

In contrast to the apical four-chamber view, on parasternal RV inflow and the parasternal short-axis views, visualized tricuspid valve leaflets can vary depending on the imaging plane of the acquired view. On parasternal long-axis RV inflow view, the displayed leaflets include the anterior leaflet and either the septal or the posterior leaflet. On parasternal short axis (PSSX), the displayed leaflets include the posterior leaflet and either the septal or the anterior leaflet.

Selected Reference

1. Huttin O, Voilliot D, Mandry D, Venner C, Juillière Y, Selton-Suty C. All you need to know about the tricuspid valve: tricuspid valve imaging and tricuspid regurgitation analysis. *Arc Cardiovasc Dis.* 2016;109:67-80.

---

**7.** Correct Answer: A. 41 mm Hg

*Rationale:* The RVSP is estimated by measuring the TR $V_{max}$ using continuous-wave spectral Doppler. In the absence of RV outflow tract (RVOT) obstruction or pulmonic stenosis, RVSP is equal to the PASP. From the tricuspid regurgitant jet velocity, RVSP is estimated using the modified Bernoulli equation. RVSP = 4 ($V_{max}$ m/s)$^2$ + RA pressure. Central venous pressure is often used as a surrogate of the right atrial pressure (RAP).

- In this patient, the RVSP = 4 (2.80)$^2$ + 10 = 41.36 mm Hg. Note that for the RVSP calculation, the TR $V_{max}$ is defined in m/s.

Selected Reference

1. Rudski LG, Lai WW, Afilalo J, et al. Guidelines for the echocardiographic assessment of the right heart in adults: a report from the American Society of Echocardiography. *J Am Soc Echocardiogr.* 2010;23(7):685-713.

---

**8.** Correct Answer: C. 50 mm Hg

*Rationale:* From the tricuspid regurgitant jet velocity, RVSP is estimated using the modified Bernoulli equation. RVSP = 4 ($V_{max}$ m/s)$^2$ + RAP. In the absence of a central venous line, RAP can be estimated by assessing the IVC size and respiratory variation. According to the American Society of Echocardiography (ASE) guidelines:

- IVC diameter <2.1 cm and collapse >50% correspond to a normal RAP of 0 to 5 mm Hg.
- An IVC diameter <2.1 cm with <50% collapse or IVC diameter >2.1 cm with >50% collapse corresponds to an intermediate RAP of 5 to 10 mm Hg.
- IVC diameter >2.1 cm with <50% collapse suggests a high RAP of 10 to 20 mm Hg.

In order to standardize reporting of RAP values, guidelines recommend using midrange values of 3 mm Hg for normal, 8 mm Hg for intermediate, and 15 mm Hg for high RAP based on IVC assessment. In this patient, the maximum TR jet velocity is obtained from the parasternal short-axis view at the level of the aortic valve. There is no RVOT obstruction. Based on the maximal IVC diameter and respiratory variation pattern, the RAP is in the intermediate range.

$$RVSP = 4 (3.25 \text{ m/s})^2 + 8 \text{ mm Hg} = 50 \text{ mm Hg}$$

Selected Reference

1. Rudski LG, Lai WW, Afilalo J, et al. Guidelines for the echocardiographic assessment of the right heart in adults: a report from the American Society of Echocardiography endorsed by the European Association of Echocardiography, a registered branch of the European Society of Cardiology, and the Canadian Society of Echocardiography. *J Am Soc Echocardiogr*. 2010;23(7):685-713. quiz 786-688.

**9.** Correct Answer: **D. 64 mm Hg**

*Rationale:* In the presence of RV outflow obstruction, such as pulmonic stenosis, RVSP will not reflect the systolic pulmonary arterial pressure. In the presence of pulmonary valve stenosis, RVSP will be greater than PASP.

- $RVSP = PASP + \Delta P_{RV\text{-}PA}$
- $RVSP = 4 (TR\ V_{max})^2 + RAP = 4 (4)^2 + 15 = 79 \text{ mm Hg}$
- $PASP = RVSP - mPG_{PV}$ (mean pressure gradient across pulmonary valve)
- $PSAP = 79 - 15 = 64 \text{ mm Hg}$

Selected Reference

1. Skinner GJ. Echocardiographic assessment of pulmonary arterial hypertension for pediatricians and neonatologists. *Front Pediatr*. 2017;5:168. doi:10.3389/fped.2017.00168.

**10.** Correct Answer: **A. Endocarditis**

*Rationale:* Based on the patient's medical history and the presence of a mobile, echo-dense mass attached to the tricuspid valve, the most likely etiology for this patient's symptoms is infective endocarditis.

Cardiac fibromas are distinct, well-demarcated, noncontractile, and solid, highly echogenic masses that are located within the myocardium. Lambl's excrescences are filiform fronds that occur at the sites of valvular closure and present primarily at the aortic valve. Echocardiographic features of pericardial mesothelioma include pericardial effusion and a tumor encasing the heart.

Selected References

1. Evangelista A, Gonzalez-Alujas MT. Echocardiography in infective endocarditis. *Heart*. 2004;90(6):614-617.
2. Mankad R, Herrmann J. Cardiac tumors: echo assessment. *Echo Res Pract*. 2016;3(4):R65-R77.

**11.** Correct Answer: **C. Overestimated**

*Rationale/Critique:* The cursor appears to be measuring too much into what appears to be Doppler noise that not seen on subsequent beats, likely resulting in an overestimation of the peak tricuspid regurgitant velocity. Also, the first beat in a series should not be measured because the beat preceding may have been a PVC or some other aberrant beat which would make the the value of the first beat erroneous. For correct estimation of the RVSP, the peak tricuspid regurgitant velocity is obtained from the highest velocity acquired from all examined views.

Selected Reference

1. Rudski LG, Lai WW, Afilalo J, et al. Guidelines for the echocardiographic assessment of the right heart in adults: a report from the American Society of Echocardiography. *J Am Soc Echocardiogr*. 2010;23(7):685-713.

**12.** Correct Answer: **B. Eustachian valve (EV)**

*Rationale:* EV is a remnant of the right valve of sinus venosus. It appears as a crescent-like fold of variable size at the posterior margin of the IVC. EV can be visible on the RV inflow tract view, apical four-chamber view, or the parasternal short-axis view at the level of the aortic valve. On echocardiographic examination, EV can be seen as a linear structure at the junction of the IVC and the RA.

Although a mass is also seen adhering to the tricuspid valve, the *arrow* in Figure 26.6 and ▶ **Video 26.12** points to the prominent EV present in this patient. Crista terminalis is a vertical ridge of smooth myocardium within the RA. Echo findings suggestive of crista terminalis include a homogenous nodular mass with adjacent myocardium, located at the posterolateral wall of RA near the superior vena cava (SVC), and the phasic change in size of the structure becoming larger during atrial systole. Pores of Kohn are interalveolar connections between adjacent pulmonary alveoli.

### Selected Reference

1. Kim MJ, Jung HO. Anatomic variants mimicking pathology on echocardiography: differential diagnosis. *J Cardiovasc Ultrasound.* 2013;21(3):103-112. doi:10.4250/jcu.2013.21.3.103.

---

**13.** Correct Answer: B. Small RA

*Rationale:* Ebstein anomaly is a congenital disorder resulting from an abnormality in the tricuspid valve. Multiple anatomic abnormalities are associated with the disorder, which include (1) abnormal downward displacement of the tricuspid valve within the right ventricle, (2) varying degrees of TR, (3) RV hypoplasia, and (4) "atrialization" of the inlet component of the right ventricle.

Cardiac rhythm disturbances are frequently observed in this patient population, including Wolff-Parkinson-White syndrome. A common clinical presentation therefore involves new-onset atrial arrhythmias or reentrant tachyarrhythmias.

### Selected Reference

1. Shiina A, Seward JB, Edwards WD, Hagler DJ, Tajik AJ. Two-dimensional echocardiographic spectrum of Ebstein's anomaly: detailed anatomic assessment. *J Am Coll Cardiol.* 1984;3(2 Pt 1):356-370.

---

**14.** Correct Answer: C. Severe

*Rationale:* The TR in this patient is graded as severe given the presence of a large central jet that occupies >50% area of the RA. The presence of a large central jet is confirmed on RV inflow view (▶ **Video 26.14**) and the apical four-chamber view (▶ **Video 26.17**).

### Selected Reference

1. Zoghbi WA, Adams D, Bonow RO, et al. Recommendations for noninvasive evaluation of native valvular regurgitation. *J Am Soc Echocardiogr.* 2017;30:303-371.

---

**15.** Correct Answer: A. Acute pulmonary embolism (PE)

*Rationale:* Acute PE is the likely cause of TR and circulatory collapse in this patient. McConnell sign can be seen on the apical four-chamber view (▶ **Videos 26.16** and **26.17**). It is characterized by akinesia of the mid-ventricular free wall and hypercontractility of the apex. McConnell sign can be seen anytime there is an acute RV failure due to various etiologies such as hemodynamically significant PE or an acute RV infarction. Clinically, the presence of hypoxia, history of malignancy, history of deep vein thrombosis, and the acute severe TR point to acute PE as the cause of hemodynamic collapse and the development of McConnell sign in this patient.

- There is absence of any vegetations making infective endocarditis unlikely. The left ventricle is hyperdynamic and no left ventricular regional wall motion abnormalities are present. Pneumonia is also unlikely given the absence of any supporting data.

### Selected Reference

1. Torbicki A. Echocardiographic diagnosis of pulmonary embolism: a rise and fall of McConnell sign?. *Eur J Echocardiogr.* 2005 Jan;6(1):2-3.

# 27 | PULMONARY VALVE DISEASES

Rachel C. Frank and Dusan Hanidziar

1. A 38-year-old man with a history of intravenous drug use is admitted to the intensive care unit (ICU) with septic shock. Computed tomography (CT) chest reveals multiple bilateral pulmonary emboli. The best windows to image the pulmonic valve with transthoracic echocardiography (TTE) include:

   A. Parasternal long-axis view tilted toward right ventricular (RV) outflow tract (RVOT)
   B. Parasternal short-axis view optimized for RVOT and pulmonary artery bifurcation
   C. Subcostal view with anterior angulation
   D. All of the above

2. You and your team are evaluating several ICU patients with TTE. You are estimating RV systolic pressure (RVSP) to assess the pulmonary artery systolic pressure. In which of the following conditions is the pulmonary artery systolic pressure not accurately estimated by calculating the RVSP?

   A. Dilated right ventricle
   B. Pulmonic stenosis
   C. Prior pulmonic valvuloplasty
   D. Prior history of pulmonary embolism

3. A 55-year-old female patient with a history of severe pulmonary hypertension is admitted to the ICU with septic shock. You are performing an echocardiogram on admission.

   Which of the following standard TTE views can best assess for pulmonic insufficiency?
   A. Parasternal long-axis RV outflow view and parasternal pulmonary artery bifurcation view
   B. Parasternal pulmonary artery bifurcation view and suprasternal long axis of aortic arch view
   C. Parasternal short-axis aortic valve/RVOT level view and apical five-chamber view
   D. Subcostal aortic valve and RVOT view and right parasternal ascending aorta view

4. Which of the following echocardiographic findings is suggestive of severe pulmonic regurgitation in the patient from **Question 3**?

   A. Dense regurgitant jet
   B. Early termination of diastolic regurgitant flow
   C. RV enlargement
   D. All of the above

5. A 35-year-old woman is intubated in the ICU following a motor vehicle accident. Her central venous pressure (CVP) is 17 cm $H_2O$. A systolic ejection murmur is heard over the left upper sternal border. A TTE is performed, and the right ventricle is noted to be hypertrophied. Accelerated velocities are noted across the pulmonic valve. Which of the following features is consistent with severe pulmonic stenosis?

    A. Peak velocity >4 m/s
    B. Peak gradient >64 mm Hg
    C. Acceleration of color Doppler below the pulmonic valve
    D. Both A and B

6. A 36-year-old female with a history of factor V Leiden deficiency and tobacco use disorder presents with hypoxemic respiratory failure. In the ICU, you are concerned about pulmonary embolism as a possible etiology of her respiratory failure. A CT pulmonary angiogram has been performed and the read is pending. Which of the following echocardiographic findings are utilized to risk-stratify the pulmonary embolism?

    A. RV hypertrophy
    B. Intraventricular septal bowing into the right ventricle
    C. McConnell sign (RV dysfunction sparing the apex)
    D. Decreased RVSP

7. Which among the following echocardiographic findings would be a contraindication to Impella RP placement?

    A. Pulmonary valve peak gradient 68 mm Hg
    B. Systolic flow reversal by color and pulse wave Doppler in the hepatic vein
    C. Pulmonary regurgitant jet equal to the width of the right ventricular outflow tract
    D. All of the above

8. A 65-year-old man is admitted to the ICU with septic shock. Prior to presentation, he reported 1 week of fevers, chills, and malaise following a wisdom tooth extraction. CT scan is obtained and is notable for septic emboli in the lungs. TTE is performed on the day of ICU admission. The tricuspid valve is not noted to have any vegetations; however, the pulmonic valve is not well visualized. On hospital day 4, he develops worsening hemodynamics with signs of RV failure. An early diastolic decrescendo murmur is best heard at the left upper sternal border, and jugular venous distention is noted as is a pulsatile liver. The lungs are clear to auscultation.

Which of the following valvular lesions and echocardiographic findings do you most likely expect to detect on repeat TTE?
A. Severe pulmonic stenosis with peak velocity >2 m/s and peak gradient >32 mm Hg
B. Severe tricuspid regurgitation with no appreciable tricuspid regurgitant flow on continuous-wave and color Doppler
C. Aortic valve mean gradient >40 mm Hg, and valve area <1 cm$^2$ consistent with severe aortic stenosis
D. Flail pulmonic valve leaflet with early diastolic termination of regurgitant jet on continuous-wave and color Doppler

9. A 19-year-old male with unknown medical history is brought into the ICU intubated after he was found unresponsive. His initial vitals are notable for hypotension, tachycardia, and fever. When you first examine him, you notice a systolic crescendo decrescendo late peaking murmur best heard at the left upper sternal border. Laboratory data are pending, cultures are obtained, and the patient is empirically treated for septic shock.

A TTE is performed. There are increased velocities when continuous-wave Doppler is applied in the parasternal short-axis view at the pulmonary artery bifurcation level (i.e., spanning from the RVOT to the pulmonary artery). What is the most likely etiology and valvular abnormality?
A. Pulmonic stenosis from congenital heart disease
B. Pulmonic regurgitation from congenital heart disease
C. Aortic stenosis
D. Tricuspid stenosis

10. A 23-year-old woman with a history of pulmonic valve stenosis status post transcatheter valve replacement is admitted to the ICU with shock. A loud systolic murmur is heard at the left upper sternal border. A TTE is performed. Due to poor acoustic windows, two-dimensional (2D) image quality is poor, but on continuous-wave Doppler there is increased velocity noted across the pulmonic valve.

This is most concerning for:
**A.** Pulmonary hypertension
**B.** Infective endocarditis resulting in stenosis
**C.** Acute pulmonic regurgitation
**D.** Acute pulmonary embolism

# Chapter 27 ▪ Answers

## 1. Correct Answer: D. All of the above

*Rationale:* The pulmonic valve may be seen in the parasternal long axis with the transducer tilted toward the RVOT and in the parasternal short axis angled toward the RVOT. The pulmonic valve may also be seen in the subcostal view with an anterior orientation. Depending on the patient's windows, the pulmonic valve can be challenging to view on 2D echocardiography. Spectral and color Doppler are tools that improve valve assessment.

### Selected References
1. Mitchell C, Rahko PS, Blauwet LA, et al. Guidelines for performing a comprehensive transthoracic echocardiographic examination in adults: recommendations from the American Society of Echocardiography. *J Am Soc Echocardiogr.* 2019;32(1):1-64.
2. Quader N, Makan M, Perez J. *The Washington Manual of Echocardiography.* 2nd ed. Wolters Kluwer; 2017.

## 2. Correct Answer: B. Pulmonic stenosis

*Rationale:* The RVSP is used as a surrogate measurement for the pulmonary artery systolic pressure in echocardiography. The RVSP is estimated using the Bernoulli equation: RVSP $= 4(V)^2+$ right atrial (RA) pressure, where $V$ is the peak velocity (m/s) of the tricuspid valve regurgitant jet and RA pressure is in mm Hg. There is institutional variation in estimating the RA pressure. Some institutions may estimate the RA pressure using changes in inferior vena cava (IVC) diameter with respiratory variation. In the setting of normal RA pressure, the IVC should collapse by >50% with inspiration (decreased intrathoracic pressure). However, other institutions use a fixed value for the RA pressure (such as at Massachusetts General Hospital where the value of 10 mm Hg is used). The Bernoulli equation and RVSP are not accurate estimates of pulmonary artery systolic pressure when there is obstruction along the RVOT such as pulmonic stenosis or a double-chamber right ventricle.

### Selected Reference
1. Rudski LG, Lai WW, Afilalo J, et al. Guidelines for the echocardiographic assessment of the right heart in adults: a report from the American Society of Echocardiography endorsed by the European Association of Echocardiography, a registered branch of the European Society of Cardiology, and the Canadian Society of Echocardiography. *J Am Soc Echocardiogr.* 2010;23(7):685-788.

## 3. Correct Answer: A. Parasternal long-axis RV outflow view and parasternal pulmonary artery bifurcation view

*Rationale:* Pulmonary insufficiency can be evaluated in the parasternal long-axis RV outflow view, parasternal pulmonary artery bifurcation view, parasternal short-axis aortic valve/RVOT level view, and subcostal aortic valve, and RVOT view. The apical, right parasternal, and suprasternal views do not show the RVOT or pulmonic valve. Both color Doppler and continuous-wave Doppler aid in the evaluation of pulmonary regurgitation.

### Selected References
1. Mitchell C, Rahko PS, Blauwet LA, et al. Guidelines for performing a comprehensive transthoracic echocardiographic examination in adults: recommendations from the American Society of Echocardiography. *J Am Soc Echocardiogr.* 2019;32(1):1-64.
2. Quader N, Makan M, Perez J. *The Washington Manual of Echocardiography.* 2nd ed. Wolters Kluwer; 2017.

**4.** Correct Answer: D. All of the above

*Rationale:* A dense regurgitant jet on continuous-wave Doppler is one echocardiographic sign of severe pulmonary regurgitation. In general, increased density of a wave on continuous-wave or color Doppler signifies a higher severity of regurgitation. Early termination of diastolic regurgitant flow is a sign of severe pulmonic insufficiency because it results in early diastolic equalization of pressure between the pulmonary artery and the right ventricle. With chronic volume overload, the RV cavity may dilate, resulting in an enlarged and often hypertrophied RV cavity; however, this may be absent in acute pulmonic regurgitation.

Selected Reference
1. Asher CR, Griffin BP. *Manual of Valvular Heart Disease.* Wolters Kluwer; 2018.

**5.** Correct Answer: D. Both A and B

*Rationale:* Patients with pulmonic stenosis have a range of clinic presentations from asymptomatic to RV failure. Continuous-wave Doppler and color Doppler are crucial in evaluating pulmonary valvular disease. Severe pulmonic stenosis is defined by peak velocity >4 m/s across the pulmonic valve and peak gradient >64 mm Hg measured by continuous-wave Doppler. Acceleration of the color Doppler below the pulmonic valve suggests subvalvular stenosis such as RVOT obstruction or double-chamber right ventricle. Other echocardiographic features associated with pulmonic stenosis include poststenotic dilation of the pulmonary artery (although this is nonspecific). The right ventricle may hypertrophy as a response to chronic pressure overload. Pulmonic stenosis is often associated with other congenital heart disease. Care should be taken to evaluate for other forms of structural heart disease in patients with pulmonic stenosis.

Selected References
1. Asher CR, Griffin BP. *Manual of Valvular Heart Disease.* Wolters Kluwer; 2018.
2. Nishimura RA, Otto CM, Bonow RO, et al. 2014 AHA/ACC guideline for the management of patients with valvular heart disease: a report of the American College of Cardiology/American Heart Association Task Force on Practice Guidelines. *J Am Coll Cardiol.* 2014;63(22):e57-e185.

**6.** Correct Answer: C. McConnell sign (RV dysfunction sparing the apex)

*Rationale:* **See Figure 27.1.** TTE may be used to look for right heart strain in the setting of pulmonary embolism and may even visualize proximal, saddle emboli in the main pulmonary artery at the pulmonary artery bifurcation view. Evidence of RV strain on echocardiogram in addition to McConnell sign includes RV fractional area of change <35%, a tricuspid annular plane systolic excursion (TAPSE) <1.6 cm, S' of <10 cm/s (obtained via tissue Doppler of the RV free wall at the tricuspid annulus) or interventricular septal bowing into the left ventricle (due to right ventricular overload). Because pulmonary embolism causes acute increases in RV afterload, the right ventricle does not have time to adapt and hypertrophy would suggest a more chronic process. The pulmonic valve may be noted to close in midsystole due to the increase in pulmonary arterial systolic pressure. As a result, there may not be a large increase in the estimated RVSP (estimated using the Bernoulli equation and the tricuspid regurgitant jet).

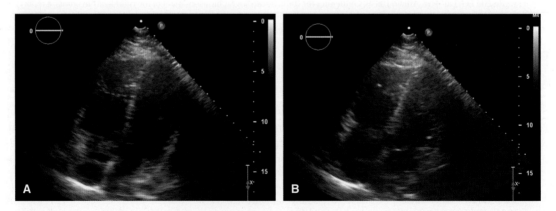

**Figure 27.1** A. Right ventricular (RV) focused view during late diastole. B. RV focused view during systole. McConnell's sign is defined as RV free wall hypokinesis with sparing of the RV apex.

Selected References

1. Dutta T, Frishman WH, Aronow WS. Echocardiography in the evaluation of pulmonary embolism. *Cardiol Rev.* 2017;25(6):309-314.
2. Quader N, Makan M, Perez J. *The Washington Manual of Echocardiography.* 2nd ed. Wolters Kluwer; 2017.

**7.** Correct Answer: D. All of the above

*Rationale:* An Impella RP is a percutaneously placed Impella device that is used for RV support. The Impella RP works by utilizing axial flow to bypass the right ventricle and deliver blood from the IVC inlet (into the right atrium) to the pulmonary artery. As a result, the device sits across the tricuspid valve and the pulmonic valve. Severe valvular disease including severe pulmonic stenosis or regurgitation, as well as severe tricuspid regurgitation or stenosis is a contraindication to Impella RP placement. The aforementioned echocardiographic parameters are all suggestive of severe valvular disease and therefore would preclude Impella RP placement. Systolic flow reversal in the hepatic vein is consistent with severe tricuspid regurgitation. Peak gradient across the pulmonic valve >65 mm Hg is consistent with severe pulmonic stenosis. A pulmonic regurgitation jet that fills the right ventricular outflow tract is consistent with severe pulmonic regurgitation. In addition, left ventricular dysfunction can be worsened when univentricular RV support is initiated prior to recognizing the degree of left ventricular dysfunction.

Selected References

1. ABIOMED product manual for Impella RP heart pump, software v6.2. 2012. https://www.accessdata.fda.gov/cdrh_docs/pdf14/H140001D.pdf.
2. Khalid N, Rogers T, Shlofmitz E, et al. Adverse events and modes of failure related to Impella RP: insights from the Manufacturer and User Facility Device Experience (MAUDE) database. *Cardiovasc Revasc Med.* 2019;20(6):503-506. doi:10.1016/j.carrev.2019.03.010.
3. Quader N, Makan M, Perez J. *The Washington Manual of Echocardiography.* 2nd ed. Wolters Kluwer; 2017.

**8.** Correct Answer: D. Flail pulmonic valve leaflet with early diastolic termination of regurgitant jet on continuous-wave and color Doppler

*Rationale:* While rare, isolated pulmonic valve endocarditis can occur. Symptoms include those associated with right-sided endocarditis including septic pulmonary emboli and infarctions, persistent bacteremia, and signs/symptoms of right-sided heart failure. The sequela of missed pulmonic valve endocarditis includes chronic bacteremia and seeding of metastatic sites of infection as well as flail pulmonic valve leaflets. Limitations of TTE in viewing the pulmonic valve include ability to visualize only one to two leaflets. If TTE windows are limited, it is reasonable to pursue a transesophageal echocardiogram or other cardiac imaging such as magnetic resonance imaging (MRI) to evaluate the valve. Of note, transesophageal imaging also has limited windows in which to image the pulmonic valve and the transesophageal probe is farther away from right-sided valves, making this a suboptimal imaging modality. Severe pulmonic stenosis is defined by peak velocity >4 m/s and peak gradient >64 mm Hg; therefore, answer A is incorrect. It would be highly unusual to have severe tricuspid regurgitation without evidence of a tricuspid regurgitant jet on continuous-wave or color Doppler. An early diastolic decrescendo murmur is not consistent with aortic stenosis, which would have a systolic ejection murmur best heard at the right upper sternal border. A mean gradient >40 mm Hg and valve area <1 cm$^2$ are consistent with severe aortic stenosis.

Selected References

1. Bhatia A. Transesophageal echocardiography evaluation of tricuspid and pulmonic valves. *Ann Card Anaesth.* 2016;19(suppl):S21-S25. doi:10.4103/0971-9784.192616.
2. Dhakam S, Jafary F. Pulmonary valve endocarditis. *Heart.* 2003;89:480.
3. Lancellotti P, Tribouilloy C, Hagendorff A, et al. European Association of Echocardiography recommendations for the assessment of valvular regurgitation. Part 1: aortic and pulmonary regurgitation (native valve disease). *Eur J Echocardiogr.* 2010;11(3):223-244.

**9.** Correct Answer: A. Pulmonic stenosis from congenital heart disease

*Rationale:* A normal pulmonic valve is a trileaflet structure consisting of three cusps. The etiology of pulmonic stenosis is most likely to be congenital. It may occur in isolation or in conjunction with other congenital heart disease including tetralogy of Fallot, transposition of the great vessels, Noonan syndrome, or Williams syndrome. Valve morphology may be abnormal with bicuspid or unicuspid valves. Other etiologies include rheumatic heart disease, carcinoid, or more rarely endocarditis. On echocardiography, thickening of the pulmonic valve and doming of the valve leaflets may be seen. Continuous-wave Doppler will show an elevated gradient across the valve. Patients who have not had consistent access to healthcare may present as adults with congenital abnormalities.

### Selected References

1. Asher CR, Griffin BP. *Manual of Valvular Heart Disease*. Wolters Kluwer; 2018.
2. Quader N, Makan M, Perez J. *The Washington Manual of Echocardiography*. 2nd ed. Wolters Kluwer; 2017.

**10.** Correct Answer: B. Infective endocarditis resulting in stenosis

*Rationale:* Transcatheter pulmonic valve replacements have been used for patients with congenital RVOT abnormalities. Unfortunately, endocarditis is a very dangerous complication. In patients who have undergone transcatheter pulmonic valve replacement, some patients present with RVOT obstruction secondary to vegetation and leading to shock. This subset of patients with fulminant presentations is not fully understood, but high suspicion and early recognition are key to ensuring there is minimal delay in diagnosis. Acute pulmonic regurgitation would demonstrate a dense regurgitant jet on continuous-wave Doppler with early termination of the diastolic regurgitant jet. Echocardiographic signs of acute pulmonary embolism include acute RV strain or failure, but there should not be increased velocities across the RVOT/pulmonic valve. Pulmonary hypertension may result in pulmonary artery dilation but should not result in increased velocities in the RVOT or across the pulmonic valve.

### Selected References

1. McElhinney DB, Sondergaard L, Armstrong AK, et al. Endocarditis after transcatheter pulmonary valve replacement. *J Am Coll Cardiol*. 2018;72(22):2717-2728.
2. Quader N, Makan M, Perez J. *The Washington Manual of Echocardiography*. 2nd ed. Wolters Kluwer; 2017.

# 28 | MECHANICAL AND BIOPROSTHETIC VALVES

Daniel S. Cormican, Stephen M. McHugh, and Timothy P. Goldhardt

1. A 49-year-old woman with a history of hepatitis C virus, asthma, and intravenous (IV) drug abuse is admitted to the intensive care unit (ICU) after presenting to the Emergency Department (ED) in septic shock. Blood cultures and urine cultures are sent and a transthoracic echocardiogram (TTE) is performed. Based on the apical view shown in **Figure 28.1**, what is the diagnosis?

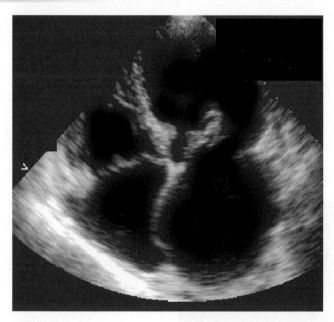

**Figure 28.1**

A. Endocarditis
B. Hypovolemia
C. Ventricular septal defect
D. Left ventricular (LV) pseudoaneurysm

2. A 78-year-old man with a past medical history (PMH) of type 2 diabetes and a prior three-vessel coronary artery bypass graft (CABG) and mechanical aortic valve replacement 18 years ago is admitted to the ICU with pneumonia and hypotension. A bedside TTE is performed and a continuous-wave Doppler (CWD) measurement through the aortic valve is shown in **Figure 28.2**.

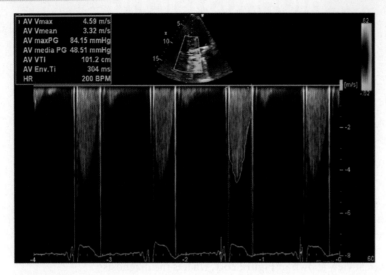

| AV Vmax | 4.59 m/s |
| AV Vmean | 3.32 m/s |
| AV maxPG | 84.15 mmHg |
| AV media PG | 48.51 mmHg |
| AV VTI | 101.2 cm |
| AV Env.Ti | 304 ms |
| HR | 200 BPM |

**Figure 28.2**

What is the diagnosis?
A. Mechanical aortic valve regurgitation
B. Mechanical aortic valve stenosis
C. Mechanical paravalvular leak
D. Normal mechanical aortic valve function

3. An 80-year-old man with a PMH of colon cancer, type 2 diabetes, and mechanical mitral valve presents to the emergency room with acute onset of shortness of breath. He has bilateral rales and his oxygen saturation is 81% on room air. He is intubated and a transesophageal echocardiography (TEE) is performed that is shown in **Figure 28.3**.

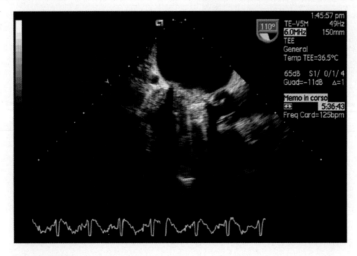

**Figure 28.3**

What is the diagnosis?
A. Cardiac tamponade
B. Patent foramen ovale
C. Mechanical mitral valve thrombosis
D. Paravalvular leak

4. A 69-year-old woman was admitted to the ICU immediately after a transcatheter aortic valve replacement (TAVR). Shortly after arrival in the ICU, she developed significant hypotension. A TEE is performed and **Figure 28.4** is obtained. What is the finding shown in Figure 28.4?

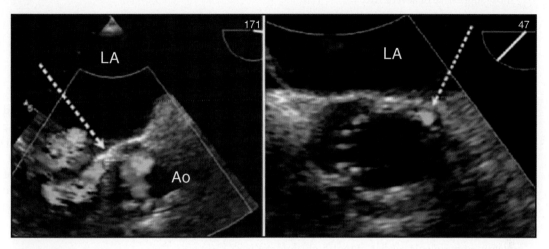

**Figure 28.4**

A. Stenosis of the TAVR valve
B. Endocarditis
C. Malpositioned valve
D. Paravalvular leak

5. A 69-year-old man with a history of a mechanical mitral valve replacement on warfarin presents to the ED with shortness of breath. His blood pressure is measured at 86/45 and his heart rate is 118 bpm. His international normalized ratio (INR) is measured at 4.3. The subcostal view from his bedside TTE is shown in **Figure 28.5A** (subcostal four-chamber view in systole) and **Figure 28.5B** (M mode through right atrium).

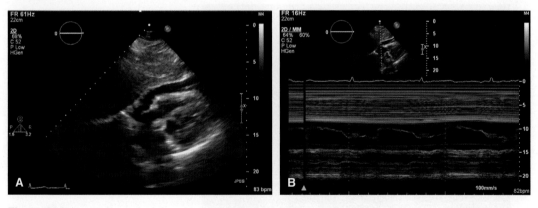

**Figure 28.5**

What is the diagnosis?
A. Cardiac tamponade
B. Pericardial tumor
C. Pulmonary embolus
D. Right ventricular failure

6. A 70-year-old gentleman with a history of bioprosthetic valve replacement in the aortic position is evaluated in the ICU for progressive dyspnea and increasing oxygen requirements. TEE is completed, and prosthetic valve aortic regurgitation (AR) is diagnosed. Which of the following TEE findings is most suggestive of severe AR?

   A. Measured regurgitant fraction of 35%
   B. Measured regurgitant volume of 35 mL/heart beat
   C. Pressure half-time of 190 ms via CWD
   D. Vena contracta measurement of 0.5 cm

7. A patient with bileaflet mechanical valve in mitral position is evaluated for progressive dyspnea and symptoms of congestive heart failure. He has been placed on epinephrine infusion at 0.08 µg/kg/min, and recent right heart catheterization showed a cardiac index of 4.1 L/min/m². His heart rate is 125 bpm and mean arterial pressure is 85 mm Hg. Echocardiographic Doppler evaluation of the mechanical valve (averaged over three separate measures) reveals peak velocity of 3.2 m/s and mean gradient of 16 mm Hg. Qualitative assessment of valve function shows normal leaflet motion without suggestion of thrombus or pannus. Which factor is most likely to be the cause of Doppler measurements consistent with prosthetic valve stenosis in this case?

   A. Supraphysiologic cardiac output/high-flow state
   B. Malalignment of Doppler beam through the valve
   C. Erroneous Doppler measurement of pulmonary vein inflow
   D. Use of pulsed-wave Doppler instead of CWD

8. A 76-year-old gentleman is evaluated due to progressive respiratory failure approximately 24 hours after undergoing aortic valve replacement for treatment of severe aortic stenosis. His blood pressure is 129/49, and heart rate is 41, with bradycardia due to heart block. TEE reveals normal biventricular systolic function without regional wall motion abnormalities (RWMA) and LV hypertrophy. The prosthetic aortic valve leaflets open appropriately and there is no echocardiographic signal of prosthetic valve stenosis. Color Doppler evaluation of the aortic valve is noted in **Figure 28.6**. Based on Figure 28.6, what is the most likely etiology of his respiratory failure?

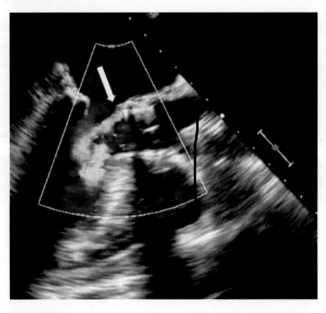

**Figure 28.6**

   A. Intravalvular AR
   B. Paravalvular AR
   C. Mitral regurgitation
   D. Aortic valve endocarditis

9. A 64-year-old woman with a history of mitral regurgitation is admitted to the cardiothoracic ICU (CTICU) immediately after mitral valve replacement; the mean arterial pressure is 50 mm Hg with infusion of high-dose norepinephrine. Her preoperative TTE is notable for severe mitral regurgitation, severe left atrial dilation, moderately dilated left ventricle and left ventricular ejection fraction (LVEF) of 50% (by visual estimate), and no RWMA. STAT bedside echocardiography shortly after arrival in the CTICU shows a well-seated bioprosthetic valve in the mitral position with normal leaflet opening and a mitral valve mean gradient of 4 mm Hg. The left ventricle is moderately-to-severely dilated, with LVEF of 20%, severe diffuse hypokinesis, and no regional dysfunction. Which pathophysiologic change most likely explains the patient's hypotension after mitral valve replacement?

 A. Increased LV afterload
 B. Inadvertent ligation of the left circumflex coronary artery
 C. Prosthetic valve stenosis
 D. Severe hypovolemia

10. An 88-year-old woman is evaluated for hypotension and oliguria 8 hours after arrival in the CTICU after mitral valve replacement to treat mixed mitral regurgitation and stenosis. The operative procedure was reportedly complex and required considerable debridement of mitral annular calcification so as to allow for appropriate valve seating. Urgent TTE imaging is technically limited; transesophageal imaging is performed (**Figure 28.7**) and reveals a large fluid collection posterior to the left atrium, with compressive effect on that chamber.

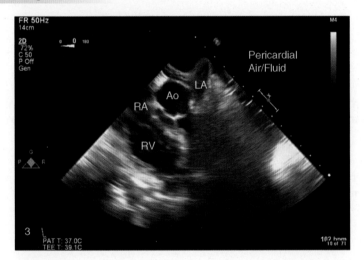

**Figure 28.7**

Which clinical situation most likely accounts for these findings?
 A. Aortotomy site bleeding
 B. Atrioventricular groove disruption (AVD)
 C. Inadequate heparin reversal after conclusion of cardiopulmonary bypass
 D. Retained foreign body

11. A 51-year-old morbidly obese male with chronic atrial fibrillation underwent an elective aortic valve replacement for critical aortic stenosis using a mechanical bileaflet tilting disc valve. He consistently fails physical therapy goals in the ICU as he reports significant shortness of breath as his limiting factor. You are concerned he may have a patient–prosthesis mismatch with the new valve. When evaluating for patient–prosthesis mismatch of a mechanical aortic valve, which of the following Doppler echocardiography methods is *least* likely to help you determine the degree (if any) of patient–prosthesis mismatch?

 A. Peak and mean gradients
 B. Doppler velocity index (DVI) or dimensionless index
 C. Effective orifice area
 D. Contour of the jet profile

**12.** An 81-year-old female underwent a transcutaneous aortic valve replacement for critical aortic stenosis under sedation. There were no intraoperative complications. A brief TTE performed by cardiology after deployment of the valve showed an LVEF of 55%, a peak prosthetic aortic jet velocity of 3.2 m/s, a DVI of 0.31, and an acceleration time (AT) of >110 ms. Of these reported parameters, which one is *most* likely to suggest severe prosthetic aortic valve stenosis and possible patient–prosthesis mismatch?

    A. LVEF 55%
    B. Peak jet velocity of 3.2 m/s
    C. DVI of 0.31
    D. AT of >110 ms

**13.** In the absence of other significant valvular disease, evaluation of LV diastolic function is *least* accurate in the presence of a prosthetic heart valve in the:

    A. Aortic position
    B. Mitral position
    C. Pulmonic position
    D. Tricuspid position

**14.** The 2D ultrasound imaging artifacts commonly caused by mechanical prosthetic valves is least likely from:

    A. Near-field clutter
    B. Shadowing
    C. Side/grating lobe
    D. Comet tail

**15.** Of the following TTE and TEE views, which one will allow you to perform the most comprehensive Doppler examination of the mitral valve in a patient with a bileaflet tilting disc mechanical mitral valve?

    A. Apical four-chamber view
    B. Parasternal long-axis view
    C. Midesophageal two-chamber view
    D. Transgastric two-chamber view

# Chapter 28 ▪ Answers

**1.** Correct Answer: A. Endocarditis

*Rationale:* Figure 28.1 shows a mass on the anterior leaflet of the mitral valve consistent with a vegetation from endocarditis. Episodes of endocarditis have been increasing in recent years and there are now up to 50,000 cases per year diagnosed in the United States. Echocardiography is key to making the diagnosis of endocarditis. TTE has been reported to have overall ~70% sensitivity, with TEE being even more sensitive and specific. Echocardiographic signs of endocarditis include valvular vegetations, paravalvular abscesses, and intracardiac fistulae. In a patient with bacteremia or sepsis with unknown source, the possibility of endocarditis should be evaluated. The TTE image shown in Figure 28.1 reveals no evidence of a ventricular septal defect or an LV pseudoaneurysm. Hypovolemia is a clinical diagnosis that can be informed by echocardiographic information. This image shows no findings suggestive of hypovolemia.

Selected Reference

1. Afonso L, Kottam A, Reddy V, Penumetcha A. Echocardiography in infective endocarditis: state of the art. *Curr Cardiol Rep.* 2017;19(12):127.

**2.** Correct Answer: B. Mechanical aortic valve stenosis

*Rationale/Critique:* Figure 28.2 shows CWD measurements through the aortic valve. Normal mean pressure gradients through a properly functioning aortic valve are <10 mm Hg. The values in this patient are significantly elevated, with a mean pressure gradient of 48.51 mm Hg. These values are most consistent with stenosis of his mechanical aortic valve. The exact cause of the stenosis cannot be determined from CWD measurement alone. In general, mechanical valves have a longer potential life span than bioprosthetic valves, but both types of valves can malfunction over time. Severe aortic stenosis can result in congestive heart failure and pulmonary edema and may have played a role in the patient's development of pneumonia. Regurgitation of the mechanical valve and a paravalvular leak both would show flow of blood backward into the left ventricle, which are not present in Figure 28.2.

Selected Reference

1. Chikwe J, Filsoufi F, Carpentier AF. Prosthetic valve selection for middle-aged patients with aortic stenosis. *Nat Rev Cardiol.* 2010;7(12):711-719.

**3.** Correct Answer: C. Mechanical mitral valve thrombosis

*Rationale:* Figure 28.3 shows a mass on the patient's mechanical mitral valve that is consistent with mechanical mitral valve thrombosis. The risk of thrombosis is approximately five times greater for prosthetic valves in the mitral position than in the aortic position. Patients with valve thrombosis may be asymptomatic with small, slowly developing thrombus, or acutely symptomatic with signs of reduced cardiac output when a large thrombus develops quickly. Echocardiographic signs of valve thrombus include an abnormal mass on the prosthetic valve, restricted valve motion, and elevated flow gradients through the valve. Management of mechanical valve thrombosis ranges from directed thrombolysis to open surgical repair.

Selected Reference

1. Lim WY, Lloyd G, Bhattacharyya S. Mechanical and surgical bioprosthetic valve thrombosis. *Heart.* 2017;103(24):1934-1941.

**4.** Correct Answer: D. Paravalvular leak

*Rationale:* The TEE image (Figure 28.4) shows a paravalvular leak around the TAVR valve. This can be seen in the long-axis view of the transcatheter valve as regurgitant flow around the posterior edge of the valve back into the LV outflow tract, and in the short-axis view of the valve as color flow during diastole at approximately 2 o'clock. Echocardiographic assessment for paravalvular leak is important after all TAVR procedures because its presence is associated with poorer long-term outcomes. Stenosis of the transcatheter aortic valve would be best evaluated with CWD measurements through the valve and is not indicated by the regurgitant flow in the images. Signs of endocarditis such as vegetations and abscesses are not present in the images and endocarditis of the valve would be essentially impossible immediately after the procedure. Finally, the valve appears to be appropriately positioned.

Selected Reference

1. Vollema EM, Delgado V, Bax JJ. Echocardiography in transcatheter aortic valve replacement. *Heart Lung Circ.* 2019;28(9):1384-1399.

**5.** Correct Answer: A. Cardiac tamponade

*Rationale:* A pericardial effusion is an abnormal collection of fluid in the pericardial sac. When an effusion begins to produce increased pressure great enough to impair filling of the heart, cardiac tamponade has developed. Pericardial effusions can occur from a wide variety of causes, including uremia, malignancy, postmyocardial infarction, and bleeding into the pericardial space. In this case, the patient's INR is significantly elevated and likely led to bleeding that eventually caused cardiac tamponade. Echocardiography is considered the preferred modality for diagnosis of cardiac tamponade. Features indicating true tamponade include compression of the right atrium and diastolic compression of the right ventricle. The compression of the right atrium typically happens during end-diastole and systole. It is important to note that, by convention, systole and diastole refer to ventricular systole and diastole. Figure 28.5A shows systolic collapse of the right atrium. Right atrial collapse for more than one-third of the duration of cardiac cycle (Figure 28.5B) is very specific for tamponade. Specifically, diastolic compression of the right ventricle is more sensitive and specific for tamponade.

Selected Reference

1. Appleton C, Gillam L, Koulogiannis K. Cardiac tamponade. *Cardiol Clin.* 2017;35(4):525-537.

**6.** Correct Answer: C. Pressure half-time of 190 ms via CWD

*Rationale:* Short pressure half-time measurements (<200 ms) in the setting of AR are reflective of rapid decay of the regurgitant jet flow, due to LV pressure equalization. Holodiastolic flow reversal in the descending aorta is thought to become more indicative of a marker of severe AR the more distal it is found, so severe regurgitation is more likely when the flow reversal is seen in the abdominal aorta as compared to the proximal descending aorta. A regurgitant volume 60 mL or more per heart beat suggests severe AR. Similarly, a regurgitant fraction of 50% or more per heart beat suggests severe AR. Vena contracta is not a component of the American Society of Echocardiography (ASE) guidelines for the assessment of prosthetic aortic valve regurgitation severity.

Selected Reference

1. Zoghbi WA, Chambers JB, Dumesnil JG, et al. Recommendations for evaluation of prosthetic valves with echocardiography and Doppler ultrasound. *J Am Soc Echocardiogr.* 2009;22:975-1014.

**7.** Correct Answer: A. Supraphysiologic cardiac output/high-flow state

*Rationale:* Measured Doppler gradients through cardiac valves are dependent on blood flow; elevated heart rates and blood flows will raise gradients. While malalignment of the Doppler flow may alter accuracy of gradients, averaging multiple measurements helps avoid single sample errors. Pulmonary vein flow is low velocity (<1 m/s) and typically has a Doppler "envelope" image that is different than that seen in Doppler mitral valve flow. Use of pulsed-wave Doppler would likely create aliasing in the setting of high flow velocities, requiring a change to CWD assessment.

Selected Reference

1. Mahmood F, Matyal R, Mahmood F, Sheu RD, Feng R, Khabbaz KR. Intraoperative echocardiographic assessment of prosthetic valves: a practical approach. *J Cardiothorac Vasc Anes.* 2018 Apr;32(2):823-837.

**8.** Correct Answer: B. Paravalvular AR

*Rationale:* The TEE image (Figure 28.6) is frozen in diastole and shows a jet of AR outside of the aortic valve stent. Based on Figure 28.6, this patient most likely had a balloon-expandable stented TAVR. The regurgitation flow is seen outside of the stent, confirming that the regurgitation is paravalvular in nature. Surgical aortic valve replacement or TAVR is associated with a certain risk of heart block. In this patient, bradycardia from heart block in conjunction with paravalvular AR potentially led to acute pulmonary edema resulting in respiratory failure. Mitral regurgitation will be seen with systole and hence cannot be commented on from this image in diastole. Also, there is no evidence of vegetations or aortic root abscess on the image suggestive of endocarditis.

Selected Reference

1. Zoghbi WA, Asch FM, Bruce C, et al. Guidelines for the evaluation of valvular regurgitation after percutaneous valve repair or replacement: a report from the American Society of Echocardiography developed in collaboration with the Society for Cardiovascular Angiography and Interventions, Japanese Society of Echocardiography, and Society for Cardiovascular Magnetic Resonance. *J Am Soc Echocardiogr.* 2019 Apr;32(4):431-475.

**9.** Correct Answer: A. Increased LV afterload

*Rationale:* LVEF may not accurately reflect forward cardiac output in patients with severe mitral regurgitation, as a considerable portion of LV stroke volume may be due to retrograde flow into the left atrium. After mitral valve surgery to decrease regurgitation, the low-pressure "outlet" of LV stroke volume is abolished, and the left ventricle must now eject blood through the aortic valve against systemic blood pressure. This relative increase in LV afterload may depress LV contractility. Mitral valve surgery can be complicated by coronary artery injury and subsequent decreases in LVEF, but concurrent RWMA are almost always noted in this situation. Prosthetic valve stenosis is typically associated with mean gradients >10 mm Hg and/or limited valve opening.

Selected Reference

1. Stephens RS, Whitman GJR. Postoperative critical care of the adult cardiac surgical patient: Part II: procedure-specific considerations, management of complications, and quality improvement. *Crit Care Med.* 2015;43:1995-2014.

**10.** Correct Answer: **B. Atrioventricular groove disruption (AVD)**

*Rationale:* AVD must be considered in all patients who have undergone mitral valve surgery, and the risk for AVD is particularly high in elderly patients who require mitral annular calcification debridement for appropriate valve intervention. The occurrence rate of AVD is fortunately low, but the condition is not always immediately evident, requires difficult surgical repair, and there is high mortality associated with AVD. Echocardiographically, fluid (blood) is seen outside the heart, and there may be compression of the left atrium or left ventricle due to this fluid collection. If color flow Doppler is used, blood flow may be seen leaving the left atrium at the atrioventricular junction. Aortotomy site bleeding can cause clinical instability and echocardiographic change, but is usually noted immediately in the operating room (OR). By convention, laboratory evaluation of heparin effect (usually via activated clotting time [ACT]) is done both pre-bypass and post-bypass in the OR; with the routine administration of protamine and reassessment of ACT prior to leaving the OR, inadequate heparin reversal is unlikely. There is no evidence of a retained foreign body in Figure 28.7.

Selected Reference

1. Kwon JT, Jung TE, Lee DH. The rupture of atrioventricular groove after mitral valve replacement in an elderly patient. *J Cardiothorac Surg.* 2014;9:28.

**11.** Correct Answer: **C. Effective orifice area**

*Rationale:* In a patient with atrial fibrillation, calculating the effective orifice area using the continuity equation will be the least accurate measurement as the velocity time integral can vary with each heartbeat. Furthermore, accurate measurement of the LV outflow tract is the greatest source of error when using the continuity equation.

Selected References

1. Quiñones MA, Otto CM, Stoddard M, Waggoner A, Zoghbi WA. Recommendations for quantification of Doppler echocardiography: a report from the Doppler Quantification Task Force of the Nomenclature and Standards Committee of the American Society of Echocardiography. *J Am Soc Echocardiogr.* 2002;15:167-184.
2. Zoghbi WA, Chambers JB, Dumesnil JG, et al. Recommendations for evaluation of prosthetic valves with echocardiography and Doppler ultrasound: a report from the American Society of Echocardiography's Guidelines and Standards Committee and the Task Force on Prosthetic Valves, developed in conjunction with the American College of Cardiology Cardiovascular Imaging Committee, Cardiac Imaging Committee of the American Heart Association, the European Association of Echocardiography, a registered branch of the European Society of Cardiology, the Japanese Society of Echocardiography and the Canadian Society of Echocardiography, endorsed by the American College of Cardiology Foundation, American Heart Association, European Association of Echocardiography, a registered branch of the European Society of Cardiology, the Japanese Society of Echocardiography, and Canadian Society of Echocardiography. *J Am Soc Echocardiogr.* 2009;22:975-1014.

**12.** Correct Answer: **D. AT of >110 ms**

*Rationale:* Based on the 2009 ASE recommendations for evaluation of prosthetic valves, of the parameters listed, only an AT of >100 ms is highly suggestive of severe prosthetic aortic valve stenosis. The peak jet velocity of 3.2 m/s can suggest stenosis, but also may be a normal value depending on the size and type of valve. A DVI of 0.31 is considered a normal value for a prosthetic aortic valve. A normal LVEF contributes little to the evaluation of potential prosthetic aortic valve stenosis in this example.

Selected Reference

1. Zoghbi WA, Chambers JB, Dumesnil JG, et al. Recommendations for evaluation of prosthetic valves with echocardiography and Doppler ultrasound: a report from the American Society of Echocardiography's Guidelines and Standards Committee and the Task Force on Prosthetic Valves, developed in conjunction with the American College of Cardiology Cardiovascular Imaging Committee, Cardiac Imaging Committee of the American Heart Association, the European Association of Echocardiography, a registered branch of the European Society of Cardiology, the Japanese Society of Echocardiography and the Canadian Society of Echocardiography, endorsed by the American College of Cardiology Foundation, American Heart Association, European Association of Echocardiography, a registered branch of the European Society of Cardiology, the Japanese Society of Echocardiography, and Canadian Society of Echocardiography. *J Am Soc Echocardiogr.* 2009;22:975-1014.

**13.** Correct Answer: B. Mitral position

*Rationale:* When evaluating LV diastolic function, obtaining accurate mitral inflow Doppler measurements (as well as lateral mitral annular tissue Doppler measurements) can be greatly affected by the presence of atrial fibrillation, moderate mitral annular calcification, any mitral stenosis or regurgitation greater than moderate severity, mitral valve repair or replacement, LV assist devices, left bundle branch block, or ventricular paced rhythms.

Selected Reference

1. Nagueh SF, Smiseth OA, Appleton CP, et al. Recommendations for the evaluation of left ventricular diastolic function by echocardiography: an update from the American Society of Echocardiography and the European Association of Cardiovascular Imaging. *J Am Soc Echocardiogr.* 2016;29:277-314.

**14.** Correct Answer: A. Near-field clutter

*Rationale:* Near-field clutter describes the poor visibility of structures commonly seen in the areas of an ultrasound image closest to the ultrasound probe. It is caused by high-amplitude oscillations of the piezo-electric elements in the probe itself leading to extra echoes in the very near field. Mechanical heart valves are well known to create comet tails, shadowing, and side/grating lobe artifacts. Comet tails are reverberation artifacts that create hyperechoic lines, or "tails," distal to the object and parallel to the sound beam. Shadowing is an attenuation artifact caused by loss of ultrasound beam transmission from either high reflection or absorption. Distal structures appear darker or even anechoic. A side lobe (from single-element transducer) or grating lobe (from array transducers) is a refraction artifact caused by weak ultrasound beams emitted outside the path of the main ultrasound beam. These weak beams bounce off hyperechoic structures and appear as duplicates of the true object, at the same level or depth and on either side of the true object.

Selected References

1. Bertrand PB, Levine RA, Isselbacher EM, et al. Fact or artifact in two-dimensional echocardiography: avoiding misdiagnosis and missed diagnosis. *J Am Soc Echocardiogr.* 2016;29(5):381-391.
2. Le HT, Hangiandreou N, Timmerman R, et al. Imaging artifacts in echocardiography. *Anesth Analg.* 2016;122(3):633-646.

**15.** Correct Answer: C. Midesophageal two-chamber view

*Rationale:* Doppler analysis (pulsed-wave Doppler, CWD, and color flow Doppler) of the mitral valve requires the ultrasound beam to be in-line with the blood flow vector being analyzed, so the parasternal long-axis and transgastric two-chamber views could not be used. Acoustic shadowing by the mechanical mitral valve, especially in the closed position during systole, can mask regurgitant jets when viewed from the apical four-chamber view (or any apical TTE view) and prohibit Doppler analysis of regurgitant jet velocities. Of the options provided, only the midesophageal two-chamber view will allow Doppler analysis of mitral inflow as well as regurgitant jets in a patient with a mechanical mitral valve.

Selected References

1. Quiñones MA, Otto CM, Stoddard M, Waggoner A, Zoghbi WA. Recommendations for quantification of Doppler echocardiography: a report from the Doppler Quantification Task Force of the Nomenclature and Standards Committee of the American Society of Echocardiography. *J Am Soc Echocardiogr.* 2002;15:167-184.
2. Zoghbi WA, Chambers JB, Dumesnil JG, et al. Recommendations for evaluation of prosthetic valves with echocardiography and Doppler ultrasound: a report from the American Society of Echocardiography's Guidelines and Standards Committee and the Task Force on Prosthetic Valves, developed in conjunction with the American College of Cardiology Cardiovascular Imaging Committee, Cardiac Imaging Committee of the American Heart Association, the European Association of Echocardiography, a registered branch of the European Society of Cardiology, the Japanese Society of Echocardiography and the Canadian Society of Echocardiography, endorsed by the American College of Cardiology Foundation, American Heart Association, European Association of Echocardiography, a registered branch of the European Society of Cardiology, the Japanese Society of Echocardiography, and Canadian Society of Echocardiography. *J Am Soc Echocardiogr.* 2009;22:975-1014.

# 29 | ENDOCARDITIS AND OTHER PATHOLOGIC AND NORMAL ANATOMIC VARIANTS

Lev Deriy, Brian Starr, Carlos E. Vazquez, Pamela Y.F. Hsu, Eli L. Torgeson, and Neal S. Gerstein

**1.** Using the transthoracic echocardiography (TTE) image(s) shown in **Figure 29.1** and ▶ **Video 29.1** the structure indicated by the *arrow* in this view is most likely a:

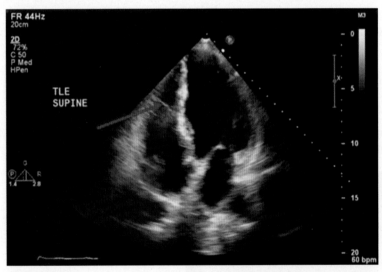

**Figure 29.1**

**A.** Thrombus
**B.** False tendon
**C.** Ebstein anomaly
**D.** Moderator band

2. TTE is taken from a 50 year-old man with no known cardiac disease.

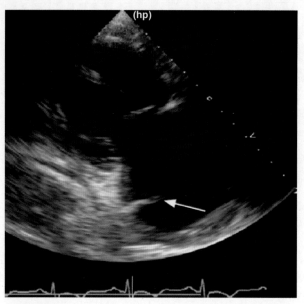

**Figure 29.2**

The structure indicated by the *arrow* in this view is most likely:
A. Superior vena cava
B. Cor triatriatum
C. Chiari network or atrial myxoma
D. Eustachian valve

3. A 35-year-old male is admitted to the intensive care unit (ICU) with a diagnosis of bacterial endocarditis of a bicuspid aortic valve. **Figure 29.3** shows the TTE obtained.

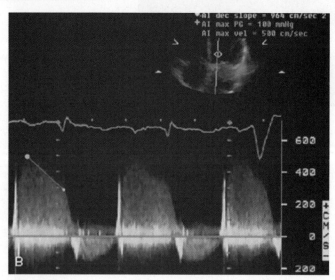

**Figure 29.3**

In Figure 29.3, the calipers over the 1st "peak" are measuring what?
A. Peak velocity of the aortic valve regurgitant jet
B. Vena contracta of the aortic valve regurgitant jet
C. Pressure half-time (PHT) of the aortic valve regurgitant jet
D. EROA—effective regurgitant orifice area

4. TTE was taken from a 45-year-old woman with antiphospholipid syndrome and history of cryptogenic strokes.

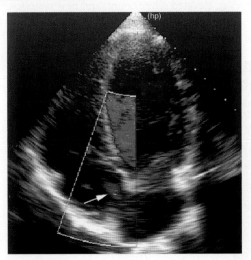

**Figure 29.4**

Based on what is seen in **Figure 29.4**, what procedure would likely benefit the patient most?
A. Coronary artery bypass surgery
B. Percutaneous device closure
C. Pulmonary thromboendarterectomy
D. Left atrial appendage ligation

5. Which of the following statements regarding the structural abnormality demonstrated in **Question 29.4** and Figure 29.4 is correct?

A. Color-flow Doppler (CFD) examination alone is the gold standard for diagnosis
B. Is found in up to 3% to 5% of the general population
C. Patients with combined patent foramen ovale (PFO) and atrial septal aneurysm (ASA) have lower risk of stroke than those with an isolated PFO
D. Implanted cardiac devices or catheters may inadvertently cross the presented pathology

6. The transesophageal echocardiography (TEE) image in **Figure 29.5** shows a 35-year-old male with a recent history of mitral valve replacement due to severe mitral regurgitation from bacterial endocarditis now readmitted to the ICU with acute hemolytic anemia.

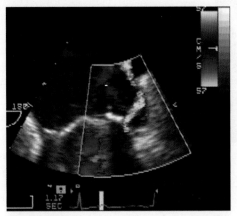

**Figure 29.5**

Figure 29.5 is obtained showing:
A. Normal leakage regurgitant jets
B. Transvalvular regurgitation
C. Paravalvular regurgitation
D. Flow from the left atrial appendage

7. A 65-year-old male with a history of permanent pacemaker implantation for sick sinus syndrome presented to the Emergency Department (ED) with fever, elevated white count, and new systolic murmur. Which of the following statements regarding the structural abnormality demonstrated in this patient's bedside TTE (**Figure 29.6**) is correct (PWi: pacing wire)?

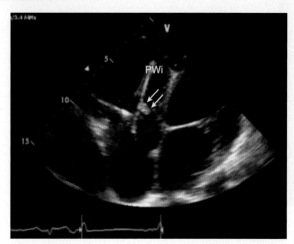

**Figure 29.6**

A. Antimicrobial prophylaxis is not indicated after initial implantation
B. TTE has higher sensitivity in establishing the diagnosis than TEE
C. Aortic and mitral valves are not affected by this pathology
D. Surgical or percutaneous removal of the pacemaker leads is indicated.

8. Subcostal TTE view is obtained from a 65-year-old male with a long history of severe emphysema requiring steroid therapy.

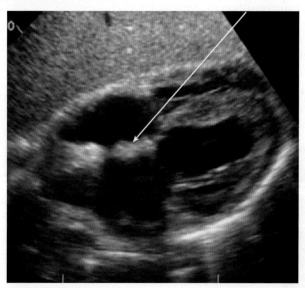

**Figure 29.7**

The structure indicated by the *arrow* in **Figure 29.7** is *most* likely:
A. Thrombus in the right atrium
B. Left atrial myxoma
C. "Coumadin ridge"
D. Lipomatous hypertrophy of the atrial septum (LHAS)

9. TTE shows an echogenic structure attached to the tricuspid valve.

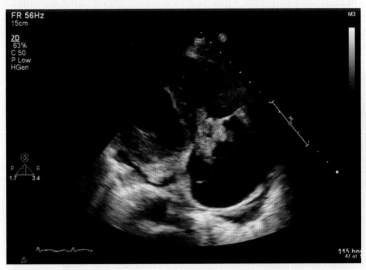

**Figure 29.8**

Of the following choices, the *most* likely diagnosis is:
A. Thrombus
B. Eustachian valve
C. Chiari network
D. Artifact shadow
E. Catheter-associated infection

10. What structure does the *arrow* in the presented TTE in **Figure 29.9** indicate?

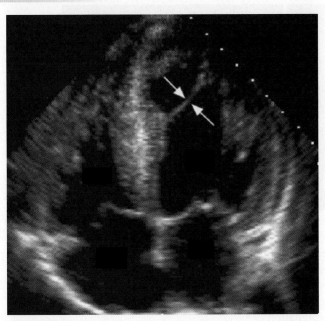

**Figure 29.9**

A. Moderator band
B. Left ventricular (LV) false tendon
C. Eustachian valve
D. Coumadin ridge, or crista terminalis

11. A 62-year-old patient is transferred to cardiothoracic ICU after three-vessel coronary artery bypass surgery. He is still intubated, on high-dose inotropic support with an epinephrine infusion with blood pressure 72/38 mm Hg and heart rate 128 bpm. The bedside TTE was performed and **Figure 29.10** was obtained showing apical five-chamber (A5C) view during early systole (**Figure 29.10A**) and mid-systole (**Figure 29.10B**) of the same beat.

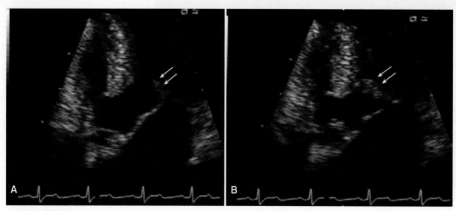

**Figure 29.10**

Which of the following is *most* likely causing this hemodynamic instability?
A. Myocardial dysfunction due to ischemia-reperfusion injury
B. Graft failure due to acute thrombosis
C. Acute pulmonary hypertension and right ventricular (RV) failure due to reaction to protamine
D. Systolic anterior motion (SAM) of the mitral valve leaflets

12. From the patient in **Question 29.11, Figure 29.11** was obtained.

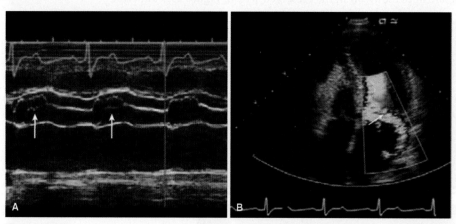

**Figure 29.11**

The *arrows* in left and right image, respectively, point to:
A. Mitral valve closure and mitral regurgitation
B. Aortic valve closure and mitral regurgitation
C. Mitral valve closure and aortic regurgitation
D. Aortic valve closure and aortic regurgitation

13. The *most* appropriate next step in the management of the patient in **Question 29.11** would be:

A. Escalate inotropic support by adding milrinone infusion
B. Insert intra-aortic balloon pump
C. Stop epinephrine and start infusion of vasoconstrictor
D. Start extracorporeal membrane oxygenation (ECMO) support

14. In the parasternal short-axis view at the level of aortic valve (**Figure 29.12**) taken from a 40-year-old patient with recent fevers and signs of acute heart failure, which of the following is a potential complication of the disease process?

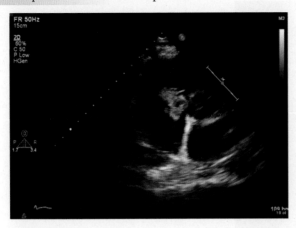

**Figure 29.12**

A. Embolic stroke

B. Acute lower extremity ischemia

C. Leaflet perforation/rupture

D. Myocardial infarction

15. In the TEE still of **Figure 29.13**, identify the structure indicated by the *arrow* from the following list of cardiac structures see in this standard TEE view.

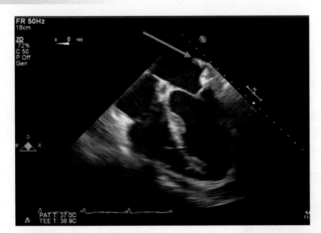

**Figure 29.13**

A. Left upper pulmonary vein

B. Coumadin ridge

C. Left atrium

D. Anterior mitral valve leaflet

E. Posterior mitral valve leaflet

16. In the TTE (**Figure 29.14**) taken from an asymptomatic 61-year-old man with no prior cardiac history after seven days of hospitalization, which of the following is the *most* likely diagnosis (see ▶ **Video 29.2**)?

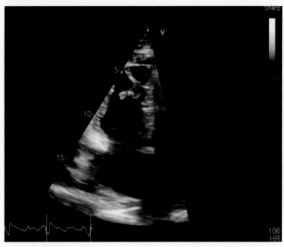

**Figure 29.14**

A. Infective endocarditis
B. Myxoma
C. Fibroelastoma
D. Moderator band–associated thrombus

17. Which of the following echocardiographic findings is an intermediate risk factor for the development of infective endocarditis?

A. Prosthetic valve
B. Prosthetic material used for native valve repair
C. Mitral valve prolapse
D. Unrepaired cyanotic congenital heart disease

18. A 73-year-old female patient is undergoing preoperative TEE examination in preparation for an elective three-vessel coronary artery bypass grafting (CABG) operation (**Figure 29.15**). The patient has a history of hypertension, diabetes, and atrial fibrillation.

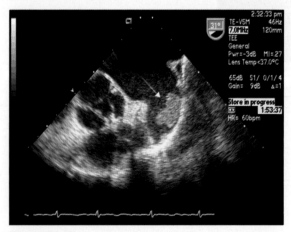

**Figure 29.15**

What is the *arrow* pointing to?
A. Thrombus in the pulmonary artery
B. Myxoma in the left atrium
C. Large mitral valve vegetation
D. Thrombus in left atrial appendage

19. **Figure 20.16** TTE was taken from a 40-year-old man with a history of intravenous drug use (IVDU) who was admitted to the ICU due to the signs and symptoms of right heart failure and an increased oxygen requirement. He was found to have methicillin-resistant *Staphylococcus aureus* (MRSA) bacteremia, a pleural effusion with likely empyema, and a peripheral wedge-shaped opacity on chest computed tomography (CT).

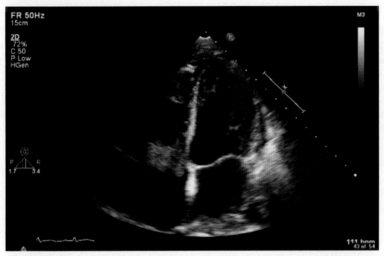

**Figure 29.16**

Which of the following echocardiographic characteristics is *most* consistent with the involved process?
A. High degree of echogenicity
B. Nonvalvular location
C. Highly mobile and oscillating
D. Smooth surface
E. Absence of tissue destruction/regurgitation

20. For Figure 29.16 in **Question 29.20**, which of the following statements regarding the demonstrated pathology is correct?

A. The greater the mobility of the endocarditis lesion, the greater the likelihood for an embolic event.
B. Endocarditis lesion size does not correlate with the risk of an embolic event.
C. Timing of antibiotics administration does not affect the risk of an embolic event.
D. Aortic valve endocarditis is at higher risk for an embolic event than a mitral valve lesion.

# Chapter 29 ▪ Answers

1. Correct Answer: D. Moderator band

*Rationale:* The moderator band (also known as the septomarginal trabecula) is a muscular structure that connects the interventricular septum with the anterolateral wall of the right ventricle. During contraction together with anterior papillary muscle it prevents the tricuspid regurgitation through applying tension on the chordae tendineae. False tendon is usually found in the left ventricle. There is a normal level of insertion of tricuspid valve, so Ebstein anomaly is incorrect. Moderator band has a myocardial-like echogenicity and contracts synchronously with the rest of the ventricle, making a diagnosis of thrombus and/or artifact very unlikely.

Selected Reference

1. Lee J-Y, Hur M-S. Morphological classification of the moderator band and its relationship with the anterior papillary muscle. Anat Cell Biol. 2019 Mar;52(1):38-42.

**2.** Correct Answer: **D. Eustachian valve**

*Rationale/Critique:* The transthoracic parasternal RV inflow view demonstrates the right atrium and right ventricle with the arrow pointing to the Eustachian valve at the cavoatrial junction. The Eustachian valve may be a nidus for thrombus or infection. Cor triatriatum is more frequently associated with the left atrium and is typically seen as a thin membrane that crosses from the atrial septum in the region of the fossa ovalis to the lateral wall of the atrium. A Chiari network is a right atrial structure typically seen as a mobile thin reticulated network of fibers originating from the Eustachian valve, occasionally fenestrated, connecting to various parts of the right atrium. An atrial myxoma is more likely to be seen as a pedunculated rounded mass more frequently arising from the septum. However, myxomas have been reported to arise from a Eustachian valve.

Selected Reference

1. Onwuanyi AE, Brown RJ, Vahedi M, Narayanan R, Nash IS, Goldman ME. Eustachian valve thrombus: critical factor in outcome of venous thromboembolism. *Echocardiography.* 2003;20(1):71-73.

**3.** Correct Answer: **C. Pressure half-time (PHT) of the aortic valve regurgitant jet**

*Rationale:* Numerous modalities exist to help quantify regurgitant jets. Figure 29.3 displays an apical four-chamber TTE view of the left ventricle with continuous-wave Doppler interrogating the aortic valve. The resulting "jets" point up or toward the probe, in this view indicating flow into the left ventricle, and in diastole, consistent with aortic regurgitation. In this case, the calipers are measuring the downward slope of the jet used for calculating the PHT. PHT more specifically measures the interval between the maximal transvalvular gradient and when it is half the maximum. Computer analysis determines PHT from the slope, with a value of <200 ms suggesting severe aortic regurgitation. PHT can be affected by LV compliance, systemic vascular resistance, and aortic compliance. Increasing LV diastolic pressure shortens PHT while the chronic adaptation to severe aortic regurgitation prolongs PHT.

Selected References

1. Cohen IS. Aortic regurgitation. In: Perrino AC, Reeves ST, eds. *A Practical Approach to Transesophageal Echocardiography.* 2nd ed. Wolters Kluwer; 2008:226-240.

2. de Marchi SF, Windecker S, Aeschbacher BC, Seiler C. Influence of left ventricular relaxation on the pressure half time of aortic regurgitation. *Heart.* 1999;82(5):607-613.

3. Zoghbi WA, Adams D, Bonow RO, et al. Recommendations for noninvasive evaluation of native valvular regurgitation: a report from the American Society of Echocardiography developed in collaboration with the society for cardiovascular magnetic resonance. *J Am Soc Echocardiogr.* 2017;30(4):303-371.

**4.** Correct Answer: **B. Percutaneous device closure**

*Rationale:* The primary variant demonstrated in this case is a PFO. Up to 40% of all ischemic strokes are considered cryptogenic, implying a stroke without a definitive etiology, and a PFO is found in half of younger patients (<60 years) with a cryptogenic stroke. PFOs are reported in up to 29% of the population. Device closure is frequently indicated in the setting of PFO history of cryptogenic strokes
There is no mention of wall motion abnormalities or other signs of coronary disease; hence, bypass surgery is not indicated. Pulmonary thromboendarterectomy is indicated in chronic thromboembolic pulmonary hypertension, which is not described in the case patient. Though stroke may be related to left atrial appendage thrombus, the case patient has no data indicating this as her source.

Selected References

1. Hagen PT, Scholz DG, Edwards WD. Incidence and size of patent foramen ovale during the first 10 decades of life: an autopsy study of 965 normal hearts. *Mayo Clin Proc.* 1984;59:17-20.

2. Kent DM, Dahabreh IJ, Ruthazer R, et al. Device closure of patent foramen ovale after stroke: pooled analysis of completed randomized trials. *J Am Coll Cardiol.* 2016;67:907-917.

3. Kerut EK, Norfleet WT, Plotnick GD, Giles TD. Patent foramen ovale: a review of associated conditions and the impact of physiological size. *J Am Coll Cardiol.* 2001;38(3):613-623.

**5.** Correct Answer: **D. Implanted cardiac devices or catheters may inadvertently cross the presented pathology**

*Rationale:* Figure 29.4 TTE demonstrates a small PFO by CFD; however, the "gold standard" for diagnosing PFO entails a bubble study while administering a Valsalva maneuver *along with* CFD. PFO and

ASA are related structural abnormalities of the atrial septum. PFOs are reported in up to 29% of the population. ASA is defined as ≥1 cm of septal excursion toward either the right or left atrium, with a base excursion ≥1.5 cm. The association between PFO and ASA is derived from the observation that in patients with a stroke history and the combined PFO and ASA abnormalities, the recurrent stroke risk is significantly higher than in those with an isolated PFO.

### Selected Reference

1. Hari P, Pai RG, Varadarajan P. Echocardiographic evaluation of patent foramen ovale and atrial septal defect. *Echocardiography*. 2015;32 Suppl 2:S110-S124.

---

**6.** Correct Answer: **C. Paravalvular regurgitation**

*Rationale:* Figure 29.5 TEE shows a mechanical valve placed into the mitral position (mid-esophageal probe position, 0-20° angulation). TEE is invaluable in helping to evaluate a newly placed valve for regurgitation, valve stenosis, and valve malposition. In the above image, an eccentrically directed paravalvular regurgitant jet (paravalvular leak [PVL]) is noted, usually caused by incomplete fixation of the prosthetic sewing ring to the native annulus, or dehiscence of the sewing ring. In the past, surgical closure was the treatment of choice for symptomatic patients with PVLs. The less invasive alternative, transcatheter PVL closure, is safe and effective, with lower procedural morbidity and mortality. However, transcatheter PVL is not available for all types of valves and anatomy and requires meticulous preprocedural planning.

Mechanical valves normally permit some "leakage regurgitant jets" preventing thrombus formation on the valve; these are generally small, symmetric, lower flow jets. Pathologic transvalvular jets in mechanical valves are often from chronic degenerative changes but can occur acutely if a valve leaflet malfunctions and will not close properly. This image can mimic flow from the left atrial appendage into the left atrium, but one can see the mechanical valve leaflet immediately adjacent to the jet. Also, the higher velocity/aliased jet with a definitive vector argues against it being flow from the left atrial appendage.

### Selected References

1. Cheung AT. Prosthetic valves. In: Perrino AC, Reeves ST, eds. *A Practical Approach to Transesophageal Echocardiography*. 2nd ed. Wolters Kluwer; 2008:257-280.
2. Cruz-Gonzalez I, Rama-Merchan JC, Rodríguez-Collado J, et al. Transcatheter closure of paravalvular leaks: state of the art. *Neth Heart J*. 2017 Feb;25(2):116-124.

---

**7.** Correct Answer: **D. Surgical or percutaneous removal of the pacemaker leads is indicated.**

*Rationale:* Infections related to implantable cardiac electronic devices (ICEDs) are increasing in incidence and can be life-threatening. An early diagnosis and appropriate management can help to decrease infection-related morbidity and mortality. TEE is preferred to visualize lead infections and also to determine whether the tricuspid valve is affected. TTE has a lower sensitivity than TEE (22%-43% vs 90%-96%). Lack of appropriate antimicrobial prophylaxis has been the most consistently identified risk factor. Valve involvement is often not limited to the tricuspid valve, with the aortic or mitral valve affected in 10% to 15% of patients. Multivalvular involvement is associated with higher mortality. Surgical or percutaneous removal of infected leads is recommended.

### Selected References

1. Saghir MK, Banerjee S, Cooper DH. Infective endocarditis. In: Rasalingam R, Majesh M, Pérez JE, eds. *The Washington Manual of Echocardiography*. Wolters Kluwer; 2012: 180–191; Chapter 14.
2. Sandoe JAT, Barlow G, Chambers JB, et al. Guidelines for the diagnosis, prevention and management of implantable cardiac electronic device infection. Report of a joint Working Party project on behalf of the British Society for Antimicrobial Chemotherapy (BSAC, host organization), British Heart Rhythm Society (BHRS), British Cardiovascular Society (BCS), British Heart Valve Society (BHVS) and British Society for Echocardiography (BSE). *J Antimicrob Chemother*. 2015;70(2):325-359. doi: 10.1093/jac/dku383

---

**8.** Correct Answer: **D. Lipomatous hypertrophy of the atrial septum (LHAS)**

*Rationale:* LHAS is usually a benign anomaly of the heart. Lipomatous infiltration involves the upper and lower portions of atrial septum, sparing the fossa ovalis, which gives a characteristic hourglass-shaped appearance. One of the rare risk factors is emphysema with chronic steroid therapy, causing a mediastinal and intracardiac deposition of adipose tissue. LHAS has been associated with various atrial arrhythmias, including atrial fibrillation and rarely sudden death.

Selected References

1. Bielicki G, Lukaszewski M, Kosiorowska K. Lipomatous hypertrophy of the atrial septum – a benign heart anomaly causing unexpected surgical problems: a case report. *BMC Cardiovasc Disord*. 2018;18:152.
2. Arnold SV. Cardiac masses. In: Rasalingam R, Majesh M,  Pérez JE, eds. *The Washington Manual of Echocardiography*. Wolters Kluwer; 2012: 251–260; Chapter 18.

## 9. Correct Answer: A. Thrombus

*Rationale:* It is important to appreciate that as a clinician, one cannot make a tissue diagnosis solely based on echocardiography. The TTE parasternal RV inflow image (Figure 29.7) clearly demonstrates an abnormality associated with the tricuspid valve. It is not an artifact but any further details about the echogenic mass are indeterminate. The differential diagnosis for a valvular-associated echogenic mass include tumor, thrombus, and vegetation. There is no visible implanted catheter, making catheter-associated infection incorrect. A Chiari network is a right atrial structure typically seen as a thin reticulated network of fibers originating from the Eustachian valve, occasionally fenestrated, connecting to various parts of the right atrium.

Selected References

1. Baddour LM, Wilson WR, Bayer AS, et al. Infective Endocarditis in Adults: Diagnosis, Antimicrobial Therapy, and Management of Complications: A Scientific Statement for Healthcare Professionals From the American Heart Association. Circulation 2015; 132:1435.
2. Habib G, Lancellotti P, Antunes MJ, et al. 2015 ESC Guidelines for the management of infective endocarditis: The Task Force for the Management of Infective Endocarditis of the European Society of Cardiology (ESC). Endorsed by: European Association for Cardio-Thoracic Surgery (EACTS), the European Association of Nuclear Medicine (EANM). *Eur Heart J.* 2015;36:3075.
3. Onwuanyi AE, Brown RJ, Vahedi M, Narayanan R, Nash IS, Goldman ME. Eustachian valve thrombus: critical factor in outcome of venous thromboembolism. *Echocardiography*. 2003;20(1):71-73.

## 10. Correct Answer: B. LV false tendon

*Rationale:* The arrow in this apical long-axis TTE (Figure 29.9) indicates an LV false tendon, which is a fibromuscular band extending across the LV cavity from the septum to the lateral wall. A moderator band would be located in a similar region but in the right ventricle. The Eustachian valve is a valve flap at the inferior vena cava–right atrial junction. A coumadin ridge is actually normal cardiac anatomy; it is a ridge of tissue separating the left atrial appendage from the left upper pulmonary vein. The crista terminalis is a vertical ridge of myocardium located at the orifice of the superior vena cava–right atrial junction.

Selected References

1. Arnold SV. Cardiac masses. In: Rasalingam R, Majesh M,  Pérez JE, eds. *The Washington Manual of Echocardiography*. Wolters Kluwer; 2012: 251–260; Chapter 18.
2. Rajiah P, MacNamara J, Chaturvedi A, Ashwath R, Fulton NL, Goerne H. Bands in the heart: multimodality imaging review. *Radiographics*. 2019:180176. doi: 10.1148/rg.2019180176. [Epub ahead of print]

## 11. Correct Answer: D. Systolic anterior motion (SAM) of the mitral valve leaflets

*Rationale:* All of these choices can contribute to post-bypass hypotension. Figure 29.10 demonstrates the anterior motion of mitral valve leaflets toward the interventricular septum during systole, causing a dynamic left ventricular outflow tract obstruction (LVOTO). The following anatomic and hemodynamic factors predispose to this condition:
- Redundant mitral valve leaflets
- Papillary muscle displacement
- Interventricular septal hypertrophy
- Chordal anomaly
- Hypovolemia
- Increased contractility
- Tachycardia
- Low peripheral vascular resistance (vasoplegia)

Selected References

1. Licker M, Diaper J, Cartier V, et al. Management of weaning from cardiopulmonary bypass after cardiac surgery. *Ann Card Anaesth*. 2012;15(3):206-223.
2. Dugar S, Latifi M, Moghekar A, Duggal A. All shock states are not the same systolic anterior motion of mitral valve causing left ventricular outflow tract obstruction in septic shock. *Ann Am Thorac Soc*. 2016;13(10):1851-1855.

**12.** Correct Answer: B. Aortic valve closure and mitral regurgitation

*Rationale:* It is important to appreciate the value of different imaging modalities, in this case M-mode and color Doppler, which can assist with accurate diagnosis. LVOTO may lead to early closure or fluttering of the aortic valve because of reduced subvalvular pressure. Mitral regurgitation with posteriorly directed jet occurs due to incomplete coaptation of the leaflets.

Selected Reference

1. Holley CL. Cardiomyopathies. In: Rasalingam R, Majesh M, Pérez JE, eds. *The Washington Manual of Echocardiography.* Wolters Kluwer; 2012 : 88–106; Chapter 8.

**13.** Correct Answer: C. Stop epinephrine and start infusion of vasoconstrictor

*Rationale:* Effective management of SAM/LVOTO should be directed at correcting the predisposing hemodynamic factors listed in explanations to **Question 29.11**. Increase in LV end-diastolic volume can be achieved by augmentation of venous return, increase in diastolic filling time, and intravascular volume expansion. Switching from an inoconstrictor (epinephrine) to a pure vasoconstrictor without inotropic properties (phenylephrine or vasopressin) reduces cardiac contractility, heart rate, and LVOT blood flow velocity. Intra-aortic balloon pump may exacerbate the SAM/LVOTO by augmenting contractility and reducing the afterload. Initiation of ECMO can be used as a last resort if all other measures to support hemodynamics fail.

Selected Reference

1. Dugar S, Latifi M, Moghekar A, Duggal A. All shock states are not the same systolic anterior motion of mitral valve causing left ventricular outflow tract obstruction in septic shock. *Ann Am Thorac Soc.* 2016;13(10):1851-1855.

**14.** Correct Answer: C. Leaflet perforation/rupture

*Rationale:* The parasternal short-axis view at the level of aortic valve demonstrates tricuspid valve endocarditis (Figure 29.12). Being a right-sided vegetation, it is very unlikely the patient's disease process would impact the systemic artery (coronary, cerebral, etc.) unless there is a right-to-left shunt (eg, PFO). **Table 29.1** lists complications of endocarditis.

**Table 29.1 Complications of Endocarditis**

| Structural | Hemodynamic |
|---|---|
| Leaflet rupture | Acute valve regurgitation |
| Flail leaflet | Valve obstruction |
| Leaflet perforation | Heart failure |
| Abscess | Intracardiac shunt |
| Aneurysm | Perivalvular regurgitation |
| Fistula | Tamponade |
| Prosthetic valve dehiscence | |
| Embolization | |
| Pericardial effusion | |

Selected References

1. Byku M, Makan M, Quader N. Infective endocarditis. In: Quader N, Makan M, Perez J, eds. *Washington Manual of Echocardiography.* 2nd ed. Wolters Kluwer, 2017:194-207.
2. Habib, G, Lancellotti, P, Antunes, MJ, et al. 2015 ESC guidelines for the management of infective endocarditis: the Task Force for the Management of Infective Endocarditis of the European Society of Cardiology (ESC). Endorsed by: European Association for Cardio-Thoracic Surgery (EACTS), the European Association of Nuclear Medicine (EANM). *Eur Heart J.* 2015;36:3075-3128.
3. Infective endocarditis. In: Armstrong W, Ryan T, eds. *Feigenbaum's Echocardiography.* 8th ed. Wolters Kluwer; 2019:347-376.

**15.** Correct Answer: B. Coumadin ridge

*Rationale:* All of these structures are those seen in a typical mid-esophageal four-chamber or two-chamber TEE view (Figure 29.13). The left upper pulmonary vein is above the coumadin ridge and the left atrial appendage is inferior to the coumadin ridge.

Selected Reference

1. Byku M, Makan M, Quader N. Infective endocarditis. In: Quader N, Makan M, Perez J, eds. *Washington Manual of Echocardiography.* 2nd ed. Wolters Kluwer, 2017:194-207.

**16.** Correct Answer: D. Moderator band–associated thrombus

*Rationale:* In this zoomed-in apical four-chamber TTE view (Figure 29.14), one notices an abnormal mobile echolucency in the mid-to-apical region of the right ventricle. Endocarditis is possible but is unlikely in an otherwise healthy patient with no fevers or risk factors for endocarditis. Myxomas are typically pedunculated mobile masses attached to the interatrial septum. This mass does not have the appearance or typical location for a myxoma. Fibroelastomas are typically located on the downstream side of valvular surfaces. Fibroelastomas are frond-like in morphology, benign, and rarely cause any hemodynamic disturbances. In a sedentary hospitalized patient, the most likely possibility is thrombus, which in this case is associated with his moderator band and possibly one or more of the RV trabeculations. The right ventricle is a relatively uncommon site for intracardiac masses and the presence of RV trabeculations can make identification of masses challenging. The most common caval or right atrium mass is a thrombus; hence, the RV would be the next most likely region for thrombus. This clinical scenario likely is more common than appreciated, with most thromboemboli passing through the right heart.

Selected References

1. Kwak YL, Shim JK. Assessment of endocarditis and intracardiac masses by TEE. *Int Anesthesiol Clin.* 2008;46(2):105-120.
2. Malik M, Shilo K, Kilic A. Papillary fibroelastoma arising from the coumadin ridge. *J Cardiovasc Thorac Res.* 2017;9(2):118-120.

**17.** Correct Answer: C. Mitral valve prolapse.

*Rationale:* Of the four listed answers, mitral valve prolapse is the only condition associated with an intermediate risk for the development of infective endocarditis; the other four choices are all four of the highest-risk variables associated with the development of endocarditis.

Selected Reference

1. Habib, G, Lancellotti, P, Antunes, MJ, et al. 2015 ESC guidelines for the management of infective endocarditis: the Task Force for the Management of Infective Endocarditis of the European Society of Cardiology (ESC). Endorsed by: European Association for Cardio-Thoracic Surgery (EACTS), the European Association of Nuclear Medicine (EANM). *Eur Heart J.* 2015;36:3075-3128.

**18.** Correct Answer: D. Thrombus in left atrial appendage

*Rationale:* TEE is an invaluable resource in evaluating cardiac function and pathology. The above image is taken from the mid-esophageal position at 30°. Several of the above answer choices seem plausible at first until it is fully determined what structures are being visualized. The white arrow points to thrombus plainly visible in the left atrial appendage (a common location for cardiac thrombi, especially in patients with atrial fibrillation). Thrombi in the left atrial appendage can lead to cerebrovascular accident.

Selected Reference

1. Jadbabaie F. Cardiac masses and embolic sources. In: Perrino AC, Reeves ST, eds. *A Practical Approach to Transesophageal Echocardiography.* 2nd ed. Wolters Kluwer; 2008:401-413.

**19.** Correct Answer: C. Highly mobile and oscillating

*Rationale:* A large endocarditis lesion on the atrial side of the tricuspid valve is presented in this image. **Table 29.2** lists positive and negative echocardiographic features demonstrative of endocarditis.

**Table 29.2 Endocarditis Features**

| Negative Feature | Positive Feature |
| --- | --- |
| High echogenicity | Low reflectance |
| Nonvalvular location | Attached to valve/upstream side |
| Smooth surface | Irregularly shaped |
| Nonmobile | Highly mobile/oscillating |
| Absence of tissue destruction/regurgitation | Tissue destruction/valve regurgitation |

Selected References

1. Habib, G, Lancellotti, P, Antunes, MJ, et al. 2015 ESC guidelines for the management of infective endocarditis: the Task Force for the Management of Infective Endocarditis of the European Society of Cardiology (ESC). Endorsed by: European Association for Cardio-Thoracic Surgery (EACTS), the European Association of Nuclear Medicine (EANM). *Eur Heart J.* 2015;36:3075-3128.
2. Infective endocarditis. In: Armstrong W, Ryan T, eds. *Feigenbaum's Echocardiography*. 8th ed. Wolters Kluwer; 2019:347-376.

**20.** Correct Answer: A. The greater the mobility of the endocarditis lesion, the greater the likelihood for an embolic event.

*Rationale/Critique:* The larger the vegetation, the greater the risk of an embolic event. Similarly, increased mobility increases the risk of an embolic event happening. Option C is incorrect because it has been shown that after beginning antibiotics, the risk of an embolic stroke due to endocarditis decreases. Embolic risk is higher with endocarditis of the mitral valve as compared to the aortic valve.

Selected References

1. Anavekar NS, Schultz JC, De Sa DD, et al. Modifiers of symptomatic embolic risk in infective endocarditis. *Mayo Clin Proc.* 2011;86(11):1068-1074.
2. Chang E, Lee KH, Yang KY, Lee YC, Perng RP. Septic pulmonary embolism associated with a peri-proctal abscess in an immunocompetent host. *BMJ Case Rep.* 2009;2009:bcr07.2008.0592. doi:10.1136/bcr.07.2008.0592.
3. Okonta KE, Adamu YB. What size of vegetation is an indication for surgery in endocarditis? *Interact Cardiovasc Thorac Surg.* 2012;15(6):1052-1056.
4. Rizzi M, Ravasio V, Carobbio A, et al. Predicting the occurrence of embolic events: an analysis of 1456 episodes of infective endocarditis from the Italian Study on Endocarditis (SEI). *BMC Infect Dis.* 2014;14:230.

# 30 | LEFT ATRIAL AND RIGHT ATRIAL SIZE, FUNCTION, AND PATHOLOGY

Bryan Simmons

1. A 67-year-old gentleman presents to the hospital with chest pain and is ultimately diagnosed with a non-ST-elevation myocardial infarction (NSTEMI). Cardiac catheterization reveals multivessel coronary artery disease and he is scheduled to undergo coronary artery bypass grafting. A preoperative transthoracic echocardiogram (TTE) demonstrates normal biventricular function as well as the following imaging shown in **Figure 30.1** and ▶ **Video 30.1.**

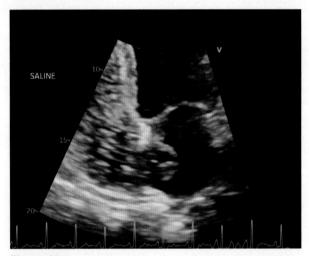

**Figure 30.1**

Based on the imaging, the patient is most likely to have which of the following?
A. Positive blood cultures
B. A patent foramen ovale (PFO)
C. A defect in the septum secundum
D. A cleft mitral valve leaflet

2. A 58-year-old female with hypertension and hyperlipidemia presents to the Emergency Department with a 2-hour history of word-finding difficulty. The patient is diagnosed with a stroke and administered tissue plasminogen activator (tPA) with resolution of her symptoms. She undergoes a TTE for evaluation of a cardioembolic etiology of her stroke. ▶ **Video 30.2** is obtained.

Based on ▶ **Video 30.2**, the patient *most* likely has which of the following?
A. A PFO
B. A ventricular septal defect
C. A transpulmonary shunt
D. An atrial septal defect (ASD)

3. A 56-year-old gentleman with a history of hypertension and obesity is admitted to the intensive care unit (ICU) with fever, hypotension, and hypoxemia. He remains hypotensive despite 30 mL/kg of intravenous (IV) fluids and IV antibiotics. He is intubated and a transesophageal echocardiogram (TEE) is performed. Interrogation of the interatrial septum is shown **in Figure 30.2**.

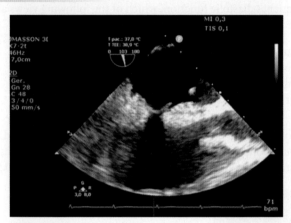

**Figure 30.2**

Which of the following would the patient *most* likely benefit from?

A. Inhaled pulmonary vasodilators
B. Vasopressors
C. Percutaneous placement of a septal occlusion device
D. Cardiac surgery consult for resection of an intracardiac mass

4. A 64-year-old female presents to the Emergency Department with a 3-week history of palpitations and a 2-day history of presyncopal episodes. Electrocardiography (ECG) reveals atrial fibrillation with rapid ventricular response. Despite attempts at rate control, the patient remains in atrial fibrillation with intermittent presyncopal episodes. She is ultimately scheduled for TEE and synchronized cardioversion. Based upon the TEE images obtained as shown in **Figure 30.3**, ▶ **Videos 30.3,** and **30.4**, which of the following is *most* accurate?

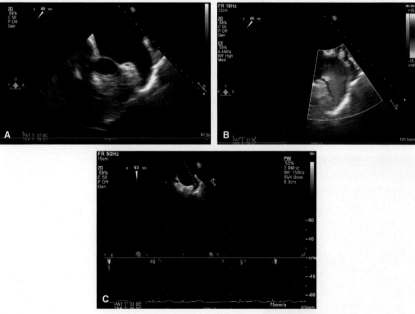

**Figure 30.3**

A. There is no clot visualized in the left atrial appendage (LAA); however, LAA exiting velocities are low and the patient may still be at risk for cardioembolic stroke following cardioversion.
B. There is a clot in the LAA. No cardioversion should be attempted.
C. There is no clot visualized in the LAA. Exiting velocities are normal. Cardioversion should be attempted.
D. TEE is not an appropriate test to evaluate LAA thrombus.

5. A 75-year-old female with a history of hypertension, obesity, and nonobstructive coronary artery disease is admitted to the ICU on postoperative day 2 following a left hip arthroplasty with new-onset atrial fibrillation and an increase in oxygen requirement. Her ECG is without significant ST changes, troponins are negative, and brain natriuretic peptide is elevated. Diastolic dysfunction is suspected and a TTE is performed. In assessing this patient's diastolic function, which of the following views and measurement methods are *most* appropriate in assessing left atrial (LA) size?

   A. Biplane method of discs, apical four-chamber and apical two-chamber views
   B. Anteroposterior (AP) linear measurement, parasternal long-axis view
   C. Area-length technique, apical four-chamber and apical two-chamber views
   D. Area via planimetry, apical four-chamber view

6. A 50-year-old female with a 2-month history of worsening dyspnea on exertion is intubated and sedated in the ICU after being admitted for a stroke. A transthoracic echocardiogram (TTE) is attempted but results in poor image quality. A transesophageal echocardiogram (TEE) is obtained (**Figure 30.4** and ▶ **Video 30.5**).

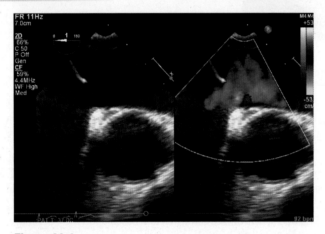

**Figure 30.4**

Which of the following is *most* likely true of the anatomic abnormality shown in Figure 30.4 and ▶ **Video 30.5**?
A. The defect is associated with partial anomalous pulmonary venous return (PAPVR)
B. There is a defect in the septum secundum
C. The defect is associated with Scimitar syndrome
D. There is a defect in the septum primum

7. A 39-year-old female is admitted to the ICU with a 3-week history of worsening shortness of breath and lower extremity swelling. A focused TTE is performed (**Figure 30.5** and ▶ **Video 30.6**). What is the structure indicated by the *arrow* in Figure 30.5?

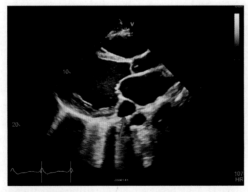

**Figure 30.5**
A. Aorta
B. Pericardial cyst
C. Left atrial appendage
D. Coronary sinus

**8.** A 57-year-old male with a history of recent lung resection for primary lung cancer 2 weeks ago is admitted to the ICU with shortness of breath. A focused bedside ultrasound is performed (**Figure 30.6** and ▶ **Video 30.7**). Which of the following is *most* likely true of the structure indicated by the *arrow* in Figure 30.6?

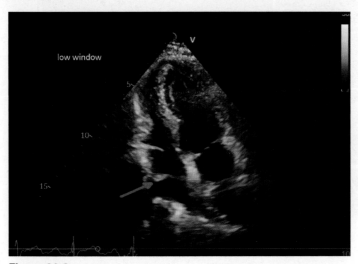

**Figure 30.6**

**A.** The structure is a remnant of fetal life
**B.** The structure is most consistent with thrombus
**C.** The structure is most consistent with a vegetation
**D.** The structure is an artifact

**9.** A 56-year-old female with a distant history of lung cancer status post resection presents with worsening orthopnea and dyspnea on exertion. As part of her workup, the patient undergoes a TTE, which is followed by a TEE. Images from both studies are shown in **Figure 30.7,** ▶ **Videos 30.8,** and ▶ **30.9.**

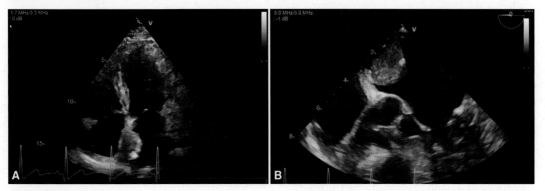

**Figure 30.7**

Which of the following is the *most* appropriate next step in her management?
**A.** Administer tPA for pulmonary embolism
**B.** Start antibiotics
**C.** Cardiac surgical consultation
**D.** The finding is a benign condition; continue working up the patient's orthopnea and dyspnea on exertion

**10.** Pulmonary venous (**Figure 30.8A**) and transmitral spectral Doppler (**Figure 30.8B**) profiles were obtained in a patient following coronary artery bypass grafting. The pulmonary artery occlusion pressure (PAOP) waveform is also shown in **Figure 30.8C**.

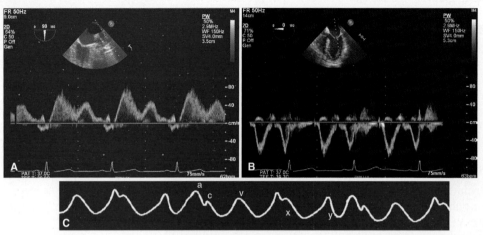

**Figure 30.8**

Which of the following statements is *most* accurate?

**A.** The a-wave on the PAOP waveform correlates with the D-wave on the pulmonary venous Doppler profile and the E-wave on the transmitral Doppler profile.

**B.** The v-wave on the PAOP waveform correlates with the D-wave on the pulmonary venous Doppler profile and the E-wave on the transmitral Doppler profile.

**C.** The y-descent on the PAOP waveform correlates with the D-wave on the pulmonary venous Doppler profile and the E-wave on the transmitral Doppler profile.

**D.** The y-descent on the PAOP waveform correlates with the S-wave on the pulmonary venous Doppler profile and the E-wave on the transmitral Doppler profile.

# Chapter 30 ▪ Answers

**1.** Correct Answer: **B. A patent foramen ovale (PFO)**

*Rationale:* ▶ **Video 30.1** demonstrates an atrial septal aneurysm (ASA), which is a redundant, mobile atrial septal tissue present in approximately 2% of the general population. Although most patients with ASAs are asymptomatic, the presence of an ASA is associated with a PFO, Chiari network, and stroke. Echocardiographic diagnosis of an ASA requires a total septal excursion (right and left) of at least 15 mm or an excursion of at least 10 mm into either chamber (right or left atrium). M-mode can be particularly useful in obtaining these measurements.

There is no clinical or echocardiographic suggestion of endocarditis that would put the patient at risk for having positive blood cultures. When the atrioventricular valves are involved, vegetations usually involve the atrial side of the valve. Vegetations are also associated with regurgitation and move in tandem with the valve leaflet. The septum secundum is the thicker portion of the interatrial septum. Primum ASDs are associated with a cleft mitral valve leaflet, an invagination of mitral valve leaflet, resulting in mitral regurgitation.

Selected References

1. Agmon Y, Khandheria BK, Meissner I, et al. Frequency of atrial septal aneurysms in patients with cerebral ischemic events. *Circulation.* 1999;99(15):1942-1944.

2. Cabanes L, Mas JL, Cohen A, et al. Atrial septal aneurysm and patent foramen ovale as risk factors for cryptogenic stroke in patients less than 55 years of age. A study using transesophageal echocardiography. *Stroke.* 1993;24(12):1865-1873.

3. Pearson AC, Nagelhout D, Castello R, Gomez CR, Labovitz AJ. Atrial septal aneurysm and stroke: a transesophageal echocardiographic study. *J Am Coll Cardiol.* 1991;18(5):1223-1229.

**2.** Correct Answer: C. A transpulmonary shunt

*Rationale:* ▶ **Video 30.2** is a bubble study. While TEE is considered the gold standard in detection of intracardiac shunts at the atrial level, bubble studies obtained with TTE are typically the initial imaging modality given the less invasive nature and acceptable sensitivity and specificity. A bubble study is commonly performed with 10 mL of agitated saline (or 8-10 mL of saline mixed with 0.5 mL of air) rapidly injected through a peripheral IV catheter. When interrogating the interatrial septum, provocative maneuvers, such as Valsalva maneuver or abdominal pressure, are provided to transiently increase right atrial pressures and elicit a right-to-left shunt. These maneuvers are released once the contrast opacifies the right atrium. The apical four-chamber view is the preferred imaging plane when a bubble study is performed. It is recommended to record at least 20 consecutive heart beats to ensure detection of transpulmonary shunts. A bubble study is positive for an intracardiac shunt if bubbles are seen in the left atrium or left ventricle within four cardiac cycles following opacification of the right atrium. Appearance of bubbles in the left-sided chambers beyond six cardiac cycles is most consistent with a transpulmonary shunt, which can be seen with pulmonary arteriovenous (AV) malformations and hepatopulmonary syndrome. With transpulmonary shunting, the contrast may be seen originating from the pulmonary veins.

The bubble study provided in the vignette illustrates a transpulmonary shunt. Contrast appears in the left atrium, but not until the tenth cardiac cycle following opacification of the right atrium.

Selected References
1. Mitchell C, Rahko PS, Blauwet LA, et al. Guidelines for performing a comprehensive transthoracic echocardiographic examination in adults: recommendations from the American Society of Echocardiography. *J Am Soc Echocardiogr.* 2019;32(1):1-64.
2. Silvestry FE, Cohen MS, Armsby LB, et al. Guidelines for the echocardiographic assessment of atrial septal defect and patent foramen ovale: from the American Society of Echocardiography and Society of Cardiac Angiography and Interventions. *J Am Soc Echocardiogr.* 2015;28(8):910-958.

**3.** Correct Answer: B. Vasopressors

*Rationale:* There are a number of benign anatomic variants involving the atria that the astute echocardiographer must know. Figure 30.2 illustrates lipomatous hypertrophy of the atrial septum (LHAS), a condition caused by adipose infiltration of the interatrial septum. The incidence of LHAS has been quoted to be as high as 7%. Echocardiographically, LHAS appears as a circumscribed, dumbbell-like structure involving the superior and inferior portions of the interatrial septum. Typically, the fossa ovalis is spared. This condition is nearly always benign and of no hemodynamic significance.

In the setting of suspected sepsis, initiation of vasopressor therapy for persistent hypotension is the most appropriate next step following source control, antibiotics, and fluid resuscitation. Percutaneous septal occlusion devices are Food and Drug Administration (FDA)-approved for transcatheter closure of a PFO to prevent recurrent stroke in patients with a history of cryptogenic stroke. There is no evidence of a PFO on the image provided, nor is there a history of cryptogenic stroke.

Selected Reference
1. Pochis WT, Saeian K, Sagar KB. Usefulness of transesophageal echocardiography in diagnosing lipomatous hypertrophy of the atrial septum with comparison to transthoracic echocardiography. *Am J Cardiol.* 1992;70(3):396-398.

**4.** Correct Answer: A. There is no clot visualized in the LAA; however, LAA exiting velocities are low and the patient may still be at risk for cardioembolic stroke following cardioversion.

*Rationale:* For patients in whom maintenance of normal sinus rhythm is desirable and conventional anticoagulation (consisting of 3-4 weeks of therapeutic anticoagulation) prior to cardioversion is not feasible, TEE can be utilized to evaluate the atria for the presence of clot. TEE is superior to TTE in this regard given the closer proximity of the TEE transducer to the atria and the higher frequency (better resolution).

Thrombus responsible for cardioembolic events most frequently arises from the LAA. In evaluating for thrombus, the LAA should be imaged in multiple planes with 2D imaging. Color flow Doppler (CFD) should be utilized to ensure the entire LAA fills with color, employing a lower Nyquist limit. Pulse-wave Doppler (PWD) is useful in measuring LAA flow velocities. As peak LAA exiting velocities fall below 40 cm/s, one must become increasingly suspicious of LAA thrombus risk. Peak LAA exiting velocities less than 20 cm/s have been clearly associated with LAA thrombus and stroke. To obtain LAA flow velocities, the PWD sample cursor should be placed 1 cm into the LAA. Note that when using TEE, LAA exiting velocities obtained with PWD travel *toward* the transducer and by convention are displayed *above* the baseline.

A common pitfall is mistaking the ligament of Marshall, or artifacts arising from this structure, as LAA thrombus. The ligament of Marshall, also known as the coumadin ridge or warfarin ridge, is the atrial tissue that separates the LAA from the left upper pulmonary vein. Imaging the LAA from multiple different planes will help avoid this problem.

In this vignette, there is no clot present in the LAA on TEE imaging. The LAA fills completely with color Doppler; however, LAA exiting velocities seen on the PWD image provided are less than 20 cm/s. As mentioned earlier, LAA exiting velocities less than 20 cm/s are associated with both clot formation and stroke.

### Selected References

1. Goldman ME, Pearce LA, Hart RG, et al. Pathophysiologic correlates of thromboembolism in nonvalvular atrial fibrillation: I. Reduced flow velocity in the left atrial appendage (The Stroke Prevention in Atrial Fibrillation [SPAF-III] study). *J Am Soc Echocardiogr.* 1999;12(12):1080-1087.
2. Klein AL, Grimm RA, Murray RD, et al. Use of transesophageal echocardiography to guide cardioversion in patients with atrial fibrillation. *N Engl J Med.* 2001;344(19):1411-1420.

**5.** Correct Answer: A. Biplane method of discs, apical four-chamber and apical two-chamber views

*Rationale:* LA enlargement is associated with a number of adverse outcomes including stroke, atrial fibrillation, diastolic dysfunction, and congestive heart failure. As mentioned in the vignette, LA size is important in assessing diastolic dysfunction with LA enlargement being one diagnostic criteria. The clinical significance of diastolic dysfunction in the ICU patient population is becoming increasingly recognized. The presence of diastolic dysfunction has been associated with failure to wean from mechanical ventilation and even mortality.

In patients with restrictive cardiomyopathies and restrictive filling patterns, LA enlargement can be quite remarkable and atrial size can approach the size of the left ventricle. Measurements of the left atrium can be obtained from a multitude of views; however, LA volume measurements are recommended by guidelines. Volume measurements more accurately reflect LA remodeling and enlargement, which can occur in all directions. The recommended technique to measure LA volume is the disc summation method (or biplane method of discs, **Figure 30.9A**) in which LA volume is approximated with a series of discs. After the volume of each disc is estimated, the discs are summed to yield a total LA volume. Note that the LAA and pulmonary veins are not included in the measurement. Also, *measurements of LA size should always be obtained at the end of left ventricular (LV) systole, when the left atrium is largest.* LA volume is indexed to body surface area (BSA) with LA enlargement defined as $>34$ mL/m$^2$. As mentioned previously, an LA indexed volume of $>34$ mL/m$^2$ is one of the diagnostic criteria for diastolic dysfunction.

Other methods for LA quantification are commonly obtained. The most commonly reported linear measurement (**Figure 30.9B**) is the LA AP diameter obtained from the parasternal long-axis view. With the aortic root in long axis, the LA is measured with a perpendicular line drawn at the level of the aortic sinus. Normal values for women are 2.7 to 3.8 cm and for men are 3.0 to 4.0 cm. Three-dimensional echocardiography has shown promise in the evaluation of LA size, but currently lacks robust standardization of normal values and is not a recommended standard at this time.

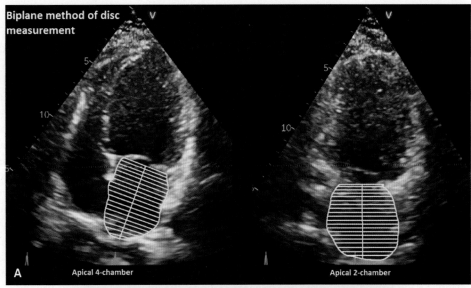

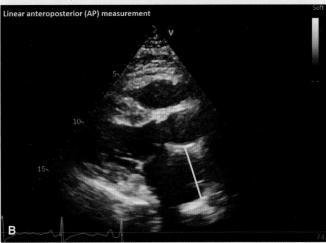

**Figure 30.9**

## Selected References

1. Barnes ME, Miyasaka Y, Seward JB, et al. Left atrial volume in the prediction of first ischemic stroke in an elderly cohort without atrial fibrillation. *Mayo Clin Proc*. 2004;79(8):1008-1014.
2. Benjamin EJ, D'Agostino RB, Belanger AJ, Wolf PA, Levy D. Left atrial size and the risk of stroke and death. The Framingham Heart Study. *Circulation*. 1995;92(4):835-841.
3. Gonzalez C, Begot E, Dalmay F, et al. Prognostic impact of left ventricular diastolic function in patients with septic shock. *Ann Intensive Care*. 2016;6(1):36.
4. Lang RM, Badano LP, Mor-Avi V, et al. Recommendations for cardiac chamber quantification by echocardiography in adults: an update from the American Society of Echocardiography and the European Association of Cardiovascular Imaging. *J Am Soc Echocardiogr*. 2015;28(1):1-39.
5. Mourad M, Chow-Chine L, Faucher M, et al. Early diastolic dysfunction is associated with intensive care unit mortality in cancer patients presenting with septic shock. *Br J Anaesth*. 2014;112(1):102-109.
6. Nagueh SF, Smiseth OA, Appleton CP, et al. Recommendations for the evaluation of left ventricular diastolic function by echocardiography: an update from the American Society of Echocardiography and the European Association of Cardiovascular Imaging. *J Am Soc Echocardiogr*. 2016;29(4):277-314.
7. Papanikolaou J, Makris D, Saranteas T, et al. New insights into weaning from mechanical ventilation: left ventricular diastolic dysfunction is a key player. *Intensive Care Med*. 2011;37(12):1976-1985.
8. Simek CL, Feldman MD, Haber HL, et al. Relationship between left ventricular wall thickness and left atrial size: comparison with other measures of diastolic function. *J Am Soc Echocardiogr*. 1995;8(1):37-47.
9. Tsang TS, Barnes ME, Bailey KR, et al. Left atrial volume: important risk marker of incident atrial fibrillation in 1655 older men and women. *Mayo Clin Proc*. 2001;76(5):467-475.
10. Tsang TS, Barnes ME, Gersh BJ, et al. Risks for atrial fibrillation and congestive heart failure in patient >/=65 years of age with abnormal left ventricular diastolic relaxation. *Am J Cardiol*. 2004;93(1):54-58.

**6.** Correct Answer: D. There is a defect in the septum primum

*Rationale:* There are a number of abnormal atrial septal communications that can go undiagnosed long into adulthood. These defects can predispose patients to paradoxical emboli and, if large enough, eventually lead to pulmonary hypertension and right heart failure. Although many abnormal atrial septal communications can be diagnosed with TTE, TEE is superior in characterization of atrial septal abnormalities given its higher resolution.

The most common atrial septal abnormality is a PFO. A PFO is not a true ASD, but instead is a potential communication between the atria that occurs due to incomplete fusion of the septum primum and septum secundum. It is a remnant of fetal circulation that allows shunting of oxygenated blood from the inferior vena cava (IVC) to the left atrium. A PFO is present in up to 25% of the population. A PFO can be diagnosed with TTE or TEE utilizing CFD or a bubble study. Contrast or CFD can often be seen traversing the interatrial septum between the thin septum primum and thicker septum secundum. The flow of contrast or color Doppler is typically parallel to the septum, distinguishing it from a secundum ASD.

A secundum ASD, or ostium secundum ASD, is the most common ASD. It is important to remember that a secundum ASD is actually a defect in the septum primum, the thin membranous portion of the interatrial septum. The defect can vary from small fenestrations to complete absence of the septum primum. Unlike a PFO, the direction of CFD or contrast across the interatrial septum is usually perpendicular to the septum. Secundum ASDs are amenable to percutaneous closure and associated with mitral valve prolapse, mitral regurgitation, and anomalous pulmonary venous return.

A primum ASD, or ostium primum ASD, is the second most common ASD. It is a defect in the inferior portion of the interatrial septum and falls within the spectrum of endocardial cushion defects. A primum ASD may also be referred to as a partial AV canal defect. Primum ASDs are associated with cleft mitral valves, trisomy 21, and conduction abnormalities. Complete and transitional AV canal defects consist of a primum ASD and inlet-type ventricular septal defect.

Other rare atrial communication abnormalities include sinus venosus defects and coronary sinus defects, although these are not true ASDs. Sinus venosus defects are abnormal communications between superior (SVC) or IVC and the pulmonary veins. With SVC-type sinus venosus defects, the right upper pulmonary vein drains anomalously into the SVC, resulting in PAPVR. This can be identified with TEE in the bicaval view appearing as a defect in the interatrial septum that occurs superior to the crista terminalis. IVC-type sinus venosus defects involve communication between the IVC and either the right lower or middle pulmonary vein (Scimitar syndrome). Coronary sinus defects are characterized as direct communication between the coronary sinus and the left atrium, commonly referred to as "unroofing" of the coronary sinus. This allows a communication between the left and right atria via the coronary sinus. Coronary sinus defects are associated with a persistent left superior vena cava (PLSVC).

### Selected References

1. Allan LD, Sharland GK. The echocardiographic diagnosis of totally anomalous pulmonary venous connection in the fetus. *Heart.* 2001;85(4):433-437.
2. Ari ME, Dogan V, Özgür S, et al. Persistent left superior vena cava accompanying congenital heart disease in children: experience of a tertiary care center. *Echocardiography.* 2017;34(3):436-440.
3. Craig RJ, Selzer A. Natural history and prognosis of atrial septal defect. *Circulation.* 1968;37(5):805-815.
4. Leachman RD, Cokkinos DV, Cooley DA. Association of ostium secundum atrial septal defects with mitral valve prolapse. *Am J Cardiol.* 1976;38(2):167-169.
5. Schneider B, Zienkiewicz T, Jansen V, Hofmann T, Noltenius H, Meinertz T. Diagnosis of patent foramen ovale by transesophageal echocardiography and correlation with autopsy findings. *Am J Cardiol.* 1996;77(14):1202-1209.
6. Silvestry FE, Cohen MS, Armsby LB, et al. Guidelines for the echocardiographic assessment of atrial septal defect and patent foramen ovale: from the American Society of Echocardiography and Society of Cardiac Angiography and Interventions. *J Am Soc Echocardiogr.* 2015;28(8):910-958.
7. Williams MR, Perry JC. Arrhythmias and conduction disorders associated with atrial septal defects. *J Thorac Dis.* 2018; 10(Suppl 24):S2940-S2944.

**7.** Correct Answer: D. Coronary sinus

*Rationale:* The structure indicated by the *arrow* in Figure 30.5 is the coronary sinus. In the parasternal long-axis view, the coronary sinus can be seen at the posterior junction of the left ventricle and left atrium. It is important not to confuse the coronary sinus with the descending thoracic aorta. The coronary sinus lies anterior to the pericardium, whereas the aorta lies posterior to the pericardium. The coronary sinus may not always be clearly visible in the parasternal long-axis view; however, in this patient the coronary sinus is dilated, which should raise concern for a PLSVC.

A PLSVC is the most common central venous anomaly occurring between 0.3% and 0.5% of the population. PLSVC represents persistence of the left anterior cardinal vein from fetal development. A PLSVC, which drains the left jugular and subclavian veins, drains into the coronary sinus and finally the right atrium. Many PLSVCs are diagnosed incidentally during left-sided central venous cannulation with the central venous catheter coursing to the left of the aortic knob on chest x-ray. PLSVC is typically accompanied by a dilated coronary sinus (>1.1 cm). Diagnosis can be confirmed with a bubble study. In cases of PLSVC, contrast injected into a left antecubital IV catheter will opacify the coronary sinus prior to opacification of the right atrium. It is important to remember that these patients are at risk for paradoxical embolic events because of commonly accompanied intracardiac shunts such as ASDs and coronary sinus ASDs.

The patient in the vignette did have a PLSVC. A venogram of the same patient shows an atrophic SVC and a PLSVC, which drains into the coronary sinus and then right atrium (**Figure 30.10** and ▶ **Video 30.10**).

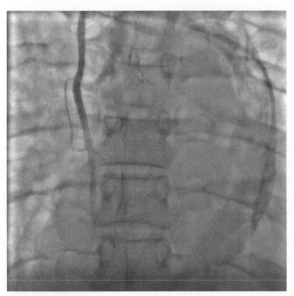

**Figure 30.10**

**Selected References**

1. Dearstine M, Taylor W, Kerut EK. Persistent left superior vena cava: chest x-ray and echocardiographic findings. *Echocardiography*. 2000;17(5):453-455.
2. Tak T, Crouch E, Drake GB. Persistent left superior vena cava: incidence, significance and clinical correlates. *Int J Cardiol*. 2002;82(1):91-93.

**8.** Correct Answer: A. The structure is a remnant of fetal life

*Rationale:* Anatomic variants are common to the atria, most of which are benign. Nonetheless, it is important to recognize these variants to avoid being led astray. The structure depicted in Figure 30.6 and ▶ **Video 30.7** in this vignette is an eustachian valve, an embryologic remnant of the right sinus venosus valve. In embryonic life, it is responsible for directing blood from the IVC through the foramen ovale. The size of the eustachian valve varies from completely absent to a long, fibrinous, mobile structure extending from the inferior cavoatrial junction. It is not clinically significant, but may be mistaken for a mass, thrombus, or vegetation.

A prominent eustachian valve should not be confused with *cor triatriatum dexter*, a rare congenital heart anomaly in which the right atrium is divided into two chambers by a thin membrane. This thin membrane is also the result of incomplete regression of the right sinus venosus valve; however, unlike a prominent eustachian valve, cor triatriatum dexter creates an obstruction to blood flow.

Other normal right atrial anatomic variants that must be distinguished from pathologic structures include the crista terminalis, Chiari network, thebesian valve, and prominent right atrial pectinate muscles. The crista terminalis is a muscular ridge dividing the IVC and SVC from the right atrium. The crista terminalis can occasionally be seen joining the eustachian valve inferiorly. Echocardiographically, a prominent crista terminalis is most frequently seen as a finger-like protrusion at the junction of the right atrium and SVC. A Chiari network, when present, is a thin, mobile, net-like structure located in the right atrium that has variable attachments to the eustachian valve, crista terminalis, right atrium, and even interatrial septum. Although thought to be benign, the presence of a Chiari network has been associated with a PFO, ASA, and arterial embolism. The thebesian valve is a thin, membranous structure at the junction of the right atrium and coronary sinus. It is rarely seen on transthoracic imaging, but can be seen occasionally with TEE. Finally, pectinate muscles can be seen in both left and right atria and when prominent can mimic masses or thrombi. Pectinate muscles are most often seen with TEE imaging as multiple, small digitated projections originating from the atrial endocardial border. These structures *do not* move independently from the atrial walls.

### Selected References

1. Moral S, Ballesteros E, Huguet M, Panaro A, Palet J, Evangelista A. Differential diagnosis and clinical implications of remnants of the right valve of the sinus venosus. *J Am Soc Echocardiogr.* 2016;29(3):183-194.
2. Schneider B, Hofmann T, Justen MH, Meinertz T. Chiari's network: normal anatomic variant or risk factor for arterial embolic events? *J Am Coll Cardiol.* 1995;26(1):203-210.

**9.** Correct Answer: C. Cardiac surgical consultation

*Rationale:* Intracardiac masses can have dramatic hemodynamic, electrical, and cardioembolic consequences. The greatest number of intracardiac masses are nonneoplastic, such as thrombi and vegetations. Neoplastic cardiac masses can be primary cardiac tumors that originate from the heart or extracardiac metastatic neoplasms that are derived from outside the heart. Extracardiac metastatic tumors are more common, particularly melanoma and lymphoma as well as lung, esophageal, and breast cancers. Primary cardiac tumors are overwhelmingly benign, such as myxomas, rhabdomyomas, fibromas, and lipomas. Recognizing common cardiac tumors that occur in adults and distinguishing them from other intracardiac masses, such as thrombi and vegetations, can have dramatic implications on treatment.

The intracardiac mass in this vignette is typical of a myxoma. Myxomas are the most common primary tumors in adulthood and typically involve the left atrium (up to at least 75% of the time), but can occur in any cardiac chamber. Patients typically present in the fourth to sixth decade of life with dyspnea, progressive congestive heart failure, systolic and diastolic murmurs, arrhythmias, or embolic phenomena. There is a slight female predominance. Myxomas can occur as part of a syndrome known as Carney complex, characterized by myxomas, endocrinopathies, and skin pigmentation.

Echocardiographically, myxomas often appear as a pedunculated mass with a smooth, lobulated, or a friable villous surface. The body of the myxoma appears nonhomogeneous and enhances with echocardiographic contrast. The stalk is usually attached to the interatrial septum near the fossa ovalis. Management of myxomas is surgical resection.

Papillary fibroelastomas are nonneoplastic endocardial growths usually attached to semilunar or atrioventricular valves. When attached to the atrioventricular valves, papillary fibroelastomas most commonly involve the atrial side. On echocardiographic imaging, fibroelastomas appear as mobile, pedunculated masses with a villous surface and homogeneous texture. Papillary fibroelastomas are often asymptomatic but can cause strokes and other embolic diseases; thus, surgical resection is often advocated.

LHAS is a benign condition of the interatrial septum characterized by adipose infiltration. Echocardiographically, LHAS is classically described as a dumbbell-shaped interatrial septum with sparing of the fossa ovalis. The texture of the interatrial septum is typically homogeneous.

Intracardiac thrombus can be of intracardiac or extracardiac origin, both of which can mimic cardiac tumors. Thrombi can be adjacent to the endocardial surface or freely floating. Intracardiac thrombi tend to form in areas of stasis. Atrial thrombi occur most frequently in the LAA, particularly in atrial fibrillation and other low-flow states such as mitral stenosis, LA enlargement, and low cardiac output. Ventricular thrombi tend to form near or adjacent to hypokinetic walls, aneurysms, or commonly the apex in dilated cardiomyopathy. With echocardiographic imaging, thrombi often appear as well-circumscribed masses that can be mobile or sessile and take a variety of different configurations. Unlike many cardiac tumors, thrombi *do not* enhance with contrast agents.

Endocarditis can also mimic cardiac tumor; however, vegetations occur predominantly in the setting of clinical sepsis. Vegetations seen in infective endocarditis have three common features. First, vegetations are frequently attached to valvular structures. When the atrioventricular valves are involved, vegetations are usually found on the atrial side. When semilunar valves are involved, vegetations are typically seen on the ventricular side. Second, vegetations are associated with valvular destruction or result in some degree of valvular regurgitation. Finally, vegetations are often accompanied by abscess formation. Vegetations themselves appear in a variety of different shapes and sizes; however, they are usually mobile, heterogeneous, and prone to embolization.

### Selected References

1. Bussani R, De-Giorgio F, Abbate A, Silvestri F. Cardiac metastases. *J Clin Pathol*. 2007;60(1):27-34.
2. Habib G, Badano L, Tribouilloy C, et al. Recommendations for the practice of echocardiography in infective endocarditis. *Eur J Echocardiogr*. 2010;11(2):202-219.
3. Maleszewski JJ, Anavekar NS, Moynihan TJ, Klarich KW. Pathology, imaging, and treatment of cardiac tumours. *Nat Rev Cardiol*. 2017;14(9):536-549.
4. McAllister HA, Hall RJ, Cooley DA. Tumors of the heart and pericardium. *Curr Probl Cardiol*. 1999;24(2):57-116.
5. Pochis WT, Saeian K, Sagar KB. Usefulness of transesophageal echocardiography in diagnosing lipomatous hypertrophy of the atrial septum with comparison to transthoracic echocardiography. *Am J Cardiol*. 1992;70(3):396-398.

**10.** Correct Answer: **C.** The y-descent on the PAOP waveform correlates with the D-wave on the pulmonary venous Doppler profile and the E-wave on the transmitral Doppler profile.

*Rationale:* LA hemodynamics are commonly utilized in the assessment of diastolic function. It is important to recognize the different components of both transmitral and pulmonary venous Doppler profiles, how they change in different physiologic or pathologic states, and how they relate to the cardiac cycle. Although this discussion is in reference to the left heart chambers, the concepts are analogous when considering the right heart chambers.

Transmitral blood flow is a diastolic phenomenon. Similar to diastole, the transmitral Doppler profile can be broken into four phases: isovolumetric relaxation time (IVRT), early filling (E-wave), diastasis, and atrial contraction (A-wave). IVRT is the period of time between aortic valve closure and opening of the mitral valve. Early filling and the E-wave begin with mitral valve opening and end with equalization of the pressures between the left ventricle and left atrium. Diastasis is the time between the end of active LV relaxation and atrial contraction. Finally, the A-wave correlates with atrial contraction. The heights of the E-wave and A-wave as well as the durations of all four phases are dependent on a number of variables (diastolic function, volume status, rhythm, etc.). In order to distinguish the E-wave from the A-wave, referencing the transmitral Doppler profile to the ECG can be helpful. Occurring in early diastole, the E-wave occurs shortly after the T-wave of the ECG. In contrast, the A-wave of the transmitral Doppler profile occurs shortly after the P-wave of the ECG. On the PAOP waveform, the a-wave correlates with the A-wave of the transmitral Doppler profile, while the y-descent correlates with the E-wave of the transmitral Doppler profile (**Figure 30.11**).

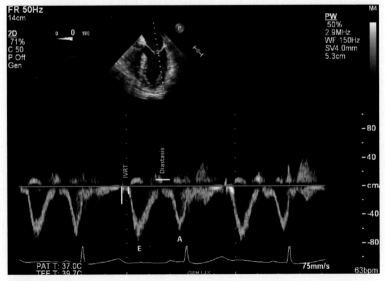

**Figure 30.11**

Whereas the transmitral Doppler profile is a depiction of how the left ventricle fills, the pulmonary venous Doppler profile illustrates how blood enters the left atrium. There are three main components of the pulmonary venous Doppler profile: systolic forward flow (S-wave), diastolic forward flow (D-wave), and an atrial reversal wave (AR-wave). The S-wave reflects the filling of the left atrium during ventricular systole (and atrial relaxation). The S-wave can sometimes be split into two components, S1 and S2. S1 occurs due to active atrial relaxation, while S2 occurs a bit later and reflects descent of the LV annulus with LV systole. The D-wave represents the forward flow of blood during diastole (after the mitral valve opens). During this time, the left atrium serves as nothing more than a conduit. As such, the D-wave on the pulmonary venous Doppler profile is a direct correlate to the E-wave on the transmitral Doppler profile. Finally, the AR-wave corresponds to blood flowing back into the pulmonary veins during atrial contraction. In reference to the ECG, the AR-, S-, and D-waves occur shortly after the P-wave, QRS, the T-wave, respectively. In reference to the PAOP tracing, the AR-wave corresponds to the a-wave, while the D-wave corresponds to the y-descent (**Figure 30.12**).

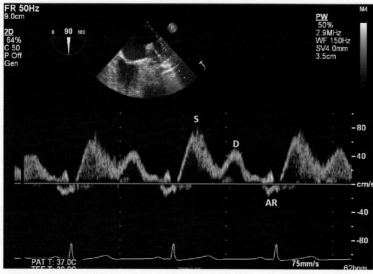

**Figure 30.12**

### Selected References

1. Appleton CP. Hemodynamic determinants of Doppler pulmonary venous flow velocity components: new insights from studies in lightly sedated normal dogs. *J Am Coll Cardiol.* 1997;30(6):1562-1574.
2. Nagueh SF, Smiseth OA, Appleton CP, et al. Recommendations for the evaluation of left ventricular diastolic function by echocardiography: an update from the American Society of Echocardiography and the European Association of Cardiovascular Imaging. *J Am Soc Echocardiogr.* 2016;29(4):277-314.
3. Nishimura RA, Abel MD, Hatle LK, Tajik AJ. Relation of pulmonary vein to mitral flow velocities by transesophageal Doppler echocardiography. Effect of different loading conditions. *Circulation.* 1990;81(5):1488-1497.

# 31 | PERICARDIAL DISEASE

David Luu, Shawn Jia, Mohammad R. Rasouli, Duncan J. McLean, Tara Ann Lenk, and Yuriy S. Bronshteyn

1. A 63-year-old female presents to the cardiothoracic intensive care unit (ICU) after an open mitral valve (MV) replacement. The patient has a history of rheumatic fever as a child, well-controlled hypothyroidism, cycles 10 miles per day, and had no coronary artery disease on left heart catheterization 3 weeks prior.

On arrival to the ICU, the patient is on 0.02 µg/kg/min of epinephrine only, and vital signs are HR 93/min, BP 101/54 (85) mm Hg, central venous pressure (CVP) 11 cm $H_2O$. Five hours postoperatively, you are called to the bedside to evaluate acute hypotension. Vital signs are HR 128/min, BP 65/39 (56) mm Hg, CVP 16 cm $H_2O$ despite epinephrine at 0.1 µg/kg/min and vasopressin at 0.04 units/min. You perform a point-of-care ultrasound, which reveals mildly dilated right atrium and right ventricle, with normal right ventricular function and left ventricular (LV) diastolic collapse.

What is the likely cause of the echocardiographic findings?

A. Perioperative myocardial infarction
B. Hypovolemic shock
C. Acute pericarditis (AP)
D. Regional cardiac tamponade

2. Which of the following signs are *not* suggestive of acute cardiac tamponade?

A. Caval plethora
B. Decrease in right ventricular diameter during inspiration
C. Reduced LV end-diastolic volume
D. Increased variation of transvalvular flow velocity over the tricuspid valve (TV)

3. A 75-year-old male presents with shortness of breath and hypotension.

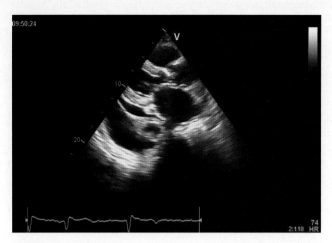

**Figure 31.1**

The parasternal long-axis view of his heart in **Figure 31.1** shows:
A. Pericardial effusion
B. Pleural effusion
C. Pericardial and pleural effusions
D. Cardiac tamponade

4. Which of the following respiratory changes to Doppler flow velocities is most likely to be found in a spontaneously breathing patient with cardiac tamponade?

A. Tricuspid inflow velocity decreases during inspiration and increases during expiration.
B. Mitral inflow velocity increases during inspiration and decreases during expiration.
C. Reversal of systolic hepatic vein flow during inspiration
D. Reversal of diastolic hepatic vein flow during expiration

5. Which echocardiographic finding is most sensitive for cardiac tamponade?

A. Inferior vena cava (IVC) plethora
B. Increased respiratory variation of mitral and TV inflows
C. Diastolic collapse of the right ventricle
D. Large pericardial effusion

6. A 55-year-old, 115 kg female presents to the emergency room with a 3-day history of positional, pleuritic chest pain and fever. She is hemodynamically stable. Her past medical history is significant for chronic steroid use secondary to lupus, type 2 diabetes mellitus, and hypertension. She recently traveled to Eastern Europe for a mission trip with her church. Cardiac auscultation is notable for an audible friction rub. Electrocardiogram (ECG) is notable for the following: (1) aVR showing for ST-segment depression and PR-segment elevation and (2) otherwise diffuse concave ST depressions. Which of the following echocardiographic findings is *most* supportive of the diagnosis of acute pericarditis?

A. A new echo-free space between the visceral and parietal pericardium present during the entire cardiac cycle
B. Tissue Doppler of MV annulus showing lateral e′ = 12 cm/sec and medial e′ = 6 cm/sec
C. Transmitral flow pattern showing E/A < 1
D. Pulmonary artery acceleration time > 120 msec

7. A 23-year-old male stabbing victim is admitted to the trauma bay with a blood-soaked bandage across his right parasternal chest area. His pulse is weak and significant pulse variation is seen on the pulse oximetry waveform. Which of the following echo findings is characteristic of cardiac tamponade in a spontaneously breathing patient?

   **A.** Biventricular collapse on inspiration
   **B.** 50% respirophasic collapsibility of the IVC
   **C.** Reduced left ventricle end-diastolic and end-systolic dimensions
   **D.** Septal bounce into the left ventricle during expiration

8. For the patient in Question 7, the team proceeds to the operating room for a pericardial window. What should be expected for the transmitral peak "E" velocity after the tamponade is relieved and positive pressure ventilation is initiated?

   **A.** Increase during inhalation, decrease during exhalation
   **B.** Increase during inhalation and exhalation
   **C.** Decrease during inhalation and exhalation
   **D.** Decrease during inhalation, increase during exhalation

9. A 65-year-old female presents with constrictive pericarditis (CP). She underwent open heart surgery 5 years ago, which was complicated by several return visits to the operating room for bleeding. In a spontaneously breathing patient, which of the following characteristics would be expected of the pulse-wave Doppler tracing of the MV?

   **A.**

   | E/A ratio | Deceleration time | Lateral e′ | Medial e′ |
   |-----------|-------------------|------------|-----------|
   | >1 | Prolonged | 12 cm/sec | 6 cm/sec |

   **B.**

   | E/A ratio | Deceleration time | Lateral e′ | Medial e′ |
   |-----------|-------------------|------------|-----------|
   | >1 | Shortened | 6 cm/sec | 12 cm/sec |

   **C.**

   | E/A ratio | Deceleration time | Lateral e′ | Medial e′ |
   |-----------|-------------------|------------|-----------|
   | <1 | Shortened | 12 cm/sec | 6 cm/sec |

   **D.**

   | E/A ratio | Deceleration time | Lateral e′ | Medial e′ |
   |-----------|-------------------|------------|-----------|
   | <1 | Prolonged | 6 cm/sec | 12 cm/sec |

10. Which of the following statements is *most* true regarding comparison between CP and cardiac tamponade?

   **A.** Ventricular interdependence is found in tamponade but *not* in CP.
   **B.** Kussmaul sign is seen in tamponade but *not* CP.
   **C.** Attenuated Y wave in central venous waveform is seen in CP but *not* tamponade.
   **D.** Both cardiac tamponade and CP are associated with increased transmitral flow velocities in spontaneously breathing patients.

11. What is the best view to see the oblique sinus during transesophageal echocardiography?

   A. Mid-esophageal ascending aorta long-axis view
   B. Mid-esophageal aortic valve long-axis view
   C. Transgastric mid-papillary short-axis view
   D. Deep transgastric long-axis view

12. Which of the following statements is *most* accurate regarding comparison of CP versus restrictive cardiomyopathy?

   A. In CP, medial e′ is usually <8 cm/sec.
   B. In spontaneously breathing patients with restrictive cardiomyopathy, reversal of hepatic vein diastolic flow is usually seen during expiration.
   C. In restrictive cardiomyopathy, lateral e′ is usually >12 cm/sec.
   D. In CP, E/e′ ratio is *inversely* related to left atrial pressure.

13. A 60-year-old female presents to the ICU with signs of dyspnea and lower extremity edema. She has no history of congestive heart failure, but had cardiac surgery 2 years ago for a valve replacement. BP is 90/50, HR 110 bpm, oxygen saturation 98% on 2 L nasal cannula. Point-of-care ultrasound shows a left pleural effusion, moderate pericardial effusion, thickened and calcified pericardium, and minimal respiratory variation of the IVC. Which of the following signs on echocardiography most likely points toward a diagnosis of CP versus cardiac tamponade?

   A. Minimal IVC collapsibility
   B. Pericardial calcification and thickness
   C. Right-sided chamber collapse
   D. Ventricular interdependence

14. A patient presents with dyspnea and hypotension and is found to have pulsus paradoxus. Which of the following statements about pulsus paradoxus is *most* accurate?

   A. Pulsus paradoxus rules in cardiac tamponade as the cause of the patient's symptoms.
   B. Across all patients, pulsus paradoxus has 90%-100% sensitivity for cardiac tamponade.
   C. Among patients with documented pericardial effusion, pulsus paradoxus >10 mm Hg increases the likelihood of tamponade threefold.
   D. Pulsus paradoxus helps differentiate cardiac tamponade from CP.

15. A patient is brought to the Emergency Department by ambulance after a motor vehicle collision. He is intubated and initial vital signs are notable for the following:

   • **HR: 150 bpm**
   • **BP: 80/40 mm Hg**
   • **Oxygen saturation: 90% (on $FiO_2 = 0.9$)**

   Vital signs improve to BP 90/40 and HR 120 after fluid challenge. Portable chest X-ray (CXR) reveals no pneumothorax, blunting of bilateral costophrenic angles, and a well-positioned endotracheal tube. Focused Assessment with Sonography in Trauma (FAST) reveals no intraperitoneal or intrapericardial fluid.
   Which of the following statements provides the *most* appropriate interpretation of the ultrasound data and next course of action?
   A. FAST examination negative, proceed to computed tomography (CT) of chest/abdomen/pelvis to evaluate for occult injury.
   B. FAST examination positive, proceed to emergent exploratory laparotomy.
   C. FAST examination indeterminate, use bedside ultrasound to evaluate the size of pleural effusions.
   D. FAST examination negative, proceed to ICU for further resuscitation.

# Chapter 31 ▪ Answers

Correct Answer: D. Regional cardiac tamponade

*Rationale:* Cardiac tamponade in the postoperative cardiac surgical patient can present atypically, as loculated effusions or localized clot can cause compression of a part of the heart. In contrast to tamponade due to a circumferential effusion, regional cardiac tamponade has a more pronounced impact on the structures that are compressed. Notably, in many cases after cardiac surgery, transthoracic windows are inadequate to rigorously screen for cardiac tamponade and transesophageal echocardiography (TEE) is required.

In this example, there is likely posterior/lateral regional tamponade as the left heart is disproportionately impacted, with LV diastolic collapse and severe hypotension.

- Perioperative myocardial infarction is likely to result in hypotension; however, the likely echocardiographic findings would be regional wall motion abnormalities in the anatomic territory of the affected vessel(s).
- Hypovolemic shock would manifest as underfilled left *and* right ventricles. In this example, the patient has a mildly dilated right atrium and ventricle, which suggests euvolemia to hypervolemia.
- Although pericarditis can occur in the postoperative cardiac surgical patient, the case described here is not typical of pericarditis. Typically, post-pericardiotomy syndrome occurs beyond a week postoperatively and is usually inflammatory and rarely due to a localized infection. A classical presentation is unexplained fever, pericardial friction rub, and a new or enlarging pericardial effusion.

## Selected References

1. Klein AL, Abbara S, Agler DA, et al. American Society of Echocardiography clinical recommendations for multimodality cardiovascular imaging of patients with pericardial disease endorsed by the Society for Cardiovascular Magnetic Resonance and Society of Cardiovascular Computed Tomography. *J Am Soc Echocardiogr.* 2013;26:965-1012.
2. Wann S, Passen E. Echocardiography in pericardial disease. *J Am Soc Echocardiogr.* 2008;21:7-13.

Correct Answer: B. Decrease in right ventricular diameter during inspiration

*Rationale:* Acute cardiac tamponade is the result of increasing external pressure placed on the cardiac chambers, usually from the accumulation of fluid in the pericardial space. However, this can occur with an open or absent pericardium such as the postoperative cardiac surgical patient with mediastinal bleeding.

- Cardiac tamponade causes caval plethora by reducing the flow of blood through the heart, which causes an elevation in pressure in both the superior vena cava (SVC) and the IVC. The accepted definition for inferior caval plethora is a <50% decrease in diameter of the IVC on inspiration.
- Although acute cardiac tamponade causes a reduction in the volume in all of the cardiac chambers through compression, the decreased intrathoracic pressure from inspiration still causes a relative increase in right ventricular diameter relative to its diameter during expiration.
- Cardiac tamponade causes a reduction in the volume of all chambers by a combination of direct compression and also secondary to a reduction in right ventricular output, which subsequently decreased filling of the left cardiac chambers, thereby reducing LV end-diastolic volume.
- Cardiac tamponade has the greatest impact on the right heart due to the relatively lower pressures compared to the left heart. During inspiration, flow is increased to the right atrium and is decreased during expiration, as is also the case in normal cardiac physiology. However, during cardiac tamponade, the difference in right heart filling between inspiration and expiration is greater. This is reflected when measuring peak transvalvular E-wave velocities across the TV during inspiration and expiration.

## Selected References

1. Himelman RB, Kircher B, Rockey DC, Schiller NB. Inferior vena cava plethora with blunted respiratory response: a sensitive echocardiographic sign of cardiac tamponade. *J Am Coll Cardiol.* 1988;12:1470-1477.
2. Klein AL, Abbara S, Agler DA, et al. American Society of Echocardiography clinical recommendations for multimodality cardiovascular imaging of patients with pericardial disease endorsed by the Society for Cardiovascular Magnetic Resonance and Society of Cardiovascular Computed Tomography. *J Am Soc Echocardiogr.* 2013;26:965-1012.

**3.** Correct Answer: C. Pericardial and pleural effusions

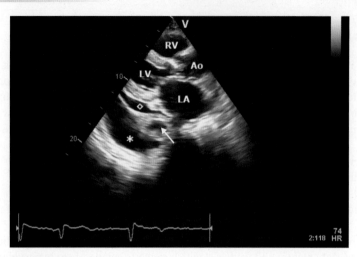

**Figure 31.2**

*Rationale:* Hypoechoic fluid between the descending aorta (**Figure 31.2,** marked by the *arrow*) and the heart supports the diagnosis of pericardial fluid (Figure 31.2, marked by ◊). Pleural fluid (Figure 31.2, marked by *) is unable to enter the potential space between the descending aorta and the heart. Both pericardial and pleural effusions are present in this image. Cardiac tamponade would be suggested by findings such as cardiac chamber collapse, MV/TV flow variation, and IVC plethora, none of which can be seen in this echocardiographic window.

Selected References

1. Foster E. Echocardiographic evaluation of the pericardium. *UpToDate.* Wolters Kluwer Accessed June 26, 2019 from https://www.uptodate.com/contents/echocardiographic-evaluation-of-the-pericardium#H27.
2. Klein AL, Abbara S, Agler DA, et al. American Society of Echocardiography clinical recommendations for multimodality cardiovascular imaging of patients with pericardial disease: endorsed by the Society for Cardiovascular Magnetic Resonance and Society of Cardiovascular Computed Tomography. *J Am Soc Echocardiogr.* 2013 Sep;26(9):965-1012.e15.

**4.** Correct Answer: D. Reversal of diastolic hepatic vein flow during expiration

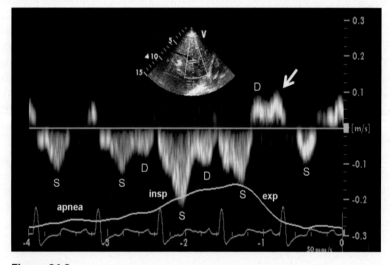

**Figure 31.3**

*Rationale:* Normally hepatic venous flow is biphasic with greater forward flow during systole than diastole. When intrathoracic pressure becomes negative during inspiration, both the peak systolic and diastolic hepatic vein flow velocities increase. As intrathoracic pressure increases during normal expiration, the systolic and diastolic hepatic venous flow is attenuated but still forward flowing. When pericardial/intracardiac pressures are increased in cardiac tamponade, overall hepatic venous flow velocities are significantly reduced (from the normal 50 to 20-40 cm/sec). Systolic hepatic vein flow now predominates because right heart pressures only decrease significantly during ventricular contraction. Diastolic hepatic vein flow reversal as observed by pulse-wave Doppler (**Figure 31.3**) may now be present during expiration.

TV inflow velocity increases with inspiration and decreases with expiration. Conversely, MV velocity increases with expiration and decreases with inspiration. This is true under normal circumstances but is greatly exaggerated with tamponade physiology. Respiratory cycle variation of >30% in either mitral or tricuspid inflow velocities strongly supports the diagnosis of tamponade so long as other signs of tamponade are present (e.g., presence of a pericardial effusion, signs of decreased cardiac output, and elevated right heart filling pressures).

### Selected References

1. Appleton CP, Hatle LK, Popp RL. Superior vena cava and hepatic vein Doppler echocardiography in healthy adults. *J Am Coll Cardiol.* 1987;10:1032-1039.
2. Klein AL, Abbara S, Agler DA, et al. American Society of Echocardiography clinical recommendations for multimodality cardiovascular imaging of patients with pericardial disease: endorsed by the Society for Cardiovascular Magnetic Resonance and Society of Cardiovascular Computed Tomography. *J Am Soc Echocardiogr.* 2013 Sep;26(9):965-1012.e15.
3. Mercé J, Sagristà-Sauleda J, Permanyer-Miralda G, Evangelista A, Soler-Soler J. Correlation between clinical and Doppler echocardiographic findings in patients with moderate and large pericardial effusion: implications for the diagnosis of cardiac tamponade. *Am Heart J.* 1999 Oct;138(4 Pt 1):759-764.

**5.** Correct Answer: **A. Inferior vena cava (IVC) plethora**

*Rationale:* IVC plethora on echocardiography is a highly sensitive sign of tamponade, expected in >90% of patients. A dilated IVC (>2.1 cm) with <50% reduction in diameter during inspiration suggests an elevated CVP that occurs with increased pericardial/intracardiac pressures. Although IVC plethora is very sensitive for tamponade, it is not specific as it can be present in numerous other disease states that do not involve the pericardium. Respiratory variation of MV/TV inflows, right heart collapse during diastole, and the presence of a large pericardial effusion are more specific for tamponade but less sensitive.

### Selected References

1. Himelman RB, Kircher B, Rockey DC, Schiller NB. Inferior vena cava plethora with blunted respiratory response: a sensitive echocardiographic sign of cardiac tamponade. *J Am Coll Cardiol.* 1988 Dec;12(6):1470-1477.
2. Klein AL, Abbara S, Agler DA, et al. American Society of Echocardiography clinical recommendations for multimodality cardiovascular imaging of patients with pericardial disease: endorsed by the Society for Cardiovascular Magnetic Resonance and Society of Cardiovascular Computed Tomography. *J Am Soc Echocardiogr.* 2013 Sep;26(9):965-1012.e15.

**6.** Correct Answer: **A. A new echo-free space between the visceral and parietal pericardium present during the entire cardiac cycle**

*Rationale:* AP refers to inflammation of the pericardial sac. In developed countries, most cases are thought to be due to a viral origin. In developing countries, cases are typically due to tuberculosis or human immunodeficiency virus (HIV). AP is a clinical diagnosis that requires at least two of the following findings:
- typical chest pain (pleuritic, worse when lying down, relieved when sitting forward)
- pericardial friction rub
- ECG changes consistent with pericarditis (i.e., the ECG changes described in this stem)
- new or worsening pericardial effusion
- elevated C-reactive protein

When AP is suspected, echocardiography helps in two ways:
1. by screening for the presence of new or worsening pericardial effusion (one of the diagnostic criteria for AP)
2. if a pericardial effusion is found, evaluating for tamponade physiology

Because of these two reasons (especially the latter), patients suspected of having AP should undergo echocardiography within ~24 hours of presentation.

This patient demonstrates a history and clinical findings highly suggestive of AP. Of the listed choices, only one (*Answer A*) is a widely accepted diagnostic criteria for AP. *Answer A* simply describes the presence of a new pericardial effusion: a new echo-free space between the visceral and parietal pericardium.

In fact, none of the other choices have relevance to the diagnosis of AP.

*Answer B* describes a situation of divergent tissue Doppler velocities along the mitral annulus: a normal lateral velocity and a subnormal medial velocity (normally, lateral e′ is ≥10 cm/sec and medial e′ ≥8 cm/sec). This can occur in patients with diastolic dysfunction. (As a side note, the opposite of this classically occurs in constrictive pericarditis: lateral mitral tissue velocities will be slow, whereas medial annulus velocities will be normal or supranormal. This occurs in CP because the lateral annulus is physically in contact with the constricted pericardium, whereas the medial mitral annulus has no physical contact with the pericardium.)

*Answer C* describes a finding classically found in the first phase of diastolic dysfunction ("impaired relaxation"). This finding has no bearing on the echocardiographic diagnosis of AP.

*Answer D* describes a normal pulmonary artery acceleration time (>120 msec). A pulmonary artery acceleration time <60 msec is associated with pulmonary hypertension. Values between 60 and 120 msec are often considered indeterminate.

**Selected References**

1. Klein AL, Abbara S, Agler DA, et al. American Society of Echocardiography clinical recommendations for multimodality cardiovascular imaging of patients with pericardial disease: endorsed by the Society for Cardiovascular Magnetic Resonance and Society of Cardiovascular Computed Tomography. *J Am Soc Echocardiogr.* 2013;26(9):965-1012.e1015.
2. Kurzyna M, Torbicki A, Pruszczyk P, et al. Disturbed right ventricular ejection pattern as a new Doppler echocardiographic sign of acute pulmonary embolism. *Am J Cardiol.* 2002;90(5):507-511.
3. Nagueh SF, Smiseth OA, Appleton CP, et al. Recommendations for the evaluation of left ventricular diastolic function by echocardiography: an update from the American Society of Echocardiography and the European Association of Cardiovascular Imaging. *Eur Heart J Cardiovasc Imaging.* 2016;17(12):1321-1360.

**7.** Correct Answer: **C. Reduced left ventricle end-diastolic and end-systolic dimensions**

*Rationale:* In a previously healthy patient with cardiac tamponade, the left ventricle will classically appear underfilled throughout the cardiac cycle (*Answer C*).

In a spontaneously breathing patient, during inspiration, cardiac tamponade classically causes small LV cavity dimensions and expansion of right ventricular (RV) chamber dimensions (*Answer A*). Classically, tamponade is associated with elevated right atrial pressures causing plethora (fixed dilation) of the IVC and hepatic veins (*Answer B*).

Ventricular interdependence is also common in both cardiac tamponade and CP. In both of these conditions, cardiac expansion is halted by the presence of a fixed "shell" of sorts around the heart, causing the interventricular septum to bounce toward whichever chamber has the most impaired filling at any given time in the respiratory cycle. In a spontaneously breathing patient, inspiration drops the intrathoracic pressure, which has the following immediate effects:

- increases preload to the right ventricle
- decreases preload to the left ventricle

In a spontaneously breathing patient experiencing cardiac tamponade, this augmented filling of the right ventricle and decreased filling of the left ventricle cause septal bulging into the left ventricle. In this patient during exhalation, the filling of the two ventricles reverses and the septum bulges away from the left ventricle (toward the right ventricle). Thus, *Answer D* is incorrect.

**Selected Reference**

1. Klein AL, Abbara S, Agler DA, et al. American Society of Echocardiography clinical recommendations for multimodality cardiovascular imaging of patients with pericardial disease: endorsed by the Society for Cardiovascular Magnetic Resonance and Society of Cardiovascular Computed Tomography. *J Am Soc Echocardiogr.* 2013;26(9):965-1012.e1015.

**8.** Correct Answer: **A. Increase during inhalation, decrease during exhalation**

*Rationale:* The patient had his tamponade relieved so he would presumably return back to normal physiology. Positive pressure inspiration normally increases early transmitral filling by compressing the pulmonary venous system, which increases left atrial pulmonary venous return. This is followed by a decrease in transmitral inflow during expiration. Transmitral peak "E" velocity is a surrogate for transmitral filling: the larger the flow from left atrium to left ventricle during diastole, the higher the peak "E" velocity.

Notably, the transmitral/transtricuspid flow patterns of tamponade during positive pressure ventilation remain poorly described. Whereas tamponade is associated with large respirophasic variation in transmitral and transtricuspid flow in spontaneously breathing patients, only a single small study to date has looked at these flow patterns when tamponade is exposed to positive pressure ventilation. This study used a tamponade model in 11 anesthetized dogs subjected to positive pressure ventilation.[2] Surprisingly, the authors found that, during positive pressure ventilation, respirophasic transmitral flow variation actually *decreased* in dogs subject to tamponade compared to when those same were free of tamponade. Further research is needed to better understand respirophasic changes in transmitral/transtricuspid flow when tamponade is combined with positive pressure ventilation.

Selected References

1. Faehnrich JA, Noone RB, Jr., White WD, et al. Effects of positive-pressure ventilation, pericardial effusion, and cardiac tamponade on respiratory variation in transmitral flow velocities. *J Cardiothorac Vasc Anesth.* 2003;17(1):45-50.
2. Klein AL, Abbara S, Agler DA, et al. American Society of Echocardiography clinical recommendations for multimodality cardiovascular imaging of patients with pericardial disease: endorsed by the Society for Cardiovascular Magnetic Resonance and Society of Cardiovascular Computed Tomography. *J Am Soc Echocardiogr.* 2013;26(9):965-1012.e1015.

**9.** Correct Answer: B.

| E/A ratio | Deceleration time | Lateral e′ | Medial e′ |
|-----------|-------------------|------------|-----------|
| > 1 | Shortened | 6 cm/sec | 12 cm/sec |

*Rationale:* A patient with CP will show a restrictive LV and RV diastolic filling pattern, similar to the pattern seen in high-grade diastolic dysfunction:

- E/A ratio > 1 (often > 2)
- short deceleration (indicating rapid equilibration of left atrial and LV pressures)

One classical finding that differentiates CP from other causes of this restrictive filling pattern is: *annulus reversus.* Normally, the early diastolic tissue velocity (e′) is higher in the lateral mitral annulus than the medial. Specifically, lateral e′ is normally ≥10 cm/sec and medial e′ is normally ≥8 cm/sec. In restrictive cardiomyopathy (e.g., amyloidosis), both of these values decline below normal and the relationship between them is preserved: medial e′ less than lateral e′. However, in CP, medial e′ is classically greater than lateral e′. This is likely because the motion of the lateral annulus is physically constrained by pericardial adhesions, whereas the medial annulus has no contact with the pericardium and maintains its freedom of movement. In fact, the medial e′ is often hyperdynamic (significantly greater than normal) in pure CP without concurrent diastolic dysfunction.

Selected Reference

1. Klein AL, Abbara S, Agler DA, et al. American Society of Echocardiography clinical recommendations for multimodality cardiovascular imaging of patients with pericardial disease: endorsed by the Society for Cardiovascular Magnetic Resonance and Society of Cardiovascular Computed Tomography. *J Am Soc Echocardiogr.* 2013;26(9):965-1012.e1015.

**10.** Correct Answer: D. Both cardiac tamponade and CP are associated with increased transmitral flow velocities in spontaneously breathing patients.

*Rationale:* In spontaneously breathing patients with either cardiac tamponade or CP, there is usually increased respirophasic, peak-to-peak variation in transmitral flow velocities. This happens due to fixed cardiac volume limiting cardiac filling during inspiration, leading to exaggerated respiratory variation during spontaneous ventilation.

Ventricular interdependence (*Answer A*) is a septal movement during the respiratory cycle due to competition between the ventricles for filling inside of a constrained space. It is seen in both CP and cardiac tamponade.

Kussmaul sign is a paradoxical increase in jugular venous pressure with inspiration. It is classically seen in CP and classically absent in cardiac tamponade (*Answer B*).

Kussmaul was also the first to describe *pulsus paradoxus.* He defined it as a slight and irregular pulse that disappears during inspiration and returns during expiration. However, pulsus paradoxus is currently defined as an inspiratory fall in systolic BP of >10 mm Hg. Pulsus paradoxus is commonly seen in cardiac tamponade and occasionally seen in CP as well.

The "Y" of the CVP tracing wave reflects diastolic flow into the right ventricle and is affected differently by CP and cardiac tamponade (*Answer C*). In CP, diastolic flow into the right ventricle is brisk up until the right ventricle reaches a certain volume wherein the shell of constricted pericardium prevents any further filling. This manifests as a brisk "Y" descent. However, in tamponade, diastolic filling is impaired from the start because the pericardial pressure is greater than the RV pressure during diastole. This manifests as attenuated "Y" descent. One well-known mnemonic is: "In tamponade, you lose your Y and you die."

Selected References

1. Klein AL, Abbara S, Agler DA, et al. American Society of Echocardiography clinical recommendations for multimodality cardiovascular imaging of patients with pericardial disease: endorsed by the Society for Cardiovascular Magnetic Resonance and Society of Cardiovascular Computed Tomography. *J Am Soc Echocardiogr.* 2013;26:965-1012.
2. Sarkar M, Bhardwaj R, Madabhavi I, Gowda S, Dogra K. Pulsus paradoxus. *Clin Respir J.* 2018;12:2321-2331.
3. Welch TD. Constrictive pericarditis: diagnosis, management and clinical outcomes. *Heart.* 2018;104:725-731.

**11.** Correct Answer: B. Mid-esophageal aortic valve long-axis view

*Rationale:* There are two pericardial sinuses: oblique and transverse. The oblique sinus is a cul-de-sac, which is located behind the left atrium and its borders are defined by the pulmonary veins and the IVC. The superior border of the oblique sinus is separated from the transverse sinus by a double reflection of serous pericardium. The oblique sinus is best seen in a mid-esophageal aortic valve long-axis view right behind the left atrium.

The transverse sinus is a passage with the following boundaries:
- anterior boundary: ascending aorta
- posteriorly: left atrium and right pulmonary artery
- medially: SVC
- laterally: main pulmonary artery

The transverse sinus can be seen in mid-esophageal ascending aorta long- and short-axis views.

Selected References
1. Klein AL, Abbara S, Agler DA, et al. American Society of Echocardiography clinical recommendations for multimodality cardiovascular imaging of patients with pericardial disease: endorsed by the Society for Cardiovascular Magnetic Resonance and Society of Cardiovascular Computed Tomography. *J Am Soc Echocardiogr.* 2013;26:965-1012.
2. Pericardium. In: Vegas A. *Perioperative Two-Dimensional Transesophageal Echocardiography.* 2nd ed. Springer Nature; 2018: 316-319.

**12. Correct Answer:** D. In CP, E/e′ ratio is *inversely* related to left atrial pressure.

*Rationale:* Doppler tissue imaging is an important tool in distinguishing CP and restrictive cardiomyopathy. CP is characterized by *annulus reversus* and *annulus paradoxus*. In a normal heart, the MV lateral e′ velocity is higher than the medial e′ velocity, whereas in CP, this relationship is reversed (*annulus reversus*), most likely because the pericardium constricts the movement of the lateral mitral annulus, whereas the medial annulus remains untethered. Thus, in CP, the medial e′ is typically >8 cm/sec, whereas the lateral e′ is typically <10 cm/sec (*Answer A*). Further, in patients with classical diastolic dysfunction due to impaired relaxation (e.g., restrictive cardiomyopathy), there is usually a linear association between E/e′ and the left atrial pressure. However, in patients with CP, this relationship is reversed (*annulus paradoxus*) because medial e′ increases progressively as the severity of constriction increases (*Answer D*).

In patients with restrictive cardiomyopathy, the lateral and medial annular velocities typically decline proportionately. Thus, medial e′ is typically <8 cm/sec and lateral e′ is typically <10 cm/sec (*Answer A*).

In patients with CP, late diastole hepatic vein flow reversal is seen during expiration due to decreased right-sided cardiac filling while this reversal is absent or minimal during inspiration. Expiration-related hepatic vein flow reversal is very specific for CP. In contrast, patients with restrictive cardiomyopathy may show hepatic vein flow reversal during inspiration (*Answer B*).

Selected References
1. Ha JW, Oh JK, Ling LH, Nishimura RA, Seward JB, Tajik AJ. Annulus paradoxus: transmitral flow velocity to mitral annular velocity ratio is inversely proportional to pulmonary capillary wedge pressure in patients with constrictive pericarditis. *Circulation.* 2001;104:976-978.
2. Klein AL, Abbara S, Agler DA, et al. American Society of Echocardiography clinical recommendations for multimodality cardiovascular imaging of patients with pericardial disease: endorsed by the Society for Cardiovascular Magnetic Resonance and Society of Cardiovascular Computed Tomography. *J Am Soc Echocardiogr.* 2013;26:965-1012.
3. Welch TD. Constrictive pericarditis: diagnosis, management and clinical outcomes. *Heart.* 2018;104:725-731.

**13.** Correct Answer: B. Pericardial calcification and thickness

*Rationale:* CP is a condition when a thickened, scarred, often calcified noncompliant pericardium limits diastolic filling of the ventricles. It is often a diagnosis that is missed and shares many clinical and echocardiographic features with cardiac tamponade. Clinically, patients present with fluid retention (ascites, leg edema, dyspnea, pleural effusions), and the two most common causes in developed countries are idiopathic and previous cardiac surgery. Like in tamponade, CP is characterized by elevated left and right heart filling pressures. Pulsus paradoxus is seen in both conditions but is not specific for either syndrome. It is more common in cardiac tamponade and seen only in about one-third of CP patients even though a pronounced inspiratory decline in the velocity of mitral inflow and an increase in tricuspid inflow are characteristic Doppler findings. The reason for this may be that the restrictive pericardium prevents transmission of the inspiratory fall in thoracic pressure into the right atrium, such that inspiration cannot increase venous return to the right heart to the extent seen with tamponade. Although ventricular interdependence is seen in both conditions (*Answer D*; septum bulges to the left with inspiration), bulging takes place more slowly in cardiac tamponade, which favors pulsus paradoxus, whereas the septum bounces rapidly so that the change in the ratio of ventricular volumes takes place abruptly in CP, which does not favor pulsus paradoxus. Both conditions also have a full, minimally respirophasic IVC with minimal collapsibility (*Answer A*).

CP is often missed clinically, perhaps because it presents subacutely (rather than acutely), is a heart failure with preserved ejection fraction mimic, and lacks the dramatic ultrasound features of cardiac tamponade. When seen, pericardial calcification and thickening seen on echocardiography or radiography is highly suggestive. Other echocardiographic features seen in CP are modest biatrial enlargement, early rapid diastolic filling (constraining effects do not happen until mid-diastole), and characteristic septal bounce. Importantly, chamber collapse, which is pathognomonic of cardiac tamponade, is not appreciated in CP (*Answer C*).

### Selected References

1. Klein AL, Abbara S, Agler DA, et al. American Society of Echocardiography clinical recommendations for multimodality cardiovascular imaging of patients with pericardial disease: endorsed by the Society for Cardiovascular Magnetic Resonance and Society of Cardiovascular Computed Tomography. *J Am Soc Echocardiogr.* 2013;26(9):965-1012.e1015.
2. Borlaug BA. Pulsus paradoxus in pericardial disease. Accessed July 31 2019, 2019. https://www.uptodate.com/contents/pulsus-paradoxus-in-pericardial-disease. Published 2019.

**14.** Correct Answer: **C. Among patients with documented pericardial effusion, pulsus paradoxus >10 mm Hg increases the likelihood of tamponade threefold.**

*Rationale:* Pulsus paradoxus is defined as an exaggeration of the normal inspiratory drop in systolic BP. In a spontaneously breathing patient, the systolic BP normally drops a small amount (10 mm Hg or less) during inspiration compared to the systolic BP between breaths because of the following sequence of events[1]:

- Inspiration lowers intrathoracic pressure relative to pressure in the rest of the body. This has differential effects on the right and left heart:
- Temporarily increases the preload and decreases the afterload of the right ventricle, immediately boosting RV stroke volume.
- Temporarily decreases the preload and increases the afterload of the left ventricle, immediately decreasing LV stroke volume.

The net effect is normally a small, immediate decrease in measured systolic BP (10 mm Hg or less). However, the inspiratory drop in systolic BP can be exaggerated (>10 mm Hg) in any of the following clinical disease states[1]:

- Pericardial syndromes: cardiac tamponade, CP;
- Nonpericardial cardiac syndromes: RV infarction, restrictive cardiomyopathy;
- Pulmonary syndromes: asthma/chronic obstructive pulmonary disease (COPD), obstructive sleep apnea, pulmonary embolism, tension pneumothorax, bilateral pleural effusions;
- Other syndromes: marked obesity, hypovolemic shock, pectus excavatum, extrinsic cardiac compression.

As the list suggests, the finding of pulsus paradoxus is *not* specific for cardiac tamponade (*Answer A*). Further, a significant percentage of patients with cardiac tamponade (25%-88%) do not exhibit pulsus paradoxus, thus the sensitivity of this finding for tamponade is generally poor when looking at all patients (*Answer B*). However, *among patients with a documented pericardial effusion*, the finding of pulsus paradoxus is highly sensitive for tamponade physiology, with one meta-analysis showing a likelihood ratio of 3.3 for tamponade in this population.

In short, the combination of (i) a documented pericardial effusion and (ii) pulsus paradoxus is *highly suggestive* of tamponade physiology. However, pulsus paradoxus can occur in a wide range of conditions aside from cardiac tamponade, including CP (*Answer D*). Thus, the finding of pulsus paradoxus without ultrasound confirmation of a pericardial effusion still leaves a broad differential diagnosis of conditions originating from the heart, lungs, and other organs.

### Selected References

1. Borlaug B. Pulsus paradoxus in pericardial disease. In: Downey B, ed. *UpToDate.* UpToDate Inc. Accessed July 6, 2019. https://www.uptodate.com.
2. Roy CL, Minor MA, Brookhart MA, Choudhry NK. Does this patient with a pericardial effusion have cardiac tamponade? *JAMA.* 2007;297(16):1810-1818.

**15.** Correct Answer: C. FAST examination indeterminate, use bedside ultrasound to evaluate the size of pleural effusions.

*Rationale:* In the setting of abdominal and/or chest trauma, the FAST examination is an important bedside tool to rapidly evaluate for intra-abdominal and/or intrapericardial hemorrhage. More recently, some practitioners have broadened the scope of the FAST examination to include evaluation of the lungs for pneumo- and hemothorax and termed this the extended FAST (eFAST).

This question stem specifically described the use of the classical FAST examination (henceforth just referred to as "FAST examination"), which omits evaluation of the lungs. Of note, the FAST examination has high specificity for detecting intra-abdominal and intrapericardial fluid. However, a single FAST examination has low sensitivity and can miss many kinds of life-threatening injuries in the chest and abdomen.

This question stem describes a high-velocity blunt trauma with resulting hypotension, hypoxemia, and possible bilateral pleural effusions (based on the CXR report). In the setting of high-impact blunt trauma and a pleural effusion (left or right), the FAST examination is uninterpretable for cardiac perforation. This is because a small percentage of patients with cardiac perforation develop concurrent pericardial perforation, resulting in cardiac bleeding directly into either pleural space or mediastinum, leaving potentially little or no blood visible in the pericardial sac. Given the patient's instability, in this case, it would be prudent to extend the ultrasound examination into the chest and evaluate the size of the suspected bilateral pleural effusions (*Answer C*). Confirmation of a large effusion would alert the trauma team to prepare for possible emergent thoracotomy to treat cardiac perforation if the patient's clinical condition deteriorates further.

The other answer choices were all suboptimal. *Answer A*: the patient's FAST examination is best described as indeterminate rather than negative and the patient appears to be too unstable to be sent for CT. *Answer B*: the FAST examination in this case is not actually positive, but rather remains indeterminate. Further, the FAST has revealed no evidence of intra-abdominal bleeding to warrant exploratory laparotomy. *Answer D*: given the potential for cardiac perforation, it seems premature to send this patient to the ICU without getting some additional information about the cause of their hypotension.

### Selected References

1. Kittaka H, Yagi Y, Zushi R, Hazui H, Akimoto H. Combination of blunt cardiac and pericardial injury presenting a massive hemothorax without hemopericardium. *Acute Med Surg.* 2015;2(4):257-259.
2. May AK, Patterson MA, Rue LW, 3rd, Schiller HJ, Rotondo MF, Schwab CW. Combined blunt cardiac and pericardial rupture: review of the literature and report of a new diagnostic algorithm. *Am Surg.* 1999;65(6):568-574.
3. McCoy CE, Langdorf MI. Traumatic Right ventricular rupture after blunt cardiac injury: CT diagnosis after false negative pericardial window on FAST due to concomitant pericardial rupture. *Clin Pract Cases Emerg Med.* 2017;1(1):65-66.
4. Scalea TM, Rodriguez A, Chiu WC, et al. Focused Assessment with Sonography for Trauma (FAST): results from an international consensus conference. *J Trauma.* 1999;46(3):466-472.
5. Schellenberg M, Inaba K, Bardes JM, et al. The combined utility of eFAST and CXR in blunt thoracic trauma. *J Trauma Acute Care Surg.* 2018 Jul;85(1):113-117.

# 32 | AORTIC AND OTHER GREAT VESSEL DISEASES

Christina Anne Jelly and Megan Henley Hicks

1. Using transthoracic echocardiography (TTE), which view(s) are *best* for examination of the ascending aorta and aortic arch?

    A. Parasternal long-axis view for both
    B. Parasternal long-axis view for the ascending aorta and apical four-chamber view for the aortic arch
    C. Suprasternal views for both
    D. Parasternal long-axis view for the ascending aorta and suprasternal views for the aortic arch

2. Measurement of the left ventricular outflow tract (LVOT) diameter should occur in which phase of the cardiac cycle and which view of TTE?

    A. Systole, parasternal short-axis view
    B. Systole, parasternal long-axis view
    C. Diastole, parasternal short-axis view
    D. Diastole, parasternal long-axis view

3. Which of the following findings is *most* suggestive of acute pulmonary embolism (PE)?

    A. Small right ventricular (RV) dimension
    B. Akinesis of the RV apex with free wall sparing
    C. Akinesis of the RV free wall with apical sparing
    D. Left ventricular dilatation

4. Which of the following mechanisms of acute aortic regurgitation (AR) is *least* likely to be associated with an acute Type A aortic dissection?

    A. Dilatation of the aortic root leading to incomplete aortic leaflet coaptation
    B. Cusp prolapse
    C. Disruption of aortic annular support resulting in a flail leaflet
    D. Aortic leaflet perforation

5. Cardiac ultrasound examination of a 56-year-old man with chest pain and a history of long-standing tobacco abuse, familial hypercholesterolemia, and poorly controlled hypertension reveals diastolic fluttering of the mitral valve in the parasternal long-axis view. What is the *most* likely underlying pathology in this patient?

    **A.** Aortic dissection
    **B.** Ascending aortic aneurysm without significant annular dilatation
    **C.** Inferior wall myocardial infarction
    **D.** Lateral wall myocardial infarction

6. Which of the measurements in **Figure 32.1** demonstrate the *best* method to measure the aortic root diameter at the level of the sinus of Valsalva in this parasternal long-axis view TTE image?

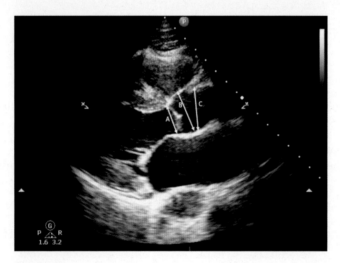

**Figure 32.1**

    **A.** Line A
    **B.** Line B
    **C.** Line C
    **D.** The sinus of Valsalva cannot be reliably measured in this view

7. Which of the following structures is indicated by the *arrow* on the parasternal short-axis view of the great vessels seen in **Figure 32.2**?

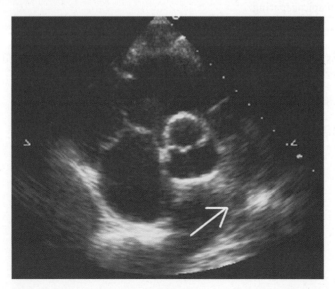

**Figure 32.2**

    **A.** RV outflow tract
    **B.** Aorta
    **C.** Superior vena cava
    **D.** Right pulmonary artery (PA)

8. A PA diameter measurement of 30 mm was obtained from a parasternal short-axis view of the great vessels in a patient presenting with respiratory distress. This finding in combination with findings of RV dilatation and a peak tricuspid regurgitant velocity of 3.5 m/s is *most* suggestive of which diagnosis?

    **A.** Acute PE
    **B.** Pulmonary edema
    **C.** Pulmonary hypertension
    **D.** Grade 1 diastolic dysfunction

9. A 36-year-old female admitted for chest pain with uncontrolled hypertension and new congestive heart failure is found to have a coarctation of the aorta. Which of the following congenital defects is *most* likely to also be noted on echo?

    **A.** Anomalous pulmonary venous return
    **B.** Cor triatriatum dexter
    **C.** Cor triatriatum sinister
    **D.** Bicuspid aortic valve

10. A 16-year-old male is involved in a high-speed motor vehicle collision with a tree while intoxicated. The patient is found to have blunt aortic injury (BAI). Where is the *most* likely location this injury would be found on echo?

    **A.** Supravalvular portion of the ascending aorta
    **B.** Aortic isthmus just distal to the left subclavian artery
    **C.** Descending thoracic aorta at the location of the diaphragm
    **D.** Aortic arch

11. A 46-year-old male with a history of hypertension presents to the emergency room after an episode of syncope. On arrival, his BP is 82/54 mm Hg and his HR is 89 bpm. His heart sounds are normal on auscultation and an electrocardiogram (ECG) demonstrates diffuse ST-segment depressions. Bedside echocardiography demonstrates a dilated aortic root, severe AR, and a linear, mobile echogenic structure prolapsing from the aortic root into the left ventricle. What is the *most* appropriate next step?

    **A.** Emergency cardiac catheterization
    **B.** Immediate surgical consultation and initiation of anti-impulse therapy
    **C.** Initiation of antibiotic therapy and referral for intensive care unit (ICU) admission
    **D.** One-liter bolus of Lactated Ringer's and continued monitoring

12. A 33-year-old female presents with severe, acute chest and back pain that began at rest. TTE is performed at bedside for a new diastolic murmur and demonstrates an aortic dissection with severe aortic insufficiency (AI). Which of the following syndromes may be associated with this diagnosis?

    **A.** Ehlers-Danlos syndrome
    **B.** Turner syndrome
    **C.** Noonan syndrome
    **D.** All of the above

13. A 66-year-old female with known history of hypertension and polycystic kidney disease presents to the emergency room with acute-onset chest pain radiating to the back concerning for aortic dissection. What is the recommended first-line imaging modality of choice?

    A. Transesophageal echocardiography (TEE)
    B. Magnetic resonance imaging (MRI)
    C. Computed tomography (CT)
    D. Transthoracic echocardiography

14. An 86-year-old female with multiple comorbidities was admitted after a mechanical fall and diagnosed with a hip fracture. She undergoes intertrochanteric fracture repair. On postoperative day 2, she develops acute-onset shortness of breath. Her shortness of breath is responsive to oxygen therapy. She has a BP of 140/95 mm Hg, HR of 82 bpm, and an SpO$_2$ of 100% on a non-rebreather. Bedside echocardiography (**Figure 32.3**) demonstrates no evidence of RV strain; however, a mobile, echogenic mass is found at the bifurcation of the right and left PAs.

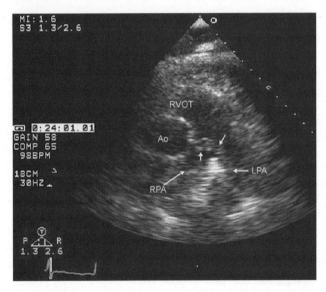

**Figure 32.3**

Assuming she remains hemodynamically stable, what is the *most* appropriate next step?
A. CT pulmonary angiography (CTPA)
B. Interventional consultation for catheter-directed thrombolysis therapy
C. Cardiac surgical referral for urgent pulmonary embolectomy
D. Administration of thrombolytic therapy and admission to the ICU

15. **Figure 32.4** was obtained from a 43-year-old male who presented with chest pain.

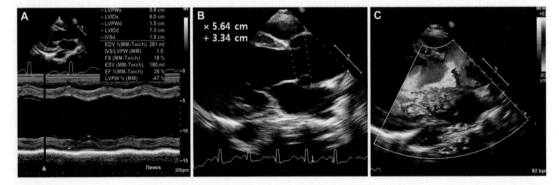

**Figure 32.4**

What is the *most* appropriate diagnosis based on these findings?
A. Aortic root aneurysm
B. Aortic dissection
C. Overriding aorta
D. Bicuspid aortic valve and ascending aortic aneurysm

16. Which of the following statements is the *most* accurate method to distinguish the true from the false lumen in a patient with aortic dissection?

    A. The dissection flap typically moves toward the false lumen in systole.
    B. The dissection flap typically moves away from the false lumen in systole.
    C. The true lumen is usually larger than the false lumen.
    D. The false lumen typically has laminar flow on color flow Doppler examination.

17. A 69-year-old female with hypertension and known ascending aortic aneurysm presents with acute-onset chest and back pain. She is hypertensive and tachycardic on arrival. Bedside echocardiography demonstrates normal left ventricular function with left ventricular hypertrophy with no evidence of AR or pericardial effusion in the parasternal long-axis and short-axis views. The echo probe is placed at the right upper sternal border and demonstrates what is shown in **Figure 32.5**.

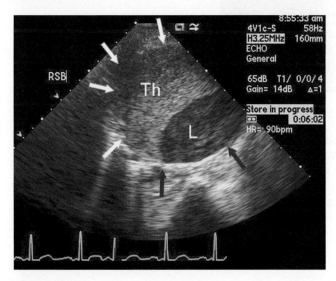

**Figure 32.5**

What is the *most* likely diagnosis?
A. Acute pulmonary embolus
B. Penetrating aortic ulcer of the ascending thoracic aorta
C. Intramural hematoma of the ascending thoracic aorta
D. Acute aortic dissection of the descending thoracic aorta

18. A suprasternal view of the aorta is shown in **Figure 32.6**.

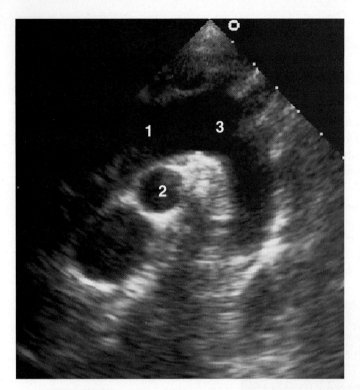

**Figure 32.6**

What is the correct identification of the structures marked in the image?
A. 1: Ascending Aorta; 2: Superior Vena Cava; 3: Descending Aorta
B. 1: LVOT; 2: Superior Vena Cava; 3: Ascending Aorta
C. 1: Descending aorta; 2: Right PA; 3: Aortic Arch
D. 1: Ascending Aorta; 2: Right PA; 3: Aortic Arch

19. A 53-year-old male with a history of hypertension and hyperlipidemia is in the postanesthesia care unit following an uneventful total knee replacement under spinal anesthesia. Bedside echocardiography is performed and is notable for a hyperdynamic left ventricle, hypovolemia, and a grossly enlarged descending thoracic aorta. His hypotension resolves with administration of 1 L of Lactated Ringer's. Based on your echocardiographic findings, he later undergoes contrast CT imaging of his chest, abdomen, and pelvis, which demonstrates descending aortic dilatation from the origin of the left subclavian to the suprarenal aorta. Based on the information provided and **Figure 32.7**, what is the *best* description of his thoracoabdominal aneurysm based on the Crawford Classification system?

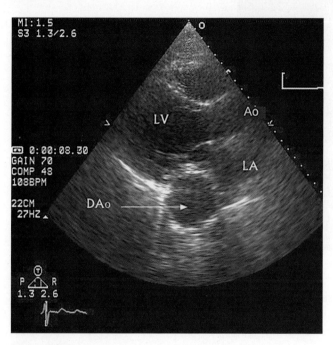

**Figure 32.7**

A. Crawford Type I
B. Crawford Type II
C. Crawford Type III
D. Crawford Type IV

20. A 37-year-old female with a history of intravenous drug use and infective endocarditis (IE) is admitted to the ICU after presenting with fevers, chills, and rigors and found to be tachycardic and hypotensive. She has blood cultures drawn and is started on broad-spectrum antibiotic therapy. Her blood cultures are positive for methicillin-resistant *Staphylococcus aureus* (MRSA) and a TTE is ordered. A parasternal short-axis view of the aortic valve is notable for the finding, indicated by the *arrow* as shown in **Figure 32.8**.

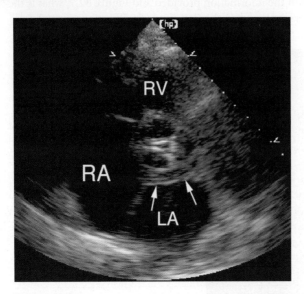

**Figure 32.8**

What is the *most* likely diagnosis based on the image provided?
A. Prosthetic aortic valve IE
B. Native aortic valve IE
C. Left atrial thrombus
D. Aortic root abscess

# Chapter 32 ▪ Answers

1. Correct Answer: D. Parasternal long-axis view for the ascending aorta and suprasternal views for the aortic arch

*Rationale:* Evaluation of the proximal ascending aorta and aortic arch using TTE is performed primarily in two views. In the parasternal long-axis view, the aortic valve, aortic root, and ascending aorta are visualized in long axis and the descending aorta is seen in short axis. Whereas the aortic arch is often a "blind spot" in TEE, the suprasternal view in TTE allows visualization of the distal ascending aorta, aortic arch, three great vessels (innominate, left carotid, and left subclavian arteries), as well as the proximal descending aorta. In addition to measurements for hemodynamic calculations and evaluation of aortic valve pathologies, aortic aneurysm, and aortic dissection, these views are also useful for evaluation of aorta atheroma and positioning of intra-aortic balloon pumps.

*Key point: The ascending aorta is best viewed in the parasternal long-axis view, whereas the aortic arch is best appreciated in the suprasternal views.*

Selected Reference
1. Evangelista A, Flachskampf FA, Erbel R, et al. Echocardiography in aortic diseases: EAE recommendations for clinical practice. *Eur J Echocardiogr.* 2010;11:645-658.

**2.** Correct Answer: B. Systole, parasternal long-axis view

*Rationale:* Measurement of the LVOT should occur during midsystole (valve leaflets open) in the parasternal long-axis view. The image should be zoomed as closely as possible to minimize error and measurements should be made parallel to the aortic valve annulus and at the level of the annulus. Error in the LVOT diameter will be exaggerated in calculations of valve area using the continuity equation, with an undermeasured LVOT diameter leading to an underestimated aortic valve area. The dimensionless index can be used as an alternative valve area calculation to avoid this error.

*Key point: LVOT diameter should be measured in midsystole in the parasternal long-axis view.*

Selected Reference

1. Baumgartner H, Hung J, Bermejo J, et al. Recommendations on the echocardiographic assessment of aortic valve stenosis: a focused update from the European Association of Cardiovascular imaging and the American Society of Echocardiography. *J Am Soc Echocardiogra.* 2017;30:372-392.

**3.** Correct Answer: C. Akinesis of the RV free wall with apical sparing

*Rationale:* Acute PE may present with RV dysfunction due to pressure overload from high pulmonary vascular resistance and obstructed PA flow. While CT angiography has become the gold standard for evaluation of PE, echocardiography is a useful adjunct for diagnosis and management. Both the McConnell sign, RV free wall motion abnormality with sparing of the apical segment, and the 60-60 sign, an RV systolic pressure <60 mm Hg and a pulmonary acceleration time <60 msec, have been found to have high specificity (100% and 94%, respectively) and high positive predictive values (100% and 90%, respectively) for RV dysfunction in the setting of PE. Mobile intracardiac thrombus and depressed tricuspid annular plane systolic excursion (TAPSE) may further support a diagnosis of RV pressure overload, and at least 25% of patients with PE will demonstrate RV dilatation.

*Key point: The McConnell sign is an echocardiographic finding described in patients with PE characterized by abnormal wall motion and depressed function of the RV free wall with normal wall motion in the apical segment. Echocardiography in general has low sensitivity for diagnosing PE, although regional wall motion abnormalities of the right ventricle that spare the apex can be suggestive of PE.*

Selected References

1. Konstantinides SV, Torbicki A, Agnelli G, et al. 2014 ESC Guidelines on the diagnosis and management of acute pulmonary embolism. *Eur Heart J.* 2014;35:3033-3080.
2. Kurzyna M, Torbicki A, Pruszczyk P, et al. Disturbed right ventricular ejection pattern as a new Doppler echocardiographic sign of acute pulmonary embolism. *Am J Cardiol.* 2002;90:507-511.

**4.** Correct Answer: D. Aortic leaflet perforation

*Rationale:* AR occurs in approximately 50% to 70% of patients with Type A aortic dissections. The severity of AR is usually explained by pathologic changes in the valve and annular structure because of the dissection in patients with anatomically normal valves. Mechanisms of AR include dilatation of the aortic root leading to incomplete aortic leaflet coaptation, aortic cusp prolapse from an asymmetric dissection depressing one or more cusps below the annulus, disruption of the aortic annular support resulting in a flail leaflet, as well as invagination or prolapse of a dissection flap through the aortic valve in diastole. Determining the mechanism and severity of AR is important for surgical decision-making in determining whether to replace the aortic valve as part of the dissection repair.

Aortic leaflet perforation more commonly results from structural deterioration of the valve, usually from aortic valve endocarditis, making it the least likely choice.

*Key point: Disruption of the aortic root due to aortic dissection often results in significant AR.*

Selected References

1. Goldstein S, Evangelista A, Abbara S, et al. Multimodality imaging of diseases of the thoracic aorta in adults: from the American Society of Echocardiography and the European Association of Cardiovascular Imaging. *J Am Soc Echocardiogr.* 2015;28:119-182.
2. Keane MG, Wiegers S, Yang E, Ferrari VA, St John Sutton MG, Bavaria JE. Structural determinants of aortic regurgitation in type A dissection and the role of valvular resuspension as determined by intraoperative transesophageal echocardiography. *Am J Cardiol.* 2000;85(5):604-610.

**5.** Correct Answer: A. Aortic dissection

*Rationale:* Diastolic fluttering of the anterior leaflet of the mitral valve may be caused by a regurgitant aortic valve jet directed toward the mitral valve. Fluttering may be noted on direct visualization using echocardiography or by using M-mode Doppler through the mitral valve leaflets. Acute aortic dissection with a retrograde dissection flap or involvement of the aortic valve annulus is likely to cause AI. In this patient, with acute chest pain and multiple risk factors for aortic dissection, the most likely mechanism for diastolic fluttering of the mitral valve is AI related to acute aortic dissection. Despite the presence of an aortic aneurysm (choice B), the absence of annular dilatation makes AI unlikely, particularly with the acute onset of symptoms described in the question. Inferior and lateral wall myocardial infarctions are unlikely to lead to AI. Other causes of diastolic fluttering include atrial fibrillation, which is characteristically of lower frequency than that associated with AI.

*Key point: Diastolic fluttering of the mitral valve is a classic finding for AI, possibly due to aortic dissection.*

Selected References

1. Louie EK, Mason TJ, Shah R, Bieniarz T, Moore AM. Determinants of anterior mitral leaflet fluttering in pure aortic regurgitation from pulsed Doppler study of the early diastolic interaction between the regurgitant jet and mitral inflow. *Am J Cardiol.* 1988;61:1085-1091.
2. Winsberg F, Gabor GE, Hernberg JG, Weiss B. Fluttering of the mitral valve in aortic insufficiency. *Circulation.* 1970;41:225-229.

**6.** Correct Answer: B. Line B

*Rationale:* Measurement of the aortic root diameter should be made perpendicular to the axis of the proximal aorta. The American Society of Echocardiography recommends measurements be performed from leading edge to leading edge, at end-diastole, and perpendicular to the long axis of the aorta, as demonstrated in Figure 32.1 (Line B). End-diastolic measurements have great reproducibility as the aortic pressure is most stable during late diastole. Other techniques for measuring the aorta include the inner edge-to-inner edge approach, although this has not shown to reproduce measurements most similar to CT and MRI compared to the leading edge-to-leading edge approach.

*Key point: Measurements of the aorta are diastolic measurement as compared to measurements of the LVOT and aortic annulus, which are systolic measurements.*

Selected Reference

1. Goldstein S, Evangelista A, Abbara S, et al. Multimodality imaging of diseases of the thoracic aorta in adults: from the American Society of Echocardiography and the European Association of Cardiovascular Imaging. *J Am Soc Echocardiogr.* 2015;28:119-182.

**7.** Correct Answer: D. Right pulmonary artery (PA)

*Rationale:* In Figure 32.2, the parasternal short-axis view of the great vessels is obtained in the left parasternal window by rotating 90° from the parasternal long-axis view and then tilting the ultrasound probe beam superiorly. A portion of the aortic valve and the ascending aorta is seen in cross section as well as the right atrium, RV outflow tract, pulmonary valve, and the main PA with the left and right PA branches in this view. The main PA diameter can be measured in this view midway between the pulmonic valve and the PA bifurcation, using an inner edge-to-inner edge technique at end-diastole. (See **Figure 32.9.**)

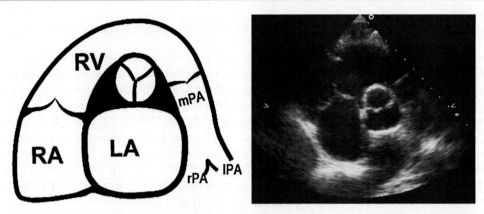

**Figure 32.9** Parasternal short-axis view of the great vessels. LA, left atrium; IPA, left pulmonary artery; mPA, main pulmonary artery; RA, right atrium; rPA, right pulmonary artery; RV, right ventricle.

### Selected References

1. Mitchell C, Rahko P, Blauwet L, et al. Guidelines for performing a comprehensive transthoracic echocardiographic examination in adults; recommendations from the American Society of Echocardiography. *J Am Soc Echocardiogr.* 2019;31(1):1-64.
2. The comprehensive echocardiographic examination. In: Armstrong WF, Ryan T, eds. *Feigenbaum's Echocardiography.* 8th ed. Wolters Kluwer; 2019:61-99.

## 8. Correct Answer: C. Pulmonary hypertension

*Rationale:* TTE is used to image the effects of pulmonary hypertension on the heart and estimate the systolic PA pressure using Doppler measurements. Echocardiographic signs suggestive of pulmonary hypertension include RV dilatation, RV hypertrophy, flattening of the intraventricular septum, enlarged right atrium, and an enlarged PA. The PA dimension is measured in end-diastole halfway between the pulmonic valve and the bifurcation of the main PA. A diameter >25 mm is considered abnormal. As the PA dilates in response to chronic volume and pressure overload, an acute PE is unlikely to lead to a finding of an enlarged PA. Pulmonary edema would not result in PA dilatation. While a peak tricuspid regurgitant velocity of 3.5 m/s would be indicative of diastolic dysfunction, this finding suggests left atrial pressure overload in the presence of normal PAs and would thus indicate more severe forms of diastolic dysfunction (Grade 2 or 3).

### Selected References

1. Augustine D, Coates-Bradshaw L, Willis J, et al. Echocardiographic assessment of pulmonary hypertension: a guideline protocol from the British Society of Echocardiography. *Echo Res Pract.* 2018;5(3) G11-G24.
2. Galie N, Humbert M, Vachiery, J, et al. 2015 ESC/ERS guidelines for the diagnosis and treatment of pulmonary hypertension: The Joint Task Force for the Diagnosis and Treatment of Pulmonary Hypertension of the European Society of Cardiology (ESC) and the European Respiratory Society. *Eur Heart J.* 2016;37(1):67-119.

## 9. Correct Answer: D. Bicuspid aortic valve

*Rationale:* Coarctation of the aorta refers to a discrete narrowing, or stricture, of a portion of the aorta, usually found distal to the left subclavian artery. Clinical presentation of coarctation depends on the location and severity of the stricture. Over time, aortic coarctation can cause reduced blood flow to the lower body, which may present as severe hypertension. A bicuspid aortic valve is present in over 50% of patients with aortic coarctation while <10% of patients with a bicuspid aortic valve have coarctation. While imaging of the coarctation is possible by TTE, CT and MRI aortography are best to determine the exact site, degree of obstruction, and the extent of collaterals which develop over time due to the restricted flow. *Key point: Coarctation of the aorta is a common congenital malformation most often associated with a bicuspid aortic valve.*

### Selected Reference

1. Goldstein S, Evangelista A, Abbara S, et al. Multimodality imaging of diseases of the thoracic aorta in adults: from the American Society of Echocardiography and the European Association of Cardiovascular Imaging. *J Am Soc Echocardiogr.* 2015;28:119-182.

**10.** Correct Answer: B. Aortic isthmus just distal to the left subclavian artery

*Rationale:* The aortic isthmus is the most common location for BAIs, accounting for 80% to 95% of aortic injuries from blunt force trauma. The next most common locations of BAIs are the supravalvular portion of the ascending aorta and the diaphragmatic portion of the descending thoracic aorta. These regions represent transition points between relatively fixed and mobile points of the aorta and have the greatest exposure to shear and hydrostatic forces during abrupt deceleration. TTE has a limited role in the assessment of aortic injury following blunt chest trauma, largely due to suboptimal echocardiographic findings. TTE may be helpful to assess for myocardial contusions and valvular pathology. TEE allows acquisition of additional data that may evaluate areas of the aorta not accessible by TTE if clinical suspicion is high and CT imaging is not feasible in unstable patients who need emergent operating room (OR) exploration. *Key point: The aortic isthmus is the most common location for BAI.*

Selected References
1. Goldstein S, Evangelista A, Abbara S, et al. Multimodality imaging of diseases of the thoracic aorta in adults: from the American Society of Echocardiography and the European Association of Cardiovascular Imaging. *J Am Soc Echocardiogr*. 2015;28:119-182.
2. Karalis DG, Victor MF, Davis GA, et al. The role of echocardiography in blunt chest trauma: a transthoracic and transesophageal echocardiographic study. *J Trauma*. 1994;36:53-58.

**11.** Correct Answer: B. Immediate surgical consultation and initiation of anti-impulse therapy

*Rationale:* The bedside echocardiography findings are suggestive of a Type A (or DeBakey I/II) aortic dissection. The finding of a mobile intimal flap prolapsing into the left ventricle in addition to aortic root dilatation and AI is highly specific for aortic dissection. Other findings that may be visualized on TTE in patients with aortic dissection include flail aortic leaflets, wall motion abnormalities, pericardial effusion or tamponade, and differential color Doppler flow patterns within the true and false lumens. While TTE has limited diagnostic value for the initial diagnosis of aortic dissection, it is safe, portable, inexpensive, quick, and highly specific. Additionally, TTE is valuable for diagnosing the complications of aortic dissection including AR and pericardial effusions.

Selected Reference
1. Solomon SD. *Essential Echocardiography: A Practical Handbook*. Humana Press Inc.; 2007.

**12.** Correct Answer: D. All of the above

*Rationale:* All of the above are factors predisposing to aortic dissection. Cystic medial degeneration (e.g., Marfan syndrome and Ehlers-Danlos syndrome) account for 5% to 9% of all aortic dissection cases. Marfan syndrome is responsible for the majority of aortic dissection in patients under the age of 40 years. Turner syndrome, Noonan syndrome, and coarctation of the aorta have also been associated with a higher risk of dissection. Other known risk factors for aortic dissection include polycystic kidney disease, bicuspid aortic valvular disease, Takayasu disease, Loeys-Dietz syndrome, and giant cell arteritis.

Selected References
1. Goldstein S, Evangelista A, Abbara S, et al. Multimodality imaging of diseases of the thoracic aorta in adults: from the American Society of Echocardiography and the European Association of Cardiovascular Imaging. *J Am Soc Echocardiogr*. 2015;28:119-182.
2. Solomon SD. *Essential Echocardiography: A Practical Handbook*. Humana Press Inc.; 2007.

**13.** Correct Answer: C. Computed tomography (CT)

*Rationale:* CT is the recommended first-line imaging modality for patients with clinical suspicion of aortic dissection. CT allows visualization of the entire aorta, including the arch vessels, mesenteric vessels, and renal arteries. CT has the quickest diagnostic times, is widely available, relatively operator independent, and is the initial test of choice in most patients presenting with symptoms concerning for aortic dissection. TEE also has high diagnostic accuracy in detecting ascending aortic dissection and can detect complications of aortic dissection including pericardial effusion, left ventricular dysfunction, coronary involvement, and AR. However, TEE is not the best choice as it is highly operator dependent and semi-invasive and may require sedation in a potentially hemodynamically unstable patient. TTE lacks sensitivity in detecting aortic dissection distal to the aortic root, and the descending thoracic aorta is imaged less easily and accurately. MRI requires a longer examination time and is not ideal in emergent or unstable clinical situations. Aortic angiography has less sensitivity than CT, TEE, and MRI and often misses intramural hematoma (IMH).

### Selected Reference

1. Goldstein S, Evangelista A, Abbara S, et al. Multimodality imaging of diseases of the thoracic aorta in adults: from the American Society of Echocardiography and the European Association of Cardiovascular Imaging. *J Am Soc Echocardiogr.* 2015;28:119-182.

---

**14.** Correct Answer: **A. CT pulmonary angiography (CTPA)**

*Rationale:* CTPA is the imaging modality of choice because it is sensitive and specific for the diagnosis of PE. Echocardiography is not the diagnostic modality of choice for the detection of acute pulmonary emboli. TTE has an estimated sensitivity between 50% and 60% with a specificity of 80% to 90% for the diagnosis of pulmonary embolus. However, if thrombus is visualized in the proximal PAs, as it is in this patient, it may be used to diagnose presumptive PE to guide emergency therapies in hemodynamically unstable patients. In patients who are hemodynamically stable, echocardiography is considered insensitive and nonspecific. This patient is hemodynamically stable and thus urgent pulmonary embolectomy is not warranted. The patient also underwent recent surgery, which is a relative contraindication to thrombolytic therapy. Serial bedside echocardiography can be used to monitor response to therapy. Typical echocardiographic findings in patients with hemodynamically significant pulmonary embolus include the following: RV strain, interventricular septum bulging into the left ventricle, dilated proximal PAs, elevated RV systolic pressure, increased tricuspid regurgitation jet severity, McConnell's sign, and elevated right atrial pressure as evidenced by a plethora of inferior vena cava with no inspiratory collapse.

### Selected References

1. Echocardiography in systemic disease and clinical problem solving. In: Armstrong WF, Ryan T, eds. *Feigenbaum's Echocardiography.* 7th ed. Wolters Kluwer; 2010:741-755.
2. Saric M, Armour AC, Arnaout MS, et al. Guidelines for the use of echocardiography in the evaluation of a cardiac source of embolism: from the American Society of Echocardiography. *J Am Soc Echocardiogr.* 2016;29:1-42.

---

**15.** Correct Answer: **A. Aortic root aneurysm**

*Rationale:* The parasternal long-axis view in Figure 32.4 demonstrates an enlarged aortic root with a diameter greater than 5 cm at the sinus of Valsalva. Aortic aneurysms are a pathologic diagnosis distinct from aortic dissection. True aortic aneurysms result from the stretching of the entire thickness of the aortic wall including the intima, media, and adventitia. The majority of thoracic aortic aneurysms (TAAs) involve the aortic root and ascending tubular aorta, as depicted in the transthoracic image. An aortic aneurysm is defined as a permanent focal dilatation of an artery having a >50% increase in diameter compared with the expected normal diameter of the artery. Aortic diameter is the principal risk factor of aortic rupture and dissection and risk increases significantly at diameters above 60 mm. Aortic root dilatation may be followed serially by TTE in most cases. Maximum aortic diameter is used to determine the timing of prophylactic surgical repair to mitigate the risk of aortic rupture and dissection.

### Selected References

1. Evangelista A, Flachskampf FA, Erbel R, et al. Echocardiography in aortic diseases: EAE recommendations for clinical practice. *Eur J Echocardiogr.* 2010;11:645-658.
2. Goldstein S, Evangelista A, Abbara S, et al. Multimodality imaging of diseases of the thoracic aorta in adults: from the American Society of Echocardiography and the European Association of Cardiovascular Imaging. *J Am Soc Echocardiogr.* 2015;28:119-182.

---

**16.** Correct Answer: **A. The dissection flap typically moves toward the false lumen in systole.**

*Rationale:* While TEE is superior for imaging in aortic dissection, TTE may often be used to differentiate the true and false lumens in these patients. The dissection flap typically moves toward the false lumen in systole as the true lumen expands from blood flow during ventricular systole. Conversely, the false lumen typically collapses during systole. The true lumen is typically smaller than the false lumen. Antegrade systolic flow is usually rapid to create brighter shades of red or blue on color flow Doppler interrogation of the true lumen. Conversely, the false lumen usually has sluggish flow as evidenced by spontaneous echo contrast or even varying degrees of thrombus formation.

Selected Reference

1. Goldstein S, Evangelista A, Abbara S, et al. Multimodality imaging of diseases of the thoracic aorta in adults: from the American Society of Echocardiography and the European Association of Cardiovascular Imaging. *J Am Soc Echocardiogr*. 2015;28:119-182.

**17.** Correct Answer: C. Intramural hematoma of the ascending thoracic aorta

*Rationale:* The high right parasternal view of the aorta is demonstrated in Figure 32.5 obtained by placing the echo probe at the right upper parasternal border. This view may be used to demonstrate pathology and flow in the ascending aorta. Echocardiographic findings of IMH include a wall thickness >7 mm with an echolucent crescent-shaped zone in the aortic wall that leads to compression of the aortic lumen. Figure 32.5 may also be consistent with an acute aortic dissection with a thrombosed false lumen; however, the ascending aorta is visualized at the right upper sternal border. Echocardiographic imaging features of IMH also include focal aortic wall thickening that is crescentic rather than concentric, preserved luminal shape with a smooth luminal border, echolucent regions in the aortic wall, and central displacement of intimal calcium. IMH is typically a more localized process than a classic aortic dissection, but given the significant risk of complications and death associated with ascending aorta IMHs with medical treatment alone, immediate surgery is usually performed. Penetrating aortic ulcers (PAUs) occur when ulceration of an atherosclerotic lesion penetrates the aortic internal elastic lamina into the aortic media. PAUs appear like a "craterlike" outpouching of the aortic wall. Clinical presentation of PAU is similar to both aortic dissection and IMH. When the ulcer penetrates into the media, it may cause an IMH to develop. The natural history of PAU is unknown, but it does not require immediate surgical repair. These patients with PAU are monitored with serial imaging studies to document disease progression.

Selected References

1. Alomari IB, Hamirani YS, Madera G, Tabe C, Akhtar N, Raizada V. Aortic intramural hematoma and its complications. *Circulation*. 2014;129:711-716.
2. Goldstein S, Evangelista A, Abbara S, et al. Multimodality imaging of diseases of the thoracic aorta in adults: from the American Society of Echocardiography and the European Association of Cardiovascular Imaging. *J Am Soc Echocardiogr*. 2015;28:119-182.
3. Mitchell C, Rahko PS, Blauwet LA, et al. Guidelines for performing a comprehensive transthoracic echocardiographic examination in adults: recommendations from the American Society of Echocardiography. *J Am Soc Echocardiogr*. 2019;32:1-64.

**18.** Correct Answer: D. 1: Ascending Aorta; 2: Right PA; 3: Aortic Arch

*Rationale:* The transthoracic image shown in Figure 32.6 is a suprasternal long-axis view of the aorta. Figure 32.6 is obtained by placing the transducer in the suprasternal notch with the index facing 12 o'clock with gradual clockwise rotation toward the left shoulder and tilted toward the plane that cuts through the right nipple and the tip of the left scapula. This view can be used to evaluate the ascending aorta, transverse arch, descending aorta, innominate artery, left common carotid artery, and the left subclavian artery. The right PA is seen in cross section. (See also **Figure 32.10**.)

Selected References

1. The echocardiographic examination. In: Armstrong WF, Ryan T, eds. *Feigenbaum's Echocardiography*. 7th ed. Wolters Kluwer; 2010:91-120.

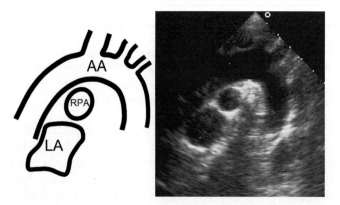

**Figure 32.10** From the suprasternal notch, the imaging plane is aligned parallel to the aortic arch (AA). The relationship among the arch, right pulmonary artery (RPA), and left atrium (LA) is demonstrated.

**19.** Correct Answer: A. Crawford Type I

*Rationale:* The transthoracic parasternal long-axis view (Figure 32.7) demonstrates dilatation of the descending aorta distal to the takeoff of the left subclavian. Like this patient, most patients with TAAs have no symptoms due to the aneurysm at the time of discovery. TTE is not the optimal imaging modality of choice for TAAs as it does not image the entire aorta and there may be significant artifact from overlying ribs. CT and magnetic resonance angiography are the preferred imaging modalities to detect TAAs. TAAs are described by the Crawford Classification as seen in **Figure 32.11**. This patient has aortic dilatation from the takeoff of the left subclavian to the suprarenal aorta, which describes a Crawford Type I TAA.

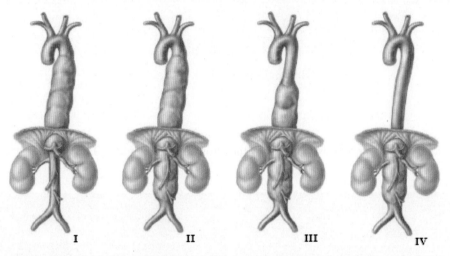

I          II          III          IV

**Figure 32.11** Crawford classification of the extent of thoracoabdominal aortic aneurysms.

Selected References
1. Conrad CF, Cambria RP. Open thoracoabdominal aortic aneurysm repair. In: Fischer JE, ed. *Fischer's Mastery of Surgery*. 7th ed. Wolters Kluwer; 2019: 2279-2327.
2. Diseases of the aorta. In: Armstrong WF, Ryan T, eds. *Feigenbaum's Echocardiography*. 7th ed. Wolters Kluwer; 2010: 633-665.

**20.** Correct Answer: D. Aortic root abscess

*Rationale:* The patient described has multiple risk factors for IE, including a prior episode of IE and active drug use. Echocardiographic features of IE include an echogenic mobile mass that has an irregular, shaggy appearance. Vegetations are usually located on the atrial side of mitral valves and the ventricular side of aortic valves, when they occur. It is not possible to diagnose IE from this still image of the aortic side of the native aortic valve alone. However, Figure 32.8 demonstrates a thickened, nonhomogeneous perivalvular cavity adjacent to the non- and left coronary cusps. Abscesses are more frequently observed in aortic valve IE and in patients with prosthetic valve IE. The diagnosis of aortic abscess is based on the presence of a thickened space at the aortic root with development of a perivalvular cavity that does not communicate with the cardiovascular lumen. The sensitivity of TTE for the diagnosis of abscess is about 50% compared to TEE that has a sensitivity of 90%.

Selected Reference
1. Habib G, Badano L, Tribouilloy C, et al. Recommendations for the practice of echocardiography in infective endocarditis. *Eur J Echocardiogr*. 2010;11:202-219.

# 33 | ISCHEMIC/NONISCHEMIC CARDIOMYOPATHIES AND CONGENITAL HEART DISEASE

Christina Anne Jelly and Ali H. Bedair

**1.** Which of the following are most likely indicated by the arrow shown in **Figure 33.1**?

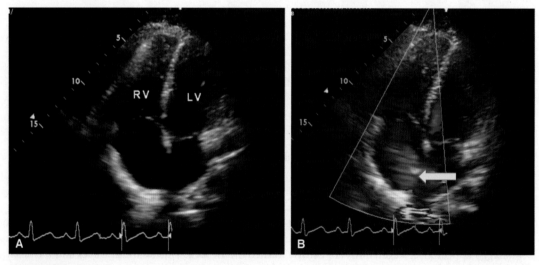

**Figure 33.1**

**A.** Sinus venosus atrial septal defect (ASD)
**B.** Ostium secundum ASD
**C.** Patent foramen ovale (PFO)
**D.** Ostium Primum ASD

**2.** What would be the *most* likely initial echocardiographic finding in a patient with an isolated secundum ASD with left-to-right shunting?

**A.** Right ventricular dilation
**B.** Right ventricular hypertrophy
**C.** Left ventricular (LV) dilation
**D.** LV hypertrophy

3. A 72-year-old male with past medical history of coronary artery disease, chronic obstructive lung disease, and heart failure with preserved ejection fraction presents after an ischemic stroke and is found to have a PFO on transthoracic echocardiography (TTE). Which of the following statements regarding PFO in patients after an ischemic stroke is *true*?

   **A.** Evidence of paradoxical embolism and a PFO after a cryptogenic stroke should prompt urgent percutaneous PFO closure for secondary stroke prevention.
   **B.** TTE is more sensitive to detect PFO compared to transesophageal echocardiography (TEE).
   **C.** Patients with cryptogenic stroke and a PFO should also be evaluated for the presence of deep venous thrombosis.
   **D.** PFO discovered incidentally at the time of cardiac surgery should prompt surgical closure at the time of surgery.

4. Which of the following echo findings is *most* commonly associated with an ostium primum ASD?

   **A.** Cleft mitral valve
   **B.** Anomalous pulmonary venous return
   **C.** Persistent left-sided superior vena cava
   **D.** Mitral valve prolapse

5. The following transthoracic parasternal long-axis and short-axis views are acquired from a patient during ventricular systole. What is the congenital cardiac lesion demonstrated in **Figure 33.2**?

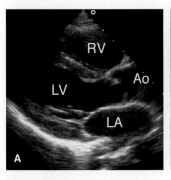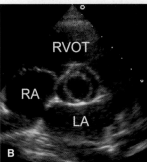

**Figure 33.2**

   **A.** Parachute mitral valve
   **B.** Ebstein anomaly
   **C.** Bicuspid aortic valve
   **D.** Atrial septal defect

6. A 74-year-old male with a known ventricular septal defect is reported to have a Qp/Qs of 2:1. It *most* likely suggests which of the following?

   **A.** Pulmonic flow is 2× systemic flow.
   **B.** Pulmonic flow is ½ of systemic flow.
   **C.** Systemic flow is 2× pulmonary flow.
   **D.** The pulmonary and systemic flows are within normal limits.

7. A 58-year-old male with no cardiovascular risk factors is admitted after a cerebrovascular accident. A paradoxical embolus is suspected, and you perform a bedside TTE. Agitated saline is injected into a peripheral intravenous (IV) to assess for PFO during a Valsalva maneuver. What is the *best* explanation for the physiologic basis for using a Valsalva maneuver to assess for PFO in patients with cryptogenic stroke?

  A. Increased intrathoracic pressure during the release phase of Valsalva leads to transient increase in left atrial (LA) pressure over right atrial (RA) pressure and may reveal right-to-left shunting.
  B. Increased intrathoracic pressure during the strain phase of Valsalva leads to transient increase in LA pressure over RA pressure and may reveal right-to-left shunting.
  C. Decreased intrathoracic pressure during the release phase of Valsalva leads to transient increase in RA pressure over LA pressure and may reveal right-to-left shunting.
  D. Increased intrathoracic pressure during the strain phase of Valsalva leads to transient increase in RA pressure over LA pressure and may reveal right-to-left shunting.

8. A parasternal long-axis view (**Figure 33.3**) demonstrates a dilated circular structure adjacent to the left atrium and mitral annulus concerning for an enlarged coronary sinus. The patient has normal biventricular function and you suspect a persistent left superior vena cava (PLSVC).

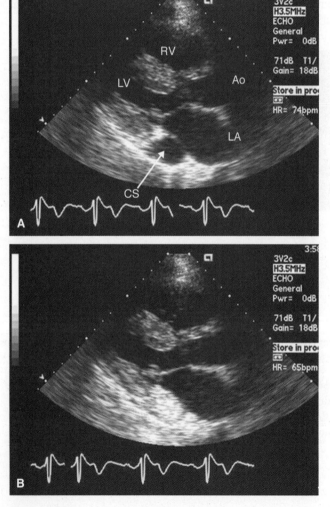

**Figure 33.3**

A PLSVC may be confirmed by injecting agitated saline into which of the following vessels and leading to visualization of bubbles in the coronary sinus prior to the right ventricle?

**A.** Right upper extremity vein

**B.** Left upper extremity vein

**C.** Right lower extremity vein

**D.** Left lower extremity vein

---

9. A 52-year-old male is involved in a motor vehicle collision and admitted to the intensive care unit (ICU) after emergent surgery for a pelvic fracture. Due to hemodynamic instability, a pulmonary artery catheter was inserted intraoperatively to help guide management. Cardiac index by thermodilution is 1.3 L/cm². The patient is treated with volume resuscitation and started on dobutamine, with marginal response. Bedside echocardiography is performed (▶ **Video 33.1**). **Figure 33.4** and ▶ **Video 33.2** show color Doppler interrogation of the parasternal long-axis view in systole.

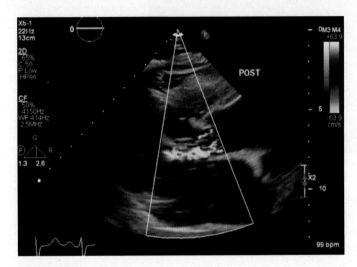

**Figure 33.4**

The tip of the anterior mitral leaflet appears to move toward the left ventricular outflow tract (LVOT) during systole with evidence of turbulent flow during systole on color Doppler interrogation. Based on the echocardiographic and hemodynamic findings, what would be the *best* management of this patient?

**A.** Switch from dobutamine to epinephrine

**B.** Avoid crystalloids and transfuse only blood products if necessary

**C.** Stop dobutamine, continue volume resuscitation, and initiate alpha-1 agonist if needed

**D.** Emergent pericardial drainage

**10.** A patient with known hypertrophic cardiomyopathy (HCM) develops hypotension in the postanesthesia care unit (PACU) after elective thyroidectomy. M-mode recording at the level of the mitral valve leaflet in the parasternal long-axis view demonstrates the following. What is the *best* description for the findings demonstrated by the *arrow* on the M-mode recording shown in **Figure 33.5**?

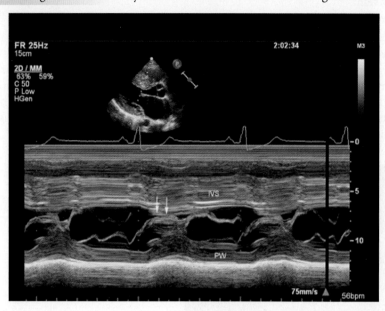

**Figure 33.5**

A. Septal to posterior wall thickness of 1:2
B. Presence of systolic anterior motion of the mitral valve
C. Diminished LV internal diastolic diameter
D. Early systolic closure of the aortic valve

**11.** A 37-year-old male with a past medical history of morbid obesity and D-transposition of the great arteries who underwent a lateral Fontan procedure at age 20 undergoes a laparoscopic sleeve gastrectomy to aid with weight loss required prior to be considered for heart transplantation. Postoperatively, he develops somnolence, hypotension, and hypoxia in the PACU. Bedside echocardiography is performed and demonstrates severe LV dilation in addition to the lateral tunnel visualized in the right atrium (**Figure 33.6**).

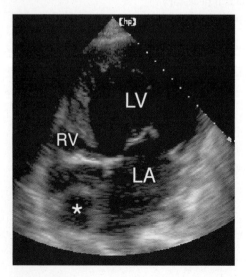

**Figure 33.6**

Which of the following statements *most* accurately describes Fontan physiology?
A. The Fontan procedure directs systemic venous return to the pulmonary veins.
B. Adequate cardiac output in Fontan patients is dependent on the transpulmonary gradient.
C. Fontan patients require high pulmonary arterial pressures to maintain adequate cardiac output.
D. Central venous pressures should be targeted at 0 to 4 mm Hg intraoperatively to maintain adequate cardiac output.

12. The two M-mode recordings (**Figure 33.7**) were obtained from patient A and patient B, both with known dilated cardiomyopathy and systolic dysfunction.

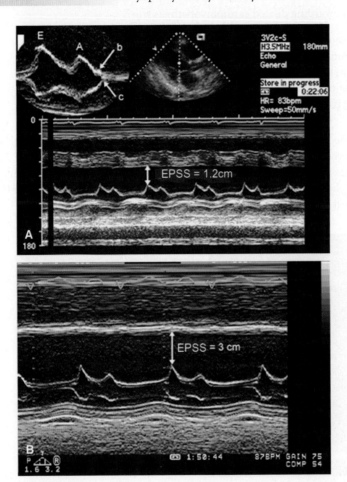

**Figure 33.7**

Which is *most* likely true based on the mitral valve E-point septal separation (EPSS) values provided for the respective patients in the M-mode recordings?
A. Patient A has significantly worse systolic dysfunction compared to patient B.
B. Patient B has significantly worse systolic dysfunction compared to patient A.
C. Patient A has significantly worse diastolic dysfunction compared to patient B.
D. Patient B has significantly worse diastolic dysfunction compared to patient A.

13. Which of the following echocardiographic findings is *most* indicative that the etiology of mitral regurgitation (MR) is due to dilated cardiomyopathy (or functional MR)?

A. Myxomatous mitral valve leaflets, prolapse of the posterior leaflet, and anteriorly directed MR jet
B. Symmetric tenting of mitral valve leaflets, dilated mitral valve annulus, and centrally directed jet of MR
C. Chordal rupture
D. Mitral leaflet perforation

14. Which of the following echocardiographic features in a patient with severe systolic dysfunction would *most* strongly suggest nonischemic dilated cardiomyopathy as the etiology?

   A. Thinned, akinetic myocardial segment with mild compensatory hypertrophy of the other segments
   B. Global hypokinesis of all segments
   C. A two-layer structure with a compacted epicardium and a noncompacted endocardial layer with a maximal end-systolic ratio of noncompacted to compacted layers of >2
   D. Biatrial enlargement with ventricular hypertrophy and evidence of severe diastolic dysfunction

15. Which of the following statements regarding dilated cardiomyopathy is *true*?

   A. Dilated cardiomyopathy is the most common indication for heart transplantation worldwide.
   B. Amyloidosis is the most common cause of dilated cardiomyopathy.
   C. The presence of diastolic dysfunction rules out dilated cardiomyopathy.
   D. Transplantation is the treatment of choice for patients with dilated cardiomyopathy as medical therapy has not shown any survival benefit.

16. A 69-year-old female with a past medical history of hypertension, chronic kidney disease, and alcohol use presents with sudden-onset, severe headache and is found to have a subarachnoid hemorrhage. She is admitted to the ICU and becomes increasingly hypotensive and tachycardic. TTE is performed and **Figure 33.8** shows the apical four-chamber view with evidence of apical ballooning as indicated by the arrows and hyperdynamic motion at the base of the heart.

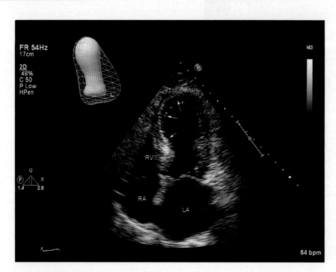

**Figure 33.8**

Which of the following statements about Takotsubo cardiomyopathy is *most* accurate?
A. Takotsubo cardiomyopathy is more common in males compared to females.
B. Elevated troponin levels rule out Takotsubo cardiomyopathy and should prompt cardiac catheterization.
C. The presence of apical ballooning is necessary for the diagnosis of Takotsubo cardiomyopathy.
D. Patients with Takotsubo cardiomyopathy are more likely to have history of neurologic or psychiatric disorder compared to patients with acute coronary syndrome (ACS).

17. Which of the following echocardiographic characteristics can help distinguish restrictive cardiomyopathy (RCM) from constrictive pericarditis (CP)?

    A. Biatrial enlargement
    B. Plethoric inferior vena cava
    C. Reduced mitral annular velocities by tissue Doppler are seen in patients with RCM but often normal in patients with CP
    D. Respirophasic variation and ventricular filling are minimal in CP but often varies by 30% to 60% in patients with RCM

18. Bedside echocardiography is performed on a patient in the ICU admitted for shortness of breath, orthopnea, and peripheral edema concerning for acute heart failure exacerbation. **Figure 33.9** shows parasternal long-axis and parasternal short-axis views obtained and demonstrates nondilated ventricles with a speckled appearance of the myocardium.

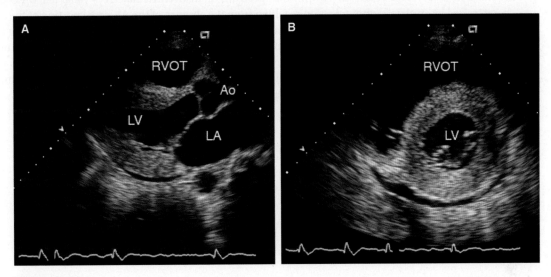

**Figure 33.9**

Which of the following causes of cardiomyopathy is *most* consistent with the echo images provided?
    A. Sarcoidosis
    B. Chagas cardiomyopathy
    C. Alcohol-induced cardiomyopathy
    D. Amyloidosis

19. Which of the following echocardiographic features is most common in patients with restrictive cardiomyopathy (RCM)?

    A. Biventricular enlargement
    B. Biatrial enlargement
    C. Decreased LV systolic function
    D. Decreased ventricular thickness

20. Which of the following is the most common echocardiographic finding suggestive of peripartum cardiomyopathy (PPCM) in a young female with no other explanation for heart failure in the peripartum period?

    A. Right ventricular dysfunction
    B. LV dysfunction with LV ejection fraction (LVEF) < 45%
    C. Severe tricuspid regurgitation
    D. Right ventricular dilation

# Chapter 33 ▪ Answers

**1.** Correct Answer: **B. Ostium secundum ASD**

*Rationale:* ASDs are the most common acyanotic congenital heart defect occurring in 0.1% of births. They are the most common cause of clinically significant intracardiac shunts, accounting for 30% to 40% of cases. Echocardiographic evaluation of ASD includes detection and quantification of size and shape of septal defects, evaluation of rims of tissue surrounding the defect, the degree of shunting and remodeling, and changes in size and function of cardiac chambers. The direction of shunting should be assessed via color flow Doppler and the presence of associated congenital defects should be evaluated.

Ostium secundum defects are the most common form of true ASDs and are defects in the septum primum tissue. Secundum ASDs are the most amenable to percutaneous closure via transcatheter techniques. Ostium primum defects are within the spectrum of atrioventricular (AV) canal defects and are characterized by an atrial communication resulting from the absence of the AV canal portion of the atrial septum, near the AV valves. Sinus venosus defects are less common and are not true ASDs, resulting from partial or complete absence of the sinus venosus septum between the superior vena cava and right upper pulmonary vein or the inferior vena cava and the right lower or middle pulmonary veins. PFO is not a true defect of atrial tissue, but rather a separation between the septum primum and septum secundum that occurs in 25% of the adult population. (See **Figure 33.10**.)

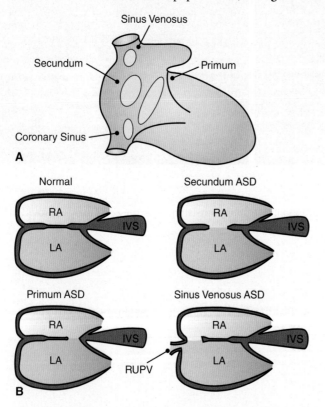

**Figure 33.10** These schematics illustrate the different types of atrial septal defect (ASD). A, The relationship of the different types of ASDs viewed from the perspective of the right heart. B, The differences among the types of ASD from a subcostal four-chamber perspective. See text for details. RUPV, right upper pulmonary vein.

**Selected References**

1. Congenital heart disease. In: Armstrong WF, Ryan T, eds. *Feigenbaum's Echocardiography*. 8th ed. Wolters Kluwer; 2019:544-607.
2. Silvestry FE, Cohen MS, Armsby LB, et al. Guidelines for the echocardiographic assessment of atrial septal defect and patent foramen ovale: from the American Society of Echocardiography and Society for Cardiac Angiography and Interventions. *J Am Soc Echocardiogr*. 2015;29:910-958.

**2.** Correct Answer: **A. Right ventricular dilation**

*Rationale:* The hemodynamic effects of ASDs are a result of the direction and magnitude of shunting between the right and left atrium. The direction and magnitude of shunting depend on the size of the defect as well as the relative compliances of the systemic vasculature, pulmonary vasculature, and the left and right ventricle. Initially, the pulmonary vasculature is able to accommodate for the increase in flow secondary to an ASD, leading to a left-to-right shunt without a substantial rise in pulmonary arterial pressure. However, over time, the continued increase in left-to-right shunt flow will lead to right ventricular dilation and then eventually pulmonary hypertension.

Right ventricular hypertrophy may result after prolonged increase in left-to-right shunt flow leading to pulmonary hypertension but would likely result after right ventricular dilation. LV dilation and LV hypertrophy would not be the expected initial echocardiographic finding in a patient with left-to-right shunting.

### Selected Reference

1. Silvestry FE, Cohen MS, Armsby LB, et al. Guidelines for the echocardiographic assessment of atrial septal defect and patent foramen ovale: from the American Society of Echocardiography and Society for Cardiac Angiography and Interventions. *J Am Soc Echocardiogr.* 2015;29:910-958.

**3.** Correct Answer: **C. Patients with cryptogenic stroke and a PFO should also be evaluated for the presence of deep venous thrombosis.**

*Rationale:* Right-to-left shunting through a PFO may lead to paradoxical emboli and can present as a cryptogenic stroke. PFOs typically close within 3 months after birth but may persist through adulthood in 25% to 30% of the population. The diagnosis of PFO relies on ultrasonography, either by echocardiography or transcranial Doppler techniques. TEE has increased sensitivity for detection of PFO compared to TTE (Choice B is incorrect), but TTE is often the initial test of choice as it is noninvasive. Presence of a PFO after cryptogenic stroke should prompt an evaluation for the presence of deep venous thrombi (Choice C is correct). Antiplatelet therapy is the initial treatment of choice for patients with cryptogenic stroke who have a PFO. Percutaneous closure devices eliminate the PFO and may be considered as a means for secondary stroke prevention. However, multiple randomized trials did not demonstrate significantly reduced rates of recurrent ischemic stroke with closure compared to medical therapy alone (Choice A is incorrect). A retrospective analysis of patients with an incidentally discovered PFO at the time of surgery demonstrated a higher risk of perioperative stroke in patients who underwent surgical closure, although there was no long-term difference in outcomes (Choice D is incorrect).

### Selected References

1. Mas JL, Derumeaux G, Guillon B, et al. Patent foramen ovale closure or anticoagulation vs. antiplatelets after stroke. *N Engl J Med.* 2017;377:1011.
2. Mathew JP, Ayoub CM, Swaminathan M. Transesophageal echocardiography for congenital heart disease. In: *Clinical Manual and Review of Transesophageal Echocardiography.* 2nd ed. The McGraw-Hill Companies, Inc.; 2010:406-439;Chapter 18.
3. Saver JL. Cryptogenic stroke. *N Engl J Med.* 2016;374:2065-2074.

**4.** Correct Answer: **A. Cleft mitral valve**

*Rationale:* Ostium primum defects are one of the several variants of common AV canal defects and result in an interatrial communication near the AV valves. Ostium primum defects are usually associated with abnormalities of the AV valves, most commonly a cleft in the anterior mitral leaflet.

Ostium secundum defects, the most common form of ASDs, are true defects in the atrial septum in the region of the fossa ovalis. The most common associated anomaly with ostium secundum defects is mitral valve prolapse. Mitral valve prolapse is the superior displacement of one or both mitral valve leaflets into the left atrium (at least 2 mm) during systole. Marked displacement of the mitral leaflet may lead to MR.

The two less common forms of ASDs are sinus venosus defects and coronary sinus defects. Sinus venosus defects are a communication between one or more of the right pulmonary veins with either the superior vena cava (superior sinus venosus defect) or inferior vena cava (inferior sinus venosus defect). Sinus venosus defects represent 4% to 11% of all ASDs and are most commonly associated with anomalous pulmonary venous return.

Coronary sinus defects are the least common form of ASDs and result from partial or complete unroofing of tissue separating the coronary sinus from the left atrium. PLSVC is associated commonly with coronary sinus septal defects and when found together is termed Raghib syndrome.

### Selected Reference

1.  Geva T, Martins JD, Wald RM. Atrial septal defects. *Lancet.* 2014;383:1921-1932.

---

### 5. Correct Answer: C. Bicuspid aortic valve

*Rationale:* The parasternal short-axis view at the level of the aortic valve demonstrates a bicuspid aortic valve.

Bicuspid aortic valves with superimposed calcific changes are a common cause of aortic stenosis. Bicuspid valves most often result from fusion of the right and left coronary cusps, as is suggested in Figure 33.2. Dilation of the aortic root and tubular ascending aorta is associated with bicuspid aortic valvular disease and may be visualized by echocardiography, but it is not suggested by Figure 33.2.

Parachute mitral valve is a congenital lesion characterized by unifocal attachment of the mitral chordae tendineae to a single papillary muscle, which may lead to mitral valve stenosis. Ebstein anomaly is a congenital anomaly of the tricuspid valve in which the tricuspid leaflets are tethered by varying degrees to the right ventricular free wall and ventricular septum leading to significant tricuspid regurgitation and a small right ventricular size.

The image above may suggest an ASD given the absence of visualized tissue between the right and left atrium in the still image. However, this may represent an artifact due to acoustic shadowing at the aortic annulus. The presence of an ASD would need to be confirmed from multiple views with or without the addition of color Doppler interrogation.

### Selected References

1.  Baumgartner H, Hung J, Bermejo J, et al. Recommendations on the echocardiographic assessment of aortic valve stenosis: a focused update from the European Association of Cardiovascular Imaging and the American Society of Echocardiography. *J Am Soc Echocardiogr.* 2017;30:372-392.
2.  Booker OJ, Nanda NC. Echocardiographic assessment of Ebstein's anomaly. *Echocardiography.* 2015;32 Suppl2:S177-S188.
3.  Jacob D, Sibert T, Ledley G, Cho S-H, Kiliddar PG. Parachute mitral valve in an adult. *J Am Coll Cardiol.* 2019;73(9_suppl 1):2769.

---

### 6. Correct Answer: A. Pulmonic flow is 2× systemic flow.

*Rationale:* The degree of shunt flow across a ventricular septal defect can be quantified with Doppler techniques. The Qp/Qs is the amount of shunt through a defect expressed as a ratio of pulmonary to systemic flow. The Qp/Qs can be assessed echocardiographically by determining LV and right ventricular stroke volumes, which are derived from the aortic and pulmonary flow velocity profiles. The Qp/QS is normally one, indicating that pulmonic flow and systemic flow are equal and thus there is no shunting. A Qp/QS over 1.5 represents a significant shunt. A Qp/Qs of 2:1 suggests that the pulmonic flow is twice the systemic flow and is indicative of a significant shunt that should be considered for interventional or surgical closure.

### Selected Reference

1.  Congenital heart disease. In: Armstrong WF, Ryan T, eds. *Feigenbaum's Echocardiography.* 8th ed. Wolters Kluwer; 2019:561-632.

---

### 7. Correct Answer: C. Decreased intrathoracic pressure during the release phase of Valsalva leads to transient increase in RA pressure over LA pressure and may reveal right-to-left shunting.

*Rationale:* Patients with cryptogenic stroke should have a TTE to assess for paradoxical embolism as a cause for cerebral ischemia. Paradoxical emboli refer to passage of a thrombus from the systemic veins to the arterial circulation via an intracardiac shunt. Paradoxical emboli most commonly occur through a PFO, which occurs in 25% to 30% of the adult population. Under normal physiologic conditions, a PFO may not lead to right-to-left shunting given the higher LA pressure compared to the RA pressure. However, right-to-left shunting may occur in patients with right-sided hypertension such as right ventricular dysfunction, tricuspid regurgitation, pulmonary hypertension, chronic obstructive pulmonary disease (COPD), and during Valsalva maneuver. The Valsalva maneuver during the strain phase causes an initial decrease in RA filling due to the increased intrathoracic pressure. After Valsalva release, the rush of blood into the right atrium causes the RA pressure to momentarily increase above the LA pressure and reverse the normal interatrial pressure gradient and may reveal right-to-left shunting. During cases of increased RA pressure, a right-to-left interatrial shunt may occur through a PFO. It is important to capture images during the strain and release phase of Valsalva maneuver.

### Selected References
1. Chung TO. Paradoxical embolism a diagnostic challenge and its detection during life. *Circulation*. 1976;53(3):565-568.
2. Rodrigues AC, Picard MH, Carbone A, et al. Importance of adequately performed Valsalva maneuver to detect patent foramen ovale during transesophageal echocardiography. *J Am Soc Echocardiogr*. 2013;26(11):1337-1343.

## 8. Correct Answer: B. Left upper extremity vein

*Rationale:* PLSVC occurs in about 0.5% of the general population and occurs in 1% to 10% of patients with congenital heart disease. It is a result of abnormal fetal development, which leads to blood draining from the junction of the left internal jugular and left subclavian veins directly into the coronary sinus. The diagnosis can be confirmed echocardiographically by injecting agitated saline contrast into a left upper extremity vein. The agitated saline will be visualized first in the coronary sinus before proceeding into the right atrium and right ventricle, thus B is the correct answer choice. Injection of agitated saline into the right upper or lower extremity veins would lead to visualization of bubbles in the right atrium before the coronary sinus. PLSVC in the absence of other congenital abnormalities is usually asymptomatic but may be discovered incidentally during pacemaker insertion or cannulation for cardiopulmonary bypass. Other causes of coronary sinus dilation also include atrial hypertension and tricuspid regurgitation.

### Selected Reference
1. Silbiger J. Echocardiographic examination of the posterior atrioventricular groove. *Echocardiography*. 2013;31:223-233.

## 9. Correct Answer: C. Stop dobutamine, continue volume resuscitation, and initiate alpha-1 agonist if needed

*Rationale:* ⊙ **Videos 33.1** and **33.2** show systolic anterior motion of the mitral valve, and flow acceleration in the LVOT during systole. This is typically seen in patients with hypertrophic obstructive cardiomyopathy (HOCM), which is the likely cause in our patient as well. HCM is inherited in an autosomal dominant pattern with variable penetrance and expression. Some of these patients develop LVOT obstruction causing decreased cardiac output. Thickening of the left ventricle (especially the interventricular septum) results in an alteration of blood flow, which pushes the anterior mitral valve leaflet into the LVOT, creating an obstruction. The obstruction results in acceleration of flow across the LVOT, further dragging the leaflet into the LVOT. Dobutamine is not required since contractility is adequate and further beta-1 agonism could worsen LVOT obstruction. Preload should be optimized as much as possible, keeping in mind that almost all HCM patients have some degree of diastolic dysfunction. An empty left ventricle will bring the anterior mitral leaflet closer to the LVOT and promote obstruction. Furthermore, augmenting afterload with agents that do not affect inotropy or chronotropy is ideal since this helps delay the rapid emptying of the left ventricle and counteracts the increased contractility. This is particularly important toward the end of systole when the ventricle is most empty and obstruction is at its worst.

### Selected Reference
1. Maron BJ. Clinical course and management of hypertrophic cardiomyopathy. *N Engl J Med*. 2018;379:655-668.

## 10. Correct Answer: B. Presence of systolic anterior motion of the mitral valve

*Rationale:* HCM leads to structural abnormalities in the mitral valve apparatus including hypertrophy of the papillary muscles and intrinsic increase in mitral leaflet area and elongation. These morphologic changes predispose the leaflet to be dragged into the LVOT due to a hyperdynamic ejection fraction. This phenomenon is called systolic anterior motion and leads to the obstructive physiology typical of HOCM. The M-mode recording with a beam directed across the mitral valve demonstrates the mitral leaflet making direct contact with the ventricular septum for more than 40% of the systolic cycle, which is highly suggestive of outflow obstruction.

Selected Reference
1. Nagueh SF, Bierig SM, Budoff MJ, et al. American Society of Echocardiography clinical recommendations for multimodality cardiovascular imaging in patients with hypertrophic cardiomyopathy. *J Am Soc Echocardiogr*. 2011;24:473-498.

**11.** Correct Answer: **B. Adequate cardiac output in Fontan patients is dependent on the transpulmonary gradient.**

*Rationale:* The Fontan procedure results in systemic venous return connected directly to the pulmonary arterial circulation (Choice A is incorrect). The driving force for cardiac output is thus dependent on a single ventricular chamber. The return of blood to the pulmonary circulation from the systemic veins is entirely passive. Thus, maintenance of the transpulmonary gradient between the central venous pressure and the common atrial pressure is paramount to maintaining cardiac output (Choice B is correct). Increases in pulmonary arterial pressures or pulmonary vascular resistance are not tolerated well in Fontan patients as this negatively affects the transpulmonary gradient and can lead to hypoxia via venovenous and intracardiac shunting. Volume status should be closely monitored to prevent elevated central pressures, which may also potentially lead to hypoxemia due to shunting through existing venovenous collaterals. Fontan patients often have increased systemic venous pressures to drive blood flow to the pulmonary circulation. Thus, decreases in preload, as may occur during positive pressure ventilation and pneumoperitoneum, are not tolerated well (Choice D is incorrect). Preservation of normoxia, normocarbia, adequate preload, and mitigating increases in pulmonary vascular resistance are important goals during the care of a Fontan patient.

Selected References
1. Congenital heart disease. In: Armstrong WF, Ryan T, eds. *Feigenbaum's Echocardiography*. 8th ed. Wolters Kluwer; 2019:544-607.
2. Gewillig M. The Fontan circulation. *Heart*. 2005;91:839-846.
3. Jolley M, Colan C, Rhodes J, DiNardo J. Fontan physiology revisited. *Anesth Analg*. 2015;121(1):172-182.

**12.** Correct Answer: **B. Patient B has significantly worse systolic dysfunction compared to patient A.**

*Rationale:* Mitral valve EPSS is defined as the minimal distance (in millimeters) between the E-point (most anterior motion of the anterior mitral leaflet during diastole) and a line tangential to the most posterior excursion of the interventricular septum within the same cardiac cycle. The internal dimension of the left ventricle is proportional to LV diastolic volume and the maximal diastolic excursion of the mitral valve is proportional to the mitral valve stroke volume. Thus, mitral valve opening becomes more restricted, as indicated by a greater separation between the E-point and the septum, as systolic function decreases and LV volume increases. A normal EPSS is ≤6 mm. A value above 7 mm is indicative of reduced systolic function but a normal value does not exclude LV dysfunction. Both EPSS values shown are above the normal range and indicative of systolic dysfunction. The EPSS value of 3 cm in patient B suggests they have significantly worse systolic function compared to patient A and thus B is the correct answer choice. EPSS is not a measure of diastolic dysfunction and thus answer choice C and D cannot be determined by the information provided.

Selected References
1. Dilated cardiomyopathy. In: Armstrong WF, Ryan T, eds. *Feigenbaum's Echocardiography*. 8th ed. Wolters Kluwer; 2019:507-537.
2. Lew W, Henning H, Schelberg H, Karliner JS. Assessment of mitral valve E point-septal separation as an index of left ventricular performance in patients with acute and previous myocardial infarction. *Am J Cardiol*. 1978;41:836-845.

**13.** Correct Answer: **B. Symmetric tenting of mitral valve leaflets, dilated mitral valve annulus, and centrally directed jet of MR**

*Rationale:* Global LV systolic function leading to LV remodeling and dilated cardiomyopathy can often cause functional MR. As the left ventricle dilates, it results in displacement of the papillary muscles and the underlying myocardium, which causes symmetric tethering of the mitral apparatus toward the apex. Ventricular remodeling may also lead to progressive mitral annular dilation. The resulting jet of MR is often centrally directed. Functional MR occurs commonly in patients with dilated cardiomyopathy who have otherwise normal mitral valve leaflets.

Answer choices A, C, and D all describe causes of MR due to abnormal leaflet motion. Answer choice A describes a patient with abnormal myxomatous mitral valve leaflets and posterior leaflet prolapse often seen in Barlow disease. Chordal rupture may occur due to myxomatous valvular disease or infective endocarditis. Mitral valve leaflet perforation is most commonly secondary to infective endocarditis.

**Selected References**
1. Dilated cardiomyopathy. In: Armstrong WF, Ryan T, eds. *Feigenbaum's Echocardiography*. 8th ed. Wolters Kluwer; 2019:507-537.
2. Zoghbi WA, Adam D, Bonow RO, et al. Recommendations for noninvasive evaluation of native valvular regurgitation: a report from the American Society of Echocardiography Developed in collaboration with the society for Cardiovascular Magnetic Resonance. *J Am Soc Echocardiogr*. 2017;30(4):303-371.

**14.** Correct Answer: **B. Global hypokinesis of all segments**

*Rationale:* The primary echocardiographic feature of dilated cardiomyopathy is LV dilation. The degree and distribution of systolic dysfunction depend on the degree of dilation as well as the etiology of cardiomyopathy. Nonischemic dilated cardiomyopathies tend to manifest with global dysfunction in all myocardial segments (Choice B is correct). Ischemic cardiomyopathy, whether dilated or not, is more commonly associated with regional hypokinesis according to coronary distribution (Choice A is incorrect). In ischemic cardiomyopathy, nonischemic myocardial segments may hypertrophy to compensate for the reduced systolic function of ischemic myocardial segments. Choice C describes LV noncompaction, a disease characterized by prominent LV trabeculae and deep intertrabecular recesses that are associated with LV dilation and systolic dysfunction. Choice D describes the echocardiographic hallmarks of restrictive cardiomyopathy (RCM), which include normal ventricular size and systolic function with evidence of diastolic stiffening leading to biatrial enlargement and severe diastolic dysfunction.

**Selected References**
1. Dilated cardiomyopathy. In: Armstrong WF, Ryan T, eds. *Feigenbaum's Echocardiography*. 8th ed. Wolters Kluwer; 2019:507-537.
2. Ihaddaden M, Mansencal N, Soulat G, Delobelle J, Arslan M, Dubourg O. Assessment of isolated left ventricular non-compaction by multimodality imaging. *Int J Cardiol*. 2013;168(2):72-73.

**15.** Correct Answer: **A. Dilated cardiomyopathy is the most common indication for heart transplantation worldwide.**

*Rationale:* Dilated cardiomyopathies are a heterogeneous group of diseases characterized by the presence of LV dilation and contractile dysfunction. Acquired causes of dilated cardiomyopathy include infection such as viral myocarditis, autoimmune diseases, peripartum cardiomyopathy (PPCM), toxicity due to ethanol, cocaine, or drugs such as antineoplastic drugs, nutritional deficiencies, and inborn errors of metabolism. Dilated cardiomyopathy is one of the most common causes of heart failure and accounts for the most common indication for heart transplantation (Choice A is correct). Amyloidosis is a common cause for RCM and does not usually result in ventricular dilation (Choice B is incorrect). Diastolic dysfunction is common in patients with severe systolic dysfunction due to dilated cardiomyopathy as cardiac remodeling and reduction in ventricular compliance lead to reduced ventricular filling (Choice C is incorrect). Angiotensin-converting enzyme (ACE) inhibitors and beta-blockers have been shown to improve survival and reduce hospital admission in patients with heart failure due to dilated cardiomyopathy (Choice D is incorrect). Mineralocorticoid antagonists, such as spironolactone, have been shown to improve survival and reduce hospital admissions when combined with ACE inhibitor and beta-blocker therapy.

**Selected References**
1. Dilated cardiomyopathy. In: Armstrong WF, Ryan T, eds. *Feigenbaum's Echocardiography*. 8th ed. Wolters Kluwer; 2019:507-537.
2. Weintraub RG, Semsarian C, Macdonald P. Dilated cardiomyopathy. *Lancet*. 2017;390:400-414.

**16.** Correct Answer: **D. Patients with Takotsubo cardiomyopathy are more likely to have history of neurologic or psychiatric disorder compared to patients with acute coronary syndrome (ACS).**

*Rationale:* Takotsubo, or stress-induced, cardiomyopathy is a transient form of cardiomyopathy characterized by systolic and diastolic LV dysfunction with a variety of wall motion abnormalities. It primarily occurs in elderly women in response to severe forms of emotional or physical stress but can also occur in the absence of an identifiable trigger (Choice A is incorrect). Troponin levels are elevated in 80% of patients with Takotsubo cardiomyopathy and cardiac enzyme elevation is generally milder compared to the degree of wall motion abnormalities. Takotsubo cardiomyopathy commonly presents with symptoms similar to ACS and may also cause elevated troponin and electrocardiographic changes suggestive of ischemia. Coronary angiography is thus necessary to rule out ACS (Choice B is incorrect) in most cases. Apical ballooning as shown in the provided echocardiographic image is identified in over 80% of patients with Takotsubo but forms of ventricular dysfunction may be observed as well (Choice C is incorrect). More than 50% of patients with Takotsubo cardiomyopathy have had a history of neurologic or psychiatric disease including subarachnoid hemorrhage, electroconvulsive therapy, head injury, stroke, anxiety, or depression (Choice D is correct).

### Selected References

1. Echocardiography in systemic disease and specific clinical presentations. In: Armstrong WF, Ryan T, eds. *Feigenbaum's Echocardiography*. 8th ed. Wolters Kluwer; 2019:692-726.
2. Templin C, Ghadri JR, Diekmann J, et al. Clinical features and outcomes of takotsubo (stress) cardiomyopathy. *N Engl J Med*. 2015;373:929-328.

**17.** Correct Answer: **C. Reduced mitral annular velocities by tissue Doppler is seen in patients with RCM but often normal in patients with CP**

*Rationale:* Both RCM and CP share the hallmark of marked reduction in LV chamber compliance. In RCM, the reduced LV compliance is due to abnormal properties of the myocardium or interstitial matrix. In CP, LV compliance is determined by the external constraint of the thickened pericardium. The restriction to diastolic filling may lead to a plethoric inferior vena cava suggesting elevated diastolic pressure in both RCM and CP (Choice B is incorrect). Impedance to diastolic filling over time leads to increased atrial pressures as a compensatory mechanism and may lead to biatrial enlargement (Choice A is incorrect). Doppler echocardiography can be used to distinguish CP from RCM.  CP is associated with pronounced respirophasic variation of ventricular filling as high as 30% to 60% (Choice D is incorrect). Respirophasic variation in RCM is usually minimal. Tissue Doppler interrogation of the mitral annulus reveals decreased excursion with RCM (E' < 8 cm/s) due to decreased ability for the myocardium to relax appropriately. The E' of the mitral annulus for patients with CP is usually normal. Patients with CP often have the finding of "annulus reversus" in which the lateral mitral annular e' velocities are lower than e' velocities from the medial annulus as the severity of constriction worsens.

### Selected References

1. Garcia MJ. Constrictive pericarditis versus restrictive cardiomyopathy? *J Am Coll Cardiol*. 2016;67:2061.
2. Pereira N, Grogan M, Dec G. Spectrum of restrictive and infiltrative cardiomyopathies. *J Am Coll Cardiol*. 2018;71:1130-1148.

**18.** Correct Answer: **D. Amyloidosis**

*Rationale:* The parasternal echocardiographic images (Figure 33.9) demonstrate a speckled, granular-appearing myocardium that is commonly associated with cardiac amyloidosis (Choice D is correct). Cardiac amyloidosis is an infiltrative disease characterized by LV and right ventricular thickening and diastolic restriction that may progress to systolic dysfunction and overt heart failure. However, the speckled, granular-appearing myocardium is not specific to amyloidosis and may also be seen in patients with HCM and end-stage renal disease. Additional findings on echocardiography in patients with cardiac amyloidosis include thickened valves, atrial septal thickening, and biatrial enlargement.

Echocardiographic findings in cardiac sarcoidosis are heterogeneous and may include a variety of findings including increased wall thickness, focal areas of hypokinesis, wall thinning, or aneurysm. Echocardiography has limited sensitivity for detecting cardiac sarcoidosis and cardiac MRI is preferred (Choice A is incorrect). Both Chagas disease and alcohol-induced cardiomyopathy are forms of dilated cardiomyopathy (Choices B and C are incorrect).

### Selected References

1. Falk RH, Quarta CC. Echocardiography in cardiac amyloidosis. *Heart Fail Rev*. 2015;20:125-131.
2. Hypertrophic and other cardiomyopathies. In: Armstrong WF, Ryan T, eds. *Feigenbaum's Echocardiography*. 8th ed. Wolters Kluwer; 2019:539-560.

**19.** Correct Answer: **B. Biatrial enlargement**

*Rationale:* RCM is characterized by impaired diastolic dysfunction often in the presence of normal ventricular size and systolic function (Choice A is incorrect). Echocardiographic findings in RCM include biatrial enlargement, normal or small LV cavity size, and abnormal diastolic function (Choice B is correct). Increased ventricular thickness is often observed in infiltrative causes of RCM such as amyloidosis and storage diseases such as hemochromatosis and glycogen storage disease. Decreased LV systolic function may occur in advanced cases of RCM but would not be the most common feature among all patients with RCM (Choice C is incorrect).

Selected Reference
1. Hypertrophic and other cardiomyopathies; In: Armstrong WF, Ryan T, eds. *Feigenbaum's Echocardiography*. 8th ed. Wolters Kluwer; 2019: 539-560.

---

**20.** Correct Answer: B. LV dysfunction with LVEF < 45%

*Rationale:* PPCM is a rare form of usually dilated cardiomyopathy that develops in the last month of pregnancy or up to 5 months postpartum with LV systolic dysfunction. PPCM is among the leading causes of maternal mortality in the United States, accounting for over 10% of cases. Independent risk factors for PPCM include advanced maternal age, preeclampsia, eclampsia, hypertension, asthma, substance abuse, and multiple gestation pregnancy. The majority of patients present post partum, predominantly during the first month after delivery with heart failure symptoms such as dyspnea on exertion, orthopnea, paroxysmal nocturnal dyspnea, and lower extremity edema. PPCM requires echocardiographic evidence of LV dysfunction with LVEF < 45% but other findings may include right ventricular dilation and dysfunction, pulmonary hypertension, LA or biatrial enlargement, functional mitral and/or tricuspid regurgitation, and intracardiac thrombus.

Selected Reference
1. Honigberg MC, Givertz MM. Peripartum cardiomyopathy. *BMJ*. 2019;364:k5287.

# 34 | MYOCARDIAL ISCHEMIA, INFARCTION, AND WALL MOTION ABNORMALITIES

Lev Deriy, Brian Starr, Carlos E. Vazquez, Pamela Y.F. Hsu, Eli L. Torgeson, and Neal S. Gerstein

1. A 79-year-old patient with a known history of coronary artery disease (CAD) was admitted to the Emergency Department (ED) with chest pain radiating to the left shoulder and diaphoresis. Which of the following findings on the initial transthoracic echocardiogram (TTE) is *most* consistent with noncardiac causes of chest pain?

   A. Severe mitral regurgitation due to torn papillary muscle
   B. Depressed left ventricular (LV) systolic function
   C. Extensive regional wall motion abnormalities (RWMAs) with multiple hypokinetic and akinetic segments
   D. Myocardial wall thickening >40% during systole
   E. Dilated right ventricle with tricuspid annular plane systolic excursion (TAPSE) <16 mm

2. Which among the following is the most specific sign/symptom of acute myocardial ischemia?

   A. Chest pain and shortness of breath
   B. T-wave abnormalities on electrocardiogram (ECG)
   C. RWMAs
   D. More than three B-lines per intercostal space on lung ultrasound

3. A 68-year-old female with a long history of insulin-dependent diabetes mellitus and hypertension arrives at the emergency room (ER) with acute onset of shortness of breath and chest discomfort. Which of the following TTE views would be the *most* helpful in evaluating distribution of all three major coronary arteries in a single view?

   A. Parasternal long-axis view
   B. Parasternal short-axis midpapillary view
   C. Apical four-chamber view
   D. Subcostal view

4. In a patient presenting with shock, which of the following ultrasound findings supports a cardiogenic etiology for the shock?

   A. LV fractional shortening of 45%
   B. More than three B-lines per intercostal space
   C. Mitral annular plane systolic excursion (MAPSE) >14 mm
   D. E/e′ ratio <8
   E. E-point septal separation (EPSS) <3 mm

5. TTE images (**Figure 34.1** and ▶ **Video 34.1**) were obtained from the patient with recent acute myocardial infarction (MI).

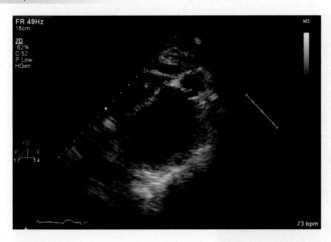

**Figure 34.1**

Which complication of acute MI is demonstrated here?
A. Cardiac tamponade
B. Papillary muscle rupture
C. Mitral regurgitation
D. Ventricular septal defect (VSD)
E. Pseudoaneurysm

6. For the patient in **Question 5**, which of the following echocardiographic findings is *most* helpful in differentiating a true aneurysm of the left ventricle from pseudoaneurysm?

A. Bidirectional flow through the narrow neck on color and spectral Doppler examination
B. Spontaneous echo contrast and thrombus in pericardial space
C. A small narrow neck connects the ventricular cavity with the pericardial space.
D. The neck diameter to maximal aneurysmal diameter ratio is >0.5.

7. Using TTE (**Figure 34.2** and ▶ **Video 34.2**), a wall motion abnormality located between the *arrows* could be caused by decreased blood flow in which coronary artery?

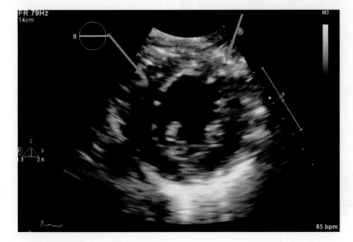

**Figure 34.2**

A. Circumflex
B. Right coronary
C. Left anterior descending (LAD)
D. Posterior descending

8. A 65-year-old male is admitted to the intensive care unit (ICU) with acute MI and cardiogenic shock. The bedside transesophageal echocardiogram (TEE) reveals mitral regurgitation (**Figure 34.3**).

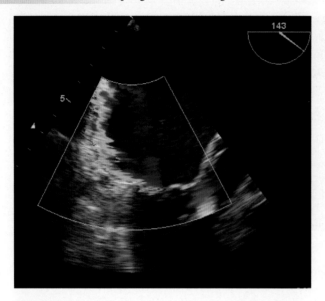

**Figure 34.3**

Which among the following parameters is least reliable for quantifying the severity of this mitral regurgitation jet?
A. Vena contracta
B. Regurgitant volume
C. Jet area
D. Pulmonary vein Doppler waveform

9. A 52-year-old male presents to the ED with chest pain. An ECG demonstrates ST changes suspicious of ischemia, and hence a troponin and TTE is ordered. What does the *asterisk* in the TTE in **Figure 34.4** denote? (See also ▶ **Video 34.3**.)

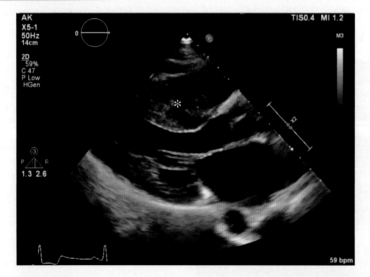

**Figure 34.4**

A. A normal interventricular septum
B. A thickened interventricular septum
C. A large interventricular hematoma
D. An aortic root abscess

10. In **Question 9**, the patient was started on inotropic support, he became profoundly hypotensive and was transferred to ICU for further management. TTE images as shown in **Figure 34.5A** and **B** were obtained.

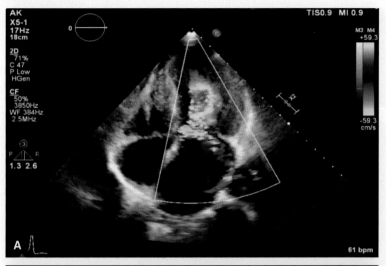

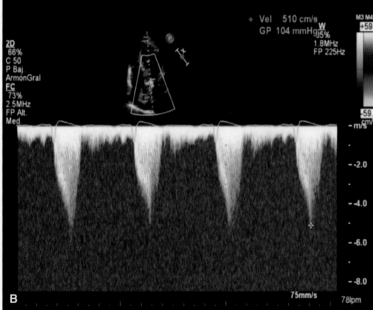

**Figure 34.5**

Which of the following echo findings would best explain the ongoing hemodynamic instability (▶ **Video 34.4**)?

A. Acute LV ischemia

B. Low systemic vascular resistance

C. Acute pulmonary embolism

D. Dynamic left ventricular outflow tract (LVOT) obstruction

E. Cardiac tamponade

11. A 75-year-old presents to the ED with symptoms of cardiac ischemia and syncope causing a hip fracture. The patient underwent a TTE and apical four-chamber view with continuous-wave Doppler image in **Figure 34.6** was obtained. What does **Figure 34.6** most likely show?

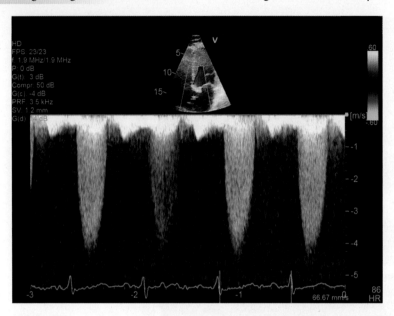

**Figure 34.6**

A. Moderate-to-severe diastolic dysfunction
B. Mild aortic stenosis
C. Severe mitral regurgitation
D. Severe aortic stenosis
E. Severe aortic regurgitation

12. An 82-year-old male with severe three-vessel CAD is admitted to the ICU with onset of hemodynamic instability status post MI a week ago. A brief TTE reveals **Figure 34.7**. The (1) *asterisk* and (2) *arrows* point to:

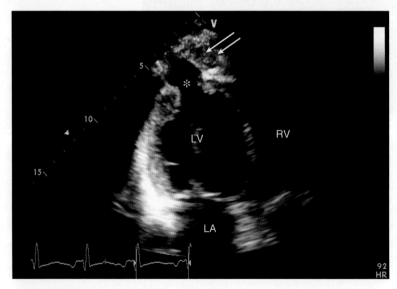

**Figure 34.7**

A. (1) Right ventricle; (2) Interventricular hypertrophy
B. (1) Right ventricle; (2) Right ventricular (RV) thrombus
C. (1) LV pseudoaneurysm; (2) Thrombus
D. (1) Left atrium; (2) Left atrial appendage thrombus
E. (1) VSD; (2) Interventricular hypertrophy

**13.** A 74-year-old man with a long history of poorly controlled hypertension is admitted to the ED with acute onset of chest pain and progressive shortness of breath. The 12-lead ECG demonstrated ST-segment elevation in: II, III, aVF. According to the American Society of Echocardiography 17-segment model of coronary perfusion territories, and assuming right coronary dominance, which of the following segments are *most* likely to be affected?

    **A.** Basal anterior
    **B.** Mid-anterolateral
    **C.** Apical septal
    **D.** Mid-anteroseptal
    **E.** Basal inferoseptal

**14.** A 67-year-old female with a history of diabetes mellitus type II, hypertension, and smoking presents to the ERD two hours after onset of left side chest pain, diaphoresis, and shortness of breath. Heart rate (HR): 97, blood pressure (BP): 85/55, SpO$_2$: 90% room air, respiratory rate (RR) 16. Physical examination reveals bilateral rales. A STAT ECG shows ST elevation in the anterior leads without reciprocal changes. A bedside TTE is performed. The apical four-chamber view is shown in **Figure 34.8** with the image frozen in systole. What is the most likely diagnosis (see also ▶ **Video 34.5**)?

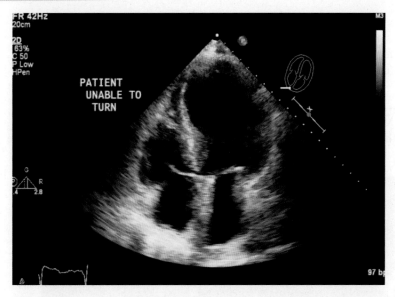

**Figure 34.8**

    **A.** Takotsubo cardiomyopathy
    **B.** Myocarditis
    **C.** Pheochromocytoma
    **D.** Pericarditis

15. What complication associated with an inferior myocardial infarction is *most* likely being demonstrated with the following four-chamber apical TTE (**Figure 34.9**)?

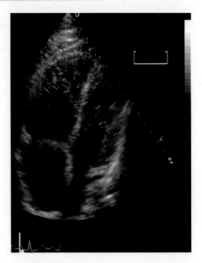

**Figure 34.9**

   **A.** Right heart failure
   **B.** LV free wall rupture
   **C.** Ventricular septal defect
   **D.** Papillary muscle rupture
   **E.** LV thrombus

16. A patient with an acute MI develops a new murmur. Given transesophageal echo image shown in **Figure 34.10**, which of the following complications of an acute MI is *most* likely responsible for the new murmur?

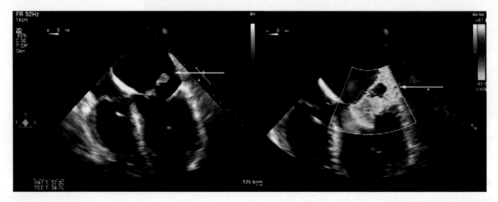

**Figure 34.10**

   **A.** Ventricular septal defect
   **B.** Papillary muscle rupture
   **C.** Pericardial effusion
   **D.** Pseudoaneurysm

17. Which of the following point-of-care ultrasound (POCUS) findings is *most* consistent with RV infarction leading to shock?

   **A.** Absence of lung sliding
   **B.** Decreased RV base descent
   **C.** A decrease in inferior vena cava (IVC) diameter of ≥50% with deep inspiration
   **D.** TAPSE of 25 mm

18. A 55-year-old male without health care maintenance arrives to the ED with crushing left-sided chest pain, diaphoresis, and shortness of breath. A point-of-care echo shows RWMAs in the areas indicated in **Figure 34.11**.

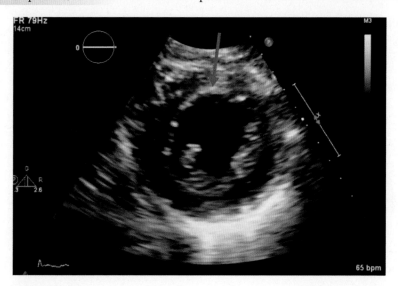

**Figure 34.11**

A stat ECG would be expected to show ST elevations in which of the following leads?
A. $V_1$-$V_2$
B. $V_3$-$V_4$
C. $V_5$-$V_6$
D. II, III, aVF
E. I, aVL

19. A 58-year-old male with a past medical history significant for hypertension, hypercholesterolemia, and diabetes type II presents to the ER with sudden onset of left-sided chest pain, diaphoresis, anxiety, and dyspnea. His vital signs are: HR: 56, BP: 95/66, RR 18, $SpO_2$: 95% on room air. Suspecting an RV acute MI, right-sided ECG leads are placed, showing 2 mm of ST elevation in $V_4R$ lead. What area of the left ventricle in the TTE in **Figure 34.12** would most likely be affected by such a presentation?

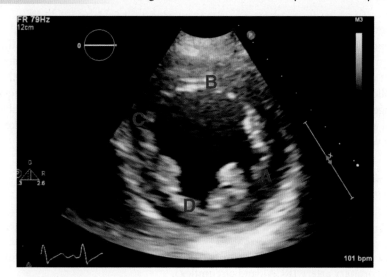

**Figure 34.12**

A. Inferolateral wall
B. Anterior wall
C. Anteroseptal wall
D. Inferior wall

20. When the patient from **Question 19** is brought to the cardiac catheterization suite for angiography and intervention, which coronary artery is most likely to be occluded?

A. Left anterior descending
B. Posterior descending
C. Circumflex
D. Left main
E. Proximal right coronary

# Chapter 34 ■ Answers

**1.** Correct Answer: **D. Myocardial wall thickening >40% during systole**

*Rationale:* Acute myocardial ischemia manifests as impairment of systolic myocardial wall motion. There are two components to this motion, endocardial excursion and wall thickening. Reduced wall thickening is a more reliable sign of myocardial ischemia than endocardial excursion, which may be affected by tethering from adjacent unaffected myocardium. The following sequence of events occurs during the ischemic cascade: diastolic dysfunction followed by systolic dysfunction (RWMAs), with subsequent development of ECG changes, symptoms, and finally a reduction in cardiac output. The myocardial wall motion can be quickly and accurately assessed by TTE, which allows the earliest diagnosis of acute myocardial ischemia.

Normal myocardial thickening is defined as >40% during systole. A myocardial thickening value >40% is not a sign of acute myocardial ischemia/infarction. Option 4 is incorrect.

Selected Reference
1. Sidebotham D. *Practical Perioperative Transesophageal Echocardiography.* 3rd ed. Oxford University Press; 2018.

**2.** Correct Answer: **C. RWMAs**

*Rationale/Critique:* Acute myocardial ischemia manifests as an impairment of systolic myocardial wall motion. There are two components to this motion: endocardial excursion and wall thickening. Wall thickening is a more reliable sign of myocardial ischemia than endocardial excursion, which may be affected by tethering from adjacent unaffected myocardium. The following sequence of events occurs with the "ischemic cascade": diastolic dysfunction followed by systolic dysfunction (RWMAs), with subsequent development of ECG changes, symptoms, and finally a reduction in cardiac output. The myocardial wall motion can be quickly and accurately assessed by TTE. Normal regional myocardial function makes an acute myocardial ischemia very unlikely.

Selected References
1. Otto C. *Echocardiography Review Guide: Companion to the Textbook of Clinical Echocardiography.* 4th ed. Elsevier; 2019.
2. Sidebotham D. *Practical Perioperative Transesophageal Echocardiography.* 3rd ed. Oxford University Press; 2018.

**3.** Correct Answer: **B. Parasternal short-axis midpapillary view**

*Rationale:* The midpapillary view allows assessment of coronary perfusion in all the three major coronary vessels (i.e., the LAD, right coronary artery [RCA], and circumflex).
1. LAD: anterior and anteroseptal segments
2. Circumflex: anterolateral and inferolateral segments
3. RCA: Inferior and inferoseptal segments
New RWMAs are an early sign of myocardial ischemia and usually precede electrocardiographic changes and angina. (See **Figure 34.13** and **Chapter 22, Figure 22.13** for further details.)

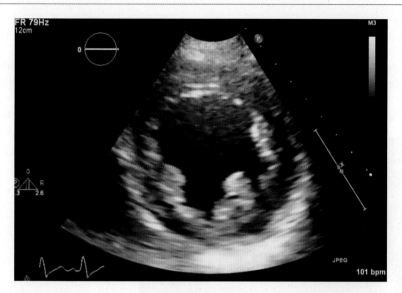

**Figure 34.13**

Selected References
1. Denault AY, Langevin S, Lessard MR, Courval JF, Desjardins G. Transthoracic echocardiographic evaluation of the heart and great vessels. *Can J Anaesth*. 2018 Apr;65(4):449-472.
2. Lang RM, Badano LP, Mor-Avi V, et al. Recommendations for cardiac chamber quantification by echocardiography in adults: an update from the American Society of Echocardiography and the European Association of Cardiovascular Imaging. *J Am Soc Echocardiogr*. 2015;28(1):1-39.e14.

**4.** Correct Answer: B. More than three B-lines per intercostal space

*Rationale:* Cardiogenic shock is one of the life-threatening complications of large acute MI. Clinically, it manifests as severe hypotension due to impaired myocardial contractility and cardiogenic pulmonary edema. Patients may have echocardiographic findings of LV systolic and/or diastolic dysfunction, and yet not manifest cardiogenic shock; none of answers A, C, and E indicate abnormal LV systolic function, and answer D can be normal LV diastolic function.

Lung ultrasound is one of the most useful noninvasive tools for early diagnosis of acute cardiogenic pulmonary edema. It has higher diagnostic accuracy than chest radiograph and auscultation.

B-lines, also called comet tails, are defined as discrete laser-like vertical hyperechoic reverberation artifacts extending from the pleural line to the bottom of the screen. Although the presence of up to two B-lines is physiologic, having at least three B-lines between two ribs in longitudinal scan defines a positive B pattern. The number of B-lines per intercostal space correlates directly with the severity of pulmonary edema.

Selected References
1. Díaz-Gómez JL, Ripoll JG, Tavazzi G, Ratzlaff RA. Perioperative lung ultrasound for the cardiothoracic anesthesiologist: emerging importance and clinical applications. *J Cardiothorac Vasc Anesth*. 2017;31:610-625.
2. Topalian S, Ginsberg F, Parrillo JE. Cardiogenic shock. *Crit Care Med*. 2008;36(1):S66-S74.

**5.** Correct Answer: E. Pseudoaneurysm

*Rationale:* LV pseudoaneurysm is the result of a contained rupture along the ventricular free wall with hemorrhage into the pericardial space that is self-contained by an organizing clot or thrombus. Although a small effusion is visible at the apex of the right ventricle, there are no signs of tamponade demonstrated in the clip. VSD and mitral regurgitation are better diagnosed with color Doppler. Papillary muscle rupture would present as a highly mobile echogenic structure attached to the mitral valve (MV). Recognition of a pseudoaneurysm is critical because of a high risk of rupture and death.

Selected Reference
1. Quader N, Makan M, Perez P, eds. *The Washington Manual of Echocardiography*. 2nd ed. Wolters Kluwer; 2017.

**6.** Correct Answer: **D.** The neck diameter to maximal aneurysmal diameter ratio >0.5

*Rationale:* LV pseudoaneurysm is the result of a rupture along the ventricular free wall with hemorrhage into the pericardial space that is self-contained by an organizing clot or thrombus. A small, narrow neck connects the ventricular cavity with the walled-off pericardial space.

Pseudoaneurysms (**Figure 34.14**) can be differentiated from true aneurysms by the following features:

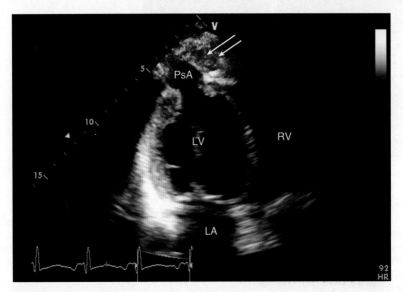

**Figure 34.14** An apical pseudoaneurysm (PsA) seen on an "off-axis" apical long-axis image. Note the narrow neck and thrombus in the pericardial space (*arrows*).

1. The neck diameter to maximal aneurysmal diameter ratio is <0.5.
2. Color and spectral Doppler show bidirectional flow through the narrowed neck.
3. The identification of spontaneous echo contrast (stasis of blood) and thrombus in the pericardial space.

Recognition of a pseudoaneurysm is critical because of a high risk of rupture and death.

Selected Reference

1. Olusesi O, Yeung M. Ischemic heart disease and complications of myocardial infarction. In: Quader N, Makan M, Perez P, eds. *The Washington Manual of Echocardiography*. 2nd ed. Wolters Kluwer; 2017:81-92.

**7.** Correct Answer: **C.** Left anterior descending (LAD)

*Rationale/Critique:* Having knowledge of coronary anatomy and perfusion is imperative for properly interpreting an echocardiography examination. Figure 34.2 in **Question 7** displays a short-axis view of the left ventricle. This view reveals information on wall motion abnormalities that can be extrapolated to coronary perfusion. Typically, the LAD coronary perfuses the anteroseptum and anterior wall; the circumflex perfuses the anterolateral and inferolateral walls; and the right coronary and posterior descending coronary perfuse the inferior and inferoseptal walls. (See also rationale for **Answer 34.3.**)

Selected Reference

1. London MJ. Diagnosis of myocardial ischemia. In: Perrino AC, Reeves ST, eds. *A Practical Approach to Transesophageal Echocardiography*. 2nd ed. Wolters Kluwer; 2008:Chapter 4.

**8.** Correct Answer: **C.** Jet area

*Rationale:* Mitral regurgitant jets can present during acute MIs, due to ischemic cardiomyopathy or papillary muscle rupture. Knowledge of the anatomy of the MV is imperative in addressing and assessing these regurgitant jets. The above image shows a mid-esophageal aortic valve long-axis view revealing an eccentric (wall hugging) regurgitant jet into the left atrium through the MV. Measuring jet area in wall hugging jets underestimates the severity of regurgitation. The regurgitant jet spreads around the wall

(Coanda effect), making the cross-sectional area of the jet in this plane appear small. Also, being adjacent to the left atrial wall could slow down the jet. Other parameters like vena contracta, regurgitant volume, and pulmonary vein flow are less affected by the eccentric nature of the jet.

### Selected Reference

1. Lamabert AS. Mitral regurgitation. In: Perrino AC, Reeves ST, eds. *A Practical Approach to Transesophageal Echocardiography.* 2nd ed. Wolters Kluwer; 2008:171-188.

**9.** Correct Answer: B. A thickened interventricular septum

*Rationale:* TTE image in **Figure 34.15** reveals a thickened interventricular septum suspicious of hypertrophic cardiomyopathy (HCM).

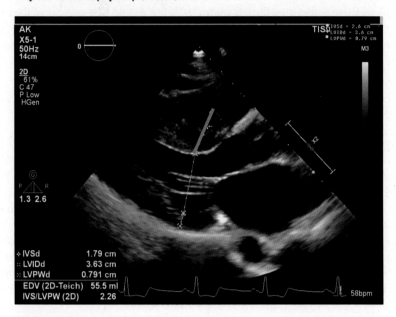

**Figure 34.15**

The normal interventricular wall diameter (IVSd) in males is <1.2 cm. IVSd >2.0 cm is consistent with severe LV wall hypertrophy. Myocardial ischemia is a recognized complication of HCM. The suggested mechanisms of myocardial ischemia in patients with HCM include structural abnormalities in arteriolar architecture, intramural vessels (myocardial bridging), imbalance of myocardial oxygen supply and demand due to hypertrophied myocardium, and impaired coronary vasodilatory reserve.

### Selected References

1. Holley CL. Cardiomyopathies. In: Rasalingam R, Majesh M, Pérez JE, eds. *The Washington Manual of Echocardiography.* Philadelphia, PA: Wolters Kluwer; 2012:89-105.
2. Gupta T, Harikrishnan P, Kolte D, et al. Outcomes of acute myocardial infarction in patients with hypertrophic cardiomyopathy. *Am J Med.* 2015;28(8):879-887.

**10.** Correct Answer: D. Dynamic LVOT obstruction

*Rationale/Critique:* HCM can predispose to a dynamic LV outflow obstruction (as opposed to a "fixed" obstruction in aortic stenosis) and remains an important cause of sudden cardiac death in young adults. The following anatomic factors predispose to this condition:

- Redundant MV leaflets
- Papillary muscle displacement
- Interventricular septal hypertrophy
- Chordal anomaly

The apical four-chamber view (Figure 34.5A) with continuous-wave Doppler interrogation of LVOT (**Figure 34.5B**) demonstrates typical late-peaking Doppler profile ("dagger" shape) indicative of a severe subvalvular obstruction with blood flow velocity of 5.1 m/s (>4.0 m/s is severe), and peak pressure gradient of 104 mm Hg (>70 mm Hg is severe). A mean pressure gradient of >40 mm Hg is also considered severe. The color flow Doppler (Figure 34.5A) confirms a high-velocity turbulent flow in LVOT and also shows eccentric mitral regurgitation both of which are consistent with dynamic LVOT obstruction.

### Selected Reference

1. Holley CL. Cardiomyopathies. In: Rasalingam R, Majesh M, Pérez JE, eds. *The Washington Manual of Echocardiography*. Wolters Kluwer; 2012:89-105.

---

**11.** Correct Answer: **D. Severe aortic stenosis**

*Rationale/Critique:* Figure 34.6 TTE image shows an apical four-chamber view with continuous-wave Doppler interrogating the aortic valve. Since the "jet" is oriented down or away from the probe, the blood is traveling through the aortic valve and exiting the left ventricle during systole. The velocity of the blood (see the Y-axis) approximates 4.5 m/s (>4.0 m/s is severe), leading to a peak gradient of 81 mm Hg (simplified Bernoulli equation: Peak gradient (mm Hg) = $4 \times$ (aortic peak velocity)$^2$). Based on this velocity, the aortic stenosis can be quantified as severe.

### Selected Reference

1. Cohen IS. Aortic Stenosis. In: Perrino AC, Reeves ST, eds. *A Practical Approach to Transesophageal Echocardiography*. 2nded. Wolters Kluwer; 2008:Chapter 12;292-312.

---

**12.** Correct Answer: **C. (1) LV pseudoaneurysm; (2) Thrombus**

*Rationale:* Ventricular pseudoaneurysms result from rupture along the ventricular free wall with hemorrhage into the pericardial space that is self-contained by an organizing clot or thrombus. A small neck connects the ventricular cavity with the walled-off pericardial space. Pseudoaneurysms differ from true aneurysms by having a neck diameter to maximal aneurysmal diameter ratio <0.5, color Doppler shows bidirectional flow through the neck, and spontaneous echo contrast (stasis of blood) and thrombus appear in the pericardial space. An apical pseudoaneurysm (Figure 34.7, *asterisk*) is seen on an "off-axis" in the apical long-axis TTE image. Figure 34.7 can be misleading as it looks similar to a short-axis transgastric TEE image or even a mid-esophageal four-chamber image, which would lead to the incorrect answer selections in the question.

### Selected Reference

1. Olusesi O, Yeung M. Ischemic heart disease and complications of myocardial infarction. In: Quader N, Makan M, Perez P, eds. *The Washington Manual of Echocardiography*. 2nd ed. Wolters Kluwer; 2017:81-92.

---

**13.** Correct Answer: **E. Basal inferoseptal**

*Rationale:* The left ventricle is divided into basal, midventricular, and apical segments. In the short axis it is divided into six segments: anterior, anterolateral, inferolateral, inferior, inferoseptal, and anteroseptal.

Knowledge of the typical distribution of coronary artery blood flow to the various myocardial segments allows confirmation in multiple views of suspected lesions. Correlation of findings to specific location(s) of coronary artery stenosis:

- LAD: Anterior, anteroseptal, apex, +/- inferoapical ("wraparound" LAD)
- Circumflex: Anterolateral, inferolateral
- RCA: Inferior, inferoseptal

Also, see rationale of **Answer 34.3.**

### Selected References

1. Lang RM, Badano LP, Mor-Avi V, et al. Recommendations for cardiac chamber quantification by echocardiography in adults: an update from the American Society of Echocardiography and the European Association of Cardiovascular Imaging. *J Am Soc Echocardiogr*. 2015;28(1):1-39.e14.
2. Otto C. *Echocardiography Review Guide: Companion to the Textbook of Clinical Echocardiography*. 4th ed. Elsevier; 2019.
3. Quader N, Makan M, Perez P, eds. *The Washington Manual of Echocardiography*. 2nd ed. Wolters Kluwer; 2017.

**14.** Correct Answer: A. Takotsubo cardiomyopathy

*Rationale:* When evaluating the patient with chest pain, it is important to consider conditions that mimic acute coronary syndrome. All of the answer choices may produce the clinical signs and symptoms, ECG changes, troponin elevations, and echocardiographic findings consistent with acute coronary syndrome. In the case of pheochromocytoma and Takotsubo cardiomyopathy, it is thought that the excessive release of catecholamines is responsible for this mimicry of acute coronary syndrome. In the presented figure, basal pronounced hypercontractility with apical ballooning is present. Less common variants of this pattern and more subtle findings have been reported.

Selected References

1. Bybee KA, Kara T, Prasad A, et al. Systematic review: transient left ventricular apical ballooning: a syndrome that mimics ST-segment elevation acute myocardial infarction. *Ann Intern Med.* 2004;141:858-865.
2. Cooper LT. Clinical manifestations and diagnosis of myocarditis in adults. https://www.uptodate.com/contents/clinical-manifestations-and-diagnosis-of-myocarditis-in-adults
3. Ripoll JG, Blackshear JL, Díaz-Gómez JL. Acute cardiac complications in critical brain disease. *Neurol Clin.* 2017;29(2):281-297.

**15.** Correct Answer: A. Right heart failure

*Rationale:* Complications of acute MI include VSD formation, papillary muscle rupture or dysfunction, ventricular free wall rupture with or without formation of a pseudoaneurysm, LV thrombus formation, and right heart failure. An LV free wall rupture most often results in acute pericardial tamponade and sudden death. In the case of the formation of a pseudoaneurysm, the defect is contained by localized pericardial adhesions, allowing for the potential of prompt diagnosis, and avoidance of death from future rupture. The echocardiographic characteristics of pseudoaneurysm are discussed in another question explanation. Additionally, a murmur is present in two-thirds of pseudoaneurysms and is described as "to and fro," although in some instances it may be indistinguishable from that of mitral regurgitation. Papillary muscle rupture and dysfunction both cause a murmur of mitral regurgitation. A VSD is often associated with hypotension in addition to the presence of a new harsh, loud, and holosystolic murmur. Right heart failure is most often associated with an inferior MI due to the overlapping blood supply. The echo image shows an enlarged right ventricle and atrium. RWMAs may be present. In addition, one might expect to see tricuspid regurgitation resulting from the altered right ventricle geometry and enlarged tricuspid annulus. See **Figure 34.16** and ▶ **Video 34.6**.

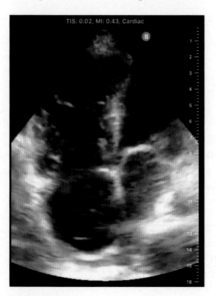

**Figure 34.16**

Selected References

1. Laham R, Simons M, Suri R. Mechanical complications of acute myocardial infarction. 2017. https://www.uptodate.com/contents/acute-myocardial-infarction-mechanical-complications
2. Naseerullah F, Baig M, Wool K, Murthy A. Left ventricle pseudoaneurysm: diagnosis by a new murmur. *J Cardiol Cases.* 2018;18(1):20-24.
3. Shapira O. Left ventricular aneurysm and pseudoaneurysm following acute myocardial infarction. 2019. https://www.uptodate.com/contents/left-ventricular-aneurysm-and-pseudoaneurysm-following-acute-myocardial-infarction

**16.** Correct Answer: B. Papillary muscle rupture

*Rationale:* Cardiogenic shock is the number one cause of mortality in patients suffering ST-elevation myocardial infarction (STEMI) and has a number of causes. Chief among them is LV failure, resulting from a large infarction. All of the answer choices may produce both a murmur and symptoms of heart failure. The echocardiographic image shows a ruptured papillary muscle. The arrow points to the chordae tendinae of the posterior medial papillary muscle, which is sensitive to ischemia due to its common singular blood supply. In one study of 251 patients from multiple centers, the etiology of cardiogenic shock after acute MI was the following: LV failure: 85%, VSD or MR: 8%, RV infarct: 2%, other: 5%.

Selected References
1. Hochman JS, Boland J, Sleeper LA, et al. Current spectrum of cardiogenic shock and effect of early revascularization on mortality. Results of an International Registry. SHOCK Registry Investigators. *Circulation.* 1995;91:873-881.
2. Laham R, Simons M, Suri R. Mechanical complications of acute myocardial infarction. 2017. https://www.uptodate.com/contents/acute-myocardial-infarction-mechanical-complications.

**17.** Correct Answer: B. Decreased RV base descent

*Rationale:* RV infarction most commonly occurs in conjunction with left ventricle inferior wall infarction as the posterior descending artery supplies this area in 85% of the population. RV dysfunction leads to decreased LV filling and consequent decreased LV cardiac output even in the absence of coexisting LV impairment. Because the atrioventricular (AV) node is supplied by the RCA in 90% of the population, arrhythmias such as bradycardia or complete AV block are often associated and may further contribute to hypotension. Presenting symptoms—chest pain, nausea, anxiety, and dizziness—are shared with LV inferior MI. Jugular venous distention and peripheral edema strongly suggest right heart involvement, and a right-sided ECG showing $V_4R > 1.0$ mm is 100% sensitive and 87% specific in these cases. In the situation of RV infarction leading to shock, characteristic echocardiographic signs include RV enlargement, RV wall motion abnormalities, decreases in RV base descent, as well as a dilatation of the IVC that does not decrease in diameter with deep inspiration. A TAPSE < 16 mm is consistent with RV dysfunction, while a TAPSE of 25 mm would be considered normal. Treatment includes optimization of preload via judicious volume administration, inotropic support, and avoidance of nitrates, diuretics, and opioids, which may compromise RV filling pressures. Absence of lung sliding would be expected in cases of pneumothorax.

Selected References
1. Goldberger JJ, Himelman RB, Wolfe CL, Schiller NB. Right ventricular infarction: recognition and assessment of its hemodynamic significance by two-dimensional echocardiography. *J Am Soc Echocardiogr.* 1991 Mar-Apr;4(2):140-146.
2. Levin T, Goldstein J. Right ventricular myocardial infarction. 2019. https://www.uptodate.com/contents/right-ventricular-myocardial-infarction

**18.** Correct Answer: B. $V_3$-$V_4$

*Rationale:* Figure 34.11 is a two-chamber view with the arrow pointing at the anterior wall. The anterior wall is represented on the ECG by leads V3-V4. In addition to ST elevation in these precordial leads, reciprocal changes of ST depression in leads II, III, in aVF may also be apparent (30% of the time). Knowing specific ECG patterns (**Table 34.1**) of change and the corresponding echocardiographic findings is valuable in diagnosing acute MI. (See also rationale in **Answer 34.3.**)

**Table 34.1 EKG Patterns**

| Anatomy | Leads | Findings |
| --- | --- | --- |
| Anterior | $V_2$-$V_4$, II, III, aVF | ST elevation ≥ 2 mm Reciprocal depression |
| Inferior | II, III, aVF aVL | ST elevation ≥ 1 mm Reciprocal depression (in 80%) |
| Right Ventricle | $V_4R$ $V_1$-$V_3$ | ST elevation diagnostic ST elevation indicative |
| Lateral | I, aVL, $V_5$, $V_6$ | ST elevation ≥ 1 mm (in precordial leads) |
| Posterior | $V_1$, $V_2$ $V_8$, $V_9$ | Reciprocal depression *only* ST elevation ≥ 0.5 mm |

Selected References

1. Lang RM, Badano LP, Mor-Avi V, et al. Recommendations for cardiac chamber quantification by echocardiography in adults: an update from the American Society of Echocardiography and the European Association of Cardiovascular Imaging. *J Am Soc Echocardiogr.* 2015;28(1):1-39.e14.

2. Stapczynski JS, ed. Missed myocardial infarction: ECG strategies to reduce the risk in emergency medicine reports. Accessed June 8, 2009. https://www.reliasmedia.com/articles/113394-missed-myocardial-infarction-ecg-strategies-to-reduce-the-risk.

**19.** Correct Answer: **D. Inferior wall**

*Rationale:* Isolated RV MI is a rare event. The right ventricle is inherently more resistant to myocardial ischemia than the left ventricle because:

- The right ventricle is a thinner walled structure that has lower oxygen requirements due to less energy consumption during the cardiac cycle,
- Receives perfusion during both systole and diastole, and
- There is often significant collateral flow from left coronary artery to RCA distributions.

It should be noted that isolated right heart infarction is possible as a result of complications of interventional procedures and cardiac surgery. A right coronary occlusion is capable of obstructing flow to the majority of the RV free wall if it occurs prior to the take-off of the RV marginal arteries. Additionally, rhythm disturbances are possible. The inferior wall of the left ventricle is supplied by the RCA in roughly 85% of the population (right dominant supply), by circumflex artery in 10% (left dominant), and by both RCA and circumflex in 5% (codominant). Wall motion abnormalities and corresponding ECG changes are most commonly seen in this area.

Selected References

1. Horan LG, Flowers NC. Right ventricular infarction: specific requirements of management. *Am Fam Physician.* 1999 Oct 15;60(6):1727-1734.

2. Jeffers JL, Parks LJ. Right ventricular myocardial infarction. [Updated 2019 Feb 28]. In: StatPearls [Internet]. StatPearls Publishing; 2019 Jan. https://www.ncbi.nlm.nih.gov/books/NBK431048/

3. Levin T, Goldstein JA. Right ventricular myocardial infarction. 2019. https://www.uptodate.com/contents/right-ventricular-myocardial-infarction

**20.** Correct Answer: **E. Proximal right coronary**

*Rationale:* See **Answer 34.19** rationale. Although the posterior descending artery supplies the inferior left ventricle in this scenario, (right dominance) the combination of both right heart infarction (see both ECG signs and supportive symptoms) with inferior infarction is most consistent with a proximal RCA occlusion.

Selected References

1. Horan LG, Flowers NC. Right ventricular infarction: specific requirements of management. *Am Fam Physician.* 1999 Oct 15;60(6):1727-1734.

2. Jeffers JL, Parks LJ. Right ventricular myocardial infarction. [Updated 2019 Feb 28]. In: StatPearls [Internet]. StatPearls Publishing; 2019 Jan. https://www.ncbi.nlm.nih.gov/books/NBK431048/

3. Levin T, Goldstein JA. Right ventricular myocardial infarction. 2019. https://www.uptodate.com/contents/right-ventricular-myocardial-infarction

# 35 | DIASTOLOGY

Archit Sharma and Sung Kim

---

**1.** The mitral inflow pattern in **Figure 35.1** is consistent with:

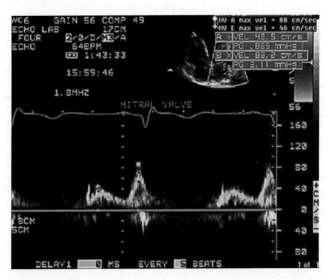

**Figure 35.1**

A. Abnormal left ventricular (LV) relaxation with elevated left atrial (LA) pressure
B. Abnormal LV relaxation with normal LA pressure
C. Restrictive LV filling
D. Pseudonormal filling
E. Normal LV filling

---

**2.** What is the best Doppler evaluative method to distinguish between restrictive pericarditis and constrictive pericarditis?

A. Mitral inflow pattern
B. Pulmonary vein flows
C. Atrial size
D. Inferior vena cava (IVC) dilatation
E. Mitral annulus e' (early diastolic) velocity with tissue Doppler imaging (TDI)

3. Which of the following statements are true about pulmonary vein flow pattern?

   **A.** Peak atrial regurgitation (AR) > 35 cm/s suggests elevated LV filling pressures.
   **B.** The pulmonary S wave is related to LV relaxation.
   **C.** The S/D ratio provides an accurate estimation of LV filling pressures in patients with preserved and reduced systolic function.
   **D.** (Pulmonary venous AR duration) – (Mitral inflow A wave duration) of less than 30 ms signifies elevated filling pressures.
   **E.** Pulmonary venous flow AR can be obtained in only 50% of patients.

4. Diastolic heart failure is often associated with LV hypertrophy and LA size. Which of the following transthoracic echocardiography (TTE) views is best to evaluate LA volume?

   **A.** Parasternal long axis
   **B.** Subcostal four-chamber view
   **C.** Apical four-chamber view
   **D.** Aortic valve view
   **E.** Parasternal left ventricle short-axis view

5. A 52-year-old male patient with a past medical history of hypertension and diabetes has the following values on the TTE:

   - Left ventricular ejection fraction (LVEF) = 58%
   - e' = 7.2 cm/s
   - E = 82.4 cm/s
   - A = 117.7 cm/s
   - Tricuspid regurgitation (TR) velocity of 3.2 m/s
   - LA volume index of 38 mL/m$^2$

   What is your assessment?
   **A.** Patient has normal diastolic function
   **B.** Patient has diastolic dysfunction
   **C.** Patient has severe TR
   **D.** Patient has severe pulmonary hypertension
   **E.** Cannot be determined with information provided

6. The pulmonary vein flow shown in **Figure 35.2** is indicative of:

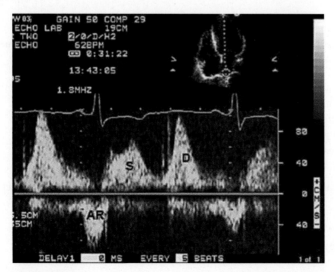

**Figure 35.2**

A. Elevated LA pressure with normal end-diastolic pressure (EDP)
B. Elevated LA pressure with elevated EDP
C. Abnormal LV relaxation with normal EDP
D. Elevated LVEDP with normal LA pressure
E. Normal LA pressure

7. Which of the following statements about impaired LV relaxation is true?

A. Impaired LV relaxation causes the mitral inflow E velocity to decrease with a longer deceleration time, representing a decreased early diastolic LV filling rate.
B. Impaired LV relaxation causes the mitral inflow E velocity to increase with a longer deceleration time, representing a decreased early diastolic LV filling rate.
C. Impaired LV relaxation causes the mitral inflow E velocity to decrease with a longer deceleration time, representing an increased early diastolic LV filling rate.
D. Impaired LV relaxation causes the mitral inflow E velocity to decrease with a shorter deceleration time, representing a decreased early diastolic LV filling rate.
E. Impaired LV relaxation causes the mitral inflow E velocity to increase with a shorter deceleration time, representing an increased early diastolic LV filling rate.

8. A 62-year-old female shows the following features on TTE:

- Deceleration time of 120 ms
- Pulmonary venous flow: S2 < D velocity
- Increased atrial reversal

These echocardiographic features can be present in which among the following conditions?
A. Constrictive pericarditis
B. Dilated cardiomyopathy
C. Restrictive cardiomyopathy
D. Ischemic cardiomyopathy
E. All of the above

9. Which of the following factors is not an independent determinant of e'?

A. Active relaxation of the left ventricle
B. Passive relaxation of the left ventricle
C. Restoring forces of the left ventricle
D. Lengthening load of the left ventricle
E. Both C and D

10. Which of the following answers correctly pairs transmitral Doppler flow velocity waveform with the phase of the cardiac cycle?

A. E wave = Rapid LV filling,   A wave = Isovolumetric contraction
B. E wave = Isovolumetric relaxation,   A wave = Rapid LV filling
C. E wave = Isovolumetric contraction,   A wave = Atrial contraction
D. E wave = Atrial contraction,   A wave = Rapid LV filling
E. E wave =  Rapid LV filling,   A wave = Atrial contraction

11. The pulmonary vein S wave may be less prominent than the D wave in the following situations except:

A. Young children
B. Atrial fibrillation
C. Moderate-to-severe mitral regurgitation (MR)
D. Elevated LA pressure
E. Abnormal LV relaxation with normal LA pressure

12. Normal pulmonary vein A-wave duration compared to mitral A-wave duration is:

    **A.** Less
    **B.** More
    **C.** Same
    **D.** Variable
    **E.** No relation between the two and diastolic failure.

13. The part of the flow curve denoted by the *arrow* in this pulmonary vein flow in **Figure 35.3** is caused by:

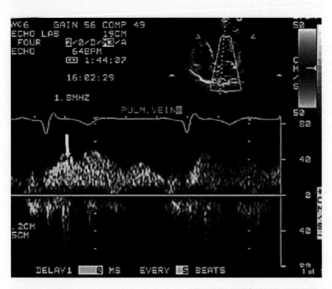

**Figure 35.3**

    **A.** LA relaxation
    **B.** Right ventricular (RV) ejection
    **C.** Mitral valve opening
    **D.** Mitral annular descent
    **E.** Mitral regurgitation

14. All of the following factors affect pulmonary vein A-wave (A-reversal) amplitude except:

    **A.** Pulmonary vein diameter
    **B.** LV end-diastolic stiffness
    **C.** Heart rate (HR)
    **D.** LA function
    **E.** Pulmonary artery pressure

15. Color Doppler M-mode (CMM) echocardiography provides information on flow propagation velocity (Vp) which is unique in that it is relatively independent of which of the following?

    **A.** Cardiac output
    **B.** LV compliance
    **C.** LA size
    **D.** Loading conditions
    **E.** Heart rate

16. Normal mitral E-wave propagation velocity by CMM inside the LV is:

    A. 10 to 30 cm/s
    B. 30 to 50 cm/s
    C. Greater than 50 cm/s
    D. Greater than 500 cm/s
    E. Less than 10 cm/s

17. Both atrial mechanical failure and high LA pressure result in a high E/A ratio. Which of the following is least likely to help in the differential diagnosis in this situation?

    A. E-wave deceleration time
    B. Amplitude and duration of AR wave
    C. Pulmonary vein S/D time velocity integral ratio
    D. Mitral annular velocity with TDI
    E. Tricuspid annular velocity with TDI

18. An abnormal LV relaxation pattern is consistent with:

    A. Mean LA pressure of 10 mm Hg and LVEDP of 22 mm Hg
    B. Mean LA pressure of 22 mm Hg and LVEDP of 10 mm Hg
    C. Mean LA pressure of 10 mm Hg and LVEDP of 12 mm Hg
    D. Mean LA pressure of 28 mm Hg and LVEDP of 30 mm Hg
    E. Mean LA pressure of 28 mm Hg and LVEDP of 40 mm Hg

19. The mitral inflow pattern in **Figure 35.4** is consistent with:

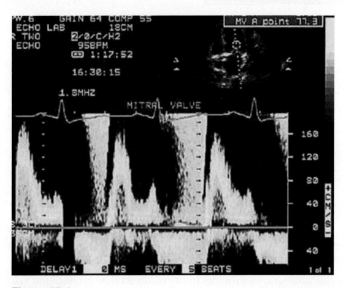

**Figure 35.4**

    A. Severe MR
    B. Prosthetic mitral valve
    C. Atrial fibrillation
    D. Severe mitral stenosis
    E. Atrial flutter

20. Which of the findings listed below is considered a classical finding on TTE in patients with amyloidosis?

   A. Interventricular septal "bounce"
   B. Increased myocardial strain
   C. Short deceleration time associated with worsening prognosis
   D. Normal LV wall thickness
   E. Increased systolic and early diastolic velocities of the mitral annulus on TDI

21. A 57-year-old male with a history of hypertensive heart disease, diabetes mellitus, and Crohn disease presents to the clinic with symptoms of fatigue and recent weight gain. A TTE is ordered. During echocardiographic Doppler evaluation of the patient's mitral inflows, patient is asked to bear down and perform a Valsalva maneuver. **Figure 35.5A** shows the Doppler tracing prior to the Valsalva and **Figure 35.5B** represents the Doppler tracing after the Valsalva.

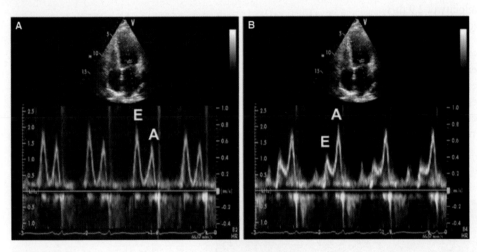

**Figure 35.5**

Choose the correct diagnosis from the options listed below.
   A. Figure 35.5A (Pseudonormal); Figure 35.5B (Grade I dysfunction)
   B. Figure 35.5A (Normal); Figure 35.5B (Pseudonormal)
   C. Figure 35.5A (Normal); Figure 35.5B (Grade I dysfunction)
   D. Figure 35.5A (Grade II dysfunction); Figure 35.5B (Normal)
   E. Figure 35.5A (Grade III dysfunction); Figure 35.5B (Normal)

22. The mitral flow pattern shown in **Figure 35.6** is suggestive of:

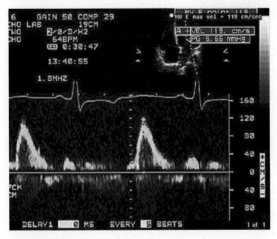

**Figure 35.6**

A. Atrial mechanical failure
B. High LA pressure
C. Normal LA pressure
D. Abnormal LV relaxation with normal LA pressure
E. Low LA pressure

23. A 61-year-old female patient with a past medical history of hypertension, asthma, and hypothyroidism has the following values on the TTE:

- LVEF = 60%
- Left atrial pressure (LAP) is normal
- e' = 5.9 cm/s
- E = 65 cm/s
- A = 120 cm/s
- TR velocity of 2.9 m/s
- LA volume index of 41 mL/m$^2$

What is your assessment?
A. Patient has normal diastolic function
B. Patient has Grade I diastolic function
C. Patient has Grade II diastolic function
D. Patient has Grade III diastolic function
E. Cannot be determined with information in the question

24. The pulsed-wave Doppler (**Figure 35.7**) in the left upper pulmonary vein is indicative of:

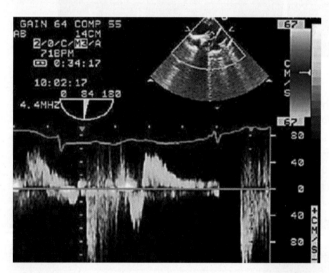

**Figure 35.7**

A. High LA pressure
B. Abnormal LV relaxation
C. Mitral stenosis
D. Severe MR
E. Normal mitral valve

25. The mitral flow profile shown in **Figure 35.8** is suggestive of:

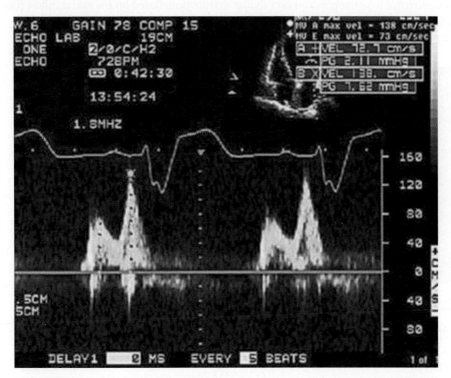

**Figure 35.8**

   **A.** Normal LV diastolic function
   **B.** Abnormal relaxation
   **C.** Pseudonormal pattern
   **D.** Restrictive pattern
   **E.** None of the above

26. What intervention can potentially change the mitral inflow pattern from **Figure 35.9A** to **Figure 35.9B**?

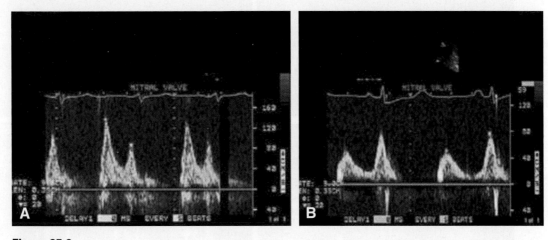

**Figure 35.9**

   **A.** Control of severe hypertension
   **B.** Diuresis
   **C.** Correction of severe anemia
   **D.** All of the above
   **E.** None of the above

27. Echocardiography for a 53-year-old male with hypertension shows a normal LV systolic function (EF = 60%), mild concentric LV hypertrophy, and no valvular dysfunction. Based on his mitral inflow pattern in **Figure 35.10**, which parameter is most helpful in confirming whether his symptoms are due to elevated filling pressures?

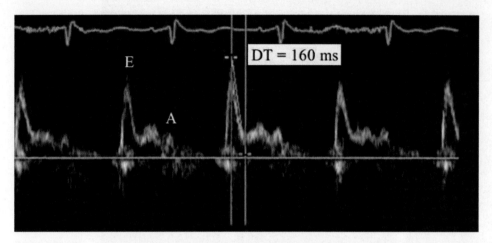

**Figure 35.10**

A. Tissue Doppler early diastolic velocity of the mitral annulus of 12 cm/s
B. LA volume index of 28 mL/m$^2$
C. Tissue Doppler–derived early diastolic velocity of the mitral annulus of 6 cm/s
D. Transmitral flow propagation velocity assessed by CMM of 60 cm/s
E. Difference in duration of pulmonary venous flow AR and mitral inflow of 15 ms

28. Out of the parts A-D displayed in **Figure 35.11**, which one best represents the tissue Doppler recordings of mitral annular velocities, with regard to Doppler settings, sampling location, gain, and filter?

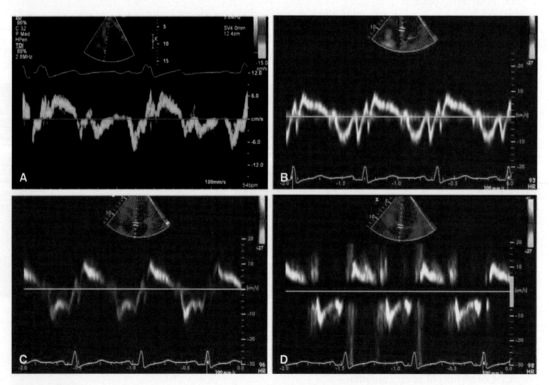

**Figure 35.11**

A. Figure 35.11A
B. Figure 35.11B
C. Figure 35.11C
D. Figure 35.11D
E. None of the above

---

29. This pulmonary vein flow pattern in **Figure 35.12** is indicative of:

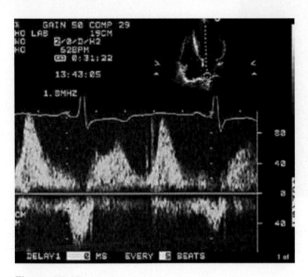

**Figure 35.12**

A. Atrial fibrillation
B. Volume depletion
C. Elevated LVEDP with normal LA pressure
D. Elevated LVEDP with high LA pressure
E. Normal LVEDP

---

30. What one of the following is the strongest determinant of mitral deceleration time?

A. LA mechanical function
B. LV operating stiffness
C. LV end-diastolic pressure
D. LA reservoir function
E. Ejection fraction

**31.** The hemodynamics shown in **Figure 35.13** for this patient potentially with a HR of 70 could be improved by:

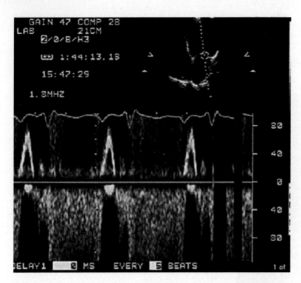

**Figure 35.13**

   **A.** Positive inotropes
   **B.** Afterload reduction
   **C.** Shortening the PR interval
   **D.** All of the above
   **E.** None of the above

**32.** When performing pulsed-wave Doppler imaging to assess mitral annular velocities, which of the following is true?

   **A.** The sample volume should be positioned at or 1 cm from insertion sites of the mitral leaflets.
   **B.** The velocity scale should be set at about 30 cm/s above and below the baseline.
   **C.** Spectral recordings are obtained while performing a Valsalva maneuver.
   **D.** Angulation up to 50° between the ultrasound and the plane of cardiac motion is acceptable.
   **E.** All of these are correct

**33.** Which statement is most correct with respect to the application of the Valsalva maneuver in the assessment of diastolic function?

   **A.** The Valsalva maneuver is specific and sensitive for differentiating stage 1 diastolic function from normal diastology.
   **B.** The lack of reversibility in E/A, after Valsalva, in patients with advanced diastolic dysfunction indicates irreversible restrictive physiology and implies a very poor prognosis.
   **C.** The Valsalva maneuver should be used in every patient when assessing diastology.
   **D.** A decrease of >50% in E/A ratio is highly specific for increased LV filling pressures.
   **E.** The Valsalva maneuver has no correlation with assessing diastolic function.

34. A 42-year-old female undergoes a heart transplantation procedure for her cardiac dysfunction due to nonischemic cardiomyopathy and in the week following the transplantation has troubles weaning from the ventilator and follow-up echocardiography is done to evaluate the transplanted heart function (**Figure 35.14A** and **B**).

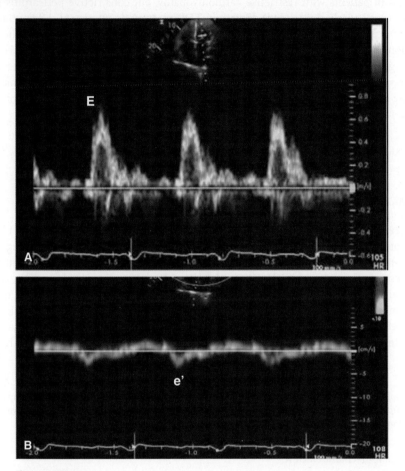

**Figure 35.14**

What would be your assessment and plan based on the echocardiographic evidence?
**A.** Patient has abnormal cardiac function and reduced filling pressures.
**B.** Patient has abnormal cardiac function and elevated filling pressures.
**C.** Patient has normal cardiac function and no intervention is needed.
**D.** None of the above is true.
**E.** No estimate about filling pressures can be made.

# Chapter 35 ▪ Answers

**1.** Correct Answer: B. Abnormal LV relaxation with normal LA pressure

*Rationale:* Abnormal LV relaxation pattern includes E/A ratio <1 (bigger A wave compared to E wave), prolonged LV isovolumic relaxation time (>100 ms), and E-wave deceleration time >250 ms.

### Selected Reference

1. Nagueh SF, Smiseth OA, Appleton CP, et al. Recommendations for the evaluation of left ventricular diastolic function by echocardiography: an update from the American Society of Echocardiography and the European Association of Cardiovascular Imaging. *Eur Heart J Cardiovasc Imaging.* 2016 Dec;17(12):1321-1360.

**2.** Correct Answer: E. Mitral annulus e' (early diastolic) velocity with tissue Doppler imaging (TDI)

*Rationale*: Mitral inflow and pulmonary venous flow do not always exhibit the typical respiratory changes. The IVC is typically dilated in both patients with constrictive and restrictive cardiomyopathy. Atrial size will usually be increased in patients with restrictive cardiomyopathy, but constrictive pericarditis will also eventually result in (particularly right-sided) dilatation. TDI can provide important differentiating information. In restrictive cardiomyopathy, myocardial relaxation (e') will be severely impaired, whereas patients with constriction usually have preserved annular vertical excursion. A septal e' velocity $\geq 7$ cm/s has been shown to be highly accurate in differentiating patients with constrictive pericarditis from those with restrictive cardiomyopathy. Since the lateral annular e' velocity could be decreased if the constrictive process involves the lateral mitral annulus, the septal e' velocity is considered more specific for this assessment.

### Selected Reference

1. Dal-Bianco JP, Sengupta, Khandheria BK. Role of echocardiography in the diagnosis of constrictive pericarditis. *J Am Soc Echocardiogr*. 2009;22(1):24-33.

**3.** Correct Answer: A. Peak AR >35 cm/s suggests elevated LV filling pressures.

*Rationale:* AR may increase with age, but AR >35 cm/s is usually consistent with elevated LV filling pressures, particularly at end diastole. The pulmonary D wave is related to LV relaxation. Young and healthy individuals can therefore exhibit large D waves indicating forceful elastic recoil of the left ventricle rather than high LA pressure. The pulmonary S wave is related to LV contractility, atrial function, atrial pressure, and MR. Mitral and pulmonary vein inflow patterns are not very reliable for assessment of LV filling pressures in patients with an overall normal systolic function. $AR_{dur} - A_{dur} >30$ ms is, therefore, a more robust marker of elevated LVEDP in this group of patients. Pulmonary venous atrial reversal can be obtained in more than 70% of patients. A commercially available contrast injection can help enhance the Doppler tracing.

### Selected Reference

1. Nagueh SF, Smiseth OA, Appleton CP, et al. Recommendations for the evaluation of left ventricular diastolic function by echocardiography: an update from the American Society of Echocardiography and the European Association of Cardiovascular Imaging. *Eur Heart J Cardiovasc Imaging*. 2016 Dec;17(12):1321-1360.

**4.** Correct Answer: C. Apical four-chamber view

*Rationale:* LA size is an important marker of the severity of LV diastolic dysfunction. An LA volume of 34 mL/m$^2$ (reflective of moderate or greater LA dilatation) has been shown to predict death and nonfatal cardiovascular events among patients without atrial fibrillation or valvular heart disease. The most accurate echocardiographic measurement of LA size is the LA volume from the transthoracic apical views.

### Selected Reference

1. Murata M, Iwanaga S, Ogawa S. A real-time three-dimensional echocardiographic quantitative analysis of left atrial function in left ventricular diastolic dysfunction. *Am J Cardiol*. 2008;102(8):1097-1102.

**5.** Correct Answer: B. Patient has diastolic dysfunction

*Rationale:* In a patient with normal EF, the following criteria can be used to determine if the patient has diastolic dysfunction:
1. Average E/e' > 14,
2. Septal e' velocity <7 cm/s or lateral e' velocity <10 cm/s,
3. LA volume index >34 mL/m$^2$,
4. TR velocity >2.8 m/s.

If more than 50% of them are positive (i.e., three or more), then the patient has diastolic dysfunction. For making determinations in patients who have a preserved EF (Figure 35.15A) versus patients who have a depressed EF or myocardial disease (Figure 35.15B), please refer to **Figure 35.15** for the algorithm delineated by the American Society of Echocardiography.

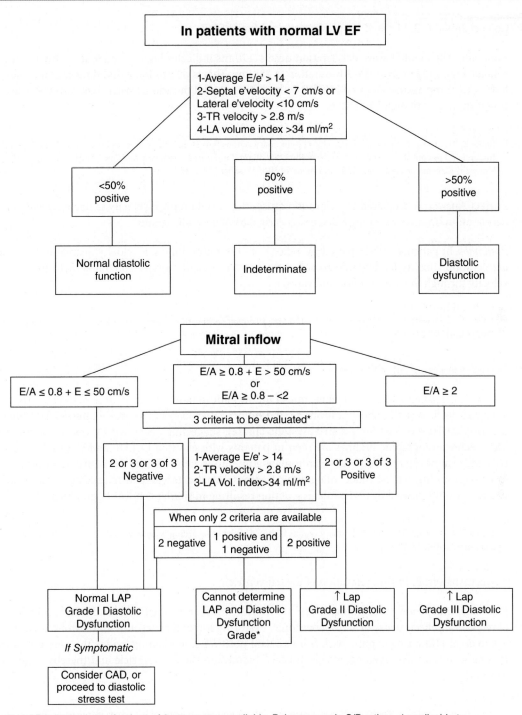

(* : LAP indeterminate if only 1 of 3 parameters available. Pulmonary vein S/D ration <1 applicable to conclude elevated LAP in patients with depressed LV EF)

**Figure 35.15**

### Selected Reference

1. Nagueh SF, Smiseth OA, Appleton CP, et al. Recommendations for the evaluation of left ventricular diastolic function by echo-cardiography: an update from the American Society of Echocardiography and the European Association of Cardiovascular Imaging. *Eur Heart J Cardiovasc Imaging.* 2016 Dec;17(12):1321-1360.

**6.** Correct Answer: B. Elevated LA pressure with elevated EDP

*Rationale:* The rapid D-wave deceleration time <170 ms indicates high LA pressure. Also, the S wave is smaller than the D wave. The AR duration is 220 ms. This is due to increased duration of atrial systole having to pump against elevated LVEDP. Pulmonary vein AR duration greater than mitral A-wave duration is indicative of high LVEDP.

Selected References
1. Buffle E, Kramarz J, Topilsky Y. Added value of pulmonary venous flow Doppler assessment in patients with preserved ejection fraction and its contribution to the diastolic grading paradigm. *Eur Heart J Cardiovasc Imaging.* 2015;16(11):1191-1197.
2. Morrissey C. Echo for diastology. *Ann Card Anaesth.* 2016;19(*suppl S1*):12-18.

**7.** Correct Answer: A. Impaired LV relaxation causes the mitral inflow E velocity to decrease with a longer deceleration time, representing a decreased early diastolic LV filling rate.

*Rationale:* In patients with impaired LV relaxation, the mitral inflow E velocity decreases with a longer deceleration time, reflecting a decreased early diastolic LV filling rate. To complement this change, A velocity through the mitral inflow increases.

Selected Reference
1. Tabata T, Thomas JD, Klein AL. Pulmonary venous flow by doppler echocardiography: revisited 12 years later. *J Am Coll Cardiol.* 2003 Apr;41(8):1243-1250.

**8.** Correct Answer: E. All of the above

*Rationale:* In patients with a restrictive mitral inflow pattern (a deceleration time <150 ms), the pulmonary venous flow (PVF) shows a lower S2 and higher D velocities (severely blunted systolic flow) and increased atrial reversals (unless atrial systolic failure), suggesting decreased LV operating compliance. These echocardiographic findings are seen in patients with elevated LVEDP and elevated LA pressure. Dilated cardiomyopathy, restrictive cardiomyopathy, and ischemic cardiomyopathy cause diastolic dysfunction resulting in these echocardiographic findings. In patients with constrictive pericarditis, LV compliance is compromised by pericardial restriction resulting in similar echocardiographic features.

Selected Reference
1. Tabata T, Thomas JD, Klein AL. Pulmonary venous flow by doppler echocardiography: revisited 12 years later. *J Am Coll Cardiol.* 2003 Apr;41(8):1243-1250.

**9.** Correct Answer: B. Passive relaxation of the left ventricle

*Rationale:* Independent determinants of e' are LV relaxation, restoring forces, and lengthening load. Rate of relaxation reflects decay of active fiber force. Restoring forces that account for diastolic suction is similar to an elastic spring coming back from a recoil position. Lengthening load is the pressure in the left atrium at mitral valve opening, which "pushes" blood into the left ventricle and thereby lengthens the ventricle.

Selected Reference
1. Nagueh SF, Smiseth OA, Appleton CP, et al. Recommendations for the evaluation of left ventricular diastolic function by echocardiography: an update from the American Society of Echocardiography and the European Association of Cardiovascular Imaging. *Eur Heart J Cardiovasc Imaging.* 2016 Dec;17(12):1321-1360.

**10.** Correct Answer: E. E wave = Rapid LV filling,   A wave = Atrial contraction

*Rationale:* In a sinus heart rhythm, two waveforms are seen on the transmitral Doppler flow velocity profile. E wave represents rapid LV filling during the early part of diastole and A wave represents atrial contraction that occurs at the end.

Selected Reference
1. Zile MR, Brutsaert DL. New concepts in diastolic dysfunction and diastolic heart failure: Part I: diagnosis, prognosis, and measurements of diastolic function. *Circulation.* 2002;105(11):1387-1393.

**11.** Correct Answer: E. Abnormal LV relaxation with normal LA pressure

*Rationale:* Young children have very compliant left ventricle, resulting in rapid early filling (mitral E wave) paralleled by an increase in D wave that might have rapid deceleration as well. As S1 is due to atrial relaxation, atrial fibrillation results in reduced S-wave amplitude. Systolic LA filling from MR will impede pulmonary vein flow in systole. High LA pressure renders the left atrium less compliant due to rightward shift of its pressure-volume curve and hence will impede atrial systolic filling, as the left atrium is a closed chamber receiving only pulmonary venous flow during systole. Abnormal LV relaxation reduces E- and D-wave amplitudes, resulting in an increase in S-wave amplitude in the absence of elevated LA pressure.

Selected Reference
1. Daneshvar D, Wei J, Merz CNB. Diastolic dysfunction: improved understanding using emerging imaging techniques. *Am Heart J.* 2010;160(3):394-404.

**12.** Correct Answer: A. Less

*Rationale:* Increased pulmonary A-wave duration compared to mitral A-wave duration indicates high LVEDP. A difference in duration of more than 30 ms is very suggestive of high LVEDP.

Selected Reference
1. Nagueh SF, Smiseth OA, Appleton CP, et al. Recommendations for the evaluation of left ventricular diastolic function by echocardiography: an update from the American Society of Echocardiography and the European Association of Cardiovascular Imaging. *Eur Heart J Cardiovasc Imaging.* 2016 Dec;17(12):1321-1360.

**13.** Correct Answer: A. LA relaxation

*Rationale:* The arrow denotes the systolic S1 wave, created by LA relaxation. Mitral annular descent and RV ejection generate the S2 wave, which follows the S1 wave. The mitral valve opening generates the diastolic D wave, which is synchronous with the mitral E wave.

Selected Reference
1. Rossvoll O, Hatle LK. Pulmonary venous flow velocities recorded by transthoracic Doppler ultrasound: relation to left ventricular diastolic pressures. *J Am Coll Cardiol.* 1993;21(7):1687-1696.

**14.** Correct Answer: E. Pulmonary artery pressure

*Rationale:* The amplitude is increased in the presence of a stiff left ventricle and reduced in LA mechanical failure. The pulmonary A wave may disappear with HRs in excess of 100/min, where flow may be entirely antegrade, and atrial contraction may produce a transient deceleration pulmonary flow without reversal. As velocity depends upon flow volume and cross-sectional area, a dilated pulmonary vein is likely to reduce the A-wave velocity and a collapsed vein in a dry patient can result in a giant A wave. Pulmonary artery pressure is least likely to have any significant effect on A-wave characteristics.

Selected Reference
1. Rossvoll O, Hatle LK. Pulmonary venous flow velocities recorded by transthoracic Doppler ultrasound: relation to left ventricular diastolic pressures. *J Am Coll Cardiol.* 1993;21(7):1687-1696.

**15.** Correct Answer: D. Loading conditions

*Rationale:* CMM echocardiography provides a way to assess the propagation velocity (Vp), which appears to be relatively independent of loading conditions and hence overcomes one of the main limitations of Doppler-based techniques. They are affected by cardiac output, LA size, LV compliance, and HR, just like other diastolic parameters. After the mitral valve opens in early diastole, there is a rapid component (phase 1), often followed by a slow component (phase 2). Finally, the last component in late diastole is associated with atrial contraction.

Selected Reference
1. Rovner A, de las Fuentes L, Waggoner AD, Memon N, Chohan R, Dávila-Román VG. Characterization of left ventricular diastolic function in hypertension by use of Doppler tissue imaging and color M-mode techniques. *J Am Soc Echocardiogr.* 2006;19(7):872-879.

**16.** Correct Answer: C. Greater than 50 cm/s

*Rationale:* Normal mitral E-wave propagation velocity is >50 cm/s.

Selected Reference
1. Vierendeels JA, Dick E, Verdonck PR. Hydrodynamics of color M-mode Doppler flow wave propagation velocity V (p): a computer study. *J Am Soc Echocardiogr.* 2002;15(3):219-224.

**17.** Correct Answer: C. Pulmonary vein S/D time velocity integral ratio

*Rationale:* High LA pressure results in short isovolumic relaxation time (IVRT), an increase in pulmonary vein AR-wave duration and amplitude, and reduced E-wave deceleration time. Mitral E/mitral annular $E_m$ ratio is a good indicator of LA pressure. The S-wave amplitude is diminished in high LA pressure due to increased LA operating stiffness during LV systole, when there is no LA emptying. Atrial mechanical failure results in diminution of pulmonary AR reversal and absence of atrial relaxation, which causes an LA suction effect and will result in diminution of S-wave amplitude.

Selected Reference
1. Nagueh SF, Smiseth OA, Appleton CP, et al. Recommendations for the evaluation of left ventricular diastolic function by echocardiography: an update from the American Society of Echocardiography and the European Association of Cardiovascular Imaging. *Eur Heart J Cardiovasc Imaging.* 2016 Dec;17(12):1321-1360.

**18.** Correct Answer: A. Mean LA pressure of 10 mm Hg and LVEDP of 22 mm Hg

*Rationale:* Abnormal relaxation generally has normal LA pressure but an elevated LVEDP because of a combination of increased contribution of LV filling during atrial systole and possibly increased LV diastolic stiffness by the same process that caused abnormal LV relaxation. Very high mean LA pressures result in pseudonormal or restrictive LV filling patterns.

Selected Reference
1. Hanrath P, Mathey DG, Bleifeld W. Left ventricular relaxation and filling pattern in different forms of left ventricular hypertrophy: an echocardiographic study. *Am J Cardiol.* 1980;45(1):15-23.

**19.** Correct Answer: A. Severe MR

*Rationale:* Presence of an A wave excludes atrial fibrillation. In mitral stenosis and prosthetic mitral valve, the E-wave deceleration will be slow. The inflow pattern shown here indicates high LA pressure typified by E/A ratio >2 and E-wave deceleration of <150 ms and is consistent with severe MR.

Selected Reference
1. Olson JJ, Costa SP, Palac RT. Early mitral filling/diastolic mitral annular velocity ratio is not a reliable predictor of left ventricular filling pressure in the setting of severe mitral regurgitation. *J Am Soc Echocardiogr.* 2006;19(1):83-87.

**20.** Correct Answer: C. Short deceleration time associated with worsening prognosis

*Rationale:* Deceleration time ≤150 ms in patients with amyloidosis has been shown to correlate with a higher risk of cardiac death over an 18-month period nearly five times greater than those patients with a deceleration time >150 ms. Similarly, 1-year cardiac survival of patients with an increased E/A ratio (≥2.1) was less than that of patients with normal or decreased E/A ratio (<2.1).

Selected Reference
1. Klein AL, Hatle LK, Taliercio CP, et al. Prognostic significance of Doppler measures of diastolic function in cardiac amyloidosis: a Doppler echocardiography study. *Circulation.* 1991;83:808-816.

**21.** Correct Answer: A. Figure 35.5A (Pseudonormal); Figure 35.5B (Grade I dysfunction)

*Rationale:* We know that Figure 35.5B is Grade I diastolic dysfunction due to the A>E pattern. The Valsalva maneuver can help distinguish normal LV filling from pseudonormal filling (and whether re-strictive LV filling is reversible or not) because a decrease in E/A ratio of >50%, not caused by E and A velocities fusion, is highly specific for increased LV filling pressures and supports the presence of diastolic dysfunction. In option A, since E>A, the pattern is either normal or pseudonormal. Valsalva maneuver leads to ventricular unloading and reduces the grade of diastolic dysfunction (reversibly) uncovering a Grade I diastolic dysfunction pattern (A>E) in Figure 35.5B. If the pattern in Figure 35.5A was normal, a Valsalva would not cause it to change to Grade I pattern.

Selected Reference

1. Nagueh SF, Smiseth OA, Appleton CP, et al. Recommendations for the evaluation of left ventricular diastolic function by echocardiography: an update from the American Society of Echocardiography and the European Association of Cardiovascular Imaging. *Eur Heart J Cardiovasc Imaging.* 2016 Dec;17(12):1321-1360.

**22.** Correct Answer: B. High LA pressure

*Rationale:* This inflow pattern shows high E/A ratio. The deceleration time is also short, suggestive of high LA pressure. In case of atrial mechanical failure, the E wave is normal, with diminished mitral A-wave amplitude.

Selected Reference

1. Nagueh SF, Smiseth OA, Appleton CP, et al. Recommendations for the evaluation of left ventricular diastolic function by echocardiography: an update from the American Society of Echocardiography and the European Association of Cardiovascular Imaging. *Eur Heart J Cardiovasc Imaging.* 2016 Dec;17(12):1321-1360.

**23.** Correct Answer: B. Patient has Grade I diastolic function.

*Rationale:* In this patient A>E, and hence this is Grade I or impaired relaxation. In a patient with normal EF, the following criteria can be used to determine the severity of the patient's diastolic dysfunction. If the patient has an E/A <0.8 and the peak E velocity is >50 cm/s, or the E/A >0.8 but <2, then additional criteria need to be evaluated. These criteria are LA volume index >34 mL/m², increased TR velocity >2.8 m/s, and average E/e' >14. If two or three of the criteria are negative, the patient has normal LAP and impaired relaxation. If only one of the criteria is positive, one negative, and one not available, the patient falls in the indeterminate category. If two or three of three are positive, the patient has a pseudonormal pattern and elevated filling pressures.

Selected Reference

1. Nagueh SF, Smiseth OA, Appleton CP, et al. Recommendations for the evaluation of left ventricular diastolic function by echocardiography: an update from the American Society of Echocardiography and the European Association of Cardiovascular Imaging. *Eur Heart J Cardiovasc Imaging.* 2016 Dec;17(12):1321-1360.

**24.** Correct Answer: D. Severe MR

*Rationale:* This is severe MR. Note the holosystolic flow reversal in the pulmonary vein that is diagnostic of severe MR. Blunting of the systolic wave signifies at least moderate MR.

Selected Reference

1. Rossvoll O, Hatle LK. Pulmonary venous flow velocities recorded by transthoracic Doppler ultrasound: relation to left ventricular diastolic pressures. *J Am Coll Cardiol.* 1993;21(7):1687-1696.

**25.** Correct Answer: B. Abnormal relaxation

*Rationale:* Abnormal relaxation is identified by an E/A ratio of <1. The E/A ratio can be lower in the elderly because of age-related LV relaxation failure, low filling pressures, more rapid HRs, and prolongation of the PR interval. In a pseudonormal pattern, the mitral inflow looks normal, but there is some other evidence of LV relaxation abnormality, such as reduced $E_m$ velocity, reduced mitral flow propagation, or increased duration of atrial systole as judged by pulmonary vein flow (AR-wave reversal duration).

Restrictive pattern is characterized by an E/A ratio of >2, E-wave deceleration of <150 ms, and isovolumic relaxation time duration of <70 ms.

Selected Reference

1. Nagueh SF, Smiseth OA, Appleton CP, et al. Recommendations for the evaluation of left ventricular diastolic function by echocardiography: an update from the American Society of Echocardiography and the European Association of Cardiovascular Imaging. *Eur Heart J Cardiovasc Imaging.* 2016 Dec;17(12):1321-1360.

**26.** Correct Answer: D. All of the above

*Rationale:* All of the interventions will improve diastolic function. Preintervention mitral flow is indicative of high LA pressure. Postintervention mitral flow is suggestive of impaired LV relaxation, which is consistent with normal or low mean LA pressure. Diastolic function will improve in response to diuresis and afterload reduction with a reduction of LV size and elimination of MR. Hypertension reduces LV ejection performance, increases LV size, and gives rise to MR due to high afterload. Due to minimal functional reserve, anemia has a serious effect on hemodynamics due to reduced oxygen-carrying capacity, creating a higher cardiac output state.

Selected Reference

1. Leite-Moreira AF. Current perspectives in diastolic dysfunction and diastolic heart failure. *Heart.* 2006;92(5):712-718.

**27.** Correct Answer: C. Tissue Doppler–derived early diastolic velocity of the mitral annulus of 6 cm/s.

*Rationale:* Elevated filling pressures in a patient with a normal EF can be confirmed with a decreased early diastolic velocity of the mitral annulus (e') <8 cm/s, an increased LA volume index >34 mL/m$^2$, a reduced CMM slope of <40 cm/s, a change in mitral inflow E/A ratio of 0.5 with the Valsalva maneuver, and a difference in duration of pulmonary venous AR and mitral inflow A-wave duration of >30 ms. Also important to note is the mitral inflow "L wave" in the image. It is the upward deflection in the Doppler envelope between E and A waves. It occurs due to continued LV filling during diastole. This presence is specific for elevated LV filling pressures, but has a low sensitivity.

Selected Reference

1. Kuwaki H, Takeuchi M, Otsuji Y. Redefining diastolic dysfunction grading: combination of E/A ≤ 0.75 and deceleration time > 140 ms and E/ε' ≥ 10. *JACC: Cardiovasc Imaging.* 2014;7(8):749-758.

**28.** Correct Answer: A. Figure 35.11A

*Rationale:* For TDI, the sampling gate needs to be placed at the annulus of the mitral valve. In Figure 35.11A, Doppler settings and sample volume location are optimal, whereas in Figure 35.11.B the sample volume is placed in the ventricular septum (not annulus). Doppler settings are suboptimal in Figure 35.11C with low gain and in Figure 35.11D with high filter.

Selected Reference

1. Nagueh SF, Smiseth OA, Appleton CP, et al. Recommendations for the evaluation of left ventricular diastolic function by echocardiography: an update from the American Society of Echocardiography and the European Association of Cardiovascular Imaging. *Eur Heart J Cardiovasc Imaging.* 2016 Dec;17(12):1321-1360.

**29.** Correct Answer: D. Elevated LVEDP with high LA pressure

*Rationale:* The D-wave velocity, which is higher than the S-wave velocity with a rapid deceleration, is indicative of high LA pressure in an adult. The AR-wave duration is markedly increased. Normally AR-wave duration is less than mitral A-wave duration and is <110 to 120 ms. Though A-wave duration is not shown, the AR-wave duration (at roughly 200 ms) is abnormal, indicating high LVEDP and causing prolonged atrial systole due to increased atrial afterload. In a hypovolemic patient, the S wave will be prominent, and the AR wave would be small; in atrial fibrillation, the AR wave is lost completely.

Selected Reference

1. Nagarakanti R, Ezekowitz M. Diastolic dysfunction and atrial fibrillation. *J Interv Card Electrophysiol.* 2008;22(2):111-118.

**30.** Correct Answer: B. LV operating stiffness

*Rationale:* E-wave deceleration time is mostly influenced by the compliance or the operating stiffness of the left ventricle. Changes in LV compliance and changes in ventricular relaxation (lusitropy) or early (instead of late) diastolic ventricular pressures will affect the deceleration time. LA mechanical function and EF are not or weakly and indirectly correlated with deceleration time.

Selected Reference
1. Ha JW, Oh JK, Tajik AJ. Diastolic stress echocardiography: a novel noninvasive diagnostic test for diastolic dysfunction using supine bicycle exercise Doppler echocardiography. *J Am Soc Echocardiogr.* 2005;18(1):63-68.

**31.** Correct Answer: D. All of the above

*Rationale:* The patient has a markedly dilated left ventricle and a short diastole despite a HR of about 70/min, very premature atrial contraction with no passive transmitral flow, with diastolic MR and prolonged systole as indicated by the systolic MR signal. All of these indicate poor systolic performance and atrioventricular dyssynchrony. Hence the hemodynamics is likely to improve with the therapies listed in the answer options.

Selected Reference
1. Galderisi M. Diastolic dysfunction and diastolic heart failure: diagnostic, prognostic and therapeutic aspects. *Cardiovasc Ultrasound.* 2005;3(1):9.

**32.** Correct Answer: A. The sample volume should be positioned at or 1 cm from insertion sites of the mitral leaflets.

*Rationale:* The sampling gate should be positioned at or 1 cm within the insertion of the mitral leaflets to cover the longitudinal excursion of the mitral annulus in both systole and diastole. Attention should be directed at Doppler spectral gain settings because annular velocities have high signal amplitude. The velocity scale should be set at about 20 cm/s above and below the zero-velocity baseline, though lower settings may be needed in severe LV dysfunction. No Valsalva maneuver is required during measurement. Minimal angulation (<20°) should be present between the ultrasound beam and the plane of cardiac motion.

Selected Reference
1. Nagueh SF, Smiseth OA, Appleton CP, et al. Recommendations for the evaluation of left ventricular diastolic function by echocardiography: an update from the American Society of Echocardiography and the European Association of Cardiovascular Imaging. *Eur Heart J Cardiovasc Imaging.* 2016 Dec;17(12):1321-1360.

**33.** Correct Answer: D. A decrease of >50% in E/A ratio is highly specific for increased LV filling pressures.

*Rationale:* A decrease ≥50% in E/A ratio with application of the Valsalva is highly specific for increased LV filling pressure. However, a smaller change does not always indicate normal diastolic function. One major limitation is that not everyone is able to perform this maneuver adequately. A decrease of 20 cm/s in mitral peak E velocity is considered an adequate effort in patients without restrictive filling. Lack of reversibility with Valsalva is imperfect as an indicator that the diastolic filling pattern is irreversible. In a busy clinical laboratory, the Valsalva maneuver can be reserved for patients in whom diastolic function assessment is not clear after measuring inflows. The Valsalva is useful to differentiate stage 2 diastolic function from normal.

Selected Reference
1. Ghazal SN. Valsalva maneuver in echocardiography. *J Echocardiogr.* 2017;15(1):1-5.

**34.** Correct Answer: B. Patient has abnormal cardiac function and elevated filling pressures.

*Rationale:* LV diastolic dysfunction has often been described as a sensitive sign of early graft rejection in heart transplant patients, since myocardial edema causes increased diastolic stiffness and elevated filling pressures, even in the presence of a normal EF. The patient has depressed diastolic function as is evidenced by the markedly reduced septal e' velocity at 2 to 3 cm/s in Figure 35.14B. Figure 35.14A also reveals a short deceleration time (DT) of mitral E velocity (<150 ms) and an abbreviated diastolic flow duration with premature termination of forward flow. All of the above findings are consistent with markedly elevated LV filling pressures, which include LVEDP.

## Selected Reference

1. Nagueh SF, Smiseth OA, Appleton CP, et al. (2016). Recommendations for the evaluation of left ventricular diastolic function by echocardiography: an update from the American Society of Echocardiography and the European Association of Cardiovascular Imaging. *Eur Heart J Cardiovasc Imaging*. 2016 Dec;17(12):1321-1360.

# 36 | MECHANICAL CIRCULATORY SUPPORT

William P. Mulvoy III

1. Which of the following echocardiography findings is not considered a contraindication prior to left ventricular assist device (LVAD) placement?

   A. Bioprosthetic aortic valve with moderate aortic regurgitation
   B. LV aneurysm
   C. Moderate pulmonic stenosis
   D. Right atrial appendage thrombus

2. A 48-year-old patient with dilated cardiomyopathy and a left ventricular ejection fraction (LVEF) of <10% presents for placement of a continuous flow LVAD as a bridge to cardiac transplantation. Upon separation from cardiopulmonary bypass, severe aortic insufficiency is visualized with no other valvular pathology. Calculate the aortic valve regurgitant blood flow given the following information:

   Heart rate = 100 bpm

   | Pulmonary artery diameter = 1.0 cm | Pulmonary artery velocity time integral (VTI) = 21.8 cm |
   | --- | --- |
   | LVAD outflow graft diameter = 1.4 cm | LVAD outflow graft VTI = 25.4 cm |

   A. 2.4 L/min
   B. 2.6 L/min
   C. 2.2 L/min
   D. 2.8 L/min

3. An LVAD inflow cannula velocity that exceeds 4 m/s measured by continuous-wave Doppler in the immediate post–cardiopulmonary bypass period is most likely indicative of which of the following?

   A. Outflow cannula obstruction by thrombus
   B. Septal inflow cannula obstruction
   C. Right ventricle failure
   D. Hypovolemia

4. Given the transthoracic echo image below (**Figure 36.1**).

This particular valvular pathology may occur in about 25% of LVAD patients, which of the following will increase the likelihood of this valvular pathology happening?

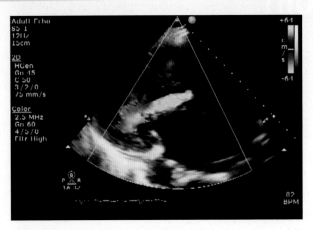

**Figure 36.1**

A. Moderate mitral valve regurgitation
B. Aortic valve that does not open
C. Presence of a bioprosthetic aortic valve
D. LV thrombus formation

5. Which of the following is not a reason to abort or stop a speed change (ramp) echocardiogram during a surveillance echocardiogram for mechanical support optimization 2 weeks post-LVAD implantation?

A. Suction event
B. Cannula flow reversal
C. Arrhythmia
D. Hypertension

6. During insertion of an Impella 2.5 the characteristic color flow Doppler signal is entirely within the LV outflow tract without appreciable Doppler signal in the proximal aorta. What is the ideal positioning depth of the Impella device inflow port in regard to distance from the aortic valve annulus?

A. 4.0 to 4.5 cm
B. 2.5 to 3.0 cm
C. 3.0 to 3.5 cm
D. 3.5 to 4.0 cm

7. A 44-year-old male patient has been on venoarterial extracorporeal membrane oxygenation (VA-ECMO) with cardiogenic shock for 8 days and the surgical team feels that he is ready for decannulation. You are performing a transesophageal echocardiogram in the cardiovascular intensive care unit (CVICU) during a preoperative "turn down" evaluation. Which of the following parameters most strongly correlates with successful weaning from VA-ECMO with a VA-ECMO flow of <1.5 L/min?

A. Mitral valve E/A > 2.1
B. Aortic valve VTI > 10 cm
C. Mitral valve lateral annulus tissue Doppler <8 cm/s
D. Pulmonary capillary wedge pressure >25 mm Hg

8. Which of the following is a good predictor of right ventricular failure following LVAD implantation?

A. Tricuspid annular plane systolic excursion of 16 mm
B. Pulmonary artery mean pressure of 15 mm Hg
C. LVEF of 10%
D. Right ventricular fractional area change (RVFAC) of 18%

9. A 26-year-old female patient with postpartum cardiomyopathy and cardiogenic shock is 7 days post implantation of an LVAD. She remains intubated and has been hypotensive requiring continuous inotropic support and now has multiple pulsatility index events and low cardiac output alarms with patient repositioning and deep breathing. Given the transesophageal echocardiography (TEE) findings in **Table 36.1**, which of the following is the most likely cause of the LVAD malfunction?

**Table 36.1. TEE Findings**

| | |
|---|---|
| LV internal dimension during diastole | 33 mm |
| LVAD inflow cannula velocity | 1.7 m/s |
| RVFAC | 43% |
| Right ventricle internal diameter during diastole | 23 mm |
| Central venous pressure (CVP) | 6 mm Hg |

   **A.** Hypotension
   **B.** Mitral valve regurgitation
   **C.** Hypovolemia
   **D.** Pulmonic valve regurgitation

10. A 51-year-old male patient in cardiogenic shock on high-dose vasopressors and VA-ECMO has just returned from the cardiac catheterization laboratory after Impella 2.5 insertion for LV decompression. The patient remains unstable and a bedside focused transthoracic echocardiogram (TTE) image is shown in **Figure 36.2**.

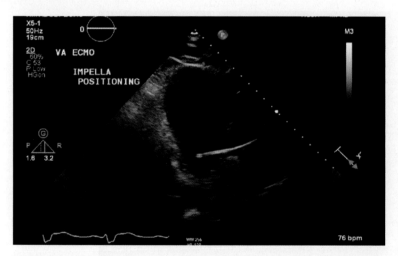

**Figure 36.2**

What is the next best step in management?

   **A.** Nothing—the Impella is in proper position
   **B.** Advance the Impella another 3 cm into the LV outflow tract (LVOT)
   **C.** Reposition the Impella as it is potentially obstructing mitral valve inflow
   **D.** Pull the Impella back 2.5 cm as it is too deep into the left ventricle

11. After placement of an Impella 2.5 via the right femoral artery in the catheterization lab, the patient is transported to the cardiothoracic ICU (CTICU). During transport the patient becomes hemodynamically unstable and an emergent TEE is performed immediately upon arrival in the CTICU **(Figure 36.3)**.

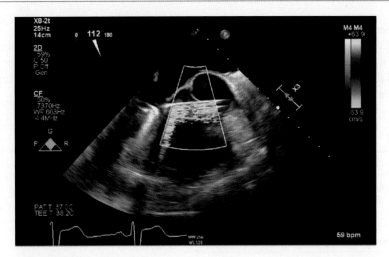

**Figure 36.3**

Based on the TEE in Figure 36.3, what is the next best step in the management of this patient?

**A.** Withdrawal of the Impella as it courses into the mitral valve chordae
**B.** Withdrawal of the Impella as it courses too far into the LV apex
**C.** Withdrawal of the Impella as it courses into the left atrium
**D.** Withdrawal of the Impella as it courses into a ventricular septal defect (VSD) as noted by color flow

12. A patient in cardiogenic shock develops acute right heart failure and the decision is made to place a percutaneous right ventricular assist device in the ICU. The surgeon appears to be struggling with wire placement and you bring up the TEE shown in **Figure 36.4**. What is your recommendation to the surgeon?

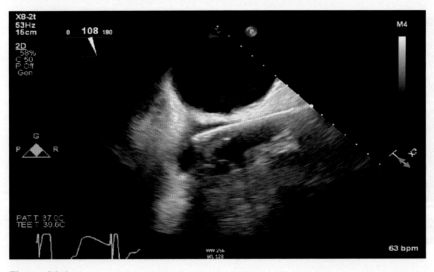

**Figure 36.4**

**A.** The wire is in the correct position
**B.** Tell the surgeon to pull the wire back as it has inadvertently passed into the inferior vena cava
**C.** Tell the surgeon to pull the wire back as it has inadvertently passed through a patent foramen ovale (PFO)
**D.** Tell the surgeon to pull the wire back as it is in the right atrial appendage

13. A 71-year-old male patient with an ejection fraction of <15% is intubated in the CVICU and for cardiac support the decision is made to place an intra-aortic balloon pump (IABP). During a transesophageal echocardiogram you see the **Figure 36.5**.

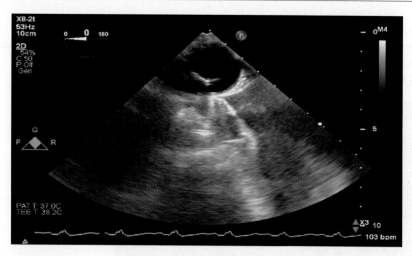

**Figure 36.5**

What is your recommendation to the cardiologist?
A. Advance the IABP 2 cm
B. Nothing—the IABP is correctly positioned
C. Remove the IABP as it is in the vena cava
D. Withdrawal of the IABP 2 cm

14. A patient is admitted to the CVICU 12 months post-LVAD placement. The patient is hypotensive and intubated. A bedside TEE is performed, and **Figure 36.6** is recorded.

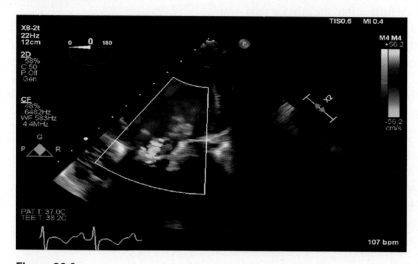

**Figure 36.6**

What factor most likely contributed to this condition?
A. Aortic valve regurgitation
B. Aortic stenosis
C. Presence of a bioprosthetic valve
D. Presence of a PFO

15. When attempting to place an Impella 2.5 [FDA 510(k), 2008] under TTE guidance, which of the following views would be best to verify proper cannula position?

A. Subcostal four-chamber view
B. Parasternal long-axis view
C. Parasternal LV short-axis view
D. Apical five-chamber view

16. A 41-year-old male patient presented with rhinovirus and was intubated for the past 7 days with progressive hypoxemia. The decision was made to place an Avalon catheter via the right internal jugular vein for veno-venous ECMO. The surgeon asks you if the cannula is properly positioned, given the TEE in **Figure 36.7**. What should you recommend?

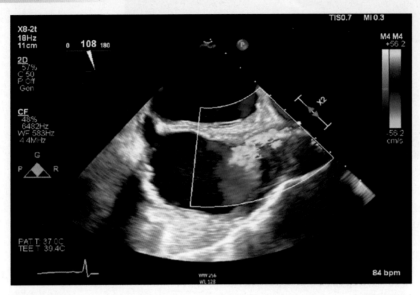

**Figure 36.7**

    **A.** Nothing—the catheter is in the correct position
    **B.** Advance the cannula further into the inferior vena cava
    **C.** Withdrawal of the cannula into the superior vena cava
    **D.** Rotate the catheter 180° and advance the cannula

17. On postoperative day 5 after LVAD implantation, a patient's CVP is 34 mm Hg and their mean pulmonary artery pressure is 38 mm Hg measured by a continuous cardiac output (CCO) Swan-Ganz catheter. The surgeon is concerned about severe right ventricular dysfunction (RVD). Which of the following parameters would be suggestive of severe RVD?

    **A.** Tricuspid annular plane systolic excursion >16 mm
    **B.** RVFAC of 15%
    **C.** Lateral tricuspid annular tissue Doppler velocity >12 mm
    **D.** Right ventricular myocardial performance index of 0.29

18. Which of the following TTE views will allow for the best assessment of an LVAD inflow cannula velocity?

    **A.** Apical three-chamber view
    **B.** Subcostal short-axis view
    **C.** Subcostal long-axis view
    **D.** Parasternal aortic valve short-axis view

19. A 54-year-old female patient is in cardiogenic shock and the decision is made to cannulate for VA-ECMO at the bedside in the CTICU. After cannulation, a focused TTE demonstrates an LV internal diameter at end diastole (LVIDd) of 65 mm and an LV internal diameter at end systole of 52 mm, with spontaneous echo contrast in the left ventricle. What should you recommend to the surgical team based on this information?

    **A.** Place an Impella device to offload the left ventricle
    **B.** Do nothing as the patient is in cardiogenic shock
    **C.** Place an IABP for additional support
    **D.** Place a percutaneous right ventricular assist device

**20.** Which of the following is not an absolute contraindication to placement of a femoral arterial IABP?

**A.** End-stage heart disease with no anticipation of recovery
**B.** Moderate aortic regurgitation
**C.** Aortic stents
**D.** Septic shock

# Chapter 36 ■ Answers

**1.** Correct Answer: D. Right atrial appendage thrombus

*Rationale:* Review of the American Society of Echocardiography Guidelines for LVAD management demonstrates multiple contraindications and/or red flags that need to be addressed prior to LVAD implantation. Table 36.1 from these guidelines discusses the echocardiography findings that must be addressed prior to separation from cardiopulmonary bypass and LVAD implantation. A bioprosthetic aortic valve with moderate aortic regurgitation needs to be repaired because once the LVAD begins to flow, the aortic regurgitation will get worse, causing a potential recirculation loop between the LVAD inflow cannula and the outflow cannula through the aortic valve. If there is an LV aneurysm, implantation of the inflow cannula may be hindered by poor tissue and/or difficulty with appropriate inflow cannula positioning. Pulmonic stenosis greater than mild should be addressed to prevent any impedance of right-sided blood flow once the LVAD is implanted. A right atrial appendage clot is not as important to address as a left atrial appendage thrombus, which could potentially embolize into the LVAD pump.

Selected Reference
1. Stainback RF, Estep JD, Agler DA, et al. Echocardiography in management of patients with left ventricular assist devices: recommendations from the American Society of Echocardiography. *J Am Soc Echocardiogr.* 2015;28(8):853-909.

**2.** Correct Answer: C. 2.2 L/min

*Rationale/Critique:* In this question the patient has two different ways that the LVAD receives blood flow. The first flow is from the right ventricular outflow tract (RVOT), thus the entire right-sided cardiac output is going into the left ventricle. The other flow into the LVAD is the regurgitant flow from the aortic valve regurgitation. To calculate the regurgitant blood flow, we need to use the following equations:

$$Q_{LVAD} = Q_{RVOT} + Q_{AI} > Q_{AI} = Q_{LVAD} - Q_{RVOT}$$

Stroke volume (SV) $= 3.14 * r^2 * VTI$

Therefore,

$$Q_{LVAD} = SV_{LVAD} * HR = 3.14 * (0.7)^2 * 25.4 \text{ cm} * 100 \text{ bpm} = 3908 \text{ mL/min} \sim \textbf{3.9 L/min}$$

$$Q_{RVOT} = SV_{RVOT} * HR = 3.14 * (0.5)^2 * 21.8 \text{ cm} * 100 \text{ bpm} = 1711 \text{ mL/min} \sim \textbf{1.7 L/min}$$

$$Q_{AI} = Q_{LVAD} - Q_{RVOT} > \textbf{QAI} = \textbf{3.9 L/min} - \textbf{1.7 L/min} = \textbf{2.2 L/min}$$

Selected References
1. Savage RM, Aronson S, Shernan SK. *Comprehensive Textbook of Perioperative Transesophageal Echocardiography.* 2nd ed. Wolters Kluwer; 2011.
2. Stainback RF, Estep JD, Agler DA, et al. Echocardiography in the management of patients with left ventricular assist devices: recommendations from the American Society of Echocardiography. *J Am Soc Echocardiogr.* 2015;28(8):853-909.

**3.** Correct Answer: B. Septal inflow cannula obstruction

*Rationale:* A peak continuous-wave Doppler flow velocity of >2.3 m/s is highly suggestive of inflow cannula obstruction regardless of the manufacturer of the LVAD. In this case the peak velocity is much greater than

2.3 m/s; the only answer that suggests inflow cannula obstruction is answer B, which is septal inflow cannula obstruction. In the immediate postcardiopulmonary bypass period, left ventricle geometry can be altered depending on the insertion, with the potential for the inflow cannula to be directed toward the interventricular septum. With the inflow cannula directed at the interventricular septum, there is potential for inflow cannula obstruction and thus turbulent blood flow. Thrombus in the outflow graft generally does not give turbulent velocities as high as 4 m/s at the inflow cannula. Hypovolemia is possible, but suction events do not cause such turbulent flows through the LVAD inflow cannula. The velocity demonstrates a significant obstruction to LVAD inflow.

Selected References

1. Chumnanvej S, Wood MJ, MacGillivray TE, Videl Melo MF. Perioperative echocardiographic examination for ventricular assist device implantation. *Anesth Analg.* 2007 Sept;105(3):583-601.
2. Denalut AY, Couture P, Vegas A, Buithieu J, Tardif JC. *Transesophageal Echocardiography Multimedia Manual a Perioperative Transdisciplinary Approach.* Taylor & Francis Group, LLC; 2005.
3. Savage RM, Aronson S, Shernan SK. *Comprehensive Textbook of Perioperative Transesophageal Echocardiography.* 2nd ed. Wolters Kluwer; 2011.

**4. Correct Answer: B. Aortic valve that does not open**

*Rationale*: New-onset aortic valve regurgitation will occur in about 25% to 33% of post-LVAD patients within 12 months of implantation. The largest risk factor for developing new-onset aortic valve regurgitation is the lack of opening of the aortic valve. The continuous negative pressure on the LV side of the aortic valve will lead to prolapse of one or multiple cusps, therefore leading to aortic valve regurgitation. It is unclear if the risk of aortic valve leaflet prolapse will be increased by the evidence of aortic valve thrombus during this time period. To minimize the development of aortic regurgitation in an aortic valve that does not open, many times the aortic valve will need to be sutured shut (**Figure 36.8**).

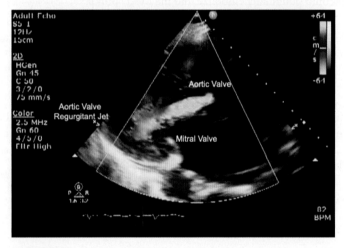

**Figure 36.8**

Selected References

1. Cowger J, Pagani FD, Haft JW, Romano MA, Aaronson KD, Kolias TJ. The development of aortic insufficiency in left ventricular assist device supported patients. *Circ Heart Fail.* 2010;3:668-674.
2. Pak SW, Uriel N, Takayama H, et al. Prevalence of de novo aortic insufficiency during long-term support with left ventricular assist devices. *J Heart Lung Transplant.* 2010;29:1172-1176.

**5. Correct Answer: C. Arrhythmia**

*Rationale*: In the case of a medical optimization examination or speed change (ramp) echocardiography examination, there are certain factors that need to be evaluated. There should always be a medically trained mechanical support staff immediately available when mechanical support adjustments are made on LVAD patients. If no staff is available, the mechanical support and/or heart failure team should be notified that an optimization or speed change echocardiogram is being performed. It is necessary to outline and define the parameters that should be evaluated during the examination. The examination should be aborted if any of the following occur: (1) completion of the test as this is an obvious reason to stop the exam; (2) a suction event (at higher speeds); (3) new symptoms—including, but not limited to—palpitations, dizziness, chest pain, shortness of breath, or headache, which may be related to hypoperfusion or hypotension; (4) hypertension; and (5) cannula flow reversal. Hypertension (mean arterial pressure

[MAP] > 85) can increase the risk of cerebral hemorrhage, stroke, renal failure, and thromboembolic events. Arrhythmias should not warrant a stop to the evaluation as these are very common post-LVAD implantation and generally do not cause the patient symptoms or the LVAD to malfunction.

### Selected Reference

1. Stainback RF, Estep JD, Agler DA, et al. Echocardiography in the management of patients with left ventricular assist devices: recommendations from the American Society of Echocardiography. *J Am Soc Echocardiogr*.2015;28(8):853-909.

## 6. Correct Answer: D. 3.5 to 4.0 cm

*Rationale*: During placement of an Impella 2.5 device the distance from the aortic valve annulus to the inflow port is ideally at a depth of 3.5 to 4.0 cm. Patient manipulation, movement, coughing, and transport have the potential to dislodge the Impella device out of the LVOT and into the proximal aorta if not properly secured after placement. Ideal placement of 3.5 to 4.0 cm from the aortic valve annulus should maintain the pump's characteristic color flow Doppler signal distal to the aortic annulus.

### Selected Reference

1. Stainback RF, Estep JD, Agler DA, et al. Echocardiography in the management of patients with left ventricular assist devices: recommendations from the American Society of Echocardiography. *J Am Soc Echocardiogr*.2015;28(8):853-909.

## 7. Correct Answer: B. Aortic valve VTI > 10 cm

*Rationale*: Controversy exists as to proper techniques to wean a patient from VA-ECMO. Current recommendations include TEE to guide weaning from VA-ECMO. Turn down studies help evaluate the extent of cardiac recovery from cardiogenic shock and improve the success of weaning by implementing a turn down TEE-driven protocol. When flows are <1.5 L/min, the three important parameters that should be evaluated are the aortic valve VTI >10 cm, the lateral mitral annulus peak systolic velocity >6 cm/s, and LVEF > 20%. Any of these three parameters correlate well with improved cardiac function. The only parameter in this question that correlates with suggested cardiac recovery and thus improved success from weaning from VA-ECMO is the aortic valve VTI >10 cm, the other answers show poor cardiac function and/or recovery with potentially elevated filling pressures, which would make weaning from VA-ECMO potentially more complicated.

### Selected References

1. Aissaoui N, El-Banayosy A, Combes A. How to wean a patient from veno-arterial extracorporeal membrane oxygenation. *Intensive Care Med*. 2015;41:902-905.
2. Aissaoui N, Luyt C-E, Leprince P, et al. Predictors of successful extracorporeal membrane oxygenation (ECMO) weaning after assistance for refractory cardiogenic shock. *Intensive Care Med*. 2011;37:1738-1745.
3. Thomas TH, Price R, Ramaciotti C, Thompson M, Megison S, Lemler MS. Echocardiography, not chest radiography, for evaluation of cannula placement during pediatric extracorporeal membrane oxygenation. *Pediatr Crit Care Med*. 2009;10:56-59.

## 8. Correct Answer: D. *Right ventricular* fractional area change (RVFAC) of 18%

*Rationale*: A normal RVFAC is >35%. Many patients who are undergoing LVAD placement have some degree of RVD, whether it be mild, moderate, or severe. LVAD success is dependent on right ventricular function postimplantation. Assuming interventricular septal interdependence is not a contributing factor post-LVAD implantation, having a pre-LVAD RVFAC of <20% is associated with a significantly increased risk of right ventricular failure. With knowledge of preimplantation RVFAC and moderate-to-severe RVD, treatment with multiple inotropic agents, inhaled pulmonary vasodilators, and possible right ventricular mechanical support may be needed.

### Selected References

1. Rudski LG, Lai WW, Afilalo J, et al. Guidelines for the echocardiographic assessment of the right heart in adults: a report from the American Society of Echocardiography endorsed by the European Association of Echocardiography, a registered branch of the European Society of Cardiology, and the Canadian Society of Echocardiography. *J Am Soc Echocardiogr*. 2010 Jul;23(7):685-713.
2. Scalia GM, McCarthy PM, Savage RM, Smedira NG, Thomas JD. Clinical utility of echocardiography in the management of implantable ventricular assist devices. *J Am Soc Echocardiogr*. 2000;13(8):754-763.

## 9. Correct Answer: C. Hypovolemia

*Rationale*: Hypovolemia in LVAD patients is generally a clinical diagnosis with a low CVP, hypotension, and increase in pulsatility events. However, focused TEE in the ICU can help guide the cause of low cardiac output and increased event alarms with direct visualization of the cardiac function. A focused TEE evaluation is vital to rule out cardiac tamponade, right ventricular failure, and inflow cannula obstruction. Given the data in the question are suggestive of low preload and low LV volume status, combined with device alarms and low cardiac output, this is highly suggestive of hypovolemia. This patient has low filling pressures on the right side of the heart combined with normal right ventricular function. With the LVAD inflow cannula velocity relatively normal, it means the device is not occluded or rather there is no evidence of inflow cannula obstruction. However, in this question when the patient moves or initiates a large deep breath, the low cardiac output alarm goes off because of relative obstruction due to hypovolemia, causing a relative positional and functional obstruction of the inflow cannula.

**Selected References**
1. Churnnanvej S, Wood MJ, MacGillivray TE, Melo ME. Perioperative echocardiographic examination for ventricular assist device implantation. *Anesth Analg.* 2007;105(3):583-601.
2. Horton SC, Khodaverdian R, Chatelain P, et al. Left ventricular assist device malfunction: an approach to diagnosis by echocardiography. *Am Coil Cardiol.* 2005;45(9):1435-1440.
3. Szymanski P, Religa G, Klisiewicz A, Baranska K, Hoffman P. Diagnosis of biventricular assist device inflow cannula obstruction. *Echocardiography.* 2007;24(4):420-424.

**10.** Correct Answer: **C. Reposition the Impella as it is potentially obstructing mitral valve inflow**

*Rationale:* **Figure 36.9** shows the apical three-chamber view. TTE demonstrates that the Impella is not properly positioned with its indicator toward the apex. In fact, looking at the image shows that the Impella is almost abutting the inferolateral wall. Its pigtail is not well visualized and not easily visualized, but based on the course of the Impella through the aortic valve, it can be assumed that it is physically in contact with the inferolateral wall. With the course of the Impella toward the inferolateral wall and in such close proximity to the anterior mitral valve leaflet, there may be concern for mitral valve obstruction caused by the Impella. Based on Figure 36.9 it appears as if the Impella may be restricting the opening of the mitral valve as the course of the Impella device is in very close proximity to the anterior leaflet of the mitral valve contributing to the hemodynamic instability.

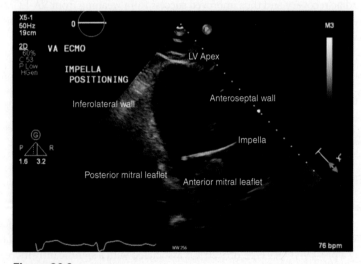

**Figure 36.9**

**Selected References**
1. Savage RM, Aronson S, Shernan SK. *Comprehensive Textbook of Perioperative Transesophageal Echocardiography.* 2nd ed. Wolters Kluwer; 2011.
2. Stainback RF, Estep JD, Agler DA, et al. Echocardiography in the management of patients with left ventricular assist devices: recommendations from the American Society of Echocardiography. *J Am Soc Echocardiogr.*2015;28(8):853-909.

**11.** Correct Answer: **A. Withdrawal of the Impella as it courses into the mitral valve chordae**

*Rationale:* **Figure 36.10** demonstrates an aortic valve long-axis TEE image. Figure 36.10 demonstrates an Impella device that is too far into the left ventricle as the color flow Doppler suggests the inflow and outflow ports are both below the aortic valve annulus. The trajectory of the Impella is toward the interventricular septum so answers B and C are both wrong as the device is not coursing in either of those directions. The color flow Doppler is not over the interventricular septum so there is no color Doppler evidence of a VSD; therefore, the correct answer is A since the trajectory of the Impella is so close to the anterior mitral valve leaflet, and one can assume that the chordae are in close proximity to the Impella causing it to course toward the interventricular septum. Also looking at the color flow Doppler and having the inflow and outflow color flow both below the aortic valve annulus, the management is complete withdrawal of the device and attempting to reposition it.

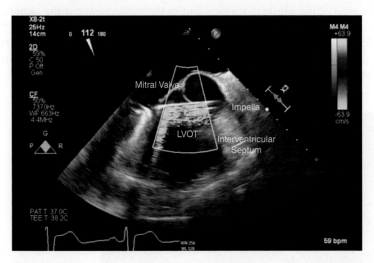

**Figure 36.10**

### Selected References

1. Savage RM, Aronson S, Shernan SK. *Comprehensive Textbook of Perioperative Transesophageal Echocardiography*. 2nd ed. Philadelphia, PA: Wolters Kluwer; 2011.
2. Stainback RF, Estep JD, Agler DA, et al. Echocardiography in the management of patients with left ventricular assist devices: recommendations from the American Society of Echocardiography. *J Am Soc Echocardiogr*.2015;28(8):853-909.

**12.** Correct Answer: **A. Do nothing as the wire is in the correct position**

*Rationale*: **Figure 36.11** is the bicaval view with focus on the superior vena cava and the right ventricular inflow. The wire is seen passing from the superior vena cava into the right ventricular inflow. In Figure 36.11 the tricuspid valve cusps are in proximity to the right atrial appendage. The wire makes an acute angle toward the tricuspid valve inflow, also confirming placement through the tricuspid valve. There is no evidence of a PFO as the interatrial septum appears intact.

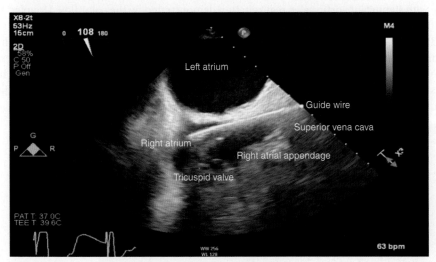

**Figure 36.11**

### Selected References

1. Savage RM, Aronson S, Shernan SK. *Comprehensive Textbook of Perioperative Transesophageal Echocardiography*. 2nd ed. Philadelphia, PA: Wolters Kluwer; 2011.
2. Stainback RF, Estep JD, Agler DA, et al. Echocardiography in the management of patients with left ventricular assist devices: recommendations from the American Society of Echocardiography. *J Am Soc Echocardiogr*.2015;28(8):853-909.

**13.** Correct Answer: D. Withdrawal of the IABP 2 cm

*Rationale*: Figure 36.5 in **Question 13** is the descending aorta short-axis view at the level of the left subclavian artery. One can see the left subclavian artery on the right side of the figure. The balloon pump may appear to be at the level of the subclavian artery, but in the aortic lumen is the radiopaque tip of the IABP. The balloon does not inflate all the way to the tip, in fact there is about a 2 to 3 cm offset from the radiopaque tip to where the balloon will occlude the lumen. Regardless, **Figure 36.12** shows the radiopaque tip at or above the level of the left subclavian artery and since the image shows the balloon deflated, it is best to maintain the echo view and withdraw the balloon until the tip is no longer visible in this view.

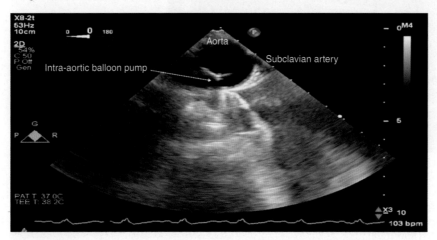

**Figure 36.12**

Selected References
1. Savage RM, Aronson S, Shernan SK. *Comprehensive Textbook of Perioperative Transesophageal Echocardiography*. 2nd ed. Wolters Kluwer; 2011.
2. Stainback RF, Estep JD, Agler DA, et al. Echocardiography in the management of patients with left ventricular assist devices: recommendations from the American Society of Echocardiography. *J Am Soc Echocardiogr*.2015;28(8):853-909.

**14.** Correct Answer: A. Aortic valve regurgitation

*Rationale*: **Figure 36.13** is of the deep transgastric view in late diastole with the aortic valve, left ventricle, and aorta visible with significant aortic valve regurgitation demonstrated by the color flow Doppler. With LVAD implantation, the aortic valve should periodically open every few beats to prevent thrombus formation. About 25% to 33% of LVAD patients without an aortic valve that opens will develop significant aortic valve regurgitation. The cause of significant regurgitation is due to the continuous negative pressure on the LV side of the aortic valve, causing prolapse of one or more of the valve leaflets. Therefore, if the aortic valve does not open, it may be sutured shut to prevent valve prolapse leading to clinically significant aortic valve regurgitation.

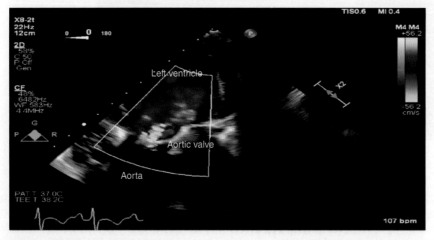

**Figure 36.13**

Selected References

1. Cowger J, Pagani FD, Haft JW, Romano MA, Aaronson KD, Kolias TJ. The development of aortic insufficiency in left ventricular assist device supported patients. *Circ Heart Fail.* 2010;3:668-674.
2. Pak SW, Uriel N, Takayama H, et al. Prevalence of de novo aortic insufficiency during long-term support with left ventricular assist devices. *J Heart Lung Transplant.* 2010;29:1172-1176.

**15.** Correct Answer: B. Parasternal long-axis view

*Rationale*: The parasternal long-axis view is the ideal view to place an Impella device into the proper position in the left ventricle. The parasternal long-axis view gives an optimal view of the left ventricle, the apex of the left ventricle, the aortic valve, and mitral valve. The apical five-chamber view and the subcostal four-chamber view do not give enough visualization of the aortic valve for proper placement across the aortic valve annulus. As for the parasternal LV short axis, one does not see anything but the walls of the right and left ventricles.

Selected References

1. Scalia GM, McCarthy PM, Savage RM, Smedira NG, Thomas JD. Clinical utility of echocardiography in the management of implantable ventricular assist devices. *J Am Soc Echocardiogr.* 2000;13:754-763.
2. Stainback RF, Estep JD, Agler DA, et al. Echocardiography in the management of patients with left ventricular assist devices: recommendations from the American Society of Echocardiography. *J Am Soc Echocardiogr.*2015;28(8):853-909.

**16.** Correct Answer: D. Rotate the catheter 180° and advance

*Rationale*: The TEE view demonstrated (**Figure 36.14**) is the modified bicaval view. Looking at the color jet we see that the outflow port of the Avalon catheter is still in the superior vena cava. More importantly, it is directed posteriorly toward the left atrium and intra-atrial septum. The ideal positioning of the Avalon outflow port is directed toward the tricuspid valve from the right atrium. By attempting to rotate the cannula 180° one can assume that the outflow port would be better directed toward the right ventricular inflow and tricuspid valve.

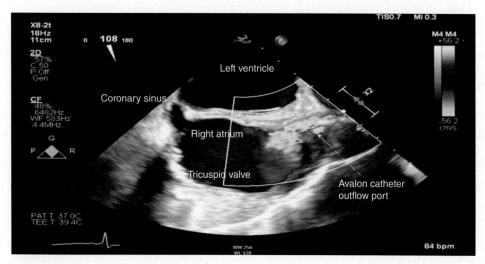

**Figure 36.14**

Selected References

1. Savage RM, Aronson S, Shernan SK. *Comprehensive Textbook of Perioperative Transesophageal Echocardiography.* 2nd ed. Wolters Kluwer; 2011.
2. Stainback RF, Estep JD, Agler DA, et al. Echocardiography in the management of patients with left ventricular assist devices: recommendations from the American Society of Echocardiography. *J Am Soc Echocardiogr.*2015;28(8):853-909.
3. Szymanski P, Religa G, Klisiewicz A, Baranska K, Hoffman P. Diagnosis of biventricular assist device inflow cannula obstruction. *Echocardiography.* 2007;24(4):420-424.

**17.** Correct Answer: B. RVFAC of 15%

*Rationale*: Normal RVFAC is >35%. The ranges for fractional area change of the right ventricle include the following: normal is >32%, mildly depressed 25% to 31%, moderately depressed 18% to 24% and severely depressed <17%. Tricuspid annular plane excursion >16 mm is considered relatively normal. Lateral tricuspid annular tissue Doppler of 12 mm is indicative of normal right ventricular function. Right ventricular myocardial performance index >0.40 is indicative of RVD. Therefore, options A, C, and D are all normal indices of right ventricular function.

Selected Reference
1. Rudski LG, Lai WW, Afilalo J, et al. Guidelines for the echocardiographic assessment of the right heart in adults: a report from the American Society of Echocardiography. *J Am Soc Echocardiogr.* 2010;23(7):685-713.

**18.** Correct Answer: A. Apical three-chamber view

*Rationale*: Of all the options presented in the question, the apical three-chamber view will allow for the best alignment of the Doppler beam in parallel with the inflow cannula. Having a Doppler beam that is parallel to the flow reduces the error associated with the Doppler equation. Remember that the Doppler equation is dependent on the cosine of the angle of incidence between the Doppler beam and direction of blood flow. With the Doppler beam parallel to the blood flow, the cosine of the angle of 0 gives the maximum value for cosine, as the cosine of 0 equals 1.

Selected References
1. Bioeffects Committee of the American Institute of Ultrasound in Medicine. American Institute of Ultrasound in medicine consensus report on potential bioeffects of diagnostic ultrasound: executive summary. *J Diagn Med Sonogr.* 2011;27(1):3-13. doi: 10.1177/8756479310394986.
2. Edelman SK. *Understanding Ultrasound Physics.* ESP; 2012.

**19.** Correct Answer: A. Place an Impella device to offload the left ventricle

*Rationale*: The TTE measurements in the question demonstrate a distended left ventricle with stasis of blood in the ventricle as a result of retrograde filling of the LV and/or inability of the LV to eject because of increased afterload. Thus, the placement of an impella device would help to offload the left ventricle to reduce the work of the left ventricle. Placing a right ventricular assist device will not help reduce the volume of blood in the left ventricle, in fact it may increase the flow to the left ventricle from the pulmonary circulation, compounding the strain on the left ventricle. Doing nothing is not an option as it is only a matter of time until complete LV failure occurs from overdistension. Finally, placing an IABP is an option, but in the case where there is evidence of overdistension and stasis of blood inside the LV chamber, direct chamber decompression is recommended, as with an Impella device.

Selected References
1. Szymanski P, Religa G, Klisiewicz A, Baranska K, Hoffman P. Diagnosis of biventricular assist device inflow cannula obstruction. *Echocardiography.* 2007;24(4):420-424.
2. Thomas TH, Price R, Ramaciotti C, Thompson M, Megison S, Lemler MS. Echocardiography, not chest radiography, for evaluation of cannula placement during pediatric extracorporeal membrane oxygenation. *Pediatr Crit Care Med.* 2009;10:56-59.

**20.** Correct Answer: D. Septic shock

*Rationale*: Moderate aortic regurgitation is worsened with IABP counterpulsations. With known grafts and/or aortic stents, placement of an IABP should be avoided since there is potential to damage the grafts or the balloon may become damaged or entangled within the aortic stents. Moreover, placement of an IABP within an aortic stent may lead to aortic dissection or transection. End-stage heart disease without recovery and/or potential bridge to mechanical support or heart transplant should preclude placement of IABP since there is a high likelihood the IABP may never be weaned off. Therefore, septic shock is actually a relative contraindication and not an absolute contraindication as the question asks.

Selected References
1. Krishna M, Zacharowski K. Principles of intra-aortic balloon pump counterpulsation. *CEACCP.* 2009;24(9):24-28.
2. Sintek MA, Gdowski M, Lindman BR, et al. Intra-aortic balloon counterpulsation in patients with chronic heart failure and cardiogenic shock: clinical response and predictors of stabilization. *J Card Fail.* 2015 Nov;21(11):868-876.

# 37 | INTRACARDIAC SHUNTS

Matthew D. Read

1. You are performing an echocardiogram on a 31-year-old woman who had a syncopal episode while playing basketball. She reports several instances of having to sit down prior to feeling like she would faint. Given the finding shown in **Figure 37.1**, which of the following is *most* likely true?

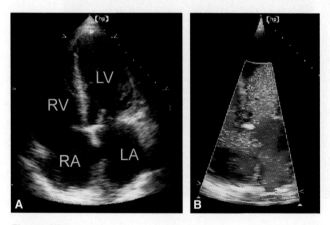

**Figure 37.1**

A. The patient has significant mitral regurgitation from a cleft leaflet.
B. The patient has a defect in the septum primum.
C. The patient has cyanosis during her presyncopal and syncopal episodes.
D. The finding shown is associated with an inlet ventricular septal defect (VSD).

2. Which image in **Figure 37.2** is most likely to be found in a patient with an atrioventricular (AV) canal defect?

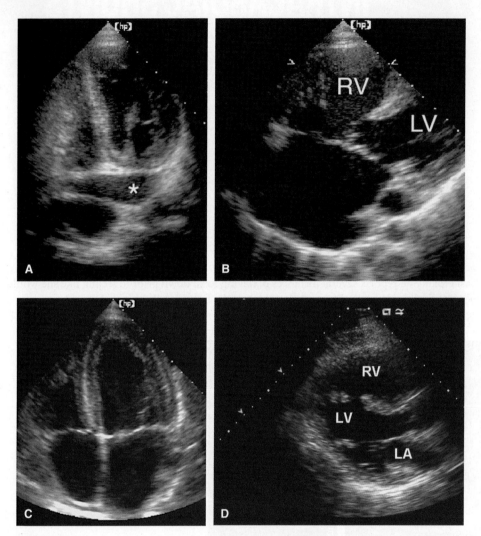

**Figure 37.2**

A. Figure 37.2A
B. Figure 37.2B
C. Figure 37.2C
D. Figure 37.2D

3. A 35-year-old man with dyspnea is undergoing echocardiographic evaluation for a systolic murmur concerning for mitral regurgitation. Which of the following intracardiac shunts is *most* likely associated with the finding shown in **Figure 37.3**?

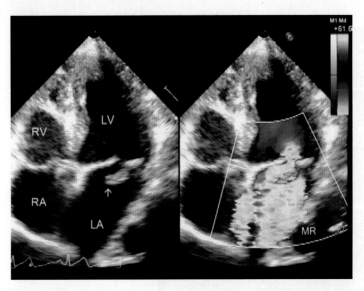

**Figure 37.3**

A. Membranous VSD
B. Ostium primum atrial septal defect (ASD)
C. Ostium secundum ASD
D. Inlet VSD

4. A 43-year-old woman is undergoing echocardiography for evaluation of hemodynamic instability and dyspnea. She is found to have severe mitral regurgitation with a cleft valve. Based on **Figure 37.4,** which of the figure parts is *most* likely to be associated with a cleft mitral valve?

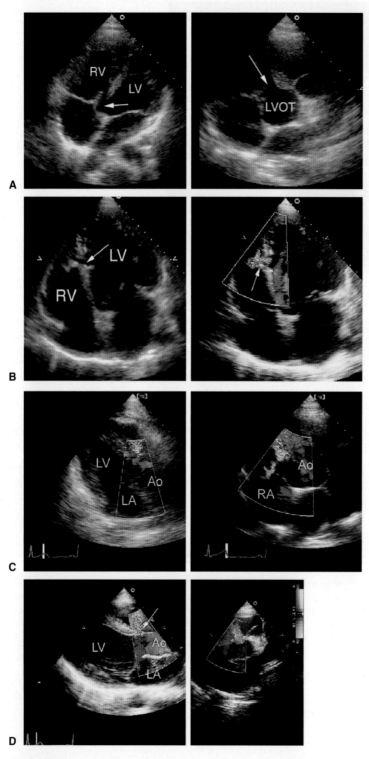

**Figure 37.4**

A. Figure 37.4A
B. Figure 37.4B
C. Figure 37.4C
D. Figure 37.4D

5. A 19-year-old woman is being evaluated for possible VSD closure. Her left ventricular outflow tract (LVOT) diameter is 2.2 cm and her right ventricular outflow tract (RVOT) diameter is 2.5 cm. The following information is also gathered: LVOT peak velocity = 92.8 cm/s, LVOT velocity time integral = 17.3 cm, RVOT peak velocity = 66.6 cm/s, and RVOT velocity time integral = 16.6 cm. What is the calculated shunt ratio?

   A. 0.8
   B. 0.9
   C. 1.1
   D. 1.2

6. A 32-year-old man has progressive exercise limitations due to lower extremity fatigue and dyspnea and has the echocardiographic finding shown in **Figure 37.5**.

   Based on Figure 37.5, which of the following is *least* likely to be true for this patient?
   A. The presence of a bidirectional shunt is indicative of Eisenmenger physiology.
   B. There is an increased risk of bacterial endocarditis.
   C. The presence of a bidirectional shunt rules out an increased LV end-diastolic volume.
   D. A continuous "machinery murmur" may not be present.

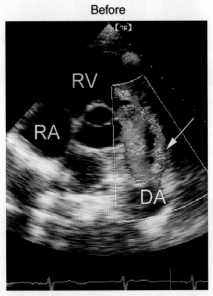

**Figure 37.5**

7. A 53-year-old man is undergoing evaluation for an ischemic cerebral vascular incident. Which of the following is *false* in a patient with patent foramen ovale (PFO)?

   A. There is an increased risk of paradoxical embolism with presence of an aneurysmal interatrial septum.
   B. The absence of bubbles in the left atrium, within three to five heartbeats, following administration of agitated saline and complete opacification of the right atrium, is diagnostic for an intact interatrial septum.
   C. It is the result of a failure of fusion between the septum primum and septum secundum.
   D. The number of bubbles present in the left atrium after a bubble study correlates with the magnitude of the defect.

8. A 37-year-old woman with a known isolated outlet VSD is having progressive dyspnea. The images below are both obtained from a parasternal long-axis view. **Figure 37.6A** is her current state, while **Figure 37.6B** is from 2 years ago.

Which of the following is *most* likely true?
A. The patient does not need surgical closure of her VSD.
B. The patient's VSD is getting larger.
C. The patient's dyspnea is caused by an increase in her RV pressure.
D. The patient now has a higher pulmonary artery (PA) blood flow.

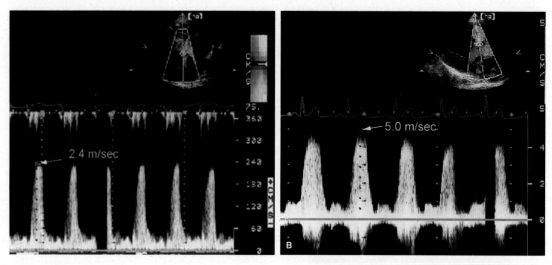

**Figure 37.6**

9. Based on **Figure 37.7**, which figure part is associated with both a sinus venosus ASD and an anomalous pulmonary venous return?

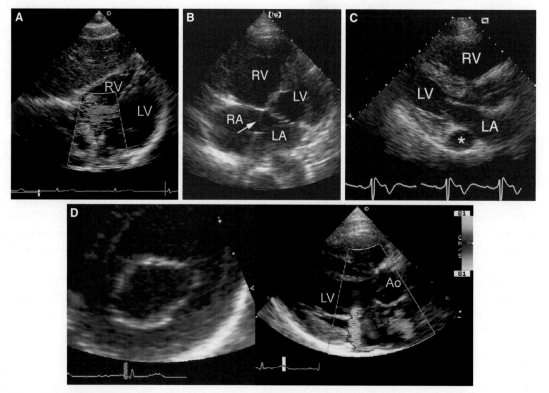

**Figure 37.7**

A. Figure 37.7A
B. Figure 37.7B
C. Figure 37.7C
D. Figure 37.7D

10. A 37-year-old woman with a known uncorrected muscular VSD is being evaluated for worsening dyspnea and cyanosis. Her arterial line blood pressure is 118/68 and central venous pressure (CVP) is 21. She does not have a left ventricular or RV outlet obstruction. Based on **Figure 37.8**, which of the following is *most* likely true?

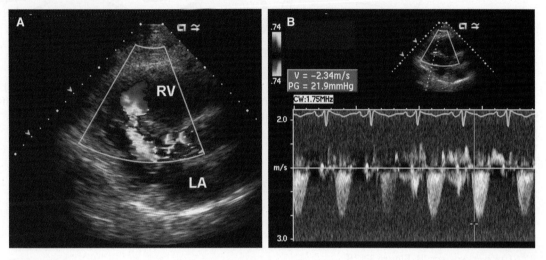

**Figure 37.8**

A. The patient should have surgical correction of her VSD.
B. The estimated RV systolic pressure (RVSP) is 96 mm Hg.
C. The patient should be given oxygen to alleviate her cyanosis.
D. The estimated pulmonary artery systolic pressure (PASP) is 140 mm Hg.

# Chapter 37 ▪ Answers

1. Correct Answer: B. It is a defect in the septum primum.

*Rationale:* Figure 37.1 shows a secundum ASD, which is a defect arising from increased apoptosis of the septum primum. While the patient may have significant mitral regurgitation, it would most likely be due to mitral valve prolapse (MVP) in the setting of a secundum ASD. A cleft mitral valve is associated with a septum primum. The patient has a left-to-right shunt as demonstrated on color Doppler imaging, thus is unlikely to have cyanosis as part of her episodes. A secundum ASD is not associated with an inlet VSD. An inlet VSD is associated with a primum ASD. **Figure 37.9** depicts the different types of ASDs.

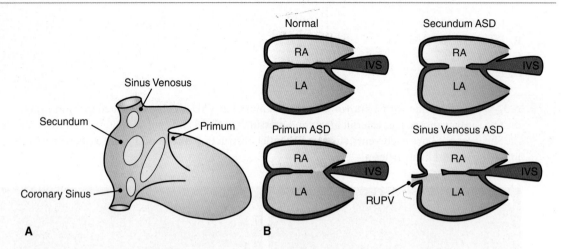

**Figure 37.9** A, A schematic of the relationship of different types of atrial septal defects (ASDs) viewed from the perspective of the right heart. B, The differences of different types of ASDs from a subcostal four-chamber perspective. IVS, interventricular septum; LA, left atrium; RA, right atrium; RUPV, right upper pulmonary vein.

### Selected References

1. Armstrong WF, Ryan T. Congenital heart diseases. In: Armstrong WF, Ryan T, eds. *Feigenbaum's Echocardiography*. 8th ed. Wolters Kluwer; 2019:544-610;Chapter 19.
2. Brickner ME. Congenital heart disease. In: Topol EJ, ed. *Textbook of Cardiovascular Medicine*. 3rd ed. Lippincott Williams and Wilkins; 2007:502-536;Chapter 30.

**2.** Correct Answer: **B. Figure 37.2B**

*Rationale:* Figure 37.2B, Choice B shows an apical four-chamber view with an ASD as well as the tricuspid and mitral valves in the same plane, a defining feature of an AV canal defect. Figure 37.2A, Choice A shows a dilated coronary sinus, in a posteriorly directed apical four-chamber view, in a patient with a persistent left superior vena cava (SVC). A persistent left SVC by itself is not a shunt; however, it may be associated with an unroofed coronary sinus or an anomalous pulmonary venous return. Figure 37.2C, Choice C shows a normal heart in the apical four-chamber view. Figure 37.2D, Choice D shows a muscular VSD, which is not a component of an AV canal.

### Selected References

1. Armstrong WF, Ryan T. The comprehensive echocardiographic examination. In: Armstrong WF, Ryan T, eds. *Feigenbaum's Echocardiography*. 8th ed. Wolters Kluwer; 2019:61-99;Chapter 4.
2. Armstrong WF, Ryan T. Congenital heart disease. In: Armstrong WF, Ryan T, eds. *Feigenbaum's Echocardiography*. 8th ed. Wolters Kluwer; 2019:544-610;Chapter 19.
3. Silvestry FE, Cohen MS, Armsby LB, et al. Atrial septal defect and patent foramen ovale: from the American Society of Echocardiography and Society for Cardiac Angiography and Interventions. *J Am Soc Echocardiogr*. 2015;28(8):910-958.
4. Stout KK, Daniels CJ, Aboulhosn JA, et al. 2018 AHA/ACC guideline for the management of adults with congenital heart disease: a report of the American College of Cardiology/American Heart Association Task Force on Clinical Practice Guidelines. *Circulation*. 2019;139:e698-e800.

**3.** Correct Answer: **C. Ostium secundum ASD**

*Rationale/Critique:* Figure 37.3 is an apical four-chamber view showing MVP, causing the patient's mitral regurgitation. MVP is associated with the presence of an ostium secundum ASD. An ostium primum ASD is associated with an inlet VSD. An AV canal exists when an ostium primum ASD and inlet VSD coexist. An isolated VSD, a partial AV canal, and complete AV canal are all part of a spectrum of lesions, collectively known as endocardial cushion defects. An ostium primum ASD is also associated with a cleft AV valve and regurgitation, in addition to trisomy 21. A membranous VSD is associated with ventricular septal aneurysms, aortic insufficiency, and aortic valve cusp prolapse into the VSD.

### Selected References

1. Armstrong WF, Ryan T. Congenital heart disease. In: Armstrong WF, Ryan T, eds. *Feigenbaum's Echocardiography*. 8th ed. Wolters Kluwer; 2019:544-610;Chapter 19.
2. Leachman R, Cokkinos D, Cooley D. Association of ostium secundum atrial septal defects with mitral valve prolapse. *Am J Cardiol*. 1976;38(2):167-169.

3. Smer A, Nanda NC, Akdogan RE, Elmarzouky ZM, Dulal S. Echocardiographic evaluation of mitral valve regurgitation. *Mini-invasive Surg*. 2020;4:52.
4. Stout KK, Daniels CJ, Aboulhosn JA, et al. 2018 AHA/ACC guideline for the management of adults with congenital heart disease: a report of the American College of Cardiology/American Heart Association Task Force on Clinical Practice Guidelines. *Circulation*. 2019;139:e698-e800.

**4.** Correct Answer: A. Figure 37.4A

*Rationale:* Figure 37.4A shows an inlet VSD (aka AV canal type) that is associated with a cleft mitral valve. An inlet VSD is part of the spectrum of endocardial cushion defects. An isolated VSD, a partial AV canal, and complete AV canal are all endocardial cushion defects.

Figure 37.4.B shows a muscular VSD (aka trabeculated).

Figure 37.4C shows a membranous VSD (aka perimembranous, conoventricular), with the left image being a modified apical two chamber showing the aorta and LVOT and VSD with left-to-right shunt just above the aortic valve, while the right image shows the VSD in the membranous region, closer to the tricuspid valve (as opposed to an outlet VSD which is closer to the pulmonic valve). A membranous VSD is the most common VSD and is associated with ventricular septal aneurysms, aortic insufficiency, and aortic valve cusp prolapse into the VSD.

Figure 37.4D shows an outlet VSD (aka infundibular, supracristal, infracristal, subarterial, subpulmonary, conal, or doubly committed juxta-arterial), seen in parasternal long axis on the left and in parasternal short axis on the right, close to the pulmonic valve (as opposed to a membranous VSD which is closer to the tricuspid valve). An outlet VSD is associated with aortic insufficiency (more so than a membranous VSD). **Figure 37.10** depicts the different types of VSDs.

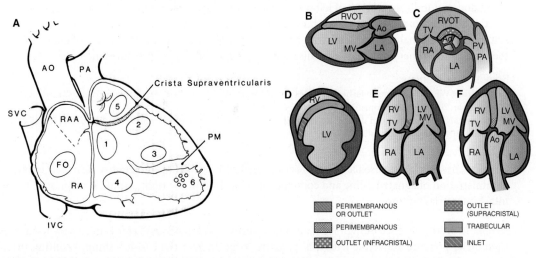

**Figure 37.10** A, Schematic of the right ventricular surface of the interventricular septum (IVS) diagramming common locations of ventricular septal defects. Region 1, membranous IVS; region 2, outflow IVS; region 3, trabecular septum; region 4, inflow septum; region 5, supracristal region; region 6, distal multiple "Swiss cheese" septal defects. B-F, Schematic depicting the locations of the various types of ventricular septal defects, which is more relative to the transthoracic views obtained. AO, aorta; FO, fossa ovalis; IVC, inferior vena cava; LA, left atrium; LV, left ventricle; MV, mitral valve; PA, pulmonary artery; PM, papillary muscle; PV, pulmonic valve; RA, right atrium; RAA, right atrial appendage; RV, right ventricle; RVOT, right ventricular outflow tract; SVC, superior vena cava; TV, tricuspid valve.

Selected References

1. Armstrong WF, Ryan T. Congenital heart disease. In: Armstrong WF, Ryan T, eds. *Feigenbaum's Echocardiography*. 8th ed. Wolters Kluwer; 2019:544-610;Chapter 19.
2. Jacobs J, Mavroudis C. Congenital heart surgery nomenclature and database project: ventricular septal defect. *Ann Thorac Surg*. 2000;69(3):25-35.
3. Stout KK, Daniels CJ, Aboulhosn JA, et al. 2018 AHA/ACC guideline for the management of adults with congenital heart disease: a report of the American College of Cardiology/American Heart Association Task Force on Clinical Practice Guidelines. *Circulation*. 2019;139:e698-e800.

**5.** Correct Answer: D. 1.2

*Rationale:* The shunt ratio for this patient is 1.2. The shunt ratio (Qp/Qs) is calculated as in the equation below:

$$\frac{Q_P}{Q_s} = \frac{SV_{right}}{SV_{left}}$$

*where*

$$SV = \pi r^2 \times VTI$$

$Q_p$ = pulmonary blood flow, $Q_s$ = systemic blood flow, $r$ = radius of outflow tract, SV = stroke volume, VTI = velocity time integral of blood flow through the outflow tract

### Selected References
1. Armstrong WF, Ryan T. Congenital heart diseases. In: Armstrong WF, Ryan T, eds. *Feigenbaum's Echocardiography*. 8th ed. Wolters Kluwer; 2019:544-610;Chapter 19.
2. Brickner ME. Congenital heart disease. In: Topol EJ, ed. *Textbook of Cardiovascular Medicine*. 3rd ed. Lippincott Williams and Wilkins; 2007:502-536;Chapter 30.

**6.** Correct Answer: C. The presence of a bidirectional shunt rules out an increased LV end-diastolic volume.

*Rationale/Critique:* Patients with a patent ductus arteriosus (PDA) have left-sided volume overload as a result of increased flow through the PAs due to the left-to-right shunt. The presence of a bidirectional shunt does not indicate absence of left-sided volume overload. Eisenmenger physiology can result from a PDA. A PDA starts as a left-to-right shunt; however, a progressive rise in PA pressures over time will result in a bidirectional shunt. Adults with an untreated PDA are at an increased risk of endocarditis. Also, the typical "machinery murmur" may disappear once the right-sided pressures increase.

### Selected References
1. Armstrong WF, Ryan T. Congenital heart diseases. In: Armstrong WF, Ryan T, eds. *Feigenbaum's Echocardiography*. 8th ed. Wolters Kluwer; 2019:544-610;Chapter 19.
2. Brickner ME. Congenital heart disease. In: Topol EJ, ed. *Textbook of Cardiovascular Medicine*. 3rd ed. Lippincott Williams and Wilkins; 2007:502-536;Chapter 30.

**7.** Correct Answer: B. The absence of bubbles in the left atrium, within three to five heartbeats, following administration of agitated saline and complete opacification of the right atrium, is diagnostic for an intact interatrial septum.

*Rationale:* In the absence of high right atrial pressures, a Valsalva maneuver is necessary to increase the right atrial pressure above the left atrial pressure to promote a right-to-left shunt, resulting in bubbles crossing the PFO. A false negative bubble study can occur in the absence of, or inappropriate timing of, the Valsalva. The Valsalva maneuver should be performed prior to injection of the agitated saline or other contrast media to allow increase of right atrial pressure prior to injection. Options A, C and D are true and hence not the answer.

### Selected Reference
1. Saric M, Armour AC, Arnaout MS, et al. Guidelines for the use of echocardiography in the evaluation of a cardiac source of embolism. *J Am Soc Echocardiogr*. 2016;29(1):1-42.

**8.** Correct Answer: C. The patient's dyspnea is caused by an increase in her RV pressure.

*Rationale:* This patient is having progressive dyspnea as a result of increased RV pressures. As RV pressure rises, the pressure gradient between the right ventricle and left ventricle decreases, resulting in a lower blood flow and lower velocity of flow across the VSD. Initially, a VSD allows a left-to-right shunt due to the LV pressure being higher than the RV pressure. This left-to-right shunt increases the amount of blood going through the pulmonary vasculature. Over time, this leads to smooth muscle hypertrophy of the pulmonary vasculature causing pulmonary hypertension. The increased pressure in the pulmonary vasculature leads to an increase in RV pressure, which will then limit flow from the left ventricle across the VSD. Eventually, a reversal of flow becoming right-to-left could develop, which is known as Eisenmenger syndrome. The patient has not yet developed Eisenmenger syndrome as the shunt is still left-to-right; however, the RV and pulmonary vasculature pressures are increasing, as evidenced by a lower velocity of flow through the shunt. A VSD should not be surgically corrected after development of Eisenmenger syndrome as it would be fatal due to lack of relief of high right-sided pressures. Current recommendations are to surgically correct a shunt to prevent development of Eisenmenger physiology. It is very unlikely that a congenital VSD would increase in size. As right-sided pressures increase from the VSD, LV volume overload is decreased due to a decrease in pulmonary vasculature blood flow.

### Selected References

1. Armstrong WF, Ryan T. Congenital heart diseases. In: Armstrong WF, Ryan T, eds. *Feigenbaum's Echocardiography*. 8th ed. Wolters Kluwer; 2019:544-610;Chapter 19.
2. Brickner ME. Congenital heart disease. In: Topol EJ, ed. *Textbook of Cardiovascular Medicine*. 3rd ed. Lippincott Williams and Wilkins; 2007:502-536;Chapter 30.

**9.** Correct Answer: **C. Figure 37.7C**

*Rationale:* Figure 37.7C shows a dilated coronary sinus in a parasternal long-axis view. A dilated coronary sinus may be associated with an unroofed coronary sinus ASD, a sinus venosus ASD, or an anomalous pulmonary venous return. A dilated coronary sinus is also present with persistent left SVC; however, a persistent left SVC in isolation is not a shunt. Figure 37.7A shows a secundum ASD that is associated with MVP. Figure 37.7B shows a primum ASD that is associated with a cleft mitral valve (shown in Figure 37.7D) and an inlet VSD. Figure 37.7D shows a cleft mitral valve in the parasternal short axis and the resulting severe mitral regurgitation in the parasternal long axis.

### Selected References

1. Armstrong WF, Ryan T. Congenital heart disease. In: Armstrong WF, Ryan T, eds. *Feigenbaum's Echocardiography*. 8th ed. Wolters Kluwer; 2019:544-610;Chapter 19.
2. Silvestry FE, Cohen MS, Armsby LB, et al. Atrial septal defect and patent foramen ovale: from the American Society of Echocardiography and Society for Cardiac Angiography and Interventions. *J Am Soc Echocardiogr*. 2015;28(8):910-958.

**10.** Correct Answer: **D. The estimated pulmonary artery systolic pressure (PASP) is 140 mm Hg.**

*Rationale:* Figure 37.8 shows a muscular VSD with a right-to-left shunt by color (Figure 37.8A) and continuous-wave Doppler (CWD) imaging (Figure 37.8B). In the absence of an LVOT obstruction, arterial systolic pressure can be used to estimate LV systolic pressure (LVSP). The same can be said for absence of an RVOT obstruction, allowing the RVSP to be used to estimate the PASP. In this case, CWD imaging shows a right-to-left shunt with a pressure gradient of 21.9 mm Hg. In order to have a right-to-left shunt, the RV pressures must be higher than the LV pressures. So adding the estimated LVSP (using arterial systolic pressure) to the pressure gradient between the ventricles will yield an estimation of the RVSP, which in the absence of an RVOT obstruction is an estimate for the PASP (i.e., 118 mm Hg + 21.9 mm Hg = 139.9 mm Hg). A VSD should not be surgically corrected after development of Eisenmenger syndrome as it would be fatal due to lack of relief of high right-sided pressures. Delivery of oxygen to a patient with a right-to-left shunt will not alleviate their cyanosis. Improvement in oxygenation will only be accomplished with decreasing the amount of shunt, in this case, by lowering the RV and PA pressures.

### Selected References

1. Armstrong WF, Ryan T. Congenital heart diseases. In: Armstrong WF, Ryan T, eds. *Feigenbaum's Echocardiography*. 8th ed. Wolters Kluwer; 2019:544-610;Chapter 19.
2. Brickner ME. Congenital heart disease. In: Topol EJ, ed. *Textbook of Cardiovascular Medicine*. 3rd ed. Lippincott Williams and Wilkins; 2007:502-536;Chapter 30.
3. Jone P-N, Ivy DD. Echocardiography in pediatric pulmonary hypertension. *Front Pediatr*. 2014;2(124):1-15.

# 38 | INTRACARDIAC MASSES, ABNORMAL STRUCTURES, NORMAL ANATOMIC VARIANTS, AND ARTIFACTS

Bhavik P. Patel and Alejandro Pino

1. In a patient with normal left ventricular function, a mass is seen on the left ventricle (see *arrow* in **Figure 38.1**), which disappears by changing the view. This mass most likely represents:

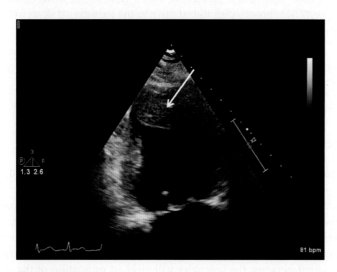

**Figure 38.1**

A. A thrombus
B. A shadowing artifact
C. A myxoma
D. A near-field clutter artifact
E. None of the above

2. The *arrow* in **Figure 38.2A** points to a left ventricular mass. After increasing the depth, seen in **Figure 38.2B**, the mass disappears.

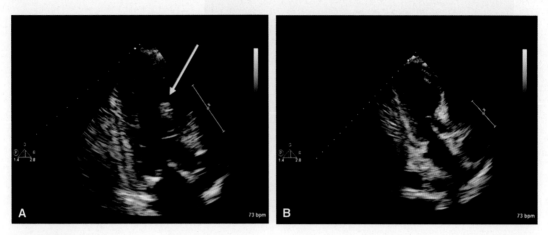

**Figure 38.2**

What does this mass most likely represent?
A. A moderator band
B. A range-ambiguity artifact (RAA)
C. A thrombus in transit
D. A side-lobe artifact
E. An acoustic shadowing artifact

3. A man presents to the emergency room with chest pain and is diagnosed with ST-segment elevation myocardial infarction. He has a transthoracic echocardiogram (TTE) that shows anterior wall akinesis and a left ventricular mass seen in **Figure 38.3**.

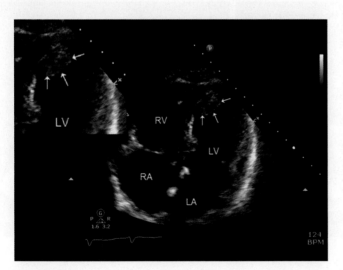

**Figure 38.3**

What is the most likely diagnosis?
A. Vegetation
B. Trabeculae
C. Thrombus
D. Myxoma
E. None of the above

4. Apical four-chamber view of a 56-year-old man is shown in **Figure 38.4**.

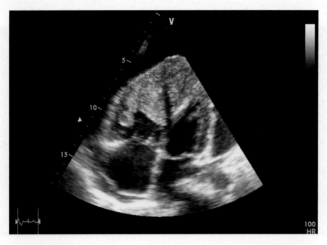

**Figure 38.4**

If the pathology is malignant in etiology, what would be the most common cause for it?
A. Rhabdomyosarcoma
B. Myxoma
C. Lymphoma
D. Metastatic disease
E. Angiosarcoma

5. Which of the following statements accurately describes the aortic valve tumor shown in echocardiogram (**Figure 38.5**)?

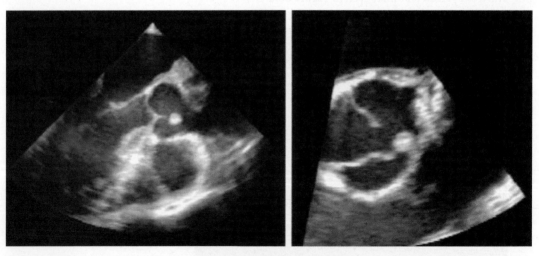

**Figure 38.5**

A. Papillary fibroelastoma (PFE) can easily be distinguished from vegetation.
B. PFE is the most common benign cardiac tumor.
C. The most common clinical manifestation of PFE is heart block.
D. PFE most commonly attaches to papillary muscles.
E. PFE accounts for the majority of valve-associated tumors.

6. Which of the following symptoms are characteristic of the tumor (*arrow*, **Figure 38.6**), most likely represented in the accompanying midesophageal four-chamber view of the heart?

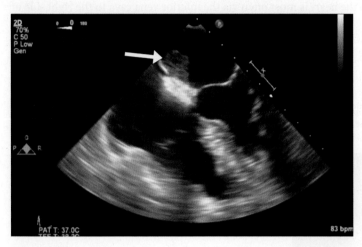

**Figure 38.6**

   **A.** Syncope and diarrhea
   **B.** Dyspnea and fevers
   **C.** Palpitations and dysphagia
   **D.** Palpitations and diarrhea
   **E.** Dyspnea and facial flushing

7. A 55-year-old woman recently diagnosed with renal cell carcinoma (RCC) presents for TTE in preparation for surgery. Parasternal long-axis view shows a mass in the right ventricle (RV; see *arrow* in **Figure 38.7**).

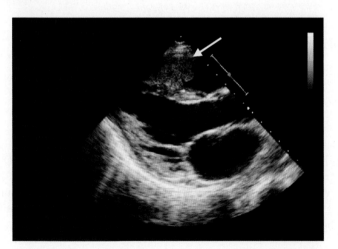

**Figure 38.7**

Which of the following statements about this mass is correct?

**A.** Thrombus is easy to distinguish from metastatic RCC on echocardiography.

**B.** Cardiac metastasis is not seen with RCC.

**C.** RCC route of metastasis to the heart is most often via the inferior vena cava to the right side of the heart.

**D.** The initial diagnosis of RCC cannot be made by detection of an intracardiac mass on echocardiography.

**E.** None of the above.

8. A 25-year-old man with no prior medical history presents after a motor vehicle accident. An echocardiogram subcostal four-chamber view is shown in **Figure 38.8**.

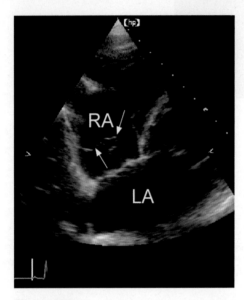

**Figure 38.8**

What does the structure highlighted by the *arrow* most likely represent?

**A.** A Chiari network

**B.** A myxoma

**C.** A thrombus

**D.** A vegetation

**E.** None of the above

9. A 38-year-old man with a history of human immunodeficiency virus (HIV) presents with a low CD4 T lymphocyte count and symptoms concerning for acquired immunodeficiency syndrome (AIDS). TTE revealed a large pericardial effusion with right atrial collapse and low-density mass at the level of auricle of the right atrium spreading toward the superior vena cava, floating in the cavity of the right atrium. Which of the following tumors has been described to affect the heart in this patient population?

**A.** Angiosarcoma

**B.** Myxoma

**C.** Kaposi sarcoma (KS)

**D.** Rhabdomyosarcoma

**E.** None of the above

10. The structure seen in the right atrium in **Figure 38.9** is most likely to be:

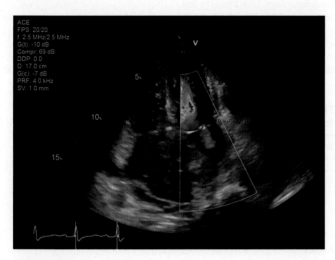

**Figure 38.9**

A. Crista terminalis
B. Chiari network
C. Eustachian valve
D. Angiosarcoma
E. Moderator band

# Chapter 38 ▪ Answers

1. Correct Answer: D. A near-field clutter artifact

*Rationale:* Near-field clutter is an artifact caused by the transducer's high-amplitude oscillations affecting or obscuring structures present in the near field. This is especially relevant when apical ventricular thrombus is suspected since the image can resemble that of a thrombus. However, unlike a thrombus, clutter is unaffected by ventricular wall motion and, at times, can appear to pass through the ventricular wall. Changing from fundamental to harmonic imaging is helpful in reducing this type of artifact, as well as side-lobe and reverberation artifacts. If there is still uncertainty, switching to other imaging planes, using contrast agents, decreasing depth, and improving near-field resolution can also reduce or eliminate this type of artifact. Cardiac myxomas are usually globular in structure, appear heterogeneous, and more commonly occur in the left atrium where the site of attachment is almost always in the region of the fossa ovalis.

Risk factors for the development of left ventricular thrombus are associated with regions of wall motion abnormality and include large infarct size, severe apical asynergy (i.e., akinesia or dyskinesia), left ventricular aneurysm, and anterior myocardial infarction. Left ventricular thrombi usually have defined margins, are seen throughout systole and diastole, are located adjacent to an area of hypokinesia or akinesia, and are seen from at least two views. **Table 38.1** summarizes some of the structures or artifacts that can mimic a thrombus in the left ventricle.

Selected References

1. Bertrand PB, Levine RA, Isselbacher EM, Vandervoort PM. Fact or artifact in two-dimensional echocardiography: avoiding misdiagnosis and missed diagnosis. *J Am Soc Echocardiogr*. 2016;29(5):381-391.
2. Brenes JC, Asher CR. Cardiac ultrasound artifacts. In: Klein AL, ed. *Clinical Echocardiography Review*. 2nd ed. Wolters Kluwer; 2018:15-29.
3. Delewi R, Zijlstra F, Piek JJ. Left ventricular thrombus formation after acute myocardial infarction. *Heart*. 2012;98:1743-1749.
4. Galiuto L, Badano L, Fox K, Sicari R, Zamorano JL. *The EAE Textbook of Echocardiography*. Oxford University Press; 2011:9.
5. Peters PJ, Reinhardt S. The echocardiographic evaluation of intracardiac masses: a review. *J Am Soc Echocardiogr*. 2006;19:230-240.

**Table 38.1  Structures or Artifacts That Can Mimic a Thrombus in the Left Ventricle**

| Normal Variants or Pathologic Structures |
| --- |
| False tendon |
| Prominent trabeculations |
| Hypertrabeculation syndrome |
| Prominent or accessory papillary muscles |
| Tumors |
| Endomyocardial fibrosis (EMF) |
| Apical hypertrophy |
| Congenital diverticula |
| Thrombus |
| Aneurysms/pseudoaneurysms |
| Noncompaction cardiomyopathy |
| **Artifact Types** |
| Reverberation |
| Near-field |
| Comet tail |
| Range ambiguity |
| Attenuation |
| Shadowing |

2. Correct Answer: B. A range-ambiguity artifact (RAA)

*Rationale:* RAA is an erroneous mapping of returning echoes into a composite picture. RAA occurs when an object outside the field of view reflects ultrasound waves that are not received until early in the next cycle. This in turn results in an appearance of deep structures closer to the transducer than they actually are. RAA can be eliminated by decreasing depth or adjusting the transducer position.

The moderator band is a conspicuous muscular ridge present in the RV and is usually noted as the most prominent trabecula, extending from the septum to the free wall. Thrombus in transit appears as a serpentine density, normally extending from the right atrium into the RV. A side-lobe artifact results when side energy lateral to the central beam of the transducer encounters a strong reflector, producing an image that appears as originating from the central beam though it is actually lateral to the true object location. An acoustic shadowing artifact occurs when there is increased attenuation by structures leading to an image that is darkened distal to the increased attenuation.

Selected References

1. Brenes JC, Asher CR. Cardiac ultrasound artifacts. In: Klein AL, ed. *Clinical Echocardiography Review*. 2nd ed. Wolters Kluwer; 2018:15-29.
2. Kremkau FW, Taylor KJ. Artifacts in ultrasound imaging. *J Ultrasound Med*. 1986 Apr;5(4):227-237.
3. Puello F, Harewood J, Lee C, Rupani N, Abe O. Thrombus in transit: the emergence of a deadly diagnosis. *Chest*. 2017 Oct;152(4):A1021.
4. Rajiah P, MacNamara J, Chaturvedi A, Ashwath R, Fulton NL, Goerne H. Bands in the heart: multimodality imaging review. *Radiographics*. 2019 Sep-Oct;39(5):1238-1263.

## 3. Correct Answer: C. Thrombus

*Rationale:* The combination of blood stasis, endothelial injury, and hypercoagulability, often referred to as Virchow's triad, is a prerequisite for thrombus formation. In myocardial infarction, regional wall akinesia or dyskinesia results in blood stasis. Prolonged ischemia leads to subendocardial tissue injury, and acute coronary syndrome can promote a hypercoagulable state. This triad can result in the formation of left ventricular thrombus.

Risk factors for the development of left ventricular thrombus include large infarct size, severe apical akinesis or dyskinesis, left ventricular aneurysm, and anterior wall myocardial infarction.

TTE is the technique used most often to help identify patients at high risk for thromboembolism and to assess the presence, shape, and size of the thrombus. It can also be used to monitor resolution of thrombus with anticoagulation. Left ventricular thrombus is defined as a discrete echodense mass in the left ventricle with defined margins that are distinct from the endocardium and seen throughout systole and diastole. It should be located adjacent to an area of hypokinesis or akinesis and seen in at least two planes. Structures such as false tendons and trabeculae can mimic a left ventricular thrombus, as can side-lobe, near-field, and reverberation artifacts. Cardiac myxomas, on the other hand, are heterogeneous globular structures attached to the endocardial surface by a stalk commonly arising from the surface of the fossa ovalis of the left atrium.

Selected References

1. Delewi R, Zijlstra F, Piek JJ. Left ventricular thrombus formation after acute myocardial infarction. *Heart*. 2012;98:1743-1749.
2. Echocardiography and coronary artery disease. In: Armstrong WF, Ryan T, eds. *Feigenbaum's Echocardiography*. 8th ed. Wolters Kluwer; 2019:427-459
3. Quien MM, Saric M. Ultrasound imaging artifacts: how to recognize them and how to avoid them. *Echocardiography*. 2018;35(9):1388-1401.

## 4. Correct Answer: D. Metastatic disease

*Rationale:* Figure 38.4 shows a right ventricular mass, likely a tumor. Cardiac tumors are rare in general, but metastasis to the heart from other primary cancers is 30 times more common. **Table 38.2** lists the primary cancers that metastasize to the heart.

**Table 38.2 Route of Spread of Tumors That Metastasize to the Heart**

| Primary Tumor | Mechanism of Spread to the Heart |
| --- | --- |
| Renal cell carcinoma | Inferior vena cava to right side of the heart |
| Breast | Hematogenous or lymphatic spread |
| Lung | Direct extension |
| Melanoma | Intracavitary or myocardial involvement |
| Lymphoma | Lymphangitic spread |
| Carcinoid | Tricuspid and pulmonic valve thickening |

There are a few primary cardiac tumors, and myxomas are the most common. These are benign tumors that usually occur in the left atrium, with the attachment site commonly at the fossa ovalis of the atrial septum. Only 25% of primary cardiac tumors are malignant, and of these, 75% are sarcomas. Malignant primary cardiac sarcomas are usually located in the right atrium and are most commonly angiosarcomas. In the left atrium, the most common malignant tumors are pleomorphic sarcomas and leiomyosarcomas.

Symptom presentation for cardiac tumors is dependent upon tumor location and size, rather than upon histologic characteristics. These include congestive heart failure from intracardiac obstruction, systemic embolization, constitutional symptoms, and arrhythmias. The pattern of heart and pericardium tumor involvement provides information important to the differential diagnosis of the cardiac condition. This determination can be made in part by diagnostic imaging, including but not limited to echocardiography.

Histopathologic determination is crucial for definitive diagnosis of a mass lesion as a type of primary tumor, a secondary metastatic neoplasm, or a nonneoplastic process. There are a number of pseudotumors that can resemble cardiac tumors. These include intracavitary thrombi or foreign bodies, intramural abscesses or hematomas, ventricular aneurysms, and coronary artery aneurysms. Cystic lesions of the pericardium are typically benign. Malignant lesions are more likely to produce pericardial adhesions, hemorrhagic pericardial effusion, or both. A solitary intramyocardial mass in the ventricular wall is likely to be a primary benign tumor, whereas multiple myocardial nodules are more likely to represent metastatic malignancy.

## Selected References

1. Armstrong WF, Ryan T. *Feigenbaum's Echocardiography*. 8th ed. Wolters Kluwer; 2019.
2. Buja LM. The multifaceted manifestations of cardiac tumors. *Tex Heart Inst J*. 2012;39(1):84-85.
3. Leja MJ, Shah DJ, Reardon MJ. Primary cardiac tumors. *Tex Heart Inst J*. 2011;38(3):261-262.

---

**5.** Correct Answer: E. PFE accounts for the majority of valve-associated tumors.

*Rationale:* PFE is the second most common type of benign cardiac tumor. Characterized as mobile and pedunculated masses, they are located predominantly on the cardiac valves. They are attached to the cardiac valves in over 80% of cases, with the aortic valve implicated in close to half of these. Only rarely do these masses attach to the endocardium or papillary muscles in the left ventricle. The most common clinical manifestation is cerebrovascular accident or transient ischemic attack. Pulmonary, mesenteric, retinal, and peripheral emboli have been reported in a minority of cases. There is a strong association between left-sided mobile PFE with a stalk and future embolic phenomena.

The real-time approach and temporal and spatial resolution of TTE make it the initial modality of choice in the diagnosis of PFE. The use of contrast in TTE may help differentiate highly vascular malignant tumors from avascular masses such as thrombi or vegetations. With contrast, malignant tumors hyperenhance, stromal tumors partially enhance, and thrombi do not enhance. Cardiac magnetic resonance imaging and computed tomography of the chest may be used to differentiate tumors from thrombi, especially when using contrast enhancement.

## Selected References

1. Gowda RM, Khan IA, Nair CK, Mehta NJ, Vasavada BC, Sacchi TJ. Cardiac papillary fibroelastoma: a comprehensive analysis of 725 cases. *Am Heart J*. 2003 Sep;146(3):404-410.
2. Hakeem H, Argenziano M, Katechis D. A left ventricular papillary fibroelastoma presenting as an acute coronary syndrome. *CASE (Phila)*. 2017;2(1):24-26.
3. Sun JP, Asher CR, Yang XS, et al. Clinical and echocardiographic characteristics of papillary fibroelastomas: a retrospective and prospective study in 162 patients. *Circulation*. 2001;103:2687-2693.

**6.** Correct Answer: **B. Dyspnea and fevers**

*Rationale:* Cardiac myxomas are the most common noncancerous primary tumors of the heart, constituting about 50% of all primary cardiac neoplasms. They usually occur in the left atrium, with the attachment site at the atrial septum. Cardiac myxomas predominantly occur in women, with an average age of onset in the sixth decade of life. The most common symptoms of cardiac myxoma are associated with obstruction due to the size and location of the tumor. Dyspnea is most common, followed by palpitations and syncope. Constitutional symptoms, such as fevers and weight loss, are also seen in approximately 15% to 20% of patients.

Carcinoid syndrome presents with symptoms such as diarrhea and facial flushing. Other symptoms include bronchospasm, hypotension, and symptoms of right-sided heart failure such as worsening dyspnea, edema, ascites, and eventual cardiac cachexia with progression of disease.

On TTE, both tricuspid and pulmonary valve leaflets and subvalvular apparatus are thickened. Excursion of the valve leaflets is reduced and eventually becomes retracted and fixed, remaining in a semiopen position. Functionally, a combination of valvular regurgitation and stenosis occurs.

### Selected References

1. Bhattacharyya S, Davar J, Dreyfus G, Caplin ME. Carcinoid heart disease. *Circulation.* 2007 Dec 11;116(24):2860-2865.
2. Burke A, Virmani R. Tumors of the heart and the great vessels. In: Rosai J, ed. *Atlas of Tumor Pathology.* 3rd ed. Fascicle 16. Armed Forces Institute of Pathology; 1996:231.
3. Hi D, Yoon A, Roberts WC. Sex distribution in cardiac myxomas. *Am J Cardiol.* 2002;90:563-565.

**7.** Correct Answer: **C. RCC route of metastasis to the heart is most often via the inferior vena cava to the right side of the heart.**

*Rationale:* Cardiac involvement in RCC commonly arises from direct tumor thrombus extension into the inferior vena cava. The second mechanism of metastasis involves tumor dissemination via hematogenous spread. Cardiac metastasis in the absence of vena cava extension is exceedingly rare, with only a few cases reported in the literature.

TTE is the first diagnostic tool for assessment of patients with suspected cardiac metastasis of RCC. In fact, echocardiography may be the method of initial RCC diagnosis in patients with predominantly cardiac symptoms. However, distinction between metastatic RCC and thrombus can be difficult to make via echocardiography due to their similar appearances. In many instances, further imaging via a modality such as cardiac magnetic resonance can be helpful to distinguish these entities.

### Selected References

1. Bouzouita M, Ben Slamaa MR, Mohameda MOS, et al. Cardiac metastasis of renal cell carcinoma, a rare location. *Prog Urol.* 2011;21:492-494.
2. Reynen K, Köckeritz U, Strasser RH. Metastases to the heart. *Ann Oncol.* 2004;15:375-381.
3. Weiner SD, Homma S. Tumors, masses, and source of emboli. In: Klein AL, ed. *Clinical Echocardiography Review.* 2nd ed. Wolters Kluwer; 2018:519-533.

**8.** Correct Answer: **A. A Chiari network**

*Rationale:* The Chiari network is a congenital remnant of the right valve of the sinus venosus and is found close to the inferior vena cava and coronary sinus, sometimes connecting these with other right atrial structures. It has been found in 2% to 3% of autopsy studies and is believed to be of little clinical consequence. However, it may at times produce diagnostic confusion; cause thromboembolism, infective endocarditis, arrhythmias; or cause a physical barrier to invasive procedures.

The echocardiographic findings of the Chiari network include a highly mobile fenestrated structure attached to the right atrium, at times confused with valve disruption, vegetation, or other mass lesion, particularly when associated with a suggestive clinical situation.

Selected References

1. Left and right atrium, and right ventricle. In: Armstrong WF, Ryan T, eds. *Feigenbaum's Echocardiography*. 8th ed. Wolters Kluwer; 2019:158-193.
2. Loukas M, Sullivan A, Tubbs RS, Weinhaus AJ, Derderian T, Hanna M. Chiari's network: review of the literature. *Surg Radiol Anat*. 2010;32(10):895-901.
3. Werner JA, Cheitlin MD, Gross BW, Speck SM, Ivey TD. Echocardiographic appearance of the Chiari network: differentiation from right-heart pathology. *Circulation*. 1981 May;63(5):1104-1109.

**9.** Correct Answer: C. Kaposi sarcoma (KS)

*Rationale:* KS is a vascular lesion of low-grade malignant potential associated with human herpesvirus-8 (HHV8) infection and presents most frequently in mucocutaneous sites. KS usually involves lymph nodes and visceral organs. Unusual locations of KS involvement include the musculoskeletal system, central and peripheral nervous system, larynx, eye, major salivary glands, endocrine organs, heart, thoracic duct, urinary system, and breast.

KS heart involvement has been reported to occur more often in patients without cutaneous disease. The epicardium (subepicardial adipose tissue) appears to be more commonly involved than the myocardium or endocardium.

In patients with AIDS, high-grade B-cell lymphomas have also been identified in cardiac tissue.

Selected Reference

1. Pantanowitz L, Dezube BJ. Kaposi sarcoma in unusual locations. *BMC Cancer*. 2008;8:190. Published 2008 Jul 7.

**10.** Correct Answer: D. Angiosarcoma

*Rationale:* Malignant primary cardiac sarcomas are usually located in the right atrium and are most commonly angiosarcomas. In the left atrium, the most common malignant tumors are pleomorphic sarcoma and leiomyosarcoma. Primary cardiac angiosarcoma is rare but is the most aggressive type of cardiac malignant tumor and can be either intracavitary or diffuse and infiltrative. When disease is confirmed, it is often in a late stage, resulting in a poor prognosis. Presenting symptoms are usually due to right heart failure or cardiac tamponade.

The crista terminalis, Chiari network, and Eustachian valve are all normal structures found in the right atrium that can be misinterpreted on two-dimensional echocardiography as pathologic.

The crista terminalis is a well-defined fibromuscular ridge formed by the junction of the sinus venosus and primitive right atrium that extends along the posterolateral aspect of the right atrial wall. Occasionally, this structure can be prominent, thus mimicking right atrial mass-like tumor, thrombus, or vegetation.

The Chiari network is a congenital remnant of the right valve of the sinus venosus, lying close to the inferior vena cava and coronary sinus, sometimes connecting these with other right atrial structures.

The Eustachian valve is an embryogenic derivative of the right valve of the sinus venosus. Although it generally disappears during fetal life, its persistence may simulate atrial tumors.

The moderator band is a normal structure found in the RV, usually noted as the most prominent trabecula, extending from the septum to the free wall.

Selected References

1. Cook AC, Yates RW, Anderson RH. Normal and abnormal fetal cardiac anatomy. *Prenat Diagn*. 2004;24:1032-1048.
2. Kodali D, Seetharaman K. Primary cardiac angiosarcoma. *Sarcoma*. 2006;2006:39130.
3. Salustri A, Bakir S, Sana A, Lange P, Al Mahmeed WA. Prominent crista terminalis mimicking a right atrial mass: case report. *Cardiovasc Ultrasound*. 2010;8:47. Published 2010 Oct 19.

# 39 | TRANSTHORACIC ECHOCARDIOGRAM VERSUS TRANSESOPHAGEAL ECHOCARDIOGRAM

Ellyn Gray and Lovkesh Arora

1. Which among the following is the most common complication following a transesophageal echocardiogram (TEE)?

   A. Dysphagia
   B. Tracheal intubation by the probe
   C. Esophageal hemorrhage
   D. Dental damage

2. A patient is in the surgical intensive care unit (ICU), status post liver transplant. Intraoperative TEE was used, and the anesthesia team reported no complications with probe placement or usage. After extubation on postoperative day 1, the patient has significant chest pain and an episode of hematemesis. All of the following can be done during use of the TEE probe to minimize the risk of this complication *except*:

   A. Maintain an unlocked position while moving the probe
   B. Minimize anteflexion and retroflexion when the probe is at the gastroesophageal junction
   C. Use a pediatric probe if there is a concern for esophageal pathology
   D. Use lower gain during imaging

3. Which of the following is an absolute contraindication for TEE?

   A. Atlantoaxial disorder
   B. Esophageal varices
   C. Esophagectomy
   D. Hiatal hernia

4. A 40-year-old male presents with diarrhea, wheezing, and new heart failure. You suspect carcinoid heart disease and want to evaluate for valvular lesions. Which of the following structures can be better visualized on transthoracic echocardiography (TTE) than TEE?

   A. Tricuspid valve
   B. Mitral valve
   C. Pulmonic valve
   D. Aortic valve

5. The TEE images shown in **Figure 39.1** were obtained to evaluate for aortic atheroma.

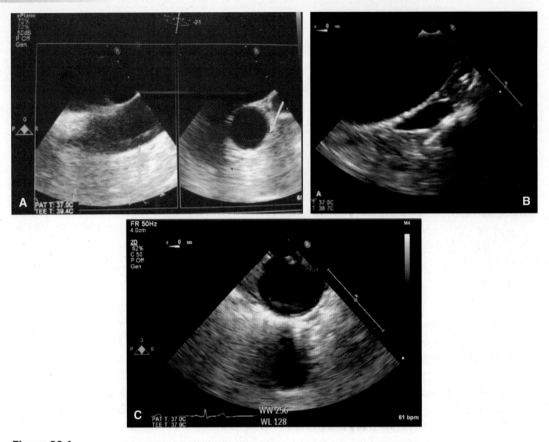

**Figure 39.1**

Which portion of the aorta is not visualized in these images?
A. Aortic arch
B. Descending aorta
C. Distal ascending aorta
D. Proximal ascending aorta

6. Your patient presented with chest pain and light-headedness and you appreciate a midsystolic murmur in the right upper sternal border. You suspect stenosis of the valve pointed out by the *red arrow* in **Figure 39.2.**

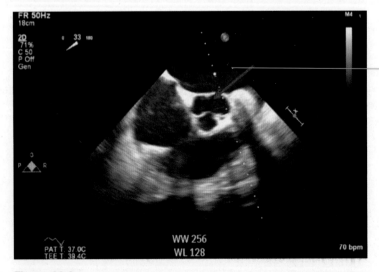

**Figure 39.2**

In which of the following views would the calculated gradient through this valve be underestimated in most patients?

**A.** Deep transgastric view
**B.** Transgastric long-axis view
**C.** Apical five-chamber view
**D.** Midesophageal long-axis view

7. A patient was admitted to the ICU with hypotension secondary to atrial fibrillation with rapid ventricular rhythm. He has a history of paroxysmal atrial fibrillation and you are considering cardioversion. You perform a TTE shown in **Figure 39.3.**

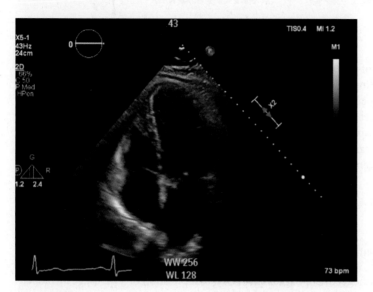

**Figure 39.3**

What additional imaging is necessary to rule out a left atrial appendage (LAA) thrombus?

**A.** Midesophageal two-chamber view
**B.** Apical four-chamber view
**C.** Midesophageal long-axis view
**D.** Parasternal long-axis view

8. A 66-year-old male presented with fevers and joint pains for 2 weeks. He recently underwent a tooth extraction. Physical examination reveals a holosystolic murmur that was not present on prior examinations. His erythrocyte sedimentation rate is markedly elevated. A painful nodule on the pad of his left index finger was also noted. You chose to do TEE over TTE due to the following advantage:

**A.** More accurate evaluation of TAPSE (tricuspid annular plane systolic excursion)
**B.** Quicker to perform
**C.** Increased sensitivity for endocarditis of the mitral valve
**D.** Improved resolution for imaging of the pulmonic valve

9. TEE is superior to TTE for imaging all the following *except*:

**A.** Atrial septal defect in adults
**B.** Right-sided infective endocarditis lesions
**C.** Aortic dissection
**D.** LAA thrombus

**10.** All of the following are important steps for proper cleaning and sterilization of the TEE probe *except*:

   **A.** Removal of organic material
   **B.** Prevent probe from drying out
   **C.** Rinsing probe with water prior to detergent
   **D.** Clean with neutral or enzymatic detergent

# Chapter 39 ▪ Answers

**1.** Correct Answer: A. Dysphagia

*Rationale:* There are numerous sites of potential injury during insertion and usage of the TEE probe. Some of the most common complications include hoarseness and lip injuries, which can occur in 12% and 13% of patients, respectively. Dysphagia occurs in 1.8% of patients. Dental injury, esophageal hemorrhage, and tracheal intubation are less likely, occurring in 0.1%, 0.03%, and 0.02% of patients, respectively. Other rare complications include bronchospasm, laryngospasm, and esophageal perforation. When obtaining patient consent for TEE, it is important to accurately portray these risks to the patient and evaluate the patient for comorbidities that put them at higher risk of complications.

Selected Reference
1. Helberath JN, Oakes DA, Shernan SK, Bulwer BE, D'Ambra MN, Eltzchig HK. Safety of transesophageal echocardiography. *J Am Soc Echocardiogr.* 2010;23(11):1115-1127.

**2.** Correct Answer: D. Use lower gain during imaging

*Rationale:* This patient possibly experienced esophageal injury as a complication of TEE usage intraoperatively. The bioeffects of ultrasound are most dependent on signal intensity. Gain settings on ultrasound create an amplification of returning ultrasound signals during imaging processing. Therefore, additional gain on ultrasound will not create an increased risk of tissue damage. In order to minimize the risk of esophageal injury during TEE, numerous precautions should be taken. Keeping the probe unlocked, especially when advancing the probe, is critical, especially if the probe is accidentally in an ante- or retroflexed position during advancement. Additionally, the gastroesophageal junction is a vulnerable portion of the esophagus that is prone to injury, particularly because manipulation of the probe at this location applies tension to relatively fixed tissues. Finally, if the patient has esophageal pathology such as an esophageal stricture or esophageal varices, but a TEE is still deemed necessary, then a pediatric probe may be considered to reduce the risk of injury.

Selected Reference
1. Helberath JN, Oakes DA, Shernan SK, Bulwer BE, D'Ambra MN, Eltzchig HK. Safety of transesophageal echocardiography. *J Am Soc Echocardiogr.* 2010;23(11):1115-1127.

**3.** Correct Answer: C. Esophagectomy

*Rationale:* According to the task force of TEE, although there are several relative contraindications to TEE, the only absolute contraindication agreed upon by the American Society of Anesthesiologists (ASA) members and consultants is previous esophagectomy or esophagogastrectomy. Only some members of the task force agree that several conditions should be absolute contraindications to TEE, including tracheoesophageal fistula, esophageal trauma, Zenker diverticulum, esophageal stricture, esophageal varices, and previous bariatric surgery. There is agreement that Barrett esophagus, hiatal hernia, unilateral vocal cord paralysis, dysphagia, and large descending aortic aneurysm are not absolute contraindications to TEE. Atlantoaxial disorders require caution during insertion of the probe to avoid excess neck extension.

Selected Reference
1. An Updated Report by the American Society of Anesthesiologists and the Society of Cardiovascular Anesthesiologists Task Force on Transesophageal Echocardiography. Practice guidelines for perioperative transesophageal echocardiography. *Anesthesiology.* 2010;112:1084-1096. doi: 10.1097/ALN.0b013e3181c51e90.

**4.** Correct Answer: C. Pulmonic valve

*Rationale:* Carcinoid syndrome most often presents with right-sided, as opposed to left-sided, valvular lesions. Due to its anterior position, the pulmonic valve is more difficult than most cardiac structures to view with TEE, which sits posterior to the heart. It can be visualized with a right ventricular inflow-outflow view and ascending aorta short-axis view; however, its resolution is often poor. On TTE, the pulmonic valve can be visualized in the parasternal short-axis view at the level of the aortic valve. A gradient across the pulmonic valve can also be obtained in this view.

The descending aorta can be visualized by TTE, most commonly in the parasternal long-axis view, lying along the posterior surface of the heart. However, a more complete evaluation and higher resolution imaging of the descending aorta is possible with TEE. This is because the TEE probe lies close to the descending aorta in the esophagus, and ultrasound signals are not interrupted by lung tissue. The tricuspid and aortic valves can be visualized well with TTE and TEE, but resolution is usually superior on TEE.

### Selected Reference

1. Denault AY, Couture EJ, Sia YT, Desjardins G. Right ventricle, right atrium, tricuspid and pulmonic valves. In: Perrino AC, Reeves ST, eds. *A Practical Approach to Transesophageal Echocardiography*. 4th ed. Wolters Kluwer; 2019:345-380.

**5.** Correct Answer: C. Distal ascending aorta

*Rationale:* Due to the location of the trachea lying in-between the esophagus and the distal ascending aorta, a blind spot exists when imaging this portion with TEE. This can interfere with identification of proper placement of the aortic cannula during cardiac surgery, as well as evaluation of an aortic disease in this region. The proximal ascending aorta can be evaluated with ascending aortic long-axis (Figure 39.1A) and short-axis views, as this portion lies below the carina. The aortic arch can be visualized with aortic arch long-axis (Figure 39.1B) and short-axis views, but the complete imaging may be partially impaired by the blind spot created by the trachea. The descending aorta is visualized in the descending aortic short-axis (Figure 39.1C) and long-axis views by rotating the TEE probe to the left. As an additional note, the right pulmonary artery can usually be visualized in the ascending aorta short-axis view; however, the view of the left pulmonary artery can be incomplete due to interruption by the left main bronchus.

### Selected References

1. Luedi MM, Phillips MC. Chapter 18: Incorrect diagnosis of a type A aortic dissection attributed to motion artifact during computer tomographic angiography: a case report. In: *100 Selected Case Reports from Anesthesia & Analgesia*. Wolters Kluwer; 2019.
2. Pruszczyk P, Torbicki A, Kuch-Wocial A, et al. Visualization of the central pulmonary arteries by biplane transesophageal echocardiography. *Exp Clin Cardiol*. 2001;6(4):206-210.
3. The comprehensive transesophageal echocardiography exam. In: Armstrong WF, Ryan T, eds. *Feigenbaum's Echocardiography*. 8th ed. Wolters Kluwer; 2019:61-99.

**6.** Correct Answer: D. Midesophageal long-axis view

*Rationale:* Figure 39.2 demonstrates the aortic valve (AV) in the AV short-axis view. To calculate an accurate gradient across the valve, the Doppler beam should be parallel with flow across the AV (i.e., as close to 0° as possible). As the angle increases between the Doppler beam and AV flow, the measured velocity across the valve will be underestimated and the calculated gradient ($4 \times$ velocity$^2$) will be further underestimated. Ideally, the beam should align within 0 to 15° of the actual jet. Echo views with the probe positioned near the apex of the heart and scanning cephalad toward the aortic valve are often the most accurate for AV gradient calculations. On TEE, the most common views for calculating the AV gradient are the deep transgastric (*Answer A*) and transgastric long-axis views, with the deep transgastric view being the most optimal for alignment of the Doppler beam. With TTE, visualization of the left ventricular outflow tract (LVOT) from the apical view (apical five-chamber view) provides the most optimal alignment. While the midesophageal long-axis view (**Figure 39.4**) allows for visualization of the LVOT and calculation of LVOT diameter, the angle between flow across the AV (green line) and the Doppler beam (white line) is larger, making calculation of the AV gradient inaccurate (*Answer B*).

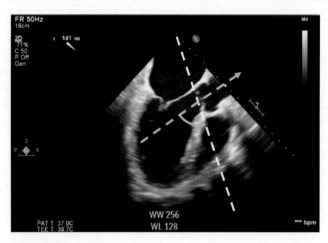

**Figure 39.4**

Selected Reference

1. Mehorta P, Cohen IS. Aortic stenosis. In: Perrino AC, Reeves ST, eds. *A Practical Approach to Transesophageal Echocardiography.* 4th ed. Wolters Kluwer; 2019:292-312.

**7.** Correct Answer: A. Midesophageal two-chamber view

*Rationale:* In the TTE image (Figure 39.3) in the question, an apical four-chamber view is displayed, which does not demonstrate visible evidence of intra-atrial or intraventricular thrombus. Prior to cardioversion, it is also critical to rule out LAA thrombus in a patient with atrial fibrillation of unknown duration. The LAA usually lies on the anterior surface of the left atrium. The midesophageal two-chamber view on TEE evaluates the left heart in an anterior-posterior direction and provides visualization of the anterior and posterior walls. By decreasing the depth with TEE and focusing on the LAA, the echocardiographer can evaluate for thrombus or spontaneous echogenic contrast in that area (indicating low-velocity blood flow). The midesophageal long-axis view shows the anteroseptal wall and the posterolateral walls and does not provide adequate visualization of the LAA. TTE has poor visualization of the LAA and is therefore poorly sensitive for LAA thrombi.

Selected Reference

1. Manning WJ, Weintraub RM, Waksmonski CA, et al. Accuracy of transesophageal echocardiography for identifying left atrial thrombi. A prospective, intraoperative study. *Ann Intern Med.* 1995 Dec 1;123(11):817-822. doi: 10.7326/0003-4819-123-11-199512010-00001. PMID: 7486462.

**8.** Correct Answer: C. Increased sensitivity for endocarditis of the mitral valve

*Rationale:* Due to superior resolution of TEE compared to TTE, the sensitivity for detection of valve leaflet vegetations is higher with TEE (over 85% vs. 60%). **Figure 39.5** demonstrates a vegetation of the mitral valve on TEE.

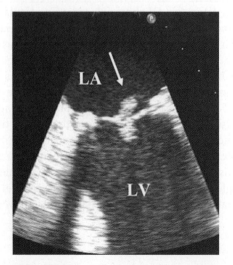

**Figure 39.5**

TAPSE is a calculation of the distance that the tricuspid annulus travels during systole, which can give an indication of right ventricular function (normal TAPSE is >16 mm). This is calculated using M-Mode over the tricuspid annulus, and for accurate measurement it requires that the annular movement be parallel to the ultrasound beam. Optimal alignment is best achieved with an apical four-chamber view in TTE.

One of the advantages of TTE in the ICU is that it is more readily available and quicker to perform on patients requiring evaluation. TEE requires more specialized equipment and the patient requires either local anesthesia or sedation to tolerate the procedure if they are awake.

Because the pulmonic valve lies in the anterior portion of the heart, imaging with TEE can have decreased resolution, and TTE can sometimes provide better imaging quality.

### Selected References

1. De Agustin JA, Zamorano JL. Mitral insufficiency. In: Garcia MJ, ed. *Noninvasive Cardiovascular Imaging: A Multimodality Approach.* Lippincott Williams & Wilkins; 2011.
2. Rudski LG, Lai WW, Afilalo J, et al. Guidelines for the echocardiographic assessment of the right heart in adults: a report from the American society of echocardiography. *J Am Soc Echocardiogr.* 2010;23(7):685-713.
3. Sapiro SM, Young E, De Guzman S, et al. Transesophageal echocardiography in diagnosis of infective endocarditis. *Chest.* 1994;105(2):377-382.

---

**9.** Correct Answer: B. Right-sided infective endocarditis lesions

*Rationale:* TEE has not been shown to be more sensitive for right heart endocarditis than TTE. Right-sided endocarditis is more commonly present in intravenous drug users, who are often young, thin patients with good transthoracic windows. These lesions also tend to be larger and therefore are more detectable on echocardiography. Additionally, right-sided lesions are more anterior and closer to the transthoracic probe. If the suspected right-sided lesion is in the setting of a cardiac device, this may interfere with transthoracic imaging and TEE may be preferred.

Atrial septal defects are often evaluated first by TTE; however, if there is a procedural intervention planned, TEE is important for detailed characterization of the defect. In pediatrics, TTE may be sufficient because echo windows are better and image quality is usually adequate for a full evaluation. TEE is more sensitive than TTE for both aortic dissection and LAA thrombi. TEE is able to provide a more complete evaluation of the aorta.

### Selected References

1. San Román JA, Vilacosta I, López J, et al. Role of transthoracic and transesophageal echocardiography in right-sided endocarditis: one echocardiographic modality does not fit all. *J Am Soc Echocardiogr.* 2012;25(8):807-814.
2. Silvestry FE, Cohen MS, Armsby LB, et al. Guidelines for the echocardiographic assessment of atrial septal defect and patent foramen ovale: from the American Society of Echocardiography and Society for Cardiac Angiography and Interventions. *J Am Soc Echocardiogr.* 2015;28:910-958.

---

**10.** Correct Answer: C. Rinsing probe with water prior to detergent

*Rationale:* After a TEE probe is used, it should first be gently wiped to remove any organic material on the probe. The probe should not be allowed to dry out, as this can make debris more difficult to remove. The probe should then be washed with a neutral or enzymatic detergent such as activated glutaraldehyde. The probe handle should be rinsed with an alcohol solution. Because of the risk of chemical burns from the detergent, it is important to thoroughly rinse the probe with preferably filtered water after (not before) detergent is used. After these steps are completed, the probe should be visually inspected for residual material and the process should be repeated if material is present.

### Selected Reference

1. Gnadinger PN. "TEE Safety." Perioperative Echocardiography Lecture Series, University of Utah; 2016.

# 40 | OBSTRUCTIVE SHOCK

Sarah Ellis and McKenzie M. Hollon

1. A 72-year-old male with a history of renal cell cancer, s/p resection, and placement of bilateral nephrostomy tubes, is admitted to the intensive care unit (ICU) with presumed urosepsis. Upon initially examining him, you note that he has a harsh systolic murmur and apply your ultrasound to his chest. You obtain imaging (shown in **Figure 40.1**). You further interrogate his aortic valve (AV) by measuring the peak velocity in the apical five-chamber view. Which of the following is the cutoff for severe aortic stenosis (AS)?

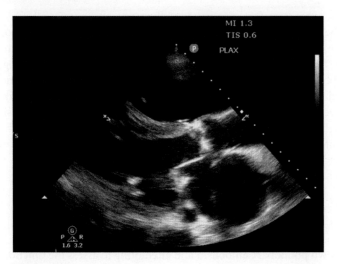

**Figure 40.1**

A. Peak velocity of >2.9 m/s
B. Peak velocity of >3.5 m/s
C. Peak velocity of >4.0 m/s
D. Peak velocity of >5.0 m/s

2. According to the current American Society of Echocardiography (ASE) guidelines, which of the following combinations of view and measurements is not recommended for echocardiographic assessment of right ventricular (RV) size?

   **A.** RV-focused apical four-chamber view with mid-cavity linear dimension measured at middle third of the RV inflow at end diastole
   **B.** RV-focused apical four-chamber view with basal linear dimension measured at the basal one-third of the RV inflow at end systole
   **C.** Parasternal long-axis view, proximal RV outflow diameter measured from the anterior RV wall to the interventricular septum
   **D.** Parasternal long-axis right ventricular outflow tract (RVOT) view, distal RVOT outflow measured just proximal to the pulmonary valve at end diastole.

3. You are called to the bedside to urgently evaluate a patient that has just arrived in the ICU. She is a 74-year-old female with a prior history of colon adenocarcinoma, previously treated with chemotherapy and radiation, and known lower extremity deep vein thrombosis (DVT). She presented to the Emergency Department (ED) 12 hours prior with shortness of breath and said she felt extremely weak. Computed tomography (CT) scan was ordered, which reported clot burden in her right and left main pulmonary arteries. She was transferred to the ICU for stabilization. You perform ultrasound and obtain a clear apical four-chamber view. Which of the following findings confirm that she has RV dilation?

   **A.** RV wall thickness >0.5 cm
   **B.** RV basal diameter of 36 mm
   **C.** Tricuspid regurgitation (TR) jet velocity >2.85 m/s
   **D.** RV mid-diameter of 48 mm

4. A 19-year-old male is admitted to the surgical ICU after presenting to the ED after a high-speed motor vehicle collision. He was taken to the operating room (OR) for an open reduction and internal fixation of his right femur and right tibia. He became acutely unstable in the OR after intramedullary nailing and transesophageal echocardiography (TEE) revealed a dilated right ventricle. The OR team also noted that he developed a petechial rash all over his upper extremities and chest. He was stabilized and taken to the CT scanner, which did not reveal pulmonary embolism. He is now in the ICU and you are using transthoracic echo to evaluate his right ventricle by measuring fractional area change (FAC). Which of the following accurately states the cutoff for abnormal RV systolic function?

   **A.** RV FAC of less than 25%
   **B.** RV FAC of less than 35%
   **C.** RV FAC of less than 45%
   **D.** RV FAC of less than 55%

5. You are evaluating a patient with known pulmonary embolism and attempting to assess the function of the right ventricle. With regard to measurement of the tricuspid annular plane systolic excursion (TAPSE), all the following are true *except*?

   **A.** TAPSE is a measurement of the circumferential systolic performance of the right ventricle
   **B.** TAPSE is influenced by the RV preload
   **C.** TAPSE measurement is dependent on the angle of incidence ($\theta$) of the Doppler cursor's perpendicular alignment with the lateral tricuspid annulus
   **D.** TAPSE only reflects the function of the basal region of the right ventricle

6. A 72-year-old male with diabetes, chronic kidney disease, hypertension, and sleep apnea is admitted to the ICU with septic shock and bacteremia presumed to be from a gangrenous foot. The following images were obtained on the day of his admission to the ICU while he was requiring high doses of vasoactive agents (**Figure 40.2A** and **B**). At that time his left ventricular outflow tract (LVOT) velocity time integral (VTI) was measured to be 12.2 cm. The AV Doppler measurements are shown in the second image, Figure 40.2B. A week later, once he had clinically improved and was weaned from inotropic support, the third image was obtained (Figure 40.2C). At the time of the second image his LVOT VTI was measured to be 22.8. What is the explanation for the change in the AV parameters between Figure 40.2B and C?

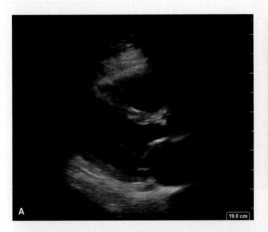
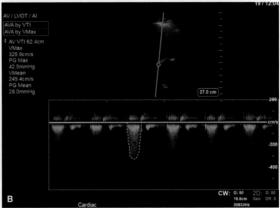
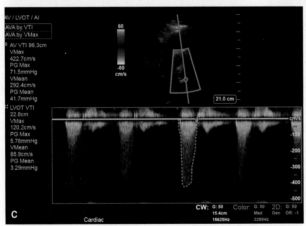

**Figure 40.2**

A. Decreased AV area
B. Improved contractility
C. AV endocarditis
D. Decreased contractility

7. Which of the following are echocardiographic features of cardiac tamponade in a spontaneously breathing patient?

A. Dilated inferior vena cava (IVC) and hepatic veins
B. Small, underfilled left ventricle
C. Respiratory variation in chamber size with increased RV and decreased LV with inspiration
D. All of the above are seen with cardiac tamponade physiology

8. A 53-year-old man with a history of coronary artery disease presents with ST-elevation myocardial infarction (STEMI) and is taken emergently to the catheterization lab for stenting, which is completed without complications, along with placement of a percutaneous ventricular assist device. About 12 hours later, he is found to have acute hemodynamic and respiratory decompensation with HR of 158 bpm, $O_2$ Sat 89%, and BP 79/46 mm Hg. He requires intubation and the initiation of high-dose vasopressors. Bedside echocardiography is shown in **Figure 40.3**, revealing a new pericardial effusion. On examination, he has marked jugular venous distention (JVD). What is the most likely diagnosis?

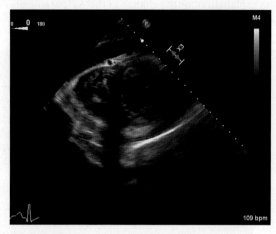

**Figure 40.3**

A. In-stent thrombosis with reinfarction
B. Cardiac tamponade
C. Retroperitoneal hemorrhage related to the femoral cannulation site of the assist device
D. Massive pulmonary embolism

9. Which of the following echocardiographic features would be most likely to rule out cardiac tamponade?

A. Large respiratory variation of transmitral Doppler inflow velocity
B. Diastolic collapse of the right atrium
C. IVC diameter of 2.2 cm
D. A distended right ventricle with depressed free wall motion

10. **Figure 40.4** shows a pulse wave spectral Doppler recording obtained from a spontaneously breathing patient in cardiac tamponade with a respirometer superimposed. What physiologic state is demonstrated by Figure 40.4?

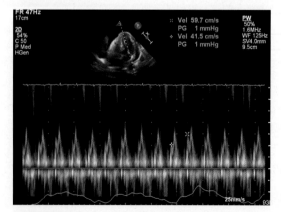

**Figure 40.4**

A. Decreased mitral transvalvular velocity with inspiration
B. Increased mitral transvalvular velocity with inspiration
C. Decreased tricuspid transvalvular velocity with expiration
D. Increased tricuspid transvalvular velocity with expiration

11. The absence of which of the following echo signs has a >90% negative predictive value for clinical cardiac tamponade?

    **A.** An effusion >1 cm in any dimension
    **B.** Absence of cardiac chamber collapse
    **C.** Evidence of exaggerated transmitral respiratory variation
    **D.** A fixed and dilated IVC

12. What is the finding in the ultrasound (**Figure 40.5**), and what pathology does it suggest?

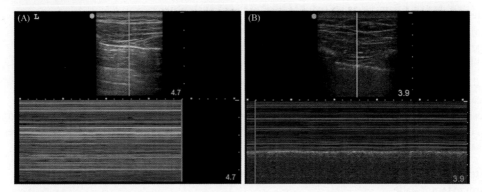

**Figure 40.5**

    **A.** Barcode sign; pneumothorax
    **B.** Lung point; pneumonia
    **C.** McConnell's sign; pulmonary embolism
    **D.** B-lines; pulmonary edema

13. In comparison to chest x-ray (CXR), which of the following is true regarding lung ultrasound?

    **A.** Lung ultrasound is more sensitive than CXR in the detection of pneumothorax
    **B.** Lung ultrasound is less sensitive than CXR in the detection of pneumothorax
    **C.** Lung ultrasound is more specific than CXR in the detection of pneumothorax
    **D.** A and C

14. A 29-year-old female who is 6 days post–cesarean section and has a known lower extremity DVT presents to the ED acutely short of breath, diaphoretic, tachycardic, and complaining of chest pain. A quick bedside scan is revealed in **Figure 40.6**. What other echocardiographic findings are most likely in this setting?

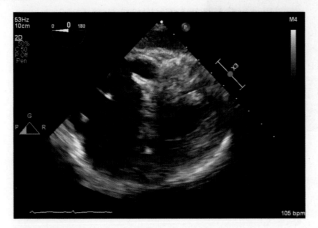

**Figure 40.6**

    **A.** High LV filling pressures
    **B.** Blunted S wave on pulmonary venous tracing
    **C.** TR jet > 2.8 m/s
    **D.** Small collapsible IVC

15. When evaluating the size of the RV in the setting of acute pulmonary embolism, which of the following is true?

    A. Moderate RV enlargement is RV:LV ratio of 0.6:1
    B. It is normal for both ventricles to appear of similar size
    C. RV function always appears depressed in the setting of RV dilation
    D. Improper probe placement can make the RV appear falsely small

16. Which of the following quantitative measures does not meet the criteria for severe AV stenosis?

    A. AV jet velocity >3.5 m/s
    B. Mean gradient >40 mm Hg
    C. Valve area derived from the continuity equation of <1.0 cm$^2$
    D. LVOT/AV velocity ratio of <0.25

17. A 38-year-old man without significant past medical history presents to the ED with acute onset of shortness of breath and hemodynamic instability after a flight home from Asia. Initial echocardiography shows a dilated right ventricle with severe hypokinesis of the free wall and relative apical hyperkinesis. What is the most likely diagnosis?

    A. Acute myocardial infarction of the left anterior descending (LAD) territory
    B. Ccardiac tamponade
    C. Pulmonary embolism
    D. Tension pneumothorax

18. A 76-year-old woman with a history of mitral valve prolapse is in the ICU after cardiotomy and mitral valve annuloplasty. Several hours after her arrival, she becomes acutely unstable and bedside echocardiography is shown in **Figure 40.7**.

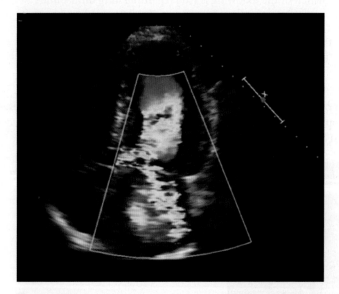

**Figure 40.7**

What is the best next step in her management?
A. Initiate an epinephrine infusion
B. Give a bolus of lactated Ringer's solution
C. Administer a gram of calcium chloride
D. Administer glucagon to reverse the effects of any beta-blockers

19. Which of the following changes in transtricuspid and transmitral flow patterns would be expected in constrictive pericarditis during spontaneous inspiration, relative to those of a normal heart?

    A. Increase in transtricuspid velocities and decrease in transmitral velocities
    B. Increase in transtricuspid velocities and increase in transmitral velocities
    C. Decrease in transtricuspid velocities and decrease in transmitral velocities
    D. Decrease in transtricuspid velocities and increase in transmitral velocities

20. Which of the following features can help to confirm a diagnosis of constrictive pericarditis as opposed to restrictive myocarditis?

    A. Elevated left atrial pressures
    B. Normal medial mitral annular tissue Doppler velocities
    C. Normal septal motion throughout the cardiac cycle
    D. LV hypokinesis

21. Which of the following is an echocardiographic feature associated with LVOT obstruction?

    A. A Y-shaped area of flow seen on color flow Doppler comprised of simultaneous LVOT turbulence and mitral regurgitation
    B. Late-peaking dagger-shaped Doppler waveform
    C. Fluttering and premature closure of one or more of the AV cusps
    D. All of the above

22. Which of the following is least likely to be considered a risk factor for dynamic LVOT obstruction?

    A. Sigmoid interventricular septum
    B. Shortened posterior mitral valve leaflet
    C. Small, hyperdynamic left ventricle
    D. Anterior displacement of the papillary muscles

23. An elderly patient with no known cardiac history presents to the ICU after fixation of a femur fracture that was sustained in a fall. On physical examination, a murmur is appreciated on auscultation at the upper left sternal border and bedside echocardiography is shown in **Figure 40.8.**

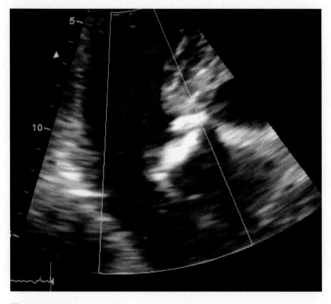

**Figure 40.8**

What are the priorities of hemodynamic management of this patient?

A. Maintenance of elevated left atrial pressure to promote filling of the hypertrophied left ventricle

B. Low-normal HR to optimize LV filling time

C. Decreasing the systemic vascular resistance to decrease the resistance to forward flow through a stenotic valve

D. A and B

E. All of the above

24. What is the best echocardiographic method to determine the significance of AS in a patient with concomitant severe reduction in LV ejection fraction?

A. Peak velocity across the AV greater than 3 m/s

B. Mean pressure gradient across the AV greater than 40 mm Hg

C. Stroke volume index less than 35 mL/m$^2$

D. Ratio of LVOT VTI to AV VTI of less than 0.25

25. Which of the following can cause the absence of lung sliding?

A. Mainstem intubation

B. Hypoventilation

C. Pneumothorax

D. All of the above

26. Which of the following is an echocardiographic finding unlikely to be seen in constrictive pericarditis?

A. Echogenic, calcified pericardium

B. Dilated IVC with minimal respiratory variation

C. Systolic blunting of pulmonary venous flow

D. Dilated left ventricle

27. The location of what structure can be used to differentiate fluid in the pericardium from a pleural effusion on echocardiography?

A. Parietal pleura

B. Descending aorta

C. Pulmonary artery (PA)

D. Right ventricle

28. In **Figure 40.9,** which of the following images is an example of severe AS?

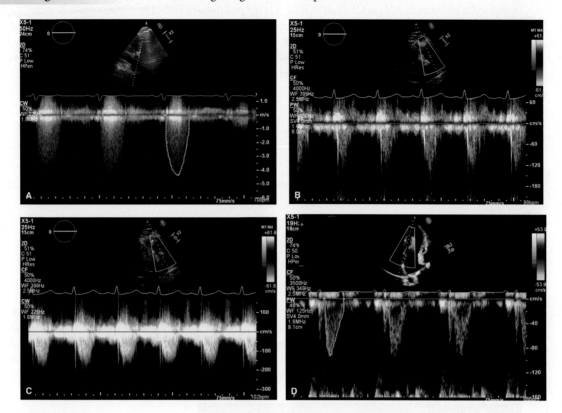

**Figure 40.9**

A. Figure 40.9A
B. Figure 40.9B
C. Figure 40.9C
D. Figure 40.9D

29. A "lung point" on ultrasound is an image of:

A. Collapsed lung within a field of fluid
B. Lung parenchyma surrounded by air
C. The point of transition from free air in the pleural space to normal lung sliding
D. Loculated pleural effusion that has become more echogenic as it consolidates

30. Which of the following is not associated with ultrasound imaging of the normal lung?

A. A-lines
B. Occasional B- or Z-lines
C. Rib shadows
D. Lung point

31. Which of the following echocardiographic features virtually excludes severe AS?

A. AV area of $>1.0$ cm$^2$ as measured by planimetry in a short-axis view of the AV
B. Normal transmitral E/A ratio
C. Absence of LV hypertrophy
D. Cusp separation of $>1.2$ cm in the long-axis view of the AV

32. A 28-year-old female smoker is admitted to the ICU after presenting to the ED with dyspnea and tachycardia and was found on CT scan to have a large pulmonary embolism. Management was initiated with catheter-based thrombolytic therapy. She has now been in the ICU for 5 days and you are attempting to estimate her PA systolic pressure with echo. You have measured her peak TR velocity to be 3 m/s and her IVC is 0.9 cm and noncollapsible. Her pulmonic valve is mildly regurgitant but has no significant stenosis. What is the PA systolic pressure?

   A. 52 mm Hg
   B. 38 mm Hg
   C. 44 mm Hg
   D. 40 mm Hg

33. Of the following echocardiographic findings, which would be expected to be seen in the setting of an acute saddle pulmonary embolism?

   A. Prolonged pulmonary ejection acceleration time
   B. Bowing of the interatrial septum to the right atrium
   C. TR peak velocity jet <2 m/s
   D. RV hypokinesis with apical sparing

34. You are called to the bedside to evaluate a patient that presented to the ED with chest pain, dyspnea, and hypotension and was intubated and started on a norepinephrine infusion in the ED. On arrival to the ICU you place a TEE probe into the esophagus and note the finding shown in **Figure 40.10** and ▶ **Video 40.1**. You begin to treat immediately. Which of the following echocardiographic signs is least likely to be useful in monitoring response to therapy in this clinical setting?

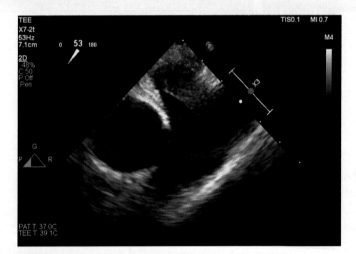

**Figure 40.10**

   A. Peak velocity of the TR jet
   B. Bowing of the interatrial septum
   C. Transmitral filling pattern
   D. Pulmonary valve acceleration time

35. What are the expected acute hemodynamic changes seen in Figure 40.10 and ▶ **Video 40.1?**

   A. Normal central venous pressure (CVP) and PA pressure with increased BP
   B. Elevated CVP with decreased PA pressure and normal BP
   C. Elevated CVP and PA pressure with decreased BP
   D. Decreased CVP, PA pressure, and BP
   E. Decreased CVP and PA pressure with normal BP

36. Which of the following echocardiographic features would be expected to be associated with a hemodynamically significant pneumothorax?

    A. Transmitral E/A ratio consistent with elevated left atrial pressure
    B. Dilated and dysfunctional left ventricle
    C. Severe TR
    D. Underfilled right ventricle

37. A 63-year-old patient presents to the ICU for workup of new-onset hepatomegaly and jaundice. Vitals: HR 105/min. BP 85/55 mm Hg. On examination, he has ascites and marked bilateral lower extremity edema. History is significant for three-vessel coronary artery bypass grafting done 10 years ago. You perform a point-of-care ultrasound examination (as shown in **Figure 40.11** and ▶ **Video 40.2**) suggesting a pericardial pathology. Which of the following echocardiographic findings support your suspicion?

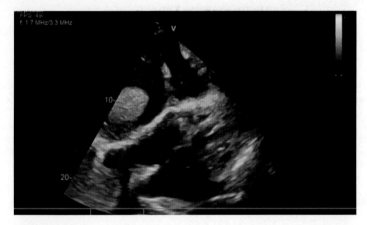

**Figure 40.11**

    A. Respiration-related ventricular septal shift
    B. Preserved or increased medial mitral annular e′ velocity
    C. Hepatic vein expiratory diastolic flow reversal
    D. All of the above

38. A 63-year-old man presents to the ED with acute onset of shortness of breath and tachycardia after a long road trip. Bilateral breath sounds are noted on auscultation. Although he is initially stable, his hemodynamics begin to decompensate. You obtain the following two loops as shown in ▶ **Videos 40.3** and **40.4**. What is the best management strategy?

    A. Rapid administration of a large bolus of intravenous (IV) fluid
    B. Treatment with a venodilator
    C. Administration of a calcium channel blocker
    D. Initiation of an inotrope such as epinephrine

39. Echocardiography is performed on a hemodynamically stable patient who has had multiple pericardial drains placed for recurrent malignant pericardial effusions. The examination demonstrates a thickened pericardium and a large anterior pericardial effusion in the presence of a dilated IVC, septal bounce, and a lateral and medial mitral annulus tissue Doppler velocities of 7 and 10 cm/s, respectively. What is the most likely diagnosis?

    A. Restrictive myocarditis
    B. Cardiac tamponade
    C. Constrictive pericarditis
    D. Aortic stenosis

# Chapter 40 ▪ Answers

**1.** Correct Answer: C. Peak velocity of >4.0 m/s

*Rationale:* The cutoff for severe AS graded by peak velocity measurement is >4.0 m/s.

Selected Reference
1. Baumgartner H, Hung J, Bermejo J, et al. Recommendations on the echocardiographic assessment of aortic valve stenosis: a focused update from the European Association of Cardiovascular Imaging and the American Society of Echocardiography. *J Am Soc Echocardiogr.* 2017;30:372-392.

**2.** Correct Answer: B. RV-focused apical four-chamber view with basal linear dimension measured at the basal one-third of the RV inflow at end systole

*Rationale:* The RV basal linear dimension should be measured in the basal one-third of the RV inflow at end diastole in the RV-focused apical four-chamber view.

Selected References
1. Lang RM, Badano LP, Mor-Avi V, et al. Recommendations for cardiac chamber quantification by echocardiography in adults: an update from the American Society of Echocardiography and the European Association of Cardiovascular Imaging. *J Am Soc Echocardiogr.* 2015;28(1):1-39.e14.
2. Rudski LG, Lai WW, Afilalo J, et al. Guidelines for the echocardiographic assessment of the right heart in adults: a report from the American Society of Echocardiography endorsed by the European Association of Echocardiography, a registered branch of the European Society of Cardiology, and the Canadian Society of Echocardiography. *J Am Soc Echocardiogr.* 2010;23(7):685-713; quiz 786-788. doi:10.1016/j.echo.2010.05.010. PMID: 20620859.

**3.** Correct Answer: D. RV mid-diameter of 48 mm

*Rationale:* The normal wall thickness of the RV is 0.5 cm or less; greater than 0.5 cm is considered RV hypertrophy. The normal range of dimensions of the RV are as follows: RV basal diameter of 25 to 41 mm, RV mid-diameter of 19 to 35 mm, and RV longitudinal diameter of 59 to 83 mm. TR jet velocity may indicate elevated right ventricular systolic pressure (RVSP) but does not provide any information about the size of the right ventricle.

Selected Reference
1. Lang RM, Badano LP, Mor-Avi V, et al. Recommendations for cardiac chamber quantification by echocardiography in adults: an update from the American Society of Echocardiography and the European Association of Cardiovascular Imaging. *J Am Soc Echocardiogr.* 2015;28(1):1-39.e14.

**4.** Correct Answer: B. RV FAC of less than 35%

*Rationale:* An RV FAC of <35% reflects abnormal RV systolic function.

Selected References
1. Lang RM, Badano LP, Mor-Avi V, et al. Recommendations for cardiac chamber quantification by echocardiography in adults: an update from the American Society of Echocardiography and the European Association of Cardiovascular Imaging. *J Am Soc Echocardiogr.* 2015 Jan;28(1):1-39.e14.
2. Rudski LG, Lai WW, Afilalo J, et al. Guidelines for the echocardiographic assessment of the right heart in adults: a report from the American Society of Echocardiography. *J Am Soc Echocardiogr.* 2010;23:685-713.

**5.** Correct Answer: A. TAPSE is a measurement of the circumferential systolic performance of the right ventricle

*Rationale:* TAPSE is a measurement of the longitudinal systolic performance of the right ventricle. It's advantages include its simplicity of measurement even in the setting of poor image quality, reproducibility, and the fact that it does not require complex echocardiography equipment or image analysis. TAPSE below 1.6 cm is considered abnormal. TAPSE incorrectly assumes that the displacement of a single segment represents the function of a complex 3D right ventricle. Additionally, TAPSE is angle dependent and may be load dependent.

Selected Reference

1. Rudski LG, Lai WW, Afilalo J, et al. Guidelines for the echocardiographic assessment of the right heart in adults: a report from the American Society of Echocardiography. *J Am Soc Echocardiogr.* 2010;23:685-713.

**6.** Correct Answer: B. Improved contractility

*Rationale:* Improved contractility. This series of images demonstrate the concept of low-flow low-gradient AS. In Figure 40.2A, the 2D appearance of the AV is hyperechoic and heavily calcified, raising suspicion for a stenotic lesion and we are told that at this time the LVOT VTI was 12 cm, indicating that the patient is in a state of low cardiac output. In Figure 40.2B, the spectral Doppler tracing demonstrates a mean pressure gradient of 28 mm Hg and a maximum velocity of 3.3 m/s, which do not meet the criteria for severe AS. We are then told that the patient recovered from his illness, and in Figure 40.2C the spectral Doppler demonstrates an LVOT VTI of 22.8 cm, which is greatly improved from 12 cm and confirms that the heart is indeed ejecting an improved stroke volume. In Figure 40.2C we can also see that his AV measurements now meet the cutoff for severe AS:pressure gradient (PG) mean of 41.7 and Vmax of 4.2 m/s. This phenomenon is termed "low-flow low-gradient AS." Essentially, when cardiac output is low, the heart is unable to generate a high enough velocity to reach the cutoff for severe AS despite the low-valve area. Once the heart has recovered contractility, the measurements reflect the true severity of AS. In states where the cardiac output is low, the severity of AS cannot be assumed by gradients alone. One viable metric is the dimensionless index, or the ratio of the LVOT VTI to the AV VTI. A value of less than 0.25 is consistent with severe AS. Another method for revealing true AS in the setting of low cardiac output is a dobutamine stress echo.

Selected Reference

1. Clavel MA, Burwash IG, Pibarot P. Cardiac imaging for assessing low-gradient severe aortic stenosis. *JACC Cardiovasc Imaging.* 2017;10(2):185-202.

**7.** Correct Answer: D. All of the above are seen with cardiac tamponade physiology

*Rationale:* When fluid accumulates in the pericardial sac, the pressure in the pericardial sac rises and tamponade physiology develops when this excessive pericardial pressure limits cardiac filling. With elevated pericardial pressures, systemic (superior vena cava [SVC] and IVC) and pulmonary venous pressures must also rise to maintain cardiac filling. As tamponade physiology develops, the gradients between the veins and the cardiac chambers diminish, resulting in less filling and lower cardiac output. The limitation of chamber filling on cardiac output is based not only on the amount of pericardial fluid, but on the pressure within the pericardial sac. This is variable among patients and because of this, cardiac tamponade is a clinical, not echocardiographic diagnosis. However, these echo findings reflect the equalization of cardiac diastolic and pericardial pressures.

Selected Reference

1. Klein AL, Abbara S, Agler DA, et al. American Society of Echocardiography clinical recommendations for multimodality cardiovascular imaging of patients with pericardial disease, endorsed by the Society for Cardiovascular Magnetic Resonance and Society of Cardiovascular Computed Tomography. *J Am Soc Echocardiogr.* 2013; 26:965-1012.

**8.** Correct Answer: B. Cardiac tamponade

*Rationale:* When tamponade is suspected, 2D echocardiography should be obtained emergently. Regardless of the effusion size, cardiac tamponade can be lethal. The symptoms and signs of tamponade depend on the etiology of the effusion and the rate of fluid accumulation within a relatively fixed pericardial space and can range from mild to severe and life threatening. Mild tamponade is usually asymptomatic, whereas when the pressure in the pericardium rises above about 15 mm Hg, symptoms including dyspnea, tachycardia, and hypotension develop due to decreasing cardiac output. Invasive cardiac procedures that can result in bleeding into the pericardium acutely can cause tamponade with as little volume as 250 mL. First line approach to treatment is removal of the effusion by echo-guided pericardiocentesis, which has been found to be relatively safe. Although imaging contributes significantly to the differential, tamponade is always a clinical diagnosis.

Selected Reference

1. Klein AL, Abbara S, Agler DA, et al. American Society of Echocardiography clinical recommendations for multimodality cardiovascular imaging of patients with pericardial disease, endorsed by the Society for Cardiovascular Magnetic Resonance and Society of Cardiovascular Computed Tomography. *J Am Soc Echocardiogr.* 2013; 26:965-1012.

**9.** Correct Answer: D. A distended right ventricle with depressed free wall motion

*Rationale:* As tamponade physiology progresses, the gradients for venous filling of the cardiac chambers are decreased and as a result the chambers are underfilled and decompressed. To compensate, venous pressures are increased, which is seen by fixed and enlarged IVC. The cyclical changes in left and right heart filling pressures with the respiratory cycle create the variation in transmitral filling patterns. Notably, the majority of pericardial effusions do not lead to tamponade physiology.

Selected Reference

1. Nagdev A, Stone MB. Point of care ultrasound evaluation of pericardial effusions: does this patient have cardiac tamponade? *Resuscitation.* 2011;82:671-673.

**10.** Correct Answer: A. Decreased mitral transvalvular velocity with inspiration

*Rationale:* The spectral Doppler displays a decreasing velocity with inspiration, a state that is characteristic of the transmitral filling pattern in a spontaneously breathing tamponade patient. In a normal state, inspiration leads to reduction in intrathoracic pressures, which create increased venous return to the right heart and a simultaneous decrease in filling of the left heart. With expiration, there is an increase in left heart filling and a decrease in right heart filling; therefore, the transmitral and transtricuspid flow have opposite respiratory variation. As ventricular interdependence develops in a tamponade state, the changes in mitral inflow velocity are much larger. A 25% inspiratory reduction in mitral peak E-wave velocity is considered diagnostic of tamponade physiology.

Selected Reference

1. Leeman DE, Levine MJ, Come PC. Doppler echocardiography in cardiac tamponade: exaggerated respiratory variation in transvalvular blood flow velocity integrals. *J Am Coll Cardiol.* 1988;11:572-578.

**11.** Correct Answer: B. Absence of cardiac chamber collapse

*Rationale:* The absence of any cardiac chamber collapse has a >90% negative predictive value for clinical cardiac tamponade. Multiple physiologic states can cause fixed and dilated IVC, as well as changes in the transmitral flow patterns. A large amount of fluid can be present in the pericardium without tamponade physiology.

Selected Reference

1. Merce J, Sagrista-Sauleda J, Permanyer-Miralda G, Evangelista A, Soler J. Correlation between clinical and Doppler echocardiographic findings in patients with moderate and large pericardial effusion: implications for the diagnosis of cardiac tamponade. *Am Heart J.* 1999;138:759-764.

**12.** Correct Answer: A. Barcode sign; pneumothorax

*Rationale:* The appearance of a "barcode sign" is the characteristic M-mode finding when there is no movement of the underlying lung tissue. Since M-mode measures the motion along one scan line over time, the appearance of straight, constant lines denotes that the structure is fixed and not moving. In contrast, when M-mode is applied to the lung during normal respiration, there are no fixed straight lines and instead there is a disjointed speckled appearance that is the M-mode equivalent of lung sliding seen on 2D ultrasound. "Barcode sign" is present in states other than pneumothorax in which the lung is not moving, including apnea, trapped lung, and prior pleurodesis.

Selected Reference

1. Husain LF, Hagopian L, Wayman D, Baker WE, Carmody KA. Sonographic diagnosis of pneumothorax. *J Emerg Trauma Shock.* 2012:5(1):76-81.

**13.** Correct Answer: D. A and C

*Rationale/Critique:* Lung ultrasound is more sensitive and specific than CXR in the detection of pneumothorax.

Selected Reference

1. Lichtenstein DA, Menu Y. A bedside ultrasound sign ruling out pneumothorax in the critically ill. *Chest.* 1995;108:1345-1348.

**14.** Correct Answer: C. TR jet $> 2.8$ m/s

*Rationale/Critique:* Figure 40.6 is a short-axis view of the left ventricle showing septal flattening and an enlarged right ventricle, indicating a state of acute RV pressure and/or volume overload. In this setting, typically RV function is reduced, the IVC is dilated, TR is elevated, and the left-sided atrial and ventricular pressures are low.

Selected Reference

1. Kurnicka K, Lichodziejewska B, Goliszek S, et al. Echocardiographic pattern of acute pulmonary embolism: analysis of 511 consecutive patients. *J Am Soc Echocardiogr.* 2016;29:907-913.

**15.** Correct Answer: D. Improper probe placement can make the RV appear falsely small

*Rationale:* The normal RV:LV ratio is 0.6:1, with the right ventricle normally appearing smaller than the left ventricle. It is possible that the RV can dilate and still maintain its functional measures, including normal FAC, ejection fraction (EF), and TAPSE. The RV will dilate in response to pressure and/or volume overload. Improper probe placement can lead to nonstandard views and inaccurate assessment of RV size.

Selected Reference

1. Rudski LG, Lai WW, Afilalo J, et al. Guidelines for the echocardiographic assessment of the right heart in adults. *J Am Soc Echocardiogr.* 2010;23:685-713.

**16.** Correct Answer: A. AV jet velocity $> 3.5$ m/s

*Rationale:* The cutoffs for quantifying severe AS are as follows: AV jet velocity of $> 4.0$ m/s, mean gradient $> 40$ mm Hg, AV area continuity $< 1.0$ cm$^2$, or LVOT/AV velocity ratio $< 0.25$.

Selected Reference

1. Baumgartner H, Hung J, Bermejo J, et al. Recommendations on the echocardiographic assessment of aortic valve stenosis: a focused update from the European Association of Cardiovascular Imaging and the American Society of Echocardiography. *J Am Soc Echocardiogr.* 2017;30:372-392.

**17.** Correct Answer: C. pulmonary embolism

*Rationale:* A dilated right ventricle with severe hypokinesis or akinesis of the free wall and relative hyperkinesis of the apex is characteristic for a large pulmonary embolism and is known as McConnell's sign. The left ventricle would most likely be underfilled and hyperdynamic. It is important to note that McConnell's sign is not specific for PE and can also be seen with other pathologies, including right coronary artery (RCA) infarctions.

Selected Reference
1. Kurnicka K, Lichodziejewska B, Goliszek S, et al. Echocardiographic pattern of acute pulmonary embolism: analysis of 511 consecutive patients. *J Am Soc Echocardiogr.* 2016;29:907-913.

**18.** Correct Answer: B. Give a bolus of lactated Ringer's solution

*Rationale:* This patient is experiencing systolic anterior motion (SAM) of the mitral valve that is causing obstruction of the LVOT as well as mitral regurgitation due to the displaced leaflet, creating the characteristic Y-shaped pattern as seen on color flow Doppler (Figure 40.7). The best steps in immediate management are to administer adequate fluid resuscitation and to decrease or discontinue any inotropes.

Selected Reference
1. Alfieri O, Lapenna E. Systolic anterior motion after mitral valve repair. *Eur J Cardiothorac Surg.* 2015;48:344-346.

**19.** Correct Answer: A. Increase in transtricuspid velocities and decrease in transmitral velocities

*Rationale:* During the respiratory cycle in a normal heart, transthoracic pressures are transmitted relatively constantly to the vasculature as well as to the chambers of the heart, such that the pressure gradient between the pulmonary veins and the left atrium and ventricle has minimal variation. This is reflected in transmitral velocities that usually have <5% variation. In constrictive pericarditis, a noncompliant pericardium leads to relative isolation of intracardiac pressures from intrathoracic pressures and thus a decrease in the gradient between the pulmonary veins and the left heart during inspiration. Because the noncompliant pericardium also causes increased ventricular interdependence, this decrease in left-sided filling is accompanied by an increase in right-sided filling and thus the expected velocities as noted in answer choice A. The opposite occurs during expiration.

Selected Reference
1. Dal-Bianco JP, Sengupta PP, Mookadam F, Chandrasekaran K, Tajik AJ, Khandheria BK. Role of echocardiography in the diagnosis of constrictive pericarditis. *J Am Soc Echocardiogr.* 2009;22:24-33.

**20.** Correct Answer: B. Normal medial mitral annular tissue Doppler velocities

*Rationale:* In restrictive myocarditis, a form of cardiomyopathy, mitral annular tissue Doppler velocities, would be expected to be decreased. In constrictive pericarditis, however, the myocardium is expected to maintain normal relaxation velocities as seen by normal or even accentuated tissue Doppler values for the mitral annulus. The lateral mitral annulus, however, may have low tissue Doppler velocity due to tethering by the fibrosed pericardium. In some cases, this leads to annulus reversus, in which medial mitral annular velocity exceeds lateral annular velocity.

Selected Reference
1. Welch TD, Ling LH, Espinosa RE, et al. Echocardiographic diagnosis of constrictive pericarditis. *Circ Cardiovasc Imaging.* 2014;7:526-534.

**21.** Correct Answer: D. All of the above

*Rationale:* All of the answer choice may be features of LVOT obstruction. The characteristic Y-shape seen on color flow Doppler occurs when there is turbulent flow through the LVOT that causes the anterior leaflet of the mitral valve to be swept into the outflow tract, leading to worsening of the obstruction as well as regurgitation through the valve. The disruption of the anterior mitral valve leaflets' normal motion leads to the formation of a posteriorly directed mitral regurgitation (MR) jet. A late-peaking dagger-shaped Doppler waveform is seen in dynamic LVOT obstruction, which peaks as the ventricle empties. Fluttering and early closure of the AV are more often seen in fixed obstruction of the LVOT.

Selected Reference

1. Nagueh SF, Bierig SM, Budoff MJ, et al. American Society of Echocardiography clinical recommendations for multimodality cardiovascular imaging of patients with hypertrophic cardiomyopathy. *J Am Soc Echocardiogr.* 2011;24:473-498.

**22.** Correct Answer: B. Shortened posterior mitral valve leaflet

*Rationale/Critique:* All of the answer choices are risk factors for the development of dynamic LVOT obstruction associated with SAM of the mitral valve, except the shortening of the posterior mitral valve leaflet. Risk factors for SAM include anterior leaflet to posterior leaflet ratio < 1.2, C-sept (shortest distance between interventricular septum and coaptation point at end systole), posterior leaflet height greater than 20 mm, and anterior leaflet height greater than 35 mm. Medical management, with volume resuscitation and discontinuation of inotropes, is often sufficient for the resolution of obstruction.

Selected Reference

1. Nagueh SF, Bierig SM, Budoff MJ, et al. American Society of Echocardiography clinical recommendations for multimodality cardiovascular imaging of patients with hypertrophic cardiomyopathy. *J Am Soc Echocardiogr.* 2011;24:473-498.

**23.** Correct Answer: B. Low-normal HR to optimize LV filling time

*Rationale/Critique:* Management of a patient with severe AS should prioritize adequate preload, a low-normal HR to optimize LV diastolic filling as well as coronary artery perfusion, and an systemic vascular resistance (SVR) that is high enough to promote coronary artery and end organ perfusion. Typically, patients with severe AS have some degree of diastolic impairment with relatively fixed LV filling. Increasing the left atrial pressure will do little to promote increased filling and instead may lead to pulmonary edema. Additionally, the stenotic AV acts as a relatively fixed afterload to the LV so decreasing the SVR will only decrease perfusion pressure, both to end organs and to the heart.

Selected Reference

1. Samarendra P, Mangione M. Aortic stenosis and perioperative risk with non-cardiac surgery. *J Am Coll Cardiol.* 2015;5:295-302.

**24.** Correct Answer: D. Ratio of LVOT VTI to AV VTI of less than 0.25

*Rationale:* This question refers to the state of low-flow low-gradient AS, in which the gradient across the valve remains low despite reduced valve area due to inability of the dysfunctional ventricle to generate "normal" flow. The dimensionless index (velocity or VTI index) is an indication of the area of the valve relative to the area of the LVOT. A value of 0.25 or less is consistent with severe stenosis.

Selected Reference

1. Baumgartner H, Hung J, Bermejo J, et al. Recommendations on the echocardiographic assessment of aortic valve stenosis: a focused update from the European Association of Cardiovascular Imaging and the American Society of Echocardiography. *J Am Soc Echocardiogr.* 2017;30:372-392.

**25.** Correct Answer: D. All of the above.

*Rationale/Critique:* All of the options listed can cause the absence of normal lung sliding on ultrasound. Lung sliding is the visualization of the visceral pleura moving along the fixed parietal pleura during normal breathing. Although the loss of lung sliding is very sensitive for pneumothorax, it is not specific and may be caused by any condition that results in abnormal inflation of the lung or of the portion of the lung that is being visualized.

Selected Reference
1. Husain LF, Hagopian L, Wayman D, Baker WE, Carmody KA. Sonographic diagnosis of pneumothorax. *J Emerg Trauma Shock.* 2012;5:76-81.

**26.** Correct Answer: D. Dilated left ventricle

*Rationale:* It is unlikely to see a dilated left ventricle in constrictive pericarditis, as the disease typically causes physical restraint of LV diastolic filling. The disease is caused by fibrosis and fusion of the pericardial layers, which may lead to an echogenic, calcified, and sometimes obviously thickened appearance on echo. The IVC will be dilated, reflecting elevated right atrial pressures, while systolic blunting of the pulmonary vein flow reflects elevated left atrial pressures. Increased ventricular interdependence seen in constrictive pericarditis leads to an abnormal motion of the interventricular septum called "septal bounce."

Selected Reference
1. Dal-Bianco JP, Sengupta PP, Mookadam F, Chandrasekaran K, Tajik AJ, Khandheria BK. Role of echocardiography in the diagnosis of constrictive pericarditis. *J Am Soc Echocardiogr.* 2009;22:24-33.

**27.** Correct Answer: B. The descending aorta

*Rationale:* In the parasternal long-axis view, fluid collection posterior to the heart may be either pericardial or pleural and can be difficult to differentiate. Visualization of the descending aorta in short axis adjacent to the mitral valve may help. Pericardial effusions will be located between the wall of the left ventricle and the aorta, while pleural effusions will be located posterior to the aorta.

Selected Reference
1. Haaz WS, Mintz GS, Kotler MN, Parry W, Segal BL. Two dimensional echocardiographic recognition of the descending thoracic aorta: value in differentiating pericardial from pleural effusions. *Am J Cardiol.* 1980;46:739-743.

**28.** Correct Answer: A. Figure 40.9A

*Rationale:* The continuous-wave spectral Doppler tracing (Figure 40.9A) is consistent with severe AS, with a peak velocity exceeding 4 m/s.

Selected Reference
1. Nagueh SF, Bierig SM, Budoff MJ, et al. American Society of Echocardiography clinical recommendations for multimodality cardiovascular imaging of patients with hypertrophic cardiomyopathy. *J Am Soc Echocardiogr.* 2011;24:473-498.

**29.** Correct Answer: C. The point of transition from free air in the pleural space to normal lung sliding

*Rationale:* The lung point is pathognomonic for the presence of a pneumothorax and refers to the point at which ultrasound evidence of normal respiration reappears, including B-lines and normal lung sliding.

Selected Reference
1. Lichtenstein DA. Lung ultrasound in the critically ill. *Ann Intensive Care.* 2014;4:1.

**30.** Correct Answer: D. Lung point

*Rationale/Critique:* The lung point is a specific finding that is pathognomonic for pneumothorax. A-lines are normal findings generated by equally spaced reflections of the highly echogenic pleura. B-lines are examples of ringdown artifacts through areas of fluid-rich lung. Occasional B-lines are normal, while large numbers of them are consistent with interstitial edema. Z-lines are another vertical reverberation artifact, which are weaker than A-lines and have no clear relationship to the pleural line.

Selected Reference
1. Lee FC. Lung ultrasound—a primary survey of the acutely dyspneic patient. *J Intensive Care.* 2016;4:57.

**31. Correct Answer: D. Cusp separation of >1.2 cm in the long-axis view of the AV**

*Rationale/Critique:* Maximal cusp separation of greater than 1.2 cm as seen in the parasternal long-axis view virtually excludes the presence of severe AS. Planimetry may be suggestive but is not a reliable method for definitively determining the presence of stenosis as effective orifice area is more important than actual orifice area and reflections of calcifications may make the valve borders difficult to determine. While a normal transmitral E/A ratio and the absence of LV hypertrophy make long-standing severe stenosis less likely, they are not determining factors. Additionally, normal transmitral E/A ratio may represent normal diastolic function or the presence of grade 2 dysfunction. A dagger-shaped continuous-wave waveform is consistent with dynamic LVOT obstruction.

Selected Reference

1. Jayaprakash K, Dilu VP, George R. Maximal aortic valve cusp separation and severity of aortic stenosis. *J Clin Diagn Res.* 2017;11:OC29-OC32.

**32. Correct Answer: C. 44 mm Hg**

*Rationale/Critique:* PA systolic pressure is estimated by the modified Bernoulli equation: 4(VTR)2 + right atrial pressure (RAP). An IVC which is small (<2.1 cm) and noncollapsible is consistent with a RAP of 8 mm Hg. $4 \times (3)^2 + 8 = 44$ mm Hg.

Selected Reference

1. Rudski LG, Lai WW, Afilalo J, et al. Guidelines for the echocardiographic assessment of the right heart in adults. *J Am Soc Echocardiogr.* 2010;23:685-713.

**33. Correct answer: D. RV hypokinesis with apical sparing**

*Rationale:* RV hypokinesis with apical sparing is known as McConnell's sign. This finding was originally described by Dr. McConnell in 1996 and has since been studied by other groups as well. Importantly, the finding of normal wall motion at the apex and abnormal wall motion in the mid–free wall can be seen in other states of RV dysfunction besides pulmonary embolism, such as RCA infarct. However, McConnell's sign does carry a reasonable sensitivity (77%), specificity (94%), and negative predictive value (96%) for acute pulmonary embolism. If the distinct pattern of regional RV dysfunction with apical sparing is noted, it should raise clinical suspicion for the diagnosis of acute pulmonary embolism.

Selected Reference

1. McConnell MV, Solomon SD, Rayan ME, Come PC, Goldhaber SZ, Lee RT. Regional right ventricular dysfunction detected by echocardiography in acute pulmonary embolism. *Am J Cardiol.* 1996;78(4):469-473.

**34. Correct Answer: C. Transmitral filling pattern**

*Rationale/Critique:* Figure 40.11 and ▶ **Video 40.1** show a large pulmonary embolism. When monitoring therapy for acute RV failure, it is useful to intermittently assess signs of elevated PA pressures or RV pressures, including peak tricuspid regurgitant velocity, signs of elevated right atrial pressure such as septal bowing or hepatic vein flow reversal. It is also useful to assess the pulmonary ejection acceleration time, which is shortened in the setting of acute PE.

Selected Reference

1. Rosenberger P, Shernan SK, Body SC, Eltzschig HK. Utility of intraoperative transesophageal echocardiography for diagnosis of pulmonary embolism. *Anesth Analg.* 2004;99:12-16.

**35. Correct Answer: C. Elevated CVP and PA pressures with decreased BP**

*Rationale:* A large saddle embolism (shown in Figure 40.10 and ▶ **Video 40.1**) will lead to elevated PA pressures, causing elevated RV, RA, and IVC pressures. Due to poor forward flow through the pulmonary vasculature from obstruction by the embolic material, the LV will be underfilled and will have a low cardiac output leading to a low mean BP. However, in the setting of a massive pulmonary embolism leading to RV failure, the PA pressures might not be as high as expected due to inability of a failing RV to generate enough contractile force against an obstructing pulmonary embolism.

Selected Reference

1. Sekhri V, Mehta N, Rawat N, Lehrman SG, Aronow WS. Management of massive and nonmassive pulmonary embolism. *Arch Med Sci.* 2012;8:957-969.

**36.** Correct Answer: D. Underfilled right ventricle

*Rationale:* Increased intrathoracic pressure from a tension pneumothorax will lead to underfilled RV and a dilated and noncollapsible IVC. The left side of the heart is also likely to be underfilled with no impact on contractility.

Selected Reference

1. Husain LF, Hagopian L, Wayman D, Baker WE, Carmody KA. Sonographic diagnosis of pneumothorax. *J Emerg Trauma Shock.* 2012. PMID: 22416161.

**37.** Correct Answer: D. All of the above

*Rationale:* The thickened and calcified pericardium and septal bounce seen in ▶ **Video 40.2** and Figure 40.11 (along with clinical presentation) raise a suspicion of constrictive pericarditis. All of the choices are independently associated findings in patients with constrictive pericarditis. Ventricular septal motion abnormalities may often be the first clue to the echocardiographer of constrictive pathology, and it is due to dissociation of intrathoracic and intracardiac pressures that occur with pericardial constriction. Inspiration leads to a decreased left-sided diastolic gradient, impairing filling of the LV. During expiration the LV has increased filling while the RV filling is decreased, which shifts the ventricular septum back to the right. This dissociation of intracardiac and intrathoracic pressures also leads to increased transmitral E velocity and shortening of deceleration time. The hepatic vein Doppler also confirms this dissociation between the intracardiac and intrathoracic and the ventricular septal shift, which leads to reduced hepatic vein forward velocity and exaggerated late diastolic reversal velocity.

Selected Reference

1. Welch TD, Ling LH, Espinosa RE, et al. Echocardiographic diagnosis of constrictive pericarditis. *Circ Cardiovasc Imaging.* 2014;7:526-534.

**38.** Correct Answer: D. Initiation of an inotrope such as epinephrine

*Rationale:* ▶ **Videos 40.3** and **40.4** demonstrate a flattened IV septum and a dilated IVC consistent with RV pressure or volume overload and concerning for RV decompensation. The most likely etiology of this patient's shortness of breath given his history and presentation is a pulmonary embolism. Given his hemodynamic instability, the best option for management would be to support the right heart pharmacologically with an inotrope until more definitive treatment could be undertaken.

Selected Reference

1. Sekhri V, Mehta N, Rawat N, Lehrman SG, Aronow WS. Management of massive and nonmassive pulmonary embolism. *Arch Med Sci.* 2012;8:957-969.

**39.** Correct Answer: C. Constrictive pericarditis

*Rationale:* None of the other diagnoses definitively applies to this patient. Normally, the lateral mitral annular velocity is greater than the medial mitral annular velocity. This patient has constrictive pericarditis as the medial mitral annular velocity is higher than the lateral mitral annular velocity due to tethering of the lateral annulus by the constricted pericardium. A normal medial mitral annular tissue Doppler would be unlikely with the myocardial dysfunction seen in restrictive myocarditis. Cardiac tamponade, while potentially a later endpoint for this patient, is a clinical diagnosis that is ruled out by hemodynamic stability and in which cardiac chamber collapse should be seen. The natural history of AS, if significant, usually includes impairment in myocardial relaxation and mitral annular tissue Doppler. LVOT obstruction is not consistent with this presentation.

Selected References

1. Klein AL, Abbara S, Agler DA, et al. American Society of Echocardiography clinical recommendations for multimodality cardiovascular imaging of patients with pericardial disease, endorsed by the Society for Cardiovascular Magnetic Resonance and Society of Cardiovascular Computed Tomography. *J Am Soc Echocardiogr.* 2013; 26:965-1012.
2. Baumgartner H, Hung J, Bermejo J, et al. Recommendations on the echocardiographic assessment of aortic valve stenosis: a focused update from the European Association of Cardiovascular Imaging and the American Society of Echocardiography. *J Am Soc Echocardiogr.* 2017;30:372-392.
3. Nagueh SF, Bierig SM, Budoff MJ, et al. American Society of Echocardiography clinical recommendations for multimodality cardiovascular imaging of patients with hypertrophic cardiomyopathy. *J Am Soc Echocardiogr.* 2011;24:473-498.

# 41 | HYPOVOLEMIC SHOCK

John C. Klick, S. Michael Roberts, Ranjit Deshpande, Lyle Gerety, Jan Kasal, and Chakradhar Venkata

1. You are called urgently to the postanesthesia care unit (PACU) to evaluate a 59-year-old male who arrived 15 minutes ago after undergoing a redo left total hip arthroplasty under general anesthesia. He appears comfortable but somnolent. He has no documented history of cardiovascular disease, but he is hypotensive with a noninvasive BP of 78/47 mm Hg. He does not have an arterial line. Estimated blood loss was approximately 1200 cc, and the resident reports that he was "well resuscitated" with a hemoglobin of 9.5 on his last blood gas 10 minutes ago. He made adequate urine in the operating room (OR) by report, and the PACU resident is now starting a phenylephrine drip. You perform a bedside ultrasound and the attached image is seen when visualizing the inferior vena cava (IVC). Left ventricular (LV) and right ventricular (RV) contractility appear hyperdynamic as shown in ▶ **Videos 41.1, 41.2, 41.3.** Based on this scenario and your imaging, what would be the next logical step in the management of this patient?

   A. Start norepinephrine
   B. Start epinephrine
   C. Administer a bolus of lactated Ringer's
   D. Give a unit of blood

2. A 22-year-old female with a history of mitral valve prolapse is involved in a motorcycle accident in which she suffered a closed head injury and extremity fractures. She arrives at your intensive care unit (ICU) after open reduction and internal fixation (ORIF) of a femur fracture. She is in sinus tachycardia at 125 bpm with a systolic BP in the high 70s (mm Hg). The anesthesiologist mentions that the patient's BP was difficult to control, requiring frequent phenylephrine boluses to which the patient would respond. There was relatively little blood loss so she did not receive much in the way of intravenous (IV) fluids. You are concerned by the BP lability and perform a bedside echocardiogram. Based on the ▶ **Video 41.4** obtained, what would be the next most appropriate step in the management of this patient?

   A. Give fluid
   B. Start epinephrine
   C. Start milrinone
   D. Insert an intra-aortic balloon pump (IABP)

3. A 68-year-old male is recovering in the ICU after undergoing an uneventful five-vessel coronary artery bypass grafting (CABG) this morning. He remains intubated. Over the past hour, he has become progressively tachycardic and hypotensive to the point where the bedside nurse asks about starting a pressor agent. You are concerned and perform a bedside transthoracic echocardiography (TTE). Windows are limited after his sternotomy, so you decide to do a transesophageal echocardiography (TEE). ▶ **Video 41.5** is obtained. While the cardiac surgeon is being paged to the bedside, which of the following choices is most appropriate for the management of this patient?

   A. Metoprolol to limit demand ischemia
   B. Emergent extracorporeal membrane oxygenation (ECMO) cannulation
   C. Start milrinone
   D. Aggressive volume resuscitation

4. A 72-year-old woman in septic shock on norepinephrine after emergent surgery for a strangulated ventral hernia is intubated in your ICU. You have been steadily escalating the pressor dose and have given quite a bit of fluid to her throughout the day. She has a history of heart failure with preserved ejection fraction (HFpEF) and you are questioning whether additional fluid might help improve her hemodynamics. You are also concerned that additional fluid may push her into heart failure. Which of the following is most appropriate to determine if she will respond to additional IV fluid?

   A. Transduce the central venous pressure (CVP) and administer fluid if CVP <15 mm Hg
   B. Place a Swan-Ganz catheter and measure a pulmonary artery occlusion pressure (PAOP) to determine LV filling pressure
   C. Use echo to determine her cardiac output (CO) and stroke volume (SV) then perform a passive leg raise (PLR) to look for an increase in SV
   D. Use echo to measure IVC collapse with mechanical respiration

5. A 78-year-old male is in your ICU with presumed urosepsis from a urinary tract infection (UTI). The patient has had multiple past admissions for congestive heart failure and has a known history of HFpEF. He is tachycardic, his BP has become more labile, and the critical care fellow has performed a bedside TTE to try to determine the cause of his instability. The parasternal short-axis view obtained is shown in ▶ **Video 41.6**. The fellow says this must be hypovolemia and wishes to give more fluid. From ▶ **Video 41.6**, what might lead you toward administering vasopressors over additional fluids?

   A. The high HR
   B. Normal end-diastolic diameter
   C. Small end-diastolic diameter
   D. Myocardial hypertrophy

6. A 74-year-old male nursing home resident is intubated in the ICU with bilateral pneumonia and acute respiratory distress syndrome (ARDS). He is currently on 6 cc/kg tidal volume with 10 cm $H_2O$ positive end-expiratory pressure (PEEP). He is in septic shock and is on norepinephrine and vasopressin infusions. He has a history of hypertension and HFpEF. Lung ultrasound examination reveals B-lines, and his chest X-ray shows pulmonary edema. His creatinine has started to rise and his urine output has drifted off. By echocardiogram, a PLR results in a 16% increase in his left-ventricular outflow tract (LVOT) velocity-time integral (VTI) so you decide to give a fluid bolus. Your ICU fellow questions the wisdom of this given that the patient already has pulmonary edema and additional fluid may worsen his oxygenation. What ultrasound tool can be used to help determine if more fluid may contribute to worsening of his pulmonary edema?

   A. Measure changes in the size of the pleural effusions using lung ultrasound
   B. Look for loss of IVC respiratory variation
   C. Use continuous-wave Doppler (CWD) of the pulmonic insufficiency (PI) jet to determine the pulmonary artery diastolic pressure (PADP)
   D. Look at the mitral E/e' as a measure of left atrial pressure

7. An otherwise healthy 20-year-old male involved in a motor vehicle collision (MVC) is brought to the ICU after ORIF of an unstable pelvic fracture. Estimated blood loss was approximately 2500 cc, and he received two units packed red blood cells (PRBCs) in the OR. He is hemodynamically unstable, requiring a phenylephrine infusion. Neuromuscular blockade was not reversed in the OR and he is receiving 8 cc/kg ideal body weight (IBW) tidal volumes. You perform a bedside TTE, and the pulsed-wave Doppler tracing from the LVOT is shown in **Figure 41.1**.

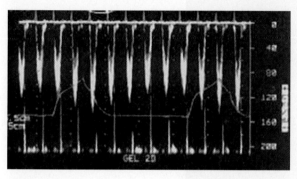

**Figure 41.1**

Based on Figure 41.1, what should be your first therapeutic maneuver to treat this patient's hypotension?
A. Change phenylephrine to norepinephrine
B. Start epinephrine
C. Place an IABP
D. 500 cc fluid bolus

8. An intubated obese 32-year-old female without other medical problems arrives from the OR intubated, in septic shock, on norepinephrine, after removal of an infected ureteral stone. You are unable to obtain good echo images on this woman.

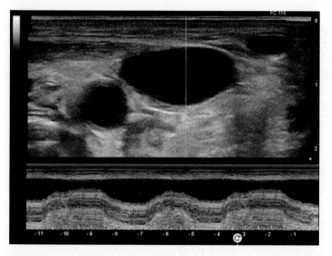

**Figure 41.2**

She is heavily sedated on AC/VC ventilation with 8 cc/kg IBW tidal volumes. She does not have central venous access, and as you scan her right internal jugular vein (IJV) to place a line you note that there is significant respiratory variation in the diameter of her IJV (**Figure 41.2**). Which of the following parameters might suggest volume responsiveness?
A. IJV collapsibility >20%
B. IJV collapsibility >10%
C. IJV distensibility >18%
D. IJV distensibility >10%

9. A 62-year-old woman with a history of HFpEF is admitted to the ICU after an MVC from which she has suffered bilateral lung contusions. Lung ultrasound (**Figure 41.3**) shows bilateral B-lines throughout both anterior lung fields. She was aggressively volume resuscitated in the Emergency Department (ED), and you are concerned she may be developing heart failure. She is hemodynamically stable, and echo confirms she has normal biventricular systolic function.

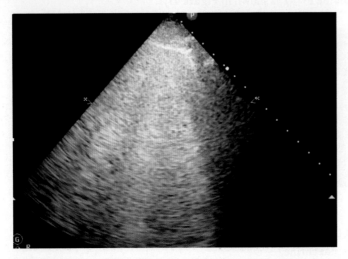

**Figure 41.3**

You question if diuresis may be beneficial to improve oxygenation. Which of the listed echo parameters may best indicate that diuresis may be beneficial in this scenario using TTE?
   A. Plethoric IVC on subcostal imaging
   B. E/e'>14
   C. Superior vena cava (SVC) collapsibility index
   D. Pulsed-wave Doppler (PWD) respiratory variation in the LVOT

10. A 55-year-old male with COVID-19 and severe ARDS is intubated in the ICU. He is intubated on low tidal-volume ventilation with 15 cm $H_2O$ PEEP. He has just been returned supine after 18 hours in the prone positiona. He has an acute kidney injury and is hypotensive on norepinephrine. TTE has confirmed that his biventricular systolic function appears normal. You are questioning whether to give additional fluid but are concerned about how poor his oxygenation is. Which of the following is the best application of echocardiography to determine if this patient will respond to additional fluid?

   A. VTI variation in the LVOT
   B. IVC distensibility
   C. Perform a PLR and look for changes in SV
   D. Measure the end-diastolic area of the left ventricle (LVEDA)

11. A 42-year-old male patient arrives intubated from the ED after being involved in an MVC. He has bilateral lung contusions and is on 90% $FiO_2$ with bilateral chest tubes. He is currently being ventilated with 6 cc/kg IBW tidal volumes and is on 12 cm $H_2O$ PEEP. Lung ultrasound shows diffuse bilateral B-lines. Echo in the ED confirmed biventricular normal systolic function. He has a pelvic fracture that will require operative intervention. On arrival, his systolic BP is in the 80s (mm Hg) and the nurse asks

to start a norepinephrine drip. What is the best way to determine whether this patient will respond to intravascular volume using TTE?

**A.** PLR maneuver to assess changes in SV
**B.** Look at IVC distensibility
**C.** Look at changes in LVOT VTI from breath to breath
**D.** Measure changes in VTI after an end-expiratory occlusion pressure

12. Twenty minutes after a laparoscopic hemicolectomy, a 72-year-old patient is found to be hypotensive (65/35 mm Hg) in the PACU, is unresponsive to a 2 L fluid bolus, and has a distended abdomen. Past medical history includes hypertension, coronary artery disease (s/p CABG), and diabetes. A brief TTE shows an LV ejection fraction of 70%, no obvious regional wall motion abnormalities, and an end-diastolic area (EDA) of 8.5 cm$^2$ in a parasternal short-axis view. The most appropriate next course of action is:

**A.** Emergent left heart catheterization
**B.** Return to OR for exploratory laparotomy
**C.** Broad-spectrum antibiotics and initiation of vasopressors
**D.** Additional 2 L fluid bolus

13. A 42-year-old male is intubated and sedated with acute pancreatitis. Despite aggressive fluid resuscitation, he remains hypotensive with low urine output. Which of the following findings are consistent with fluid responsiveness in a patient on positive pressure ventilation?

**A.** An ejection fraction of 70% with "kissing" papillary muscles
**B.** A change in PWD peak velocity through the LVOT of 14% between inhalation and exhalation
**C.** Consistent mitral inflow velocities throughout the respiratory cycle
**D.** An ejection fraction of 25% with a dilated left ventricle

14. A 23-year-old male presents to the trauma bay with multiple gunshot wounds to the abdomen and is taken immediately to the OR. Massive transfusion via a rapid transfusion device is initiated as the bleeding is controlled. Which of the following would be an indicator of over-transfusion when administering a 500 mL fluid bolus?

**A.** RV dilation without a change in BP
**B.** A decrease in peak mitral E-wave velocity variation during inspiration and expiration
**C.** Increased VTI in the LVOT
**D.** Increased lateral mitral annular systolic velocity (s')

15. A 16-year-old male became unresponsive during football practice in July. He arrived at the ED without obvious trauma, hypotensive, with a temperature of 41 °C, a Glasgow Coma Scale (GCS) of 8. He is intubated and aggressive fluid resuscitation and active cooling have been initiated. Which of the following is an indicator of further need for fluid resuscitation?

**A.** SV calculated via LVOT VTI of 80 mL with a HR of 90 bpm
**B.** IVC diameter of 1.2 cm during expiration and 1.4 cm during inspiration
**C.** Hyperdynamic left ventricle with an ejection fraction of 70%
**D.** Peak LVOT velocity of 1.2 cm/s during expiration and 0.8 cm/s during inspiration

16. Which one of the following parameters can be used to calculate mean pulmonary artery pressures in **Figure 41.4?**

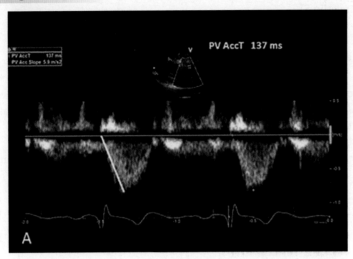

**Figure 41.4**

A. Peak velocity of early transpulmonary flow
B. Speed of early tissue relaxation velocity
C. Pulmonary artery VTI acceleration time
D. CWD assessment of the tricuspid regurgitation jet

17. A 79-year-old male is booked for an ORIF of a femur fracture. His past medical history is significant for hypertension controlled on hydrochlorothiazide. As a newly trained anesthesiologist proficient in bedside ultrasound, you perform an echocardiogram after hearing a prominent systolic murmur. The parasternal long-axis view is shown in ▶ **Video 41.7.** You plan a standard induction with propofol and use rocuronium as a neuromuscular blocker. Postintubation, the BP drops from 150/90 mm Hg to 90/50 and HR increases from 50 to 90 bpm. Which of the following agents would you use to manage his hypotension?

A. Ephedrine
B. Phenylephrine
C. One liter fluid bolus
D. Epinephrine

18. Which of the following dynamic parameters in ▶ **Video 41.8** would point toward a patient that is responsive to fluid?

A. SVC collapsibility > 36%
B. IVC collapsibility >36%
C. SVC collapsibility > 12%
D. IVC collapsibility > 12%

19. A morbidly obese 58-year-old male comes to the OR for a robotic prostatectomy. As a part of your physical examination you perform a surface echo and note plethora of the IVC. Doppler interrogation of the hepatic veins is shown in **Figure 41.5**.

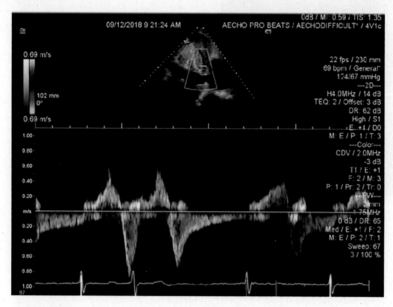

**Figure 41.5**

Which of the following valvular conditions does this patient have?
A. Mitral regurgitation
B. Mitral stenosis
C. Tricuspid regurgitation
D. Tricuspid stenosis

20. Which of the following views will be optimal to assess the LVOT velocities?

A. Apical five chamber
B. Apical four chamber
C. Subcostal five chamber
D. Subcostal four chamber

21. Which of the following conditions can lead to what is shown in ▶ **Video 41.9**?

A. RV volume overload
B. LV failure
C. Aortic stenosis
D. Cardiac tamponade

22. What is the most likely cause of hypotension followed by cardiac arrest on administration of propofol to this patient for intubation (see ▶ **Video 41.10**)?

A. Aortic stenosis
B. LV failure
C. Dynamic LVOT obstruction
D. Aortic dissection

**23.** Estimate the CVP from IVC in **Figure 41.6** and ▶ **Video 41.11**.

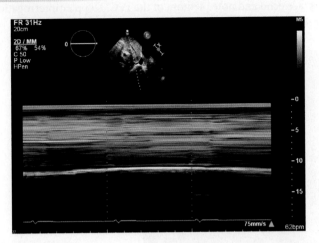

**Figure 41.6**

A. >10
B. 5-10
C. <5
D. Cannot be estimated

**24.** A 24-year-old male presents to the ICU after a MVC. He complains of abdominal pain and chest pain with a positive seat-belt sign. Shortly after his arrival, he becomes profoundly hypotensive. A PLR maneuver is performed as a TTE examination is being performed. Which of the following findings during PLR is most consistent with fluid responsiveness?

A. RV dilation and reduced tricuspid annular plane systolic excursion (TAPSE)
B. Increased stroke distance through the LVOT using PWD by 20%
C. Anterior wall hypokinesis
D. A circumferential 2 cm pericardial effusion

**25.** A 71-year-old man with coronary artery disease, diabetes, and chronic obstructive lung disease is hypotensive in the PACU following bilateral iliac stenting for claudication and rest pain. He is tachycardic and somnolent. Point-of-care ultrasound is performed, generating **Figures 41.7A and B** shortly after being intubated and then ventilated with 8 cc/kg IBW tidal volume.

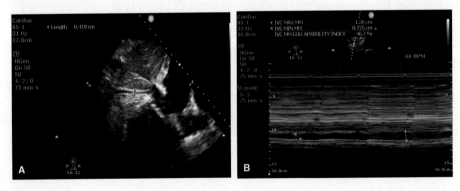

**Figure 41.7**

What is the most appropriate next step in his management?
A. Administer epinephrine at 5 μg/min
B. Administer phenylephrine at 50 μg/min
C. Administer crystalloid bolus and check hematocrit
D. Administer PRBCs and check hematocrit

**26.** A 21-year-old otherwise healthy man is in surgical ICU postoperative day 2 following craniectomy for severe head trauma after an unhelmeted snowmobile crash. He is in undifferentiated shock and has become progressively more hypotensive over 12 hours, now on vasopressin and phenylephrine. He is passively mechanically ventilated at 8 cc/kg tidal volumes by IBW. Point-of-care ultrasound reveals **Figures 41.8A-C**.

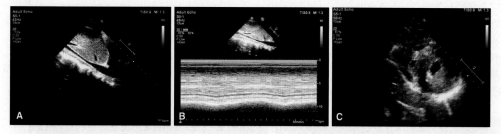

**Figure 41.8**

What is the most appropriate next step in his management?
**A.** Add an inotrope
**B.** Volume expansion with crystalloid
**C.** Add RV afterload reduction
**D.** Perform pericardiocentesis

**27.** An otherwise healthy 25-year-old man is admitted to the ED after falling 12 feet from a ladder. He is intubated and passively mechanically ventilated. He is receiving 50 µg/min phenylephrine to maintain a stable mean arterial pressure (MAP) of 65. He is tachycardic at 120 bpm. Urgent point-of-care ultrasound examination reveals **Figures 41.9A-F**.

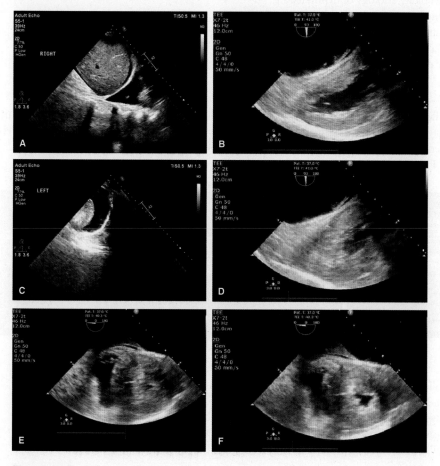

**Figure 41.9**

What is the most appropriate next step in his management?
A. Obtain two large-bore IVs and rapidly infuse fluid volume
B. Perform needle thoracostomy at 2nd intercostal space on the left
C. Perform emergent bedside needle pericardiocentesis
D. Epinephrine and administer thrombolytics given concern for pulmonary embolism (PE)

28. A 64-year-old previously healthy woman is intubated and ventilated with lung protective ventilation following respiratory failure and ARDS related to COVID-19 viral pneumonia. She exhibits narrow pulse pressure tachycardia at 125 bpm and BP 76/40 and is receiving 5 μg/min norepinephrine to maintain a MAP of 50. Prior to intubation she reported a 6-day prodrome with fatigue, lethargy, and nausea/poor appetite. Urgent point-of-care ultrasound examination using TEE to evaluate causes of hypotension reveals **Figures 41.10A** and **B**:

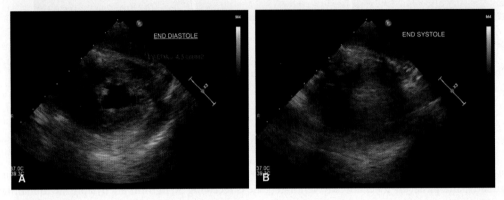

**Figure 41.10**

What is the most likely etiology of hypotension?
A. Tension pneumothorax
B. Pericardial tamponade
C. Hypovolemia
D. Left anterior descending (LAD) occlusion

29. An 81-year-old woman is admitted from an assisted living facility with septic shock following perforation of the sigmoid bowel secondary to stercoral colitis. She has gram-negative bacteremia and requires stress steroids and vasopressin and norepinephrine to achieve an MAP of 60. She is passively mechanically ventilated with tidal volumes of 8 cc/kg of IBW. Point-of-care echocardiography is performed and **Figures 41.11A-C** are gathered.

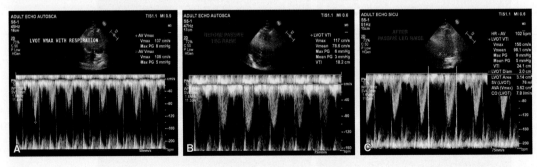

**Figure 41.11**

Which of the following statements is true with respect to these data?
A. Late peaking LVOT VTI is suggestive of systolic anterior motion (SAM) of mitral valve
B. These findings suggest volume overload and would support diuresis
C. These findings support the use of IV fluid to enhance CO
D. Wide variability in LVOT $V_{max}$ with respiration suggests tamponade

30. You are called to evaluate a 55-year-old otherwise healthy woman who is tachycardic and hypotensive following a high-speed MVC. She is awake and alert and is tachypneic, but breathing spontaneously with SpO$_2$ in the high 90s.

    Which of the following elements of a point-of-care ultrasound examination would be most useful in determining whether she is likely to be hypovolemic?
    **A.** Measurement of IVC distensibility index
    **B.** Measurement of SVC collapsibility index
    **C.** Measurement of aortic blood flow variability
    **D.** Measurement of SV/CO with PLR

31. A 52-year-old man was admitted to trauma ICU after a motor vehicle accident. He sustained bilateral rib fractures, splenic and liver lacerations, and pelvic fractures. He underwent bilateral chest tube placements, left lower lobectomy, exploratory laparotomy for splenectomy, and liver laceration repair. He required multiple blood products in the ED and in the OR. Twenty-four hours after ICU admission, the patient's hemodynamics worsen, requiring escalating doses of norepinephrine. There was no significant increase in the drainage from chest tubes or abdominal wound vacuum–assisted closure. The patient is mechanically ventilated with no spontaneous breathing activity. A point-of-care ultrasound was performed (● **Videos 41.12, 41.13, 41.14, 41.15**).

    Which of the following interventions would most likely improve the patient's hemodynamics?
    **A.** Reexploration of abdomen to look for the source of bleeding
    **B.** Initiation of dobutamine to improve CO
    **C.** Administration of crystalloid boluses to improve SV
    **D.** Addition of phenylephrine to improve LV outflow gradient

32. TTE will be of limited value in measuring which of the following to assess fluid responsiveness in a mechanically ventilated patient with hypotension?

    **A.** Respiratory variation of aortic blood flow peak velocity
    **B.** Respiratory variation of LVOT VTI
    **C.** Respiratory variation of IVC diameter
    **D.** Respiratory variation of SVC diameter

33. A 51-year-old man was brought to the ED after a motor vehicle accident. Total body computed tomography (CT) scan was notable for left-sided rib fractures, thoracic vertebra (T12) burst fracture with spinal canal compromise, and a small amount of fluid around the spleen. He underwent repair of the thoracic spine fracture and was admitted to the ICU postoperatively. Due to ongoing shock in the ICU, a point-of-care ultrasound was done to guide shock management (● **Videos 41.16** and **41.17**). What is the best course of action to improve the patient's hemodynamics?

    **A.** Check for fluid responsiveness to determine further volume administration
    **B.** Resuscitate with crystalloids and blood products
    **C.** Add norepinephrine to improve vasoplegia
    **D.** Perform lung ultrasound to rule out tension pneumothorax

34. Which of the following echocardiographic monitoring parameters is highly suggestive of hypovolemia and can be measured periodically to assess response to therapeutic interventions?

    **A.** Small mitral annular plane systolic excursion (MAPSE)
    **B.** Small LV internal diameter in diastole
    **C.** Decreased LV relative wall thickness
    **D.** Increased transmitral E/A ratio

**35.** A 60-year old woman was admitted to ICU for sepsis from aspiration pneumonia. She is mechanically ventilated, with intermittent spontaneous breathing activity assisted by the ventilator. She remained hypotensive despite 3 L of crystalloid administration. Critical care echocardiogram images from subcostal view (▶ **Video 41.18**) and apical views before (**Figure 41.12A**) and after (**Figure 41.12B**) a PLR maneuver are shown.

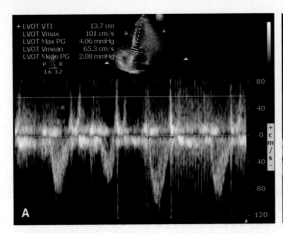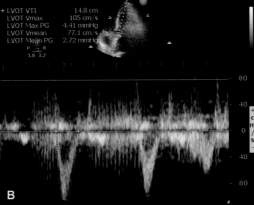

**Figure 41.12**

Which of the following statements is most accurate?
A. Patient's SV will increase with additional fluid boluses
B. Patient needs initiation of vasoactive agent to improve hemodynamics
C. Further administration of fluid will result in increased extravascular lung water
D. Additional information is needed to determine the appropriateness of PLR maneuver

**36.** Which of the following statements is most accurate when using IVC to guide fluid therapy in a mechanically ventilated patient with no spontaneous breathing activity?

A. IVC collapses with ventilator-induced passive insufflation and distends with exhalation
B. IVC diameter and its changes during ventilator-induced breaths can be used to estimate right atrial pressure (RAP)
C. Changes in IVC diameter with ventilator-induced breaths can be used to guide fluid administration
D. IVC distensibility index can be used to assess fluid responsiveness in patients with intra-abdominal hypertension

# Chapter 41 ▪ Answers

**1.** Correct Answer: **C. Administer a bolus of lactated Ringer's**

*Rationale:* This patient has undergone a redo joint replacement surgery that can be associated with significant blood loss and hypovolemia. His LV and RV contractility are hyperdynamic, obviating any need for inotropic support such as epinephrine. The almost complete collapse of the IVC with resting tidal ventilation suggests a preload deficit. This patient needs volume, but the hemoglobin of 9.5 in a patient without active ischemia or any documented history of cardiovascular disease is not an indication for blood transfusion. A bolus of a balanced crystalloid such as lactated Ringer's makes the most sense in this scenario.

Selected Reference
1. Boyd JH, Sirounis D, Maizel J, Slama M. Echocardiography as a guide to fluid management. *Crit Care*. 2016;20:274.

**2. Correct Answer: A. Give fluid**

*Rationale:* This patient has SAM of the mitral valve. While certain pathologies of the mitral valve predispose to SAM, anybody can develop it if hypovolemic enough and extremely hyperdynamic. Rather than closing appropriately in systole, the anterior leaflet of the mitral valve can get sucked into the LVOT and cause obstruction of the aortic outflow tract. The management consists of first giving fluid to allow the ventricle to expand in diastole. This way the anterior mitral leaflet will not be as close to the LVOT in the next systolic beat and less likely to get pulled into the LVOT. Other strategies are to administer beta-blockers and pure vasoconstrictors to make the ventricle less hyperdynamic and to create a higher afterload to prevent the anterior mitral leaflet from being sucked into the LVOT. Anything that decreases the LV afterload (such as an IABP) or increases the contractility of the ventricle (such as epinephrine and milrinone) can exacerbate SAM. The fact that this patient is developing SAM after a procedure with very little blood loss should prompt a search for another unrecognized source of bleeding.

Selected Reference

1. Kapoor MC. Systolic anterior motion of the mitral valve in hypovolemia and hyperadenergic states. *Indian J Anaesth.* 2014;58(1):7-8.

**3. Correct Answer: D. Aggressive volume resuscitation**

*Rationale:* This patient has cardiac tamponade (focal to left atrium) after his open heart procedure. Unlike the generalized global effusion that is usually seen with "medical" pericardial tamponade, tamponade after cardiac surgery can often be a localized phenomenon and requires redo sternotomy. In the meantime, every effort needs to be made to maintain CO while preparing to open the chest. This means keeping the ventricles "full, fast and forward." Aggressive volume resuscitation should commence to overcome the extrinsic pressure on the heart to allow it to fill, while a high HR will help maximize the limited CO. An epinephrine infusion would also help with contractility and increase HR. It is important to note that these are temporizing measures until the chest is reopened and the localized tamponade drained. Milrinone is not ideal in the setting of an acutely hypotensive patient, as it might worsen the hypotension. ECMO will not fix the underlying problem, while metoprolol may well result in cardiac arrest. TEE will be far more sensitive than TTE for the detection of a localized fluid collection after cardiac surgery.

Selected Reference

1. Khanna S, Maheshwari K. Hemopericardium and acute cardiac tamponade-images in anesthesiology. *Anesthesiology.* 2018;128:1006.

**4. Correct Answer: C. Use echo to determine her cardiac output (CO) and stroke volume (SV) then perform a passive leg raise (PLR) to look for an increase in SV**

*Rationale:* Dynamic measures of volume responsiveness are far more accurate than static pressure-based readings, which have been demonstrated time and again to not correlate with volume responsiveness. Especially given the history of HFpEF, performing a PLR allows the autotransfusion of roughly 300 cc of blood into the right side of the heart. Measuring at least a 12% change in the SV or the LVOT VTI by echo is consistent with a patient who will respond to volume administration with an increase in the CO. Changes in IVC diameter as a measure of volume responsiveness have only been validated in the setting of independently breathing patients or patients who are paralyzed on mechanical ventilation with >8 cc/kg tidal volumes.

Selected Reference

1. Miller A, Mandeville J. Predicting and measuring fluid responsiveness with echocardiography. *Echo Res Pract.* 2016;3(2):G1-G12.

**5.** Correct Answer: B. Normal end-diastolic diameter

*Rationale:* It cannot be emphasized enough that clinical decisions should rarely, if ever, be based on a single image. Still, ▶ **Video 41.6** can lead you to obtain other images that may or may not support your initial suspicion. This patient is tachycardic, hypotensive, and hyperdynamic. The initial thought is that the patient must be hypovolemic. However, one needs to look closer. Pause the video and scroll through it slowly. A low systemic vascular resistance (SVR) state, such as sepsis, can often present the same way. However, in this short-axis view, if the patient is euvolemic but with a low SVR state, the end-diastolic diameter will generally be normal. A hypovolemic heart will not fill and thus will have a decreased end-diastolic diameter. Of course, the patient could be both hypovolemic and have a low SVR state and thus more specific measures of volume status should be obtained.

Selected Reference
1. McLean AS. Echocardiography in shock management. *Crit Care.* 2016;20:275.

**6.** Correct Answer: D. Look at the mitral E/e' as a measure of left atrial pressure

*Rationale:* This patient is showing signs of end-organ dysfunction that may benefit from additional volume administration and you have echocardiographic evidence that the patient should be volume responsive. However, just because a patient is volume responsive does not mean the patient absolutely needs to receive volume. The very valid concern here is that additional fluid may worsen this patient's pulmonary edema, and we know that ARDS lungs tend to do better when they are dry. The concern is that additional volume will create cardiogenic pulmonary edema via a rise in the left atrial pressure. E/e' is an accepted measure to reflect the left atrial pressure. This involves measuring mitral inflow velocity with PWD and tissue Doppler at the mitral annulus. An E/e' > 14 indicates an elevated left atrial pressure and additional fluid has a significant chance of worsening this patient's oxygenation. In a patient on low tidal-volume ventilation on significant PEEP, the IVC respiratory variation will be very insensitive for intravascular volume. Use of CWD on a PI jet can be used to determine the PADP, but this is a cheap surrogate for the actual left atrial pressure (LAP), which is what we really want to know.

Selected Reference
1. Militaru C, Deliu R, Donoiu I, Alexandru DO, Military CC. Echocardiographic parameters in acute pulmonary edema. *Curr Health Sci J.* 2017;43(4):345-350.

**7.** Correct Answer: D. 500 cc fluid bolus

*Rationale:* While we want to avoid making clinical decisions based on only one image, Figure 41.1 shows respiratory variation in VTI in the LVOT in this paralyzed patient taking large tidal volumes and is highly suggestive that he will be volume responsive. Greater than 12% change in the peak velocities with respiration is highly sensitive and specific for volume responsiveness.

Selected Reference
1. Feissel M, Michard F, Mangin I, Ruyer O, Faller JP, Teboul JL. Respiratory changes in aortic blood velocity as an indicator of fluid responsiveness in ventilated patients with septic shock. *Chest.* 2001;119(3):867-873.

**8.** Correct Answer: C. IJV distensibility >18%

*Rationale:* In a passively mechanically ventilated patient, IJV distensibility >18% prior to volume challenge has about 80% sensitivity and 85% specificity for identification of volume responsiveness.

Selected Reference
1. Guarracino F, Ferro B, Forfori F, Bertini P, Magliacano L, Pinsky MR. Jugular vein distensibility predicts fluid responsiveness in septic patients. *Crit Care.* 2014;18:647.

**9.** Correct Answer: B. E/e'>14

*Rationale:* A plethoric IVC certainly helps suggest that the patient is not severely hypovolemic but does not really help us decide about volume overload. The same applies to SVC collapsibility, and it requires

TEE to reliably obtain. Variation in the peak Doppler velocity in the LVOT may also help with the determination of volume responsiveness, but not necessarily if the patient may respond to diuresis. The E/e' ratio is the ratio of the E-wave using PWD through the mitral valve to the tissue Doppler e' wave on the mitral annulus. An E/e' velocity ratio >14 is highly correlated with an elevation in left atrial pressure. A low E/e' gives the intensivist more confidence that the pulmonary edema is noncardiogenic in origin.

Selected Reference

1. Militaru C, Deliu R, Donoiu I, Alexandru DO, Military CC. Echocardiographic parameters in acute pulmonary edema. *Curr Health Sci J.* 2017;43(4):345-350.

**10.** Correct Answer: **C. Perform a PLR and look for changes in SV**

*Rationale:* A PLR causes the autotransfusion of approximately 300 cc of blood into the right side of the heart (**Figure 41.13**). A significant change in SV of >12% or so is consistent with the patient being volume responsive. Performing the PLR avoids giving a potentially detrimental fluid bolus and allows the intensivist to predict in advance if the patient should respond to fluid. VTI variation in the LVOT and IVC distensibility are really only applicable in the setting of tidal volumes over 8 cc/kg IBW. This patient with ARDS requires low tidal-volume ventilation so these measures would not be valid. The EDA by echo has limited sensitivity to assessment of volume responsiveness by itself.

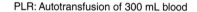

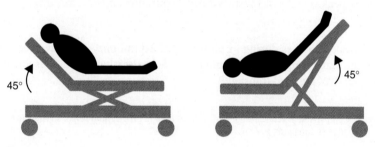

PLR: Autotransfusion of 300 mL blood

**Figure 41.13**

Selected Reference

1. Monnet X, Rienzo M, Osman D, et al. Passive leg raising predicts fluid responsiveness in the critically ill. *Crit Care Med.* 2006;34(5):1402-1407.

**11.** Correct Answer: **D. Measure changes in VTI after an end-expiratory occlusion pressure**

*Rationale:* While a PLR is a valuable tool to assess response to volume, this patient's pelvic fractures would not make it a wise option to perform IVC distensibility. Changes in LVOT VTI have only been validated in the setting of large tidal volumes >8 cc/kg, which is not applicable to this patient with bilateral lung contusions. In this patient, an end-expiratory occlusion maneuver can be performed. An increase in CO >4% after an end-expiratory occlusion reliably predicts fluid responsiveness.

Selected Reference

1. Jozwiak M, Depret F, Teboul JL, et al. Predicting fluid responsiveness in critically ill patients by using combined end-expiratory and end-inspiratory occlusions with echocardiography. *Crit Care Med.* 2017;45:e1131-e1138.

**12.** Correct Answer: **D. Additional 2 L fluid bolus**

*Rationale:* Low EDA < 10 cm² from a parasternal short-axis view is consistent with decreased preload, likely due to intra-abdominal hemorrhage in this patient. While fluid resuscitation should be initiated at that moment, a focused assessment with sonography in trauma (FAST) examination should also be performed to look for free fluid in the abdomen, suggestive of bleeding that might necessitate a return trip to the OR.

Selected Reference

1. Miller A, Mandeville J. Predicting and measuring fluid responsiveness with echocardiography. *Echo Res Pract.* 2016;3:G1-G12.

**13.** Correct Answer: B. A change in PWD peak velocity through the LVOT of 14% from systolic beat to beat

*Rationale:* Changes in PWD flow through the LVOT >12% have been shown to predict fluid responsiveness and an increase in cardiac index >15%. It is important to keep in mind that this is only valid in patients mechanically ventilated at a tidal volume >8 cc/kg IBW and without spontaneous breathing efforts.

Selected Reference
1. Feissel M, Michard F, Mangin I, Ruyer O, Faller JP, Teboul JL. Respiratory changes in aortic blood velocity as an indicator of fluid responsiveness in ventilated patients with septic shock. *Chest.* 2001;119:867-873.

**14.** Correct Answer: A. RV dilation without a change in BP

*Rationale:* RV dilation without increases in SV are an indicator of over-transfusion. Septal flattening indicated RV volume overload. Iatrogenic RV failure secondary to overaggressive rapid volume administration is an important consideration.

Selected References
1. Feneley M, Gavaghan T. Paradoxical and pseudoparadoxical interventricular septal motion in patients with right ventricular volume overload. *Circulation.* 1986;74:230-238.
2. Miller A, Mandeville J. Predicting and measuring fluid responsiveness with echocardiography. *Echo Res Pract.* 2016;3:G1-G12.

**15.** Correct Answer: D. Peak LVOT peak velocity of 1.2 cm/s during expiration and 0.8 cm/s during inspiration

*Rationale:* Changes in LVOT peak velocities during inspiration and expiration >12% have been shown to be more sensitive and specific than changes in IVC diameter >8% in assessing for fluid responsiveness when tidal volumes of >8 cc/kg IBW are used transiently.

Selected Reference
1. Vignon P, Repesse X, Begot E, et al. Comparison of echocardiographic indices used to predict fluid responsiveness in ventilated patients. *Am J Respir Crit Care Med.* 2017;195:1022-1032.

**16.** Correct Answer: C. Pulmonary artery VTI acceleration time

*Rationale:* Right ventricular outflow tract (RVOT) acceleration time (RVAT) is measured from the beginning of the flow to the peak flow velocity. It is important that the marker is placed at the peak first and then tracked back to the onset of flow, as the aim is to measure time taken to peak velocity and not the propagation. A value of >130 ms is normal, while <100 ms is highly suggestive of pulmonary hypertension. Mean pulmonary pressure is calculated by the formula: $mPAP = 90 - (0.62^*AT_{RVOT})$. While not a direct measure of volume responsiveness, elevated mean pulmonary artery pressures may make the intensivist more wary of giving excessive fluids due to concern for RV volume overload.

Selected Reference
1. Parasuraman S, Walker S, Loudon BL, et al. Assessment of pulmonary artery pressure by echocardiography—a comprehensive review. *Int J Cardiol Heart Vasc.* 2016;12:45-51.

**17.** Correct Answer: B. Phenylephrine

*Rationale:* In hypotensive patients with aortic stenosis (AS), phenylephrine is the drug of choice. LV afterload is relatively fixed due to the stenotic valve; increasing SVR will have minimal effect on myocardial work; also increasing the diastolic pressure will increase the coronary perfusion pressure and thus myocardial oxygen delivery. Phenylephrine will also decrease HR by its reflex bradycardia action, improve diastolic filling of the left ventricle, and thereby increase SV. Severe aortic stenosis is not a volume-depleted state unless there are other variables to also suggest hypovolemia.

Selected Reference
1. Samarendra P, Mangione MP. Aortic stenosis and perioperative risk with noncardiac surgery. *J Am Coll Cardiol.* 2015;65(3):295-302.

**18.** Correct Answer: A. SVC collapsibility >36%

*Rationale:* SVC collapsibility >36% is very sensitive and specific for hypovolemia in patients on passive mechanical ventilation with >8 cc/kg IBW tidal volumes. TEE is required to image the SVC reliably. Mechanical ventilation will cause distension of the IVC, as it is not an intrathoracic structure. Collapsibility >50% is usually necessary in the spontaneously ventilating patient to suggest volume responsiveness.

Selected Reference
1. Vieillard-Baron A, Chergui K, Rabiller A, et al. Superior vena caval collapsibility as a gauge of volume status in ventilated septic patients. *Intensive Care Med.* 2004;30(9):1734-1739.

**19.** Correct Answer: C. Tricuspid regurgitation

*Rationale:* Significant tricuspid regurgitation can cause a plethoric IVC, making respiratory variation in the size of the IVC to gauge volume status very unreliable. PWD interrogation of the hepatic veins shows reversal of the S wave, consistent with severe tricuspid regurgitation.

Selected Reference
1. Zoghbi WA, Adams D, Bonow RO, et al. Recommendations for noninvasive evaluation of native valvular regurgitation: a report from the American Society of Echocardiography Developed in Collaboration with the Society for Cardiovascular Magnetic Resonance. *J Am Soc Echocardiogr.* 2017;30(4):303-371.

**20.** Correct Answer: A. Apical five chamber

*Rationale:* The apical five-chamber view allows the PWD beam to align in the direction of flow in the LVOT. Determination of the VTI, in combination with the calculated LVOT area, allows one to calculate the SV. Changes in SV can be used to guide fluid resuscitation.

Selected Reference
1. Mercado P, Maizel J, Beyls C, et al. Transthoracic echocardiography: an accurate and precise method for estimating cardiac output in the critically ill patient. *Crit Care.* 2017;21:136.

**21.** Correct Answer: A. RV volume overload

*Rationale/Critique:* This parasternal short-axis TTE (▶ **Video 41.9**) shows flattening of the interventricular septum during diastole, consistent with high RV volume overload, and implies that additional fluid resuscitation is not going to be helpful. Flattening of septum during RV systole implies RV pressure overload.

Selected Reference
1. Alaverdian A, Cohen RI. The right ventricle in critical illness. *Open Crit Care Med J.* 2010;3:38-42.

**22.** Correct Answer: C. Dynamic LVOT obstruction

*Rationale:* This patient likely has hypertrophic cardiomyopathy based on the hypertrophic left ventricle seen in ▶ **Video 41.10**. Acute decreases in LV afterload or hypovolemia may lead to SAM of the mitral valve, causing dynamic LVOT obstruction and hemodynamic collapse. Aggressive volume administration is the mainstay of treatment, along with beta-blockade and increasing SVR.

Selected Reference
1. Oxlund CS, Poulsen MK, Jensen PB, Veien KT, Møller JE. A case report: hemodynamic instability due to true dynamic LVOT obstruction and systolic anterior motion following resuscitation: reversal of haemodynamics on supportive veno-arterial extracorporeal membrane oxygenation. *Eur Heart J Case Rep.* 2018;2(4):yty134.

**23.** Correct Answer: C. <5

*Rationale:* An IVC demonstrating >50% collapse with respiration with a diameter <2.1 cm is consistent with a very low CVP <5 mm Hg

Selected Reference

1. Ilyas A, Ishtiaq W, Assad S, et al. Correlation of IVC diameter and collapsibility index with central venous pressure in the assessment of intravascular volume in critically ill patients. *Cureus.* 2017;9(2):e1025.Published online 2017 Feb 12.

**24.** Correct Answer: B. Increased stroke distance through the LVOT using PWD by 20%

*Rationale:* PLR mobilizes approximately 300 mL of blood volume. Increases in LVOT stroke distance (or VTI) ≥12% correlates well with fluid responsiveness.

Selected Reference

1. Mielnicki W, Dyla A, Zawada T. Utility of transthoracic echocardiography (TTE) in assessing fluid responsiveness in critically ill patients – a challenge for the bedside sonographer. *Med Ultrason.* 2016;18:508-514.

**25.** Correct Answer: C. Administer crystalloid bolus and check hematocrit

*Rationale:* This patient was assessed in the PACU and determined to be hypovolemic. Ultimately, the patient was taken back to the OR where the angiogram (**Figure 41.14**) was obtained, revealing a large blush of contrast, diagnostic of arterial bleed.

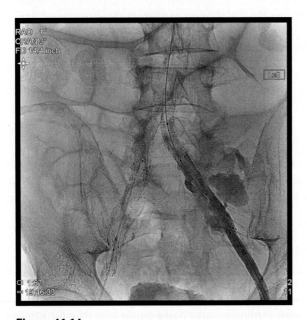

**Figure 41.14**

In Figure 41.7A the stem illustrates a very small IVC from the subcostal window, measuring <0.5 cm in diameter. While clinicians should not use the IVC as a sole indicator of volume responsiveness, IVC ultrasound may be useful at extremes and when taken into context with pretest probability and other tools assessing likelihood of volume tolerance and responsiveness. Additionally, an IVC this small warrants further scanning to ensure that what is being measured is in fact the IVC.

Figure 41.7B depicts the application of M-mode to measure the IVC distensibility index. Ideally the sweep speed is reduced to visualize the changes in IVC diameter over multiple respiratory cycles. This assessment takes advantage of heart and lung interactions, where passive positive pressure mechanical inspiration dilates IVC to a greater degree in fluid-responsive patients. IVC distensibility >18% using MaxD – MinD/MinD * 100 (or >12% using MaxD – MinD/MeanD * 100) predicts fluid responsiveness.

Limitations to this technique include that it requires passive synchrony with mechanical ventilation at >8 cc/kg of IBW and the absence of RV failure. Furthermore, conditions affecting system compliance can create error (eg, abdominal compartment syndrome).

Answer choices A and B are incorrect because while pressors and inotropes might be temporizing, the patient requires fluid resuscitation. Answer choice D is wrong because while the ultrasound and examination findings suggest hypovolemia, they are not diagnostic of acute blood loss.

### Selected References

1. Barbier C, Loubieres Y, Schmit C, et al. Respiratory changes in inferior venacava diameter are helpful in predicting fluid responsiveness in ventilated septic patients. *Intensive Care Med.* 2004;30:1740-1746.
2. Feissel M, Michard F, Faller JP, Teboul JL. The respiratory variation in inferior vena cava diameter as a guide to fluid therapy. *Intensive Care Med.* 2004;30(9):1834-1837.
3. Mikkelsen M, Gaieski D, Johnson N, Manaker S, Finlay G. *Novel Tools for Hemodynamic Monitoring in Critically Ill Patients with Shock.* Literature review current through May 2020; last updated: Mar 24, 2020. www.uptodate.com

**26.** Correct Answer: **B. Volume expansion with crystalloid**

*Rationale:* This patient was evaluated with ultrasound for undifferentiated hypotension. Figures 41.8A-C reveal multiple findings consistent with hypovolemia, including a small, collapsible IVC and a small EDA by body surface area in the parasternal short-axis view. Biventricular contractility is excellent, and there is no pericardial effusion, making answer choices A, C, and D incorrect. While dynamic parameters should be used preferentially over static parameters to predict fluid responsiveness in ICU patients, a very small IVC can be used, at extremes, as supporting evidence of hypovolemia and potential fluid responsiveness.

### Selected References

1. Feissel M, Michard F, Faller JP, Teboul JL. The respiratory variation in inferior vena cava diameter as a guide to fluid therapy. *Intensive Care Med.* 2004;30(9):1834-1837.
2. Yanagawa Y, Sakamoto T, Okado Y. Hypovolemic shock evaluated by sonographic measurement of the inferior vena cava during resuscitation in trauma patients. *J Trauma.* 2007;63:1245-1248.

**27.** Correct Answer: **A. Obtain two large-bore IVs and rapidly infuse fluid volume**

*Rationale:* Figures 41.9A-F reveal free intra-abdominal fluid as well as intrathoracic fluid in the right chest (spine sign on right, fluid under diaphragm bilaterally). Furthermore, the LVEDA is visually small at end diastole, with the appearance of pseudohypertrophy, and there is near-complete obliteration of the cavity at end systole, which also provides supporting evidence of hypovolemia. Given the history, this is suspicious for multiple sites of traumatic bleeding (chest and abdomen) until proven otherwise. There is no clear evidence of left pneumothorax based on Figures 41.9A-F shown (B is incorrect). There is no clear evidence of pericardial fluid or tamponade (C is incorrect). The right ventricle also appears small and underfilled; there is no role for thrombolytics, which could be quite harmful in this case (D is incorrect).

### Selected References

1. Di Segni E, Preisman S, Ohad DG, et al. Echocardiographic left ventricular remodeling and pseudohypertrophy as markers of hypovolemia. An experimental study on bleeding and volume repletion. *JASE.* 1997;10:926-936.
2. Michard F, Teboul JL. Predicting fluid responsiveness in ICU patients: a critical analysis of the evidence. *Chest.* 2002;121(6):2000-2008. doi:10.1378/chest.121.6.2000.
3. Mikkelsen M, Gaieski D, Johnson N, Manaker S, Finlay G. *Novel Tools for Hemodynamic Monitoring in Critically Ill Patients with Shock.* Literature review current through May 2020; last updated: Mar 24, 2020. www.uptodate.com

**28.** Correct Answer: **C. Hypovolemia**

*Rationale:* While dynamic parameters should be used preferentially over static parameters to predict fluid responsiveness in ICU patients, midpapillary LVEDA can be used at extremes as supporting evidence of hypovolemia. To be clear, there is not a great deal of value of LVEDA index measurements in discriminating between patients who are responders and nonresponders to fluid bolus, and there is marked overlap of baseline individual LVEDA values in both groups of patients. However, in at least one study, there was a significant relationship between baseline LVEDA index and the percentage of increase in SV in response to volume administration. *Severe* hypovolemia can be recognized by a hypercontractile left ventricle with a very small EDA, especially in the right clinical context. It should be noted that isolated low end-systolic area (ESA) is more suggestive of a low SVR state, which might be present with or without hypovolemia.

Therefore, small LVEDA indices <5.5 cm/m² (body surface area) can be consistent with relative hypovolemia at extremes (TTE normal values: 13 ± 2 cm²/m²), especially with the appearance of "pseudohypertrophy." In this author's opinion, this is best utilized with high pretest probability (ie, with a clinical scenario that is also consistent with hypovolemia).

Answers A, B, and D are incorrect because tension pneumothorax is extremely unlikely if bilateral lung slide is present at the most superior portion of the chest in the supine patient, there is no evidence of pericardial effusion, and there is no regional wall motion abnormality.

### Selected References

1. Di Segni E, Preisman S, Ohad DG, et al. Echocardiographic left ventricular remodeling and pseudohypertrophy as markers of hypovolemia. An experimental study on bleeding and volume repletion. *JASE*. 1997;10:926-936.
2. Leung JM, Levine EH. Left ventricular end-systolic cavity obliteration as an estimate of intraoperative hypovolemia. *Anesthesiology*. 1994;81(5):1102-1109.
3. Michard F, Teboul JL. Predicting fluid responsiveness in ICU patients: a critical analysis of the evidence. *Chest*. 2002;121(6):2000-2008. doi:10.1378/chest.121.6.2000.

**29.** Correct Answer: C. These findings support the use of IV fluid to enhance CO

*Rationale:* Figure 41.11A shows aortic blood flow variability during a respiratory cycle. The fact that passive mechanical ventilation cyclically increases intrathoracic pressure, decreasing preload and decreasing SV, can be utilized to predict fluid responsiveness. Fluctuations in SV associated with ventilator cycling are greater in the hypovolemic patient than in the completely resuscitated patient.

Evidence supports greater likelihood of fluid responsiveness if the value of the following equation is >12%:

Vpeak(LVOT)max – Vpeak(LVOT)min/Vpeak(LVOT)mean * 100

The major limitation of using variation in the VTI to identify preload sensitivity is that, similar to assessments of IVC change over a respiratory cycle, it requires the patient to be passively mechanically ventilated. In addition, since the degree of variation of SV depends on the tidal volume, the patient should be receiving 8 mL/kg tidal volume (temporarily). An irregular HR invalidates the measurement. In addition, this method for assessment of preload sensitivity has not been validated in patients with impaired RV function.

In this case, VTI was also measured before and after PLR. PLR provides a temporary "test dose" of volume expansion by redistributing blood in the lower extremities to the central compartment.

Increase of VTI by >12.5% following PLR predicts an increase in SV of 15% or more after volume expansion, with a sensitivity of 77% and a specificity of 100%. One major benefit of the PLR technique is that it also predicts preload sensitivity in patients with spontaneous respiratory effort. Limitations include that certain patients have contraindications to such a maneuver (eg, neurosurgical patients with intracranial hypertension), and that the experiment can be confounded if the maneuver causes pain (artificially increasing HR/CO). See **Figure 41.15** for an excellent description of how to perform this maneuver.

While a late peaking VTI envelope created by CWD through the aortic valve would be suggestive of SAM, this finding is not present here (answer A is wrong). There is no evidence of volume overload among the findings (answer B is wrong). Wide variability in transmitral and/or trans-tricuspid filling velocities can be seen in tamponade, but variability in LVOT Vmax with respiration is used to assess fluid responsiveness, as earlier (answer D is wrong).

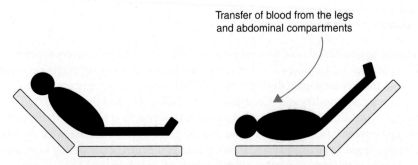

Transfer of blood from the legs and abdominal compartments

**Figure 41.15** Passive leg maneuver for fluid responses. After starting with the head elevated to 45°, rapidly repositioning the patient with legs elevated to 30 to 45° allows autotransfusion of blood from the legs into the thorax. An increase in cardiac output suggests that the patient might be fluid responsive.

## Selected References

1. Feissel M, Michard F, Mangin I, Ruyer O, Faller JP, Teboul JL. Respiratory changes in aortic bloodflow velocity as an indicator or fluid responsiveness in ventilated patients with septic shock. *Chest.* 2001;119(3):867-873.
2. Lamia B, Ochagavia A, Monnet X, Chemla D, Richard C, Teboul JL. Echocardiographic prediction of volume responsiveness in critically ill patients with spontaneously breathing activity. *Intensive Care Med.* 2007;33(7):1125-1132.
3. Maizel J, Airapetian N, Lorne E, Tribouilloy C, Massy Z, Slama M. Diagnosis of central hypovolemia by using passive leg raising. *Intensive Care Med.* 2007;33:1133-1138.
4. Mikkelsen M, Gaieski D, Johnson N, Manaker S, Finlay G. *Novel Tools for Hemodynamic Monitoring in Critically Ill Patients with Shock.* Literature review current through May 2020; last updated: Mar 24, 2020. www.uptodate.com
5. Monnet X, Rienzo M, Osman D, et al. Passive leg raising predicts fluid responsiveness in the critically ill. *Crit Care Med.* 2006;34(5):1402-1407.
6. Narasimhan M, Koenig SJ, Mayo PH. Advanced echocardiography for the critical care physician: Part 2. *Chest.* 2014 Jan;145(1):135-142.

**30.** Correct Answer: D. Measurement of SV/CO with PLR

*Rationale:* This patient is awake and breathing spontaneously and in fact is tachypneic. One of the major limitations of measurement of IVC distensibility index, SVC collapsibility index, and aortic blood flow variability across cycles of respiration is that all of these measurements are validated only for patients who are passively receiving mechanical ventilation. In fact, many of these measurements might inappropriately suggest fluid responsiveness if inappropriately applied to a spontaneously breathing patient. Therefore, answers A, B, and C would not be particularly useful for this patient and are incorrect choices.

### Selected References

1. Barbier C, Loubieres Y, Schmit C, et al. Respiratory changes in inferior venacava diameter are helpful in predicting fluid responsiveness in ventilated septic patients. *Intensive Care Med.* 2004;30:1740-1746.
2. Feissel M, Michard F, Faller JP, Teboul JL. The respiratory variation in inferior vena cava diameter as a guide to fluid therapy. *Intensive Care Med.* 2004;30(9):1834-1837.
3. Maizel J, Airapetian N, Lorne E, Tribouilloy C, Massy Z, Slama M. Diagnosis of central hypovolemia by using passive leg raising. *Intensive Care Med.* 2007;33:1133-1138.
4. Monnet X, Rienzo M, Osman D, et al. Passive leg raising predicts fluid responsiveness in the critically ill. *Crit Care Med.* 2006;34(5):1402-1407

**31.** Correct Answer: C. Administration of crystalloid boluses to improve SV

*Rationale:* The patient's ultrasound images show hyperdynamic LV function with small LVEDA (▶ Videos **41.12** and **41.13**), very small IVC with respiratory variation (▶ Video **41.15**) suggestive of hypovolemia. Hence administration of volume will improve the hemodynamics in this scenario. As this patient had significant trauma including liver laceration, hemoperitoneum is in the differential. ▶ Video **41.14** shows no fluid collection in the hepatorenal space (Morrison pouch), and the patient did not have increased output from abdominal wound drains, ruling out the need for abdominal surgery (choice A). There is no role of dobutamine to improve cardiac contractility as the left ventricle is hyperdynamic from hypovolemic state. Hyperdynamic LV function from hypovolemia can cause dynamic LVOT obstruction from SAM of the mitral valve leaflet, especially in the presence of LV hypertrophy. Addition of pure alpha-agonist vasoactive agents like phenylephrine can reduce this dynamic gradient by increasing LV afterload. However, correction of hypovolemia should be undertaken first to improve the dynamic LVOT obstruction (if present), before adding a vasoactive agent. ▶ Videos **41.12** and **41.13** do not suggest SAM; hence, choice D is incorrect. IVC was imaged via the right lateral transhepatic view, as the abdominal surgical dressings precluded obtaining a subcostal view.

Although static indices of fluid responsiveness like LVEDA and IVC diameter are not good predictors of volume responsiveness, extreme values of these parameters are useful in clinical practice. The collapse of LV walls at end systole (kissing walls) in parasternal long-axis view and obliteration of LV area at end systole in the short-axis view are seen in severe hypovolemia. An LVEDA of <10 cm$^2$ or LVEDA index (LVEDA/body surface area) of <5.5 cm$^2$/m$^2$ is highly suggestive of a hypovolemic state. An IVC diameter of <13 mm predicted fluid responsiveness with 80% specificity (specificity increased to 90% if the diameter is <10 mm), whereas an IVC diameter of >25 mm predicted absence of fluid responsiveness with 80% specificity (increased to 90% if the diameter is >27 mm) in a large cohort of mechanically ventilated patients with circulatory failure. The ability of IVC diameter to guide fluid management may be limited in patients with high intra-abdominal pressure (≥12 mm Hg). Although the end-expiratory diameter of IVC may be helpful in fluid management, it should be used in conjunction with other dynamic indices to predict fluid responsiveness. When evaluating IVC diameter variations, care must be taken to ensure the IVC does not translate out of the imaging plane during respiratory efforts, mistakenly identifying as IVC collapse.

This patient responded well to crystalloid fluid boluses and transfusion of one unit of red blood cells. Sepsis was considered in the differential due to chest radiograph findings and increased sputum production. Blood cultures grew *Enterobacter*, and sputum cultures grew multiple gram-negative organisms. This patient likely had hypovolemia from hemorrhagic shock and intraoperative volume losses and decreased vasomotor tone (relative hypovolemia) from sepsis.

### Selected References

1. Diaz-Gomez L, Nikravan S, Conlon T. *Comprehensive Critical Care Ultrasound.* 2nd ed., Section II. Society of Critical Care Medicine; 2020.
2. McLean AS. Echocardiography in shock management. *Crit Care.* 2016;20:275.
3. Vieillard-Baron A, Evrard B, Repesse X, et al. Limited value of end-expiratory inferior vena cava diameter to predict fluid responsiveness: impact of intra-abdominal pressure. *Intensive Care Med.* 2018;44:197-203.

---

**32.** Correct Answer: D. Respiratory variation of SVC diameter

*Rationale:* Fluid or preload responsiveness is the ability of a patient to increase CO with the administration of fluid bolus. Dynamic indices are better predictors than static indices (eg, CVP) in assessing fluid responsiveness. It is essential to keep in mind that these indices are less useful when fluid responsiveness is extremely likely, for example, un-resuscitated hemorrhagic shock or the initial phase of septic shock.

Critical care echocardiography is a valuable tool to measure static and dynamic indices of preload responsiveness. The above question refers to use of TTE to measure dynamic indices of fluid responsiveness. Respiratory variation of SV can be measured by placing the sample volume of PWD at the LVOT and measuring VTI in apical five-chamber view (choice B). Respiratory cycle–induced changes in peak aortic blood flow velocity measured with PWD at the level of the aortic valve or LVOT can be used as a surrogate for changes in SV (choice A). Respiratory variation in the IVC diameter can be assessed with the transthoracic echo probe in the subcostal view (choice C). However, assessment of SVC requires TEE; hence, choice D is the correct answer.

Respiratory variation of SV cannot be used to predict fluid responsiveness in the presence of spontaneous breathing, cardiac arrhythmias, RV dysfunction, poor lung compliance, or low tidal-volume ventilation. Respiratory variability of vena cava diameter to predict preload responsiveness has similar limitations except that it can be used in patients with cardiac arrhythmias. The threshold values for respiratory variations of IVC diameter to predict fluid responsiveness varied from 8% to 50% across the studies. In spontaneously breathing patients, IVC collapses with inspiration, while SVC distends. It is vice versa in patients on mechanical ventilation: IVC distends with positive pressure inspiration while the SVC collapses. In a large prospective study of mechanically ventilated patients with circulatory failure, respiratory variations in the peak velocity of LVOT blood flow had the best sensitivity (79%) to predict fluid responsiveness, whereas respiratory variations of SVC diameter had the best specificity (84%) to predict fluid responsiveness.

### Selected References

1. Monnet X, Marik PE, Teboul JL. Prediction of fluid responsiveness: an update. *Ann. Intensive Care.* 2016;6:111.
2. Vignon P, Repesse X, Begot E, et al. Comparison of echocardiographic indices used to predict fluid responsiveness in ventilated patients. *Am J Respir Crit Care Med.* 2017;195:1022-1032.

---

**33.** Correct Answer: B. Resuscitate with crystalloids and blood products

*Rationale:* The patient in this clinical vignette has normal to hyperdynamic LV function (parasternal short axis was the only view available for this patient). Hyperdynamic LV function in this patient who sustained trauma could be due to hypovolemia (bleeding), reduced vasomotor tone (spinal shock, sepsis), or from obstruction (tension pneumothorax). Besides echocardiography, additional ultrasound images are valuable to determine the etiology of shock in this scenario. The abdominal ultrasound (▶ **Videos 41.16** and **41.17**) shows fluid collection in hepatorenal space, suggesting this patient's shock is most likely from bleeding and hypovolemia. Hence the patient should be resuscitated with fluid and blood products. Assessing for preload responsiveness is not necessary as the clinical scenario is suggestive of bleeding and hypovolemia. Moreover, the question stem does not provide additional details that may preclude the feasibility and validity of parameters to assess for preload responsiveness in this patient. Obtaining a CT scan in hemodynamically unstable patients with trauma is not recommended, especially with a positive FAST examination (fluid/blood in Morrison pouch). It is important to note that blood can accumulate in Morrison pouch even if the spleen is the injured organ. Tension pneumothorax is a possibility due to rib fractures in this patient, and a lung ultrasound can rule out this possibility. However, volume and blood products should be administered first to improve the patient's hemodynamics based on the information given in **Question 41.33**.

### Selected Reference

1. Diaz-Gomez L, Nikravan S, Conlon T. *Comprehensive Critical Care Ultrasound*. 2nd ed., Section III. Society of Critical Care Medicine; 2020.

---

**34.** Correct Answer: B. Small LV internal diameter in diastole

*Rationale:* Cardiac chamber size is decreased in the hypovolemic state, and the chamber dimensions can be measured serially to assess volume status in critically ill patients. A small left ventricular internal diameter at end diastole (LVIDD) is suggestive of hypovolemia. It is best measured in the parasternal long-axis view using either 2D or M-mode, 1 cm distal to mitral valve annulus at the mitral valve leaflet tips. A small LV internal diameter in end systole (LVIDS) is also seen in hypovolemia. However, this finding can be seen with low SVR and increased inotropic state. In the hypovolemic state, LVIDD and LVIDS are decreased; however, LVIDD remains normal while LVIDS is decreased in low SVR states (eg, sepsis). Reference ranges for LVIDD are 3.9 to 5.3 cm in women and 4.2 to 5.9 cm in men. Changes in LVIDD can be measured serially to assess response to fluid administration.

MAPSE is a linear method to assess LV systolic function. A decreased MAPSE (<1 cm) is suggestive of decreased LV ejection fraction, but this is not suggestive of hypovolemia. LV relative wall thickness is used to categorize increased LV mass as either concentric or eccentric hypertrophy and to identify concentric remodeling. Doppler parameters, including the trans-mitral E/A ratio, are useful in the fluid management in ICU and OR settings. The mitral E-wave represents the gradient between the left atrium and left ventricle in early diastole, and it is preload dependent. The mitral A-wave represents the left atrium–left ventricle gradient during late diastole and is affected by LV diastolic function and left atrial compliance. Although absolute numbers of E/A ratio may be of limited value, a change in E/A ratio from a lower value (eg, <1) to a higher value (eg, >2) during fluid resuscitation may suggest limiting further fluid administration. VTI of the LVOT is a surrogate for SV, and it is diminished in hypovolemia. Besides hypovolemia, there are other conditions (eg, decreased LV or RV function, or tamponade) in which SV (and LVOT VTI) will be decreased. LVOT VTI can be measured serially to assess response to therapeutic interventions (eg, fluid administration). In a post hoc analysis of sepsis patients who underwent TEE within 12 hours of septic shock, following three echocardiographic features were highly suggestive of hypovolemia: an aortic VTI <16 cm (reflecting low LV SV), mitral E-wave <67 cm/s (reflecting low LV filling pressure), and SVC collapsibility index >39% (predictive of fluid responsiveness).

### Selected References

1. Geri G, Vignon P, Aubry A, et al. Cardiovascular clusters in septic shock combining clinical and echocardiographic parameters: a post hoc analysis. *Intensive Care Med.* 2019;45:657-667.
2. Porter TR, Shillcutt SK, Adams MS, et al. Guidelines for the use of echocardiography as a monitor for therapeutic intervention in adults: a report from the American Society of Echocardiography. *J Am Soc Echocardiogr.* 2015;28:40-56.

---

**35.** Correct Answer: B. Patient needs initiation of vasoactive agent to improve hemodynamics

*Rationale:* Figures 41.12A and B show the measurement of VTI of the LVOT before and after PLR maneuver. VTI is obtained by placing the sampling window of the PWD in the outflow tract of the left ventricle. PLR induces transfer of venous blood into the thorax (autotransfusion), and the resultant increase in preload can be used to evaluate fluid responsiveness. The patient in this clinical vignette had a VTI of 13.7 cm at baseline, which changed to 14.8 after PLR maneuver, corresponding to an 8% increase. An increase in the VTI of 10% to 15% during PLR predicts the response to volume expansion with excellent results. The patient had a small IVC (<2.1 cm) with no significant respiratory variation. Despite the small IVC diameter, lack of changes in IVC diameter with ventilator-induced breaths suggests the patient is fluid unresponsive, and further fluid administration may not improve her SV. Hence choice B is the correct answer.

As the patient is not fluid responsive based on the dynamic indices, further fluid administration may not improve the SV (hence choice A is incorrect). Although further fluid administration may increase extravascular lung water, additional information is needed before coming to this conclusion. Lung ultrasound will be valuable for assessing fluid tolerance in this scenario by evaluating for the replacement of A-lines with B-lines. This finding indicates development of interstitial edema and suggests that the patient has reached the limit of fluid tolerance. As this additional information is not provided in the question stem, choice C is not an accurate statement. PLR has been shown to predict fluid responsiveness in various conditions, including patients on mechanical ventilator support, spontaneous breathing, arrhythmias, ARDS patients with poor lung compliance, or ventilated patients with low tidal volumes (choice D is not correct). PLR may be unreliable in intra-abdominal hypertension and contraindicated in intracranial hypertension and unstable pelvic fractures. It is crucial to keep the echo probe in the same location for pre- and postassessment of VTI after a PLR maneuver.

### Selected References

1. Lichtenstein D. Fluid administration limited by lung sonography: the place of lung ultrasound in assessment of acute circulatory failure (the FALLS-protocol). *Expert Rev Respir Med.* 2012;6(2):155-162.
2. Shi R, Monnet X, Teboul JL. Parameters of fluid responsiveness. *Curr Opin Crit Care.* 2020; 26(3):319-326.

**36.** Correct Answer: C. Changes in IVC diameter with ventilator-induced breaths can be used to guide fluid administration

*Rationale:* Assessment of IVC diameter and its changes in response to respirations have been used to screen for hypovolemia, predict fluid responsiveness, and assess potential intolerance to further fluid administration. Multiple studies have explored the ability of changes in IVC diameter to predict fluid responsiveness, and the cutoff values to predict fluid responsiveness have varied significantly across the studies. When the IVC is underfilled, the vessel compliance is high, so significant respiratory variations in IVC diameter suggest hypovolemia and predict fluid responsiveness. IVC collapses with inspiration in spontaneously breathing patients and distends with positive pressure breath in mechanically ventilated patients. IVC collapsibility index in spontaneously breathing patients and IVC distensibility index in patients on mechanical ventilator support are used to predict fluid responsiveness. Different studies used different methods to calculate these indices, but it is primarily calculated as the change in IVC diameter divided by either end-expiratory IVC diameter or the average IVC diameter. A recent systematic review reported a mean IVC distensibility index threshold of 15% (range 12%-21%) predicted fluid responsiveness with 85% specificity in mechanically ventilated patients, and a mean IVC collapsibility index threshold of 41% (range 40%-42%) predicted fluid responsiveness with a specificity >80% (range 80%-97%) in spontaneously breathing patients.

It is essential to be aware of limitations to the use of IVC diameter or its respiratory variations in estimating volume status or predicting fluid responsiveness. Use of high levels of PEEP and/or low tidal volumes during mechanical ventilation, RV dysfunction, increased intra-abdominal pressure, local mechanical factors (eg, IVC filter, ECMO cannula) may affect the IVC diameter and interfere with its changes during respiration. In some patients, marked translational motion of IVC with inspiration may cause misalignment of the ultrasound scanning plane, leading to overestimation of IVC collapsibility. In this situation, interrogation of IVC in the short axis may be useful to confirm respiratory-induced changes in IVC diameter.

IVC diameter and the degree of collapse in the diameter with inspiration can be used to estimate RAP in spontaneously breathing patients. In patients who are on mechanical ventilation, inspiratory collapse will not occur; hence it should not be used to estimate RAP in this setting. However, a small IVC diameter of 12 mm can correspond to RAP <10 mm Hg in patients on mechanical ventilation. A small and collapsed IVC is also suggestive of hypovolemia in this setting.

### Selected References

1. Bentzer P, Griesdale DE, Boyd J, MacLean K, Sirounis D, Ayas NT. Will this hemodynamically unstable patient respond to a bolus of intravenous fluids? *JAMA.* 2016;316(12):1298-1309.
2. Jue J, Chung W, Schiller NB. Does this inferior vena cava size predict right atrial pressures in patients receiving mechanical ventilation? *J Am Soc Echocardiogr.* 1992;5(6):613-619.
3. Rudski LG, Lai WW, Afilalo J, et al. Guidelines for the echocardiographic assessment of the right heart in adults: A report from the American Society of Echocardiography. *J Am Soc Echocargiogr* 2010;23:685-713.
4. Via G, Tavazzi G, Price S. Ten situations where inferior vena cava ultrasound may fail to accurately predict fluid responsiveness: a physiologically based point of view. *Intensive Care Med.* 2016;42:1164-1167.

# 42 | DISTRIBUTIVE, VASODILATORY, NEUROGENIC, AND SEPTIC

Gregory Mints and Tanping Wong

1. A 76-year-old woman with a history of ischemic cardiomyopathy with known severely decreased left ventricular (LV) systolic function presents with 1 day of nausea, vomiting, right flank pain, fevers, and chills. In the emergency room she is confused. Her temperature is 39 °C, BP is 80/60 mm Hg, HR is 110 bpm, respiratory rate (RR) is 22 breaths/min, and her arterial oxygen saturation is 99% by pulse oximetry while breathing room air. Her physical examination is significant for clear lungs and warm, well-perfused extremities. Initial laboratory studies were significant for blood white cell count (WBC) of $18 \times 10^9$/L with 90% neutrophils, lactate of 3 mmol/L, and creatinine of 1.4 mg/dL. Urinalysis was significant for 50 WBC per high-power field (HPF). The patient is started on ceftriaxone for pyelonephritis and resuscitated with 3 L of intravenous (IV) normal saline. Four hours later, the patient's BP is 90/64 mm Hg, HR is 106 bpm, RR is 24 breaths/min, and arterial oxygen saturation is 99% by pulse oximetry while breathing room air. She is now obtunded. She does not appear to be in respiratory distress, and her extremities remain warm and well-perfused and lungs are still clear to auscultation. Her serum lactate is now 3.8 mmol/L. Bedside ultrasound images are shown in **Figures 42.1, 42.2,** and **42.3 (▶ Videos 42.1, 42.2,** and **42.3).**

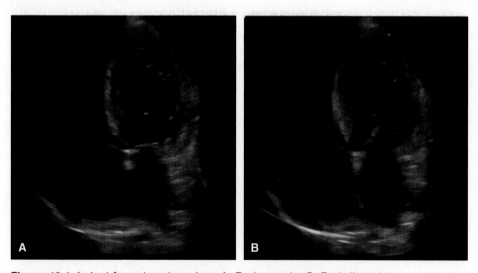

**Figure 42.1** Apical four-chamber view. A. End-systole. B. End-diastole.

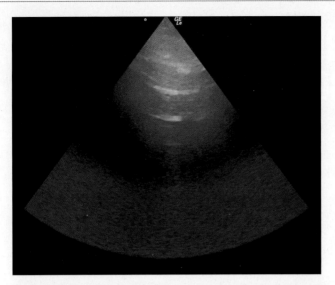

**Figure 42.2** Lung ultrasound. Anterior chest wall bilaterally.

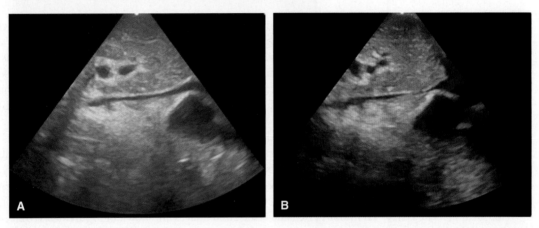

**Figure 42.3** Subcostal inferior vena cava (IVC) view. A. IVC expiration. B. IVC inspiration.

Which of the following statements is most accurate?
A. The patient is in cardiogenic shock.
B. The patient is likely to tolerate additional IV fluids.
C. It is impossible for a patient like this to have high stroke volume (SV) and cardiac output (CO).
D. None of the above.

2. An 86-year-old man is transferred from a nursing home with fever, cough, and hypoxemia. On presentation, his temperature is 39 °C, BP is 90/60 mm Hg, HR is 112 bpm, RR is 36 breaths/min, arterial oxygen saturation is 90% on 100% non-rebreather mask. His physical examination is notable for crackles in the right middle and lower lung fields. Laboratory studies show a blood WBC of $32 \times 10^9/L$, lactate of 2.4 mmol/L, and creatinine of 1.2 mg/dL. Admission chest X-ray shows right middle and right lower lobe consolidations. The patient is intubated for hypoxic respiratory failure secondary to multifocal pneumonia, given 4 L IV fluids, and started on vancomycin and piperacillin/tazobactam. The next hospital day, the patient's BP is 92/66 mm Hg and his HR is 110 bpm. Bedside ultrasound images are shown in **Figures 42.4, 42.5, 42.6A, 42.6B,** and **42.7** (▶ **Videos 42.4, 42.5, 42.6A, 42.6B,** and **42.7**).

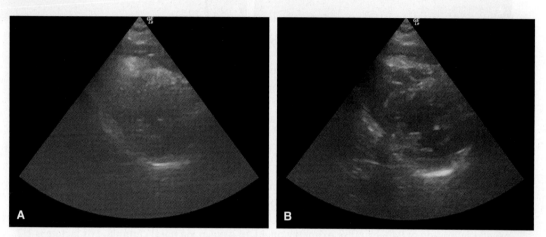

**Figure 42.4** Parasternal short-axis view. A. End-systole. B. End-diastole.

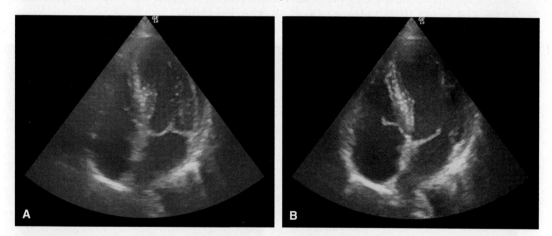

**Figure 42.5** Apical four-chamber view. A. End-systole. B. End-diastole.

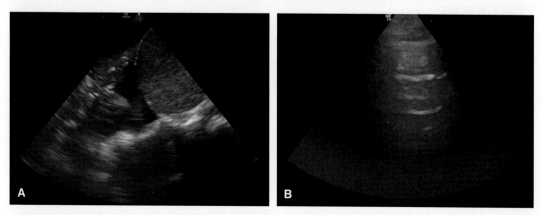

**Figure 42.6** A. Right lower lung field. Coronal plane, posterior axillary line. B. Lung ultrasound. Anterior chest wall bilaterally.

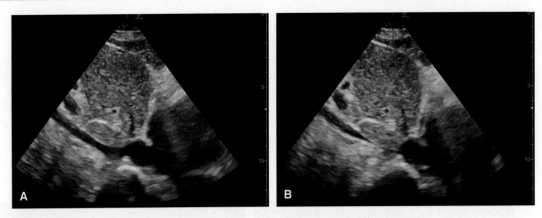

**Figure 42.7** Subcostal inferior vena cava view. A. Inspiration. B. Expiration.

Which of the following statements is most accurate?
A. The patient is in pulmonary edema and should not be given additional IV fluids.
B. Given unreliability of the inferior vena cava (IVC) parameters in ventilated patients, invasive monitoring is needed for estimation of intracardiac pressures and volume status.
C. The patient is likely fluid responsive.
D. Positive pressure ventilation (PPV) is expected to decrease IVC size and increase its collapsibility.

3. A 72-year-old man with renal cell carcinoma presents with neutropenic fever and is found to have left lower lobe pneumonia. He is started on broad-spectrum antibiotics and given 3 L of IV fluids. He remains hypotensive with BP of 80/60 mm Hg, HR of 120 bpm, RR of 24 breaths/min, and arterial oxygen saturation of 94% by pulse oximetry on 4 L of oxygen via nasal cannula. His lactate is 1.2 mmol/L, and creatinine is 1.0 mg/dL. Bedside ultrasound is performed and shown in **Figures 42.8A, 42.8B, 42.9,** and **42.10** (▶ **Videos 42.8A, 42.8B, 42.9,** and **42.10**).

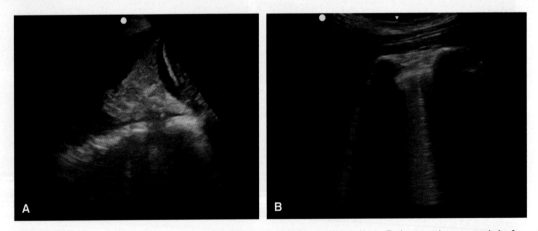

**Figure 42.8** A. Left lower lung. Coronal plane, posterior axillary line. B. Lung ultrasound. Left anterior chest wall.

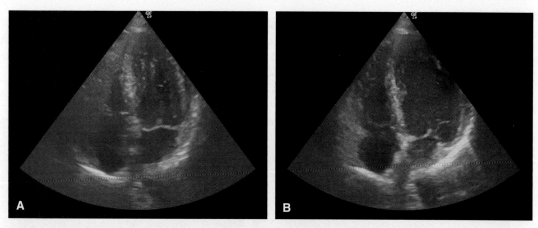

**Figure 42.9** Apical four-chamber view. A. End-systole. B. End-diastole.

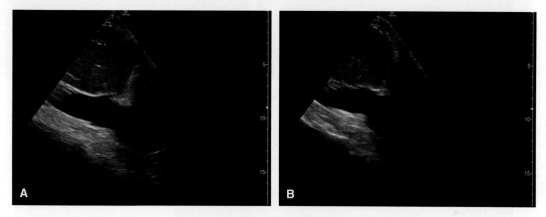

**Figure 42.10** Subcostal inferior vena cava view. A. Expiration. B. Inspiration.

What is the best next step in the management of this patient?
A. Give additional IV fluids.
B. Start vasopressors.
C. Start anticoagulation for pulmonary embolism.
D. Pericardiocentesis for presence of tamponade.

4. Which of the following statements is accurate about velocity-time integral (VTI)?

A. It is a derivative of velocity, that is, acceleration.
B. It is a linear measure, that is, its units are centimeter or meter.
C. It assumes that aortic outflow tract is a cylinder, circular in cross-section.
D. In an average size person with the HR between 65 and 80 normal VTI is 40 ± 4.

5. A 70-year-old woman with hypertension and obesity is brought in by ambulance to the emergency room from her dentist's office with undifferentiated shock. She is afebrile; her arterial BP is 80/40 mm Hg, HR is 52 bpm. She is in respiratory distress with an RR of 30 breaths/min and is wheezing. Arterial oxygen saturation is 99% on room air. Aortic outflow diameter measured in parasternal short-axis (PSAX) view is 1.8 cm. PSAX view is shown in **Figure 42.11** and ▶ **Video 42.11**.

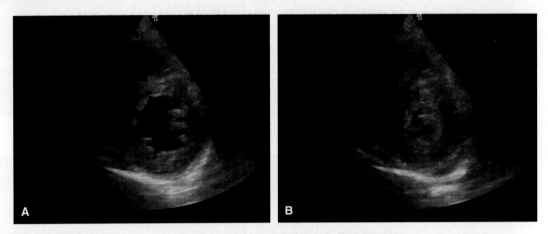

**Figure 42.11** Parasternal short-axis view. A. End-diastole. B. End-systole.

Pulse-wave Doppler of aortic ejection is shown in **Figure 42.12**.
VTI is calculated to be 23.2 cm. IVC was small and completely collapsing on inspiration. Lung ultrasound with A-line pattern in all lung fields.

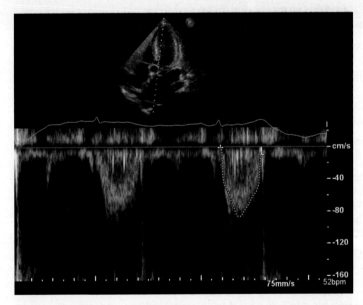

**Figure 42.12** Pulse-wave Doppler of aortic ejection. Velocity-time integral = 23.2 cm.

Which one of the following best describes the patient's physiology?
A. Cardiogenic physiology is solely responsible for this patient's shock.
B. Distributive physiology is solely responsible for this patient's shock.
C. The patient has a combination of cardiogenic and distributive physiology.
D. Neither cardiogenic nor distributive physiology is contributing to this patient's shock physiology.

6. A 63-year-old man fell from ladder and was admitted to the intensive care unit (ICU) from the Emergency Department. His injury burden included splenic injury, T4 level paraplegia from spinal cord injury, T4 level burst vertebral fracture, and bilateral calcaneal injury. He received 2 L of Lactated Ringer's in the Emergency Department for hypotension. His past medical history is significant for heart failure with reduced ejection fraction (EF). He arrives in the ICU for initial stabilization before going to the operating room for decompression and fixation of the thoracic vertebral column. On arrival to the ICU, his vitals are BP 80/40 mm Hg, HR 53 bpm, RR 18 breaths/min, and temperature 97 °F. Point of care ultrasound images are shown in **Figure 42.13** and ▶ **Video 42.12**.

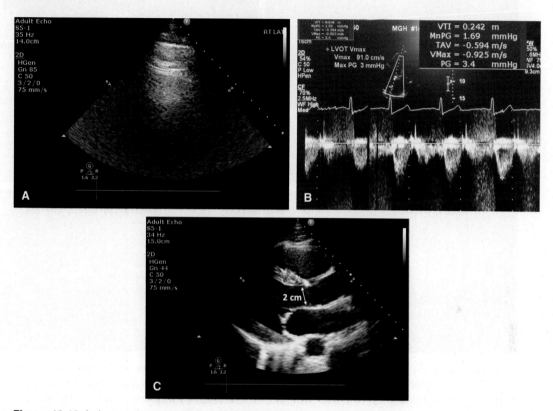

**Figure 42.13** A. Lung ultrasound. B. Apical five-chamber view. C. Parasternal long-axis view. (See ▶ **Video 42.12** for parasternal short-axis view.)

What is the most appropriate next step in his management?
A. Dobutamine
B. 1 L fluid bolus
C. Norepinephrine
D. Phenylephrine

7. A patient presents to the Emergency Department with urosepsis. His past medical history is significant for diastolic heart failure. He received 2 L Lactated Ringer's in the Emergency Department for hypotension and then was transferred to the ICU. On arrival to the ICU, he continues to be hypotensive and is mildly short of breath. Vitals: BP 80/40 mm Hg, HR 114 bpm, RR 24 breaths/min, SpO$_2$ 94% on 3 L NC. The following point-of-care ultrasound (POCUS) images are obtained and shown in **Figure 42.14** and ▶ **Video 42.13**.

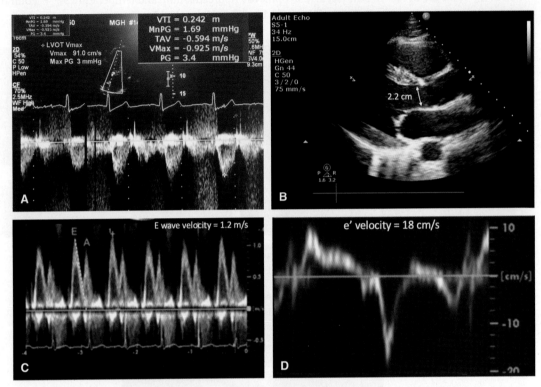

**Figure 42.14** Apical five-chamber view with pulse wave Doppler in the left ventricular outflow tract. B. Parasternal long-axis view. C. Apical four-chamber view with pulse-wave Doppler in mitral inflow. D. Apical four-chamber view with tissue Doppler at lateral mitral annulus.

What is the next best step in management based on these findings?
A. Diuresis
B. Fluid bolus
C. Milrinone
D. Norepinephrine

# Chapter 42 ▪ Answers

---

**1.** Correct Answer: B. The patient is likely to tolerate additional IV fluids.

*Rationale:* This patient with premorbid cardiomyopathy and decreased LV systolic function presents with septic shock secondary to pyelonephritis. After initial fluid resuscitation, her BP remains low, with signs of organ hypoperfusion. The presence of A-line pattern on lung ultrasound suggests that left atrial pressure (LAP) is not elevated. Correlation between IVC static and dynamic parameters is imperfect and is affected by extraneous factors, such as intra-abdominal pressure, spontaneous (vs. mechanical) ventilation, inspiratory effort, and premorbid fitness. Nonetheless, a very small IVC that is completely collapsing on inspiration suggests that right atrial pressure (RAP) is not elevated.

Utility of using static and/or dynamic IVC parameters to predict volume responsiveness in shock is disputed. Nonetheless, normal/low LAP and RAP suggest that this patient is likely to be fluid tolerant. The concept of fluid tolerance, as opposed to fluid responsiveness, is central to understanding of shock management. Fluid responsiveness is the increase in 10% to 15% of CO when you give a 500 cc bolus of fluids or do passive leg raise. Fluid intolerance is when IV fluids are no longer helpful and may cause harm. In patients with sepsis and vasodilation, even if they are persistently hypotensive and tachycardic, at some point, fluids will no longer increase the CO because the flat portion of the Starling curve is reached and continuing to give fluids has been shown to increase mortality.

**Selected References**
1. Dipti A, Soucy Z, Surana A, Chandra S. Role of inferior vena cava diameter in assessment of volume status: a meta-analysis. *Am J Emerg Med.* 2012;30(8):1414-1419.
2. Jankowich M, Gartman E. *Ultrasound in the Intensive Care Unit.* Humana Press, Springer; 2015.
3. Lichtenstein DA, Mezière GA, Lagoueyte JF, Biderman P, Goldstein I, Gepner A. Lung ultrasound as a bedside tool for predicting pulmonary artery occlusion pressure in the critically ill. *Chest.* 2009; 136:10141-1020.
4. Orso D, Paoli I, Piani T, Cilenti FL, Cristiani L, Guglielmo N. Accuracy of ultrasonographic measurements of inferior vena cava to determine fluid responsiveness: a systematic review and meta-analysis. *J Intensive Care Med.* 2020;35(4):354-363.

---

**2.** Correct Answer: C. The patient is likely fluid responsive.

*Rationale:* In spontaneously breathing patients air enters the lungs because of negative intrathoracic pressure generated during inspiration. This same negative intrathoracic pressure sucks blood from the abdominal IVC into the thorax and the right atrium (RA), causing decrease in IVC size on inspiration. In patients on PPV air instead is forced into the lungs by an external device and, if the patient is "passive on the ventilator," increases intrathoracic pressure on inspiration. This increase in intrathoracic pressure is transmitted to the RA and causes decrease in blood return from the IVC. Consequently, PPV reverses the relationship between the phases of respiratory cycle and IVC size, with decrease in IVC occurring during expiration instead of inspiration. In addition, essentially all PPV includes positive end-expiratory pressure (PEEP), which means that at its lowest (during expiration) intrathoracic pressure is still higher than in spontaneously breathing persons (in whom end-expiratory pressure is zero). This elevation of intrathoracic pressure tends to increase IVC size (a static parameter) and to alter the relationship between RAP and IVC size.

Multiple studies have failed to consistently identify a single cutoff of static and/or dynamic IVC parameters in distinguishing patients with shock who are fluid responsive from those who are not. Despite that, if one allows for a "gray zone" that is diagnostically noninformative, studies support the use of IVC size at its extremes. A very small IVC in a patient who is passive on a ventilator strongly suggests low RAP. Even though RAP is not synonymous with fluid responsiveness, it is often a useful marker when more sophisticated methods are not available.

In addition, in this patient lung ultrasound A-pattern suggests that the patient is not in pulmonary edema and can likely tolerate additional IV fluids, that is, is likely to be fluid tolerant.

**Selected References**
1. Jankowich M, Gartman E. *Ultrasound in the Intensive Care Unit.* Human Press; 2015.
2. Via G, Tavazzi G, Price S. Ten situations where inferior vena cava ultrasound may fail to accurately predict fluid responsiveness: a physiologic based point of view. *Intensive Care Med.* 2016;42:1164-1167.

3. Viellard-Baron A, Evrard B, Repesse X, et al. Limited value of end-expiratory inferior vena cava diameter to predict fluid responsiveness impact of intra-abdominal pressure. *Intensive Care Med.* 2018;44:197-203.

**3.** Correct Answer: B. Start vasopressors

*Rationale:* This patient is likely in distributive shock from sepsis. In a patient with sepsis with capillary leak, once preload has been optimized, further fluid is unlikely to further increase CO but may cause edema and end-organ dysfunction. Despite the poor evidence correlating IVC size and collapsibility in predicting fluid responsiveness, the presence of a plethoric IVC with no respiratory variability strongly suggests that this patient is fluid intolerant. This patient does not have other evidence of obstructive shock associated with a plethoric IVC given the normal right ventricle size and lack of pericardial effusion. The B-lines seen can represent pulmonary edema, but may also be seen in a patient with multifocal pneumonia.

Selected References
1. Muller L, Bobbia X, Toumi M, et al. Respiratory variation of inferior vena cava diameter to predict fluid responsiveness in spontaneously breathing patients with acute circulatory failure: need for a cautious use. *Crit Care.* 2012;16(5):R188.
2. Orso D, Paoli I, Piani T, Cilenti FL, Cristiani L, Guglielmo N. Accuracy of ultrasonographic measurements of inferior vena cava to determine fluid responsiveness: a systematic review and meta-analysis. *J Intensive Care Med.* 2020;35(4):354-363.

**4.** Correct Answer: B. It is a linear measure, that is, its units are centimeter or meter.

*Rationale:* As the name suggests, VTI is a time integral of velocity and is, therefore, the area under the velocity graph. Recall that acceleration is a derivative of velocity over time and velocity is a derivative of the distance over time. Conversely, velocity is a time integral of acceleration and distance is a time integral of velocity. VTI is therefore the *distance* that a column of blood travels during the time of systolic ejection. It is measured in linear units: centimeter or meter. Multiplying that traveled distance by the area of the column of blood (i.e., by the cross-sectional area of the LV outflow tract [LVOT]) yields volume of blood moved during systolic ejection—that is, an SV. Multiplying SV by HR yields CO, and indexing CO to body surface area results in cardiac index. VTI measurement makes no assumptions about the geometry of the LVOT, but estimation of the LVOT cross-sectional area does. The standard method measures the diameter ($d$) of the LVOT and assumes that its cross-section is circular in shape. Consequently, the area of LVOT is calculated as. In reality, LVOT is oval rather than circular in shape, which introduces an error into the area estimation.

VTI by itself, without accounting for the size of the LVOT tract and the HR, should be interpreted with caution. Normal CO is 4 to 8 L/min. With the HR 65-80 this translates into the normal SV range of approximately 60 to 100 mL/beat. On average, LVOT diameter is 2.1 ± 0.4 cm, which translates into an area of 3.6 ± 1.3 cm². Therefore, the normal range of VTI in a person with an average size LVOT is 18 to 28 cm or 23 ± 5 cm.

Selected Reference
1. Sarti A, Lorini FL. *Echocardiography for Intensivists.* Springer; 2012.

**5.** Correct Answer: C. The patient has a combination of cardiogenic and distributive physiology.

*Rationale:* Salient features of the case include shock, hyperdynamic LV with EF of 100% and bradycardia, and IVC is small and completely collapsing on inspiration.

The first impression is that the patient must be in distributive or hypovolemic shock based on the low RAP and hyperdynamic LV, which is squeezing all the blood during systole that it can. However, it is important to remember that CO and SV are not equivalent.

$$A_{LVOT} = 3.14 \times \frac{1.8^2}{4} = 2.5 \text{ cm}^2$$

$$SV = VTI \times A_{LVOT} \times 23.2 \times 2.5 = 58 \text{ cc}$$

$$CO = SV \times HR = 58 \times 52 = 3 \text{ L/min}$$

SV in this patient is estimated to be 58 cc, which is within the normal limits, though it is not appropriately increased in the context of hypotension. However, CO is certainly inadequate at 3 L/min. This combination of findings suggests bradycardia as at least a contributing factor in the patient's presentation.

Generally, patients with pure distributive shock have high CO. However, if inotropic and/or chronotropic cardiac response is impaired, the heart may not be able to adequately compensate for the need for increase in CO imposed by vasodilation. This combination can be seen in patients with intrinsic conduction disease or those on beta-blockers who experience concomitant vasodilation because of shock, anaphylaxis, etc. Transient vagotonia may result in both cardiodepressant and vasodilatory physiology and present similarly to the described patient. In this case the patient was on chronic high-dose beta-blocker therapy and had an anaphylactic reaction to the local anesthetic (administered at the dentist's office).

### Selected References

1. Jankowich M, Gartman E. *Ultrasound in the Intensive Care Unit.* Humana Press, Springer; 2015.
2. Sarti A, Lorini FL. *Echocardiography for Intensivists.* Springer; 2012.

---

**6.** Correct Answer: C. Norepinephrine

*Rationale:* Based on his history and injury burden, the differentials for shock in this case are neurogenic (given level of spinal cord injury), hypovolemic (splenic injury), and cardiogenic (heart failure with reduced EF). SV can be calculated from these images using the equation:

$$SV = VTI_{LVOT} \times \pi \, (d/2)^2$$

$$SV = 24.2 \text{ cm} \times 3.14 \times (2 \text{ cm}/2)^2 = 76 \text{ mL}$$

(SV—stroke volume, $VTI_{LVOT}$—velocity-time integral at left ventricular outflow tract, *d*—diameter of LVOT)

The normal to high SV (76 mL) rules out hypovolemic and cardiogenic shock. Also, the A-line profile on lung ultrasound (absence of pulmonary edema) argues against cardiogenic shock. The moderately reduced LVEF seen on the mid-papillary short-axis view of the left ventricle is likely preexisting, given the history of heart failure with reduced EF. A normal SV in the setting of shock suggests a distributive etiology of the shock. In this patient, the most likely etiology of distributive shock is neurogenic. The high thoracic (above T6) injury and low HR support the diagnosis of neurogenic shock. Since the patient already received initial fluid resuscitation in the Emergency Department and the SV is adequate, this primarily is a vasomotor tone incompetence. Hence, the next best step is a norepinephrine infusion. An additional fluid bolus of 1 L might not yield results given the normal SV suggesting presence of adequate preload.

Neurogenic shock results from interruption of autonomic pathways in the spinal cord (sympathetic nervous system pathways) leading to reduced vasomotor tone. It is usually accompanied by bradycardia. Vasoactive agents that will increase vascular tone and HR are recommended (e.g., norepinephrine). Guidelines recommend maintaining a higher mean arterial pressure of >85 mm Hg, although there are limited data supporting it. Hence, in this patient norepinephrine is the next best step. Although additional fluids might also help, presence of adequate SV argues against it. Also, empiric fluid administration is not preferred in a patient with a history of heart failure, given risk of precipitating congestive heart failure. Dobutamine is primarily an inotrope and is not beneficial in the setting of distributive shock. Phenylephrine is a pure alpha-agonist and hence will not increase the HR, and potentially can cause reflex bradycardia. Hence, it is not the first-line option in our patient with bradycardia.

### Selected References

1. Grigorean VT, Sandu AM, Popescu M, et al. Cardiac dysfunctions following spinal cord injury. *J Med Life.* 2009 Apr-Jun;2(2):133-145.
2. Yue JK, Tsolinas RE, Burke JF, et al. Vasopressor support in managing acute spinal cord injury: current knowledge. *J Neurosurg Sci.* 2019 Jun;63(3):308-317. doi: 10.23736/S0390-5616.17.04003-6. Epub 2017 Mar 1.

**7.** Correct Answer: D. Norepinephrine

*Rationale:* We can calculate this patient's CO using the following equation:

$$CO = SV \times HR = VTI_{LVOT} \times \pi \, (d/2)^2 \times HR = 24.2 \times 3.14 \times (2.2 \text{ cm}/2)^2 \times 114 = 10.5 \text{ L/min}$$

(CO—cardiac output, SV—stroke volume, VTI$_{LVOT}$—velocity-time integral at left ventricular outflow tract, *d*—diameter of LVOT, HR—heart rate)

A CO of 10.5 L/min rules out cardiogenic shock and hypovolemia. Hence, options milrinone and fluid bolus are incorrect. Presence of B-lines on lung ultrasound and clinical respiratory insufficiency suggest pulmonary edema. This could be either cardiogenic or noncardiogenic. The history of diastolic heart failure and recent 2 L fluid bolus raise the concern for cardiogenic pulmonary edema. On the other hand, urosepsis and associated endothelial dysfunction can lead to noncardiogenic pulmonary edema. This can be differentiated by measuring echocardiographic surrogates for pulmonary capillary wedge pressure, LV end-diastolic pressure, or LAP. The images provided allow us to calculate E/e', which is 6.7 in this case. An E/ e' <14 suggests normal pulmonary capillary wedge pressure and argues against cardiogenic pulmonary edema, and hence no further diuresis is needed. High CO in the setting of hypotension supports a diagnosis of distributive shock (likely from urosepsis). In this patient with distributive shock, maintaining the mean arterial pressure above 65 mm Hg with vasopressors (like norepinephrine) is essential to maintain end-organ perfusion.

Selected Reference
1. Mitter SS, Shah SJ, Thomas JD. A test in context: E/A and E/e' to assess diastolic dysfunction and LV filling pressure. *J Am Coll Cardiol.* 2017 Mar 21;69(11):1451-1464. doi: 10.1016/j.jacc.2016.12.037.

# 43 | CARDIOGENIC SHOCK

Negmeldeen Mamoun, Rasesh Desai, and J. Mauricio Del Rio

1. A 24-year-old male with a history of pulmonary sarcoidosis was admitted to the intensive care unit (ICU) with severe respiratory distress due to suspected pneumonia, which required urgent intubation. The patient was hypotensive after intubation, a transesophageal echocardiogram (TEE) was performed, and significant findings are shown (▶ Videos 43.1 and 43.2):

   After reviewing ▶ Videos 43.1 and 43.2, please select the finding less consistent with the visualized images:
   A. Moderate right ventricular (RV) dilation
   B. Tricuspid annular plane systolic excursion (TAPSE) measurement of <17 mm
   C. Tricuspid lateral annular systolic velocity measurement of <9.5 cm/s
   D. Right atrial (RA) dilation
   E. Interventricular septum (IVS) flattening

2. A 72-year-old female in the cardiothoracic ICU (CTICU) after thoracoabdominal aortic aneurysm repair develops bilateral lower extremity weakness. The neurologic insult and the associated emotional stress are followed by supraventricular tachycardia and hypertension; 5 mg of intravenous (IV) metoprolol is administered, which precipitates severe refractory hypotension. The patient is resuscitated appropriately, and a bedside transthoracic echocardiogram (TTE) is done. Significant findings are shown in ▶ Videos 43.3, 43.4, 43.5, 43.6.

   Which among the following statements is least associated with the suspected diagnosis?
   A. Left ventricular (LV) systolic wall motion abnormalities that are beyond a single coronary artery distribution
   B. Absence of coronary artery disease (CAD) or angiographic evidence of plaque rupture
   C. Managed with supportive therapy, with most patients recovering within 1 to 4 weeks
   D. It is crucial to augment cardiac output (CO) with catecholamines to avoid tissue hypoperfusion.
   E. Typically observed in postmenopausal women in Western countries following an emotional or physical stress

3. A 63-year-old female with a history of CAD was admitted to the surgical ICU (SICU) after failing extubation at the end of a total hip arthroplasty surgery that was complicated by bleeding and multiple blood transfusions. The intensivist performed a TTE at the bedside in order to estimate the patient's CO. Left ventricular outflow tract (LVOT) diameter was measured as 1.9 cm (**Figure 43.1A**), and LVOT velocity time integral (VTI) was measured as 26.6 cm (**Figure 43.1B**).

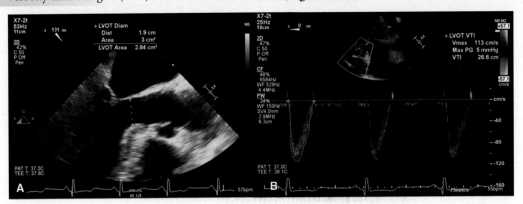

**Figure 43.1**

What is the patient's calculated cardiac index (CI) if the HR was 72 bpm and the patient's body surface area (BSA) is 1.94 m²?

A. 1.9 L/min/m²
B. 2.3 L/min/m²
C. 2.8 L/min/m²
D. 2.0 L/min/m²
E. 3.1 L/min/m²

4. A 73-year-old male with a history of aortic stenosis (AS) was admitted to the ICU in cardiogenic shock in the setting of atrial fibrillation with rapid ventricular response. The patient was electrically cardioverted into sinus rhythm, and a TTE was performed to assess the severity of AS. Interrogation with continuous wave Doppler (CWD) across the aortic valve (AV) showed an AV VTI of 112 cm (**Figure 43.2A**), and a pulsed-wave Doppler (PWD) across the LVOT showed an LVOT VTI of 26 cm (**Figure 43.2B**). The two-dimensional (2D) assessment of the LVOT revealed a diameter of 2 cm (**Figure 43.2C**).

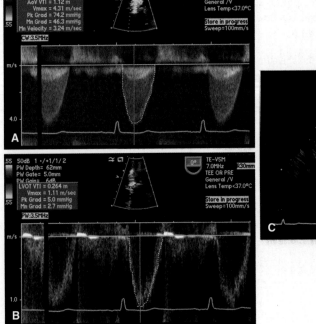

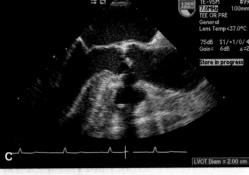

**Figure 43.2**

What is the calculated AV area for this patient?
A. 1 cm$^2$
B. 0.72 cm$^2$
C. 0.89 cm$^2$
D. 1.2 cm$^2$
E. 0.58 cm$^2$

5. A 76-year-old female with a past medical history of hypertension and diabetes presented to the emergency room (ER) with severe mitral regurgitation (MR). She was transferred to the ICU where she became progressively hypotensive, not responsive to IV fluids and boluses of phenylephrine. The patient was intubated emergently and given multiple boluses of 100 μg epinephrine with increasing HR but worsening hypotension, a TEE examination was performed immediately, and significant findings are shown in ▶ **Videos 43.7, 43.8, 43.9, 43.10**.

Which one of the following steps in the management of this patient likely will increase hemodynamic instability?
A. Administering more IV fluids
B. Administering more phenylephrine
C. Administering beta-blockers
D. Administering epinephrine boluses
E. Reverse Trendelenburg position

6. A 64-year-old retired nurse presented with chest pain that started when he was lifting weights at home. Computed tomography (CT) scan at an outside hospital showed extensive aortic dissection from the aortic root to the iliac bifurcation. The patient became hypotensive during transfer, with altered mental status and was intubated emergently. On admission to the ICU, the patient continued to be hemodynamically unstable despite fluid resuscitation, inotropic and vasopressor support. TEE was performed to guide further management and significant findings are shown in ▶ **Videos 43.11** and **43.12**.

Which of the following is *not* an echocardiographic criterion for the diagnosis of cardiac tamponade?
A. The presence of a pericardial effusion
B. Evidence of elevated RA pressure such as dilated inferior vena cava (IVC)
C. Respirophasic variability in the transmitral Doppler velocities of <30%
D. RA indentation/inversion during ventricular systole
E. RV indentation/inversion during ventricular diastole

7. A 37-year-old athletic male was running a marathon when he collapsed. Initially, the event was suspected to be a heat stroke at the scene. Cardiopulmonary resuscitation (CPR) was started once it was recognized that it was a cardiac arrest, and the patient was ultimately placed on veno-arterial (VA) extracorporeal membrane oxygenation (ECMO) via peripheral cannulation due to postcardiac arrest cardiogenic shock. In the CTICU, a TEE was performed due to lack of pulsatility on the arterial line tracing despite being on a high dose of inotropic support. The left ventricle appeared distended, as evident in ▶ **Videos 43.13** and **43.14**.

Please select the least effective measure to decrease LV distension.
A. Placing an intra-aortic balloon pump (IABP)
B. Placing a percutaneous Impella® 2.5 assist device
C. Left atrial (LA) venting via atrial septostomy
D. Switching VA-ECMO to veno-arterial-venous (VAV)-ECMO
E. Pulmonary artery (PA) drainage

8. A 63-year-old male with a history of a large renal cell carcinoma develops abrupt shortness of breath. The patient becomes markedly hypotensive and hypoxemic. The patient is intubated emergently, and a TEE is performed. Significant findings are shown in ▶ **Videos 43.15, 43.16, 43.17**.

Which of the following statements is characteristic of the suspected diagnosis?
A. McConnell sign is pathognomonic for pulmonary embolism (PE).
B. The patient has preserved RV size and function.
C. Echocardiography cannot confirm the diagnosis.
D. Echocardiography is the gold standard test for diagnosis.
E. RV dilation/dysfunction predicts worse prognosis.

9. A 48-year-old male who suffers a cardiac arrest is emergently peripherally cannulated for VA-ECMO support. Subsequently, echocardiography is performed showing LV distension. A percutaneously inserted Impella® 2.5 assist device is placed to decrease LV distension and reduce the risk of aortic root thrombosis secondary to lack of pulsatility. TEE is performed the next day to guide management and significant findings are shown in ▶ **Videos 43.18** and **43.19**.

Which of the following statements is *true* about Impella® device placement?
A. The catheter's inlet area should be into the left ventricle about 2 cm from the AV annulus.
B. The catheter's outlet area should be proximal to the aortic root.
C. Impella's flow makes it impossible for clots to form in the aortic root.
D. Severe aortic insufficiency (AI) is a contraindication to Impella® device placement.
E. All types of Impella® assist devices can be placed percutaneously.

10. A 69-year-old male with ischemic cardiomyopathy presents to the hospital with heart failure with reduced ejection fraction (left ventricular ejection fraction [LVEF] 15%). The patient undergoes left ventricular assist device (LVAD) HeartMate III placement. On the first postoperative day, he continues to have low CO with multiple suction events, prompting the intensivist to perform a TEE. Significant findings are shown in ▶ **Videos 43.20, 43.21, 43.22**.

Among the following situations, which one is the least associated with suction events during LVAD support?
A. Decreased preload (e.g., bleeding or hypovolemia)
B. Decreased afterload (e.g., vasoplegia or hypotension)
C. RV failure
D. Decreased LVAD pump speed
E. Mispositioned LVAD inflow cannula

11. A 68-year-old man undergoes an emergent coronary artery bypass graft (CABG) surgery under cardiopulmonary bypass (CPB). The patient develops severe coagulopathy requiring massive transfusion and transient shock during the immediate postoperative period. Despite resolution of the hemodynamic instability, there is progressive oliguria. The central venous pressure (CVP) is 25 mm Hg, pulmonary capillary wedge pressure (PCWP) is 12 mm Hg, and the CI is within normal limits. Compared with baseline, the serum creatinine level has increased. While the patient is on mechanical ventilation, the plateau airway pressure is 38 cm $H_2O$ and tidal volume is ~300 mL. What is the most appropriate next diagnostic step in this situation?

A. Perform a TEE examination
B. Perform chest, abdomen, and pelvis CT scan
C. Determine intra-abdominal pressure
D. Perform diagnostic laparoscopy or laparotomy
E. Perform a decubitus abdominal X-ray

12. A 76-year-old man undergoes a surgical aortic valve replacement (SAVR) via median sternotomy. The immediate postoperative period is complicated by coagulopathy and significant bleeding requiring multiple blood products transfusions. On postoperative day 4, the patient complains of progressive dyspnea at rest for several hours. In addition, the patient develops oliguria. Pertinent additional data include the following:

- Mean arterial pressure (MAP): 61 mm Hg
- HR: 112 bpm
- Respiratory rate (RR): 29 breaths/min
- CVP: 18 mm Hg

What is the *best* next course of action?
A. To obtain a comprehensive TEE
B. To obtain a CT scan of the chest
C. To obtain a portable chest X-ray
D. To obtain a focused bedside TTE
E. Perform a mediastinal exploration

13. Echocardiography has an essential role during management of patients under ECMO support. As a modality to support decision making and to guide management, the use of echocardiography has the *greatest* impact in which of the following situations?

A. For evaluation of the insertion site for peripheral ECMO cannulation
B. For determination of cannula sizes prior to cannulation
C. For monitoring during venovenous ECMO support weaning
D. For diagnosis and management of complications such as cannula malposition, cardiac tamponade, or intracardiac thrombus formation
E. For routine patient management in the ICU

14. A 66-year-old female with a past medical history of chronic systolic and diastolic heart failure presents in exacerbation with dyspnea now at rest, increase in lower extremity edema, fatigue, and increased jugular venous distension (**Figure 43.3**).

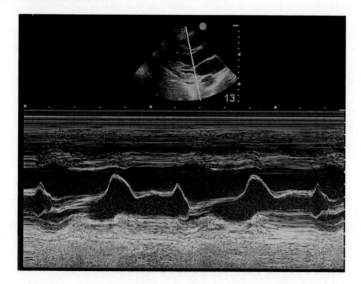

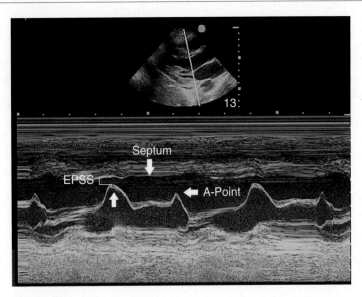

**Figure 43.3**

Which of the following echocardiographic values for systolic function correlates with a reduced LVEF?
A. Mitral valve (MV) annular plane systolic excursion of 11 mm
B. E-point septal separation (EPSS) of 10 mm
C. dP/dT of 1400 mm Hg/s
D. Fractional shortening of 37%
E. LV wall thickening >30% of diastolic thickness

15. A 23-year-old male presents 4 hours after a bonfire incident to the burn ICU with 35% total body surface area (TBSA) burns to his legs, abdomen, and chest. There are no other major injuries per his primary and secondary surveys. He arrives to the ICU with the following vital signs:

   - HR: 135 bpm
   - BP: 88/38 mm Hg, RR: 24 breaths/min
   - Arterial $O_2$ saturation ($SaO_2$): 96%

   A TTE is performed at the bedside to evaluate his volume status and biventricular cardiac function. Given the patient's recent burn injuries, his current hemodynamic profile is characterized by the following TTE pattern during passive leg raise testing:
   A. Increase in VTI/stroke volume (SV) by <12.5% during passive leg raise and decreased systolic function
   B. Increase in VTI/SV by <12.5% during passive leg raise and hyperdynamic systolic function
   C. Increase in VTI/SV by >12.5% during passive leg raise and decreased systolic function
   D. Increase in VTI/SV by >12.5% during passive leg raise and hyperdynamic systolic function
   E. Increase in VTI/SV by <12.5% during passive leg raise and decreased systolic function

16. A 75-year-old female with a past medical history of poorly controlled diabetes mellitus type II, chronic obstructive pulmonary disease (COPD), hypertension, hyperlipidemia, history of recurrent COPD exacerbations, and prior myocardial infarctions is found down in her nursing home and is unresponsive with severe hypotension. She arrives intubated and sedated with the following vital signs:

   - Temperature: 38.3 °C
   - HR: 107 bpm
   - BP: 77/38 mm Hg
   - RR: 16 breaths/min
   - $SaO_2$: 97% on 50% $FiO_2$

   Chest X-ray shows diffuse bilateral infiltrates. TTE is performed as part of her diagnostic workup and reveals severely reduced biventricular systolic function. Which of the following additional echocardiographic findings would support a diagnosis of septic cardiomyopathy over cardiogenic shock?

**A.** E/A ratio of 1.5 and normal pulmonary vein Doppler flow profile
**B.** RV diastolic collapse
**C.** LV dP/dT of 560 mm Hg/s
**D.** RV longitudinal myocardial velocity (S') of 7.5 mm/s
**E.** Inferior vena Cava diameter < 22 mm

17. A 57-year-old male with a past medical history of hypertension, hyperlipidemia, diabetes mellitus type II, COPD secondary to smoking, and chronic kidney disease stage III presents to the Emergency Department after 2 hours of severe substernal chest pressure. Which one of the following values is the lower limit of normal mitral annular plane systolic excursion (MAPSE), below which the LV systolic function is impaired?

    **A.** 16 mm
    **B.** 12 mm
    **C.** 8 mm
    **D.** 6 mm
    **E.** 20 mm

18. A 68-year-old male with a past medical history of CAD treated with percutaneous coronary intervention (PCI) several years ago and known cardiomyopathy presents with increased dyspnea at rest, jugular venous distension, and lower extremity edema. Vital signs are as follows:

    - HR: 102 bpm
    - BP: 85/43 mm Hg
    - RR: 18 breaths/min
    - $SaO_2$: 93% on 3 L of $O_2$ via nasal cannula

    TTE reveals a dP/dT of 557 mm Hg/s on the left ventricle and 187 mm Hg/s in the right ventricle. Based on this information, which of the following interventions would be appropriate for this patient?
    **A.** IV fluids
    **B.** IV fluids and vasopressor agents
    **C.** Inotropic agents
    **D.** Beta-blockers and afterload reduction
    **E.** Calcium channel blockers

19. A 73-year-old female with a past medical history of hypertension and osteoarthritis presents with new-onset dyspnea, fatigue, and chest tightness shortly after the funeral of her husband of 50 years. Which of the following findings may be visualized by echocardiographic examination in patients with Takotsubo cardiomyopathy?

    **A.** Presence of LV apical ballooning and hyperdynamic LV basal segments not limited to any single coronary distribution
    **B.** Evidence of RV dysfunction
    **C.** Presence of LVOT obstruction and acute MR
    **D.** Pericardial effusion
    **E.** All of the above

20. A 49-year-old female presents with 2 months of progressive dyspnea on exertion and lower extremities swelling accompanied by recurrent nausea and anorexia. Her past medical history is significant for morbid obesity and deep venous thrombosis 5 years prior. Upon admission to the ER an N-terminal pro-brain natriuretic peptide (NT-proBNP) level of 650 pg/mL was obtained. Which of the following echocardiographic parameters would support the diagnosis of RV failure?

    **A.** RV fractional area change (FAC) 62%
    **B.** TAPSE 18 mm
    **C.** IVC diameter 2.4 cm and no respiratory collapse
    **D.** Peak tricuspid regurgitation (TR) jet velocity 1.8 m/s
    **E.** RV basal diameter < 30mm

21. A 41-year-old male is admitted to an ICU after a syncopal episode. During the last week, the patient has been complaining of progressive fatigue, malaise, fever, and chills in the setting of a recent respiratory infection. As per his family, he has no significant past medical history. The initial vital signs are as follows:

    - BP: 82/44 mm Hg
    - HR: 122 bpm
    - RR: 26 breaths/min
    - $SaO_2$: 93% on 4 L of $O_2$ via nasal cannula

    An electrocardiogram (ECG) shows sinus tachycardia and the initial chest X-ray demonstrates bilateral pulmonary edema. Which of the following echocardiographic parameters would support the initial diagnosis of cardiogenic instead of septic shock?
    A. LVEF 75%
    B. LVOT VTI: 23 cm
    C. Mitral inflow E/A ratio: 3 and E/e' ratio: 18
    D. Dynamic LVOT obstruction
    E. LV End-diastolic diameter < 3 cm

22. A 29-year-old male patient with cystic fibrosis and advanced secondary lung disease presents with dyspnea at rest, generalized edema, and jaundice. Upon physical examination, there is systemic hypotension, cold extremities with decreased capillary refill, and anasarca. Laboratory studies are remarkable for lactic acidemia, elevated serum creatinine, alkaline phosphatase, and total bilirubin. The initial workup includes echocardiography (▶ **Video 43.23**).

    According to the visualized part of the examination, which of the following echocardiographic findings is most closely associated with the presence of severe RV dysfunction in this patient with RV failure?
    A. Leftward IVS motion at end-diastole
    B. Leftward IVS motion at end-systole
    C. RV end-diastolic area/LV end-diastolic area > 1 and paradoxical IVS motion
    D. Severe RV hypertrophy

23. According to the echocardiographic findings evident in ▶ **Video 43.24**, which mechanism is responsible for the limited LV compliance and diastolic filling?

    A. Severe RV hypertrophy
    B. Elevated ventricular interdependence
    C. Increased RV pressure overload
    D. Increased RV volume overload
    E. RA dilation with leftward displacement of the interatrial septum

24. Echocardiography is used for evaluation of patients with an acute presentation of shock, in order to establish or to confirm the diagnosis and to guide management and response to therapeutic interventions. In this setting, which of the following echocardiographic indices is the *most* reliable surrogate for the estimation of CO?

    A. Estimated LVEF
    B. LV fractional shortening (FS)
    C. LVOT VTI
    D. E-point septal separation
    E. LV dP/dT > 1200 mm Hg/s

25. Which one of the following parameters is *not* an echocardiographic finding present in patients with significant pulmonary hypertension?

    A. Estimated systolic pulmonary artery pressure (sPAP) > 40 mm Hg
    B. Early diastolic pulmonic regurgitant (PR) jet velocity <2.0 m/s
    C. RV outflow tract (RVOT) PWD profile mid-systolic notch
    D. PA acceleration time <105 ms by RVOT PWD interrogation

# Chapter 43 ■ Answers

---

**1.** Correct Answer: **A. Moderate RV dilation**

*Rationale:* For qualitative assessment, the right ventricle should be evaluated in multiple tomographic planes. The right ventricle is most often compared with the left ventricle either visually or by comparing RV and LV end-diastolic areas. In any four-chamber view, a diastolic ventricular ratio of 0.6 to 1 signifies moderate RV dilation, while a ratio ≥1 like in our patient signifies severe RV dilation. Global visual assessment of RV function has been shown to be inaccurate. The consensus recommendation is to perform quantitative assessment of RV function, where TAPSE measurement of <17 mm or tricuspid lateral annular systolic velocity measurement of < 9.5 cm/s is highly suggestive of RV systolic dysfunction.

RV dilation and dysfunction are often accompanied by other findings easily identified by echocardiography, including RA or IVC dilation, TR, and IVS flattening leading to "D-shaped" LV geometric distortion. Leftward motion of the IVS during systole is suggestive of pressure overload, whereas leftward motion during diastole is suggestive of volume overload.

## Selected References

1. Lang RM, Badano LP, Mor-Avi V, et al. Recommendations for cardiac chamber quantification by echocardiography in adults: an update from the American Society of Echocardiography and the European Association of Cardiovascular Imaging. *J Am Soc Echocardiogr.* 2015;28(1):1-39.e14.
2. Ling LF, Obuchowski NA, Rodriguez L, Popovic Z, Kwon D, Marwick TH. Accuracy and interobserver concordance of echocardiographic assessment of right ventricular size and systolic function: a quality control exercise. *J Am Soc Echocardiogr.* 2012;25(7):709-713.
3. Schneider M, Binder T. Echocardiographic evaluation of the right heart. *Wien Klin Wochenschr.* 2018;130(13-14):413-420.

---

**2.** Correct Answer: **D. It is crucial to augment cardiac output (CO) with catecholamines to avoid tissue hypoperfusion.**

*Rationale:* Takotsubo cardiomyopathy was named after the Japanese octopus trap that has a shape similar to the systolic apical ballooning of the left ventricle that occurs in the most common and typical variant of the disease. Echocardiography detects the typical wall motion abnormalities that include akinetic mid- and apical LV segments with preservation of basal segment function. The pathogenesis of Takotsubo cardiomyopathy is probably multifactorial, but excess catecholamines have been postulated as a contributing mechanism. The disease is typically observed in postmenopausal women in Western countries following an emotional or physical stress, possibly causing catecholamine-induced direct myocardial toxicity or microvascular spasm. Since catecholamines are postulated as a contributing factor, catecholamine administration should be avoided.

The diagnosis of Takotsubo cardiomyopathy is challenging, especially that its initial presentation resembles acute coronary syndrome (ACS). The Mayo Clinic diagnostic criteria are most commonly used, where all four criteria are required to establish the diagnosis. Those criteria include:

- Transient LV systolic wall motion abnormalities that extend beyond a single coronary artery distribution
- Absence of CAD or angiographic evidence of plaque rupture
- New ECG abnormalities or modest increase in troponin
- Ruling out of pheochromocytoma and myocarditis

Takotsubo cardiomyopathy is usually managed with supportive therapy, and most patients recover within 1 to 4 weeks. It is usually referred to as a reversible self-limiting cardiomyopathy, and the dramatic recovery of cardiac function might give the impression that it is a benign disorder. However, 21.8% of patients with Takotsubo cardiomyopathy were reported to develop serious in-hospital complications. Indeed, people who recover usually achieve full recovery, but this highlights the importance of early recognition and proper management in the acute phase of the disease to avoid and treat complications.

Selected References
1. Prasad A. My approach to takotsubo (stress) cardiomyopathy. *Trends Cardiovasc Med.* 2015;25(8):751-752.
2. Templin C, Ghadri JR, Diekmann J, et al. Clinical features and outcomes of takotsubo (stress) cardiomyopathy. *N Engl J Med.* 2015;373(10):929-938.

**3.** Correct Answer: C. 2.8 L/min/m$^2$

*Rationale:* CO measurement is a cornerstone of hemodynamic assessment in critically ill patients. Hemodynamic evaluation utilizes 2D echocardiography and PWD. The SV across a reference point such as the LVOT can be calculated as the product of two variables: (1) cross-sectional area (CSA) of that reference point and (2) VTI measured at the same reference point using PWD. For example, SV is equal to the CSA of the LVOT multiplied by the LVOT VTI. The CO is then obtained by multiplying the SV by the HR, and CI by dividing CO by the patient's BSA.

$$SV \ (cm^3) = CSA \ (cm^2) \times VTI \ (cm)$$

$$SV_{LVOT} = CSA_{LVOT} \times VTI_{LVOT}$$

$$SV_{LVOT} = \pi r^2 \times VTI_{LVOT}$$

$$SV_{LVOT} = 3.14 \times (D/2)^2 \times VTI_{LVOT}$$

$$SV_{LVOT} = 3.14 \times (1.9/2)^2 \times 26.6 = 75 \ cm^3$$

$$CO = SV_{LVOT} \times HR$$

$$CO = 75 \times 72 = 5.4 \ L/min$$

$$CI = CO/BSA$$

$$CI = 5.4/1.94 = 2.8 \ L/min/m^2$$

The SV can be calculated by measuring the LVOT diameter (in the parasternal long-axis view by using TTE or midesophageal long-axis view when performing TEE) and the LVOT VTI (in the apical five-chamber or apical three-chamber views using TTE or the deep transgastric or transgastric long-axis views during TEE examination). The ability to quantify LV SV becomes especially useful in the ICU, where serial measurements of SV would allow goal-directed titration of inotropic support and help guide volume resuscitation.

Selected Reference
1. Porter TR, Shillcutt SK, Adams MS, et al. Guidelines for the use of echocardiography as a monitor for therapeutic intervention in adults: a report from the American Society of Echocardiography. *J Am Soc Echocardiogr.* 2015;28(1):40-56.

**4.** Correct Answer: B. 0.72 cm$^2$

*Rationale:* 2D echocardiography can often provide important clues to the AV anatomy and morphology, including the number of leaflets and commissures, mobility, and calcification. Functional evaluation by using color flow Doppler (CFD) and spectral Doppler can assess the level of obstruction—whether it is valvular, subvalvular, or supravalvular and the severity.

Severe AS can contribute to hemodynamic instability in the ICU. Level 1 recommendations from the American Society of Echocardiography (ASE) and European Association of Echocardiography (EAE) state that grading AS is appropriate and recommended using peak AV jet velocity, mean aortic transvalvular pressure gradient, and aortic valve area (AVA) in all patients with AS. Severe AS is diagnosed in the presence of preserved LV systolic function, by the presence of one or more of the following: (a) peak AV velocity of ≥4 m/s, (b) mean AV gradient of ≥40 mm Hg, and (c) AVA of <1 cm$^2$. However, if LV function is impaired, the former two parameters may underestimate the degree of stenosis, making AVA calculation using continuity equation more accurate because it is not flow dependent.

To calculate AVA using the continuity equation, measurements are commonly taken at the AV annulus (AVA = A1, $VTI_{AV}$ = V1) and within the LVOT ($CSA_{LVOT}$ = A2, $VTI_{LVOT}$ = V2):

$$A1 = A2 \times (V2/V1)$$

$$AVA = (CSA_{LVOT} \times VTI_{LVOT})/VTI_{AV}$$

$$AVA = (\Leftrightarrow \times (LVOT/2)^2 \times VTI_{LVOT})/VTI_{AV}$$

Selected Reference

1. Baumgartner H, Hung J, Bermejo J, et al. Recommendations on the echocardiographic assessment of aortic valve stenosis: a focused update from the European Association of Cardiovascular Imaging and the American Society of Echocardiography. *J Am Soc Echocardiogr.* 2017;30(4):372-392.

**5.** Correct Answer: **D. Administer epinephrine boluses**

*Rationale:* Dynamic LVOT obstruction can cause hemodynamic instability in critically ill patients. It typically occurs in patients with either hypertrophic obstructive cardiomyopathy (HOCM) or anterior mitral leaflet redundancy. Dynamic LVOT obstruction should always be suspected in patients who do not respond to inotropic support. 2D echocardiography can demonstrate a hypertrophic and hyperdynamic left ventricle with a small cavity. Doppler interrogation can show turbulent flow in the LVOT along with significant pressure gradients, possibly with acute MR caused by systolic anterior motion of the anterior mitral leaflet. Hemodynamic instability in such cases can be managed by stopping inotropic support, fluid resuscitation, slowing the HR, and increasing systemic vascular resistance with α-agonists.

Selected Reference

1. Costachescu T, Denault A, Guimond JG, et al. The hemodynamically unstable patient in the intensive care unit: hemodynamic vs. transesophageal echocardiographic monitoring. *Crit Care Med.* 2002;30(6):1214-1223.

**6.** Correct Answer: **C. Respirophasic variability in the transmitral Doppler velocities of <30%**

*Rationale:* In a patient with hypotension or dyspnea, echocardiographic evidence that supports the diagnosis of cardiac tamponade typically requires at least the following three key findings:

1. The presence of a pericardial effusion
2. Evidence of elevated RA pressure (e.g., dilated IVC and/or hepatic veins)
3. Small LV chamber dimensions in systole and diastole

A small percentage of patients with tamponade physiology (<10%) will actually have low or normal RA pressure ("low-pressure tamponade") and thus will fail to show IVC dilation. In such cases, other echocardiographic signs of chamber compression and/or ventricular interdependence should be looked for, including the following additional signs:

- RA chamber indentation/inversion during ventricular systole
- RV chamber indentation/inversion during ventricular diastole
- Respirophasic shifting of the IVS ("septal bounce") due to ventricular interdependence, where an external constraint prevents filling of the heart, forcing the ventricles to compete with one another during diastole, with each side of the heart filling more in a specific part of the respiratory cycle
- Exaggerated respirophasic variability in the Doppler velocities of transmitral (>30%) and/or transtricuspid (>40%) blood flow

Selected Reference

1. Klein AL, Abbara S, Agler DA, et al. American Society of Echocardiography clinical recommendations for multimodality cardiovascular imaging of patients with pericardial disease: endorsed by the Society for Cardiovascular Magnetic Resonance and Society of Cardiovascular Computed Tomography. *J Am Soc Echocardiogr.* 2013;26(9):965-1012.e1015.

**7.** Correct Answer: D. Switching VA-ECMO to veno-arterial-venous (VAV)-ECMO

*Rationale:* Echocardiography is helpful during all phases of VA-ECMO support. A baseline examination prior to initiation of support can correct reversible causes of hemodynamic instability and confirm the need for support. Echocardiography can guide cannulation, confirm proper position of cannulas, and detect complications associated with cannulation such as tamponade or dissection. Patients on VA-ECMO are monitored with echocardiography to evaluate LV size to ensure adequate unloading and avoid LV distension. If the LV is distended, distension can be improved by increasing inotropic support, placement of IABP or Impella 2.5, LV venting either directly or by venting proximal to the LV such as LA venting via atrial septostomy or PA drainage. Switching to VAV-ECMO is performed in peripherally cannulated patients with respiratory failure due to concerns of cerebral hypoxemia. Biventricular function is periodically evaluated to detect recovery of myocardial function. AV opening is evaluated especially in peripheral cannulation, where risk of aortic root thrombosis is increased if the AV is closed.

A position paper by the ECMO Network and the Extracorporeal Life Support Organization (ELSO) recommended including a physician trained in echocardiography in the team caring for patients on ECMO support.

### Selected References

1. Abrams D, Garan AR, Abdelbary A, et al. Position paper for the organization of ECMO programs for cardiac failure in adults. *Intensive Care Med.* 2018;44(6):717-729.
2. Douflé G, Roscoe A, Billia F, Fan E. Echocardiography for adult patients supported with extracorporeal membrane oxygenation. *Crit Care.* 2015;19:326.

**8.** Correct Answer: E. RV dilation/dysfunction predicts worse prognosis

*Rationale:* PE is a life-threatening condition that requires timely diagnosis and treatment. Although the most definitive diagnostic test is computerized tomographic pulmonary angiography (CTPA) scan, echocardiography can provide clinically useful data in many cases. In contrast to CTPA, echocardiography requires neither renally injurious IV contrast nor the transfer of potentially unstable patients to a remote location.

Echocardiography can provide both qualitative and quantitative data of value in the workup of suspected PE. First, in a patient with hemodynamic compromise, the finding of normal RV size and function practically rules out PE as the cause of hypotension. Conversely, the finding of RV dilation/dysfunction in PE is associated with a much worse prognosis, with some studies showing a doubling of the 3-month mortality compared to patients with PE and normal RV size/function.

Unfortunately, echocardiography by itself rarely confirms a definitive diagnosis of PE. Specifically, echocardiography only can rule in PE when it reveals a clot "in transit" in the right heart, including the IVC, RA, right ventricle, or PA. Because the majority of patients with PE will not demonstrate a clot "in transit" at the time of echocardiography, substantial efforts have been dedicated to determining ultrasound findings that reliably differentiate PE from other causes of RV dysfunction. For instance, it was once thought that McConnell sign was pathognomonic for PE. McConnell sign specifically describes a pattern of RV dysfunction characterized by hypokinesis of the RV free wall basal and midsegments with relative normo- or even hyperkinesis of the RV free wall apical segment. This pattern likely occurs in PE because increased RV afterload disrupts most RV function while the apical segment of the RV free wall appears to be mobile due to its physical connection to a preserved or hyperkinetic left ventricle. Although this finding can indeed be seen in PE, case reports and case series have shown that this sign is neither sensitive nor specific for PE, and it has been observed in other conditions that disrupt RV function, including RV infarct, acute respiratory distress syndrome (ARDS), and pulmonary fibrosis.

Therefore, echocardiography is an important bedside tool in the workup of patients suspected of having a PE. Although echocardiography can only rarely "rule in" PE, it can still be useful by rapidly providing information at the bedside to narrow the differential diagnosis of shock and risk-stratify patients who have PE diagnosed by CTPA.

### Selected Reference

1. Konstantinides SV, Meyer G, Becattini C, et al. 2019 ESC Guidelines for the diagnosis and management of acute pulmonary embolism developed in collaboration with the European Respiratory Society (ERS). *Eur Heart J.* 2019;41(4):543-603.

**9.** Correct Answer: D. Severe aortic insufficiency (AI) is a contraindication to Impella® device placement.

*Rationale:* Hemodynamic instability in critically ill patients with Impella® device requires urgent echocardiographic examination to rule out catheter migration. For proper placement, the catheter's inlet area should be into the left ventricle about 3.5 to 4 cm from the annulus, which allows the outlet area to be in the ascending aorta distal to the AV annulus and the aortic root. Echocardiography can also diagnose complications encountered with the Impella® device such as interference with AV closure causing severe AI or interference with the MV apparatus causing severe MR.

The Impella® 2.5 and Impella® CP devices can be inserted via standard percutaneous catheterization procedure through the femoral artery, into the ascending aorta, across the AV and into the left ventricle. In contrast, the Impella® 5.0 and 5.5 devices (that deliver flow up to 5.0 and 6 L/min, respectively) can only be inserted via femoral arterial cut down or through surgical access into the axillary artery.

Selected References
1. Impella®. The World's Smallest Heart Pump. Accessed November 17, 2019. http://www.abiomed.com/impella.
2. Pappalardo F, Contri R, Pieri M, Colombo A, Zangrillo A. Fluoroless placement of Impella: a single center experience. *Int J Cardiol.* 2015;179:491-492.

**10.** Correct Answer: D. Decreased LVAD pump speed

*Rationale:* Echocardiography is used for ICU management of patients supported with LVAD in order to evaluate RV size compared to that of LV, RV contractility, RA and LA size, position of IVS, shunting from right to left, degree of TR, AV opening, inflow and outflow cannula positions, and optimization of LVAD pump speed.

Suction events can result from:

- Decreased preload caused by bleeding, hypovolemia, or pericardial effusion
- Decreased afterload caused by hypotension, sepsis, or vasoplegia
- RV failure
- Excessive LVAD speed

All those factors can result in a collapsed left ventricle with leftward shift of the IVS, which distorts the RV geometry and worsens TR, with subsequent worsening of RV function. Suction events can be mitigated by lowering LVAD speed.

Hypotension or loss of arterial pulsatility in patients with LVAD can be caused by several factors, most of which can be diagnosed with echocardiography. These include hypovolemia, RV failure, LVAD-associated continuous AI, LVAD-related MR, inflow cannula malposition or obstruction, outflow graft kinking or thrombosis, and LVAD pump malfunction.

Selected References
1. Ammar KA, Umland MM, Kramer C, et al. The ABCs of left ventricular assist device echocardiography: a systematic approach. *Eur Heart J Cardiovasc Imaging.* 2012;13(11):885-899.
2. Stainback RF, Estep JD, Agler DA, et al. Echocardiography in the management of patients with left ventricular assist devices: recommendations from the American Society of Echocardiography. *J Am Soc Echocardiogr.* 2015;28(8):853-909.

**11.** Correct Answer: C. Determine intra-abdominal pressure

*Rationale:* The presence of intra-abdominal hypertension (intra-abdominal pressure >12 mm Hg) is common in cardiac surgical patients (33%-46%). Importantly, intra-abdominal hypertension in postoperative cardiac surgical patients is associated with acute kidney injury. The risk factors in cardiac surgical patients include positive fluid balance and low CO/shock. Importantly, this entity can overlap with postoperative cardiogenic shock. Thus, it can be difficult to discriminate those diagnoses and to rule out associated problems such as postoperative cardiac tamponade. The clinical picture of abdominal compartment syndrome includes progressive intra-abdominal hypertension with elevated airway pressure, low tidal volume, and an isolated increase in CVP along with progressive development of acute kidney injury.

The diagnosis is confirmed by measurement of an elevated intra-abdominal pressure. It is a fast, reliable, and noninvasive procedure performed at the bedside that will rule out the diagnosis. Performing an abdominal CT scan carries the risks of transporting an unstable patient outside of the ICU and potentially delaying therapeutic intervention. In contrast, TEE evaluation is considered when intra-abdominal hypertension is ruled out and in order to evaluate the presence of cardiogenic shock. More importantly, TEE is the diagnostic modality of choice to confirm the diagnosis of postoperative cardiac tamponade and an emergent surgical exploration is only considered when the diagnosis is formally established. In a similar fashion, during this situation a diagnostic laparotomy or laparoscopy is not warranted unless there is evidence of acute abdomen or mesenteric/visceral ischemia or necrosis.

Selected References
1. Dalfino L, Sicolo A, Paparella D, Mongelli M, Rubino G, Brienza N. Intra-abdominal hypertension in cardiac surgery. *Interact Cardiovasc Thorac Surg.* 2013 Oct;17(4):644-651.
2. Mazzeffi MA, Stafford P, Wallace K, et al. Intra-abdominal hypertension and postoperative kidney dysfunction in cardiac surgery patients. *J Cardiothorac Vasc Anesth.* 2016 Dec;30(6):1571-1577.

**12.** Correct Answer: D. To obtain a focused bedside TTE

*Rationale:* This question addresses the clinical suspicion and confirmatory diagnosis of delayed pericardial tamponade after open cardiac surgery. In the clinical scenario, the patient presents with common risk factors for cardiac tamponade in such a setting (valvular surgery, postoperative coagulopathy, bleeding, and multiple transfusions). There are also common signs and symptoms of postoperative cardiac tamponade (dyspnea, tachycardia, hypotension, oliguria, and elevated CVP). The clinical picture is nonspecific, and diagnosis needs confirmation in order to proceed with therapeutic intervention.

Echocardiography is the method of choice to confirm the clinical diagnosis. In this acute setting, a focused cardiac ultrasound at the bedside in order to specifically look for pericardial effusion or evidence of cardiac tamponade should be attempted first and if imaging is inconclusive or technically difficult (i.e., postoperative patients, decubitus position, obese body habitus, chronic obstructive lung disease, or mechanical ventilation), a TEE examination is necessary. Nevertheless, TTE may fail to visualize early postoperative pericardial effusions in cardiac surgical patients.[1] Performing a comprehensive TTE in those circumstances is likely unnecessary and could delay a therapeutic intervention. In addition, such examination is out of the scope of critical care echocardiography and would require a level of expertise usually not available in the ICU at all times.

Although TEE is more sensitive, specific, and suitable to demonstrate regional tamponade—a common finding in delayed postoperative pericardial tamponade, it is also invasive, requires sedation/anesthesia with risk of aspiration, and could potentially increase hemodynamic instability. Therefore, it is not usually recommended as first choice. Otherwise, a CT scan would be useful but carries the risk of delaying diagnosis and removing patients from the controlled environment of the ICU to a remote location. Chest X-ray in this situation can present with widened mediastinum. Nonetheless, such a finding does not provide confirmation of diagnosis.

Selected References
1. Floerchinger B, Camboni D, Schopka S, Kolat P, Hilker M, Schmid C. Delayed cardiac tamponade after open heart surgery—is supplemental CT imaging reasonable? *J Cardiothorac Surg.* 2013 Jun;8:158.
2. Price S, Prout J, Jaggar SI, Gibson DG, Pepper JR. "Tamponade" following cardiac surgery: terminology and echocardiography may both mislead. *Eur J Cardiothorac Surg.* 2004 Dec;26(6):1156-1160.

**13.** Correct Answer: D. For diagnosis and management of complications such as cannula malposition, cardiac tamponade, or intracardiac thrombus formation

*Rationale:* ECMO/extracorporeal life support (ELS) constitute a group of highly specialized vital support technologies derived from CPB that are used to support critically ill patients in cardiac, respiratory, or cardiorespiratory failure.

The impact on the outcome of these support modalities has been widely studied in the pediatric population. Recently, there is a rapid expansion of ECMO/ELS use in adult populations. Echocardiography is an essential tool during management of patients supported by ECMO/ELS. Although there is evidence of the applicability and usefulness of diverse echocardiographic modalities in such patients at diverse stages of care, the most significant impact of echocardiography in management of patients supported with ECMO is for the detection and monitoring of complications.

Selected Reference

1. Platts DG, Sedgwick JF, Burstow DJ, Mullany DV, Fraser JF. The role of echocardiography in the management of patients supported by extracorporeal membrane oxygenation. *J Am Soc Echocardiogr.* 2012 Feb;25(2):131-141.

**14.** Correct Answer: **B. EPSS of 10 mm**

*Rationale:* There are multiple techniques that can be used to evaluate LV function. EPSS is a measurement of the distance from the anterior MV leaflet to the septal wall in the parasternal long-axis view using M-mode (Figure 43.3). This distance has been shown to correlate with LV contractility and LVEF. An EPSS of >7 mm has been shown to correlate with an LV contractility and LVEF <50%. All other options are associated with normal LVEF.

Selected References

1. McKaigney CJ, Krantz MJ, La Rocque CL, Hurst ND, Buchanan MS, Kendall JL. E-point septal separation: a bedside tool for emergency physician assessment of left ventricular ejection fraction. *Am J Emerg Med.* 2014;32(6):493-497.
2. Silverstein JR, Laffely NH, Rifkin RD. Quantitative estimation of left ventricular ejection fraction from mitral valve E-point to septal separation and comparison to magnetic resonance imaging. *Am J Cardiol.* 2006;97(1):137-140.

**15.** Correct Answer: **C. Increase in VTI/SV by >12.5% during passive leg raise and decreased systolic function**

*Rationale:* Burn shock is a unique combination of hypovolemic shock and cardiogenic shock. In the first 24 to 36 hours after a significant thermal injury, burn shock is manifested by intravascular volume depletion, low PA occlusion pressures, elevated systemic vascular resistance, and depressed CO.

After 36 to 48 hours, burn shock is described by the occurrence of a hyperdynamic and vasoplegic state characterized by high CO and low systemic vascular resistance. Low intravascular volume remains throughout both phases. An increase in the VTI/SV by 12.5% during passive leg raise has been shown to predict fluid responsiveness with an increase in CO and SV after fluid bolus.

Selected References

1. Lamia B, Ochagavia A, Monnet X, Chemla D, Richard C, Teboul JL. Echocardiographic prediction of volume responsiveness in critically ill patients with spontaneously breathing activity. *Intensive Care Med.* 2007 Jul;33(7):1125-1132.
2. Latenser BA. Critical care of the burn patient: the first 48 hours. *Crit Care Med.* 2009 Oct;37(10):2819-2826.
3. Maizel J, Airapetian N, Lorne E, Tribouilloy C, Massy Z, Slama M. Diagnosis of central hypovolemia by using passive leg raising. *Intensive Care Med.* 2007 Jul;33(7):1133-1138.
4. Soussi S, Dépret F, Benyamina M, Legrand M. Early hemodynamic management of critically ill burn patients. *Anesthesiology.* 2018 Sep;129(3):583-589.

**16.** Correct Answer: **A. E/A ratio of 1.5 and normal pulmonary vein Doppler flow profile**

*Rationale:* Differentiating various forms of shock is a recurrent dilemma in the ICU. Timely implementation of therapy is dependent on appropriately diagnosing and identifying the underlying etiology. Septic cardiomyopathy is not only difficult to manage but difficult to diagnose and distinguish from cardiogenic shock, especially in clinical scenarios where patients have risk factors for both. The major distinguishing factor between septic cardiomyopathy and "classic" cardiogenic shock is that septic shock is associated with normal or low LV filling pressures. This is due not only to relative intravascular volume depletion but also to LV dilation secondary to the effects of circulating endotoxin. Also, unlike classic cardiogenic shock, septic cardiomyopathy is almost always reversible, assuming resolution of sepsis.

Selected References

1. Beesley SJ, Weber G, Sarge T, et al. Septic cardiomyopathy. *Crit Care Med.* 2018 Apr;46(4):625-634.
2. Ehrman RR, Sullivan AN, Favot MJ, et al. Pathophysiology, echocardiographic evaluation, biomarker findings, and prognostic implications of septic cardiomyopathy: a review of the literature. *Crit Care.* 2018 May;22(1):112.
3. Martin L, Derwall M, Al Zoubi S, et al. The septic heart: current understanding of molecular mechanisms and clinical implications. *Chest.* 2019 Feb;155(2):427-437.
4. Vieillard-Baron A. Septic cardiomyopathy. *Ann Intensive Care.* 2011 Apr;1(1):6.

**17.** Correct Answer: C. 8 mm

*Rationale:* MAPSE has been suggested as a parameter of LV function. While still sparsely used, MAPSE has been correlated with decreased LV systolic function and low values have been associated with increased morbidity and mortality in critically ill patients similar to patients with heart failure. A MAPSE value <8 mm has been shown to correlate to decreased LV systolic function.

### Selected References
1. Bergenzaun L, Ohlin H, Gudmundsson P, Willenheimer R, Chew MS. Mitral annular plane systolic excursion (MAPSE) in shock: a valuable echocardiographic parameter in intensive care patients. *Cardiovasc Ultrasound.* 2013 May;11:16.
2. Borde DP, Joshi S, Asegaonkar B, et al. Mitral annular plane systolic excursion: a simple, reliable echocardiographic parameter to detect left ventricular systolic dysfunction in patients undergoing off-pump coronary artery bypass grafting with transesophageal echocardiography. *J Cardiothorac Vasc Anesth.* 2019 May;33(5):1334-1339.

**18.** Correct Answer: C. Inotropic agents

*Rationale:* There are multiple echocardiographic methods and parameters for the evaluation of cardiac function. In a patient with signs and symptoms of heart failure and the echocardiographic values depicted in **Question 43.18**, the most likely clinical scenario is that the patient is in cardiogenic shock and would benefit from inotropic support.

The dP/dT is an echocardiographic parameter obtained by analysis of the mitral regurgitant or TR jet during isovolumetric contraction, in order to evaluate LV or RV contractile function, respectively.

The LV dP/dT can be estimated by assessing the time interval between the MR velocities of 1 and 3 m/s in the spectral CWD envelope of the MR jet. The RV dP/dT uses the time interval between the 1 and 2 m/s velocities on the TR jet CWD envelope. This dP/dT index is thought to be a relatively afterload-independent measure of ventricular contractility. Normal values for dP/dT are >1200 mm Hg/s for the left ventricle and >400 mm Hg/s for the right ventricle.

### Selected References
1. Chengode S. Left ventricular global systolic function assessment by echocardiography. *Ann Card Anaesth.* 2016 Oct;19(Suppl):S26-S34.
2. Rudski LG, Lai WW, Afilalo J, et al. Guidelines for the echocardiographic assessment of the right heart in adults: a report from the American Society of Echocardiography endorsed by the European Association of Echocardiography, a registered branch of the European Society of Cardiology, and the Canadian Society of Echocardiography. *J Am Soc Echocardiogr.* 2010 Jul;23(7):685-713.

**19.** Correct Answer: E. All of the above

*Rationale:* The classic findings of Takotsubo cardiomyopathy include apical ballooning of the left ventricle and hyperdynamic LV basal segments. These findings are not limited to any single coronary distribution. However, there is a wide spectrum of other findings that are often also present in patients with Takotsubo cardiomyopathy. Frequently, the hyperdynamic base of the left ventricle often leads to systolic anterior motion of the anterior MV leaflet, resulting in acute LVOT obstruction and MR. Other frequently associated echocardiographic findings include the presence of RV dysfunction, intraventricular thrombus, and pericardial effusion.

### Selected References
1. Chockalingam A, Xie GY, Dellsperger KC. Echocardiography in stress cardiomyopathy and acute LVOT obstruction. *Int J Cardiovasc Imaging.* 2010 Jun;26(5):527-535.
2. Izumo M, Akashi YJ. Role of echocardiography for takotsubo cardiomyopathy: clinical and prognostic implications. *Cardiovasc Diagn Ther.* 2018 Feb;8(1):90-100.

**20.** Correct Answer: C. IVC diameter 2.4 cm and no respiratory collapse

*Rationale:* The clinical picture depicted in **Question 43.20** is suggestive of RV failure. This clinical vignette aims to identify echocardiographic parameters that can be used to confirm the diagnosis of RV failure suggested by the clinical scenario and supported by elevated levels of NT-proBNP. All provided options correspond to echocardiographic parameters used to evaluate RV function. However, the only parameter that is elevated above the recommended threshold to suggest RV dysfunction is option C. Elevation in RA pressure provides indirect evidence of significant RV dysfunction. In the absence of an invasive CVP measurement, RA pressure can be estimated by the IVC diameter and the presence and degree of its inspiratory collapse in spontaneously ventilating patients.

The IVC diameter can be measured in a subcostal window. The measurement is taken perpendicular to the long axis, at end-expiration and at a location proximal to the hepatic vein opening into the IVC, near (from 0.5 to 3.0 cm) the RA-IVC junction. An IVC diameter >2.1 cm with <50% respiratory collapse during a sniff maneuver suggests an elevated RA pressure of 15 mm Hg (range 10-20 mm Hg). Such a parameter provides a more adequate estimation in cases of high or low RA pressures. It is less accurate when estimating intermediate values.

The abnormal values for the other mentioned parameters that would support the diagnosis of RV dysfunction are RV FAC <35%; TAPSE or tricuspid annular motion (TAM) ≤16 mm; TR jet peak velocity >2.8 m/s.

### Selected References

1. Rudski LG, Lai WW, Afialo J, et al. Guidelines for the echocardiographic assessment of the right heart in adults: a report from the American Society of Echocardiography endorsed by the European Association of Echocardiography, a registered branch of the European Society of Cardiology, and the Canadian Society of Echocardiography. *J Am Soc Echocardiogr.* 2010;23:685-713.
2. Siegel RJ. Noninvasive evaluation of right atrial pressure. *J Am Soc Echocardiogr.* 2013;26:1033-1042.

**21.** Correct Answer: C. Mitral inflow E/A ratio: 3 and E/e' ratio: 18

*Rationale:* The depicted scenario is compatible with shock from an unknown etiology. In this particular situation, the presence of an infection and the absence of other comorbidities could suggest septic shock as a high possibility in the differential diagnosis. However, this real-life patient presented with acute-onset *de novo* cardiogenic shock secondary to viral myocarditis in the setting of an Influenza type A viral infection. This clinical vignette demonstrates the significant challenge posed by and the need to accurately differentiate the shock etiology. Determination of the proper pathophysiology and mechanism of shock is essential to carry out effective management and to minimize morbidity and mortality. In addition, it is possible to encounter patients in shock from combined mechanisms or from multifactorial etiologies. Therefore, echocardiography is recommended as a first-choice modality to diagnose and manage the patient in shock.

Although it is possible to find patients with septic cardiomyopathy, the initial presentation of septic shock is more likely that of a predominantly vasodilatory state with hyperdynamic ventricular function. In this setting, patients can have an elevated CO and an overestimated LVEF due to vasodilation and relative hypovolemia. As a consequence, in such a hyperdynamic state with an elevated LVEF, dynamic LVOT obstruction can occur. In a similar fashion, an LVOT VTI >20 cm is considered normal (values >18 cm correlate with adequate SV).

Cardiogenic shock is defined as hypotension associated with signs of hypoperfusion, despite adequate or elevated filling pressures. Therefore, during its initial presentation, the hallmark feature that differentiates cardiogenic shock from other etiologies is the presence of elevated filling pressures. Doppler echocardiography modalities—using both TTE and TEE—can estimate LV end-diastolic pressure (LVEDP) and LA pressure (LAP) in a wide range of pathologies, with adequate correlation with invasive measurements. The analysis of mitral inflow velocities provides the most basic measurements. The mitral inflow starts with the early diastolic filling (E wave) and is later followed by the late diastolic filling provided by the atrial contraction (A wave). The mitral inflow E/A ratio and the deceleration time (DT) of the E wave are both related to LAP and LV diastolic function. Whereas an increased E/A ratio in patients with myocardial disease is associated with increased LAP, a decrease in DT is associated with decreased LV distensibility and increased LV filling pressure. An E/A ratio ≥ 2 and an E wave DT < 120 ms accurately estimate LAP > 20 mm Hg.

With the use of tissue Doppler imaging (TDI), the measurement of mitral annulus early diastolic peak velocity (e') allows a rapid estimation of LAP. In particular, mitral E/e' ratio is a dimensionless parameter that is directly related to LAP. A mitral E/e' ratio ≥ 14 is closely correlated with elevated LVEDP.

### Selected References

1. Andersen OS, Smiseth OA, Dokainish H, et al. Estimating left ventricular filling pressure by echocardiography. *J Am Coll Cardiol.* 2017 Apr;69(15):1937-1948.
2. Nagueh SF. Non-invasive assessment of left ventricular filling pressure. *Eur J Heart Fail.* 2018 Jan;20(1):38-48.
3. Ponikowski P, Voors AA, Anker SD, et al. 2016 ESC Guidelines for the diagnosis and treatment of acute and chronic heart failure: the task force for the diagnosis and treatment of acute and chronic heart failure of the European Society of Cardiology (ESC). Developed with the special contribution of the Heart Failure Association (HFA) of the ESC. *Eur J Heart Fail.* 2016;18:891-975.

**22.** Correct Answer: C. RV end-diastolic area/LV end-diastolic area >1 and paradoxical IVS motion

*Rationale:* This patient presents with acute heart failure in the setting of an advanced chronic lung disease. The clinical presentation is compatible with cardiogenic shock secondary to RV failure. The echocardiographic findings corroborate the morphologic and functional RV changes secondary to end-stage lung disease and correspond to cor pulmonale.

All of the answer choice options are visualized and evident in ▶ **Video 43.23**. Also, all of them can be present in patients with RV dysfunction. Nonetheless, the findings that are most closely associated with cor pulmonale are: RV end-diastolic area/LV end-diastolic ratio > 1 and paradoxical IVS motion. These particular findings are correlated with severe RV dysfunction and are evidence of severe RV dilation resulting in increased interventricular interdependence with limited LV filling and ultimately low systemic CO. The RV end-diastolic area/LV end-diastolic area ratio is normally <0.6. A ratio of 0.6 to 1 indicates mild RV dilation. In contrast, a ratio >1 is characteristic of severe RV dilation.

From a different point of view, increased RV afterload results in a more vigorous and prolonged RV contraction producing a paradoxical motion of the IVS. In this circumstance, at end-systole while the left ventricle relaxes, RV contraction is maintained and the pressure overload reverses the interventricular trans-septal gradient, displacing the IVS toward the LV cavity. Thereafter, as long as diastolic pressure is equal to or higher in the right ventricle than in the left ventricle—as result of volume overload—the IVS stays displaced toward the left ventricle during diastole. During the next cycle, in early systole, LV pressure elevation increases the interventricular trans-septal gradient—overcoming RV pressure and bringing the IVS toward the left ventricle until the next end-systole.

From the previous discussion, it is evident that both leftward IVS motion at end-diastole (suggestive of RV volume overload) and the leftward IVS displacement at end-systole (from RV pressure overload) can each be seen in patients at different stages of RV dysfunction and from diverse etiologies. Likewise, the presence of severe RV hypertrophy by itself does not imply or is evidence of RV failure.

Selected References
1. Arrigo M, Ruschitzka F, Huber LC, et al. Right ventricular failure: pathophysiology, diagnosis and treatment. *Card Fail Rev.* 2019;5(3):140-146.
2. Jardin F, Dubourg O, Bourdarias JP. Echocardiographic pattern of acute cor pulmonale. *Chest.* 1997 Jan;111(1):209-217.

**23.** Correct Answer: B. Elevated ventricular interdependence

*Rationale:* ▶ **Video 43.24** contains multiple echocardiographic findings that are evidence of important morphologic and functional changes in the right heart and are compatible with significant RV dysfunction. Some of those changes include severe RA dilation with leftward displacement of the interatrial septum throughout the cardiac cycle. There are also tricuspid annular dilation and TV leaflet restriction; severe RV dilation and severe RV hypertrophy; decreased global RV systolic function; and paradoxical IVS motion. In addition, the IVS is bulging into the left ventricle during all the cardiac cycle and LV filling is significantly restricted. The leftward displacement of the IVS and the paradoxical IVS motion are evidence of elevated ventricular interdependence.

The ultimate mechanism responsible for the effects of RV size and function changes on the left ventricle is the so-called *ventricular interdependence*. As a consequence of such a mechanism, changes in size, geometry, volume, pressure, and overall function of each ventricle affect the other. This ventricular interdependence happens because the right and left ventricle share the IVS and are encircled by common myocardial fibers (responsible for systolic ventricular interdependence); additionally, both ventricles are contained in a single, common cavity—the pericardial sac. The latter accounts for diastolic ventricular interdependence.

In the presence of RV volume overload without pulmonary hypertension, there is impaired LV diastolic compliance and decreased LVEF without intrinsic alteration in contractility. In contrast, the occurrence of RV pressure overload leads to decreased LV compliance, initially with preservation of LVEF. However, with time, there is progressive LV atrophic remodeling and compromised LV systolic function.

Selected References
1. Naeije R, Badagliacca R. The overloaded right heart and ventricular interdependence. *Cardiovasc Res.* 2017 Oct;113(12):1474-1485.
2. Sanz J, Sánchez-Quintana D, Bossone E, Bogaard HJ, Naeije R. Anatomy, function, and dysfunction of the right ventricle: JACC state-of-the-art review. *J Am Coll Cardiol.* 2019 Apr;73(12):1463-1482.

**24.** Correct Answer: C. LVOT VTI

*Rationale:* All the options presented correspond to parameters that are correlated to LV contractility and can provide indirect assessment of LV systolic function. Nonetheless, the only one among those parameters that has shown close correlation with actual invasive CO measurement is the LVOT VTI.

Qualitative LVEF estimation by 2D echocardiography has an adequate correlation with quantitative and/or volumetric LVEF evaluation. However, the presence of a normal LVEF does not imply a normal CO. Conversely, a decreased LVEF does not necessarily correlate with low CO. The determination of LV FS has demonstrated adequate association with LVEF. In a similar fashion, EPSS distance has been shown to correlate with LV contractility and LVEF. An EPSS of >7 mm has been shown to correlate with LV contractility and an LVEF <50%.

### Selected References

1. Chengode S. Left ventricular global systolic function assessment by echocardiography. *Ann Card Anaesth.* 2016 Oct;19(Supplement):S26-S34.
2. Mercado P, Maizel J, Beyls C, et al. Transthoracic echocardiography: an accurate and precise method for estimating cardiac output in the critically ill patient. *Crit Care.* 2017 Jun;21(1):136.

**25.** Correct Answer: B. Early diastolic pulmonic regurgitant (PR) jet velocity <2.0 m/s

*Rationale:* All parameters in **Question 43.25** are used to assess the probability of elevated PAP or pulmonary hypertension. However, early diastolic PR jet velocity <2.2 m/s is the cutoff that has been shown to correlate with elevated PA pressures.

The most commonly used method to estimate sPAP is CWD interrogation of the TR jet and determination of the peak TR systolic velocity (TRV). The sPAP is estimated by applying the equation: $sPAP = (4 \times TRV^2) + RA$ pressure. The RA pressure can be measured or estimated as explained in a prior item. It is important to note that RA estimation can induce significant error in the sPAP estimation. All other parameters and their depicted values correspond to the recommended limits above which there is high probability of elevated PAP and the presence of significant pulmonary hypertension.

### Selected References

1. Augustine DX, Coates-Bradshaw LD, Willis J, et al. Echocardiographic assessment of pulmonary hypertension: a guideline protocol from the British Society of Echocardiography. *Echo Res Pract.* 2018 Sep;5(3):G11-G24.
2. D'Alto M, Bossone E, Opotowsky AR, Ghio S, Rudski LG, Naeije R. Strengths and weaknesses of echocardiography for the diagnosis of pulmonary hypertension. *Int J Cardiol.* 2018 Jul;263:177-183.

# 44 | VARIOUS PROTOCOLS: FATE, FEEL, FEER, FAST

Nibras Bughrara, Radwan Safa, Stephanie Cha, and Aliaksei Pustavoitau

1. A 76-year-old, 85-kg man with a past medical history of chronic obstructive pulmonary disease, coronary artery disease status post coronary artery bypass 3 years ago, and essential hypertension developed undifferentiated shock on postoperative day 2 after hip repair for femoral neck fracture and was transferred to the intensive care unit (ICU). On examination, no hematoma was apparent, postoperative wound had no drainage, and initial hemoglobin concentration was 8.6 g/dL, unchanged from 12 hours ago. Subcostal four-chamber (▶ Video 44.1; **Figure 44.1**) and lung (▶ Video 44.2; **Figure 44.2**) views were obtained upon arrival to the ICU. Despite intravenous administration of 2.5 L of balanced crystalloid solution, the patient remained hypotensive with mean arterial pressure consistently in the 50 to 55 mm Hg range, at which point repeated lung views were obtained (**Figure 44.3**; ▶ Video 44.3).

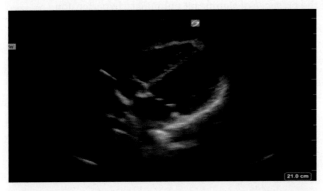

**Figure 44.1**

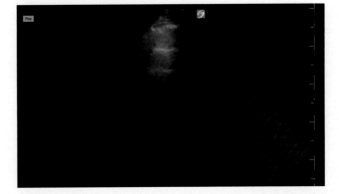

**Figure 44.2**

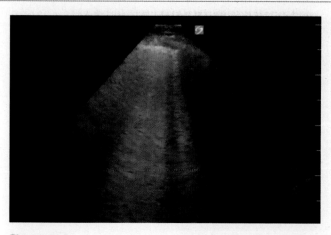

**Figure 44.3**

At this point, what is the most likely diagnosis?
A. Obstructive shock
B. Cardiogenic shock
C. Hypovolemic shock
D. Distributive shock

2. A 55-year-old, 160-cm, 142-kg woman with a past medical history of essential hypertension, obstructive sleep apnea poorly compliant with home continuous positive airway pressure therapy, and mild pulmonary hypertension on postoperative day 1 after sigmoid colectomy for adenocarcinoma developed progressive somnolence. Earlier in the day, she required adjustment in hydromorphone patient-controlled analgesia to optimize postoperative pain control. Rapid response team was activated when she became unarousable. On assessment, the patient has agonal breathing, receiving supplemental oxygen via non-rebreather facemask with blood oxygen saturation 86%. The patient receives intravenous naloxone 0.4 mg with no improvement in respiratory effort and subsequently is endotracheally intubated using indirect laryngoscopy with a 7.0 tube with subglottic suctioning port. Tube position is confirmed by the presence of end-tidal carbon dioxide exhalation, auscultation, and visualization of tube advancement during videolaryngoscopy. Postintubation and bag valve ventilation for 5 minutes, blood oxygen saturation remains in the 80% to 85% range. Bilateral lung ultrasound is performed and upper lung fields are shown in ▶ **Video 44.4** and **Figure 44.4** (right lung) and ▶ **Video 44.5** and **Figure 44.5** (left lung).

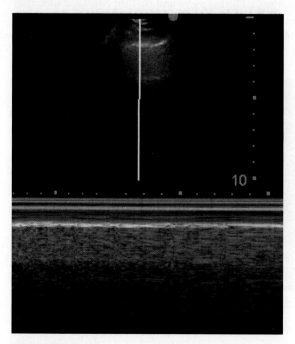

**Figure 44.4**

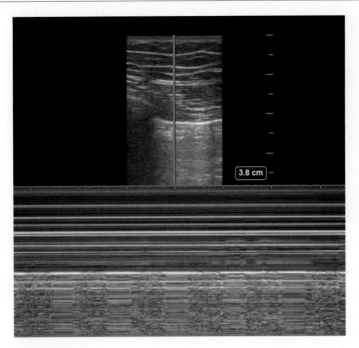

**Figure 44.5**

What is the next best intervention to improve oxygenation?
A. Advance endotracheal tube
B. Withdraw endotracheal tube
C. Administer furosemide
D. Perform needle thoracostomy

3. A 68-year-old man is admitted to the surgical ICU following right carotid endarterectomy. His past medical history is significant for coronary artery disease status post drug-eluting stent to the left anterior descending artery 2 years ago, essential hypertension, and a remote history of cigarette smoking. Two hours postoperatively, he develops sinus tachycardia with hypotension followed by pulseless ventricular tachycardia requiring defibrillation. He converts to normal sinus rhythm without pulse, and cardiopulmonary resuscitation (CPR) is performed. Epinephrine is administered according to Advanced Cardiac Life Support (ACLS) protocol. During pulse and rhythm checks, a subcostal four-chamber view is performed to assess for reversible causes of cardiac arrest. At 20 minutes, cardiac ultrasound images are obtained (▶ **Video 44.6; Figure 44.6**), which are similar to the ones obtained during the prior pulse and rhythm check.

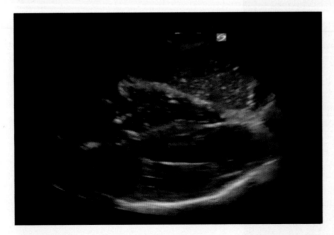

**Figure 44.6**

What is the most feasible course of action at this time?

**A.** Administer tissue plasminogen activator

**B.** Consult cardiology for emergent left heart catheterization

**C.** Consider cessation of resuscitative efforts

**D.** Perform emergent pericardiocentesis

4. A 24-year-old unrestrained man was involved in a motor vehicle accident. He is transported to the Emergency Department following a prolonged extrication. On arrival, initial survey reveals a combative patient with marked bruising over the sternum and anterior chest, a grossly deformed left lower extremity, and a forehead laceration. Vital signs include:

- Temperature: 35.3 °C
- Blood pressure (BP): 84/56 mm Hg
- Heart rate (HR): 122 beats per minute
- Respiratory rate (RR): 28 breaths per minute

▶ **Videos 44.7** and **44.8** and **Figures 44.7** and **44.8** reveal beside ultrasound findings.

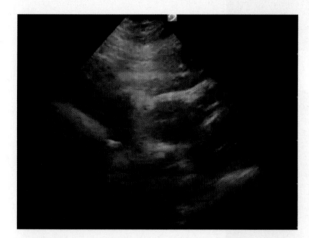

**Figure 44.7**

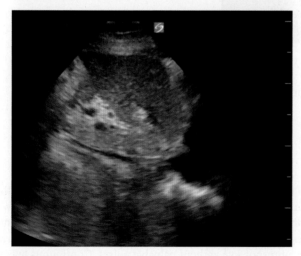

**Figure 44.8**

What is the next best step in caring for this patient?

**A.** Emergent bedside pericardiocentesis

**B.** Proceed to operating room

**C.** Ultrasound of the hepatorenal recess

**D.** Trauma computed tomography panscan

5. A 42-year-old woman with a long history of scleroderma is undergoing a right heart catheterization under moderate sedation. During the procedure, she becomes unresponsive to verbal or tactile stimuli and becomes progressively hypoxemic and hypotensive requiring emergent intubation. Vital signs are: BP 74/43, HR 110, SpO$_2$ 82% on non-rebreather face mask, RR 7. Bedside imaging reveals ▶ **Videos 44.9** and **44.10** and **Figures 44.9** and **44.10**.

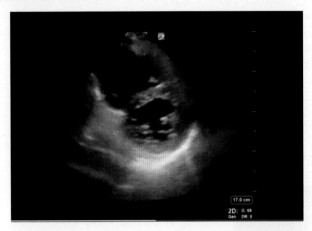

**Figure 44.9**

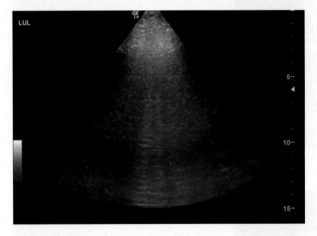

**Figure 44.10**

What is the next best step in her management?
A. Thrombolytic therapy
B. Initiation of inotropic therapy
C. Initiation of extracorporeal life support
D. Fluid administration

6. A 64-year-old man is postoperative day 16 from a coronary artery bypass surgery, complicated by the development of heparin-induced thrombocytopenia and acute right lower extremity thrombus now on warfarin therapy. Current international normalized ratio (INR) is 4.5. While preparing for emergent thrombectomy, he receives two units of fresh frozen plasma in rapid succession. Shortly afterward, he has a witnessed event in which he becomes unresponsive without palpable pulses. Continuous telemetry demonstrates sinus rhythm. CPR is initiated. Which of the following is an appropriate next step in his management?

A. Immediate defibrillation
B. Immediate performance of subcostal ultrasound
C. Performance of subcostal ultrasound following five cycles of CPR
D. Emergent chest reexploration

7. A 54-year-old man with pancreatic adenocarcinoma is undergoing an endoscopic retrograde cholangiography and has developed a sudden decrease in end-tidal $CO_2$ reading, while the blood pressure cuff cannot register blood pressure. Pulses are nonpalpable, telemetry reveals sinus tachycardia, RR is 12, $SpO_2$ 100% on controlled mechanical ventilation. Following 15 minutes of CPR, bedside ultrasound is shown in ▶ **Video 44.11** and **Figure 44.11**.

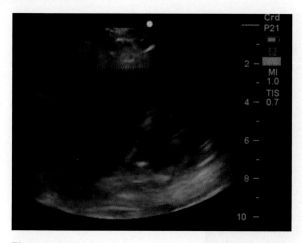

**Figure 44.11**

Which of the following statements is true?
A. Ultrasound should be repeated each cycle of CPR for no longer than 12 seconds.
B. Alternative ultrasound views should be attempted on subsequent cycles of CPR.
C. Ultrasound gel should not be used given its risk for skin burns during defibrillation.
D. CPR should be terminated due to high unlikelihood of return of spontaneous circulation.

8. A 57-year-old woman struck on the left side by a vehicle traveling in excess of 45 mph initially required large-volume transfusion, preperitoneal packing, and embolization of her right iliac artery in interventional radiology suite on presentation. On hospital day 6 she returned to the operating room for external fixation of a pelvic fracture. At the end of the procedure she abruptly became profoundly hypoxic and hypotensive with poor response to intravenous fluid boluses and suddenly progressed to cardiac arrest. After initiating CPR, focused cardiac ultrasound was obtained during the pulse check period (▶ **Video 44.12; Figure 44.12**). The patient has no palpable pulse and has no cardiac activity on the monitor.

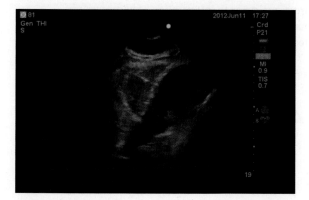

**Figure 44.12**

What is the most appropriate next step in her management?
A. Administer normal saline bolus
B. Administer 200 J biphasic direct current shock
C. Perform endotracheal intubation
D. Perform pericardiocentesis

9. A 57-year-old man sustained gunshot wounds to the neck and abdomen. He was emergently taken to the operating room for surgical exploration and control of bleeding. Upon arrival to the operating room, he suddenly developed cardiac arrest. After 2 minutes of CPR, chest compressions were paused for pulse and rhythm check, meanwhile subcostal cardiac view was attempted and recorded in 5 seconds (▶ **Video 44.13; Figure 44.13**).

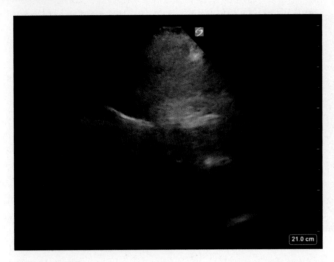

21.0 cm

**Figure 44.13**

The monitor showed normal sinus rhythm, no pulse was appreciated. Given the findings, what is the most appropriate next step in his management?
A. Attempt parasternal view
B. Perform endotracheal intubation
C. Immediately resume chest compressions
D. Administer available red blood cells

10. A 56-year-old man develops cardiac arrest after a left hemicolectomy while in postanesthesia care unit. Between cycles of CPR focused cardiac ultrasound is performed. According to the Focused Echocardiographic Evaluation in Life support (FEEL) protocol, when should the sonographer first place the ultrasound probe on the patient's chest?

A. Any time during the 2-minute cycle, while chest compressions are being performed.
B. Near the end of the 2 minutes of compressions, prior to interruption of compressions.
C. At the end of 2 minutes of compressions, during the rhythm/pulse check.
D. During the rhythm/pulse check, after team members are unable to find a palpable pulse.

# Chapter 44 ▪ Answers

1. Correct Answer: D. Distributive shock

*Rationale:* ▶ **Video 44.1** and Figure 44.1 show a normal heart and no pericardial effusion. ▶ **Video 44.2** and Figure 44.2 show an A-profile in the lung field. According to the Fluid Administration Limited by Lung Sonography (FALLS) protocol, obstructive shock is ruled out using a subcostal four-chamber view, demonstrating the absence of pericardial effusion and acute right ventricular (RV) enlargement, and lung views all showing lung sliding. Because lung views demonstrate A-profile at the time of evaluation, cardiogenic shock is ruled out and the assumption is made that pulmonary artery occlusion pressure is lower than or equal to 18 mm Hg (threshold for forming pulmonary edema). At this time the assumption is made that the patient is fluid tolerant (FALLS-responder), not bleeding based on clinical examination and laboratory value of hemoglobin, and receives intravenous fluids until lung A-profile switches to B-profile (▶ **Video 44.3**; Figure 44.3), consistent with interstitial pulmonary edema. Now the patient reaches FALLS-endpoint and intravenous fluid therapy is discontinued. Distributive shock is the only diagnosis as other types of shock are either ruled out (obstructive and cardiogenic) or corrected (hypovolemic), and the patient should receive an infusion of vasoactive medication.

### Selected Reference

1. Lichtenstein D. FALLS-protocol: lung ultrasound in hemodynamic assessment of shock. *Heart Lung Vessel.* 2013;5(3):142-147.

---

**2.** Correct Answer: B. Withdraw endotracheal tube

*Rationale:* ▶ **Video 44.4** and Figure 44.4 show both lung pulse and lung sliding with isolated B-lines. ▶ **Video 44.5** and Figure 44.5 reveal only lung pulse with isolated B-lines. This patient developed opioid-induced respiratory depression which in the setting of preexisting obstructive sleep apnea led to severe hypercapnia and respiratory arrest, requiring endotracheal intubation. Auscultation in general, and particularly in this patient, with morbid obesity (this patient's body mass index is 55.5 kg/m$^2$) is not as accurate as lung ultrasound to confirm tracheal versus bronchial positioning of endotracheal tube. When evaluating patients with respiratory failure, a systematic approach is advocated, with Bedside Lung Ultrasound in Emergency (BLUE) protocol being commonly accepted clinically. In this patient, ultrasound demonstrated both lung pulse and lung sliding on the right and only lung pulse on the left, which ruled out pneumothorax and was consistent with endobronchial intubation, requiring withdrawal of the endotracheal tube until lung sliding could be appreciated on both sides of the chest. The presence of isolated B-lines is not consistent with pulmonary edema, which requires the presence of at least three B-lines in each lung view.

### Selected References

1. Lichtenstein DA, Mezière GA. Relevance of lung ultrasound in the diagnosis of acute respiratory failure: the BLUE protocol. *Chest.* 2008;134(1):117-125.
2. Ramsingh D, Frank E, Haughton R, et al. Auscultation versus point-of-care ultrasound to determine endotracheal versus bronchial intubation: a diagnostic accuracy study. *Anesthesiology.* 2016;124(5):1012-1020.
3. Volpicelli G, Elbarbary M, Blaivas M, et al. International evidence-based recommendations for point-of-care lung ultrasound. *Intensive Care Med.* 2012;38(4):577-591.

---

**3.** Correct Answer: C. Consider cessation of resuscitative efforts

*Rationale:* ▶ **Video 44.6** shows cardiac standstill. Figure 44.6 shows absence of cardiac tamponade. In patients with pulseless electrical activity (PEA), two goals of resuscitative efforts include high-quality CPR and identifying reversible causes of cardiac arrest. Cardiac causes of PEA include acute RV failure, tamponade, left ventricular failure, and hypovolemia. While cardiac ultrasound can establish prognosis by identifying lack of cardiac motion and identify reversible causes of cardiac arrest, it may prolong pauses between cycles of CPR. Training is required to incorporate cardiac ultrasound safely into the workflow of ACLS protocols, and is the basis of Focused Echocardiographic Evaluation in Resuscitation (FEER) management. In this case, after prolonged CPR, the patient demonstrates no observable cardiac motion during two separate pauses, highly suggestive of irreversible arrest, and cessation of resuscitative effort should be considered. There is no evidence of pulmonary embolism as the right ventricle is not dilated. Left heart catheterization is not indicated in a patient without cardiac activity. There is no pericardial effusion and no evidence of tamponade to warrant pericardiocentesis.

### Selected Reference

1. Breitkreutz R, Walcher F, Seeger FH. Focused echocardiographic evaluation in resuscitation management: concept of an advanced life support-conformed algorithm. *Crit Care Med.* 2007;35(suppl 5):S150-S161.

---

**4.** Correct Answer: C. Ultrasound of the hepatorenal recess

*Rationale:* ▶ **Video 44.7** and Figure 44.7 show subcostal view with a small pericardial effusion without evidence of tamponade. ▶ **Video 44.8** and Figure 44.8 show a subcostal view of inferior vena cava (IVC) with IVC diameter less than 1 cm. Initial assessment of the hypotensive trauma patient should include an evaluation for intraperitoneal free fluid, which is an important factor determining operating room triage. Historically, diagnostic peritoneal lavage (DPL) was used to assess for intraperitoneal fluid, despite a high associated complication rate. The Focused Assessment with Sonography for Trauma (FAST) examination evolved as an ultrasound-guided protocol for the evaluation of intraperitoneal fluid and was first adopted in North America in the 1990s. With a relatively high sensitivity and specificity for detecting hemoperitoneum, and the ability to rapidly evaluate a trauma patient at the bedside, the FAST examination revolutionized the assessment of the traumatically injured patient. The views obtained in the FAST examination include the right upper quadrant, left upper quadrant, pelvic, and subxiphoid/subcostal. The FAST examination was later modified to the extended FAST examination (eFAST) to include lung views evaluating for pneumothorax. The hepatorenal recess (also known as Morison pouch), imaged in the right upper quadrant, is the most dependent portion of the peritoneal cavity in a supine patient and is the view with the highest likelihood of detecting hemoperitoneum. Pericardiocentesis is not indicated as there is no evidence of tamponade. This patient is unstable and if there is evidence of hemoperitoneum on FAST examination, this patient should proceed directly to the operating room, not the computed tomography scanner.

### Selected Reference

1. Boulanger BR, McLellan BA, Brenneman FD, et al. Emergent abdominal sonography as a screening test in a new diagnostic algorithm for blunt trauma. *J Trauma.* 1996;40(6):867-874.

---

**5.** Correct Answer: **B. Initiation of inotropic therapy**

*Rationale:* The FALLS protocol describes a protocol for the management of acute circulatory failure. First, simple cardiac and lung sonography should assess for obstructive etiologies of shock, including tamponade, pulmonary embolism, or pneumothorax (A′ profile demonstrated). Next, cardiac and lung sonography should evaluate for cardiogenic shock. Figure 44.9 and ▶ **Video 44.9** demonstrate pronounced biventricular systolic dysfunction, with notable RV dilatation and hypertrophy, and absence of pericardial effusion. This is likely a chronic process given the history of long-standing scleroderma and consequent pulmonary hypertension, exacerbated by the consequences of sedation, including hypotension and hypoventilation. ▶ **Video 44.10** and Figure 44.10 demonstrate B-profile consistent with pulmonary edema and biventricular failure. Inotropic therapy and limitation of fluid administration are therefore most appropriate. This patient may also require endotracheal intubation and positive pressure ventilation until hemodynamically stable. While this patient may be at risk for pulmonary embolism, RV dilatation alone does not confirm this diagnosis. Initiation of extracorporeal life support may be indicated if the patient is unresponsive to initial resuscitative therapies.

### Selected Reference

1. Lichtenstein DA. BLUE-protocol and FALLS-protocol: two applications of lung ultrasound in the critically ill. *Chest.* 2015;147(6):1659-1670.

---

**6.** Correct Answer: **C. Performance of subcostal ultrasound following five cycles of CPR**

*Rationale:* The Focused Echocardiographic Evaluation in Peri-Resuscitation and Life Support (FEER/FEEL) protocol has demonstrated a capacity to change clinical management in the vast majority of patients presenting in shock or cardiac arrest. Following identification of PEA, FEER is encouraged following the first five cycles of CPR and may be repeated serially. Subcostal imaging is recommended given its high yield for diagnostic quality imaging and relative ease of performance. Defibrillation is not indicated given absence of shockable rhythm. While emergent chest reexploration may be indicated in patients within 10 days of cardiac surgery, no special recommendations are made for those presenting beyond this time frame, and so standard ACLS algorithm should be followed.

### Selected References

1. Breitkreutz R, Price S, Steiger H, et al. Focused echocardiographic evaluation in life support and peri-resuscitation of emergency patients: a prospective trial. *Resuscitation.* 2010;81(11):1527-1533.
2. Breitkreutz R, Walcher F, Seeger FH. Focused echocardiographic evaluation in resuscitation management: concept of an advanced life support-conformed algorithm. *Crit Care Med.* 2007;35(suppl 5):S150-S161.
3. Bughrara N, Herrick SL, Leimer E, Sirigaddi K, Roberts K, Pustavoitau A. Focused cardiac ultrasound and the periresuscitative period: a case series of resident-performed echocardiographic assessment using subcostal-only view in advanced life support. *A A Pract.* 2020;14(10):e01278. doi:10.1213/XAA.0000000000001278
4. Dunning J, Levine A, Ley J, et al. The Society of Thoracic Surgeons Expert Consensus for the resuscitation of patients who arrest after cardiac surgery. *Ann Thorac Surg.* 2017;103(3):1005-1020.

**7.** Correct Answer: B. Alternative ultrasound views should be attempted on subsequent cycles of CPR

*Rationale:* The ultrasound image obtained (Figure 44.11; ▶ **Video 44.11**) is of poor quality but does demonstrate spontaneous cardiac motion. Following the FEEL protocol, ultrasound should be performed following the first five cycles of CPR. While subcostal imaging is recommended, alternative ultrasound views should be attempted if initial imaging is nondiagnostic or of poor quality. Ultrasound gel should be used for image optimization but can conduct electricity and risk skin burns if present during defibrillation attempts, so should be appropriately cleaned from the body prior to defibrillation. Finally, while cardiac standstill is consistently associated with low likelihood of return of spontaneous circulation or survival, imaging in this case does not show standstill.

### Selected References

1. Breitkreutz R, Walcher F, Seeger FH. Focused echocardiographic evaluation in resuscitation management: concept of an advanced life support-conformed algorithm. *Crit Care Med.* 2007;35(suppl 5):S150-S161.
2. Tsou, P, Kurbedin J, Chen Y, et al. Accuracy of point-of-care focused echocardiography in predicting outcome of resuscitation in cardiac arrest patients: a systematic review and meta-analysis. *Resuscitation.* 2017;114:92-99.

**8.** Correct Answer: B. Administer 200 J biphasic direct current shock

*Rationale:* ▶ **Video 44.12** demonstrates fine ventricular fibrillation while Figure 44.12 demonstrates absence of dilated RV and absence of tamponade. Focused cardiac ultrasound incorporated in a protocolized fashion into the management of cardiac arrest can provide diagnostic and prognostic information pertinent to cardiac motion and reversible cardiac causes of the arrest. In this patient, despite lack of electrical cardiac activity (asystole), cardiac ultrasound demonstrated fine ventricular fibrillation. Defibrillation with 200 J biphasic direct current shock is indicated next. While both administering boluses of saline and endotracheal intubation are likely to be required, timely defibrillation is the intervention that improves chances of survival in patients with ventricular fibrillation, as survival decreases with each minute delay. This patient does not have pericardial tamponade; thus, pericardiocentesis is not indicated.

### Selected References

1. Atkinson P, Bowra J, Milne J, et al. International Federation for Emergency Medicine Consensus Statement: sonography in hypotension and cardiac arrest (SHoC): an international consensus on the use of point of care ultrasound for undifferentiated hypotension and during cardiac arrest. *CJEM.* 2017;19(6):459-470.
2. Chan PS, Krumholz HM, Nichol G, Nallamothu BK; American Heart Association National Registry of Cardiopulmonary Resuscitation Investigators. Delayed time to defibrillation after in-hospital cardiac arrest. *N Engl J Med.* 2008;358(1):9-17.
3. Querellou E, Meyran D, Petitjean F, et al. Ventricular fibrillation diagnosed with trans-thoracic echocardiography. *Resuscitation.* 2009;80(10):1211-1213.

**9.** Correct Answer: C. Immediately resume chest compressions

*Rationale:* The ultrasound image (Figure 44.13; ▶ **Video 44.13**) obtained does not provide conclusive information and is of poor quality. During CPR high-quality chest compressions with minimal interruptions for rhythm and pulse check are the mainstay of patient management. Identification and treatment of reversible causes of cardiac arrest, particularly in PEA, is another major goal of resuscitation. Focused cardiac ultrasound is a tool that allows identification of obstructive causes of arrest (pulmonary embolism, pericardial tamponade, coronary thrombosis) and hypovolemia. Ultrasound can further be used to identify pneumothorax. To incorporate ultrasound safely into resuscitation, training is required to minimize interruptions in chest compressions. Thus, immediate resumption of chest compressions is a must, and a plan for proper use of ultrasound during subsequent pulse/rhythm check should be formulated; no other views should be attempted during the current pulse/rhythm check. This patient is likely bleeding and will require blood transfusion; however, blood transfusion does not replace chest compressions in a patient with cardiac arrest. Similarly, while endotracheal intubation is likely required, it must happen in the context of ongoing resuscitation.

### Selected References

1. Breitkreutz R, Price S, Steiger H, et al. Focused echocardiographic evaluation in life support and peri-resuscitation of emergency patients: a prospective trial. *Resuscitation.* 2010;81(11):1527-1533.
2. Breitkreutz R, Walcher F, Seeger FH. Focused echocardiographic evaluation in resuscitation management: concept of an advanced life support-conformed algorithm. *Crit Care Med.* 2007;35(suppl 5):S150-S161.
3. Bughrara N, Herrick SL, Leimer E, Sirigaddi K, Roberts K, Pustavoitau A. Focused cardiac ultrasound and the periresuscitative period: a case series of resident-performed echocardiographic assessment using subcostal-only view in advanced life support. *A A Pract.* 2020;14(10):e01278. doi:10.1213/XAA.0000000000001278

**10.** Correct Answer: B. Near the end of the 2 minutes of compressions, prior to interruption of compressions

*Rationale:* To minimize interruption in chest compressions, focused cardiac ultrasound is performed during pulse/rhythm check. The ultrasound probe is positioned into subcostal space prior to discontinuation of chest compressions, so that as soon as the last chest compression is performed, the sonographer can record images. Ultrasound is performed while the team leader is counting down 10 seconds, and the probe should come off the chest as soon as chest compressions are resumed. Ultrasound gel should be wiped off the skin to avoid a faulty electrical arc if cardioversion/defibrillation is needed and to avoid sliding of hands of the person performing chest compressions. All other choices do not correctly state the optimal timing and will either result in prolonging interruptions (choice D) or will not result in optimal image acquisition due to either limited time (choice C) or ongoing chest compressions (choice A).

Selected References

1. Breitkreutz R, Price S, Steiger H, et al. Focused echocardiographic evaluation in life support and peri-resuscitation of emergency patients: a prospective trial. *Resuscitation.* 2010;81(11):1527-1533.
2. Breitkreutz R, Walcher F, Seeger FH. Focused echocardiographic evaluation in resuscitation management: concept of an advanced life support-conformed algorithm. *Crit Care Med.* 2007;35(suppl 5):S150-S161.

# 45 | CARDIAC ARREST AND PERI-ARREST

Genevieve Staudt, Ryan Lefevre, Frederick Wilhelm Lombard,
Robert Deegan, and Susan Eagle

1. A 55-year-old woman with hypertension and obesity has become increasingly short of breath since undergoing colon resection 12 hours ago. On physical examination, the patient has a harsh systolic murmur heard at the upper left sternal border. Based on the continuous-wave Doppler through the left ventricular (LV) outflow tract (LVOT) on transthoracic echocardiogram (TTE) (**Figure 45.1**), which of the following is the most likely diagnosis?

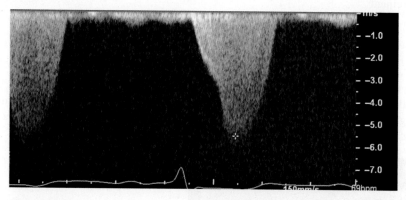

**Figure 45.1**

A. Aortic stenosis
B. Hypertrophic cardiomyopathy
C. Takotsubo cardiomyopathy
D. Mitral stenosis

2. A 72-year-old woman is admitted to the cardiovascular intensive care unit (ICU) following a mitral valve leaflet repair for severe mitral regurgitation (MR). She had an arterial BP of 81/40, HR 101, SaO$_2$ 99%, central venous pressure (CVP) 9 mm Hg, and pulmonary arterial pressure 46/21. An echocardiogram shows severe MR, LV ejection fraction >55%, and a peak gradient of 50 mm Hg on continuous-wave Doppler across the LVOT (**Figure 45.2**).

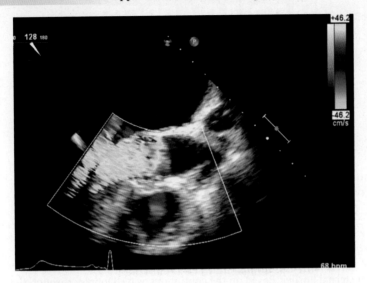

**Figure 45.2**

What is the next most appropriate step?
A. Mitral valve replacement
B. Furosemide
C. Intravenous fluid
D. Milrinone

3. A 78-year-old woman underwent placement of a drug-eluting stent in her left anterior descending (LAD) artery for an ST-elevation myocardial infarction. Five days later, she developed acute severe dyspnea and is intubated. Her vital signs are: BP 61/32, HR 125, SaO$_2$ 82%. Which of the following lesions is identified on the transesophageal echocardiogram (TEE) transgastric short-axis view (**Figure 45.3**)?

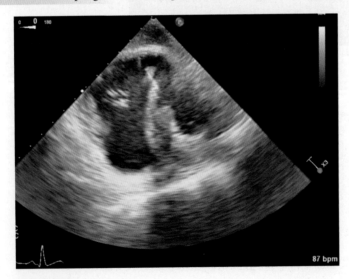

**Figure 45.3**

A. Ventricular septal defect
B. Atrial septal defect
C. Cardiac tamponade
D. LV aneurysm

4. A 42-year-old man underwent an emergency laparotomy following a motor vehicle crash. On the fourth day of hospitalization, the patient had an acute hemodynamic deterioration with a BP 62/41, HR 145, $SaO_2$ 91%. A TEE was performed to rule out a pulmonary embolism (PE). There is normal biventricular function, but a finding in the right pulmonary artery (RPA) was noted and is indicated by the *arrow*. Based on the TEE findings (**Figure 45.4**), which of the following is the most appropriate management strategy?

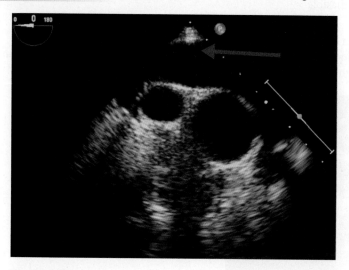

**Figure 45.4**

A. Surgical pulmonary embolectomy
B. Catheter-directed fibrinolysis
C. Intravenous tissue plasminogen activator
D. No intervention for PE

5. A 57-year-old man is admitted to the cardiac ICU following a surgical aortic valve replacement. He developed a progressive lactic acidosis and hypotension during the next 6 hours. The TTE revealed the findings noted in **Figure 45.5**. Vital signs are: BP 75/41, HR 127, pulmonary arterial pressure 42/22, CVP 19 mm Hg.

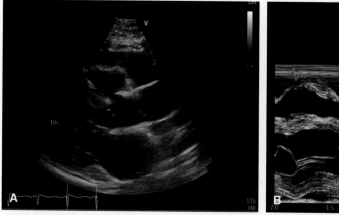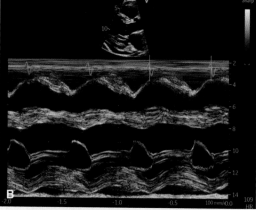

**Figure 45.5**

What finding on M-mode imaging will best guide his management?
A. Presence of pericardial effusion
B. Right ventricular (RV) collapse in diastole
C. Reduced LV wall motion
D. Reduced excursion of aortic valve leaflets

6. Which of the following echocardiographic findings is most commonly associated with cardiac tamponade?

    A. Right atrial collapse during systole
    B. Right ventricle collapse during systole
    C. Right atrial collapse during diastole
    D. Left ventricle collapse during diastole

7. A 62-year-old woman received an LV assist device (LVAD) for nonischemic cardiomyopathy. Four hours into the postoperative period, the mean arterial BP decreases from 70 to 35 mm Hg. Based on the TEE findings (**Figure 45.6**), which of the following is the next best management strategy?

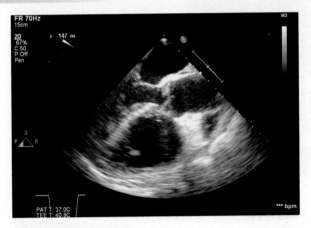

**Figure 45.6**

    A. Decrease LVAD pump speed
    B. Inhaled nitric oxide
    C. Milrinone
    D. Diuresis

8. A 72-year-old woman is intubated in the ICU for respiratory distress. Following intubation, the patient loses pulses and undergoes cardiopulmonary resuscitation (CPR) for 5 minutes before return of spontaneous circulation. The peri-arrest TEE reveals **Figure 45.7** and ▶ **Video 45.1**.

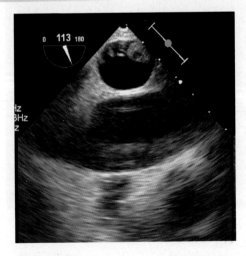

**Figure 45.7**

Which additional echocardiographic finding is most likely?
    A. Collapsed inferior vena cava (IVC)
    B. Rightward intra-atrial septum bowing
    C. D-shaped interventricular septum
    D. LV dilation

9. A 42-year-old man with hypoxic respiratory failure is intubated and subsequently arrests. Emergency femoral cannulation for venoarterial extracorporeal membrane oxygenation (ECMO) support is initiated. Which standard TEE image is most useful for guiding positioning of the femoral venous cannula?

    **A.** Midesophageal bicaval

    **B.** Midesophageal RV inflow-outflow

    **C.** Midesophageal four chamber

    **D.** Deep transgastric

10. A 69-year-old woman undergoes cardiac catheterization for an ST-elevation myocardial infarction. During the coronary intervention, she suffers a cardiac arrest for 4 minutes before return of spontaneous circulation. A mechanical support device is placed in the catheterization laboratory. The TEE (**Figure 45.8**) is most consistent with which of the following mechanical support devices?

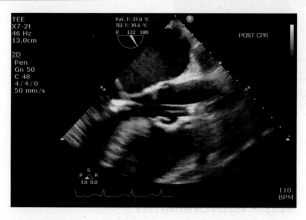

**Figure 45.8**

    **A.** Percutaneous LVAD

    **B.** Intra-aortic balloon pump (IABP)

    **C.** ECMO

    **D.** HeartMate III LVAD

11. A 68-year-old man with obesity, chronic obstructive pulmonary disease (COPD), and acute on chronic heart failure is intubated and mechanically ventilated for hypoxic respiratory failure. On the second day of hospitalization, he has an acute desaturation to 78%. The lung ultrasound (**Figure 45.9**) is most consistent with which of the following?

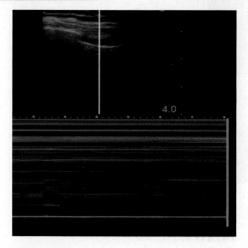

**Figure 45.9**

    **A.** Pleural effusion

    **B.** Pneumonia

    **C.** Pulmonary edema

    **D.** Pneumothorax

12. A 52-year-old man with a non-ST-elevation myocardial infarction suddenly decompensates hemodynamically. A TTE is performed (**Figure 45.10**). The *arrow* pointing to an area of severe hypokinesis is consistent with which coronary artery distribution?

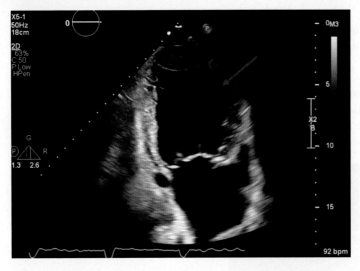

**Figure 45.10**

A. Right coronary artery
B. Left circumflex coronary artery
C. Left anterior descending coronary artery
D. Obtuse marginal coronary artery

13. A 65-year-old woman is admitted to the surgical ICU following a small bowel resection. She remains intubated and mechanically ventilated. On postoperative day 2, she develops hemodynamic instability and has the following vitals: BP 61/32, HR 137, and $SaO_2$ 91%. Based on the TEE (**Figure 45.11**), which of the following is the most appropriate management strategy?

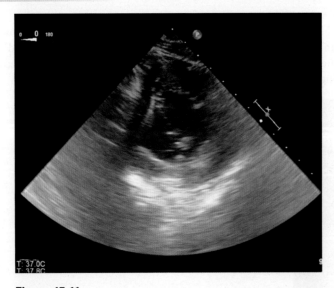

**Figure 45.11**

A. Milrinone
B. Fluid administration
C. Epinephrine
D. Metoprolol

14. A 59-year-old man with a history of coronary artery disease and drug-eluting stents is admitted to the ICU after sustaining severe burns to his upper body. On the second day of hospitalization, the patient arrests, but has return of spontaneous circulation following CPR. TTE (**Figure 45.12**) demonstrates severe focal hypokinesis (*arrow*).

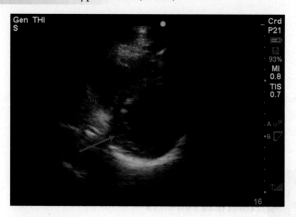

**Figure 45.12**

This area is within the distribution of which of the following coronary arteries?
A. Left anterior descending coronary artery
B. Obtuse marginal coronary artery
C. Left circumflex coronary artery
D. Right coronary artery

15. A 68-year-old woman with a history of ischemic cardiomyopathy and prior four-vessel coronary artery bypass grafting is admitted to the ICU with acute systolic heart failure. She is intubated, sedated, and has the following vital signs: BP 67/34, HR 121, SaO$_2$ 98%. A femoral IABP is inserted emergently and a TEE is utilized for balloon positioning. Which of the following is the correct location of the distal end of the balloon on TEE?

A. 2 cm distal to left subclavian artery
B. 3 cm distal to the aortic valve
C. 5 cm proximal to the LVOT
D. 1 cm proximal to the left renal artery

16. A 68-year-old man with a history of hypertension and chronic systolic heart failure is admitted to the ICU following a splenectomy after a motor vehicle crash. On postoperative day 1, the patient becomes profoundly hypotensive and intravenous fluids are administered. To determine fluid responsiveness, pulsed-wave Doppler should be performed on which part of the echocardiogram shown in **Figure 45.13**?

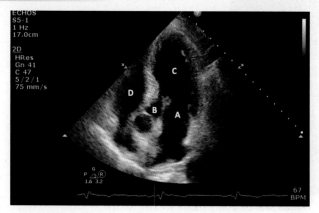

**Figure 45.13**

A. A
B. B
C. C
D. D

17. A 79-year-old woman presents to the surgical ICU following a colectomy for colon cancer. Twelve hours postoperatively, she develops new-onset atrial fibrillation and profound hypotension. Despite intubation and synchronized cardioversion, she remains in atrial fibrillation and is hypotensive. Which of the following findings on TTE most likely predicts fluid responsiveness?

    A. RV end-diastolic area
    B. Stroke volume variation
    C. IVC diameter
    D. LV end-diastolic area

18. A 29-year-old woman with a history of preeclampsia is postpartum day 1 following a cesarean section. Since delivery, she has had increased dyspnea and tachycardia for which she was admitted to the surgical ICU. Based on the TTE image shown in **Figure 45.14**, which of the following is the most appropriate management strategy?

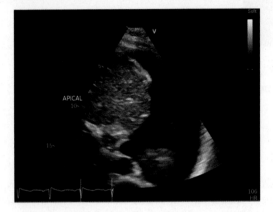

**Figure 45.14**

    A. Pericardiocentesis
    B. Thoracostomy tube
    C. Therapeutic paracentesis
    D. Intravenous heparin

19. A 55-year-old man with a history of coronary artery disease is admitted to the ICU with acute onset of chest pain. He received a drug-eluting stent 3 months ago, but has not been taking his prescribed clopidogrel. His initial BP is 110/62 with a HR of 102. Shortly after admission he acutely decompensated, was emergently intubated, and was started on norepinephrine. A transesophageal echo reveals **Figure 45.15**.

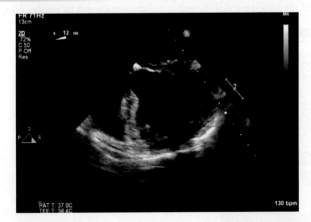

**Figure 45.15**

Which of the following associated findings is *most* likely present?
    A. Coandă effect seen on color flow Doppler
    B. Mitral inflow mean gradient of 11 mm Hg
    C. Tricuspid regurgitation (TR) jet peak velocity of 1.25 m/s
    D. Vegetation on the aortic valve

20. A 34-year-old woman is admitted to the ICU with acute dyspnea. Her oxygen saturation is 91% on room air. She notes 2 days of right lower extremity swelling. A computed tomography (CT) angiogram demonstrates a large saddle PE. A transthoracic echo would *most* likely reveal which of the following findings?

   A. IVC collapse with inspiration
   B. Tricuspid annular plane systolic excursion (TAPSE) of 1.2 cm
   C. LV fractional area change of 20%
   D. Mid-RV diameter of 2.7 cm

21. A 56-year-old man is admitted to the Emergency Department with substernal chest pain. A serum troponin-I level is obtained and is elevated. A TEE (**Figure 45.16**) shows severe hypokinesis of the highlighted segment.

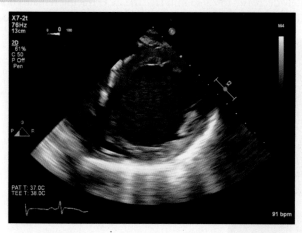

**Figure 45.16**

Which of the following is the *most* likely abnormality to be seen on electrocardiogram (ECG)?
   A. ST-elevation in leads II, III, and aVF
   B. ST-elevation in leads V1-V4
   C. ST-elevation in leads aVL, V5, V6
   D. Diffuse ST-elevation

22. A 43-year-old woman is admitted to the ICU after a mitral valve repair. Upon moving to the ICU bed she becomes acutely bradycardic and hypotensive. A coronary gas embolism is suspected. A TEE is performed and **Figure 45.17** is obtained.

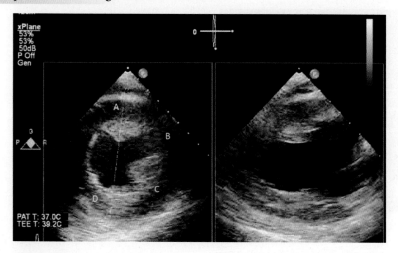

**Figure 45.17**

Which of the following walls is *most* likely to be hypokinetic?
   A. A
   B. B
   C. C
   D. D

23. Which of the following outcomes is true regarding the use of TTE in the management of critically ill patients with sepsis?

A. TTE leads to decreased fluid administration.
B. TTE leads to no change in 28-day mortality.
C. TTE leads to increased use of inotropic support.
D. TTE leads to decreased maximum norepinephrine doses.

24. A 28-year-old primigravida woman at 38 weeks gestation is admitted in active labor. An epidural catheter is placed and infused with ropivacaine, with successful analgesia obtained. Three hours into labor, she becomes acutely tachypneic, hypoxemic, and hypertensive. An emergency cesarean section is performed for fetal bradycardia. During the surgery, her BP acutely decreases to 75/43 mm Hg. The ECG tracing remains normal. A TEE is performed and **Figure 45.18** and ▶ **Video 45.2** transgastric short-axis images are obtained.

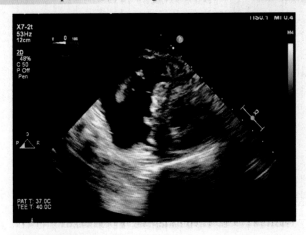

**Figure 45.18**

Which of the following is the *most* likely reason for her acute decompensation?
A. Maternal hemorrhage
B. High spinal anesthetic level
C. Local anesthetic systemic toxicity
D. Amniotic fluid embolism

25. A 62-year-old woman is admitted with acute onset of tearing chest pain. A TEE reveals **Figure 45.19**.

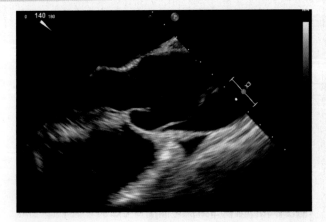

**Figure 45.19**

Which of the following is *least* likely to be an associated finding?
A. Aortic valve pressure half-time of 220 ms
B. Pulsus paradoxus on arterial line waveform
C. ST depressions in ECG leads II, III, aVF
D. LVOT/aortic valve dimensionless index of 0.21

26. A 43-year-old man with a history of hypertension and acute-onset chest pain becomes hemodynamically unstable. A transesophageal echo probe is placed and **Figure 45.20** is obtained.

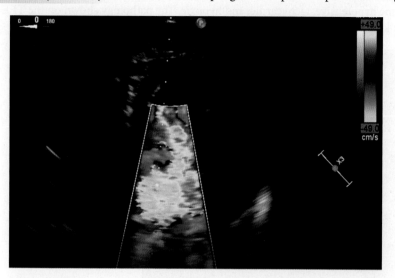

**Figure 45.20**

Which of the following associated findings is *least* likely true?
A. Widened pulse pressure
B. Effective regurgitant orifice area of 0.1 cm²
C. Antegrade cardioplegia will be ineffective.
D. Holodiastolic flow reversal in his descending aorta

27. A 78-year-old woman develops acute respiratory failure, which requires emergent intubation. She subsequently arrests, but has return of spontaneous circulation following two rounds of CPR. A TEE is performed and **Figure 45.21** is obtained.

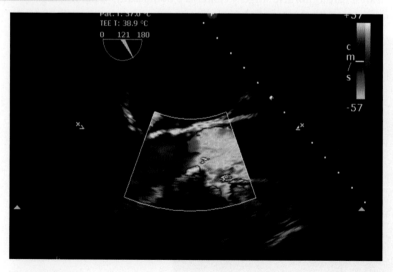

**Figure 45.21**

Which of the following findings is *most* likely?
A. Aortic valve area of 1.6 cm²
B. Aortic valve mean pressure gradient of 15 mm Hg
C. Dimensionless index of 0.21
D. Aortic valve peak velocity of 2.8 m/s

28. A 62-year-old man with a history of type II diabetes, hypertension, and obesity is in the ICU following a motor vehicle crash. The patient was hemodynamically stable on 2 L O$_2$ nasal cannula until hospital day 2, when he suddenly became hypotensive, tachycardic, and hypoxic. The pathology shown on the TEE (**Figure 45.22**) is most likely associated with which of the following?

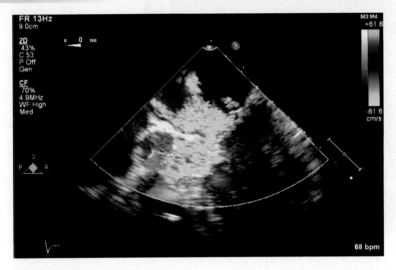

**Figure 45.22**

A. Holodiastolic aorta flow reversal
B. Systolic pulmonary vein flow reversal
C. Systolic hepatic vein flow reversal
D. Diastolic pulmonary artery flow reversal

29. A 43-year-old man with a bicuspid aortic valve and a history of cocaine abuse develops new-onset chest pain. A TTE identifies a Stanford Type A aortic dissection. The patient is diaphoretic, unable to lie flat, and the BP is 74/31. The nearest cardiothoracic surgery center is 2 hours away. What findings on TTE (**Figure 45.23**) are most consistent with tamponade?

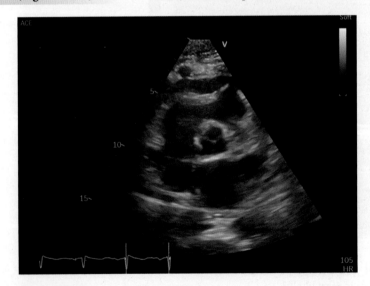

**Figure 45.23**

A. IVC collapse during inspiration
B. RV collapse in diastole
C. Increase in mitral peak E-wave velocity with inspiration
D. RA collapse in diastole

30. A 57-year-old previously healthy woman is admitted to the ICU following a motor vehicle crash, where she sustained multiple facial and rib fractures. Her vital signs are BP 77/43, HR101, respiratory rate (RR) 21, SaO$_2$ 99% on 2 L O$_2$ nasal cannula. The TTE (**Figure 45.24**) is most consistent with which of the following?

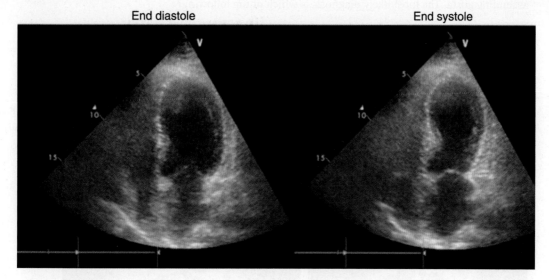

**Figure 45.24**

   A. Takotsubo cardiomyopathy
   B. Pulmonary embolism
   C. Pericardial effusion
   D. Aortic dissection

31. A 64-year-old male with new-onset chest pain and shortness of breath is taken to the cardiac catheterization lab emergently. ECG shows ST-elevation in leads II, III, and aVF. **Figure 45.25** and ▶ **Video 45.3** are most consistent with which of the following?

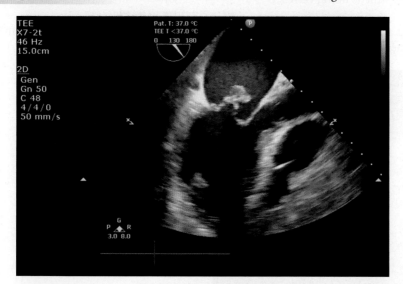

**Figure 45.25**

   A. Atrial myxoma
   B. Posterior leaflet restriction due to inferior wall ischemia
   C. Infective endocarditis with flail posterior leaflet
   D. Ruptured posteromedial papillary muscle (PPM)

32. A 27-year-old woman is recovering in the ICU after sustaining multiple injuries in a motor vehicle crash. Her right internal jugular central line is removed while sitting upright, she subsequently coughs violently and loses consciousness. She is intubated emergently and a TEE shows air bubbles in the ascending aorta. The most likely diagnosis is which of the following?

    **A.** Traumatic retrograde Type A aortic dissection
    **B.** Patent foramen ovale with air embolism
    **C.** Inadvertent internal carotid line placement
    **D.** Vasovagal syncope

33. A 54-year-old woman is admitted to the ICU with new-onset atrial fibrillation with rapid ventricular rate. The patient's BP is 62/33, pulse is 133, and SaO$_2$ is 95%. The patient is intubated and mechanically ventilated. A TEE is performed to rule out thrombus in the left atrial (LA) appendage prior to cardioversion. **Figure 45.26** and ▶ **Video 45.4** are most consistent with what pathology?

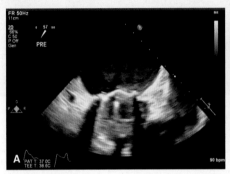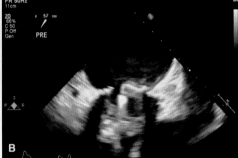

**Figure 45.26**

    **A.** Perforated bioprosthetic mitral valve leaflet
    **B.** Immobile mechanical mitral valve leaflet
    **C.** Dehiscence of a mechanical mitral valve
    **D.** Dehiscence of a bioprosthetic mitral valve

34. A 72-year-old woman is admitted for respiratory failure and is urgently intubated. A chest ultrasound is performed to evaluate her hypoxia. **Figure 45.27** is most consistent with which of the following?

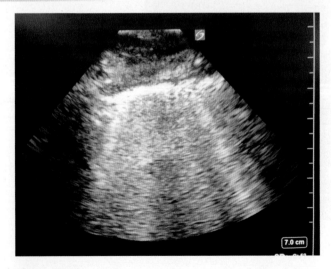

**Figure 45.27**

    **A.** Pleural effusion
    **B.** COPD
    **C.** Pneumothorax
    **D.** Pulmonary edema

**35.** A 78-year-old man who is postoperative day 2 from a total hip joint replacement develops hypoxia and hypotension. His pulse is 100, BP is 100/60, and the CVP is 18. On TEE, the peak TR velocity is 350 cm/s. What is the *best* estimate of pulmonary arterial systolic pressure (PASP)?

A. 67 mm Hg
B. 49 mm Hg
C. 31 mm Hg
D. 120 mm Hg

# Chapter 45 ▪ Answers

**1.** Correct Answer: **B. Hypertrophic cardiomyopathy**

*Rationale:* Continuous-wave Doppler pattern for LVOT obstruction seen in hypertrophic cardiomyopathy is described as "dagger shaped," with gradual increase in velocity in early systole with acceleration to peak velocity in mid-systole. LV pressure outflow gradient may be estimated using modified Bernoulli equation: $\Delta P = 4v^2$, where $\Delta P$ = pressure gradient in mm Hg and $v$ = maximal flow velocity in m/s. The continuous-wave Doppler pattern of aortic stenosis, which is a fixed rather than dynamic lesion, demonstrates a more rounded appearance with a peak in early to mid-systole. Mitral stenosis will present with a low-pitched diastolic murmur best heard at the apex, rather than a systolic murmur as demonstrated with our patient. Echocardiographic evaluation of mitral stenosis includes visualization of a laminar, high-velocity jet at the level of the narrowing. Distally, the flow pattern will become disorganized with multiple directions of blood flow. Takotsubo cardiomyopathy is an acute, stress-induced cardiomyopathy characterized by reversible ballooning of the LV apex. Patients will present with low cardiac output and symptoms that mimic acute coronary syndromes. Echocardiographic examination will not reveal increased gradient across the LVOT.

### Selected References
1. Chatterjee D. Mitral valve disease : clinical features focusing on auscultatory findings including auscultation of mitral valve prolapse. *Eur Soc Cardiol.* 2019;16:1-10.
2. Maron MS, Rowin EJ, Maron BJ. How to image hypertrophic cardiomyopathy. *Circ Cardiovasc Imaging.* 2017;10:1-15.
3. Panza JA, Petrone RK, Fananapazir L, Maron BJ. Utility of continuous wave doppler echocardiography in the noninvasive assessment of left ventricular outflow tract pressure gradient in patients with hypertrophic cardiomyopathy. *J Am Coll Cardiol.* 1992;19:91-99.
4. Salustri A, Almaghrabi A. Mitral valve disease: correlation between the most important echocardiographic parameters and hemodynamics. *e-J Cardiol Pract.* 2019;16(24):1-20.
5. Wahab A, Wahab S, Panwar R, Alvi S. Takotsubo cardiomyopathy or broken heart syndrome. *Iran Cardiovasc Res J.* 2010;4:33-34.

**2.** Correct Answer: **C. Intravenous fluid**

*Rationale:* Systolic anterior motion (SAM) of the mitral valve is characterized by the anterior displacement of the anterior leaflet of the mitral valve during systole, leading to LVOT obstruction and MR (**Figure 45.28**). SAM occurs in 4% to 5% of patients following mitral valve repair. Predisposing factors include redundant leaflet tissue, a short distance between ventricular septum and mitral valve coaptation point or coaptation-septum (CS) distance following repair, and a nondilated, hyperdynamic ventricle. SAM may present with varying clinical significance. Many patients are asymptomatic removed for brevity while other patients may have pulmonary congestion and hemodynamic collapse due to LVOT obstruction and severe MR.

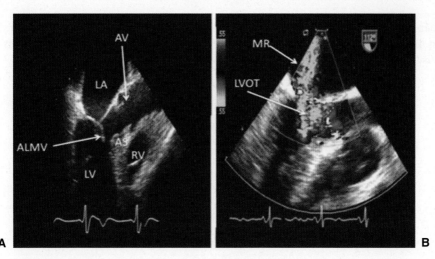

**Figure 45.28** Systolic anterior motion (SAM) resulting in left ventricular outflow tract LVOT) obstruction (A) and severe, posteriorly directed mitral regurgitation (B). ALMV, anterior leaflet mitral valve; AS, anteroseptal wall; AV, aortic valve; LA, left atrium; LV, left ventricle; MR, mitral regurgitation; RV, right ventricle.

The patient in this question is demonstrating hemodynamic and echocardiographic signs of moderate to severe SAM, characterized by low cardiac output, severe MR, and LVOT obstruction. Once the diagnosis of SAM has been made, treatment can be initiated. Reduced inotropic support and volume loading are first-line medical therapy for SAM and associated LVOT obstruction. Volume loading serves to both distend the LV dimensions and to enhance the CS distance. Administration of the diuretic furosemide would worsen intravascular volume depletion. Initiation of milrinone would potentiate the hyperdynamic cardiac condition, which may lead to increased severity of symptoms. Mitral valve replacement may be necessary in the event of severe SAM refractory to medical management, but is not a first-line therapy.

### Selected References

1. Manabe S, Kasegawa H, Arai H, Takanashi S. Management of systolic anterior motion of the mitral valve: a mechanism-based approach. *Gen Thorac Cardiovasc Surg*. 2018;66:379-389.
2. Sternik L, Zehr KJ. Systolic anterior motion of the mitral valve after mitral valve repair: a method of prevention. *Texas Hear Inst J*. 2005;32:47-49.

**3.** Correct Answer: A. Ventricular septal defect

*Rationale:* Ventricular septal rupture (VSR) is a dramatic complication following an acute myocardial infarction (AMI). Post-MI VSR occurs when the acutely infarcted tissue at the myocardial infarct border zone ruptures or tears. Incidence of post-MI VSR has a bimodal distribution with peaks within the first 24 hours and again between 3 and 5 days, but can occur as late as 2 weeks following an acute MI. The majority of cases of myocardial rupture are associated with complete occlusion of a major coronary artery.[2] Other risk factors include older age, female sex, history of hypertension, nonsmoker, and anterior infarction.[3]

With the increased use of percutaneous intervention, the incidence of post-MI VSR has decreased, but the associated mortality rate remains high (94% with conservative medical management and 47% with surgical management). Patients with post-MI VSR may present with the abrupt onset of dyspnea, hypotension, and development of a new murmur. Acute decompensation is due to pulmonary edema, biventricular failure, and cardiogenic shock.

Echocardiography may be used to detect VSR. Two-dimensional color Doppler can detect flow through the defect and is particularly helpful if the septal defect is small or the communicating tract takes a tortuous path (**Figure 45.29**).

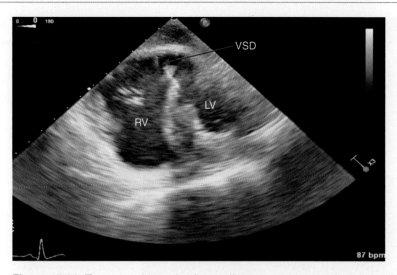

**Figure 45.29** Transesophageal echocardiogram, transgastric short-axis midpapillary left view, showing a postinfarct ventricular septal defect. LV, left ventricle; RV, right ventricle; VSD, ventricular septal defect.

### Selected References

1. Crenshaw BS, Granger CB, Birnbaum Y, et al. Risk factors, angiographic patterns, and outcomes in patients with ventricular septal defect complicating acute myocardial infarction. *Circulation.* 2000;101:27-32.
2. Evrin T, Unluer EE, Kuday E, et al. Bedside echocardiography in acute myocardial infarction patients with hemodynamic deterioration. *J Natl Med Assoc.* 2018;110:396-398.
3. Manabe S, Kasegawa H, Arai H, Takanashi S. Management of systolic anterior motion of the mitral valve: a mechanism-based approach. *Gen Thorac Cardiovasc Surg.* 2018;66:379-389.
4. Suder B, Janik Ł, Wasilewski G, et al. Post-myocardial infarction ventricular septal defect. Is it better to operate on a fresh infarction or to wait? A case study. *Kardiochirurgia i Torakochirurgia Pol.* 2016;13:39-41.

**4.** Correct Answer: **D. No intervention for PE**

*Rationale:* Figure 45.4 shows a near-field clutter artifact, which is created by high-amplitude reflections from the piezoelectric crystals themselves. While challenging, it may be distinguished from a true structure by its hazy appearance and ill-defined borders. Additionally, artifacts should not produce interruption of color Doppler flow or sonographic contrast, as seen with true structures. The ability to distinguish between artifact and thrombus is critical as this distinction may help to guide therapy and avoid unnecessary invasive treatment.

PE is an unfortunate perioperative complication following major surgical procedures and is one of the leading causes of intraoperative cardiac arrest. While a CT pulmonary angiogram is the definitive diagnostic test, TEE has been shown to detect PE in over 50% of patients and may be beneficial in the hemodynamically unstable patient. Indirect signs of PE on TEE include RV dilation with hypokinesis, a D-shaped interventricular septum indicative of RV pressure overload, and severe TR. Importantly, these findings are not specific for PE. Additionally, McConnell sign is an echocardiographic finding with a distinct pattern of RV dysfunction characterized by RV free wall akinesis with preserved apical function, which is characteristic of acute PE. These indirect echocardiographic signs of PE are of great clinical value as some studies indicate that direct visualization of thromboemboli is as low as 26%.[6] **Figure 45.30** and the aforementioned findings may also help to differentiate between acute and chronic PE.

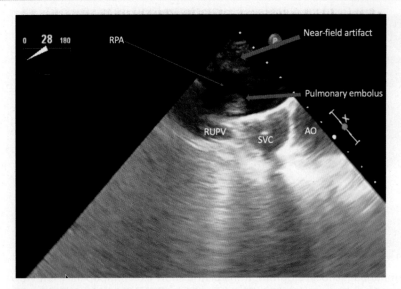

**Figure 45.30** Pulmonary embolism in the right pulmonary artery; slightly above is a near-field artifact commonly visualized in the RPA at the level of the superior vena cava. AO, aorta; RPA, right pulmonary artery; RUPV, right upper pulmonary vein; SVC, superior vena cava.

### Selected References

1. De Vos L, De Herdt V, Timmermans F. Misdiagnosis or missed diagnosis: digging out the "near-field clutter" artifact in a patient with stroke. *CASE*. 2020;4:2-6.
2. Lau G, Ther G, Swanevelder J. McConnell's sign in acute pulmonary embolism. *Anesth Analg*. 2013;116:982-985.
3. Liang Y, Alvis B, Rice MJ, Shaw AD, Deitte LA, Eagle S. A near-field clutter artifact mimicking pulmonary thrombus during transesophageal echocardiography. *Anesth Analg*. 2016;123:831-833.
4. Pamnani A, Skubas NJ. Imaging artifacts during transesophageal echocardiography. *Anesth Analg*. 2014;118:516-520.
5. Pruszczyk P, Torbicki A, Kuch-Wocial A, Szulc M, Pacho R. Diagnostic value of transesophageal echocardiography in suspected hemodynamically significant pulmonary embolism. *Heart*. 2001;85:628-634.
6. Rosenberger P, Shernan S, Weissmuller T, Eltzschig HK. Role of intraoperative transesophageal echocardiography for diagnosis and managing pulmonary embolism in the perioperative period. *Anesth Analg*. 2005;100:292-293.

**5.** Correct Answer: B. RV collapse in diastole

*Rationale:* Figure 45.5 is a transthoracic parasternal long-axis view (PLAX) demonstrating collapse of the right ventricle during diastole. Bedside echocardiography is an excellent initial imaging modality when cardiac tamponade is suspected and is recommended by the American College of Cardiology, the American Heart Association, and the American Society of Echocardiography (ASE). A focused examination for cardiac tamponade should include determination of size and extent of the pericardial effusion, collapsibility of cardiac chambers, ventricular interdependence with respiration, dilation of the IVC with limited respiratory variation, and a septal "bounce." Among these findings, RA collapsibility for over one-third of the cardiac cycle is perhaps the most reliable sign of cardiac tamponade with a near 100% specificity and 94% sensitivity. M-mode echocardiography may be used to assess RV collapse, which will occur in diastole and persist as long as pericardial pressures are higher than RV filling pressures. A greater duration of RV collapse corresponds to more significant tamponade.

Beck's triad consisting of hypotension, jugular venous distention and muffled heart sounds is present in only a minority of those with cardiac tamponade. Sinus tachycardia is a compensatory mechanism to allow at least partial maintenance of cardiac output. Pulsus paradoxus is a drop in systemic BP by >10 mm Hg with inspiration and occurs due to exaggerated ventricular interdependence. Increased RV filling during inspiration leads to bulging of the RV into the LV resulting in decrease in LV filling and SV.

### Selected References

1. Cheitlin MD, Armstrong WF, Aurigemma GP, et al. ACC/AHA/ASE 2003 guideline update for the clinical application of echocardiography: Summary article: a report of the American College of Cardiology/American Heart Association Task Force on Practice Guidelines (ACC/AHA/ASE Committee to Update the 1997 Guidelines for the Clinical Application of Echocardiography). *Circulation*. 2003;108:1146-1162.

2. Beck C. Two cardiac compression triads. *J Am Med Assoc*. 1935;104:714.
3. Fitchett D, Sniderman A. Inspiratory reduction in left heart filling as a mechanism of pulsus paradoxus in cardiac tamponade. *Can J Cardiol*. 1990;6:348.
4. Gillam LD, Guyer DE, Gibson TC, King ME, Marshall JE, Weyman AE. Hydrodynamic compression of the right atrium: a new echocardiographic sign of cardiac tamponade. *Circulation*. 1983;68:294-301.
5. Pérez-Casares A, Cesar S, Brunet-Garcia L, Sanchez-de-Toledo J. Echocardiographic evaluation of pericardial effusion and cardiac tamponade. *Front Pediatr*. 2017;5:1-10.

**6.** Correct Answer: A. Right atrial (RA) collapse during systole

*Rationale:* RA inversion/collapse beginning at end-diastole and continuing through some portion of systole has a 100% sensitivity for cardiac tamponade (**Figure 45.31**). When the duration of RA collapse is greater than one-third of the cardiac cycle, the specificity of this finding for tamponade increases to 94%. Collapse of the left atrium may occur with cardiac tamponade but is much less common than RA collapse. Collapse of the RV free wall occurs during diastole because of increases in pericardial pressure. With moderate increases in pericardial pressure, this may be observed in expiration only, but as the effusion increases in severity, collapse may be seen throughout the respiratory cycle. Collapse of the left ventricle is much less common due to its thick wall, but may be seen with a loculated pericardial effusion around the posterior wall, which can be seen following cardiac surgery.

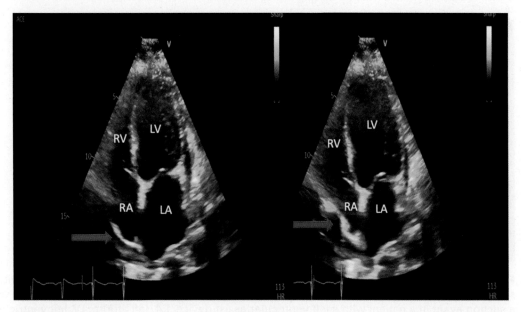

**Figure 45.31** Transthoracic echocardiography apical four-chamber view showing right atrial (RA) collapse during systole (*arrow*). LA, left atrium; LV, left ventricle; RV, right ventricle.

Selected References
1. Gillam LD, Guyer DE, Gibson TC, King ME, Marshall JE, Weyman AE. Hydrodynamic compression of the right atrium: a new echocardiographic sign of cardiac tamponade. *Circulation*. 1983;68:294-301.
2. Gillebert C, Van Hoof R, Van De Werf F, Piessens J, De Geest H. Abnormal wall movements of the right ventricle and both atria in patients with pericardial effusion as indicators of cardiac tamponade. *Eur Heart J*. 1986;7:437-443.
3. Leeman DE, Levine MJ, Come PC. Doppler echocardiography in cardiac tamponade: exaggerated respiratory variation in transvalvular blood flow velocity integrals. *J Am Coll Cardiol*. 1988;11:572-578.
4. Pérez-Casares A, Cesar S, Brunet-Garcia L, Sanchez-de-Toledo J. Echocardiographic evaluation of pericardial effusion and cardiac tamponade. *Front Pediatr*. 2017;5:1-10.

**7.** Correct Answer: A. Decrease LVAD pump speed

*Rationale:* LVADs are the most common mechanical circulatory assist devices used for severe heart failure. They may be utilized as a bridge to transplant, recovery or decision-making, or as destination therapy in those not eligible for transplantation.

The TEE (**Figure 45.32**) demonstrates RV dilation and a small, decompressed LV cavity. These findings are suggestive of a suction event. Suction events occur when the speed of the LVAD pump is excessive relative to LV filling. This results in exaggerated LV offloading and collapse of the LV cavity upon itself and the inflow cannula. Causes of suction events include low intravascular volume, RV failure, tamponade, and inflow cannula obstruction.

Echocardiographic evaluation will demonstrate a significant reduction in LV size. Evaluation of the right ventricle for signs of failure is critical as this may lead to LV underfilling and will alter long-term management. Examination of inflow cannula position should also occur as malposition of cannulas may predispose to suction events.

Immediate treatment of suction events includes slowing the device speed and administering volume. Further measures should be targeted at underlying causes of suction events including RV dysfunction. This may be treated with inotropic support such as epinephrine, nitric oxide, or placement of an RV assist device. If cannula position is an issue, surgical repositioning may be indicated.[2]

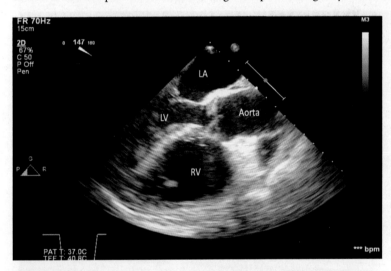

**Figure 45.32** Transesophageal echocardiogram, midesophageal long-axis aorta view, showing a severely dilated right ventricle and a decompressed left ventricle. This scenario is consistent with a suction event in a patient with a left ventricular assist device. LA, left atrium; LV, left ventricle; RV, right ventricle.

### Selected References

1. Flores AS, Essandoh M, Yerington GC, et al. Echocardiographic assessment for ventricular assist device placement. *J Thorac Dis.* 2015;7:2139-2150.
2. Sen A, Larson JS, Kashani KB, et al. Mechanical circulatory assist devices: a primer for critical care and emergency physicians. *Crit Care.* 2016.20:1-20.
3. Slaughter MS, Pagani FD, Rogers JG, et al. Clinical management of continuous-flow left ventricular assist devices in advanced heart failure. *J Hear Lung Transplant.* 2010;29:S1-S39.

**8.** Correct Answer: C. D-shaped interventricular septum

*Rationale/Critique:* The echocardiographic image shown in Figure 45.7 is a midesophageal ascending aorta long-axis view. In this view, the RPA is seen in short axis in the near field with a long-axis view of the ascending aorta visualized behind. A large intravascular thrombus is seen in the RPA.

Accompanying echocardiographic findings of hemodynamically significant pulmonary emboli include RV hypokinesis, RV dilation, severe TR, and D-shaped interventricular septum. The D-shaped appearance of the left ventricle occurs due to ventricular interdependence where RV pressure or volume overload leads to mechanical flattening of the interventricular septum and bulging into the left ventricle. This alters the geometry of the left ventricle in a deleterious manner, resulting in impaired LV function.

Selected References

1. Kapoor P, Muralidhar K, Nanda N, et al. An update on transesophageal echocardiography views 2016: 2D versus 3D tee views. *Ann Card Anaesth.* 2016;19:S56-S72.
2. Lau G, Ther G, Swanevelder J. McConnell's sign in acute pulmonary embolism. *Anesth Analg.* 2013;116:982-985.
3. Liang Y, Alvis B, Rice MJ, Shaw AD, Deitte LA, Eagle S. A near-field clutter artifact mimicking pulmonary thrombus during transesophageal echocardiography. *Anesth Analg.* 2016;123:831-833.
4. Ma C, Cohen J, Tolpin D. Right ventricular dysfunction and the "D"-shaped left ventricle. *Anesthesiology.* 2020;132:155.

**9.** Correct Answer: A. Midesophageal bicaval

*Rationale:* TEE is a useful imaging modality when initiating ECMO support, both for positioning of cannulas and to promptly recognize complications, such as pericardial effusion or aortic dissection. With femoro-femoral VA ECMO cannulation, the drainage (venous) cannula is positioned near the IVC/RA junction and the reinjection (arterial) cannula is generally positioned in the distal descending aorta. The midesophageal bicaval view is used to guide femoral venous cannulation as it provides visualization of the IVC, superior vena cava (SVC), right atrium, and tricuspid valve (TV). During placement, the echocardiographer should visualize the guidewire in both the IVC and SVC to ensure that it has not migrated into the right ventricle, across an atrial septal defect, or into the coronary sinus. Optimal position of the cannula tip is in the RA just beyond the cavoatrial junction. If the cannula remains too shallow it may abut the wall of the IVC, while deep insertion risks damage to cardiac structures including the interatrial septum or TV.

Selected References

1. Douflé G, Roscoe A, Billia F, Fan E. Echocardiography for adult patients supported with extracorporeal membrane oxygenation. *Crit Care.* 2015;19:1-10.
2. Hahn RT, Abraham T, Adams MS, et al. Guidelines for performing a comprehensive transesophageal echocardiographic examination: recommendations from the American Society of Echocardiography and the Society of Cardiovascular Anesthesiologists. *J Am Soc Echocardiogr.* 2013;26:921-964.
3. Pavlushko E, Berman M, Valchanov K. Cannulation techniques for extracorporeal life support. *Ann Transl Med.* 2017 Feb 5;5(4):70.

**10.** Correct Answer: A. Percutaneous LVAD

*Rationale:* A variety of mechanical support devices are used for the treatment of severe heart failure. These devices can be divided into three main categories: paracorporeal where the pump is located outside the body, intracorporeal with the pump inside the body, and percutaneous devices, which are small pumps inserted percutaneously.

The Impella device is a short-term, percutaneous support device that can be used for either LV or RV failure. When used for LV support, it is placed retrograde across the aortic valve via the femoral or axillary artery. The device pumps blood from the left ventricle to the ascending aorta at a rate of up to 2.5 L/min, thereby offloading the left ventricle and augmenting cardiac output. When visualized on echocardiogram, the inlet should be located 3 to 4 cm below the aortic valve and the inlet area should not contact the interventricular septum or the anterior leaflet of the mitral valve. For optimal position, the outlet should be 1.5 to 2 cm above the sinuses of Valsalva (**Figure 45.33**).

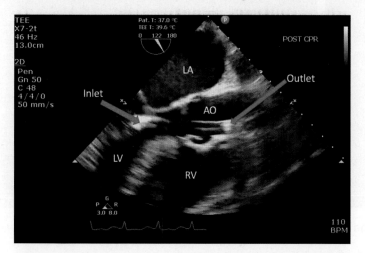

**Figure 45.33** Percutaneous support device in a postcardiac arrest patient. The inlet portion of the device can be visualized in the left ventricle and the outlet portion in the ascending aorta. AO, aorta; LA, left atrium; LV, left ventricle; RV, right ventricle.

The IABP is positioned in the thoracic aorta with the tip distal to the left subclavian artery and the proximal portion above the takeoff of the renal arteries. ECMO cannulas will be seen on echocardiography as described in **Question 9**.

HeartMate III LVAD is a durable, intracorporeal mechanical assist device. It is implanted surgically, not percutaneously. Echocardiographic assessment will reveal the inflow cannula positioned in the LV apex and the outflow cannula located in either the ascending or descending aorta.

### Selected References

1. Mukku V, Cai Q, Gilani S, Fujise K, Barbagelata A. Use of Impella ventricular assist device in patients with severe coronary artery disease presenting with cardiac arrest. *Int J Angiol*. 2012;21:163-166.
2. Sen A, Larson JS, Kashani KB, et al. Mechanical circulatory assist devices: a primer for critical care and emergency physicians. *Crit Care*. 2016;20:1-20.
3. Sponga S, Benedetti G, Livi U. Short-term mechanical circulatory support as bridge to heart transplantation: paracorporeal ventricular assist device as alternative to extracorporeal life support. *Ann Cardiothorac Surg*. 2019;8:143-150.
4. Stainback RF, Estep JD, Agler DA, et al. Echocardiography in the management of patients with left ventricular assist devices: recommendations from the American Society of Echocardiography. *J Am Soc Echocardiogr*. 2015;28:853-909.

**11.** Correct Answer: D. Pneumothorax

*Rationale:* Lung ultrasound is an increasingly utilized point-of-care technique to evaluate acute respiratory failure. Lung ultrasound relies upon the interpretation of artifacts as lung parenchyma is largely composed of air with rapidly dispersed ultrasound waves. In normal lung tissue, the pleura is the only visualized structure that will appear as a hyperechoic horizontal line. Lung sliding is the phenomenon by which the pleural line moves in synchrony with respiration.[3] Lung sliding can be confirmed using M-mode, which will demonstrate a stratified, motionless pattern above the pleura and a sandy pattern representing movement of the lung below the pleura. A-lines are hyperechoic, horizontal lines that represent normal reverberation artifacts from the pleura. They occur at regular intervals and are a sign of air within the lung parenchyma. B-lines are a reverberation artifact that appear as hyperechoic vertical lines arising from the pleural line and extend to the bottom of the screen without fading. The presence of multiple B-lines is a sign of pathology as they occur when there is increased density of the lung parenchyma due to excessive fluid or collagen content. Consolidation of the lung parenchyma, whether due to infection, infarction, fluid collection, atelectasis, or mass, will appear as a solid structure, similar to liver tissue and often referred to as hepatization.

Pneumothorax manifests with absent lung sliding, confirmed with the "stratosphere" or "barcode" sign in M-mode, which indicates absence of motion (**Figure 45.34A**). This is in contrast to the "seashore" sign that has clear contrast between immobile chest wall above the pleura and dynamic lung tissue below the pleura (**Figure 45.34B**). A lung point is the transition point between normal lung tissue and an area of pneumothorax with the absence of lung sliding and B-lines.

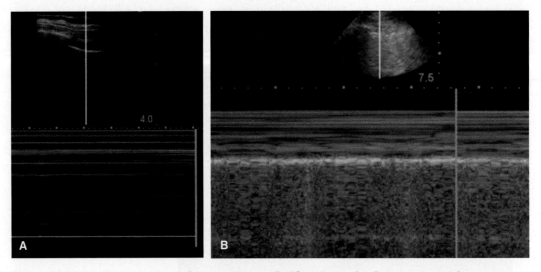

**Figure 45.34** A. "Barcode sign": Pneumothorax. B. "Seashore sign"—no pneumothorax.

A pleural effusion will appear as an anechoic or hypoechoic area between two layers of pleura.[2] Pneumonia manifests as an area of parenchymal consolidation. With large areas of consolidation, air bronchograms may be present as branching, echogenic structures. B-lines may be present in nearby tissue, often as a manifestation of inflammatory edema. Complicated pneumonia may have associated pleural effusion. The presence of B-lines demonstrates pulmonary edema.

### Selected References

1. Gargani L, Volpicelli G. How I do it: lung ultrasound. *Cardiovasc Ultrasound.* 2014;12:1-10.
2. Lichtenstein D. Lung ultrasound in the critically ill. *Ann Intensive Care.* 2014;4:2-12.
3. Saad MM, Kamal J, Moussaly E, et al. Relevance of B-Lines on lung ultrasound in volume overload and pulmonary congestion: clinical correlations and outcomes in patients on hemodialysis. *CardioRenal Med.* 2018;8:83-91.
4. Ziskin MC, Thickman DI, Goldenberg NJ, Lapayowker MS, Becker JM. The comet tail artifact. *J Ultrasound Med.* 1982;1:1-7.

## 12. Correct Answer: C. LAD coronary artery

*Rationale:* TTE may be used to rapidly identify regional wall motion abnormalities (RWMA) in patients with suspected acute coronary syndrome. Evaluation of the left ventricle in PLAX, parasternal short-axis view (PSAX), and apical four-chamber view (A4C) allows the echocardiographer to identify RWMAs in the territories of all three major coronary arteries. An anterior wall abnormality suggests involvement of the LAD artery, a lateral wall abnormality suggests involvement of the circumflex artery (CX), and an inferior wall abnormality suggests involvement of the RCA. This is a simplification of the 17-segment evaluation based on the ASE guidelines (see Figure 22.13), but does allow for more rapid evaluation of RWMAs.

Figure 45.10 is an apical two-chamber view with an arrow pointing to the anterior wall, which is supplied by the LAD artery.

### Selected References

1. Frenkel O, Riguzzi C, Nagdev A. Identification of high-risk patients with acute coronary syndrome using point-of-care echocardiography in the ED. *Am J Emerg Med.* Elsevier Inc. 2014;32:670-672.
2. Gibson R, Bishop H, Stamm R, Crampton RS, Beller GA, Martin RP. Value of early two dimensional echocardiography in patients with acute myocardial infarction. *Am J Cardiol.* 1982;49:1110-1119.
3. Lang RM, Badano LP, Mor-Avi V, et al. Recommendations for cardiac chamber quantification by echocardiography in adults: an update from the American Society of Echocardiography and the European Association of Cardiovascular Imaging. *J Am Soc Echocardiogr.* 2015;28:1-39.

## 13. Correct Answer: C. Epinephrine

*Rationale:* Figure 45.11 shows a transgastric midpapillary short-axis view on TEE. The interventricular septum is flattened and bulging into the left ventricle, often described as a D-shaped ventricle (▶ **Video 45.2**). This alters the geometry of the left ventricle, restricting its ability to fill adequately during diastole and leading to impaired ventricular function. This finding is consistent with RV pressure or volume overload, as may be seen with PE or pulmonary hypertension. The clinical scenario of a postoperative patient raises the suspicion for a thromboembolic event.

Immediate therapy should focus on treating hemodynamic compromise and supporting the struggling right ventricle. While fluid administration is often part of the initial treatment for undifferentiated shock, in patients with known RV dysfunction, fluid administration may lead to increased RV end-diastolic pressure (RVEDP), thereby worsening RV coronary perfusion pressure and placing the right ventricle at risk for ischemia. Medical therapy should be directed by enhancing RV function through increased inotropy and increased mean arterial pressure without dramatically increasing pulmonary vascular resistance. While milrinone will enhance inotropy, it will also lead to peripheral vasodilation and worsen systemic hypotension. Metoprolol would result in a deleterious drop in HR with subsequent decrease in cardiac output; therefore, epinephrine is the best treatment choice.

### Selected References

1. Ma C, Cohen J, Tolpin D. Right ventricular dysfunction and the "D"-shaped left ventricle. *Anesthesiology.* 2020;132:155.
2. Sekhri V, Mehta N, Rawat N, Lehrman SG, Aronow WS. Management of massive and non-massive pulmonary embolism. *Arch Med Sci.* 2012;8:957-969.

**14.** Correct Answer: D. RCA

*Rationale:* TTE may be used to rapidly identify RWMA in patients with suspected acute coronary syndrome. Evaluation of the left ventricle in PLAX, PSAX, and A4C allows the echocardiographer to identify RWMAs in the territories of all three major coronary arteries. An anterior wall abnormality suggests involvement of the LAD artery, a lateral wall abnormality suggests involvement of the CX, and an inferior wall abnormality suggests involvement of the RCA.[2] The figure demonstrates typical distributions of LAD, CX, and RCA based on ASE guidelines (see Figure 22.13).

Figure 45.12 is a PSAX with an *arrow* pointing to the inferior aspect of the left ventricle, which is supplied by the RCA.

### Selected References

1. Frenkel O, Riguzzi C, Nagdev A. Identification of high-risk patients with acute coronary syndrome using point-of-care echocardiography in the ED. *Am J Emerg Med.* Elsevier Inc. 2014;32:670-672.
2. Gibson R, Bishop H, Stamm R, Crampton RS, Beller GA, Martin RP. Value of early two dimensional echocardiography in patients with acute myocardial infarction. *Am J Cardiol.* 1982;49:1110-1119.
3. Lang RM, Badano LP, Mor-Avi V, et al. Recommendations for cardiac chamber quantification by echocardiography in adults: an update from the American Society of Echocardiography and the European Association of Cardiovascular Imaging. *J Am Soc Echocardiogr.* 2015;28:1-39.

**15.** Correct Answer: A. 2 cm distal to left subclavian artery

*Rationale:* IABPs are frequently used for hemodynamic support in patients with cardiogenic shock or during high-risk coronary intervention. They may be inserted percutaneously via the femoral, subclavian, or axillary artery. The balloon inflates during diastole simultaneously with aortic valve closing, resulting in increased propulsion of blood from thoracic aorta to peripheral circulation. The balloon rapidly deflates with opening of the aortic valve in systole, resulting in a decrease in afterload. The decrease in afterload is thought to decrease myocardial oxygen consumption due to a decrease in LV wall stress. Optimal positioning of the tip of the IABP places it 2 to 3 cm distal to the left subclavian (**Figure 45.35**). This positioning supports optimal coronary flow while minimizing the risk of decreased perfusion to aortic arch vessels. The proximal end of the balloon should terminate above the renal arteries in order to avoid renal ischemia.

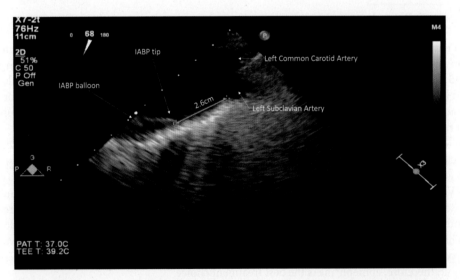

**Figure 45.35** Transesophageal echocardiogram showing an intra-aortic balloon pump (IABP) in the descending aorta, appropriately positioned 2 to 3 cm distal to the left subclavian artery.

### Selected References

1. Hyson E, Ravin C, Kelley M, Curtis AM. Intraaortic counterpulsation balloon: radiographic considerations. *Am J Roentgenol.* 1977;128:915-918.
2. Weber KT, Janicki JS. Intraaortic balloon counterpulsation: a review of physiological principles, clinical results, and device safety. *Ann Thorac Surg.* 1974;17:602-636.

**16.** Correct Answer: B. B

*Rationale:* There are several static and dynamic parameters that may be assessed via echocardiography to estimate a patient's volume status and fluid responsiveness. A hyperdynamic left ventricle with small end-diastolic area ($<10$ cm$^2$ in the PSAX) along with obliteration of the LV cavity during systole is very suggestive of hypovolemia. SV variation with respiration is used to determine volume responsiveness in mechanically ventilated patients. SV may be estimated by first obtaining the velocity-time integral (VTI, area under the curve using pulsed-wave Doppler) of the LVOT. The VTI measures the stroke distance, or how far a column of blood moves with each contraction. Next, the echocardiographer measures the LVOT diameter at the same level at which the VTI was obtained. Using the formula below it is possible to calculate the SV:

$SV= VTI \times CSA$, where SV=stroke volume, VTI=velocity-time integral, CSA=cross-sectional area, $\pi r^2$

Variation of $>12\%$ predicts fluid responsiveness.[2] When threshold variability is increased to $>15\%$, the predictive value achieves sensitivity and specificity of $>90\%$.[3]

When using TTE, VTI is obtained using the apical five-chamber view (A5C) while the PLAX is best to obtain LVOT diameter (**Figure 45.36**).

There are several limitations to the use of SV variation to predict fluid responsiveness. First, the patient must be in sinus rhythm to obtain accurate VTI calculation. Second, mechanical ventilation with high tidal volume ventilation ($>8$ cc/kg ideal body weight) is required with deep sedation or paralysis as spontaneous respiratory effort may lead to SV variability. Finally, patients must have a closed chest and normal intra-abdominal pressure.

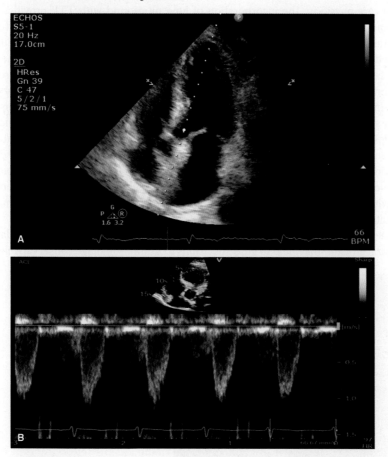

**Figure 45.36**

Selected References

1. Chew MS. Haemodynamic monitoring using echocardiography in the critically ill: a review. *Cardiol Res Pract.* 2012;2012:139537.
2. Miller A, Mandeville J. Predicting and measuring fluid responsiveness with echocardiography. *Echo Res Pract.* 2016;3:G1-G12.
3. Slama M, Masson H, Teboul JL. Respiratory variations of aortic VTI: a new index of hypovolemia and fluid responsiveness. *Am J Physiol Circ Physiol.* 2002;283:1729-1733.

**17.** Correct Answer: C. IVC diameter

*Rationale:* The size and variability of the IVC over the respiratory cycle provides helpful information when determining fluid responsiveness. In a spontaneously breathing patient, the size of the IVC immediately distal to the hepatic vein correlates closely with right atrial pressure (RAP). This relationship is no longer present when the patient is mechanically ventilated as the increase in intrathoracic pressure with positive pressure ventilation leads to a dilated IVC. However, if the IVC remains small (<10 mm) in the mechanically ventilated patient, they are likely to be fluid responsive. IVC diameter variation is most accurate in mechanically ventilated patients and variability >12% suggests fluid responsiveness. Patients with an elevated RAP lose this variability.

When taken as a single static measurement, RV or LV end-diastolic area does not have the same predictive value of fluid responsiveness as other available choices. That said, the echocardiographic triad of a small left ventricle, small right ventricle, and obliteration of the LV cavity in systole is highly suggestive of hypovolemia.

SV variation loses accuracy if the patient is not in normal sinus rhythm.

### Selected References
1. Chew MS. Haemodynamic monitoring using echocardiography in the critically ill: a review. *Cardiol Res Pract*. 2012;2012:139537.
2. Jardin F, Vieillard-Baron A. Ultrasonographic examination of the venae cavae. *Intensive Care Med*. 2006;32:203-206.
3. Miller A, Mandeville J. Predicting and measuring fluid responsiveness with echocardiography. *Echo Res Pract*. 2016;3:G1-G12.

**18.** Correct Answer: B. Thoracostomy tube

*Rationale:* For the critical care physician, the incorporation of lung ultrasound with TTE provides substantial benefit in evaluating patients with acute respiratory failure. When evaluating for a pleural effusion in a supine patient, the transducer should be placed longitudinally at the posterior axillary line with the orientation marker directed cephalad. When evaluating the right lung with the correct orientation, the liver will be opposite the orientation marker, which in the image above is evident on the left side of the screen (**Figure 45.37**). The diaphragm appears as an echogenic, curvilinear structure forming the boundary between the liver and the lung, or in this case the effusion. Layers of the chest wall, including dermis and intercostal muscle, may be seen in the near-field of the ultrasound image. The lung appears at the far-field of the image as a small, collapsed structure due to compression from a large pleural effusion. The pleural effusion itself appears as a hypoechoic or anechoic space bordered by pleura and lung tissue. The quality of the pleural effusion may provide information regarding its etiology. Anechoic (completely black) effusions are generally a transudate while any echogenicity makes the effusion exudative. Effusions may be homogeneous or be complex in nature, with areas of septation. The amount of fluid involved in the pleural effusion may be estimated based on lung ultrasound using the formula below:

$V = 20 \times Sep$ (mm), where $V$ = volume of pleural effusion and Sep = distance between pleural layers. Quantification of the pleural effusion may help to guide decisions to drain or manage conservatively.

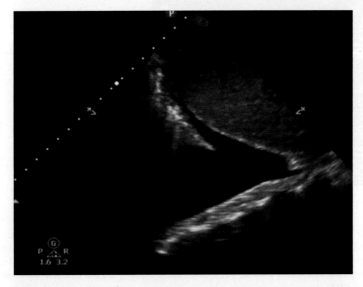

**Figure 45.37** Transthoracic echocardiography image of a large pleural effusion compressing the right lung.

Selected References

1. Balik M, Plasil P, Waldauf P, et al. Ultrasound estimation of volume of pleural fluid in mechanically ventilated patients. *Intensive Care Med.* 2006;32:318-321.
2. Díaz-gómez JL, Via G, Ramakrishna H. Focused cardiac and lung ultrasonography: implications and applicability in the perioperative period. *Rom J Anaesth Intensive Care.* 2016;23:41-54.
3. Gargani L, Volpicelli G. How I do it: lung ultrasound. *Cardiovasc Ultrasound.* 2014;12:1-10.
4. Picano E, Scali MC, Ciampi Q, Lichtenstein D. Lung ultrasound for the cardiologist. *JACC Cardiovasc Imaging.* 2018;11:1692-1705.

**19.** Correct Answer: A. Coandă effect seen on color flow Doppler

*Rationale:* Figure 45.15 demonstrates a ruptured chord leading to a flail mitral valve leaflet. This will often lead to an eccentric jet of MR that travels along the wall of the left atrium. When a fluid jet flows along a convex surface, it is referred to as the Coandă effect and is important to know because the MR is more severe than it may appear by color jet size. A mitral inflow gradient of 11 mm Hg is suggestive of severe mitral stenosis, not regurgitation. A TR jet peak velocity of 1.25 m/s would suggest a PASP of 6.25 mm Hg + CVP (via the modified Bernoulli equation of $4*v^2$, where $v$=velocity in m/s). Someone with an acute ruptured chord leading to hypotension and hypoxemia is likely to have significant pulmonary hypertension. While this lesion could reflect a vegetation, **Figure 45.38** is characteristic of a flail chord and the patient's history makes ischemia much more likely than infection.

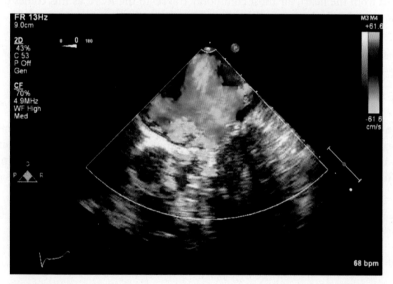

**Figure 45.38**

Selected References

1. Ginghina C. The Coandă effect in cardiology. *J Cardiovasc Med.* 2007;8(6):411-413.
2. Morales DC, Uretsky S, Koulogiannis K, et al. Flail mitral leaflet or presence of the Coanda effect are not invariably associated with severe mitral regurgitation as assessed by MRI. *J Am Coll Cardiol.* 2016;67(13 suppl):1836.

**20.** Correct Answer: B. TAPSE of 1.2 cm

*Rationale:* The expected echocardiographic findings of an acute large PE revolve around RV dysfunction, as the thrombus itself can often not be visualized directly. Other findings include RV free wall hypokinesis or even akinesis, with relative sparing of the RV apex (McConnell sign), which is specific for RV dysfunction. Of the given choices, a TAPSE of 1.2 cm is most suggestive of RV dysfunction (normal >1.5-1.8). IVC collapse with inspiration would suggest right-sided hypovolemia; however, patients with RV dysfunction typically have right-sided congestion. An LV fractional area change of 20% suggests LV dysfunction. Patients with acute RV failure often have RV dilation; however, a mid-RV diameter of 2.7 cm is normal.

Selected Reference

1. Lu SY, Dalia AA, Cudemus G, Shelton KT. Rescue echocardiography/ultrasonography in the management of combined cardiac surgical and medical patients in a cardiac intensive care unit. *J Cardiothorac Vasc Anesth.* 2020;34(10):2682-2688.

**21.** Correct Answer: **A. ST-elevation in leads II, III, and aVF**

*Rationale:* This patient is experiencing an AMI. The indicated segment on this TEE (Figure 45.16) is the inferoseptal segment. This is most likely supplied by the RCA assuming the patient has right dominant coronary circulation (posterior descending artery [PDA] supplied by RCA). This is true in most patients (70%) and therefore is the most correct answer. A small percentage of patients can have the PDA supplied by the CX or even the LAD artery.

Selected References
1. Lang RM, Badano LP, Mor-Avi V, et al. Recommendations for cardiac chamber quantification by echocardiography in adults: an update from the American Society of Echocardiography and the European Association of Cardiovascular Imaging. *J Am Soc Echocardiogr.* 2015;28(1):1-39 e14.
2. Schiller N, Shah P, Crawford M, et al. Recommendations for quantitation of the left ventricle by two-dimensional echocardiography. American Society of Echocardiography Committee on Standards, Subcommittee on Quantitation of Two-Dimensional Echocardiograms. *J Am Soc Echocardiogr.* 1989;2:358-367.

**22.** Correct Answer: **A. A**

*Rationale/Critique:* **Question 22** involves a coronary gas embolism, which is a risk following an open valve repair. Once ejected from the heart, air most commonly travels to the RCA, as this comes off the anterior surface of the aorta and is the highest point in a supine patient.

Selected Reference
1. Fuentes-García DJ. Hernández-Palazón: intracoronary air embolism detected by transoesophageal echocardiography for aortic valve replacement. *Br J Anaesth.* 2009;102(5):718-719.

**23.** Correct Answer: **C. TTE leads to increased use of inotropic support**

*Rationale:* TTE is becoming popular in the critical care setting due to the variety of clinical parameters that can be assessed. A recent database analysis of septic patients found that TTE use led to an increase in fluid administration, increased use of dobutamine, and increased peak dose (but earlier weaning) of norepinephrine. This study also found a statistically significant decrease in mortality when TTE was used.

Selected Reference
1. Feng M, McSparron JI, Kien DT. Transthoracic echocardiography and mortality in sepsis: analysis of the MIMIC-III database. *Intensive Care Med.* 2018;44(6):884-892.

**24.** Correct Answer: **D. Amniotic fluid embolism**

*Rationale:* Amniotic fluid embolism is a rare, but serious and potentially fatal event. Even if recognized and treated early, maternal mortality remains high. This embolic event causes acute pulmonary hypertension, which leads to respiratory distress. Systemic BP may be maintained early in the disease process despite reduced cardiac output due to compensatory vasoconstriction. RA and RV dilation on echocardiography is commonly seen due to the abrupt increase in pulmonary vascular resistance.

Maternal hemorrhage would be associated with underfilled right-sided chambers on echocardiography. A high spinal anesthetic level can cause respiratory distress and hypotension, but is unlikely to cause acute pulmonary hypertension and RV failure. Local anesthetic systemic toxicity can cause cardiac disturbances; however, this would most likely present as dysrhythmias and the ECG was normal in this patient.

Selected Reference
1. Shechtman M, Ziser A, Markovits R, Rozenberg B. Amniotic fluid embolism: early findings of transesophageal echocardiography. *Anesth Analg.* 1999;89(6):1456-1458.

**25.** Correct Answer: **D. LVOT/aortic valve dimensionless index of 0.21**

*Rationale:* Figure 45.19 demonstrates a Stanford Type A aortic dissection with the flap visible in the ascending aorta. An aortic valve pressure half-time of 220 ms is suggestive of severe aortic insufficiency. This can happen in an aortic dissection due to aortic valve annular dilation or because the dissection flap prolapses into the aortic valve and impairs coaptation. Pulsus paradoxus is suggestive of cardiac tamponade, which can occur if the dissection extends into the pericardial space. ST depressions in leads II, III, and aVF are suggestive of inferior (likely RCA) ischemia and can occur if the dissection flap extends down into a coronary artery. An LVOT/aortic valve dimensionless index is suggestive of severe aortic stenosis but is not typically seen in acute aortic dissections.

**Selected Reference**

1. Evangelista A, Maldonado G, Gruosso D, et al. The current role of echocardiography in acute aortic syndrome. *Echo Res Pract.* 2019;6(2):R53.

**26.** Correct Answer: B. Effective regurgitant orifice area of 0.1 cm²

*Rationale:* Figure 45.20 shows a long-axis view of the aortic valve and ascending aorta. The color flow Doppler image shows significant aortic insufficiency likely due to the dissection. Severe aortic insufficiency can cause widening of the arterial pulse pressure. A vena contracta of >6 mm corresponds with severe aortic insufficiency. Diastolic flow reversal in the descending aorta is another finding of severe aortic insufficiency. An effective regurgitant orifice area of 0.1 cm² would correspond with mild-to-moderate aortic insufficiency.

**Selected Reference**

1. Evangelista A, Maldonado G, Gruosso D, et al. The current role of echocardiography in acute aortic syndrome. *Echo Res Pract.* 2019;6(2):R53.

**27.** Correct Answer: C. Dimensionless index of 0.21

*Rationale:* Figure 45.21 shows the long-axis view of the aortic valve. This image is in ventricular systole (evidenced by the ECG trace and a closed mitral valve); however, the aortic valve leaflets are not widely opened, suggesting aortic stenosis. Figure 45.21 shows turbulence in the ascending aorta, which is also suggestive of significant aortic stenosis. A valve area of 1.6 cm², a mean gradient of 15 mm Hg, and a peak velocity of 2.8 m/s all correspond with mild aortic stenosis. A dimensionless index of 0.21 corresponds to severe stenosis and is therefore the most correct choice.

**Selected Reference**

1. Samarendra P, Mangione MP. Aortic stenosis and perioperative risk with noncardiac surgery. *J Am Coll Cardiol.* 2015;65(3):295-302.

**28.** Correct Answer: B. Systolic pulmonary vein flow reversal

*Rationale:* Figure 45.22 is a modified (cropped) midesophageal five-chamber view showing severe MR. Systolic pulmonary vein flow reversal on echocardiography (**Figure 45.39**) is pathognomonic of severe MR. Holo-diastolic aorta flow reversal is indicative of severe aortic regurgitation. Systolic hepatic vein flow reversal is associated with severe TV regurgitation. Diastolic pulmonary artery flow reversal may be seen with severe pulmonary valve insufficiency. Patients with diabetes, hypertension, and obesity are at risk for coronary artery disease. This patient group is at increased risk for an AMI due to increased myocardial demand following a major injury. AMI is often associated with mitral valve regurgitation due to geometric changes in the left ventricle and papillary muscles as well as involvement of the subvalvular apparatus of the mitral valve itself.

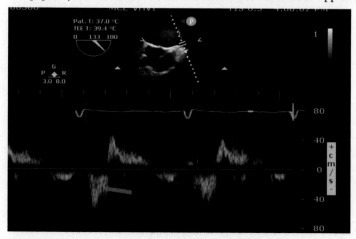

**Figure 45.39** Pulsed-wave Doppler of right upper pulmonary vein on transesophageal echocardiography reveals systolic flow reversal (*arrow*) indicative of severe mitral regurgitation.

**Selected Reference**

1. Seiler C, Aeschbacher BC, Meier B. Quantitation of mitral regurgitation using the systolic/diastolic pulmonary venous flow velocity ratio. *J Am Coll Cardiol.* 1998 May;31(6):1383-1390.

**29.** Correct Answer: B. RV collapse in diastole

*Rationale:* Acute Type A aortic dissection is a life-threatening complication resulting most often from chronic hypertension. Up to a third of Type A dissections rupture into the pericardial space, causing a pericardial effusion, which may lead to tamponade and shock. Pericardial tamponade may be diagnosed using bedside echocardiography. Presence of a pericardial effusion with chamber collapse during the cardiac cycle on TTE is pathognomonic for tamponade. RA collapse longer than one-third of the cardiac cycle, typically in systole, has a high sensitivity and specificity for tamponade. RV collapse is generally seen during diastole (**Figure 45.40**). These findings are best noted using the subcostal or A4C view. Other TTE findings include: a >25% decrease in mitral peak E-wave velocity with inspiration, dilation, or plethora of the IVC with reduced collapsibility on inspiration.

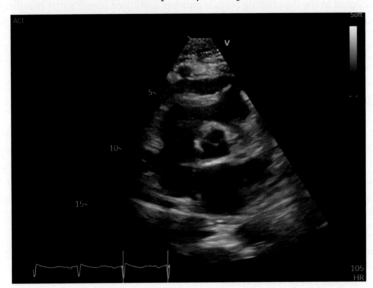

**Figure 45.40** Transthoracic echocardiogram, parasternal short-axis view at level of aortic valve with pericardial effusion and compression of the right ventricular outflow tract (*arrow*), consistent with tamponade.

### Selected References

1. Maisch B, Seferović PM, Ristić AD, et al. Guidelines on the diagnosis and management of pericardial diseases executive summary; The Task force on the diagnosis and management of pericardial diseases of the European society of cardiology. *Eur Heart J.* 2004 Apr;25(7):587-610.
2. Perez-Casares A, Cesar S, Brunet-Garcia L, Sanchez-de-Toledo J. Echocardiographic evaluation of pericardial effusion and cardiac tamponade. *Front Pediatr.* 2017;5:1-10.

**30.** Correct Answer: A. Takotsubo cardiomyopathy

*Rationale/Critique:* Figure 45.24 shows an apical view of the left ventricle, which appears normal. However, the A5C and PLAX views show ballooning of the mid- and distal segments with severe LV dysfunction.

Takotsubo cardiomyopathy, also known as "broken heart syndrome" or stress cardiomyopathy, is a condition of acute LV failure due to physical or emotional stress. Most cases occur in postmenopausal women. Takotsubo cardiomyopathy is characterized by preserved basal segments with dyskinesis or "ballooning" of the mid- and distal LV segments (**Figure 45.41A-C** and ▶ **Video 45.5A-C**) in the absence of occlusive coronary artery lesions. Treatment is primarily supportive as the cardiomyopathy typically resolves within 3 weeks.

PE would be characterized by a severely dilated right ventricle. The right ventricle in this image is of normal size. There is no evidence of a pericardial effusion or aortic dissection in Figure 45.41.

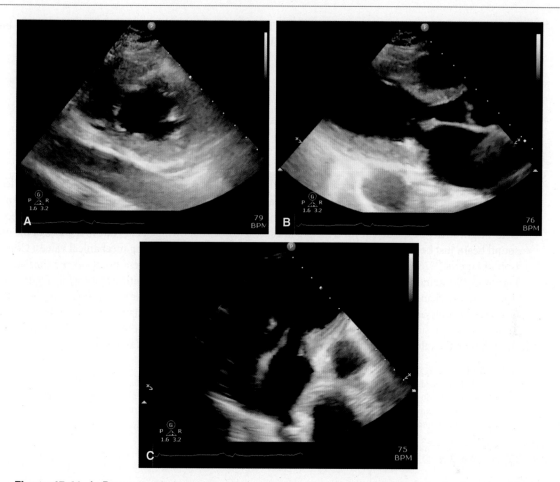

**Figure 45.41** A. Parasternal short-axis view showing normal basal left ventricular function. B. Parasternal long-axis view, showing a contracting basal segment with dilated, dyskinetic mid-left ventricular segments. C. Apical five-chamber view, again showing contracting basal segment with dilated, dyskinetic mid-left ventricular segments.

Selected Reference

1. Akashi YJ, Goldstein DS, Barbaro G, Ueyama T. Takotsubo cardiomyopathy a new form of acute, reversible heart failure. *Circulation.* 2008;118:2754-2762.

---

**31.** Correct Answer: **D. Ruptured posteromedial papillary muscle (PPM)**

*Rationale/Critique:* The appearance of this mitral valve resembles that of a posterior leaflet with a vegetation due to endocarditis (Figure 45.25). However, the ECG findings suggest that the patient has an ischemic rather than infective process. The PPM originates from the inferior wall where it meets the septum. In contrast to the anterolateral papillary muscle, which has dual blood supply, the PPM derives its blood flow from a single coronary in 63% of the population, making it more vulnerable to ischemic complications. Atrial myxomas are typically attached to the LA side of the interatrial septum and not the mitral valve leaflets.

Selected References

1. Harari R, Bansal P, Yatskar L, Rubinstein D, Silbiger JJ. Papillary muscle rupture following acute myocardial infarction: anatomic, echocardiographic, and surgical insights. *Echocardiography.* 2017;34(11):1702-1707.
2. Voci P, Bilotta F, Caretta Q, Mercanti C, Marino B. Papillary muscle perfusion pattern. A hypothesis for ischemic papillary muscle dysfunction. *Circulation.* 1995;91(6):1714-1718.

---

**32.** Correct Answer: **B. Patent foramen ovale with air embolism**

*Rationale:* Improper central line removal technique can lead to an air embolism, which is more likely when the CVP is low, such as in the upright position. Coughing, which can be triggered by venous air embolism, may result in dramatic swings in intrathoracic pressure and potentially right-to-left shunting in at-risk individuals, such as in those with a PFO.

There are case reports of traumatic retrograde Type A dissections. However, the presentation of blunt aortic injuries is usually acute with a high mortality and should not cause air embolism.[2]

### Selected References

1. Lombard FW, Welsby IJ, Booth JV. Systemic air embolism during off-pump coronary artery bypass surgery. *J Cardiothorac Vasc Anesth.* 2003;17(3):403-404.
2. Tsukioka K, Kono T, Takahashi K, Kehara H, Urashita S, Komatsu K. A case of traumatic retrograde type A aortic dissection accompanied by multiorgan injuries. *Ann Vasc Dis.* 2018;11(1):138-142.

## 33. Correct Answer: B. Immobile mechanical mitral valve leaflet

*Rationale:* The diagnosis of a struck mitral valve leaflet is most easily identified on TEE. While one leaflet readily opens and closes, the other is held stationary. This diagnosis may also be made with the still images based on imaging artifacts associated with a mechanical valve. A mirror image artifact appears as a second, echo-bright structure located beyond the prosthesis. Acoustic shadowing occurs due to the loss of the ultrasound beam just beyond the prosthesis, an anticipated finding when imaging mechanical valves. Comparison of Figure 45.26A and B demonstrates that they were captured at different points in the cardiac cycle. Figure 45.26A demonstrates both leaflets in the closed position, consistent with systole, while Figure 45.26B demonstrates a change in leaflet position consistent with diastolic opening. While the valve should be fully open, it is clear that only one valve leaflet is open to allow for ventricular filling. Spontaneous echo contrast is present in the left atrium, suggesting significant impairment of forward flow across the valve, and there appears to be thrombus on the valve. Stuck mitral valve leaflet can lead to either MR or mitral stenosis.

### Selected References

1. Bach DS. Transesophageal echocardiographic (TEE) evaluation of prosthetic valves. *Cardiol Clin.* 2000;18:751-771
2. Nishimura RA, Otto CM, Bonow RO, et al. 2014 AHA/ACC guideline for the management of patients with valvular heart disease: executive summary: a report of the American College of Cardiology/American Heart Association Task Force on Practice Guidelines. *Circulation.* 2014;129:2440-2492.

## 34. Correct Answer: D. Pulmonary edema

*Rationale/Critique:* Figure 45.27 shows multiple B-lines, which are ultrasound reverberation artifacts originating from contrast between air-filled and water-containing structures. Normal lung parenchyma has very few B-lines, less than three per field. For an examination to be positive for pulmonary edema, there has to be at least two positive scans (more than three B-lines/field) for each lung.

B-lines are not specific for any one condition, they merely diagnose loss of lung aeration due to interstitial fluid. This may be observed in cardiogenic pulmonary edema, lung contusion, acute respiratory distress syndrome, pneumonia, and pulmonary fibrosis.

### Selected References

1. Cardinale L, Priola AM, Moretti F, Volpicelli G. Effectiveness of chest radiography, lung ultrasound and thoracic computed tomography in the diagnosis of congestive heart failure. *World J Radiol.* 2014;6(6):230-237.
2. Dietrich CF, Mathis G, Blaivas M, et al. Lung B-line artefacts and their use. *J Thorac Dis.* 2016;8(6):1356-1365.

## 35. Correct Answer: A. 67 mm Hg

*Rationale:* In the absence of pulmonary stenosis, PASP will be equal to right ventricular systolic pressure (RVSP), which may be determined using the modified Bernoulli equation. In order to estimate the RVSP using echocardiography, the peak gradient of TR must be obtained using continuous-wave Doppler. RVSP may then be estimated using the formula:

$$RVSP = 4(Peak\ TR\ Velocity\ in\ m/s)^2 + CVP$$

In this equation, CVP is used as a surrogate for RAP. If CVP data are not available, a RAP estimate of 10 mm Hg is generally accepted, although it may not be accurate based on clinical picture. Average normal range of RVSP varies by age, in a 50- to 75-year-old the average RVSP is between 15 and 45 mm Hg. This patient has an elevated RVSP and PASP, which raises concern for acute PE.

### Selected Reference

1. Armstrong DWJ, Tsimiklis G, Matangi MF. Factors influencing the echocardiographic estimate of right ventricular systolic pressure in normal patients and clinically relevant ranges according to age. *Can J Cardiol.* 2010;26:35-39.

# 46 | E-FAST

Layne Alan Madden, Maxwell A. Hockstein and Deepa M. Patel

1. A patient presents after a rollover motor vehicle crash. On initial assessment, he has a Glasgow coma scale (GCS) score of 15, BP of 120/60 mm Hg, and HR of 130 bpm. His physical examination is notable for chest wall and diffuse abdominal tenderness, with bruising noted in the mid-abdomen. An extended focused assessment with sonography for trauma (eFAST) is performed and shows no peritoneal or pericardial free fluid, and no hemothorax or pneumothorax. Chest and pelvis radiographs also show no acute abnormalities. Thirty minutes later, his HR has increased to 155 bpm, and his BP has decreased to 90/50 mm Hg. What is the *most appropriate* next step in his management?

   **A.** Pain control and observation
   **B.** Repeat eFAST examination
   **C.** Computed tomography (CT) of the chest, abdomen, and pelvis with intravenous (IV) contrast
   **D.** Exploratory laparotomy

2. A patient presents with a 3 cm stab wound near the left costovertebral angle. Which of the following statements is *most* true regarding the interpretation of the eFAST examination in this patient?

   **A.** eFAST is highly sensitive but not specific for retroperitoneal injury
   **B.** eFAST is highly sensitive but not specific for splenic injury
   **C.** eFAST is highly specific but not sensitive for splenic injury
   **D.** eFAST is highly specific but not sensitive for retroperitoneal injury

3. The following suprapubic image (**Figure 46.1**) is obtained while performing a FAST examination on a young man who sustained injuries in a motorcycle crash. What is indicated by the arrow in Figure 46.1?

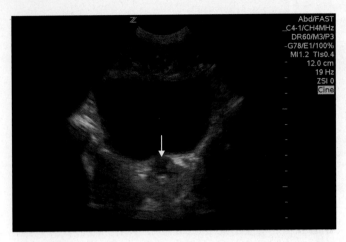

**Figure 46.1**

A. Free fluid
B. Prostate
C. Seminal vesicles
D. Rectum

4. Which of the following is the *best* way to improve sensitivity of detecting free fluid when using the suprapubic view?

A. Obtain the images while the bladder is full
B. Place a Foley catheter
C. Place the patient in Trendelenburg position
D. Scan in short-axis or transverse view only

5. A 23-year-old man is evaluated in the Emergency Department (ED) after being ejected from a motorcycle during a collision with another vehicle. Which standard view in the eFAST examination has the highest sensitivity for the detection of peritoneal free fluid?

A. Right upper quadrant (RUQ)—hepatorenal
B. Left upper quadrant (LUQ)—splenorenal
C. Longitudinal suprapubic (bladder)
D. Transverse suprapubic (bladder)

6. A 45-year-old woman is involved in a high-speed motor vehicle collision resulting in significant front-end damage to the vehicle. Her HR is 105 bpm and BP 120/78 mm Hg. Secondary survey reveals bruising over the lower abdomen, as well as RUQ tenderness. Radiographs of the chest and pelvis are negative for acute findings, and the eFAST is normal. What is the *most appropriate* next step in her management?

A. CT of the abdomen and pelvis with IV contrast
B. Diagnostic peritoneal lavage (DPL)
C. Exploratory laparotomy
D. Pain control and observation

7. A 33-year-old man is an unrestrained driver in a motor vehicle collision. Paramedics found the driver in the back seat. The patient's HR is 125 bpm and BP is 80/50 mm Hg. Portable chest x-ray demonstrates several right-sided rib fractures without pneumothorax. The pelvis x-ray is normal. The hepatorenal view from the eFAST examination is shown in **Figure 46.2** and ▶ **Video 46.1**. What is the *best* next step in his management?

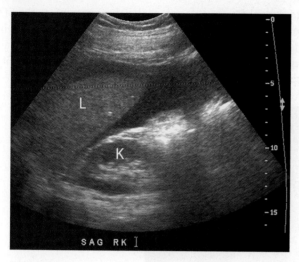

**Figure 46.2**

A. CT abdomen and pelvis with IV contrast
B. Blood transfusion and exploratory laparotomy
C. Diagnostic peritoneal lavage
D. Transfuse 2 units of packed red blood cells and reassess the patient

8. A 34-year-old woman presents with a gunshot wound to her right flank. Her airway is patent, and she has diminished breath sounds on the right. Her vital signs show HR 96 bpm, BP 110/85 mm Hg, respiratory rate (RR) 26/min, and SpO$_2$ 93% on a non-rebreather mask at 15 LPM. An eFAST is performed, and the initial RUQ (hepatorenal) view is shown in **Figure 46.3**. What is the most appropriate next step in her management?

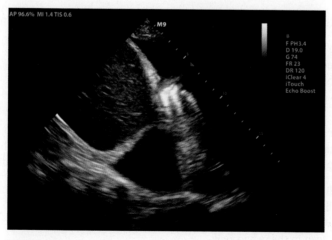

**Figure 46.3**

**A.** Exploratory laparotomy
**B.** Placement of right-sided thoracostomy tube
**C.** Endotracheal intubation
**D.** CT scan of the chest to confirm the suspected diagnosis

9. A 46-year-old man with a history of end-stage renal disease on peritoneal dialysis presents to the ED one day after a minor motor vehicle collision. He is now complaining of delayed-onset neck pain. His vital signs are normal, he has no external signs of injury, his abdominal examination is nontender, and he is neurovascularly intact. A medical student performed an eFAST examination for practice and it is shown in **Figure 46.4**. What is the most appropriate next step in his management?

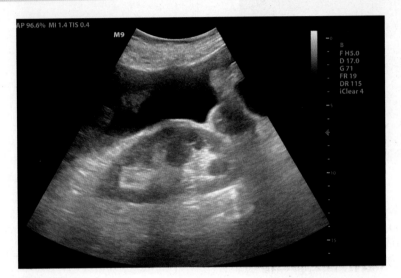

**Figure 46.4**

**A.** CT abdomen and pelvis with IV contrast
**B.** DPL using his peritoneal dialysis catheter
**C.** Admit for observation and serial abdominal examinations
**D.** Discharge home with close outpatient follow-up

10. Which of the following statements is correct with regard to optimizing the LUQ (splenorenal window)?

**A.** The splenorenal window is more anterior and inferior compared to the hepatorenal window
**B.** The probe marker should be directed toward the patient's left hip
**C.** The subphrenic space is not visible due to air artifact from the left lung
**D.** Imaging can be improved by having the patient take a deep breath

11. A 30-year-old woman presents after a low-speed rear-end motor vehicle collision, complaining of abdominal pain. She has normal vital signs and a normal physical examination. Her eFAST is notable for trace free fluid seen only in the pelvic view. What is the *most likely* explanation for this free fluid?

**A.** Fluid from intraperitoneal bleeding
**B.** Ascitic fluid from undiagnosed liver dysfunction
**C.** Physiologic fluid, since she is a woman of childbearing age
**D.** Physiologic fluid, since it is only seen in the pelvic view

12. Gain must be adjusted to avoid a false-negative suprapubic view during an eFAST. What is the name of the artifact that can cause fluid to be missed in this view?

**A.** Posterior acoustic enhancement
**B.** Mirror image
**C.** Comet tail
**D.** Reverberation

13. A 25-year-old man presents with a gunshot wound to the chest. He has a BP of 80/40 mm Hg, HR of 120 bpm, and is unconscious. He is intubated and an eFAST examination is performed. **Figure 46.5** shows the right anterior hemithorax in M-mode. Based on this image, what is the *most* appropriate diagnosis?

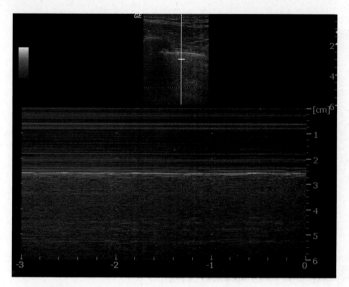

**Figure 46.5**

A. Right mainstem endotracheal tube
B. Absence of a right-sided pneumothorax
C. A right-sided hemothorax
D. Presence of right sided pneumothorax

14. A 24-year-old woman is admitted for febrile neutropenia and anemia after chemotherapy 10 days ago. She has a history of acute myeloid leukemia (AML) and has cardiomyopathy due to a chemotherapeutic agent. Upon arrival to the intensive care unit (ICU), she has a HR of 120 bpm, mean arterial pressure (MAP) of 60 mm Hg, and temperature of 39°C. Based on the left apical thoracic ultrasound in **Figure 46.6**, which finding is *most* correct?

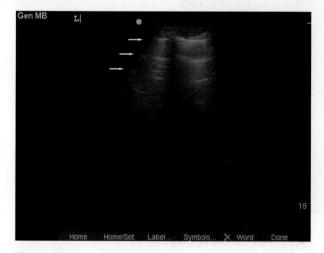

**Figure 46.6**

A. Evidence of pulmonary edema
B. Absence of artifacts seen on this ultrasound
C. Absence of a pneumothorax
D. Absence of fluid overload

15. A 58-year-old woman with an unknown past medical history is admitted to the ICU for acute hypoxemic respiratory failure. Her echocardiographic windows are difficult to obtain but her lung ultrasound is displayed in **Figure 46.7** and ▶ **Video 46.2**. Which of the following statements regarding the patient is *most* correct?

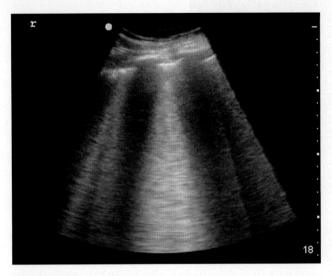

**Figure 46.7**

A. She is likely volume responsive
B. She requires a tube thoracostomy
C. She likely has a high left atrial pressure
D. She has a pneumothorax

16. A 41-year-old man is admitted to the ICU for acute-on-chronic liver failure. He has noted worsening dyspnea over the past 2 months. Which of the following is *most* correct regarding the ultrasound image shown in **Figure 46.8**?

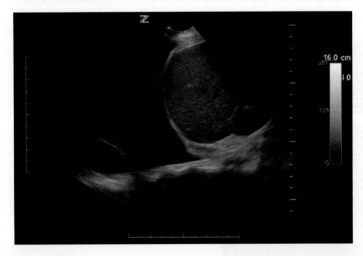

**Figure 46.8**

A. Pulmonary edema is present
B. The spine is not normally visualized in this view
C. Ascites is present
D. The diaphragm is seldom visualized in this view

17. A 25-year-old woman presents to the ED after a high-speed motor vehicle collision. She is intubated, hypotensive, and tachycardic. Which of the following therapies is *most* appropriate given the apical left-sided thoracic ultrasound demonstrated in ▶ **Video 46.3** and **Figure 46.9**?

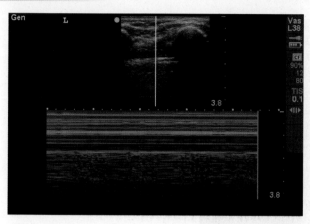

**Figure 46.9**

A. Tube thoracostomy
B. Increase positive end-expiratory pressure (PEEP)
C. Antibiotics
D. Pericardiocentesis

18. Which of the following may decrease the sensitivity of right heart findings in suspected pericardial tamponade?

A. Hypovolemia
B. Tachycardia
C. Hypothermia
D. Pulmonary hypertension

19. A 44-year-old man is admitted to the cardiac care unit (CCU) complaining of dyspnea. He notes a history of "thyroid problems" but has not been to an endocrinologist in many years. He is hemodynamically stable and complains of dyspnea on exertion. Which of the following is *most* true regarding the echocardiogram shown in **Figure 46.10,** ▶ **Video 46.4,** and ▶ **Video 46.5**?

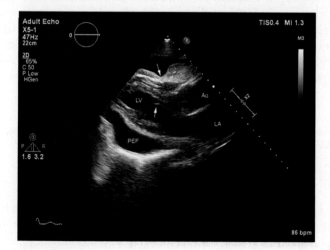

**Figure 46.10**

A. There is a pleural effusion
B. There is a pericardial effusion with evidence of tamponade physiology
C. There is a pericardial effusion without evidence of tamponade physiology
D. There is a no pericardial or pleural effusion

20. A 33-year-old woman is admitted to the ICU with dyspnea and hypotension. She has a history of end-stage renal disease but has missed her last two dialysis sessions. A point-of-care ultrasound is obtained and M-mode is performed. Which of the following is *most* true regarding the image shown in **Figure 46.11**?

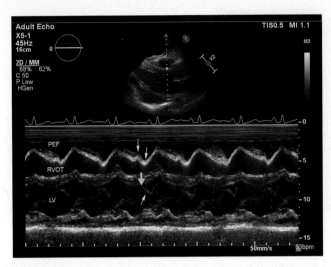

**Figure 46.11**

A. The patient has hypovolemic shock
B. The patient has left ventricular (LV) systolic dysfunction
C. The patient has tamponade physiology
D. The patient has right ventricular (RV) strain

# Chapter 46 ▪ Answers

**1.** Correct Answer: B. Repeat eFAST examination

*Rationale:* Although the first FAST scan was negative, the sensitivity for free fluid detection increases with serial examinations, especially when there are signs of potential ongoing bleeding. In one study, the sensitivity increased from 69% to 85%. This patient would go to the operating room if the eFAST examination was positive, but if the repeat examination does not show hemoperitoneum, other sources of hypotension must be pursued (e.g., retroperitoneal bleeding, cardiogenic shock). If he was stabilized, a CT scan could be performed to evaluate for surgical pathology, but with worsening hypotension it would not be a safe option at this point. Pain may be a cause for tachycardia, but would not address the hypotension.

Selected Reference

1. Nunes LW, Simmons S, Hallowell MJ, Kinback R, Trooskin S, Kozar R. Diagnostic performance of trauma US in identifying abdominal or pelvic free fluid and serious abdominal or pelvic injury. *Acad Radiol.* 2001; 8:128-36.

**2.** Correct Answer: C. eFAST is highly specific but not sensitive for splenic injury

*Rationale:* The sensitivity of eFAST to evaluate for retroperitoneal hemorrhage is quite low, with a high false-negative rate. The sensitivity of eFAST to detect abdominal free fluid from splenic injury is around 70%, with a specificity >95%. In the setting of penetrating trauma, sonographic evaluation for pneumothorax, pericardial effusion, hemothorax, and hemoperitoneum, eFAST has excellent specificity. However, ultrasound evaluation for retroperitoneal injury, isolated bowel, or peritoneal injury is limited by very low sensitivity.

Selected Reference

1. Netherton S, Milenkovic V, Taylor M, Davis P. Diagnostic accuracy of eFAST in the trauma patient: a systematic review and meta-analysis. *CJEM.* 2019:1-12.

**3.** Correct Answer: B. Prostate

*Rationale:* All of these structures can be seen posterior to the bladder. The prostate is a rounded single structure that can often be seen impinging upon the bladder. Seminal vesicles are anechoic, symmetric, tubular structures that can be confused for free fluid. In contrast to free fluid, they do not layer and track along adjacent structures. Bowel can take various forms on ultrasound, depending on the pathology, but the rectum would be posterior to the prostate in Figure 46.1. In addition, posterior acoustic enhancement may cause increased signal behind an anechoic structure like the bladder, which may obscure small volumes of peritoneal fluid. For all of these reasons, imaging in more than one plane is recommended.

### Selected References

1. Boyd JS, Rupp JD, Ferre RM. Emergency ultrasound. In: Knoop KJ, Stack LB, Storrow AB, Thurman R, eds. *The Atlas of Emergency Medicine,* 4th ed. McGraw-Hill; Accessed October 11, 2019. http://accessemergencymedicine.mhmedical.com.proxy.library.emory.edu/content.aspx?bookid=1763&sectionid=125439068.
2. Cosby KS, Kendall JL. *Practical Guide to Emergency Ultrasound,* 2nd ed. Lippincott Williams & Wilkins; 2013.
3. Fritz DA. Emergency bedside ultrasound. In: Stone C, Humphries RL, eds. *Current Diagnosis & Treatment: Emergency Medicine,* 8th ed. McGraw-Hill; Accessed October 11, 2019. http://accessemergencymedicine.mhmedical.com.proxy.library.emory.edu/content.aspx?bookid=2172&sectionid=165057390.

**4.** Correct Answer: A. Obtain the images while the bladder is full

*Rationale:* Evaluation of free fluid in the suprapubic view can be improved if images are obtained while the bladder is full and before a Foley is placed, because this improves the acoustic window. Trendelenburg positioning could improve the detection of fluid in the RUQ or LUQ views, as free fluid would pool in the upper quadrants. Conversely, reverse Trendelenburg positioning may improve the sensitivity of detecting fluid in the pelvis. Scanning in multiple orientations increases the likelihood of detecting an abnormality and distinguishing artifacts.

### Selected References

1. Beard RE, Odom SR. Focused assessment with sonography in Trauma (FAST). In: Brown SM, et al, eds. *Comprehensive Critical Care Ultrasound.* Society of Critical Care Medicine; 2015:139-149.
2. Richards JR, McGahan JP. Focused Assessment with Sonography in Trauma (FAST) in 2017: what radiologists can learn. *Radiology.* 2017;283(1):30-48. https://doi.org/10.1148/radiol.2017160107.

**5.** Correct Answer: A. Right upper quadrant (RUQ)—hepatorenal

*Rationale:* In a supine patient, the hepatorenal space (Morison's pouch) is the most dependent portion of the upper abdomen. A complete sonographic view of this space should include the diaphragm and adjacent pleural space, the caudal tip of the liver, and the inferior pole of the kidney. The sensitivity for detection of peritoneal free fluid depends on the mechanism of trauma and pretest probability, but ranges between 70% and 95%. If there are no contraindications, sensitivity can further be optimized by placing the patient in a Trendelenburg position.

### Selected References

1. Gleeson T, Blehar D. Point-of-care ultrasound in trauma. *Semin Ultrasound CT MR.* 2018;39(4):374-383.
2. Lobo V, Hunter-Behrend M, Cullnan E, et al. Caudal edge of the liver in the right upper quadrant (RUQ) view is the most sensitive area for free fluid on the FAST exam. *West J Emerg Med.* 2017;18(2):270-280.

**6.** Correct Answer: A. CT of the abdomen and pelvis with IV contrast

*Rationale:* This patient has experienced blunt traumatic injury and has objective findings of a "positive seat-belt sign" as well as tachycardia. The clinician should not be falsely reassured by a negative abdominal FAST examination when there is a high pretest probability of significant intra-abdominal injury. Sensitivity for the detection of peritoneal free fluid in a normotensive patient can be as low as 70%, while the sensitivity of CT scan for intra-abdominal injury is ~97%.

### Selected Reference

1. Savatmongkorngul S, Wongwaisayawan S, Kaewlai R. Focused assessment with sonography for trauma: current perspectives. *Open Access Emerg Med.* 2017;9:57-62.

---

**7.** Correct Answer: B. Initiate a blood transfusion and take the patient for exploratory laparotomy

*Rationale:* In an unstable trauma patient with a positive eFAST, the next step in management should be to transfer the patient to the operating room for exploratory laparotomy. It would be reasonable to begin transfusion of blood products in this unstable patient; however, waiting for reassessment of clinical response would be inappropriate and may delay definitive treatment. Similarly, CT scan would delay the necessary intervention to identify and repair a hemodynamically significant source of intra-abdominal bleeding. DPL is used sparingly for equivocal eFAST examination findings, or if it is unclear whether the observed fluid is blood (e.g., ascites).

Selected References
1. Bowra J. Positive FAST—RUQ—Morrison's Pouch. *The POCUS Atlas.* Accessed December 3, 2020. https://www.thepocusatlas .com/trauma/g6302hr5hk6l2cu7vgvwu4yf57y9jn.
2. Britt LD, Andrew B. *Peitzman. Acute Care Surgery.* Wolters Kluwer Health/Lippincott Williams & Wilkins; 2012. Print.
3. Richards J, McGahan J. Focused Assessment with Sonography in Trauma (FAST) in 2017: what radiologists can learn. *Radiology.* 2017;283(1):30-48.

---

**8.** Correct Answer: B. Placement of right-sided thoracostomy tube

*Rationale:* Penetrating injuries to the thoracoabdominal region require evaluation for injuries to both intrathoracic as well as intra-abdominal structures. Hemothorax may be identified when examining the upper quadrants of the abdomen during an eFAST examination. CT scan of the chest may be appropriate, but the hemothorax should be addressed immediately since the patient has a clinically significant injury. There is no indication for emergent laparotomy in this hemodynamically stable patient until further workup is completed. There is no apparent indication for immediate endotracheal intubation.

Selected References
1. Mowery N, Gunter O, Collier B, et al. Practice management guidelines for management of hemothorax and occult pneumothorax. *J Trauma Inj Infect Crit Care.* 2011;70(2):510-518.
2. Pariyadath M, Snead G. Emergency ultrasound in adults with abdominal and thoracic trauma. In: Post, TW, ed. *UpToDate,* Waltham, MA; 2019.

---

**9.** Correct Answer: D. Discharge home with close outpatient follow-up

*Rationale:* Though the published specificity for eFAST approaches 100%, several conditions can lead to false positives. Ascites, ventriculoperitoneal shunt overflow, peritoneal dialysate, massive volume resuscitation, or ovarian cyst rupture may all lead to "positive" eFAST examinations. For this patient on peritoneal dialysis, a sonographic evaluation of the abdomen to rule out hemoperitoneum is an inappropriate test. If the clinician has a high suspicion for intra-abdominal injury, a CT scan of the abdomen and pelvis with IV contrast should be performed. In this scenario, the patient is presenting after a low-mechanism motor vehicle collision, has normal vital signs, and a reassuring physical examination, so no further testing is necessary.

Selected References
1. Pariyadath M, Snead G. Emergency ultrasound in adults with abdominal and thoracic trauma. In: UpToDate, Post, TW, ed. *UpToDate,* Waltham, MA; 2019.
2. Richards J, McGahan J. Focused Assessment with Sonography in Trauma (FAST) in 2017: what radiologists can learn. *Radiology.* 2017;283(1):pp. 30-48.

---

**10.** Correct Answer: D. Imaging can be improved by having the patient take a deep breath

*Rationale:* Since the spleen is generally smaller than the liver, the dependent recess of the LUQ is typically more posterior and cephalad compared to the RUQ, consistent with the relative position of the left kidney compared to the right. The probe marker should be directed toward the head with the transducer along the posterior axillary line, while visualizing the subphrenic, splenorenal, and perisplenic spaces. Rotation of the imaging plane (clockwise, usually about 15°) to be parallel with the rib spaces may help minimize shadowing. If the patient is able to participate, holding a breath at deep inhalation may help minimize interference from rib shadowing.

Selected Reference
1. Bloom B, Gibbons R. Focused Assessment with Sonography for Trauma (FAST). *StatPearls [Internet].* 2019;PMID 29261902.

**11.** Correct Answer: C. Physiologic fluid since she is a woman of childbearing age

*Rationale:* A small amount of free fluid (up to 50 mL) in the pelvic view can be a normal finding in women of childbearing age. In trauma patients, fluid more than 50 mL should be considered pathologic and would require additional workup. There is no visible physiologic free fluid in men. In an asymptomatic patient with normal vital signs, additional evaluation is not warranted. Ascites not previously diagnosed is an unlikely cause for this finding. The location of fluid is gravity-dependent, thus in an upright or recumbent patient, even a small volume of peritoneal fluid or blood may collect in the pelvis.

Selected Reference

1. Richards J, McGahan J. Focused Assessment with Sonography in Trauma (FAST) in 2017: what radiologists can learn. *Radiology.* 2017;283(1):30-48.

**12.** Correct Answer: A. Posterior acoustic enhancement

*Rationale:* Posterior acoustic enhancement causes areas deep to fluid-filled structures (such as the bladder) to appear brighter and may make it hard to visualize a small volume of free fluid as a result. Reverberation artifact is a result of the ultrasound beam going back and forth between two strong reflectors (e.g., the ultrasound probe and pleura). Reverberation artifact between thickened pleural layers causes comet tail artifacts seen on lung ultrasound in the setting of pulmonary edema. A mirror image artifact results in duplication of objects from strong reflectors (e.g., the appearance of liver in the thorax from a strong reflection from the diaphragm).

Selected Reference

1. Prabhu SJ, Kanal K, Bhargava P, Vaidya S, Dighe MK. Ultrasound artifacts: classification, applied physics with illustrations, and imaging appearances. *Ultrasound Q.* 2014;30(2):145-157.

**13.** Correct Answer: B. Absence of a right-sided pneumothorax.

*Rationale:* This is called a seashore sign that reliably excludes pneumothorax at the location being scanned. The "waves" from the "sea" in the upper part of Figure 46.5 represent the static tissue above the pleural line. The "sand" on the "shore" in the lower part of Figure 46.5 represents lung parenchyma adjacent to the visceral pleura, which is aerated and moving. The "sea" and the "shore" are divided by the pleural line. The pleural line, arguably the most important landmark in thoracic ultrasound, should appear glistening, or like "ants-on-a-log" (termed "lung sliding"), which represents pleural motion. If there is no pleural motion (i.e., absence of lung sliding) in M-mode, there will be a "barcode" sign instead of a "seashore." In addition, patients with pneumothoraces can have A-lines but lack B-lines. A lack of pleural movement may suggest a mainstem intubation, which is not seen here. There is no evidence of hemothorax seen in Figure 46.5, but fluid is most likely to collect inferiorly and posteriorly first, so this area should be evaluated when there is clinical suspicion. Figure 46.5 does not provide information necessary to make a determination about obstructive lung disease.

Selected References

1. Cosby KS, Kendall JL. *Practical Guide to Emergency Ultrasound.* 2nd ed. Lippincott Williams & Wilkins; 2013.
2. Husain L, Hagopian L, Wayman D, Baker WE, Carmody KA. Sonographic diagnosis of pneumothorax. *J Emerg Trauma Shock;* 2012;5(1):76. *Medknow,* Accessed November 3, 2019. doi:10.4103/0974-2700.93116.

**14.** Correct Answer: D. Absence of fluid overload

*Rationale:* A-lines (Figure 46.6, *white arrows*) are reverberation artifacts that appear as hyperechoic lines at predictable distances on the image (the distance is akin to pleural line) and represent a strong reflection from the pleura from aerated lung or pneumothorax. The presence of A-lines in Figure 46.6 does not exclude pneumothorax. B-lines are continuous vertical artifacts starting at the pleural line and extending to the edge of the image (not seen here), which represent an interstitial syndrome that includes pulmonary edema, pneumonia, pulmonary fibrosis, and acute respiratory distress syndrome (ARDS). In the absence of B-lines, significant pulmonary edema and fluid overload are unlikely.

Selected References

1. Cosby KS, Kendall JL. *Practical Guide to Emergency Ultrasound.* 2nd ed. Lippincott Williams & Wilkins; 2013.
2. Lichtenstein DA. BLUE-protocol and FALLS-protocol: two applications of lung ultrasound in the critically ill. *Chest.* 2015;147(6):1659-1670.

**15.** Correct Answer: C. She likely has a high left atrial pressure

*Rationale:* The ultrasound in Figure 46.7 demonstrates numerous B-lines. B-lines (comet tails, lung rockets) are a reverberation artifact extending from a thickened pleural space to the edge of the image, which suggests interstitial pulmonary edema—either hydrostatic (e.g., congestive heart failure [CHF]) or inflammatory (e.g., pneumonia). In a normal lung, patients may have less than three B-lines per field. The higher the density of B-lines, the more edema is present in the visualized interstitium. The presence of B-lines rules out pneumothorax.

### Selected References
1. Bowra J, Browne D, Knights J. B-lines - pulmonary edema. *The POCUS Atlas.* Accessed December 3, 2020. https://www.thepocusatlas.com/lung/9kalmbf8y6j0nrspwvv876nyem83t5.
2. Cosby KS, Kendall JL. *Practical Guide to Emergency Ultrasound.* 2nd ed. Lippincott Williams & Wilkins; 2013:75-83.
3. Vignon P, Repessé X, Vieillard-Baron A, et al. Critical care ultrasonography in acute respiratory failure. *Crit Care*; 2016;20(1).

**16.** Correct Answer: B. The spine is not normally visualized in this view

*Rationale:* The left side of Figure 46.8 demonstrates a large pleural effusion. Given the history of liver disease, the patient very likely has a hepatic hydrothorax. Pleural effusions manifest as an anechoic collection abutting the diaphragm. In normal thoracic ultrasound, air in the lung prevents the spine from being visualized. In the setting of pleural effusion, lung is replaced with fluid, which serves as an anechoic window and allows for visualization of the thoracic spine, the "spine sign." There is no visible ascites below the diaphragm in Figure 46.8. There is insufficient lung parenchyma visible to determine if there are B-lines to suggest pulmonary edema. Compared to CT chest, lung ultrasound has a sensitivity of 73.7% and a specificity of 92.9% for clinically relevant pleural effusions.

### Selected References
1. Cosby KS, Kendall JL. *Practical Guide to Emergency Ultrasound.* 2nd ed. Lippincott Williams & Wilkins; 2013.
2. Dickman E, Terentiev V, Likourezos A, et al. Extension of the thoracic spine sign. *J Ultrasound Med.* 2015;34(9):1555-1561. *Wiley*, doi:10.7863/ultra.15.14.06013. Accessed November 3, 2019.

**17.** Correct Answer: A. Tube thoracostomy

*Rationale:* Figure 46.9 demonstrates lung point, seen in pneumothorax. When M-mode is applied over a pneumothorax, a "lung point" can be appreciated. The lung point is the "edge" of the pneumothorax where the lung makes contact with the chest wall. Note that there is an alternating pattern of barcode sign and seashore sign with inspiration and expiration. This finding confirms pneumothorax. Increasing PEEP in a patient with a pneumothorax may lead to hypotension. Antibiotics would be indicated if there was a concern for pneumonia. Figure 46.9 does not suggest a pericardial effusion.

### Selected References
1. Cosby KS, Kendall JL. *Practical Guide to Emergency Ultrasound.* 2nd ed. Lippincott Williams & Wilkins; 2013.
2. Husain L, Hagopian L, Wayman D, et al. Sonographic diagnosis of pneumothorax. *J Emerg Trauma Shock.* 2012;5(1):76. *Medknow*, Accessed November 3, 2019. doi:10.4103/0974-2700.93116.
3. Liang Liu, Emory University School of Medicine, Atlanta, Georgia.

**18.** Correct Answer: D. Pulmonary hypertension

*Rationale:* Systolic right atrial collapse and diastolic RV collapse are important findings in tamponade physiology readily appreciated on echocardiography. Because the walls of the right heart are thinner and more compliant than those of the left heart, they are impacted more easily by higher intrapericardial pressure. Hypovolemia and tachycardia will exaggerate these findings as there will be less intracavitary volume to distend the walls. If the patient has a history of pulmonary hypertension, the right heart walls will likely be hypertrophied from chronically high afterload. Therefore, the right heart walls will be more resilient in the setting of high intrapericardial pressure. In this setting, more echocardiographic parameters should be obtained to address clinical concern for tamponade. Hypothermia does not have a significant effect on hemodynamic echocardiographic observations related to tamponade.

### Selected References
1. Goldstein SA, Kronzon I, Khandheria BK, Mor-Avi V. *ASE's Comprehensive Echocardiography,* 2nd ed., Elsevier Health Sciences; 2016.
2. Plotnick GD, Rubin DC, Feliciano Z, Ziskind AA. Pulmonary hypertension decreases the predictive accuracy of echocardiographic clues for cardiac tamponade. *Chest.* 1995 Apr;107(4):919-924.

**19.** Correct Answer: B. There is a pericardial effusion with tamponade physiology

*Rationale:* The most striking feature of this parasternal long image as shown in Figure 46.10 is right ventricular outflow tract (RVOT) compression ("scalloping") by a pericardial effusion, which can be seen both anteriorly and posteriorly, distinguishing it from a pleural effusion. Note that the aortic valve is closed (and the mitral valve is open) and therefore, this is RVOT collapse during *diastole*. Because the patient has normal hemodynamics, this is very likely early tamponade.

Selected References

1. Al Chalaby S, Mortimer A. Pericardial Tamponade. *The POCUS Atlas.* Accessed December 3, 2020.https://www.thepocusatlas.com/echocardiography/pericardial-tamponade.
2. Alerhand S. Cardiac Tamponade. *The POCUS Atlas.* Accessed December 3, 2020. https://www.thepocusatlas.com/echocardiography/2017/11/15/cardiac-tamponade.
3. *Feigenbaums Echocardiography,* 8th ed. Lippincott, Williams & Wilkins; 2019.

**20.** Correct Answer: C. The patient has tamponade physiology

*Rationale:* One of the hallmarks of the diagnosis of pericardial tamponade is the motion of the RV free wall during diastole. Diastole can be appreciated by noting the opening of the mitral valve (anterior leaflet creates an "E-point" [yellow arrow, Figure 46.11]) or the accompanying electrocardiographic (ECG) tracing. At the same time, it is noted that the RVOT is compressed in diastole by increased pericardial pressure—this is tamponade physiology. Though somewhat insensitive, RV collapse during early diastole is highly specific for tamponade. Hypovolemia may exacerbate tamponade physiology, but is not the most significant finding here. There is no suggestion of decreased systolic function and the mitral valve E-point septal separation (anterior leaflet of mitral valve is near the septum in diastole) suggests the opposite (high ejection fraction [EF]). There is no suggestion of RV dysfunction from this view.

Selected Reference

1. Armstrong WF, Ryan T. *Feigenbaum's Echocardiography,* 8th ed. Lippincott, Williams & Wilkins; 2019.

# 47 | HYPOXEMIA

Allison C. Ferreira and Andrew T. Young

1. A 26-year-old woman is admitted to the intensive care unit (ICU) following intubation for hypoxemia, which developed during a thyroidectomy. She has decreased left-sided breath sounds, and ultrasound of the chest reveals absent lung sliding in the left apex and left base. M-mode over the apex reveals a "bar code" sign. No lung point is identified, but lung pulse and short vertical artifacts are present. Which of the following is the *most* likely diagnosis?

   A. Left apical pneumothorax
   B. Right mainstem bronchial intubation
   C. Left recurrent laryngeal nerve injury
   D. Obstruction of the right upper lobe bronchus

2. Which of the following characteristics can distinguish motion artifact due to movement of the hand or probe from a true lung point?

   A. Motion extending through the upper ("sea") portion of the M-mode image
   B. Motion extending into the lower ("beach") portion of the M-mode image
   C. More than three B-line artifacts present within a single rib space
   D. Indistinct pleural line and difficulty identifying the superior and inferior ribs

3. Which of the following is true regarding B-lines in thoracic ultrasound?

   A. B-lines are typically a late-stage finding in pulmonary disease.
   B. The number of B-lines is closely related to the patient's pulmonary capillary occlusion pressure (PCOP).
   C. The presence of up to five B-lines per rib space is considered normal.
   D. Coalescent B-lines correspond to ground-glass opacities on computed tomography (CT) scans.

4. Which of the following ultrasonography signs is present in **Figure 47.1**?

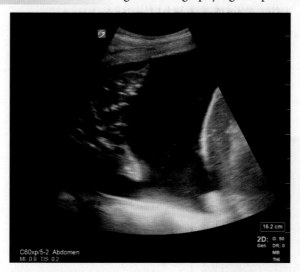

**Figure 47.1**

A. Coalescent B-lines (B2 sign)
B. Thoracic spine sign
C. Curtain sign
D. Stratosphere sign

5. A 63-year-old woman with unknown medical history presents with chest pain and dyspnea. Her heart rate is 100 bpm, the blood pressure 91/68, and the respiratory rate 32 breaths/min. Her oxygen saturation is 89% on room air, and her temperature is 37.6 °C. Ultrasound of the chest is notable for two B-lines and the presence of lung sliding on all examined rib spaces. The right leg is edematous, and the right common femoral vein is not compressible. Which is the *most* appropriate next step in her management?

A. Obtain CT angiogram
B. Initiate diuretic and nitroglycerin therapy
C. Initiate broad-spectrum intravenous antibiotic therapy
D. Perform urgent decompressive needle thoracostomy

6. A 68-year-old man with a history of smoking, chronic kidney disease, and heart failure is noted to have exertional dyspnea, cough, and an oxygen saturation of 88% on room air. Ultrasound examination of the right lung base is shown in **Figure 47.2** and ▶ **Video 47.1**. The remainder of the ultrasound examination is normal. Which of the following treatments is *most* appropriate?

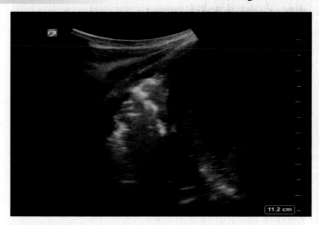

**Figure 47.2**

**A.** Needle thoracostomy
**B.** Broad-spectrum intravenous antibiotics
**C.** CT angiogram
**D.** Diuretics and noninvasive positive-pressure ventilation (NIPPV)

7. An 85-year-old man is admitted after a motor vehicle crash. He is complaining of dyspnea, left chest pain, and has an oxygen saturation of 88% despite supplemental oxygen. The blood pressure is 105/73, and the heart rate is 122. Breath sounds are reduced over the left chest. Ultrasound of the left chest is shown in **Figure 47.3**. Which of the following is the *most* appropriate next step?

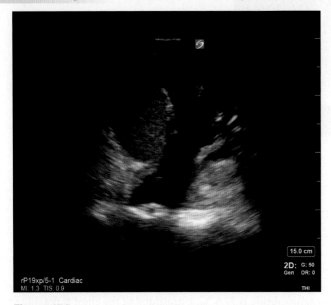

**Figure 47.3**

**A.** Thoracentesis with real-time ultrasound guidance
**B.** Large-bore chest tube placement
**C.** Broad-spectrum antibiotics
**D.** Decompressive needle thoracostomy

8. A 36-year-old man with acute intoxication, altered mental status, and emesis was intubated by paramedics. In the Emergency Department, he remains hypoxemic and cyanotic. An ultrasound of the anterior neck demonstrates an anterior, midline hypoechoic structure and a second hypoechoic structure, posterolateral to the first. There is no lung sliding bilaterally but there are B-lines at the bases. What is the *most* appropriate next step in management?

**A.** Perform bilateral decompressive needle thoracostomies
**B.** Withdraw the endotracheal tube (ETT) from the right mainstem
**C.** Extubate and then reintubate the patient
**D.** Obtain an X-ray to assess the ETT position

9. A 68-year-old man with a history of smoking, chronic cough, and chronic kidney disease presents with progressively worsening shortness of breath since running out of his inhalers several weeks ago. His cough is vigorous but nonproductive. His oxygen saturation is 94% on room air. Ultrasound examination of the chest reveals no lung sliding but a lung pulse and short vertical artifacts are present. A lung point is not identified. A-lines are present throughout. Which of the following is the *most* appropriate next step?

   A. Administer antibiotics, inhaled mucolytics, and chest physiotherapy
   B. Initiate NIPPV and prepare for endotracheal intubation
   C. Administer inhaled bronchodilators and systemic corticosteroids
   D. Place a small-bore chest tube into the left anterior second intercostal space

10. An 83-year-old man with dementia and chronic obstructive pulmonary disease is admitted for acute on chronic congestive heart failure. He improves with diuretic therapy, but on hospital day 4 he develops progressive tachypnea, tachycardia, and an increasing oxygen requirement. Blood pressure and heart rate are normal, temperature is 38.2 °C. His brain natriuretic peptide (BNP) is 20 pg/mL after an admission level of 400 pg/mL. There are rhonchi noted over the right basal lung fields. Which of the following is *most* likely to be found on ultrasound examination of the right chest?

   A. Lung point
   B. B-lines
   C. Pleural effusion
   D. Distended inferior vena cava

11. A 35-year-old man with inflammatory bowel disease undergoes placement of a right subclavian central line for total parenteral nutrition (TPN) administration. Following the procedure he complains of dyspnea. Which of the following is *most* likely to be found on ultrasound examination of the chest?

   A. Right lung pulse
   B. Right B-lines
   C. Right lung point
   D. Right curtain sign

12. A 77-year-old woman is on mechanical ventilation for respiratory failure. She undergoes insertion of a right internal jugular central venous catheter. During the procedure, the patient requires increasing oxygen to maintain a saturation above 92%. A chest ultrasound reveals small bilateral pleural effusions. Right anterior B-lines are noted, but there is no lung sliding (B'-profile). No identifiable lung point is noted and the right base is consolidated. The heart is hyperdynamic, without signs of right ventricular (RV) pressure or volume overload. Which of the following is the *most* appropriate next step in her management?

   A. Placement of right-sided chest tube
   B. Obtain a CT angiogram
   C. Advance the ETT
   D. Perform a recruitment maneuver

13. A 56-year-old man presents to the emergency room with dyspnea, cough, and hypoxemia. Ultrasound examination of the chest reveals biventricular enlargement, hypokinesis of the left heart, and diffuse, bilateral, coalescent B-lines. Which of the following is *least* likely to improve the patient's acute symptoms?

   A. Broad-spectrum antibiotics
   B. Diuretic therapy
   C. Dobutamine infusion
   D. Hemodialysis with ultrafiltration

14. A 17-year-old woman presents to the hospital after falling down an embankment several hours ago. She has had persistent dyspnea. Her blood pressure is 108/72, pulse is 107, and oxygen saturation on nasal cannula oxygen is 92%. Ultrasound examination of the chest is shown in **Figure 47.4**. What is the *most* appropriate next step?

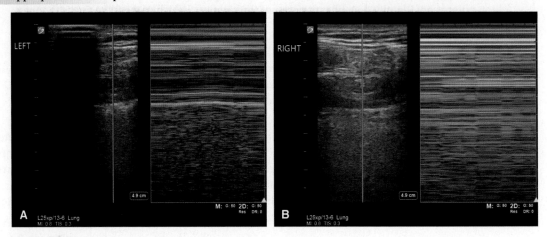

**Figure 47.4**

    **A.** Perform decompressive needle thoracostomy
    **B.** Initiate NIPPV
    **C.** Administer inhaled bronchodilators and systemic corticosteroids
    **D.** Place a small-bore chest tube

15. A 68-year-old man with systolic heart failure and chronic kidney disease was admitted with exertional dyspnea and lower extremity edema after returning from a vacation abroad. His symptoms improved with diuresis, but he still requires supplemental oxygen. Ultrasound of the left chest is shown in **Figure 47.5**. Which of the following interventions is *most* appropriate?

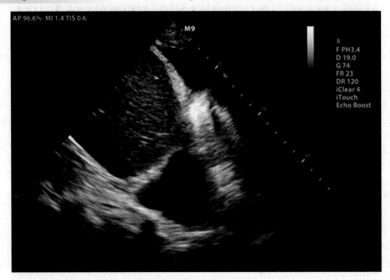

**Figure 47.5**

    **A.** Perform left-sided thoracentesis
    **B.** Initiate hemodialysis with ultrafiltration
    **C.** Place a left-sided chest tube
    **D.** Initiate NIPPV

# Chapter 47 ▪ Answers

**1.** Correct Answer: B. Right mainstem bronchial intubation

*Rationale:* Any pathophysiologic condition in which the visceral and parietal pleura no longer slide against each other will result in an absence of lung sliding (and therefore the barcode sign on M-mode) on thoracic ultrasound. Other differential diagnoses include bullous pulmonary disease, over-distension from mechanical ventilation, or adhesions. The single most specific ultrasound finding for pneumothorax is the lung point sign, the point of transition between presence and absence of lung sliding, but lack of a lung point does not rule out a pneumothorax. Lung pulse is perceptible cardiac motion observed through the pleural line, usually in the absence of sliding. This sign is equivalent to lung sliding since the "pulse" is created by movement between the two pleurae. The presence of lung pulse, lung sliding, or short vertical artifacts has a high negative predictive value for pneumothorax. Right upper lobe obstruction may create a lack of lung sliding at the apex but not at the base.

### Selected References

1. Ahn, JH, Kwon E, Lee SY, Hahm TS, Jeong JS. Ultrasound-guided lung sliding sign to confirm optimal depth of tracheal tube insertion in young children. *Br J Anaesth.* 2019 Sep;123(3):309-315.
2. Alrajab S, Youssef AM, Akkus NI, Caldito G. Pleural ultrasonography versus chest radiography for the diagnosis of pneumothorax: review of the literature and meta-analysis. *Crit Care.* 2013 Sep 23;17(5):R208.
3. Goffi A, Kruisselbrink R, Volpicelli G. The sound of air: point-of-care lung ultrasound in preoperative medicine. *Can J Anaesth.* 2018 Apr;65(4):399-416.
4. Lichtenstein DA. BLUE-protocol and FALLS-protocol: two applications of lung ultrasound in the critically ill. *Chest.* 2015 Jun;147(6):1659-1670.
5. Volpicelli G, Elbarbary M, Blaivas M, et al. International evidence-based recommendations for point-of-care lung ultrasound. *Intensive Care Med.* 2012 Apr;38(4):577-591.

**2.** Correct Answer: A. Motion extending through the upper ("sea") portion of the M-mode image

*Rationale:* Motion of the probe or hand will translate throughout the entire M-mode image back to the probe and will not behave differently at the interface between visceral and parietal pleura, as indicated by the arrowhead in **Figure 47.6**. A true lung point will demonstrate transition between "sea" and "beach" patterns only below the pleural line. B-lines are visible in 2D ultrasound and represent an interstitial syndrome when present in excess in most clinical scenarios. When superior and inferior ribs are difficult to identify and artifacts do not originate from the pleural line, subcutaneous emphysema is often present.

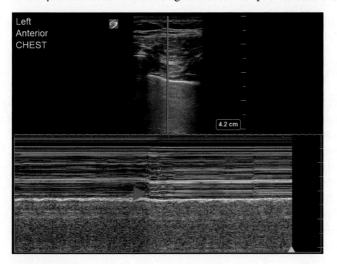

**Figure 47.6**

### Selected Reference

1. Volpicelli G, Elbarbary M, Blaivas M, et al. International evidence-based recommendations for point-of-care lung ultrasound. *Intensive Care Med.* 2012 Apr;38(4):577-591.

**3.** Correct Answer: D. Coalescent B-lines correspond to ground-glass opacities on computed tomography (CT) scans.

*Rationale:* B-lines that are coalescent or too numerous to count, the so-called "B2" pattern, correspond to areas of ground-glass appearance on chest CT. The number and density of B-lines correlate with the clinical severity of the patient's pulmonary interstitial syndrome, as well as right heart pressures; however, in the absence of left heart failure, it does not correlate with pulmonary capillary wedge pressures. B-lines can be used to anticipate progression of hypoxemic respiratory failure, as they typically precede the onset of significant symptomatic disease. More than three B-lines per rib space is considered abnormal and is correlated to the degree of extravascular lung water.

Selected References
1. Gargani L. Lung ultrasound: a new tool for the cardiologist. *Cardiovasc Ultrasound.* 2011 Feb 27;9:6.
2. Lichtenstein DA. BLUE-protocol and FALLS-protocol: two applications of lung ultrasound in the critically ill. *Chest.* 2015 Jun;147(6):1659-1670.
3. Noble VE, Murray AF, Capp R, Sylvia-Reardon MH, Steele DJR, Liteplo A. Ultrasound assessment for extravascular lung water in patients undergoing hemodialysis. Time course for resolution. *Chest.* 2009 Jun;135(6):1433-1439.
4. Platz E, Lattanzi A, Agbo C, et al. Utility of lung ultrasound in predicting pulmonary and cardiac pressures. *Eur J Heart Fail.* 2012 Sep;14:1276-1284.
5. Volpicelli G, Elbarbary M, Blaivas M, et al. International evidence-based recommendations for point-of-care lung ultrasound. *Intensive Care Med.* 2012 Apr;38(4):577-591.

**4.** Correct Answer: B. Thoracic spine sign

*Rationale:* In a normal patient, the aerated lung causes near-complete reflection of the ultrasound beam above the diaphragm. Visualization of the vertebral bodies—the "thoracic spine sign"—occurs because ultrasound waves are transmitted through a pleural effusion and allows for visualization of the vertebral bodies. B-lines, also called lung rockets or comet-tail artifacts, are laser-like vertical reverberation artifacts originating from the pleural line, extending to the bottom of Figure 47.1, and moving synchronously with lung sliding. They represent interlobar septal thickening, often due to extravascular lung water. A curtain sign is observed in normal lungs when, at full inspiration, the descent of lung and diaphragm obscures the liver or spleen. The bar code or stratosphere sign is an M-mode finding in the absence of pleural sliding.

Selected References
1. Dickman E, Terentiev V, Likourezos A, Derman A, Haines L. Extension of the thoracic spine sign: a new sonographic marker of pleural effusion. *J Ultrasound Med.* 2015 Sep;34(9):1555-1561.
2. Goffi A, Kruisselbrink R, Volpicelli G. The sound of air: point-of-care lung ultrasound in preoperative medicine. *Can J Anaesth.* 2018 Apr;65(4):399-416.
3. Volpicelli G, Elbarbary M, Blaivas M, et al. International evidence-based recommendations for point-of-care lung ultrasound. *Intensive Care Med.* 2012 Apr;38(4):577-591.

**5.** Correct Answer: A. Obtain CT angiogram

*Rationale:* This patient has a normal pulmonary ultrasound examination. Hypoxemia in the setting of a normal pulmonary examination should lead to a venous ultrasound to evaluate for the presence of deep venous thrombosis. In the setting of symptoms consistent with pulmonary embolism, as in this case, a CT angiogram is appropriate. Right heart strain on cardiac ultrasound may also support this diagnosis. Initiation of anticoagulation or thrombolysis may also be appropriate, subject to clinical course and clinician judgment. Acute decompensated heart failure requiring nitroglycerin drip will typically manifest with diffuse bilateral B-lines. Unilateral B-lines, hyperechoic areas, or dense consolidations of the visualized lung segments may suggest pneumonia and support use of antibiotics. The absence of lung sliding in the setting of hypotension would be expected with tension pneumothorax and a lung point may not be visualized due to the size of the pneumothorax.

Selected References
1. Lichtenstein DA. BLUE-protocol and FALLS-protocol: two applications of lung ultrasound in the critically ill. *Chest.* 2015 Jun;147(6):1659-1670.
2. Staub, LJ, Mazzali Biscaro RR, Kaszubowski E, Maurici R. Lung ultrasound for the emergency diagnosis of pneumonia, acute heart failure, and exacerbations of chronic obstructive pulmonary disease/asthma in adults: a systematic review and meta-analysis. *J Emerg Med.* 2019 Jan;56(1):53-69.

**6.** Correct Answer: B. Broad-spectrum intravenous antibiotics

*Rationale:* Figure 47.2 and ▶ **Video 47.1** demonstrate dense consolidation of the lung with hypere-choic areas, which correspond to air bronchograms on chest X-ray. Figure 47.2 and ▶ **Video 47.1** also show an irregular inferior border between normally aerated and abnormally aerated lung segments (the shred sign). These findings support the diagnosis of pneumonia, and antibiotics would be indicated. Nee-dle thoracostomy is performed in the setting of a tension pneumothorax, but there is no ultrasound evi-dence of a pneumothorax on Figure 47.2. Pulmonary edema requiring diuretics and NIPPV will typically demonstrate diffuse, bilateral B-lines, which are not seen here. CT angiography is used to diagnose a pulmonary embolism, but the ultrasound findings and the clinical scenario are not consistent with pul-monary edema.

Selected References
1. Copetti R, Soldati G, Copetti P. Chest sonography: a useful tool to differentiate acute cardiogenic pulmonary edema from acute respiratory distress syndrome. *Cardiovasc Ultrasound.* 2008 Apr 29;6:16.
2. Goffi A, Kruisselbrink R, Volpicelli G. The sound of air: point-of-care lung ultrasound in preoperative medicine. *Can J Anaesth.* 2018 Apr;65(4):399-416.
3. Lichtenstein DA. BLUE-protocol and FALLS-protocol: two applications of lung ultrasound in the critically ill. *Chest.* 2015 Jun;147(6):1659-1670.

**7.** Correct Answer: B. Large-bore chest tube placement

*Rationale:* Hypoxemia after blunt chest trauma may be due to pneumothorax, hemothorax, hypoventila-tion due to pain (splinting), pulmonary contusion, or mechanical inefficiency (flail chest). The ultrasound (Figure 47.3) demonstrates a large volume of pleural fluid, consistent with hemothorax and compressive atelectasis of the adjacent lung segments. Mobile particles or septa are also highly suggestive of exudate or hemothorax. Figure 47.3 is also notable for the thoracic spine sign, in which the thoracic vertebrae are visible. Traumatic hemothorax should be drained as part of the initial resuscitation. Needle thoracostomy would be indicated for decompression in tension pneumothorax, but not tension hemothorax. Thora-centesis is indicated for draining simple rather than hemorrhagic or purulent fluid and would not be performed acutely during a trauma resuscitation. Antibiotics may be indicated, but they will not address the patient's acute hypoxemia.

Selected References
1. Copetti R, Soldati G, Copetti P. Chest sonography: a useful tool to differentiate acute cardiogenic pulmonary edema from acute respiratory distress syndrome. *Cardiovasc Ultrasound.* 2008 Apr 29;6:16.
2. Lichtenstein DA. BLUE-protocol and FALLS-protocol: two applications of lung ultrasound in the critically ill. *Chest.* 2015 Jun;147(6):1659-1670.
3. Yang PC, Luh KT, Chang DB, Wu HD, Yu CJ, Kuo SH. Value of sonography in determining the nature of pleural effusion: analysis of 320 cases. *AJR Am J Roentgenol.* 1992 Jul;159(1):29-33.

**8.** Correct Answer: C. Extubate and then reintubate the patient

*Rationale:* In the setting of an esophageal intubation, the esophagus will be visible on ultrasound as a hypoechoic structure due to distention and the air-filled ETT. This is referred to as the "double trachea" or "double tract" sign and is shown in **Figure 47.7**. The next best step is extubation and either immediate reintubation or, if unable, mask ventilation. Absence of lung sliding is present when visceral and pari-etal pleura move alongside one another, but will not be seen in a variety of clinical situations including pneumothorax, pleural adhesions, apnea, mainstem intubation, or esophageal intubation. Awaiting X-ray confirmation is not appropriate given the other available data and the patient's condition.

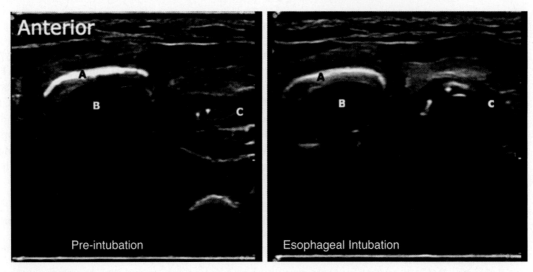

**Figure 47.7**

Selected References

1. Boretsky KR. Images in anesthesiology: point-of-care ultrasound to diagnose esophageal intubation: "the double trachea." *Anesthesiology.* 2018;129(1):190.
2. Chou HC, Tseng WP, Wang CH, et al. Tracheal rapid ultrasound exam (T.R.U.E.) for confirming endotracheal tube placement during emergency intubation. *Resuscitation.* 2011 Oct;82(10):1279-1284.
3. Gottlieb M, Holladay D, Peksa GD. Ultrasonography for the confirmation of endotracheal tube intubation: a systematic review and meta-analysis. *Ann Emerg Med.* 2018 Dec;72(6):627-636.

**9.** Correct Answer: **C. Administer inhaled bronchodilators and systemic corticosteroids**

*Rationale:* The absence of lung sliding is not specific for pneumothorax, and the presence of a lung pulse and short vertical artifacts suggests apposition of the pleural surfaces. The lung pulse is a subtle movement of the pleural line synchronous with the pulse. This finding is present in normal as well as consolidated lungs, but is not seen in the setting of a pneumothorax. Bullous emphysema is an example of a pulmonary disease where lung sliding may be undetectable because of minimal movement at the bulla. Administration of bronchodilators and systemic steroids is the first indicated intervention in a chronic obstructive pulmonary disease exacerbation. The absence of B-lines is inconsistent with infection or pulmonary edema so there is no indication for positive-pressure ventilation at this time.

Selected References

1. Goffi A, Kruisselbrink R, Volpicelli G. The sound of air: point-of-care lung ultrasound in preoperative medicine. *Can J Anaesth.* 2018 Apr;65(4):399-416.
2. Retief J, Chopra M. Pitfalls in the ultrasonographic diagnosis of pneumothorax. *J Intensive Care Soc.* 2017 May;18(2):143-145.
3. Volpicelli G, Elbarbary M, Blaivas M, et al. International evidence-based recommendations for point-of-care lung ultrasound. *Intensive Care Med.* 2012 Apr;38(4):577-591.

**10.** Correct Answer: **B. B-lines**

*Rationale:* Comprehensive lung ultrasound can be useful for rapid assessment of acute hypoxemic respiratory failure. Pneumonia will present with focal interstitial findings, such as focal or unilateral B-lines or lung consolidation. Cardiogenic pulmonary edema is less likely in this case given the normal BNP and unilateral findings on lung auscultation. Pulmonary edema causes diffuse interstitial findings, such as bilateral B-lines. A lung point is pathognomonic for pneumothorax but is not suggested by the history. A pleural effusion typically causes decreased breath sounds and, in cardiogenic pulmonary edema, would be expected to be bilateral. A parapneumonic effusion is unlikely to have developed so acutely. A distended inferior vena cava may be seen in cardiogenic causes of hypoxemia, such as heart failure or tamponade, but are not suggested here.

Selected References

1. Copetti R, Soldati G, Copetti P. Chest sonography: a useful tool to differentiate acute cardiogenic pulmonary edema from acute respiratory distress syndrome. *Cardiovasc Ultrasound.* 2008 Apr 29;6:16.
2. Lichtenstein DA. BLUE-protocol and FALLS-protocol: two applications of lung ultrasound in the critically ill. *Chest.* 2015 Jun;147(6):1659-1670.
3. Staub, LJ, Mazzali Biscaro RR, Kaszubowski E, Maurici R. Lung ultrasound for the emergency diagnosis of pneumonia, acute heart failure, and exacerbations of chronic obstructive pulmonary disease/asthma in adults: a systematic review and meta-analysis. *J Emerg Med.* 2019 Jan;56(1):53-69.

**11.** Correct Answer: **C. Right lung point**

*Rationale:* Lung sliding can be seen during respiration when the parietal and visceral pleura move relative to one another. This is lost during pneumothorax due to intervening air and loss of pleural contact. The lung point is the position in the chest where the pleura come in contact again, and sliding is seen intermittently as the point of contact moves during the respiratory cycle. This finding is pathognomonic with pneumothorax. B-lines are produced by interstitial processes such as pulmonary edema and are mutually exclusive with pneumothorax. The lung pulse is a subtle movement of the pleural line synchronous with the pulse but would not be present in a pneumothorax. The curtain sign is a normal finding seen at the bases when the aerated lung obscures the view of the liver or spleen.

Selected References

1. Lichtenstein D. Lung ultrasound in the critically ill. *Curr Opin Crit Care.* 2014 Jun;20(3):315-322.
2. Lichtenstein D, Mezière G, Biderman P, Gepner A. The "lung point": an ultrasound sign specific to pneumothorax. *Intensive Care Med.* 2000 Oct;26(10):1434-1440.
3. Volpicelli G, Elbarbary M, Blaivas M, et al. International evidence-based recommendations for point-of-care lung ultrasound. *Intensive Care Med.* 2012 Apr;38(4):577-591.

**12.** Correct Answer: **D. Perform a recruitment maneuver**

*Rationale:* Lung ultrasound can be useful in excluding a number of acute pathologies. The presence of B-lines, which are long, well-defined, hyperechoic tails originating from the pleural line, excludes pneumothorax. Lung sliding may be lost in interstitial syndromes such as pneumonia but B-lines are present (B'-profile). Unlike the presence of a lung point, which is very specific for a pneumothorax, loss of lung sliding occurs in several conditions. Small pleural effusions would not be expected to cause hypoxemia. A hyperdynamic heart is consistent with septic shock and makes massive or submassive pulmonary embolism unlikely, especially without signs of RV strain. Although absent lung sliding may be seen in endobronchial intubation, advancement of the ETT would not be indicated. The Trendelenburg position can lead to hypoventilation and/or atelectasis, especially in obese patients, and this may be relieved by recruitment maneuvers.

Selected References

1. Lichtenstein DA. BLUE-protocol and FALLS-protocol: two applications of lung ultrasound in the critically ill. *Chest.* 2015 Jun;147(6):1659-1670.
2. Lichtenstein D, Mezière G, Biderman P, Gepner A. The comet-tail artifact: an ultrasound sign ruling out pneumothorax. *Intensive Care Med.* 1999 Apr;25(4):383-388.
3. Staub, LJ, Mazzali Biscaro RR, Kaszubowski E, Maurici R. Lung ultrasound for the emergency diagnosis of pneumonia, acute heart failure, and exacerbations of chronic obstructive pulmonary disease/asthma in adults: a systematic review and meta-analysis. *J Emerg Med.* 2019 Jan;56(1):53-69.

**13.** Correct Answer: **A. Broad-spectrum antibiotics**

*Rationale:* The presence of diffuse, bilateral B-lines suggests the presence of global interstitial syndrome, such as acute cardiogenic pulmonary edema, which is further suggested by the cardiac findings. The number of B-lines correlates with the degree of extravascular lung water. Appropriate therapies for cardiogenic pulmonary edema are directed at the heart and include diuresis, inotropic therapies, and, if indicated (such as in oliguric renal failure), hemodialysis and ultrafiltration. There is no indication for antibiotics in this patient since pneumonia is unlikely.

Selected References

1. Copetti R, Soldati G, Copetti P. Chest sonography: a useful tool to differentiate acute cardiogenic pulmonary edema from acute respiratory distress syndrome. *Cardiovasc Ultrasound.* 2008 Apr 29;6:16.

2. Noble VE, Murray AF, Capp R, Sylvia-Reardon MH, Steele DJR, Liteplo A. Ultrasound assessment for extravascular lung water in patients undergoing hemodialysis. Time course for resolution. *Chest.* 2009 Jun;135(6):1433-1439.

3. Staub, LJ, Mazzali Biscaro RR, Kaszubowski E, Maurici R. Lung ultrasound for the emergency diagnosis of pneumonia, acute heart failure, and exacerbations of chronic obstructive pulmonary disease/asthma in adults: a systematic review and meta-analysis. *J Emerg Med.* 2019 Jan;56(1):53-69.

**14.** Correct Answer: D. Place a small-bore chest tube

*Rationale:* The patient has absent lung sliding on the right side, consistent with pneumothorax, without clinical findings consistent with tension pneumothorax. The characteristic "seashore" sign is seen in the left chest (Figure 47.4A), with static structures superficial to the pleural line ("waves" or "sea," subcutaneous tissue) and motion effect ("beach" or "sand," subpleural artifact) due to differential movement of the visceral and parietal pleura. The "bar code" or "stratosphere" sign on the right (Figure 47.4B) shows static subpleural structures, which may be seen in several conditions including pneumothorax. Given this patient's clinical scenario, placement of a small-bore chest tube on the right side is appropriate. If there are concerns for coexisting hemothorax, then a large-bore chest tube may be more appropriate. Positive-pressure ventilation is not clinically indicated at this time. Bronchodilators and corticosteroids are not indicated in this patient.

### Selected References

1. Alrajab S, Youssef AM, Akkus NI, Caldito G. Pleural ultrasonography versus chest radiography for the diagnosis of pneumothorax: review of the literature and meta-analysis. *Crit Care.* 2013 Sep 23;17(5):R208.

2. Lichtenstein DA. BLUE-protocol and FALLS-protocol: two applications of lung ultrasound in the critically ill. *Chest.* 2015 Jun;147(6):1659-1670.

3. Volpicelli G, Elbarbary M, Blaivas M, et al. International evidence-based recommendations for point-of-care lung ultrasound. *Intensive Care Med.* 2012 Apr;38(4):577-591.

**15.** Correct Answer: A. Perform left-sided thoracentesis

*Rationale:* The patient has persistent left-sided pleural effusion with the ongoing oxygen requirement. There is a positive thoracic spine sign, with visible thoracic vertebral bodies, consistent with clinically significant pleural effusion. The fluid is homogeneous and hypoechoic, consistent with transudate. Simple thoracentesis is appropriate. He has otherwise responded to diuretic therapy, making hemodialysis inappropriate; reaccumulation is not anticipated and thus a chest tube is also not indicated. He has no clinical indication for positive-pressure ventilation as he is adequately supported with supplemental oxygen.

### Selected References

1. Volpicelli G, Elbarbary M, Blaivas M, et al. International evidence-based recommendations for point-of-care lung ultrasound. *Intensive Care Med.* 2012 Apr;38(4):577-591.

2. Yang PC, Luh KT, Chang DB, Wu HD, Yu CJ, Kuo SH. Value of sonography in determining the nature of pleural effusion: analysis of 320 cases. *AJR Am J Roentgenol.* 1992 Jul;159(1):29-33.

# 48 | MECHANICAL CIRCULATORY SUPPORT AND CANNULATION STRATEGIES

Shu Y. Lu and Adam A. Dalia

1. According to the American Society of Echocardiography (ASE) guidelines, prior to the implantation of a left ventricular (LV) assist device (LVAD), which of the following is considered a "red-flag" finding on transthoracic echocardiogram (TTE)?

   A. Trace mitral stenosis
   B. Normal right ventricular (RV) systolic
   C. Presence of a moderator band
   D. LV apical aneurysm

2. Which of the following statements is correct regarding LV function and LVAD implantation?

   A. A qualifying condition for LVAD implantation as a destination therapy is LV ejection fraction <40%.
   B. A severely decreased LV ejection fraction is the only clinical parameter used for determining referral for an LVAD.
   C. RV ejection fraction is not a component for clinical risk stratification and suitability for an LVAD.
   D. Use of microbubble contrast agents to improve precision of LV ejection fraction measurement before LVAD implantation is strongly recommended.

3. Which of the following statements regarding LV internal dimension at end-diastole (LVIDd) in patients with an LVAD is true?

   A. A comparison of the preoperative LVIDd to the postoperative LVIDd is the primary clinical measure of the degree of LVAD-mediated left ventricle unloading.
   B. LVIDd should be measured from 2D parasternal short axis.
   C. LVIDd is decreased in most patients who are considered for an LVAD.
   D. A smaller LV cavity prior to LVAD implantation is associated with a decreased 30-day mortality rate after LVAD implantation.

4. Which of the following echocardiographic signs is least suggestive of RV dysfunction in a patient scheduled for an LVAD implantation?

   A. Tricuspid annular plane systolic excursion (TAPSE) <17 mm
   B. RV fractional area change (FAC) <35%
   C. RV dilatation
   D. Mild tricuspid regurgitation

5. Which of the following findings is an anatomic contraindication to the placement of an Impella LVAD?

    **A.** Mild aortic insufficiency
    **B.** RV thrombus
    **C.** Presence of a mechanical aortic valve (AV)
    **D.** AV area $<1.0$ cm$^2$

6. Aortic insufficiency (aortic regurgitation [AR]) is noted in the TTE examination of a patient scheduled for placement of a HeartMate III. Which of the following statements is correct?

    **A.** AR is a normal finding among LVAD candidates and is not clinically important.
    **B.** Surgical closure of the valve is an option and has little consequence once the HeartMate III is inserted.
    **C.** AR pressure half-time method is recommended for quantifying AR prior to LVAD implantation.
    **D.** AR can cause a "blind" loop of flow between LVAD, ascending aorta, and back into the left ventricle.

7. After implantation of a HeartMate III a transesophageal echocardiogram (TEE) is performed and shows **Figure 48.1** and ▶ **Video 48.1**.

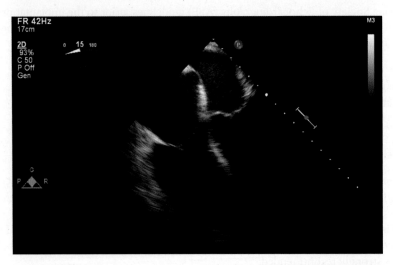

**Figure 48.1**

Which of the following statements is true?
**A.** The image demonstrates a normal interventricular septum (IVS).
**B.** The patient likely has elevated LV filling pressure.
**C.** The patient may benefit from an increase in HeartMate pump speed.
**D.** The patient may benefit from starting an inhaled pulmonary vasodilator.

8. After implantation of a HeartMate III LVAD, **Figure 48.2** and ▶ **Video 48.2** were obtained during a TEE.

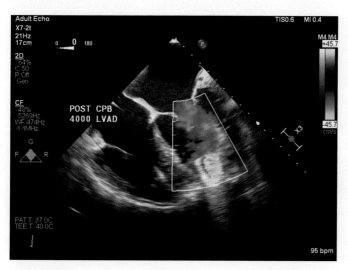

**Figure 48.2**

Based on the color Doppler profile, which of these statements is correct?
A. There is no evidence of mechanical obstruction.
B. There is bidirectional flow in the inflow cannula.
C. There is an artifact of the impeller.
D. The profile cannot be used to determine inflow velocity.

9. After implantation of a HeartMate II, you are asked to assess the inflow cannula via echocardiography. Which of the following statements is *most* correct?

A. Inflow cannula velocity can only be assessed using continuous-wave Doppler.
B. Continuous-wave Doppler for the assessment of the inflow cannula velocity is unaffected by mitral inflow.
C. Continuous-wave Doppler interrogation of a properly aligned inflow cannula should reveal low-velocity (<1.5 m/s) flow.
D. The inflow cannula should be in direct contact with the IVS.

10. Which of the following statements is correct regarding the outflow cannula of an HeartMate II?

A. The outflow graft peak systolic velocity should be >2 m/s.
B. Doppler interrogation of the outflow graft is performed coaxially to the direction of flow.
C. The outflow cannula cannot be visualized using TTE or TEE.
D. The distal outflow graft to aorta anastomosis is often not visible with TEE.

11. In comparison to preimplantation echocardiography images, postimplantation images in a patient with a new centrifugal LVAD (CF-LVAD) is most likely to demonstrate which of the following?

A. Increase in LV size
B. Decrease in LV cardiac output
C. Decrease in mitral regurgitation
D. Masking of a patent foremen ovale (PFO) shunt

**12.** This Impella 5.5 inlet (shown in **Figure 48.3** and ▶ **Video 48.3**) was measured to be 6 cm below the AV, what is the next best step for positioning?

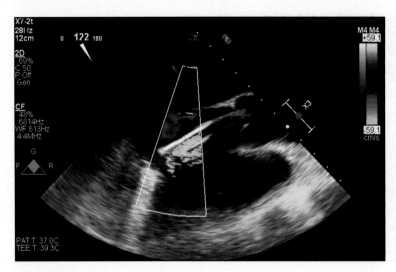

**Figure 48.3**

   **A.** The Impella should be advanced into the ventricle.
   **B.** The Impella should be withdrawn from the ventricle.
   **C.** The Impella should be redirected away from the mitral valve.
   **D.** The Impella should be replaced due to a damaged inlet.

**13.** Which of the following statements on TTE views in patients with a CF-LVAD device is *false*?

   **A.** Apical views can be used to assess IVS position.
   **B.** The apical views allow for assessment of the heart without artifacts from the LVAD device.
   **C.** The apical four-chamber view can be used to assess the inflow cannula of the LVAD.
   **D.** Long-axis view of the ascending aorta can be used to assess the outflow cannula of the LVAD.

**14.** Echocardiographic "red flags" for LVAD dysfunction include which of the following?

   **A.** No change in LVIDd with RAMP study
   **B.** Midline position of the IVS
   **C.** AV opens with every other beat
   **D.** Increased mitral regurgitation

**15.** A patient who underwent HeartMate III placement 2 days ago is noted to have a "low-flow" alarm. You perform a bedside echo and obtain ▶ **Video 48.4**. Which of the following statements is *most* correct?

   **A.** There is a thrombus in the inflow cannula of the LVAD.
   **B.** This complication can be corrected with volume removal.
   **C.** This complication is a result of a "suction event."
   **D.** This complication can be corrected by increasing the LVAD rotations per minute (RPM).

**16.** Which of the following statements regarding LVAD function is *most* correct?

   **A.** In a patient with an LVAD, AV opening can be assessed using color M-mode at a sweep of 25 to 50 mm/s.
   **B.** The presence of aortic insufficiency is uncommon after LVAD implantation.
   **C.** Persistent AV opening in a patient with an LVAD is associated with aortic root thrombus.
   **D.** An increase in LVAD pump speed can lead to sudden AV opening, increasing the risk of thromboembolism.

17. Which of the following statements is *most* correct regarding the use of TEE to assist in the placement of venovenous extracorporeal membrane oxygenation (VV-ECMO) cannulas?

   A. The midesophageal four-chamber views provide excellent visualization of the inferior vena cava (IVC), superior vena cava (SVC), tricuspid valve (TV) and right atrium (RA).
   B. The cannula tips should be located in the vena cava, 1.5 cm from the caval-atrial junction.
   C. Although correct cannula position is important, malposition of VV-ECMO cannulas is not associated with recirculation.
   D. The interatrial septum and the tricuspid valve can be damaged if the VV-ECMO cannulas are advanced too far.

18. A TTE of a patient on peripheral venoatrial (VA)-ECMO support demonstrates a nonopening AV and distended left ventricle. Which of the following is the *most* appropriate next step in management?

   A. Optimize native RV output
   B. Place an Impella device for LV decompression
   C. Increase VA-ECMO flow
   D. Place an RVvent

19. Which of the following is the best echocardiographic view to assess for proper placement of an Impella device?

   A. TEE midesophageal AV short axis
   B. TEE midesophageal AV long axis
   C. TTE apical five chamber
   D. TTE parasternal short axis

20. A TTE performed on a hypotensive patient with an LVAD demonstrates a decrease in LV size, a decrease in RV size, and a midline IVS. What is the clinical diagnosis that best explains the patient's hypotension?

   A. LVAD suction event
   B. Hypovolemia
   C. RV failure
   D. Tamponade

# Chapter 48 ▪ Answers

1. Correct Answer: D. LV apical aneurysm

*Rationale:* All LVAD candidates should be screened for structural and functional abnormalities that preclude LVAD implantation. Optimal candidate selection is one of the determinants for operative and long-term success of an LVAD. A TTE is generally the first-line imaging modality used to screen for structural and functional abnormalities. However, in some situations, a patient may require an urgent or emergent surgical LVAD placement. In these situations, a TEE can be used. In addition to performing a comprehensive examination, the ASE suggests to focus on high-risk or "red-flag" findings that may impact successful LVAD implantation.

**Left Ventricle and IVS**
- Small LV size
- LV thrombus
- LV aneurysm
- Ventricular septal defect

## Right Ventricle
- RV dilatation
- RV dysfunction

## Atria, Interatrial Septum
- LA appendage thrombus
- PFO
- Atrial septal defect (ASD

## Valvular Abnormalities
- Any prosthetic valve
  - Mild aortic insufficiency (AI)
- Moderate or severe mitral stenosis (MS)
- Moderate or severe tricuspid regurgitation (TR)
  - Mild tricuspid stenosis (TS)
- Moderate or severe pulmonic regurgitation (PR)
  - Mild pulmonic stenosis (PS)

## Other
- Congenital abnormalities
- Aortic pathology
- Mobile mass
- Shunts

### Selected Reference

1. Stainback RF, Estep JD, Agler DA, et al. Echocardiography in the management of patients with left ventricular assist devices: recommendations from the American Society of Echocardiography. *J Am Soc Echocardiogra.* 2015;28(8):853-909.

**2.** Correct Answer: D. Use of microbubble contrast agents to improve precision of LV ejection fraction measurement before LVAD implantation is strongly recommended.

*Rationale/Critique:* According to the Centers for Medicare and Medicaid, qualifying conditions for LVAD implantation as a destination therapy include an LV ejection fraction of <25% (A). While LV ejection fraction is a component of clinical risk scoring tools (Seattle Heart Failure Model, Heart Failure Survival Score) that can be used to calculate a patient's expected survival times and suitability for LVAD, it is not the only clinical parameter used to determine whether a patient gets referred for an LVAD (B and C). Calculating an accurate ejection fraction can be difficult among LVAD candidates. The ASE recommends either the biplane method of disk (modified Simpson's rule) from two-dimensional images or three-dimensional assessment for determining LV ejection fraction. The ASE also recommends using microbubble contrast agents when indicated to improve endocardial definition and precision of LV ejection fraction measurement (D).

### Selected References

1. Aaronson KD, Schwartz JS, Chen TM, Wong KL, Goin JE, Mancini DM. Development and prospective validation of a clinical index to predict survival in ambulatory patients referred for cardiac transplant evaluation. *Circulation.* 1997;95(12):2660-2667.1.
2. Patel CB, Cowger JA, Zuckermann A. A contemporary review of mechanical circulatory support. *J Heart Lung Transplant.* 2014;33(7):667-674.

**3.** Correct Answer: A. Comparison of the preoperative LVIDd to the postoperative LVIDd is the primary clinical measure of the degree of LVAD-mediated left ventricle unloading

*Rationale:* LVIDd is an important parameter for LVAD candidates and patients who have undergone LVAD implantation. The LVIDd is best measured from parasternal long-axis TTE images (B). Prior to LVAD implantation, LVAD candidates often have increased LVIDd (C). Special consideration should be focused on patients whose preoperative LVIDd is small (<63 mm) as data suggest that it is associated with increased 30-day morbidity and mortality after LVAD implantation (D). Comparison of the preoperative LVIDd to the postoperative LVIDd is the primary clinical measure of the degree of LVAD-mediated LV unloading (A).

Selected Reference
1. Topilsky Y, Oh JK, Shah DK, et al. Echocardiographic predictors of adverse outcomes after continuous left ventricular assist device implantation. *JACC Cardiovasc Imaging.* 2011;4(3):211-222.

## 4. Correct Answer: D. Mild tricuspid regurgitation

*Rationale:* It is important to assess RV function when evaluating patients for LVAD. Failure of the right ventricle in the perioperative period is the leading cause of morbidity and mortality following placement of an LVAD. Preoperative clinically severe RV dysfunction may prompt biventricular mechanical support devices as this may lead to better outcomes in this population. Echocardiographic signs of RV dysfunction include TAPSE <17 mm, RV FAC <35%, RV dilatation, and moderate or greater tricuspid regurgitation.

Selected References
1. Rudski LG, Lai WW, Afilalo J, et al. Guidelines for the echocardiographic assessment of the right heart in adults: a report from the American Society of Echocardiography: endorsed by the European Association of Echocardiography, a registered branch of the European Society of Cardiology, and the Canadian Society of Echocardiography. *J Am Soc Echocardiogr.* 2010;23(7):685-713.
2. Slaughter MS, Pagani FD, Rogers JG, et al. Clinical management of continuous-flow left ventricular assist devices in advanced heart failure. *J Heart Lung Transplant.* 2010 Apr;29(4 suppl):S1-S39.

## 5. Correct Answer: C. Presence of a mechanical AV

*Rationale/Critique:* According to the manufacturer, Abiomed, the Impella is contraindicated for use in patients with a mural thrombus in the left ventricle, mechanical AV or heart constrictive device, AV stenosis/calcification (equivalent to an orifice area of 0.6 cm$^2$ or less), moderate-to-severe aortic insufficiency (echocardiographic assessment graded as $\geq$ +2), severe peripheral arterial disease precluding placement of the Impella System, significant right heart failure, combined cardiorespiratory failure, presence of an atrial or ventricular septal defect, LV rupture, and cardiac tamponade.

Selected Reference
1. Impella® left-side devices indication & safety information. Accessed February 29, 2020. http://www.abiomed.com/important-safety-information.

## 6. Correct Answer: D. When present at HeartMate III implantation, AR can enable a "blind" loop of flow between LVAD, ascending aorta, and back into the left ventricle.

*Rationale:* LVADs, including CF-LVADs such as the HeartMate III, lead to a reduction in LV diastolic filling pressure and an increase in central aortic pressure. This physiologic change worsens AR. It is estimated that AR occurs in 25% to 30% of patients with continuous-flow LVAD. Significant AR can lead to ineffective LVAD output due to the recycling of regurgitant blood from the outflow graft in the proximal aorta back into the LV inflow cannulas (D).

Among patients with preexisting AR, AR generally worsens after LVAD implantation. As a result, moderate or severe AR is a contraindication for continuous-flow LVAD (A). Vena contracta width, and jet width/LV outflow tract width are recommended to assess AR severity (C). While surgical closure of the AV can eliminate AR after LVAD implantation, this can leave the patient with no means of LV ejection in the event of LVAD failure (B).

Selected Reference
1. Bouabdallaoui N, El-Hamamsy I, Pham M, et al. Aortic regurgitation in patients with a left ventricular assist device: a contemporary review. *J Heart Lung Transplant.* 2018;37(11):1289-1297.

## 7. Correct Answer: D. The patient may benefit from starting an inhaled pulmonary vasodilator.

*Rationale:* After LVAD implantation, the preload to the right ventricle increases secondary to an increase in LV cardiac output. As a result, the output of the right ventricle has to increase to match the LVAD work. Unfortunately, early RV dysfunction after LVAD initiation is not uncommon. Rapid increases in RV preload, cardiopulmonary bypass, and underlying RV dysfunction can all contribute to RV dysfunction after LVAD initiation. Furthermore, LVAD implantation can lead to a leftward IVS shift that alters RV geometry and further exacerbates RV dysfunction. The echo image demonstrates RV dysfunction, which echocardiographically presents as an enlarged right ventricle, a left shifted IVS, small left ventricle, and RV hypokinesis (A). Due to a decrease in RV cardiac output and small left ventricle, the LV filling pressure is decreased (B). Increasing LVAD pump speed can result in a "suction event," a condition in which a segment of the LV myocardium partially occludes the inflow cannula and reduces pump inflow, further worsening the patient's hemodynamics (C). Often, post-LVAD implantation RV dysfunction can be treated with RV afterload reduction by using agents such as inhaled pulmonary vasodilators (D, ▶ **Video 48.5**).

### Selected Reference

1. Flores AS, Essandoh M, Yerington GC, et al. Echocardiographic assessment for ventricular assist device placement. *J Thorac Dis.* 2015;7(12):2139.

---

**8.** Correct Answer: **A. There is no evidence of mechanical obstruction.**

*Rationale:* Traditionally, perioperative echocardiographic assessment of LVAD patients includes assessment of flow around the inflow and outflow cannula. Utilizing color flow Doppler can assist in determining the presence or absence of a mechanical obstruction (A) based on turbulence of flow (notice the lack of mosaicism near the inflow cannula in Figure 48.2) (C). The blue noted on color Doppler indicates flow away from the probe and there is no bidirectional flow noted near the inflow cannula (B). This color Doppler flow allows for the assessment of flow direction, flow velocity, and mechanical obstruction (D).

### Selected Reference

1. Stainback RF, Estep JD, Agler DA, et al. Echocardiography in the management of patients with left ventricular assist devices: recommendations from the American Society of Echocardiography. *J Am Soc Echocardiogra.* 2015;28(8):853-909.

---

**9.** Correct Answer: **C. Continuous-wave Doppler interrogation of a properly aligned inflow cannula should reveal low-velocity (<1.5 m/s) flow.**

*Rationale:* In HeartMate and HeartWare devices, appropriately positioned inflow cannulas should lie near or within the LV apex and are directed toward the mitral valve. Significant angulation of the inflow cannula can cause direct contact between the inflow cannula and the septum, which can cause ventricular arrhythmias and/or cannula obstruction and may necessitate surgical revision. Inflow cannula velocity can be assessed using pulsed-wave and continuous-wave spectral Doppler. Spectral Doppler profile should yield low-velocity (<1.5 m/s) and unidirectional laminar flow. In some cases, blood flow from normal mitral valve inflow or AR can contaminate spectral Doppler assessment of the inflow cannula.

### Selected References

1. Chivukula VK, Beckman JA, Prisco AR, et al. Left ventricular assist device inflow cannula angle and thrombosis risk. *Circ Heart Fail.* 2018;11(4):e004325.1.
2. Rasalingam R, Johnson SN, Bilhorn KR, et al. Transthoracic echocardiographic assessment of continuous-flow left ventricular assist devices. *J Am Soc Echocardiogr.* 2011;24(2):135-148.

---

**10.** Correct Answer: **B. Doppler interrogation of the outflow graft should be performed coaxially to the direction of flow.**

*Rationale:* Outflow cannulas can be visualized by both TTE and TEE. Whereas the proximal outflow graft is not visible with TEE, the distal portion of the outflow cannula attached to the aorta can be visualized in the majority of patients. For optimal assessment of outflow graft velocity, spectral Doppler interrogation should be performed coaxially to the direction of flow. Both pulsed-wave Doppler and continuous-wave Doppler can be used to assess outflow graft flow. Outflow graft peak systolic velocity should be <2 m/s. Velocity >2 m/s should warrant further investigation as it may suggest possible obstruction.

### Selected References

1. Rasalingam R, Johnson SN, Bilhorn KR, et al. Transthoracic echocardiographic assessment of continuous-flow left ventricular assist devices. *J Am Soc Echocardiogr.* 2011;24(2):135-148.
2. Stainback RF, Estep JD, Agler DA, et al. Echocardiography in the management of patients with left ventricular assist devices: recommendations from the American Society of Echocardiography. *J Am Soc Echocardiogra.* 2015;28(8):853-909.

**11.** Correct Answer: C. Decrease in mitral regurgitation

*Rationale:* Placement of a CF-LVAD increases LV cardiac output, which decreases LV size, LV pressure, and mitral regurgitation. One should be aware that a malpositioned LVAD can worsen mitral regurgitation. This decrease in LV pressure coupled with an increased ascending aorta pressure from the LVAD outflow cannula can lead to worsening aortic insufficiency. After initiation of the LVAD, particular attention should be focused on the interatrial septum as the decrease in left-sided pressure coupled with an increase in right-sided pressure can unmask a PFO with right-to-left shunt. This can present clinically as a decrease in arterial oxygen saturation.

Selected References
1. Kapur NK, Conte JV, Resar JR.. Percutaneous closure of patent foramen ovale for refractory hypoxemia after HeartMate II left ventricular assist device placement. *J Invasive Cardiol.* 2007;19(9):E268-E270.
2. Stainback RF, Estep JD, Agler DA, et al. Echocardiography in the management of patients with left ventricular assist devices: recommendations from the American Society of Echocardiography. *J Am Soc Echocardiogra.* 2015;28(8):853-909.

**12.** Correct Answer: B. The Impella should be withdrawn from the ventricle.

*Rationale/Critique:* The Impella 5.5, as the name suggests, should have the inlet orifice placed no more than 5.5 cm from the AV. It is important to properly position the Impella and maintain proper Impella position to prevent recirculation or inappropriate LV decompression. Impella position is best assessed in the TTE parasternal long-axis window or the TEE midesophageal long-axis window. The inflow portion of the Impella should be roughly 5 cm below the AV and the outflow portion of the Impella should be 1.5 to 2 cm above the sinus of Valsalva. Furthermore, the Impella should be turned away from the mitral valve, pointed to the LV apex, and free from mitral valve subannular structures. The color Doppler of the inlet may appear turbulent due to high speeds, but this does not indicate a damaged inlet orifice.

Selected References
1. Cardozo S, Ahmed T, Belgrave K. Impella induced massive hemolysis: reemphasizing echocardiographic guidance for correct placement. *Case Rep Cardiol.* 2015;2015:464135.
2. Leverett LB, Hellums JD, Alfrey CP, Lynch EC. Red blood cell damage by shear stress. *Biophys J.* 1972;12(3):257–273.

**13.** Correct Answer: B. The apical views allow for assessment of the heart without artifacts from the LVAD device.

*Rationale:* Patients with CF-LVAD devices often receive postimplantation echocardiography, which can be routine LVAD surveillance echocardiography or LVAD problem-focused echocardiography. During an echo examination of a patient with a CF-LVAD, it is important to comment on the IVS position. This can be assessed in multiple views but TTE apical four-chamber view or the TEE midesophageal four-chamber view allows for good visualization of the IVS (A). A leftward shift of the IVS can be due to elevated RV pressure, reduced LV preload, or excess LVAD speed. A rightward shift of the IVS can be due to elevated LV pressure, inadequate LVAD speed, pump dysfunction, increased LV afterload, or severe AR. The inflow cannula of a CF-LVAD can be adequately imaged in the standard TTE parasternal and apical views (C). However, it is important to remember that spectral Doppler assessment of the inflow cannula in the apical four chamber may be contaminated by low-velocity diastolic AR flow or mitral inflow (B). In contrast to the inflow cannula, assessment of the outflow cannula may require atypical TTE windows such as the high left parasternal long-axis view in order to visualize the outflow cannula anastomosis to the aorta (D).

Selected Reference
1. Stainback RF, Estep JD, Agler DA, et al. Echocardiography in the management of patients with left ventricular assist devices: recommendations from the American Society of Echocardiography. *J Am Soc Echocardiogra.* 2015;28(8):853-909.

**14.** Correct Answer: D. Increased mitral regurgitation

*Rationale/Critique*: During postimplantation TTE assessment of an LVAD patient, it is important to assess for echocardiographic "red flags," which may suggest possible LVAD dysfunction or thrombosis. Possible echocardiographic findings that may suggest inflow cannula obstruction, outflow graft torsion, device failure, or improper VAD speeds include:

- Dilated left ventricle
- Decreased or obliterated right ventricle
- IVS shifted toward the right ventricle
- AV opening with every beat
- Increased mitral regurgitation
- Peak outflow cannula velocity >2 m/s
- Blunted change in LVIDd during RAMP study

### Selected References

1. Estep JD, Vivo RP, Cordero-Reyes AM, et al. A simplified echocardiographic technique for detecting continuous-flow left ventricular assist device malfunction due to pump thrombosis. *J Heart Lung Transplant*. 2014;33(6):575-586.
2. Stainback RF, Estep JD, Agler DA, et al. Echocardiography in the management of patients with left ventricular assist devices: recommendations from the American Society of Echocardiography. *J Am Soc Echocardiogra*. 2015;28(8):853-909.

**15.** Correct Answer: C. This complication is a result of a "suction event."

*Rationale*: ▶ **Video 48.4** demonstrates a small left ventricle, a midline IVS, and a normal size right ventricle. These findings are consistent with hypovolemia causing a suction event. A suction event occurs when there is reduced filling of the pump (reduced preload), which increases negative pressure within the left ventricle. When this occurs, the LV wall is "sucked over" and covers the pump's inflow cannula causing a decrease in LVAD outflow and an alarm. Treatment with a fluid bolus can correct the problem. The problem can also be temporarily resolved with decreasing the LVAD RPM. However, this may not produce adequate cardiac output for perfusion.

### Selected Reference

1. Sen A, Larson JS, Kashani KB, et al. Mechanical circulatory assist devices: a primer for critical care and emergency physicians. *Crit Care*. 2016;20(1):153.

**16.** Correct Answer: A. In a patient with an LVAD, AV opening can be assessed using color M-mode at a sweep of 25 to 50 mm/s.

*Rationale*: TTE or TEE examination of a patient with an LVAD should include evaluation of the AV and degree of AV opening. The degree of AV opening is influenced by LVAD speed, native LV function, volume status, and afterload. It is recommended that the LVAD speed be set to allow for at least intermittent AV opening. Whether the AV opens has clinical implications as a persistently closed AV is associated with aortic root thrombus, a potential source of thromboembolism especially during LVAD pump speed changes. The frequency of AV opening can be accurately assessed by recording multiple cardiac cycles at a slow M-mode speed (25-50 mm/s). In addition to assessing for AV opening, assessment of the AV in a patient with an LVAD should also include a comment on the severity of aortic insufficiency as new-onset AR occurs in approximately 25% to 33% of patients 12 months after LVAD implantation. Worsening AR can impair LVAD performance and is associated with an increase in morbidity and mortality. Persistent AV closure is a risk factor for de novo AR after LVAD implantation even without the presence of aortic root thrombus.

### Selected References

1. Cowger J, Pagani FD, Haft JW, et al. The development of aortic insufficiency in left ventricular assist device-supported patients. *Circ Heart Fail*. 2010;3(6):668-674.
2. Stainback RF, Estep JD, Agler DA, et al. Echocardiography in the management of patients with left ventricular assist devices: recommendations from the American Society of Echocardiography. *J Am Soc Echocardiogra*. 2015;28(8):853-909.
3. Toda K, Fujita T, Domae K, Shimahara Y, Kobayashi J, Nakatani T. Late aortic insufficiency related to poor prognosis during left ventricular assist device support. *Ann Thorac Surg*. 2011;92(3):929-934.

**17.** Correct Answer: D. Interatrial septum and the tricuspid valve can be damaged if the VV-ECMO cannulas are advanced too far.

*Rationale:* During VV-ECMO, the blood is drained from and returned to the patient's venous system (**Figure 48.4**). Traditionally VV-ECMO uses a femoral vein cannula for drainage and the internal jugular vein for venous return, with the tips of the cannulas at the respective caval-atrial junctions (B). Correct position of the cannulas is important to prevent recirculation of the oxygenated blood between the two cannulas (C). Furthermore, inserting the cannulas too deep into the atria can result in damage to the interatrial septum and tricuspid valve (D). Under TEE visualization, the caval-atrial junctions of the IVC and SVC are best visualized in the midesophageal bicaval view (A).

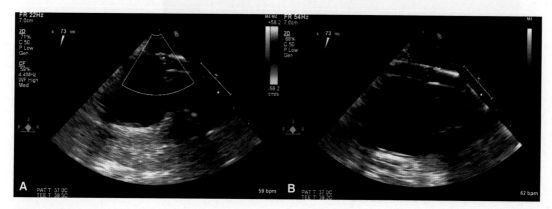

**Figure 48.4**

Selected Reference

1. Douflé G, Roscoe A, Billia F, Fan E. Echocardiography for adult patients supported with extracorporeal membrane oxygenation. *Crit Care.* 2015;19(1):326.

**18.** Correct Answer: B. Place an Impella device for LV decompression

*Rationale:* VA-ECMO can provide short-term mechanical support for patients in cardiogenic shock. In peripheral VA-ECMO, blood is drained from the venous system via a cannula inserted in the femoral vein with tips in the RA. The blood is returned via an arterial cannula in the femoral artery with the tip in the common iliac artery. The flow of the arterial return cannula creates retrograde flow toward the AV, resulting in higher afterload on the heart. This marked increase in afterload leads to LV distension, increased LV wall stress, and increased myocardial oxygen demands, which can all impair LV recovery. Furthermore, distended left ventricle and elevated LV pressures will result in increased left atrial and pulmonary pressures, leading to pulmonary edema. For these reasons, it is important to ensure the left ventricle is decompressed in a patient on peripheral VA-ECMO. This can be accomplished by improving native LV cardiac output, inserting an Impella device, or by placing an LV vent (B).

Selected Reference

1. Kapoor PM. Echocardiography in extracorporeal membrane oxygenation. *Ann Card Anaesth.* 2017;20(suppl 1):S1.

**19.** Correct Answer: B. TEE midesophageal AV long axis

*Rationale:* Proper Impella positioning is best visualized with the left ventricle and aorta in long axis (**Figure 48.5**). Either the TTE parasternal long axis or the TEE midesophageal AV long axis provides the best window to assess Impella positioning (b).

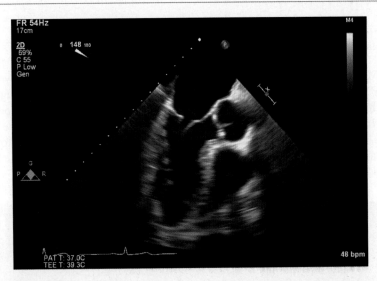

**Figure 48.5**

Selected Reference

1.  Stainback RF, Estep JD, Agler DA, et al. Echocardiography in the management of patients with left ventricular assist devices: recommendations from the American Society of Echocardiography. *J Am Soc Echocardiogra*. 2015;28(8):853-909.

**20.** Correct Answer: B. Hypovolemia

*Rationale/Critique:* See **Table 48.1**.

**Table 48.1 Physiologic Changes noted on Echocardiography**

|                          | Hypovolemia | RV failure      | Tamponade | Hypertensive crisis |
| ------------------------ | ----------- | --------------- | --------- | ------------------- |
| **LV size**              | Decreased   | Decreased       | Decreased | Increased           |
| **RV size**              | Decreased   | Increased       | Decreased | No change           |
| **Interatrial septal shift** | Midline | Leftward shift  | Midline   | Midline             |

Selected References

1.  Keller SP. Management of peripheral venoarterial extracorporeal membrane oxygenation in cardiogenic shock. *Crit Care Med*. 2019;47(9):1235-1242.
2.  Platts DG, Sedgwick JF, Burstow DJ, Mullany DV, Fraser JF. The role of echocardiography in the management of patients supported by extracorporeal membrane oxygenation. *J Am Soc Echocardiogra*. 2012;25(2):131-141.

# 49 | PREDICTING AND MEASURING FLUID RESPONSIVENESS

Aranya Bagchi

1. A 75-year-old man presents to the Emergency Department complaining of fever and shortness of breath. Laboratory evaluation reveals white blood cell (WBC) count of 21,000/mm$^3$ and a serum lactate level of 4.2 mmol/L. Chest X-ray demonstrates a left lower lobe infiltrate. During these tests, his BP drops to 80/60 mm Hg and he becomes somnolent. A bolus of 30 mL/kg of lactated Ringer's solution is rapidly administered, and repeat BP measurement is 82/65 mm Hg. His oxygen saturation is also noted to decrease from 94% to 89% while on 2 L oxygen by nasal cannula. Point-of-care lung ultrasound (▶ Video 49.1) shows a representative image of his anterior lung fields—ultrasound findings were identical bilaterally.

What is the *most appropriate* next step?
A. Repeat 30 mL/kg intravenous fluid bolus
B. Provide supplemental oxygen via non-rebreather mask
C. Begin infusion of dopamine
D. Begin infusion of norepinephrine

2. You are evaluating the patient in **Question 1** to determine additional interventions. Which of the following findings would be the most reliable indicator to *withhold* further fluid administration?

A. A central venous pressure (CVP) of 8 cm H$_2$O
B. An inferior vena cava (IVC) maximal diameter of 2.3 cm, with >50% variation in respiration, measured by point-of-care ultrasound (POCUS)
C. No change in the velocity-time integral (VTI) obtained at the left ventricular (LV) outflow tract (LVOT) following a passive leg raise maneuver
D. An ejection fraction (EF) of 45% by point-of-care echocardiography

3.  A patient with septic shock is sedated and mechanically ventilated in the intensive care unit (ICU) and is becoming progressively more hypotensive. The patient's arterial line tracing shows >30% pulse pressure variation. A rapid, focused, POCUS examination is performed to further investigate the cause of the pulse pressure variation. Which of the following ultrasound findings would argue *against* additional fluid resuscitation as the next step in care?

    A.  End-systolic effacement of LV walls ("kissing ventricle") at the mid-papillary level on a parasternal short-axis window and an IVC with a maximum diameter of 0.8 cm
    B.  The presence of pericardial fluid in the subcostal long-axis view and a finding of diastolic inversion of the right ventricular (RV) free wall
    C.  An S' velocity at the tricuspid annulus of 6 cm/s and diastolic flattening of the interventricular septum in the parasternal short-axis mid-papillary view
    D.  All the above findings suggest volume responsiveness

4.  A 64-year-old man presents with fevers, hypotension, and altered mental status. Blood cultures have grown methicillin-resistant *Staphylococcus aureus* (MRSA). An echocardiogram reveals a large vegetation on his mitral valve (see ▶ **Video 49.2**), with moderate to severe mitral regurgitation. He is deeply sedated and mechanically ventilated.

    A pulmonary artery catheter is placed, and the pulmonary capillary wedge pressure (PCWP) is noted to be 16 mm Hg. With point-of-care echocardiography, the VTI at the LVOT is noted to vary by 25% with respiration. His blood lactate concentration is 7 mmol/L, and he is oliguric. Which of the following statements is *most* accurate?

    A.  Given his oliguria and lactic acidosis, renal replacement therapy with continuous venovenous hemofiltration (CVVH) should be initiated.
    B.  A PCWP of 16 mm Hg contraindicates further volume administration, as it is likely to induce pulmonary edema.
    C.  Epinephrine would be preferred over the combination of norepinephrine and dobutamine to support his cardiac output and BP.
    D.  Given a VTI variation of 25%, his cardiac output is likely to increase with a fluid bolus.

5.  A 47-year-old woman is admitted to the ICU with septic shock and is intubated and mechanically ventilated. She is hypoxemic, with a P:F ratio of 125. A central line has been placed, and she is receiving norepinephrine and vasopressin to support her BP. Her CVP is 10 mm Hg. With POCUS, her maximal aortic velocity variation by pulsed-wave Doppler is 18%, and lung ultrasound shows bilateral consolidations. Which of the following statements is *most* true regarding her management?

    A.  A crystalloid bolus of 500 mL over 15 minutes is likely to increase her cardiac output.
    B.  Diuresis should be initiated to improve her oxygenation.
    C.  A CVP of 10 mm Hg predicts a lack of fluid responsiveness.
    D.  CVP readings have very little clinical utility in modern critical care medicine.

6.  A 70-year-old woman presents to the Emergency Department with a 2-day history of high fever, flank pain, and dysuria. She has a history of paroxysmal atrial fibrillation (AF) and elevated body mass index (BMI). An electrocardiogram (ECG) shows AF with a rapid ventricular response (HR 134 bpm), and she becomes diaphoretic and hypotensive soon after arrival. POCUS shows normal RV function and moderately depressed LV function. Her lactate is 3.2 mmol/L. A resident prepares to administer a crystalloid bolus of 1 L, but is stopped by the attending physician, who points out that with her reduced LV ejection fraction (LVEF), rapid volume administration may precipitate pulmonary edema and may require intubation. Which of the following maneuvers would *most* reliably predict a beneficial effect from volume administration?

    A.  A 25% variation between her maximum and minimum IVC diameter on ultrasound assessment
    B.  An increase of 15% in her pulse pressure on performing a passive leg raising test
    C.  A change in pulse pressure of more than 10% with respiration
    D.  A measured CVP of 5 mm Hg

7. A 42-year-old man with severe H1N1 influenza and acute respiratory distress syndrome (ARDS) is intubated and ventilated in the ICU. Lung-protective ventilator settings (tidal volume <8 mL/kg, plateau pressures <30 cm $H_2O$, and appropriate positive end-expiratory pressure [PEEP]) are used. However, to maintain a plateau pressure <30 cm $H_2O$, the tidal volume is reduced to 5 mL/kg ideal body weight, and the respiratory rate (RR) is increased to 24 breaths/min. The patient is sedated and paralyzed to eliminate ventilator–patient dyssynchrony. Assessment of the patient's fluid responsiveness is carried out by measuring the IVC diameter at end-inspiration and end-expiration, calculating the IVC collapsibility index, which is found to be 0% (**Figure 49.1**).

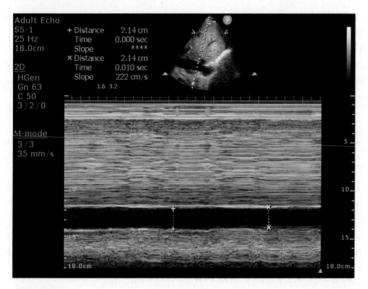

**Figure 49.1**

Which of the following statements is *most* accurate regarding intravascular volume management for this patient?

A. An IVC collapsibility index <12% indicates a lack of fluid responsiveness. Therefore, this patient should not get any additional fluid.

B. Colloid-based resuscitation fluids are preferred in patients with ARDS, because increasing the oncotic pressure decreases pulmonary edema.

C. The IVC collapsibility index has not been validated in patients being ventilated with the tidal volumes being used in this case.

D. The IVC collapsibility index corresponds to the CVP and does not predict the likelihood of fluid responsiveness.

8. A 24-year-old woman presents to the Emergency Department after a motor vehicle collision. She is awake and coherent, but clearly in significant pain, specifically in her left flank area. Her BP is 105/40 mm Hg, and her HR is 95 bpm. A POCUS examination shows an IVC with a maximum diameter of 1.5 cm, which collapses completely on inspiration, and some fluid is seen in the splenorenal space (see ▶ **Videos 49.3** and **49.4**).

Based on this ultrasound examination, which of the following statements about the patient's volume status and management is *most* accurate?

A. She is likely to be volume responsive and should get 1 L crystalloid infused rapidly over 15 minutes.

B. She is likely to be volume responsive, but should not get rapid volume resuscitation.

C. She is not likely to be volume responsive and should get maintenance crystalloid infusion at 100 mL/h.

D. She is not likely to be volume responsive and should not get fluid (bolus or maintenance).

9. Which of the following statements is *most* true regarding the measurement of superior vena cava (SVC) diameter variation with respiration as an indicator of volume responsiveness in intubated, mechanically ventilated patients?

   A. Transesophageal echocardiography (TEE) is required to assess the SVC.
   B. It is *less* specific than pulse pressure variation in predicting volume responsiveness.
   C. It can be used effectively in spontaneously breathing patients.
   D. All of the above.

10. A 46-year-old African American man with a history of heart failure with reduced EF presents to the Emergency Department with 2 days of fever, dysuria, left flank pain, and foul-smelling urine. He reports dizziness when getting up from his bed that morning. His temperature is 39°C, BP 80/55 mm Hg, HR 110 bpm, RR 28/min, and SpO$_2$ 95% on room air. Serum lactate is elevated (5.4 mmol/L). A presumptive diagnosis of pyelonephritis with severe sepsis is made. Given his history of heart failure, a point-of-care echocardiographic examination is performed, and some of the clips are shown (▶ **Videos 49.5** and **49.6**).

    Based on the patient's history and ultrasound findings, which of the following statements is *most* accurate?
    A. Given the severely reduced LVEF demonstrated in these images, fluid resuscitation is contraindicated due to the risk of precipitating pulmonary edema.
    B. The images demonstrate mildly reduced LV systolic function, and the patient should receive 30 mL/kg crystalloid bolus as recommended by the Surviving Sepsis Guidelines.
    C. Severely reduced LV systolic function does not, contraindicate fluid resuscitation, but the volume of fluid used should be carefully determined by repeated assessment of volume responsiveness to minimize the risk of complications.
    D. The patient should be started on dobutamine to improve LV systolic function.

11. A patient with severe ARDS is paralyzed and mechanically ventilated with tidal volumes of 6 mL/kg ideal body weight. The patient's lung compliance is poor (19 mL/cm H$_2$O), and P:F ratio is 95 mm Hg. Bedside echocardiography is performed to measure the VTI from an apical five-chamber view. While performing an end-expiratory occlusion test (EEOT), the VTI is noted to increase by 15%. Which of the following statements is *most* true when considering the EEOT?

    A. Poor lung compliance makes the EEOT invalid in this population.
    B. End-expiratory occlusion is a static maneuver and therefore not very useful in predicting fluid responsiveness.
    C. An EEOT should be carried out for 5 seconds to determine fluid responsiveness.
    D. Combining EEOT with an end-inspiratory occlusion test (EIOT) can improve the sensitivity of the technique when using echocardiography.

12. A clinician is performing point-of-care echocardiography on an intubated, ventilated patient with septic shock. The patient is being ventilated on volume-controlled ventilation using 6 mL/kg ideal body weight, but is relatively lightly sedated and "overbreathing" the ventilator. The patient is on 10 μg/min of norepinephrine but has warm extremities with bounding pulses. The clinician is trying to determine whether the patient should be given a fluid bolus. Which of the following findings would be *most* reliable to predict fluid responsiveness based on the current literature?

    A. The IVC diameter at end-inspiration is 1.8 cm, and at end-expiration is 1.3 cm.
    B. The LVEF is 65%.
    C. The VTI at the LVOT increases by 20% with a passive leg raise.
    D. There is >10% variation in the maximal LVOT velocity with respiration.

13. Which of the following statements is *most* true regarding the least significant change (LSC) that can be reliably measured by echocardiography when measuring VTI changes under dynamic conditions, such as with mechanical ventilation?

    **A.** The LSC in measuring the VTI in two sequential examinations is the same whether a single operator performs both examinations or the examinations are performed by different operators.

    **B.** The LSC in the VTI that can be reliably measured by a single operator is about 11%.

    **C.** The LSC in the VTI that can be measured by a single observer is lower in mechanically ventilated patients than in spontaneously breathing patients.

    **D.** In most clinical situations, a change in VTI of 5% can be reliably detected by echocardiography.

14. When considering fluid management questions, POCUS is typically used to assess fluid responsiveness. However, POCUS can also be helpful in identifying patients who have systemic venous congestion and would benefit from fluid removal. One such index that can be clinically useful is the portal venous pulsatility index (PVPI). Which of the following statements about the PVPI is *most* true?

    **A.** Since IVC measurements provide a reliable estimation of right atrial pressure (RAP) in mechanically ventilated patients, there is no need to assess PVPI if a reliable RAP estimate can be obtained.

    **B.** The portal vein is typically assessed from the subxiphoid view using a cardiac (phased-array) probe.

    **C.** The portal vein is only pulsatile in patients with severe cirrhosis and portal hypertension.

    **D.** The portal vein is typically nonpulsatile—a PVPI >50% is a useful indicator of systemic congestion and RV dysfunction.

15. A 64-year-old man with severe ARDS (P:F ratio 92 mm Hg) is intubated, sedated, and paralyzed, mechanically ventilated with volume control ventilation. To reduce plateau and driving pressure, his tidal volume has been reduced to 5 mL/kg ideal body weight. In order to assess whether he is fluid responsive, a point-of-care echocardiogram is performed to measure the changes in VTI with respiration. The percent change in the VTI is noted to be 6%. Which of the following statements is *most* true?

    **A.** Since the patient's VTI variation is <10%, he is unlikely to be fluid responsive.

    **B.** No technique for evaluating fluid responsiveness has been shown to be reliable in patients being ventilated with <6 mL/kg ideal body weight.

    **C.** The combination of low tidal volumes and poor lung compliance in this patient makes VTI variation with respiration relatively unpredictable.

    **D.** None of the above.

16. The following statements regarding the use of esophageal Doppler probes for goal-directed resuscitation in the operating room are true *except*:

    **A.** Studies suggest that the use of esophageal Doppler probes during major surgery to guide resuscitation can reduce the incidence of postoperative complications.

    **B.** An increase in the stroke distance in the esophageal Doppler signal after a fluid challenge suggests improving cardiac output.

    **C.** The esophageal Doppler signal detects flow in the ascending aorta and therefore reflects the total LV stroke volume.

    **D.** Esophageal Doppler signals can be used to diagnose aortic regurgitation and pericardial tamponade.

17. A 67-year-old woman with a history of heart failure with reduced EF and elevated BMI ($42 \, kg/m^2$) is admitted to an ICU with acute decompensated heart failure. Her temperature is 36°C, HR 95 bpm, BP 105/75 mm Hg, RR 105/min, and $SpO_2$ 84% on room air. On physical examination, she is noted to have cool extremities with 2+ pitting edema and crackles at both lung bases. POCUS shows severely depressed LV function, mildly depressed RV function, and pathologic "B-lines" in bilateral anterior lung fields. She is intubated for increasing hypoxemia and started on an epinephrine infusion to support her cardiac output and BP. Renal replacement therapy with CVVH is initiated for severe volume overload and diuretic resistance. Which of the following statements is *most* true regarding the assessment of her volume status with ultrasound?

   A. Volume removal will increase her stroke volume, by reducing LV size and bringing the heart to a more physiologic position on the Starling curve.
   B. The number and severity of B-lines will decrease as fluid is removed.
   C. Chest X-ray is more sensitive than lung ultrasound when assessing extravascular lung water (EVLW).
   D. B-lines are specific for the presence of EVLW.

18. After intubation, the PEEP is increased from 5 to 10 cm $H_2O$. **Figure 49.2** shows cardiac output in the patient and case discussed in **Question 17**, before (**Figure 49.2A**) and after (**Figure 49.2B**) the increase in PEEP.

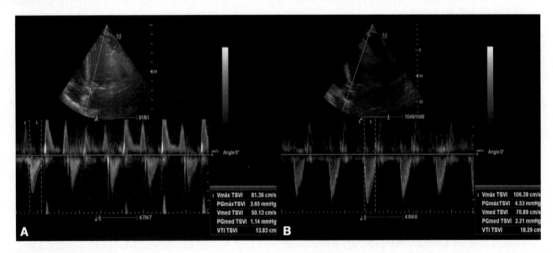

**Figure 49.2**

This change in cardiac output is best explained by which of the following effects of a higher PEEP?
   A. An increase in RV preload
   B. A decrease in LV afterload
   C. A decrease in systolic BP
   D. None of the above

19. A 50-year-old woman with a history of asymptomatic severe aortic stenosis is undergoing a radical cholecystectomy for gallbladder cancer. Given the urgent need for surgery, a decision is made to proceed without treating her aortic stenosis. She is anesthetized, paralyzed, and mechanically ventilated. Monitoring includes a radial arterial catheter in place for BP monitoring and TEE. Her mean arterial pressure is 66 mm Hg, urine output is >0.5 mL/kg/h, and a blood gas analysis shows a pH of 7.48, $PaCO_2$ of 42 mm Hg, and $PaO_2$ of 160 mm Hg (on 40% oxygen). Interrogation of the peak aortic velocity using continuous-wave Doppler shows 20% variation with respiration. Which of the following would be the *best* next step in her management?

    A. No change in the current management.
    B. Administer 1 L crystalloid bolus because a 20% change in aortic velocity with respiration is an indicator that the patient would increase her cardiac output in response to volume.
    C. Administer a unit of packed red blood cells because the high aortic velocity variation might indicate occult blood loss.
    D. Start an infusion of dobutamine to increase cardiac output.

20. Which of the following statements is *most* true regarding the use of brachial artery peak velocity variation to determine fluid responsiveness?

    A. The angle between the plane of brachial arterial blood flow and the incident ultrasound beam should not exceed 30°.
    B. This method of assessment is most accurate when the patient is passively ventilated with tidal volumes >8 mL/kg.
    C. This technique has been shown to be effective in patients with atrial fibrillation.
    D. Continuous-wave Doppler provides superior results due to the high velocity of blood flow in the brachial artery.

21. Doppler interrogation of the carotid arteries can provide easy-to-perform indices of volume responsiveness. In this context, all of the following are true *except*:

    A. Carotid corrected flow time (CFT) increases in response to volume administration and decreases after volume removal during dialysis.
    B. Carotid blood flow (CBF) can increase in response to a passive leg raise test in patients who are fluid responsive.
    C. CBF may be a better marker of cardiac output than CFT, which may correlate with volume status.
    D. These indices have been shown to remain accurate even in the presence of carotid disease.

**22.** A 72-year-old woman is admitted to the Emergency Department with urosepsis. Her temperature is 37°C, BP 110/50 mm Hg, HR 110 bpm, RR 18/min, and SpO$_2$ 95% on room air. She is confused and has a serum lactate of 4.0 mmol/L. After rapid administration of 30 mL/kg of lactated Ringer's solution, her arterial oxygen saturation begins to fall, while she remains hypotensive, and her extremities are cool and mottled. Cardiac ultrasound and representative lung ultrasound images are shown (**Figure 49.3;** ▶ **Videos 49.7** and **49.8**). She has an E/e' ratio of 18, and the mean gradient across the mitral valve is 2 mm Hg.

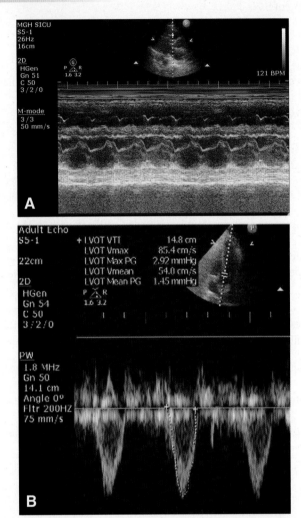

**Figure 49.3** A. Parasternal long-axis view, showing M-mode across the mitral valve. B. Apical five-chamber view showing VTI through the LVOT. LVOT, left ventricular outflow tract; VTI, velocity-time integral.

Which of the following is *most* true regarding these findings?

**A.** New-onset B-lines, together with a normal EF, indicate noncardiogenic pulmonary edema.

**B.** This patient would benefit from diuresis to improve oxygenation.

**C.** B-lines are strongly correlated with a PCWP of >18 mm Hg.

**D.** Vasopressor therapy would be preferred over additional fluid boluses.

23. Based on the patient's echocardiographic findings in **Question 22**, which of the following is *most* accurate with regard to her cardiac function?

    A. The patient has dynamic LVOT obstruction and would benefit from additional intravascular volume.
    B. She has cardiogenic pulmonary edema due to LV diastolic dysfunction.
    C. Her pulmonary edema is due to severe mitral stenosis.
    D. Both systolic and diastolic function are normal, and her pulmonary edema is due to ARDS.

24. A 64-year-old 70 kg man presents with cholangitis and septic shock. His temperature is 39°C, BP 80/60 mm Hg, HR 140 bpm, RR 38/min, and $SpO_2$ 99% on room air. He is conscious but drowsy, has cool extremities, is diaphoretic, and has a lactate of 9.4 mmol/L. Images from a point-of-care echocardiography examination are shown in **Figure 49.4;** ▶ **Videos 49.9** and **49.10.**

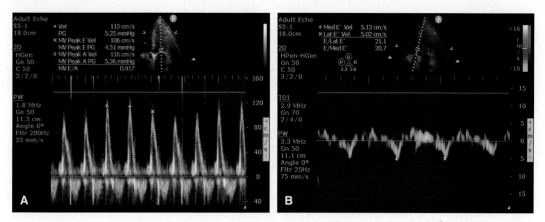

Figure 49.4 A. Transmitral Flow. B. Tissue Doppler imaging through the mitral annulus.

    An arterial blood gas (ABG) shows a pH of 7.38, $PaO_2$ of 84 mm Hg on room air, and a $PaCO_2$ of 18 mm Hg. A 30 mL/kg bolus of lactated Ringer's solution is administered, blood cultures are drawn, and antibiotics are started. Which of the following would be the *most* appropriate next step in his management?
    A. Initiation of an intravenous esmolol infusion to slow his HR and improve diastolic filling time
    B. Start phenylephrine because he clearly has sepsis, and his tachycardia precludes an agent with beta agonism, such as norepinephrine
    C. Repeat a bolus of lactated Ringer's solution
    D. Institute mechanical circulatory support for his severe shock

25. An 81-year-old woman is transferred to the ICU for management of acute hypotension. She has a known history of RV dysfunction and obstructive sleep apnea, and had been admitted to the surgical ward with a mechanical fall resulting in a pubic ramus fracture. She developed AF with a rapid ventricular response, for which she was treated with a diltiazem bolus and infusion, shortly after which she became bradycardic to 52 bpm and hypotensive (80/50 mm Hg). She was given 1 L crystalloid bolus, and repeat BP is unchanged. On arrival to the ICU, she is awake and anxious. Her extremities are cool. Point-of-care echocardiography is shown in ▶ **Videos 49.11** and **49.12.**

    Which of the following actions would be the *most* appropriate next step in her management?
    A. Administer a fluid bolus for hypotension.
    B. Start an inopressor (e.g., epinephrine) to maintain systemic BP and support RV inotropy.
    C. Perform pulmonary artery catheterization at the bedside and use data from it to guide fluid and vasoactive medication management.
    D. Initiate inhaled nitric oxide via a high-flow nasal cannula.

26. A 35-year-old African American man with elevated BMI is post-op day 1 after a HeartMate 3™ LV assist device (LVAD) placement. He is sedated and intubated and has been given multiple volume boluses overnight for hypotension and low LVAD flow alarms. During morning rounds, his CVP is noted to be 24 mm Hg, and his mean arterial pressure is 58 mm Hg. A point-of-care echocardiogram is shown in ▶ **Video 49.13**.

What is the *most* appropriate next step in his management?
A. Provide an additional intravenous fluid bolus.
B. Perform a passive leg raise test, using a 10% increase in mean arterial pressure as a criterion for additional volume resuscitation.
C. Decrease the speed of the LVAD and start an epinephrine infusion.
D. Contact the surgical team for the placement of a right ventricular assist device to treat severe RV failure.

27. A 26-year-old previously healthy woman presents to the Emergency Department with fever and altered mental status for 2 days. Her temperature is 38.9°C, BP 70/50 mm Hg, HR 110 bpm, RR 22/min, and $SpO_2$ 95% on room air. Her husband notes that she has been vomiting frequently. While performing a POCUS examination, the resident concludes that the IVC diameter is 1.8 cm and does not vary with respiration (▶ **Video 49.14**).

Which of the following is *most* true about this image?
A. The lack of variation of the IVC in this young hypotensive patient suggests that she may have some form of obstructive shock, such as pericardial tamponade and tension pneumothorax.
B. The lack of IVC collapse with respiration makes it likely that this patient will not be fluid responsive.
C. The resident has in fact imaged the abdominal aorta instead of the IVC because the IVC diameter is extremely low in this hypotensive and hypovolemic patient.
D. None of the above.

28. The passive leg raise maneuver is an effective method to identify fluid-responsive patients by giving them an "autotransfusion." Which of the following methods has *not* been validated to determine whether a passive leg raise increases cardiac output?

A. LVOT VTI
B. Arterial pulse pressure variation
C. Stroke volume
D. IVC diameter

29. **Figures 49.5A-C** show three M-mode images of the IVC in spontaneously breathing patients that correspond to different estimates of CVP.

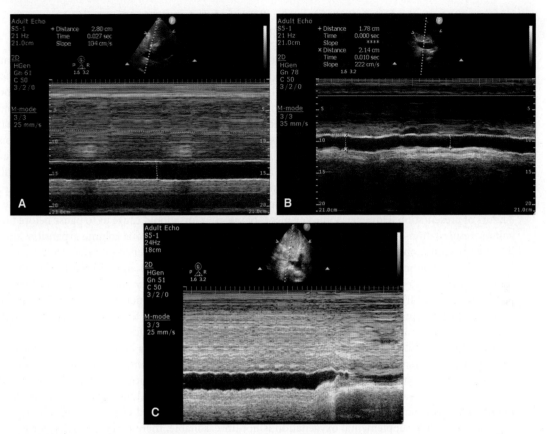

**Figure 49.5** A. End-inspiratory diameter 2.8 cm, end-expiratory diameter 2.8 cm. B. End-inspiratory diameter 1.78 cm, end-expiratory diameter 2.14 cm. C. End-inspiratory diameter 0.2 cm, end-expiratory diameter 1.8 cm.

The measurements at end-inspiration and end-expiration are described in the figure legends. Which of the following statements is *most* accurate regarding interpretation of these images?

A. The patient shown in Figure 49.5A has RV failure based on a complete lack of variation of the IVC with respiration.

B. The patient in Figure 49.5B is not fluid responsive based on his IVC collapsibility index.

C. The patient in Figure 49.5C will likely increase his cardiac output with a fluid bolus.

D. Imaging the IVC can only provide useful information in sedated and paralyzed patients.

30. A subcostal view can be occasionally challenging to obtain, either because of recent surgery with incision site dressings that obscure the subxiphoid region or because of an acutely tender abdomen or bowel gas. Under these circumstances, which of the following statements is *most* true regarding visualization of the IVC and the abdominal aorta?

A. The IVC and abdominal aorta can be imaged from the right flank.

B. If the subcostal view is not possible, assessment of the IVC and/or the abdominal aorta should not be attempted.

C. Dynamic changes in IVC diameter are consistent and agree across multiple sites of IVC measurement.

D. None of the above.

# Chapter 49 ▪ Answers

**1.** Correct Answer: D. Begin infusion of norepinephrine

*Rationale:* Intravascular volume resuscitation is a core competency among healthcare providers managing acutely ill patients. Unfortunately, there are few definitive answers to questions such as *when* to infuse fluids and *how much* to administer to a hypotensive patient. Furthermore, increasing evidence of harm from over-resuscitation suggests that a more judicious approach to volume resuscitation may be appropriate. There is no single monitor or metric that is invariably predictive—thus, integrating data from different sources is often the most useful approach. Ultrasound-guided fluid resuscitation, in the context of other commonly used indices of predicting fluid responsiveness, may help guide volume resuscitation. This patient presented with severe sepsis (life-threatening organ dysfunction caused by a dysregulated host response to infection). Volume resuscitation is recommended as the initial intervention to improve perfusion by the Surviving Sepsis Guidelines, specifically, at least 30 mL/kg of crystalloid within the first 3 hours of presentation. However, some key pieces of information should cause us to pause before further volume resuscitation—the fact that his BP has not changed after intravenous volume expansion, and that his oxygen saturation is decreasing (Option A is incorrect). In the absence of a detailed past medical history (history of heart failure or chronic kidney disease, for example) and without further examination, it is difficult to define whether his desaturation is from pulmonary edema (either cardiogenic or noncardiogenic) or from decreased alveolar ventilation in the setting of increasing drowsiness and respiratory fatigue. The presence of a bilateral anterior B-line profile on lung ultrasound suggests significant extravascular lung water (EVLW). A bilateral B-line profile has been suggested to correlate with a PCWP >18 mm Hg, but this is not invariably true. While it is possible to have a bilateral B-line profile in noncardiogenic pulmonary edema, given his decreasing oxygen saturation and clear evidence of worsening EVLW, starting the patient on norepinephrine (the initial vasoactive medication of choice in severe sepsis or septic shock) is reasonable while a more detailed assessment is carried out regarding further therapy. Dopamine is associated with worse outcomes for sepsis when compared to norepinephrine (Option C is incorrect). While supplemental oxygenation is not unreasonable, there is no indication for a non-rebreathing mask—the degree of hypoxemia (SpO$_2$ 89% on room air) does not warrant a non-rebreather (Option B is incorrect).

## Selected References

1. Bentzer P, Griesdale DE, Boyd J, MacLean K, Sirounis D, Ayas NT. Will this hemodynamically unstable patient respond to a bolus of intravenous fluid? *JAMA* 2016;316:1298-1309.
2. De Backer D, Aldecoa C, Njimi H, Vincent JL. Dopamine versus norepinephrine in the treatment of septic shock: a meta-analysis. *Crit Care Med.* 2012;40(3):725-730.
3. De Backer D, Biston P, Devriendt J, et al. Comparison of dopamine and norepinephrine in the treatment of shock. *N Engl J Med.* 2010;362(9):779-789.
4. Lichtenstein DA, Meziere GA, Lagoueyte J-F, Biderman P, Goldstein I, Gepner A. Lung ultrasound as a bedside tool for predicting pulmonary artery occlusion pressure in the critically ill. *Chest.* 2009;136:1014-1020.
5. Picano E, Pellikka PA. Ultrasound of extravascular lung water: a new standard for pulmonary congestion. *Eur Heart J.* 2016;37:2097-2104.
6. Price S, Platz E, Cullen L, et al. Echocardiography and lung ultrasonography for the assessment and management of acute heart failure. *Nat Rev Cardiol.* 2017;14:427-440.
7. Rhodes A, Evans LE, Alhazzani W, et al. Surviving sepsis campaign: international guidelines for the management of sepsis and septic shock: 2016. *Crit Care Med.* 2017;45:486-552.
8. Singer M, Deutschman CS, Seymour CW, et al. The third international consensus definitions for sepsis and septic shock (sepsis 3). *JAMA.* 2016;315(8):801-810.
9. Volpicelli G, Skurzak S, Boero E, et al. Lung ultrasound predicts well extravascular lung water but is of limited usefulness in the prediction of wedge pressure. *Anesthesiology.* 2014;121:320-327.

**2.** Correct Answer: C. No change in the velocity-time integral (VTI) obtained at the left ventricular (LV) outflow tract (LVOT) following a passive leg raise maneuver

*Rationale:* Frequent assessment of the patient's clinical status should drive fluid administration, particularly as over-resuscitation has been shown to be associated with adverse consequences. A CVP of 8 cm $H_2O$ does not discriminate effectively between patients that will or will not benefit from additional intravascular volume expansion. The value of respiratory variation in IVC diameter in spontaneously breathing patients to determine fluid responsiveness is unclear. The EF by itself is not particularly useful in identifying patients who will increase their cardiac output following a fluid bolus. The change in the VTI at the LVOT in response to a passive leg raise maneuver can be used to predict volume responsiveness, by "autotransfusing" intravascular volume from the lower extremities into the central circulation and evaluating the change in stroke volume. Since the LVOT diameter remains constant in a given patient, stroke volume is directly proportional to the LVOT VTI. Given the information available, the absence of an increase in the VTI in response to passive leg raise predicts a lack of volume responsiveness (**Figure 49.6**). In this context, additional intravascular volume is unlikely to provide a hemodynamic benefit and more likely to exacerbate deleterious effects.

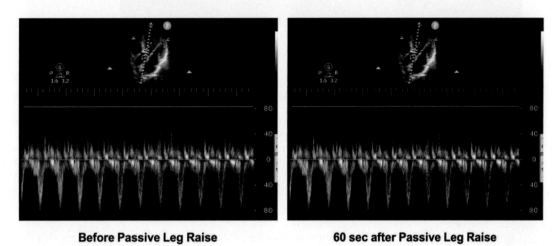

**Before Passive Leg Raise**          **60 sec after Passive Leg Raise**

**Figure 49.6**

### Selected References

1. Airapetian N, Maizel J, Alyamani O, et al. Does inferior vena cava respiratory variability predict fluid responsiveness in spontaneously breathing patients? *Crit Care.* 2015;19:400.
2. Marik PE, Cavallazzi R. Does the central venous pressure predict fluid responsiveness? An updated meta-analysis and a plea for some common sense. *Crit Care Med.* 2013;41:1774-1781.
3. Vignon P, Repessé X, Bégot E, et al. Comparison of echocardiographic indices used to predict fluid responsiveness in ventilated patients. *Am J Respir Crit Care Med.* 2017;195:1022-1032.

**3.** Correct Answer: C. An S' velocity at the tricuspid annulus of 6 cm/s and diastolic flattening of the interventricular septum in the parasternal short-axis mid-papillary view.

*Rationale:* The findings in Option A are consistent with significant intravascular hypovolemia, which could present as pulse pressure variation and would likely respond to volume resuscitation. Echocardiographic features described in Option B are consistent with pericardial tamponade. Rapid volume expansion is a key supportive measure while definitive management (drainage or evacuation of the effusion) is being arranged, particularly in hypotensive patients (systolic BP <100 mm Hg). The findings described in Option C are consistent with RV dysfunction and volume overload of the right ventricle. RV dysfunction can also present with pulse pressure variation due to ventricular interdependence. One well-validated echocardiographic marker of RV systolic function is tissue Doppler interrogation (TDI) of the tricuspid annulus velocity (S'). An S' velocity <10 cm/s is consistent with RV dysfunction (**Figure 49.7**). In the setting of RV dysfunction, further fluid administration should be undertaken with caution, if at all. A focused point-of-care echocardiography examination can rapidly differentiate between these three key causes of pulse pressure variation and, if available, should be considered in the evaluation of all hemodynamically unstable patients.

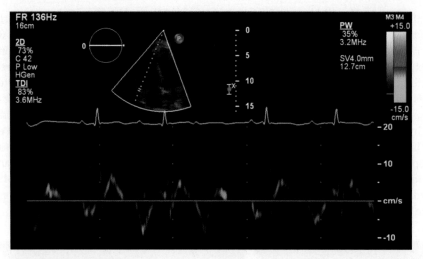

**Figure 49.7**

## Selected References

1. Magder S. Further cautions for the use of ventilatory-induced changes in arterial pressures to predict volume responsiveness. *Crit Care.* 2010;14(5):197.
2. Mahjoub Y, Pila C, Friggeri A, et al. Assessing fluid responsiveness in critically ill patients: false-positive pulse pressure variation is detected by Doppler echocardiographic evaluation of the right ventricle. *Crit Care Med.* 2009;37:2570-2575.
3. Rudski LG, Lai WW, Afilalo J, et al. Guidelines for the echocardiographic assessment of the right heart in adults: a report from the American Society of Echocardiography endorsed by the European Association of Echocardiography, a registered branch of the European Society of Cardiology, and the Canadian Society of Echocardiography. *J Am Soc Echocardiogr.* 2010;23(7):685-713.
4. Sagrista-Sauleda J, Angel J, Sambola A, Permanyer-Miralda G. Hemodynamic effects of volume expansion in patients with cardiac tamponade. *Circulation.* 2008;117:1545-1549.

**4.** Correct Answer: D. Given a VTI variation of 25%, his cardiac output is likely to increase with a fluid bolus.

*Rationale:* Although the patient is oliguric and has lactic acidosis, there is not enough information to determine whether renal replacement therapies should be initiated immediately (Option A). If, for instance, his cardiac output improves with a fluid bolus, his lactic acidosis may decrease and urine output increase. A PCWP of 16mm Hg does not reliably discriminate between volume responders and nonresponders (Option B). It is important to remember that the static indices of volume status (e.g., PCWP, CVP, or EF) are of very limited value in defining patients who are volume responsive. Dynamic indices of fluid responsiveness, on the other hand, look at the effect of a physiologic perturbation of venous return and its influence on cardiac output. This may involve respirophasic variation or assessing response to small fluid boluses or passive leg raising, among others. Variation in LVOT VTI >20% with controlled respiration predicts volume responsiveness, although the sensitivity of this finding may be reduced in patients being ventilated with low tidal volumes (<8 mL/kg); however, lower tidal volumes are likely to *underestimate* volume responsiveness. It is unclear whether epinephrine is better than a combination of norepinephrine and dobutamine (Option C). The CATS trial addressed this question in patients with septic shock and found that the two approaches were largely equivalent, with the exception of a higher incidence of lactic acidosis with epinephrine.

## Selected References

1. Annane D, Vignon P, Renault A, et al. Norepinephrine plus dobutamine versus epinephrine alone for management of septic shock: a randomised trial. *Lancet.* 2007;370:676-684.
2. Bentzer P, Griesdale DE, Boyd J, MacLean K, Sirounis D, Ayas NT. Will this hemodynamically unstable patient respond to a bolus of intravenous fluid? *JAMA* 2016;316:1298-1309.
3. De Backer D, Fagnoul D. Intensive care ultrasound: VI. Fluid responsiveness and shock assessment. *Ann Am Thorac Soc.* 2014 11:129-136.
4. Marik PE, Monnet X, Teboul JL. Hemodynamic parameters to guide fluid therapy. *Ann Intensive Care.* 2011;1:1.

**5.** Correct Answer: A. A crystalloid bolus of 500 mL over 15 minutes is likely to increase her cardiac output.

*Rationale:* Although many critical care physicians use the CVP to make decisions regarding fluid administration, the CVP is a poor tool for this purpose (Option C). Like measuring changes in VTIs with respiration, changes in maximal aortic velocity >12% can predict fluid responsiveness, that is, an increase in cardiac output by 10-15% in response to a crystalloid bolus. An additional advantage of this technique is that it is quicker to measure the maximal velocity compared to tracing the VTI envelope. Although initiating diuresis (Option B) in patients on vasopressors who are grossly volume overloaded is not unreasonable, in the absence of those indications diuresis is often initiated after patients are no longer vasopressor dependent, as in the Fluid and Catheter Treatment Trial (FACTT). While the CVP is not particularly helpful in identifying patients who are fluid responsive, it can be very helpful in many contexts, including as a measure of RV dysfunction.

**Selected References**

1. Cannesson M, Pestel G, Ricks C, Hoeft A, Perel A. Hemodynamic monitoring and management in patients undergoing high risk surgery: a survey among North American and European anesthesiologists. *Crit Care.* 2011;15:R197.
2. Feissel M, Michard F, Mangin I, Ruyer O, Faller JP, Teboul JL. Respiratory changes in aortic blood velocity as an indicator of fluid responsiveness in ventilated patients with septic shock. *Chest.* 2001;119:867-873.
3. National Heart, Lung, and Blood Institute Acute Respiratory Distress Syndrome (ARDS) Clinical Trials Network, Wiedemann HP, Wheeler AP, Bernard GR, et al. Comparison of two fluid-management strategies in acute lung injury. *N Engl J Med.* 2006;354:2564-2575.

**6.** Correct Answer: B. An increase of 15% in her pulse pressure on performing a passive leg raising test.

*Rationale:* Many of the dynamic indices of fluid responsiveness require stable ventilation with large tidal volumes (>8 mL/kg) to induce a sufficient perturbation in venous return that can reliably modify cardiac output. Similarly, most tests require the patient to be in a sinus rhythm. An important exception is the passive leg raising test, which has been shown to accurately predict fluid responsiveness in a broad range of patient conditions, including assisted or spontaneous ventilation, reduced lung compliance, and arrhythmias.

Ideally, the passive leg raise maneuver should be coupled with a measure of cardiac output or its surrogate (such as the VTI or aortic maximum velocity). If the expertise to measure VTI is unavailable, the pulse pressure variation (>12%) is an acceptable alternative. It is important to keep in mind that while changes in pulse pressure induced by passive leg raising are relatively specific, they are not very sensitive, which is why a metric of cardiac output is preferable.

Both IVC diameter variation (Option A) and pulse pressure changes with respiration (Option C) are not well-validated in spontaneously breathing patients and AF, although at least one study suggests that IVC diameter variation may remain valid in patients with dysrhythmias. While IVC collapse of >40-50% in spontaneously breathing patients is a specific predictor of fluid responsiveness, IVC collapsibility has poor sensitivity in this population, limiting its overall value. In any case, the IVC variation in this example is only 25%. As discussed earlier, CVP is not very useful in predicting volume responsiveness. It is also worth emphasizing that, while the respiratory variation in pulse pressure is not accurate in spontaneously breathing patients or in patients with arrhythmias, pulse pressure variation in response to passive leg raise may be. Note that, since this patient has AF, the change in pulse pressure should be averaged over a few heartbeats to improve accuracy.

**Selected References**

1. Bortolotti P, Colling D, Colas V, et al. Respiratory changes of the inferior vena cava diameter predict fluid responsiveness in spontaneously breathing patients with cardiac arrhythmias. *Ann Intensive Care.* 2018;8(1):79.
2. Monnet X, Bleibtreu A, Ferré A, et al. Passive leg raising and end-expiratory occlusion tests perform better than pulse pressure variation in patients with low respiratory system compliance. *Crit Care Med.* 2012;40:152-157.
3. Monnet X, Marik P, Teboul JL. Passive leg raising for predicting fluid responsiveness: a systematic review and meta-analysis. *Intensive Care Med.* 2016;42:1935-1947.
4. Monnet X, Rienzo M, Osman D, et al. Passive leg raising predicts fluid responsiveness in the critically ill. *Crit Care Med.* 2006;34:1402-1407.

**7.** Correct Answer: C. The IVC collapsibility index has not been validated in patients being ventilated with the tidal volumes being used in this case.

*Rationale:* The IVC collapsibility index is defined as: [(Maximum IVC diameter – Minimum IVC diameter)/Minimum IVC diameter] or [(Maximum IVC diameter – Minimum IVC diameter)/Mean IVC diameter]. Depending on which method is used, the cutoff values for predicting volume responsiveness are 18% or 12%, respectively. Importantly, both studies were among mechanically ventilated patients with tidal volumes >8 to 10 mL/kg ideal body weight. In patients being ventilated by small tidal volumes, as in this case, the sensitivity of the index is much lower. Therefore, the IVC collapsibility index cannot be used to reliably evaluate volume responsiveness in this patient and is likely to underestimate volume responsiveness. Early studies of IVC diameter variation were conducted in spontaneously breathing patients with the purpose of estimating CVP and are the source of the American Society of Echocardiography's guidelines for estimating CVP. However, in sedated ventilated patients with large tidal volumes and a lack of spontaneous breathing, the IVC index is a reasonable predictor of fluid responsiveness. There is no convincing evidence that colloid-based resuscitation is superior to crystalloid-based resuscitation in ARDS.

Selected References

1. Barbier C, Loubières Y, Schmit C, et al. Respiratory changes in inferior vena cava diameter are helpful in predicting fluid responsiveness in ventilated patients. *Intensive Care Med.* 2004;30:1740-1746.
2. Feissel M, Michard F, Faller JP, Teboul JL. The respiratory variation in inferior vena cava diameter as a guide to fluid therapy. *Intensive Care Med.* 2004;30(9):1834-1837.

**8.** Correct Answer: B. She is likely to be volume responsive, but should not get rapid volume resuscitation.

*Rationale:* This patient has a mechanism for intra-abdominal hemorrhage. The fluid in the lienorenal (or splenorenal) space, together with her mechanism of injury, raises the suspicion of splenic injury. Given this predisposition to hypovolemia, an IVC maximal diameter of 1.5 cm is consistent with hypovolemia, and she would likely be volume responsive. However, the principles of damage control resuscitation advise against volume resuscitation, as long as perfusion to critical organs is maintained.

Selected References

1. Cap AP, Pidcoke HF, Spinella P, et al. Damage control resuscitation. *Mil Med.* 2018;183(suppl_2):36-43.
2. Schmidt GA, Koenig S, Mayo PH. Shock: ultrasound to guide diagnosis and therapy. *Chest.* 2012;142(4):1042-1048.

**9.** Correct Answer: A. Transesophageal echocardiography (TEE) is required to assess the SVC.

*Rationale:* Like the IVC, variations in SVC diameter can also be used to predict volume responsiveness. Although the SVC can be visualized by transthoracic echocardiography (TTE), it is inconsistently visible, and TTE-based SVC evaluation has not been well studied. SVC variation using transesophageal echo (Option A) has been well-validated in mechanically ventilated patients. It is more sensitive and specific than either IVC diameter variation or pulse pressure variation (Option B). Like the IVC collapsibility index, it is not well-validated in patients on assisted breathing modes (Option C).

Selected Reference

1. Vignon P, Repessé X, Bégot E, et al. Comparison of echocardiographic indices used to predict fluid responsiveness in ventilated patients. *Am J Respir Crit Care Med.* 2017;195(8):1022-1032.

**10.** Correct Answer: C. Severely reduced LV systolic function does not, contraindicate fluid resuscitation, but the volume of fluid used should be carefully determined by repeated assessment of volume responsiveness to minimize the risk of complications.

*Rationale*: This patient presents with signs and symptoms consistent with the current definition of sepsis, but also has a documented history of heart failure with a reduced EF. POCUS examination shows severely decreased LVEF in apical three-chamber and apical two-chamber views (▶ **Videos 49.5** and **49.6**).

However, poor LV systolic function or high filling pressures (central venous or pulmonary capillary wedge) do not preclude fluid administration (Option A). Nonetheless, the tolerance of patients with poor LV function for large volumes of fluid may be limited. The best response would be to administer relatively small fluid boluses (250-500 mL) and reassess for evidence of fluid responsiveness (Option C). The videos show severely reduced LV systolic function, so Option B is incorrect. There is not enough data to determine whether this patient will need an inotrope such as dobutamine, certainly not as the next step in management (Option D).

### Selected References

1. Singer M, Deutschman CS, Seymour CW, et al. The third international consensus definitions for sepsis and septic shock (sepsis 3). *JAMA*. 2016;315(8):801-810.
2. Vincent JL, Weil MH. Fluid challenge revisited. *Crit Care Med*. 2006;34(5):1333-1337.

**11.** Correct Answer: D. Combining EEOT with an end-inspiratory occlusion test (EIOT) can improve the sensitivity of the technique when using echocardiography.

*Rationale:* The EEOT is based on the principle that a sustained (>15 seconds) interruption in positive pressure ventilation can increase venous return and consequently increase cardiac output in volume-responsive patients. Conversely, in volume-replete patients, there is a minimal difference in venous return with interruption of ventilation, and therefore no change in cardiac output. In practice, EEOT can be performed with a prolonged expiratory hold in sedated and paralyzed patients. The EEOT has been shown to be useful in patients with poor lung compliance, unlike pulse pressure variation (Option A). It is not a static maneuver, as it relies on altering venous return in response to intrathoracic pressure changes (Option B). Combining EEOT with EIOT allows the incorporation of the decrease in VTI with a sustained inspiratory hold. EIOT is maintained for 15 seconds (as with EEOT), with 1 minute between measurements. If the total change in VTI (increase with EEOT + decrease with EIOT) is >13%, the patient is likely to be fluid responsive (see **Figure 49.8**). While the test can be carried out in patients who have some spontaneous respiratory activity, the patient should be able to tolerate a 15-second breath-hold without taking a spontaneous breath. In practice, this limits its use in spontaneously breathing patients.

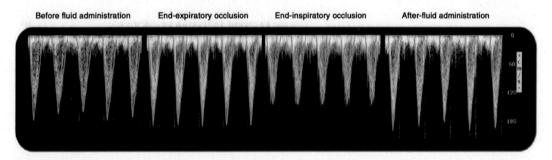

**Figure 49.8** Change in velocity-time integral (VTI) at baseline, during an end-expiratory hold, and after end-inspiratory occlusion.

### Selected References

1. Jozwiak M, Depret F, Teboul JL, et al. Predicting fluid responsiveness in critically ill patients by using combined end-expiratory and end-inspiratory occlusions with echocardiography. *Crit Care Med*. 2017;45:e1131-e1138.
2. Monnet X, Osman D, Ridel C, Lamia B, Richard C, Teboul JL. Predicting volume responsiveness by using the end-expiratory occlusion in mechanically ventilated intensive care unit patients. *Crit Care Med*. 2009;37:951-956.

**12.** Correct Answer: C. The VTI at the LVOT increases by 20% with a passive leg raise.

*Rationale:* The passive leg raise test has proven to be useful in identifying fluid responsiveness in patients under a diverse set of conditions. To be most effective, the passive leg raise should be coupled with measurement of cardiac output. One of the ways to do this is to acquire an LVOT VTI by echocardiography before and after the maneuver. It should be noted that although this is a well-validated method, it requires advanced echocardiographic skills. While the IVC distensibility index is approximately 33% for this patient, the IVC index has not been validated in patients on assisted (but not passive) ventilation. Similarly, changes in LVOT maximal velocity have not been shown to be predictive in patients on assisted ventilation. The EF can appear normal in patients with severe diastolic dysfunction and low stroke volume, as well as with severe valvular regurgitant lesions, and adds little value in predicting fluid responsiveness.

### Selected Reference
1. Brun C, Zieleskiewicz L, Textoris J, et al. Prediction of fluid responsiveness in severe preeclamptic patients with oliguria. *Intensive Care Med.* 2013;39(4):593-600.

**13.** Correct Answer: B. The LSC in the VTI that can be reliably measured by a single operator is about 11%.

*Rationale:* For most dynamic measures of fluid responsiveness, measuring cardiac output or its surrogates (such as VTI) is more reliable than measuring the pulse pressure variation. Since the echocardiographic assessments of VTI are commonly used to assess fluid responsiveness, it is important to assess the accuracy, precision, and the LSC that can be reliably detected. There is a paucity of studies that address this question; however, recent work by Jozwiak, et al. has provided some guidance. The authors found that sequential measurements of VTI were able to detect a smaller change in the VTI when the examinations were performed by the same operator than when different operators performed the examinations (Option A is incorrect). The median LSC that can be detected by a single examiner was found to be 11% (Option B is correct). Interestingly, the LSC was similar for both spontaneously breathing and mechanically ventilated patients (Option C is incorrect). Finally, given that the LSC in sequential VTI measurements is around 11%, smaller changes are unlikely to be reliably detected by echocardiography (Option D is incorrect).

### Selected References
1. Jozwiak M, Mercado P, Teboul JL, et al. What is the lowest change in cardiac output that transthoracic echocardiography can detect? *Crit Care.* 2019;23(1):116.
2. Monnet X, Marik P, Teboul JL. Passive leg raising for predicting fluid responsiveness: a systematic review and meta-analysis. *Intensive Care Med.* 2016;42(12):1935-1947.

**14.** Correct Answer: D. The portal vein is typically nonpulsatile—a PVPI >50% is a useful indicator of systemic congestion and RV dysfunction.

*Rationale:* Systemic congestion can have detrimental effects on organ function, inducing acute kidney injury and congestive hepatopathy. In ventilated patients, the value of IVC measurements in inferring CVP measurements can be poor (Option A is incorrect). Assessing portal venous pulsatility can be a valuable technique for detecting systemic venous congestion and RV dysfunction. The portal vein can be imaged with a 2.5 to 5 MHz transducer (cardiac or abdominal) at the posterior axillary line, allowing the IVC, the hepatic vein, and the portal vein to be visualized (Option B is incorrect). The walls of the portal vein are relatively more hyperechoic than the walls of the hepatic vein. Blood flow in the portal vein is normally nonpulsatile, and significant pulsatility (a PVPI >50%) indicates RV dysfunction or systemic congestion (Option D). While other causes of portal hypertension (cirrhosis, portal venous thrombosis) can also cause a high PVPI, cardiac dysfunction (e.g., tricuspid regurgitation) can also be a cause (Option C is incorrect). (See **Figure 49.9.**)

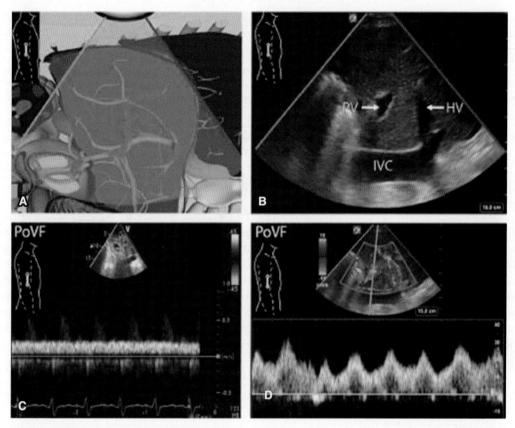

**Figure 49.9** Measurement of portal venous pulsatility. The figure shows the identification of the portal vein by ultrasound in a simulated model (A) and in an actual patient (B). A normal profile of portal vein flow is shown in (C), while an exaggerated portal venous pulsatility index consistent with systemic congestion is shown in (D).

### Selected References

1. Beaubien-Souligny W, Bouchard J, Desjardins G, et al. Extracardiac signs of fluid overload in the critically ill cardiac patient: a focused evaluation using bedside ultrasound. *Can J Cardiol.* 2017;33(1):88-100.
2. Denault AY, Azzam MA, Beaubien-Souligny W. Imaging portal venous flow to aid assessment of right ventricular dysfunction. *Can J Anaesth.* 2018;65(11):1260-1261.
3. Jue J, Chung W, Schiller NB. Does inferior vena cava size predict right atrial pressures in patients receiving mechanical ventilation? *J Am Soc Echocardiogr.* 1992;5(6):613-619.
4. Styczynski G, Milewska A, Marczewska M, et al. Echocardiographic correlates of abnormal liver tests in patients with exacerbation of chronic heart failure. *J Am Soc Echocardiogr.* 2016;29(2):132-139.

**15.** Correct Answer: C. The combination of low tidal volumes and poor lung compliance in this patient makes VTI variation with respiration relatively unpredictable.

*Rationale:* This patient has severe ARDS with low lung compliance, reflected in the need to reduce his tidal volumes to 5 mL/kg to keep plateau pressure and driving pressure within recommended limits. In such patients, airway pressure changes may not be reliably transmitted from the lung parenchyma to the extrapulmonary intrathoracic space, and therefore have unpredictable effects on preload. Because of this, the effects of changes in cardiac output, VTI, or pulse pressure variation with respiration can be unpredictable (Option C is correct). Therefore, the lack of significant VTI variation with respiration is not sufficient to define this patient as being fluid unresponsive (Option A is incorrect). It is important to recognize that the test retains its specificity—a large VTI variation would imply volume responsiveness in the setting of poorly compliant lungs/small tidal volumes. A number of dynamic indices of fluid responsiveness lose sensitivity in the setting of low-tidal-volume ventilation/poor lung compliance. Those which do not rely on changes in intrathoracic pressure, such as passive leg raise, do not. Measuring the change in VTI in response to a passive leg raise maneuver is a good technique to assess fluid responsiveness in this situation (Option B is incorrect).

### Selected References

1. Charron C, Fessenmeyer C, Cosson C, et al. The influence of tidal volume on the dynamic variables of fluid responsiveness in critically ill patients. *Anesth Analg.* 2006;102(5):1511-1517.
2. De Backer D, Fagnoul D. Intensive care ultrasound: VI. Fluid responsiveness and shock assessment. *Ann Am Thorac Soc.* 2014 11:129-136.
3. Monnet X, Marik PE, Teboul JL. Prediction of fluid responsiveness: an update. *Ann Intensive Care.* 2016;6(1):111.
4. Vignon P, Repessé X, Bégot E, et al. Comparison of echocardiographic indices used to predict fluid responsiveness in ventilated patients. *Am J Respir Crit Care Med.* 2017;195(8):1022-1032.

**16.** Correct Answer: **C. The esophageal Doppler signal detects flow in the ascending aorta and therefore reflects the total LV stroke volume.**

*Rationale:* The esophageal Doppler probe is placed transorally into the esophagus to a depth of about 35 to 40 cm, capturing the flow signal from the descending thoracic aorta (Option C is false, and therefore the correct answer). Therefore, only a part of the LV stroke volume is accessible, and manufacturers use algorithms to extrapolate that value into the cardiac output. The use of these probes in goal-directed resuscitation during major surgery has been found to reduce the incidence of postoperative complications in some studies (Option A). The stroke distance on the Doppler signal is directly proportional to the stroke volume (Option B), and changes in the morphology of the Doppler signal can be used to detect aortic regurgitation and cardiac tamponade (Option D).

### Selected References

1. Singer M. Oesophageal Doppler. *Curr Opin Crit Care.* 2009;15(3):244-248.
2. Wakeling HG, McFall MR, Jenkins CS, et al. Intraoperative oesophageal Doppler guided fluid management shortens postoperative hospital stay after major bowel surgery. *Br J Anaesth.* 2005; 95:634-642.

**17.** Correct Answer: **B. The number and severity of B-lines will decrease as fluid is removed.**

*Rationale:* There remains some controversy regarding the shape and significance of the Starling curve, as it relates to cardiac filling pressure and stroke volume. A decrease in preload will not increase stroke volume. This would involve the presence of a "descending" limb on the higher-pressure side of the Starling curve. However, many investigators have shown that at steady state, this descending limb does *not* exist. Furthermore, the presence of a descending limb would imply an unstable clinical condition, where increasing filling pressures lead to decreasing stroke volumes in a vicious cycle. Therefore, Option A is incorrect. B-lines across lung fields can be quantified by counting the number of B-lines per zone scanned and multiplying by the number of zones. Investigators have shown that the number of B-lines decreases significantly after volume removal with hemodialysis (Option B). Lung ultrasound has been shown to be more sensitive than chest X-ray in detecting EVLW, not less (Option C). While B-lines typically are associated with EVLW, "dry" B-lines may also be seen in diseases associated with pulmonary fibrosis, such as systemic sclerosis (Option D).

### Selected References

1. Elzinga G. "Starling's Law of the Heart" a historical misinterpretation. *Basic Res Cardiol.* 1989;84(1):1-4.
2. Enghard P, Rademacher S, Nee J, et al. Simplified lung ultrasound protocol shows excellent prediction of extravascular lung water in ventilated intensive care patients. *Crit Care.* 2015;19(1):36.
3. Gargani L, Doveri M, D'Errico L, et al. Ultrasound lung comets in systemic sclerosis: a chest sonography hallmark of pulmonary interstitial fibrosis. *Rheumatology.* 2009;48:1382-1387.
4. Katz AM. The descending limb of the starling curve and the failing heart. *Circulation.* 1965;32:871-875.
5. Noble VE, Murray AF, Capp R, Sylvia-Reardon MH, Steele DJR, Liteplo A. Ultrasound assessment for extravascular lung water in patients undergoing hemodialysis. Time course for resolution. *Chest.* 2009;135:1433-1439.

**18.** Correct Answer: B. A decrease in LV afterload

*Rationale:* The use of PEEP supports a failing left ventricle by decreasing transmural wall stress. Since PEEP increases pleural pressure, transmural pressure for a given systolic pressure is reduced by the Laplace relationship (wall stress = $PR/2h$, where $P$ = transmural pressure, $R$ = ventricular radius, and $h$ = wall thickness). It is also thought that by creating a pressure gradient between the intrathoracic and extrathoracic aorta, systemic afterload is reduced by the increase in intrathoracic pressure. Conversely, PEEP can cause a decrease in RV preload and thus reduce cardiac output. However, patients in decompensated heart failure are typically *hyper*volemic, and PEEP does not have much of a deleterious effect on RV preload in those patients (Option A). The aim of noninvasive ventilation and PEEP in acute decompensated heart failure is primarily to improve oxygenation (alveolar recruitment) and augment LV function (decrease afterload). Defining optimal PEEP in patients with heart failure can be challenging. However, studies dating back to the 1970's suggest that the PEEP associated with the best lung compliance is also the least likely to cause impaired hemodynamics or hypotension. There is no reason to limit PEEP to a specific value (such as 10 cm $H_2O$), particularly in obese patients, such as in this case (Option C).

Selected References
1. Alviar CL, Miller PE, McAreavey D, et al. Positive pressure ventilation in the cardiac intensive care unit. *J Am Coll Cardiol.* 2018;72(13):1532-1553.
2. Suter PM, Fairley B, Isenberg MD. Optimum end-expiratory airway pressure in patients with acute pulmonary failure. *N Engl J Med.* 1975;292:284-289.

**19.** Correct Answer: A. No change in the current management.

*Rationale:* Not all patients who are fluid responsive need fluid. As long as the patient appears to be well-perfused, there is no need to increase cardiac output by volume resuscitation (Option A). A 20% change in aortic velocity is a good indicator of volume responsiveness in this paralyzed, mechanically ventilated patient, and if she becomes hypotensive or hypoperfused (e.g., decreasing urine output, increasing acidemia or lactate) volume administration would be indicated (Option B), but that is not the case here. Administration of blood products should be guided by multiple considerations, including volume of blood lost, ongoing hemorrhage, and the patient's ability to tolerate acute anemia (Option C). Initiation of dobutamine is also not indicated, as there is no evidence of hypoperfusion. Moreover, dobutamine may lower her BP without increasing her cardiac output (due to the limited flow rate through her aortic valve), which could lead to a vicious cycle of worsening LV systolic function. Therefore, Option D is also incorrect.

Selected Reference
1. Vignon P, Repessé X, Bégot E, et al. Comparison of echocardiographic indices used to predict fluid responsiveness in ventilated patients. *Am J Respir Crit Care Med.* 2017;195:1022-1032.

**20.** Correct Answer: B. This method of assessment is most accurate when the patient is passively ventilated with tidal volumes >8 mL/kg.

*Rationale:* For brachial artery Doppler measurements to be most accurate as a marker of volume responsiveness, the patient should be in sinus rhythm and not have spontaneous respiratory effort (Option B). Unlike echocardiographic measurements, it is permissible to use the angle correction feature of the ultrasound machines up to incident angles of 60°, as these values are normalized to flow at the same angle, eliminating the requirement for flow to be in-line with the Doppler beam. In echo measurements, since absolute values are important, the use of angle correction is discouraged (Option A). Brachial artery peak velocity variation is calculated as follows:

$$\Delta V = 100 \times \frac{\text{Peak velocity max} - \text{Peak velocity min}}{\left[\dfrac{\text{Peak velocity max} + \text{Peak velocity min}}{2}\right]}.$$

A value >10% has been suggested to correlate with volume responsiveness, though further validation is needed. Like with pulse pressure variation, the presence of AF renders brachial arterial velocities difficult to interpret (Option C). Continuous-wave Doppler measures the highest velocity of flow in the path of the ultrasound wave, while pulsed-wave Doppler measures the velocity at a user-defined area. Since brachial artery velocity signals depend on measuring the velocity of flow in a very specific region, continuous-wave Doppler is not useful here (Option D).

### Selected Reference

1. Monge Garcia MI, Gil Cano A, Diaz Monrove JC. Brachial artery peak velocity variation to predict fluid responsiveness in mechanically ventilated patients. *Crit Care.* 2009;13:R142.

---

**21.** Correct Answer: D. These indices have been shown to remain accurate even in the presence of carotid disease.

*Rationale:* Measurements of flow through the carotid arteries are easy to obtain with POCUS without extensive training, and have been studied for their utility in determining volume responsiveness. Two parameters that have been studied specifically include CBF and CFT. CBF is defined as the VTI of flow in the carotid arteries multiplied by the carotid artery area. CFT is defined as the systolic flow time divided by the square root of the total cycle time, where the systolic flow time is the time from the systolic upstroke to the start of the dicrotic notch. Firm conclusions regarding the value of carotid ultrasonography in assessing volume responsiveness are not appropriate at this time, but some investigators have suggested that a change in CFT with passive leg raise can predict volume responsiveness. CFT seems to be more closely correlated to volume status (total intravascular volume) than CBF, which is better correlated with cardiac output. Importantly, the utility of these indices in the presence of carotid artery disease has not been established. (See also **Figure 49.10**.)

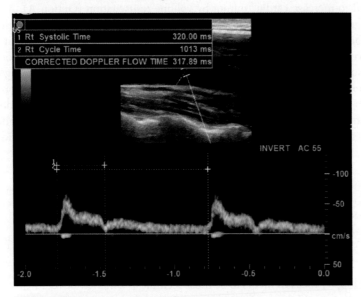

**Figure 49.10** Assessment of carotid flow time.

### Selected References

1. Barjaktarevic I, Toppen WE, Hu S, et al. Ultrasound assessment of the change in carotid corrected flow time in fluid responsiveness in undifferentiated shock. *Crit Care Med.* 2018;46(11):e1040-e1046.
2. Blehar DJ, Glazier S, Gaspari RJ. Correlation of corrected flow time in the carotid artery with changes in intravascular volume status. *J Crit Care.* 2014;29(4):486-488.
3. Ma IWY, Caplin JD, Azad A, et al. Correlation of carotid blood flow and corrected carotid flow time with invasive cardiac output measurements. *Crit Ultrasound J.* 2017;9(1):10.
4. Marik PE, Levitov A, Young A, Andrews L. The use of bioreactance and carotid Doppler to determine volume responsiveness and blood flow redistribution following passive leg raising in hemodynamically unstable patients. *Chest.* 2013;143:364-370.

**22.** Correct Answer: D. Vasopressor therapy would be preferred over additional fluid boluses.

*Rationale:* This patient presents with septic shock and has received initial volume resuscitation of 30 mL/kg of crystalloid. The appearance of new B-lines suggests increasing EVLW, either cardiogenic or noncardiogenic. The normal EF does not rule out a cardiogenic cause of pulmonary edema. Heart failure with preserved ejection fraction (HFpEF), dynamic LVOT obstruction, or mitral stenosis could all produce high left atrial pressures leading to cardiogenic pulmonary edema (Option A). Although patients with noncardiogenic pulmonary edema may be volume responsive, the appearance of new B-lines should prompt an analysis of the risks and benefits of further fluid administration, rather than continuing empiric administration. The fluid administration limited by lung sonography (FALLS) protocol suggests limiting volume resuscitation with the appearance of B-lines, although this has not been prospectively validated. Although some studies have suggested that the presence of anterior B-lines is strongly correlated with a PCWP >18 mm Hg, more recent data do not support that interpretation. The presence of B-lines suggests increased EVLW, without discriminating between cardiogenic or noncardiogenic causes (Option C). Given the information from cardiac and lung ultrasound examination, starting a pressor like norepinephrine is the preferred course. Diuresis in the presence of shock and a need for vasopressors may cause harm (Option B), unless there is clear evidence of hypervolemia. There is some evidence that the pattern of B-lines may help differentiate cardiac from noncardiac pulmonary edema (the presence of subpleural consolidations and a coarse, irregular pleural line favoring noncardiogenic pulmonary edema), but these findings require more validation before they are adopted into routine clinical practice.

### Selected References

1. Copetti R, Soldati G, Copetti P. Chest sonography: a useful tool to differentiate acute cardiogenic pulmonary edema from acute respiratory distress syndrome. *Cardiovasc Ultrasound.* 2008;6:16.
2. Lichtenstein D, Karakitsos D. Integrating lung ultrasound in the hemodynamic evaluation of acute circulatory failure (the fluid administration limited by lung sonography protocol). *J Crit Care.* 2012;27:533.e11-e19.

**23.** Correct Answer: B. She has cardiogenic pulmonary edema due to LV diastolic dysfunction.

*Rationale:* A patient with a normal or hyperdynamic left ventricle under conditions of sympathetic stimulation and relative hypovolemia (such as seen in septic shock) may induce dynamic LVOT obstruction. Identification of dynamic LVOT obstruction is important because the management of this condition (volume expansion and the use of pure vasopressors) is different than the management described. However, the lack of evidence of systolic anterior motion on the M-mode images at the mitral valve and the lack of a "dagger-shaped" LVOT VTI argue against this cause (Option A). This patient has severe diastolic dysfunction, suggested by E/e' >15 (it is 18 here). Lanspa, et al. have shown that using an E/e' >14 in critically ill patients is a good indicator of diastolic dysfunction (Option B). The low mean gradient across the mitral valve argues against the presence of significant mitral stenosis (Option C). The high E/e' ratio is consistent with a high left atrial pressure, making it likely that the patient's pulmonary edema is at least partially cardiogenic, therefore Option D is incorrect.

### Selected References

1. Lanspa MJ, Gutsche AR, Wilson EL, et al. Application of a simplified definition of diastolic function in severe sepsis and septic shock. *Crit Care.* 2016;20:243.
2. Ritzema JL, Richards AM, Crozier IG, et al. Serial Doppler echocardiography and tissue Doppler imaging in the detection of elevated directly measured left atrial pressure in ambulant subjects with chronic heart failure. *JACC Cardiovasc Imaging.* 2011;4:927-934.

**24.** Correct Answer: C. Repeat a bolus of lactated Ringer's solution

*Rationale:* This patient presents with mixed septic and cardiogenic shock. His echo is consistent with systolic and diastolic dysfunction, but he remains well-oxygenated on room air and has a bilateral "A"-line profile on lung ultrasound, arguing against significant pulmonary edema. Administering another crystalloid bolus is therefore the next best step (Option C). Although he has a normal pH and $PaO_2$, he is maintaining a normal pH by significant hyperventilation (his $PaCO_2$ is only 18 mm Hg) to compensate for his metabolic acidosis. As his respiratory effort diminishes (he is becoming drowsier), he will be unable to compensate for his acidosis and risks becoming severely acidemic. The presence of impaired ventricular function with dilated atria is a clue to diastolic dysfunction, supported by his E/e' ratio of 20 (see **Question 23**). Attempting to improve diastolic filling by slowing his HR with esmolol may prove counterproductive, as patients with severe diastolic dysfunction and poor contractility are often HR-dependent (Option A). Using phenylephrine as a primary pressor in a patient with impaired contractility may maintain arterial pressures initially, but at the expense of arterial flow, leading to worsening hypoperfusion. It is safer to use agents that increase both inotropy and vascular tone such as norepinephrine or epinephrine, even in patients with tachycardia (Option B). Norepinephrine is also the first-line vasoactive medication recommended by the surviving sepsis campaign guidelines. Mechanical circulatory support (e.g., venoarterial extracorporeal membrane oxygenation [VA-ECMO]) for severe septic shock in adults is controversial, with most centers reporting poor outcomes. While not contraindicated, it is not the immediate next step in management (Option D).

### Selected References

1. Rhodes A, Evans LE, Alhazzani W, et al. Surviving sepsis campaign: international guidelines for the management of sepsis and septic shock: 2016. *Crit Care Med.* 2017;45:486-552.
2. Ro SK, Kim WK, Lim JY, Yoo JS, Hong SB, Kim JB. Extracorporeal life support for adults with refractory septic shock. *J Thorac Cardiovasc Surg* 2018;156:1104-1109.e1.
3. Tsang TS, Barnes ME, Gersh BJ, Bailey KR, Seward JB. Left atrial volume as a morphophysiologic expression of left ventricular diastolic dysfunction and relation to cardiovascular risk burden. *Am J Cardiol.* 2002;90:1284-1289.

**25.** Correct Answer: B. Start an inopressor (e.g., epinephrine) to maintain systemic BP and support RV inotropy

*Rationale:* Acute RV failure is a hemodynamic emergency. Management involves volume status optimization, maintenance of systemic arterial pressure, minimizing pulmonary vascular resistance, and supporting RV inotropy. Although traditional teaching emphasizes volume administration as part of the initial management of patients with RV failure, the presence of diastolic flattening of the interventricular septum, together with a dilated, nonvariable IVC, suggests high venous pressures and RV overload. Further fluid administration may not be helpful and could possibly impair RV function even more (Option A). The concept that most patients with acute RV failure respond to volume loading is not accurate, and the ultrasound findings shown here argue against further volume loading. The presentation here is most consistent with RV volume overload, compounded by negative inotropy and negative chronotropy caused by the diltiazem. Starting an inopressor such as epinephrine would help provide chronotropy and inotropy to support the right ventricle, as well as increased systemic pressure. RV function can be improved by increasing *systemic* arterial pressure, which improves RV function by multiple mechanisms: improving blood flow to the right coronary artery, keeping the interventricular septum (a major contributor to RV function) in a more physiologic position, and improving LV function, allowing ventricular interdependence to improve RV function (Option B). While pure inotropes (such as dobutamine or milrinone) can be used in selected cases of acute RV dysfunction, the presence of hypotension in this case argues against their use, as they may exacerbate hypotension. Although the use of a pulmonary artery catheter can help in the management of patients with RV failure, this patient is unstable, and the echocardiographic findings can guide initial management (Option C), particularly if the patient is a candidate for mechanical circulatory support. Similarly, using an inhaled pulmonary vasodilator such as nitric oxide or epoprostenol (if available) may improve RV function by decreasing RV afterload, but it is not the most appropriate next step and may worsen pulmonary function in some cases (e.g., pulmonary venous hypertension) (Option D).

### Selected References

1. Harjola VP, Mebazaa A, Čelutkienė J, et al. Contemporary management of acute right ventricular failure: a statement from the Heart Failure Association and the Working Group on Pulmonary Circulation and Right Ventricular Function of the European Society of Cardiology. *Eur J Heart Fail* 2016;18(3):226-241.
2. Hrymak C, Strumpher J, Jacobsohn E. Acute right ventricle failure in the intensive care unit: assessment and management. *Can J Cardiol.* 2017;33:61-71.
3. Konstam MA, Kiernan MS, Bernstein D, et al. Evaluation and management of right-sided heart failure: a scientific statement from the American Heart Association. *Circulation.* 2018;137(20):e578-e622.
4. Vieillard-Baron A, Naeije R, Haddad F, et al. Diagnostic workup, etiologies and management of acute right ventricle failure: A state-of-the-art paper. *Intensive Care Med.* 2018;44(6):774-790.

**26.** Correct Answer: C. Decrease the speed of the LVAD and start an epinephrine infusion

*Rationale:* Using echocardiography as an adjunct to the physical examination speeds the diagnosis of issues like suboptimal LVAD speed settings and can also help to correct the problem expeditiously. In this case, the LVAD speed appears to have been set too high, causing too much decompression of the left ventricle and a shift of the interventricular septum to the left, causing RV dilation, worsening tricuspid regurgitation, and RV function. Decreasing the LVAD speed and supporting systemic BP and RV inotropy with epinephrine would be the appropriate management (Option C). Hypovolemia is a common cause of hypotension in patients with LVADs—however, it is essential to exonerate less common, but potentially more serious causes of hypotension (e.g., pericardial tamponade and RV dysfunction). The passive leg raise test has not been validated in patients with LVADs (Option B). Given that the primary problem is acute RV dysfunction, a volume bolus will only serve to overload the RV further, and not correct the underlying problem (Option A). Inappropriately high LVAD speeds have induced an acute deterioration of RV function, but this is promptly correctable with adjustments to LVAD speed—there is no indication at this point to place an RV assist device (Option D). (See also ▶ **Video 49.15.**)

Selected Reference

1. Slaughter MS, Pagani FD, Rogers JG, et al. Clinical management of continuous-flow left ventricular assist devices in advanced heart failure. *J Heart Lung Transplant* 2010;29(4 suppl):S1-S39.

**27.** Correct Answer: C. The resident has in fact imaged the abdominal aorta instead of the IVC because the IVC diameter is extremely low in this hypotensive and hypovolemic patient.

*Rationale:* This patient has fever, poor oral intake, gastrointestinal (GI) volume losses for at least 24 hours, and presents with significant hypotension, making it very likely that she is hypovolemic from a combination of high insensible fluid loss, poor oral intake, and GI losses. ▶ **Video 49.14** captures the abdominal aorta, not her IVC. Because of the very narrow caliber of her IVC, the resident has missed the IVC and focused on the abdominal aorta (see the two clips below—they are from the same patient). To avoid making such errors, it is advisable to include some of the following practices while scanning patients' IVCs: (1) ensure that the IVC can be seen draining into the right atrium, and that the hepatic vein drains into the IVC; (2) always attempt to identify both the IVC and the aorta—in the typical subcostal approach to the IVC, the aorta is found by angling the probe so that the ultrasound beam scans to the left of the patient's vertebral column while the IVC is to the right of the vertebral column; and (3) rotate the probe clockwise by approximately 90° to see both the aorta and the IVC in short axes simultaneously. These practices add minimal time to the POCUS examination, but helps reduce the chances of errors in identifying the IVC. (See also ▶ **Video 49.16.**)

**28.** Correct Answer: D. IVC diameter

*Rationale:* The best method to monitor the change in cardiac output in response to a passive leg raise is by a direct measure of cardiac output. In the absence of a measure of cardiac output, arterial pulse pressure variation has been used, but these measures generally result in lower sensitivity and specificity compared to cardiac output-based methods. Use of IVC diameter measurements has not been studied in this context—a change in IVC diameter with leg raising may indicate a change in loading conditions, but not necessarily changes in cardiac output (Option D). The IVC distensibility index (as measured by Barbier, et al.) has been found to correlate positively with a change in cardiac output after fluid infusion, but this was reported in the context of change in IVC diameter with passive mechanical ventilation, not passive leg raise.

Selected References

1. Barbier C, Loubières Y, Schmit C, et al. Respiratory changes in inferior vena cava diameter are helpful in predicting fluid responsiveness in ventilated septic patients. *Intensive Care Med.* 2004;30:1740-1746.
2. Monnet X, Bataille A, Magalhaes E, et al. End-tidal carbon dioxide is better than arterial pressure for predicting volume responsiveness by the passive leg raising test. *Intensive Care Med.* 2013;39:93-100.
3. Monnet X, Rienzo M, Osman D, et al. Passive leg raising predicts fluid responsiveness in the critically ill. *Crit Care Med.* 2006;34:1402-1407.

**29.** Correct Answer: C. The patient in Figure 49.5C will likely increase his cardiac output with a fluid bolus.

*Rationale:* Examining the IVC in spontaneously breathing patients does provide useful clinical information that should be interpreted within the appropriate clinical context, and it is not true that IVC imaging is only of value in sedated and paralyzed patients (Option D is incorrect). A dilated, unvarying IVC may be seen in RV failure—however, it may be seen in other conditions as well (significant volume overload, pericardial tamponade, etc.), and should not be used to infer the state of RV function in isolation (Option A is incorrect). The patient in Figure 49.5B has an IVC collapsibility index of ~17% based on the data provided, while the patient in Figure 49.5C has an IVC collapsibility index of almost 90%. Most studies suggest that IVC collapsibility indices of 40% to 50% or greater are likely to respond to fluid boluses by increasing cardiac output. However, the studies also agree on the relatively poor sensitivity of the IVC measurements—in other words, it is difficult to exclude fluid responsiveness in patients with an IVC collapsibility index of <40%. Thus, while the patient in Figure 49.5B is unlikely to be a fluid responder, the possibility cannot be excluded (Option B is incorrect). In this situation (and as a general rule), it is helpful to use more than one metric to make predictions of fluid responsiveness.

Selected References
1. Airapetian N, Maizel J, Alyamani O, et al. Does inferior vena cava respiratory variability predict fluid responsiveness in spontaneously breathing patients? *Crit Care.* 2015;19:400.
2. Muller L, Bobbia X, Toumi M, et al.; AzuRea group. Respiratory variations of inferior vena cava diameter to predict fluid responsiveness in spontaneously breathing patients with acute circulatory failure: need for a cautious use. *Crit Care.* 2012;16(5):R188.
3. Preau S, Bortolotti P, Colling D, et al. Diagnostic accuracy of the inferior vena cava collapsibility to predict fluid responsiveness in spontaneously breathing patients with sepsis and acute circulatory failure. *Crit Care Med.* 2017;45(3):e290-e297.

**30.** Correct Answer: A. The IVC and abdominal aorta can be imaged from the right flank.

*Rationale:* The IVC and the abdominal aorta can be visualized from the right flank in patients in whom the subcostal view is not accessible. The probe is placed with its long axis along the midaxillary line, with the marker pointing cephalad, by convention. Using the liver as an acoustic window, the hepatorenal space (Morison's pouch) can be identified as an ultrasonic landmark, as with a Focused Assessment Sonography in Trauma (FAST) examination. Once identified, the probe is angled so that the ultrasound beam is directed ventrally until the IVC can be visualized traveling through the liver across the diaphragm, entering the right atrium. The abdominal aorta is seen deep to the IVC (to the patient's left). ▶ **Videos 49.17** and **49.18** demonstrate this view. In ▶ **Video 49.17**, the IVC is collapsed, while in the ▶ **Video 49.18**, it is seen more easily. While this view can be very useful in qualitatively evaluating the IVC and its variations with respiration, the measurements obtained from this approach do not necessarily agree with measurements from the standard subcostal approach and have not been rigorously validated.

Selected Reference
1. Finnerty NM, Panchal AR, Boulger C, et al. Inferior vena cava measurement with ultrasound: what is the best view and best mode? *West J Emerg Med.* 2017;18(3):496-501.

# 50 | CLINICAL APPLICATIONS OF DIASTOLOGY

Gregory Mints

1. In **Figure 50.1**, what is being measured in this zoomed-in apical four-chamber view with a focus on the mitral valve (MV) from a patient with normal left ventricular (LV) systolic function?

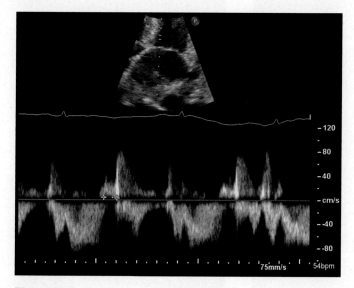

**Figure 50.1**

A. E-wave velocity
B. E-wave deceleration time (E-DT)
C. Isovolumic relaxation time (IVRT)
D. A-wave duration ($A_{dur}$)

2. A 49-year-old man with known nonischemic dilated cardiomyopathy presents with shortness of breath (SOB). Cardiac ultrasound is performed (**Figure 50.2** and ▶ **Video 50.1**).

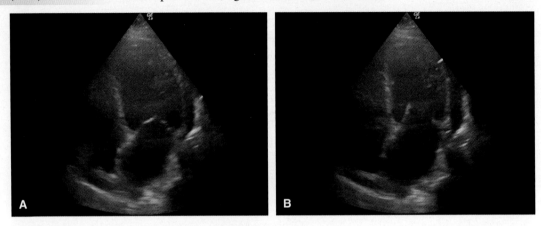

**Figure 50.2** A. End-diastole. B. End-systole.

Based on **Figure 50.3**, which of the following mitral inflow patterns corresponds to the best state this patient may hope to attain, that is, the state of the lowest left atrial (LA) pressure (LAP)? (*In answering this question please disregard the variable heart in the shown Doppler tracings.*)

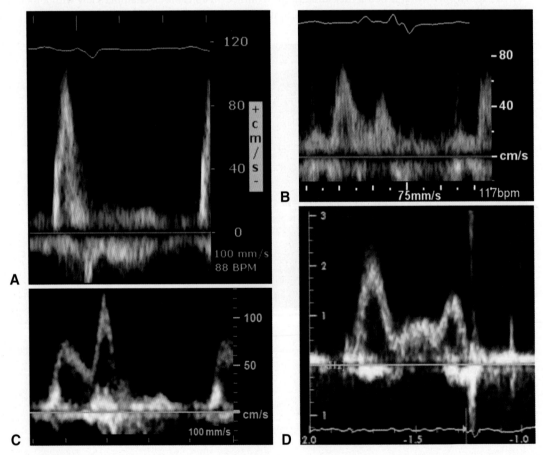

**Figure 50.3**

A. Figure 50.3A
B. Figure 50.3B
C. Figure 50.3C
D. Figure 50.3D

3. For the following five patients, based on the information provided, determine whether LA pressure is likely to be normal or elevated.

1. A 20-year-old athlete with E/A = 3 and lateral e' of 14 cm/s
2. A deconditioned 60-year-old man with normal systolic function and E/A = 0.3
3. A 50-year-old obese woman with long-standing arterial hypertension (HTN), left ventricular hypertrophy (LVH), but normal LV systolic function and E/A = 3
4. A 70-year-old man with normal LV systolic function, E/A = 1.4, and lateral e' of 7 cm/s
5. A 45-year-old woman with type 2 diabetes mellitus (DM2), HTN, normal LV systolic function, E/A = 1.6, and medial e' of 10 cm/s

Choose the option which annotates each patient with their expected LA pressure.

A. 1—normal, 2—elevated, 3—normal, 4—normal, 5—elevated
B. 1—normal, 2—normal, 3—elevated, 4—elevated, 5—normal
C. 1—normal, 2—elevated, 3—elevated, 4—elevated, 5—normal
D. 1—normal, 2—normal, 3—elevated, 4—normal, 5—normal

4. Which of the following is true about normal ranges for diastolic function parameters as given in the American Society of Echocardiography (ASE) guidelines?

A. The norms are age specific.
B. The norms listed are for healthy young adults. When interpreting study results, it is important to remember that abnormal values may just be older age-related and not related to any pathology.
C. The norms listed are for a healthy elderly population. When interpreting study results, it is important to remember that "supra-normal" values may be younger age-related and not related to any pathology.
D. There are no norms listed. All values are interpretable only in dynamics within each individual.

5. Transition between which two stages of diastolic dysfunction (**Figure 50.4**) corresponds to the transition from the left ventricle being filled by "pull," that is, by the suctioning effect of the relaxing left ventricle, to being filled by "push," that is, filling by increase in the LA pressure?

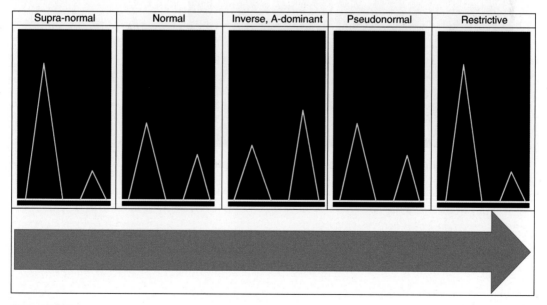

**Figure 50.4**

A. Between supra-normal and normal
B. Between normal and inverse, A-dominant (grade I)
C. Between inverse, A-dominant (grade I), and pseudonormal (grade II)
D. Between pseudonormal (grade II) and restrictive (grade III)

6. A 60-year-old woman with a history of left breast cancer for which she received radiation therapy (XRT) to the left chest wall and chemotherapy (which included an anthracycline) presents with subacute dyspnea on exertion which now occurs with minimal activity. Lung examination is significant for bibasilar crackles. Jugular venous pressure (JVP) is elevated to the angle of the jaw and there is significant lower extremity edema to the knees bilaterally. There are no murmurs appreciated.

Apical four-chamber view (**Figure 50.5** and ▶ **Video 50.2**), mitral inflow Doppler tracings (**Figure 50.6**), and tissue Doppler of the mitral annulus (**Figure 50.7**) are obtained.

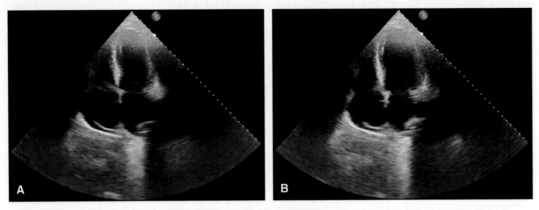

**Figure 50.5** Apical four-chamber view. A. End-systole. B. End-diastole.

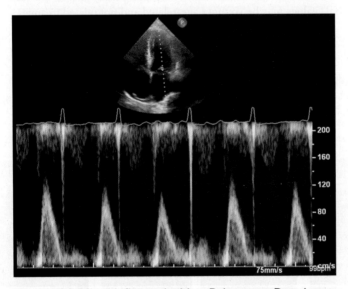

**Figure 50.6** Mitral inflow velocities. Pulse-wave Doppler.

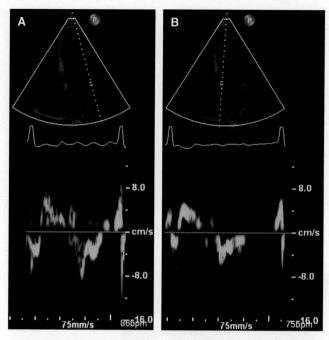

**Figure 50.7** Mitral annular tissue Doppler.

Which of the following is the most likely diagnosis?
A. Constrictive pericarditis
B. Restrictive filling pattern
C. Diastolic heart failure with grade III diastolic dysfunction
D. None of the above

7. A 63-year-old man with known ischemic cardiomyopathy and chronic obstructive pulmonary disease (COPD) as well as interstitial fibrosis is admitted for SOB 3 days after Thanksgiving. Patient's pulmonary fibrosis has been stable for many years. His COPD has manifested mostly as chronic bronchitis with acute exacerbations three to four times per year. Patient is not receiving home oxygen therapy. At baseline he can walk four city blocks before he needs to rest because of dyspnea.

Patient reports being compliant with his medication regimen but admits to violating his dietary restrictions during the Thanksgiving festivities. On presentation to the Emergency Department he was tachypneic with respiratory rate (RR) of 26 breaths/min. His arterial BP was 110/50 mm Hg, and arterial oxygen saturation by pulse oximeter was 93% while breathing room air. His extremities were warm and well perfused. Lung examination was significant for bilateral crackles half the way up and mild diffuse wheezing. Lung ultrasound showed confluent B-lines bilaterally. There were no murmurs but an S3 gallop was heard at the apex with the bell of the stethoscope. JVP was elevated to the angle of the jaw. The patient received two 100 mg doses of intravenous furosemide 6 hours apart with significant improvement in his symptoms. When you meet the patient the next day, he appears more comfortable, with an RR of 16 breaths/min. He reports no SOB at rest but still reports significant dyspnea on ambulation from his room to the bathroom. On lung auscultation, there are mild diffuse wheezes with good air entry, and crackles are still present half the way up bilaterally. His JVP is normal at 7 cm $H_2O$. Laboratory studies are unremarkable, except for serum creatinine, which, while elevated on admission, has now returned to the baseline. "Dry weight" is not available.

Lung ultrasound still shows confluent B-lines bilaterally. Cardiac ultrasound shows inferior vena cava (IVC) of 1.5 cm in diameter, which collapses by 60% on inspiration. Parasternal short-axis (PSAx) view (**Figure 50.8** and ▶ **Video 50.3**) and mitral inflow pattern (**Figures 50.9** and **50.10**) are obtained.

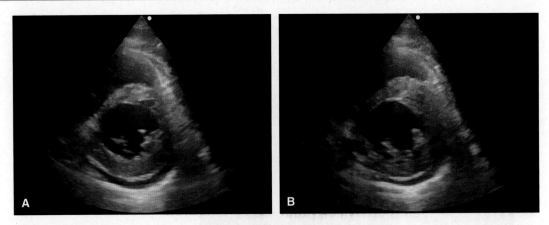

**Figure 50.8** Parasternal short-axis view. A. End-systole. B. End-diastole.

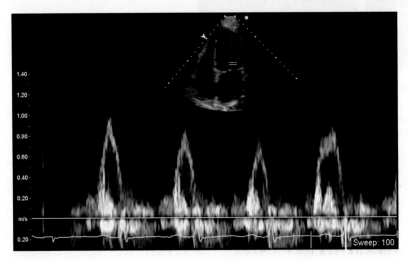

**Figure 50.9** Mitral inflow velocities. Pulse-wave Doppler.

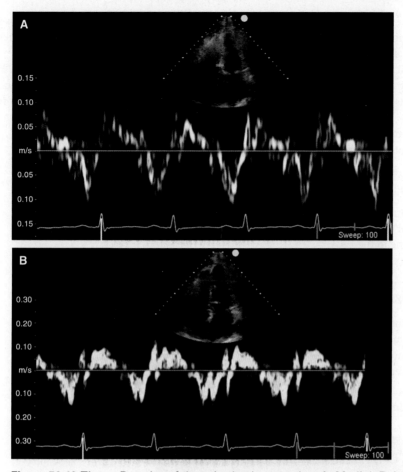

**Figure 50.10** Tissue Doppler of the mitral valve annulus. A. Medial. B. Lateral.

Based on the sonographic parameters, what is most likely to be correct about this patient's LAP and utility of further diuresis?

A. This patient is clinically euvolemic and his left filling pressures are as good as they can possibly get. He should receive only his usual maintenance diuretics.

B. This patient still has elevated left filling pressures. He may benefit from further diuresis.

C. This patient has constrictive physiology and further diuresis is contraindicated.

D. This patient is over-diuresed already and is unlikely to tolerate further diuresis.

8. The patient described in **Question 7** has now received three additional days of diuresis. He has improved significantly but is still dyspneic on walking from his room to the nurses station. Mitral inflow velocities by pulse-wave Doppler (PWD) on repeat cardiac ultrasound are shown in **Figure 50.11**.

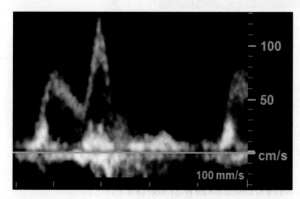

**Figure 50.11** Mitral inflow velocities by pulse-wave Doppler.

Patient's JVP is now 5 cm H$_2$O. IVC is 1 cm but collapses <50% on inspiration. Serum creatinine is still normal. Lung examination is unchanged and is still significant for diffuse mild wheezes and crackles half-way up bilaterally. Based on the sonographic parameters, what is most likely to be correct?

A. This patient is clinically euvolemic and his left filling pressures are as good as they will ever get. He should receive only his usual maintenance diuretics. Etiology of his dyspnea is likely noncardiac.

B. This patient still has elevated left filling pressures that have not been optimized. He may benefit from further diuresis.

C. This patient has constrictive physiology and further diuresis is contraindicated.

D. This patient will not tolerate further diuresis based on the low right filling pressures.

9. Where should the Doppler sampling volume be positioned while assessing mitral inflow velocities?

A. At the center of the MV opening
B. At the tips of the MV in the left ventricle
C. Under the MV plane in the LA
D. At the area of the greatest flow determined by color Doppler

10. Which of the following is most likely to result in overestimation of mitral inflow velocity?

A. Imperfect alignment of the Doppler interrogation line with the blood flow during diastole
B. Coexisting severe mitral regurgitation (MR)
C. Coexisting severe aortic stenosis (AS)
D. Coexisting aortic regurgitation (AR)

11. Spectral Doppler tracings were obtained from a patient who presented with SOB (**Figure 50.12**).

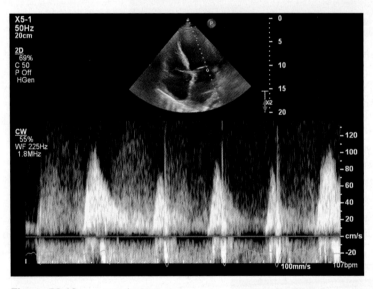

**Figure 50.12**

Assuming that the goal was to obtain mitral inflow velocity tracing, what technical errors were made in this case?

A. Continuous-wave Doppler (CWD) was used instead of PWD
B. Sample volume was positioned below the valve in the LA instead of the right atrium above the valve leaflets of the MV in the left ventricle
C. Apical four-chamber view was used instead of apical five-chamber view
D. Tissue Doppler was used instead of PWD

**12.** A 70-year-old man with moderate obesity and history of arterial HTN and benign prostatic hypertrophy presents with a urinary tract infection. He does not have any history of coronary heart disease, congestive heart failure (CHF), or any pulmonary disease. On admission, the patient's HR was 110 bpm. Arterial BP was 150/80 mm Hg, which is his baseline. He was thought to be dehydrated due to poor oral intake in the preceding few days and received 2 L intravenous normal saline. The next morning the patient is noted to be tachypneic to 22 breaths/min. His HR is 80 bpm, and BP is 155/85 mm Hg. Crackles are noted at bilateral bases. Acute pulmonary edema secondary to excessive intravenous crystalloid is suspected. Apical four-chamber view (**Figure 50.13** and ▶ **Video 50.4**) and spectral Doppler recordings (**Figures 50.14** and **50.15**) are obtained.

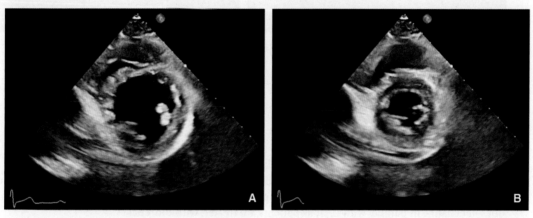

**Figure 50.13** Parasternal short-axis view. A. End-diastole. B. End-systole.

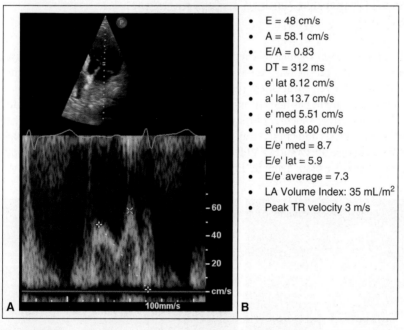

- E = 48 cm/s
- A = 58.1 cm/s
- E/A = 0.83
- DT = 312 ms
- e' lat 8.12 cm/s
- a' lat 13.7 cm/s
- e' med 5.51 cm/s
- a' med 8.80 cm/s
- E/e' med = 8.7
- E/e' lat = 5.9
- E/e' average = 7.3
- LA Volume Index: 35 mL/m$^2$
- Peak TR velocity 3 m/s

**Figure 50.14** Mitral inflow velocities (A) and measurements (B).

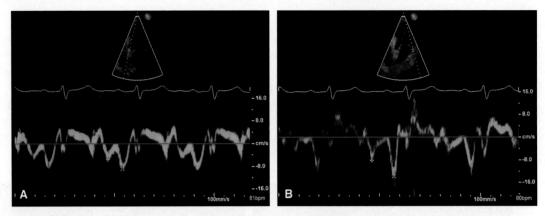

**Figure 50.15** Tissue Doppler of the mitral annulus. A. Medial. B. Lateral.

Which of the following is the most accurate statement regarding this patient's diastolic function?
A. Normal diastolic function
B. Grade I diastolic dysfunction
C. Grade II diastolic dysfunction
D. Grade III diastolic dysfunction

13. The 2016 ASE diastolic function evaluation guidelines have drawn a number of criticisms. Which of the parameters used in the ASE document as a staple of evaluation for the presence of diastolic dysfunction does *not* change in parallel with LAP, as patients are treated with diuretics?

A. E
B. E/e'
C. Tricuspid regurgitant (TR) peak flow velocity
D. LA volume index (LAVI)

14. A 40-year-old woman presents with dyspnea on exertion. She has no history of heart or lung disease. Until 6 months prior to presentation she was exercising regularly and had no physical limitations. She was then involved in a motor vehicle accident (pedestrian struck) and sustained an ankle fracture. Since the trauma the patient has had chronic pain in the ankle, was not able to return to her exercise routine, and has led a rather sedentary lifestyle. Physical examination is unremarkable, and so are the electrocardiogram (ECG) and chest X-ray. PSAx view (**Figure 50.16** and ▶ **Video 50.5**), apical four-chamber view (**Figure 50.17** and ▶ **Video 50.6**), mitral inflow velocity spectral Doppler (**Figure 50.18**), and mitral annular tissue Doppler images (**Figure 50.19**) are obtained.

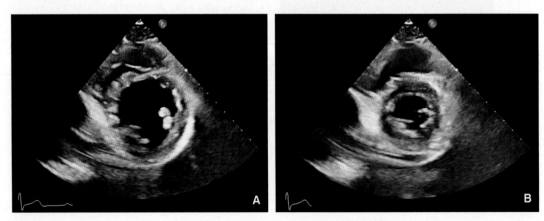

**Figure 50.16** Parasternal short-axis view. A. End-diastole. B. End-systole.

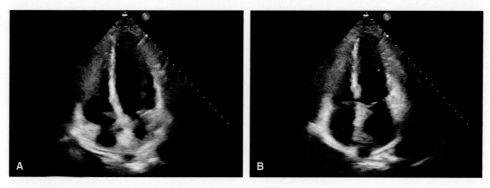

**Figure 50.17** Apical four-chamber view. A. End-diastole. B. End-systole.

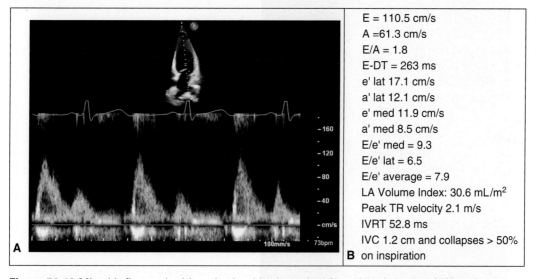

E = 110.5 cm/s
A =61.3 cm/s
E/A = 1.8
E-DT = 263 ms
e' lat 17.1 cm/s
a' lat 12.1 cm/s
e' med 11.9 cm/s
a' med 8.5 cm/s
E/e' med = 9.3
E/e' lat = 6.5
E/e' average = 7.9
LA Volume Index: 30.6 mL/m$^2$
Peak TR velocity 2.1 m/s
IVRT 52.8 ms
IVC 1.2 cm and collapses > 50%
on inspiration

**Figure 50.18** Mitral inflow velocities obtained in the apical four-chamber view (A), and measurements (B).

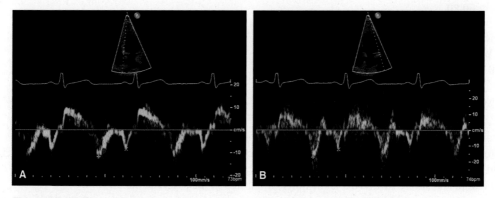

**Figure 50.19** Tissue Doppler of the mitral annulus. A. Medial. B. Lateral.

Which of the following is true?

**A.** IVRT of 52.8 ms is normal but is sufficient to exclude the diagnosis of diastolic dysfunction.

**B.** E-DT of 253 ms is elevated (>160 ms) and suggests diastolic dysfunction, but is not sufficient for the diagnosis.

**C.** Peak tricuspid regurgitant velocity (TR $V_{max}$) of 2.1 m/s is suggestive of pulmonary arterial HTN, which, in the absence of lung disease, can be presumed to be secondary to elevated LAP. It is, however, insufficient to make the diagnosis.

**D.** E/e' < 10 and e' > 10 are suggestive of diastolic dysfunction. It is, however, by itself insufficient to make the diagnosis.

**E.** e' lateral > e' medial, which is normal and, in this case, is sufficient to exclude constriction.

**15.** Based on the case presented in **Question 14,** which of the following best describes the patient's diastolic function?

   **A.** Normal diastolic function
   **B.** Grade I diastolic dysfunction
   **C.** Grade II diastolic dysfunction
   **D.** Grade III diastolic dysfunction

**16. Figure 50.20** shows a spectral graph of tissue Doppler recording obtained from the lateral aspect of the mitral annulus from the case presented in **Question 14.**

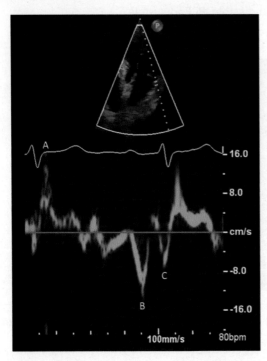

**Figure 50.20**

Which labeled wave is the E-wave?
   **A.** A
   **B.** B
   **C.** C
   **D.** None of the above

**17.** According to the latest 2016 ASE guidelines, one of the first steps in assessing severity of diastolic dysfunction is identification of special cases in which such assessment is either not possible or differs from the standard, such as mitral stenosis (MS), severe mitral annular calcification (MAC), atrial fibrillation, and severe MR. What is the other initial step in the assessment?

   **A.** Evaluation for the presence of myocardial disease, such as decreased LV systolic function, LVH, and known diastolic dysfunction
   **B.** Measurement of mitral inflow E- and A-waves and their ratio (E/A)
   **C.** Measurement of IVRT and E-DT
   **D.** Measurement of A-wave duration

18. A 50-year-old moderately obese man with a history of arterial HTN presents with dyspnea on exertion. He has no history of lung disease and has no signs of heart failure at rest. Echo and Doppler images are obtained (**Figures 50.21, 50.22, 50.23,** and **50.24,** ▶ **Videos 50.7** and **50.8**). LAVI was calculated to be 35 mL/m².

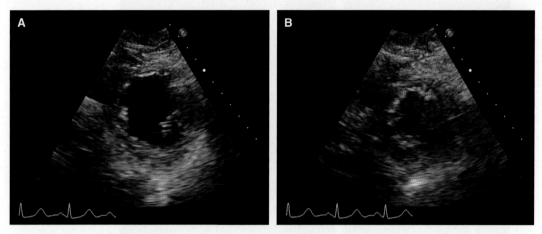

**Figure 50.21** Parasternal short-axis view. A. End-diastole. B. End-systole.

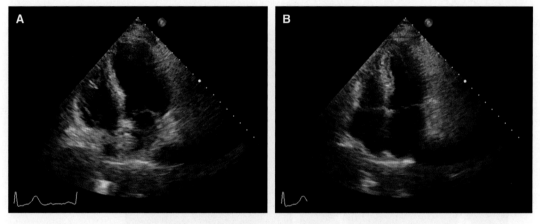

**Figure 50.22** Apical four-chamber view. A. End-diastole. B. End-systole.

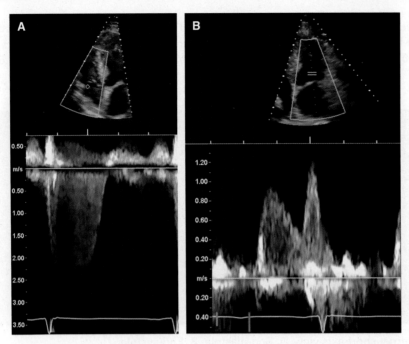

**Figure 50.23** A. Tricuspid regurgitation continuous-wave Doppler. A4 view. B. Mitral inflow pulse-wave Doppler. A4 view.

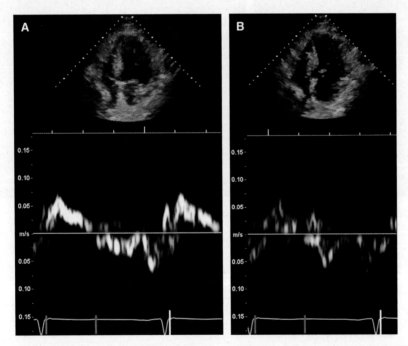

**Figure 50.24** A. Tissue Doppler imaging (TDI) septal mitral annulus. B. TDI lateral mitral annulus.

What can be said about this patient's diastolic function?
**A.** Diastolic function is normal
**B.** Grade I diastolic dysfunction
**C.** Grade II diastolic dysfunction
**D.** Grade III diastolic dysfunction
**E.** Diastolic function is indeterminate

19. A 54-year-old woman with obesity, arterial HTN but no known cardiac history is admitted for SOB and is diagnosed with viral pneumonia due to COVID-19. She is requiring oxygen supplementation at 2 L/min with ambulation to maintain arterial oxygen saturation by pulse oximetry of 92%, but none at rest. She is normotensive and appears comfortable at rest. On ultrasound her left and right ventricular (RV) size and function are normal and there are no significant valvular lesions. Mild LVH is noted. In addition to conventional Doppler parameters, pulmonary vein (PV) Doppler was obtained (**Figure 50.25**).

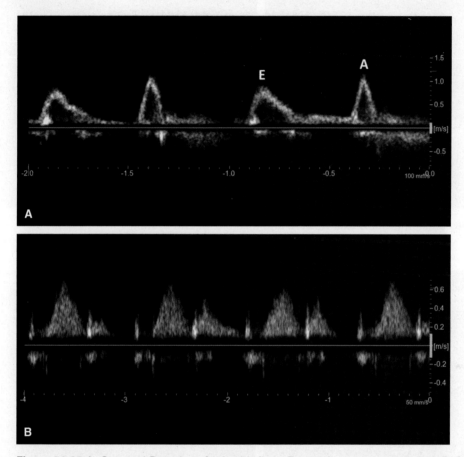

**Figure 50.25** A. Spectral Doppler of mitral inflow. E- and A-waves are labeled. B. Spectral Doppler of pulmonary venous flow obtained from the superior medial pulmonary vein in the apical four-chamber view.

What can be said about this patient's LV diastolic function and LV filling pressures?
A. Diastolic function is normal with normal LV filling pressures
B. Grade I diastolic dysfunction with normal LV filling pressures
C. Grade II diastolic dysfunction with elevated LV filling pressures
D. Grade III diastolic dysfunction with elevated LV filling pressures

**20.** A 62-year-old man with acute respiratory distress syndrome secondary to COVID-19 pneumonia is being considered for extubation. He has a history of arterial HTN with LVH and DM2. He is awake and able to follow commands. He has been initiating spontaneous breaths on PS 5/5 for 10 minutes with adequate tidal volumes and RR of 20. His oxygen saturation is 95% on $F_iO_2$ of 0.3. Ultrasound and Doppler images are obtained (**Figures 50.26, 50.27,** and **50.28,** ▶ **Videos 50.9** and **50.10**).

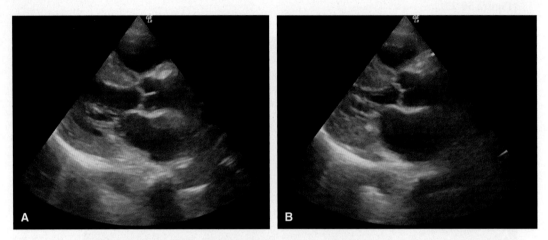

**Figure 50.26** Parasternal short-axis view. A. End-diastole. B. End-systole.

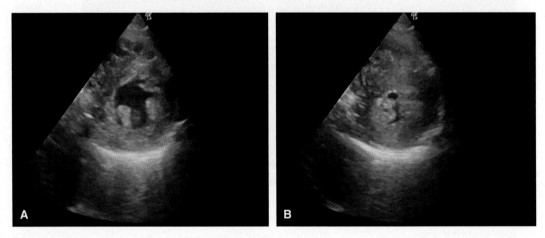

**Figure 50.27** Parasternal short-axis view. A. End-diastole. B. End-systole.

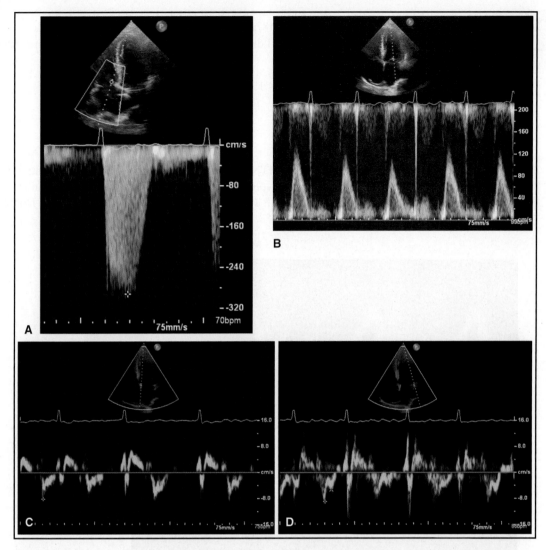

**Figure 50.28** A. Continuous-wave Doppler through the tricuspid valve. A4 view. B. Pulse-wave Doppler through the mitral inflow tract. A4 view. C. Tissue Doppler imaging (TDI) of the septal mitral annulus. D. TDI of the lateral mitral annulus.

What can be said about this patient's diastolic function?

**A.** Diastolic function is normal

**B.** Grade I diastolic dysfunction

**C.** Grade II diastolic dysfunction

**D.** Grade III diastolic dysfunction

**21.** Based on the cases presented in **Question 20**, which of the following is true?

**A.** There is a strong correlation between E/e′ and mean LAP, as estimated invasively by pulmonary artery capillary wedge pressure (PCWP).

**B.** 2016 ASE guidelines are able to classify the absolute majority of critical care patients into high or low estimated LAP groups.

**C.** Elevated LAP as estimated echocardiographically (e.g., by E/e′) predicts failure to extubate.

**D.** 2016 ASE guidelines are highly accurate in classifying critical care patients as having or not having elevated LAP (with PCWP being the reference standard).

22. By the 2016 guidelines E/A > 2, average E/e' > 14, and TR peak velocity > 2.8 m/s are used as indicators of a restrictive filling pattern (grade III diastolic dysfunction) and elevated LAP. What other parameters are indicative of restrictive filling?

    A. $T_{E-e'}$ is prolonged and IVRT/$T_{E-e'}$ > 2, E-DT <150 ms, and IVRT <70 ms
    B. Prominent L-wave of mitral inflow
    C. Late diastolic MR
    D. All of the above

23. A 79-year-old man with obesity, DM2, arterial HTN, chronic kidney disease (CKD), chronic atrial fibrillation, and COPD presents with SOB and hypoxemia. Chest X-ray shows diffuse patchy infiltrates. Polymerase chain reaction (PCR) confirms positivity for COVID-19. Selected ultrasound and Doppler images are obtained (**Figures 50.29** and **50.30**).

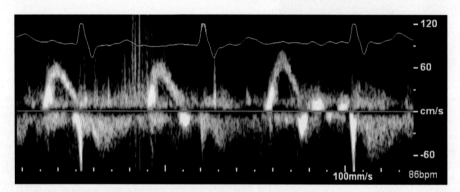

**Figure 50.29** Mitral inflow velocity spectral pulse-wave Doppler.

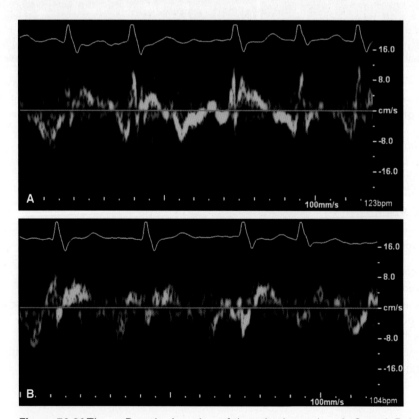

**Figure 50.30** Tissue Doppler imaging of the mitral annulus. A. Septal. B. Lateral.

LV systolic function was moderately decreased. LA was severely dilated, and TR $V_{max}$ was 3.1 m/s. There were no significant valvular abnormalities. He is in atrial fibrillation.

Selected Doppler measurements are given below:

- E = 7.5 m/s
- E-DT = 108 ms
- TR $V_{max}$ = 3.1 m/s
- e' lateral = 0.08 m/s
- e' septal = 0.08 m/s
- E/e' = 94

Which one of these statements about this patient is correct?

**A.** In patients like this, LV filling pressures cannot be predicted by any echocardiographic parameters available in routine clinical practice

**B.** Severe LA dilatation is highly suggestive of elevated LV filling pressures

**C.** Very high E/A in this case suggests restrictive filling pattern

**D.** Short E-DT is consistent with high LV filling pressures

---

**24.** An 89-year-old woman with a history of arterial HTN, DM2, and 100 pack-years of cigarette smoking presents with dyspnea during activities of daily living.

Selected cardiac ultrasound and Doppler images are obtained (**Figures 50.31, 50.32, 50.33, and 50.34** and ▶ **Video 50.11**). LV systolic function is severely decreased, but there are no hemodynamically significant valvular abnormalities.

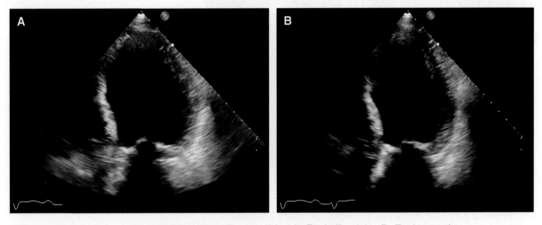

**Figure 50.31** Apical four-chamber view. Zoomed in. A. End-diastole. B. End-systole.

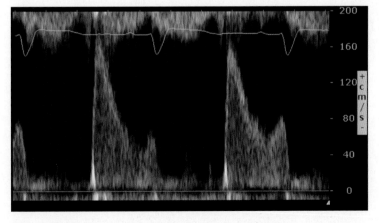

**Figure 50.32** Mitral inflow velocity spectral Doppler.

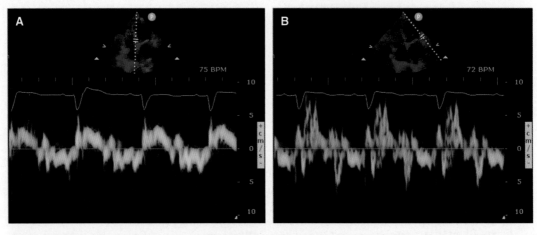

**Figure 50.33** A. Mitral annular tissue Doppler imaging (TDI). Medial. B. Mitral annular TDI. Lateral.

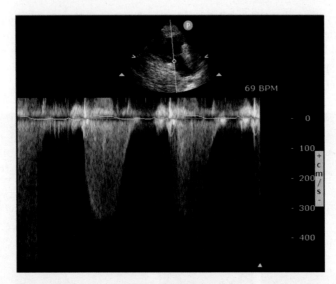

**Figure 50.34** Right ventricular inflow view. Continuous-wave Doppler.

What can be said about this patient's LV filling pressures?

**A.** In patients with severe MAC, E/e' is unreliable.

**B.** In patients with severe MAC, LV filling pressures cannot be reliably estimated.

**C.** E/e' is >15 in this patient with reduced LV systolic function, therefore LV filling pressures are likely elevated.

**D.** This patient has normal LV filling pressures.

**25.** An 86-year-old woman with a history of arterial HTN is admitted to the hospital with dyspnea on exertion, which developed over a period of 1 week. Ten days prior to admission the patient developed nasal congestion and rhinorrhea, followed by dry cough. She has not been febrile and has not had any diarrhea or change in her olfaction. She has never had a similar episode in the past and has been fully compliant with her medications and diet. On admission the patient's RR is 26 breaths/min, arterial BP is 200/110 mm Hg, and HR is 60 bpm. Arterial oxygen saturation by pulse oximetry is 92% while breathing room air. JVP is normal by physical examination. Lung auscultation reveals diffuse crackles in all lung fields. There is no lower extremity edema. Nasal swab is positive for severe acute respiratory syndrome coronavirus (SARS-CoV)-2. (See also **Figure 50.35**.)

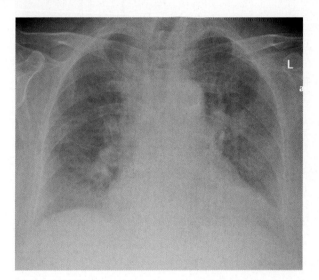

**Figure 50.35** Anteroposterior portable radiograph of the chest on admission.

Bedside cardiac ultrasound showed a hyperdynamic left ventricle and normal RV size and function. There was mild MR. IVC was 1.5 cm and collapsed to 0.5 cm on inspiration. There was not enough tricuspid regurgitation (TR) to estimate peak TR velocity. Mitral inflow velocity spectral Doppler tracing is shown in **Figure 50.36**.

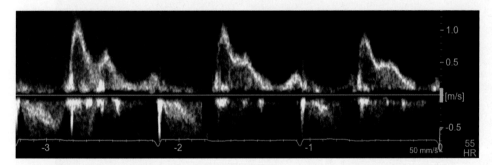

**Figure 50.36** Pulse-wave Doppler of mitral inflow obtained in the apical four-chamber view.

Select one true statement about this patient:
**A.** The findings are suggestive of elevated LV filling pressures, and therefore diastolic CHF may be contributing to her symptoms.
**B.** The findings are suggestive of normal LV filling pressures, and therefore her symptoms are likely all due to viral pneumonia.
**C.** There is not enough information to make any conclusions regarding patient's LV filling pressures.
**D.** The observed pattern of mitral inflow is virtually always pathologic.

26. A 46-year-old man presented with new-onset dyspnea on minimal exertion and palpitations. He was found to be in atrial fibrillation. He was also found to have severely decreased LV systolic function. He was treated with beta-blockers and intravenous diuretics. On hospital day 2 he underwent a successful direct current (DC) cardioversion. His ECG (**Figure 50.37**) and mitral inflow spectral Doppler tracing (**Figure 50.38**) are obtained.

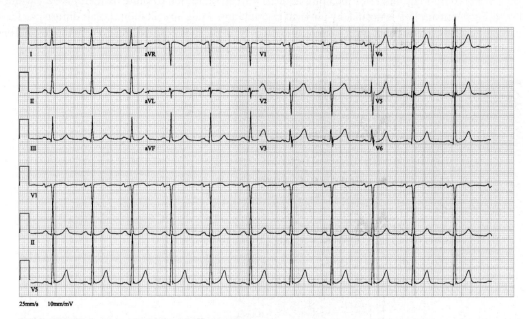

25mm/s    10mm/mV

**Figure 50.37** A 12-lead electrocardiogram.

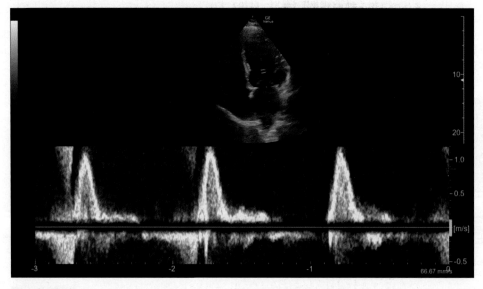

**Figure 50.38**

Which of the following is correct about this patient?

A. Patient is still in atrial fibrillation

B. Patient has E>>A, that is, a restrictive filling pattern, and likely has significantly elevated LV filling pressures

C. PV tracing is likely to show a normal Ar-wave

D. None of the above

27. In which of the following conditions can the standard approach to evaluation of diastolic function be used?

    **A.** Significant AS
    **B.** Restrictive cardiomyopathy
    **C.** Significant MS
    **D.** Significant MAC
    **E.** Significant MR
    **F.** Atrial fibrillation

28. **Figure 50.39** was obtained from a patient with diastolic dysfunction.

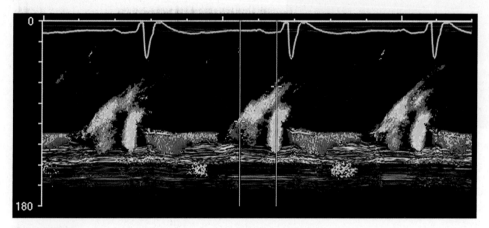

**Figure 50.39**

What modality is being used and for what purpose?
**A.** Color Doppler of mitral inflow. Direction of inflow jet is being visualized.
**B.** Color Doppler of the MR jet. Presence of systolic MR is being sought.
**C.** M-mode through the MV. Presence of diastolic L-wave is being sought.
**D.** Color M-mode (CMM). Mitral inflow propagation velocity is being assessed.

29. A 76-year-old man with a previous history of coronary artery bypass grafting, peripheral vascular disease, HTN, and diabetes was admitted for acute severe dyspnea at rest. On physical examination, the patient was diaphoretic and tachypneic with bilateral lung crackles. Initial echocardiogram revealed normal LV ejection fraction of 57%, but with a low stroke volume index of 30 mL/m$^2$, normal wall motion, mild LVH, moderate biatrial enlargement, and normal RV size and function. AR was present. A BP of 155/57 mm Hg was recorded.

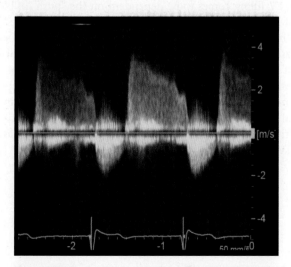

**Figure 50.40** Continuous-wave Doppler through the aortic valve obtained in the apical five-chamber view.

What is the significance of the notching of the AR CWD spectral recording shown in **Figure 50.40**?

**A.** It suggests that LV end-diastolic pressure (EDP) is elevated.
**B.** It suggests that there is a concomitant AS present.
**C.** It suggests that AR is severe.
**D.** It suggests that the MV is stenotic because the anterior leaflet is pushed in by the AR jet.

30. **Figure 50.41** is a PWD recording of mitral inflow.

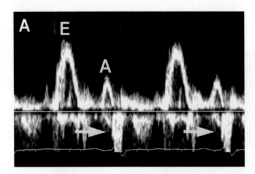

**Figure 50.41**

Which Doppler finding associated with increased LVEDP is indicated by the *arrows*?

**A.** A-dip
**B.** B-bump
**C.** L-wave
**D.** Diastolic MR

# Chapter 50 ▪ Answers

1. Correct Answer: C. Isovolumic relaxation time (IVRT)

*Rationale:* IVRT is the time from the beginning of diastole (aortic valve closure) to the beginning of rapid filling (E) phase of LV diastolic filling. Like many other indices of diastolic function, IVRT has a biphasic course as diastolic dysfunction progresses. Normal IVRT is 70 to 90 ms. Initially, as LV diastolic relaxation becomes impaired and delayed, IVRT lengthens and in grade I dysfunction IVRT is typically >90 ms. As diastolic dysfunction progresses LV filling comes to be dependent on the "push" of blood from the LA instead of the normal "pull" of an actively relaxing left ventricle. As LV filling pressure (i.e., mean LAP) rises, MV opens earlier in the cardiac cycle and IVRT shortens back into the normal range in grade II dysfunction. In grade III diastolic dysfunction (restrictive filling pattern) IVRT further shortens and falls below 70 ms. In this patient IVRT is 130 ms, which is consistent with grade I diastolic dysfunction. IVRT is not one of the main parameters for identification of diastolic dysfunction, but may nonetheless be useful in some cases. IVRT is measured by positioning the PWD sampling volume in between the mitral and aortic valves in the apical five-chamber view, so that the aortic ejection velocity and mitral inflow velocity can be measured from the same recording. The time interval from the cessation of aortic flow to the beginning of mitral flow is IVRT.

All other answer options involve parameters also used in assessment of diastolic function, but all the listed parameters are obtained from mitral inflow velocity recordings which are obtained in the A4 view by positioning the PWD sample volume in the left ventricle right at the tips of the mitral leaflets. In contrast, IVRT is obtained closer to the aorta, in order to catch both aortic ejection as well as the mitral inflow.

On spectral Doppler graphs velocity is plotted on the Y-axis and time on the X-axis. E-wave velocity is its height, not its duration (**Figure 50.42**).

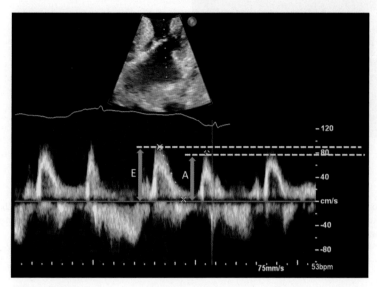

**Figure 50.42**

Deceleration time refers to E-wave deceleration and is measured as shown in **Figure 50.43.**

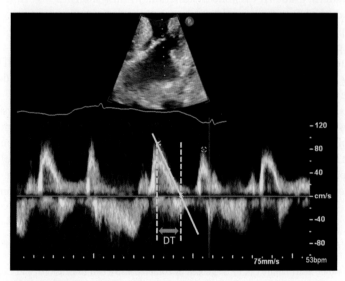

**Figure 50.43**

A-wave duration measurement is shown in **Figure 50.44.**

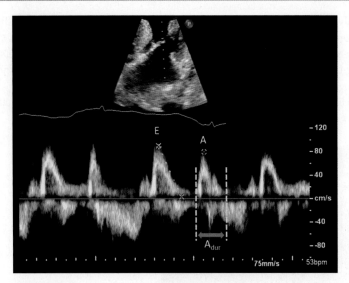

**Figure 50.44**

Selected References

1. Nagueh SF, Smiseth OA, Appleton CP, et al. Recommendations for the evaluation of left ventricular diastolic function by echocardiography: an update from the American Society of Echocardiography and the European Association of Cardiovascular Imaging. *J Am Soc Echocardiogr.* 2016 Apr;29(4):277-314. doi:10.1016/j.echo.2016.01.011.
2. Oh JK. Assessment of diastolic function. *In*: Oh JK, Kane GC, Seward JB, Tajik AJ, eds. *The Echo Manual.* 4th ed. Wolters Kluwer; 2019.

**2.** Correct Answer: **C. Figure 50.3C**

*Rationale:* All answer options offer a different spectral (PWD) graph of mitral inflow.

Answer A shows a restrictive pattern, grade III diastolic dysfunction. In this pattern E >> A. In this case, A-wave is essentially absent, despite the presence of atrial contraction.

Answer B shows a normal or pseudonormal (grade II) inflow pattern. Here E/A is > 0.8 but <2.0. Whether the pattern is normal or pseudonormal depends on clinical circumstances.

Answer D shows a relatively rare pattern featuring a third diastolic inflow wave—the L-wave. This is generally a sign of elevated filling pressures and can be seen in combination with grade II or grade III patterns. It is thought to always be abnormal.

The most important learning point of this question is that it is assumed that all patients with systolic dysfunction also have diastolic dysfunction. The truth of this statement has been debated, but it remains a useful general principle applicable to the absolute majority of patients. Assuming this is correct, no patient with systolic dysfunction can have a normal filling pattern regardless of volume status. If the normal pattern is excluded, then any E-predominant mitral inflow must represent pseudonormalization. The "best" or most normal filling pattern a patient with systolic CHF can hope to achieve is an A-dominant (grade I) pattern of mitral inflow.

Selected References

1. Kerut EK, McIlwain EF, Plotnick GD. *Handbook of Echo-Doppler Interpretation*, 2nd ed. Futura, an imprint of Blackwell Publishing; 2004.
2. Oh JK, Hatle L, Tajik AJ, Little WC. Diastolic heart failure can be diagnosed by comprehensive two-dimensional and Doppler echocardiography. *J Am Coll Cardiol.* 2006 Feb 7;47(3):500-506. doi:10.1016/j.jacc.2005.09.032. Epub 2006 Jan 18.
3. Sharon M. Kay, Sidney University. Purrrfect Echo chic @sharonmkay. Accessed April 23, 2021. http://twitter.com/sharonmkay/status/380264241267093504. Posted Sep 18, 2013.

**3.** Correct Answer: B. 1—normal, 2—normal, 3—elevated, 4—elevated, 5—normal

*Rationale:* Determination of diastolic function is complex and may depend on many echo-derived parameters. However, a three-step procedure is able to classify most patients correctly.

First, patients should be classified as having or not having LV *systolic* dysfunction. In the second step, in patients with normal systolic function, mitral inflow pattern will be able to place a patient on the continuum of diastolic function, albeit with some ambiguity. Finally, e' velocity will allow for the final classification into diastolic function categories. Note that this is *not* an algorithm recommended in the latest ASE guidelines, but is an easier to understand, pathophysiology-based approach. (See also **Figure 50.45**.)

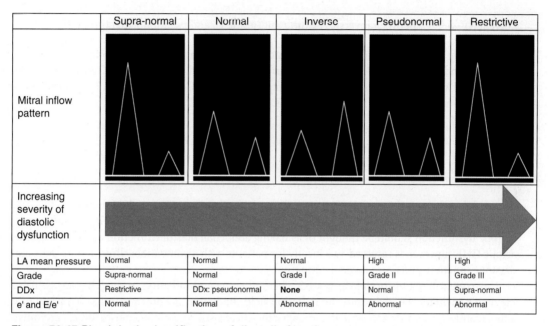

|  | Supra-normal | Normal | Inverse | Pseudonormal | Restrictive |
|---|---|---|---|---|---|
| Mitral inflow pattern |  |  |  |  |  |
| Increasing severity of diastolic dysfunction |  |  |  |  |  |
| LA mean pressure | Normal | Normal | Normal | High | High |
| Grade | Supra-normal | Normal | Grade I | Grade II | Grade III |
| DDx | Restrictive | DDx: pseudonormal | **None** | Normal | Supra-normal |
| e' and E/e' | Normal | Normal | Abnormal | Abnormal | Abnormal |

**Figure 50.45** Physiologic classification of diastolic function.

Differentiation between supra-normal and restrictive and between normal and pseudonormal patterns is made based on tissue Doppler parameters (e' and E/e').

Among patients with disordered diastolic function, transition from grade I to grade II is characterized by transition from normal to elevated LA pressure and from "pull" to "push" filling physiology.

1—LAP is **normal**. Patient has a restrictive (grade III) vs "supra-normal" pattern. LV diastolic fx is supra-normal (likely normal for her age), as evidenced by high e'. Therefore, she likely has a supra-normal filling pattern and normal LAP.

2—LAP is **normal**. Patient likely has grade I diastolic dysfunction. This pattern does not have a differential diagnosis and is always abnormal.

3—LAP is **elevated**. Patient likely has grade III diastolic dysfunction (restrictive filling pattern). The phenotype suggests that the patient is not fit and has multiple features predictive of diastolic dysfunction.

4—LAP is **elevated**. This E/A pattern is consistent with both pseudonormal and normal filling patterns. In this case normal diastolic function is ruled out by abnormally low e', therefore this patient has grade II diastolic dysfunction.

5—LAP is **normal**. Patient has a normal vs pseudonormal filling pattern. Diastolic fx is normal as evidenced by normal e', therefore this patient likely has a normal filling pattern and normal LAP.

**Selected Reference**

1. Oh JK, Kane GC, Seward JB, Tajik AJ, eds. *The Echo Manual.* 4th ed. Wolters Kluwer; 2019.

4. Correct Answer: C. The norms listed are for a healthy elderly population. When interpreting study results, it is important to remember that "supra-normal" values may be younger age-related and not related to any pathology.

*Rationale:* The norms listed are for a healthy elderly population. When interpreting study results, it is important to remember that "supra-normal" values may be younger age-related and not related to any pathology.

Selected Reference

1. Oh JK, Kane GC, Seward JB, Tajik AJ, eds. *The Echo Manual.* 4th ed. Wolters Kluwer; 2019.

5. Correct Answer: C. Between inverse, A-dominant (grade I), and pseudonormal (grade II)

*Rationale:* Up until and including grade I diastolic dysfunction the filling is thought to occur by active relaxation and suctioning effect of the left ventricle on the blood, that is, by "pull." After that the left ventricle is rigid and filling occurs by the LA pushing blood into it. Consequently, LAP is typically normal up until pseudonormal (grade II) pattern develops.

Selected Reference

1. Oh JK, Kane GC, Seward JB, Tajik AJ, eds. *The Echo Manual.* 4th ed. Wolters Kluwer; 2019.

6. Correct Answer: B. Restrictive filling pattern

*Rationale:* As the apical four-chamber view shown in Figure 50.5, LV systolic function in this case is severely depressed. This automatically rules out diastolic CHF as a sole diagnosis. In fact, *all* patients with systolic dysfunction should be thought of as having abnormal diastolic function as well. Diagnosis of diastolic CHF, however, is reserved specifically for patients with a compatible clinical syndrome, abnormal diastolic function, and *normal* systolic function.

This patient has a history of cardiotoxic chemotherapy and radiation to the left chest, which almost inevitably includes the heart into the radiation field. Radiation is known to cause a variety of cardiac abnormalities, including accelerated coronary atherosclerosis, constrictive pericarditis, cardiomyopathy, and valvulopathies. In any patient with a history of radiation to the chest who presents with a syndrome of CHF, constrictive pericarditis must be kept in the differential. Even though echo diagnosis of constriction is complex, tissue Doppler of mitral annulus (Figure 50.7) offers a relatively simple assessment. In a normal heart, the lateral part of the mitral annulus, being part of the free wall, moves faster than the medial, and lateral e' will be greater than medial. In contrast, in constrictive pericarditis, the lateral annulus is tethered to the pericardial sac, resulting in lateral e' being less than medial, which is sometimes referred to as "annulus reversus." In this case, $e'_{lateral} > e'_{medial}$, making constriction unlikely.

Filling pattern in this case shows E>>A. This pattern is called "restrictive filling" and indicates very elevated LA pressures. It can be seen in patients with either grade III diastolic dysfunction or systolic dysfunction. Restrictive filling is not to be confused with restrictive cardiomyopathy, which too may result in a restrictive filling pattern, but is a term reserved for a particular type of cardiomyopathy.

Selected References

1. Oh JK. Assessment of diastolic function. *In*: Oh JK, Kane GC, Seward JB, Tajik AJ, eds. *The Echo Manual.* 4th ed. Wolters Kluwer; 2019.
2. Rygiel K. Cardiotoxic effects of radiotherapy and strategies to reduce them in patients with breast cancer: an overview. *J Cancer Res Ther.* 2017 Apr-Jun;13(2):186-192. doi:10.4103/0973-1482.187303.
3. Welch TD, Ling LH, Espinosa RE, et al. Echocardiographic diagnosis of constrictive pericarditis: Mayo Clinic criteria. *Circ Cardiovasc Imaging.* 2014 May;7(3):526-534. doi:10.1161/CIRCIMAGING.113.001613. Epub 2014 Mar 14.

7. Correct Answer: B. This patient still has elevated left filling pressures. He may benefit from further diuresis.

*Rationale:* This patient has a restrictive filling pattern (E>>A), suggestive of significantly elevated left-sided filling pressures. Though there is no guarantee that the patient will tolerate further diuresis, normal serum creatinine and normal RV filling pressures (as assessed by IVC and JVP) suggest that he is currently not "over-diuresed," that is, there is no evidence that his cardiac output (and end-organ perfusion) have diminished after decrease in preload following diuretics. Consequently, it is not unreasonable to attempt further diuresis in this patient who is still symptomatic. Recall that the theoretical best inflow pattern in patients with decreased systolic function, who are presumed to always have diastolic dysfunction as well, is the "inverse" (E<A) corresponding to grade I diastolic dysfunction. There are certainly other ways of gauging LAP by ultrasound, the main one being lung ultrasound pattern. A pattern effectively rules out elevated LV filling pressures as a cause of dyspnea. In this patient, however, lung auscultation and ultrasound are noninformative, because of the coexisting parenchymal lung disease. There is no evidence of constriction and lateral e' is greater than medial (i.e., annulus reversus is absent).

**Selected Reference**

1. Oh JK. Assessment of diastolic function. *In*: Oh JK, Kane GC, Seward JB, Tajik AJ, eds. *The Echo Manual*. 4th ed.  Wolters Kluwer; 2019:168-201.

**8.** Correct Answer: A. This patient is clinically euvolemic and his left filling pressures are as good as they will ever get. He should receive only his usual maintenance diuretics. Etiology of his dyspnea is likely noncardiac.

*Rationale:* The patient has an inverse filling pattern characteristic of impaired diastolic relaxation (grade I diastolic dysfunction). This is the "best" filling pattern a patient with impaired systolic function can attain. Recall that systolic dysfunction always is presumed to imply the presence of diastolic dysfunction. Consequently, it is not possible for a patient with impaired systolic function to have normal filling, regardless of loading conditions. In fact, a "normal" filling pattern in this patient would indicate that it is in fact not normal but is "pseudonormal" and would suggest that in the absence of contraindications, further diuresis may be attempted. This patient's LV filling pressures have now likely been optimized. As always, if tolerated, reduction of afterload in CHF is indicated.

Normal right filling pressure is zero, and therefore right atrial pressures (RAPs) in the range described in this case are not by themselves a contraindication to continuing diuresis.

Importantly, evidence of normal LV filling pressures suggests that other, noncardiac, etiologies should be sought in order to explain the patient's dyspnea.

**Selected Reference**

1. Oh JK. Assessment of diastolic function. *In*: Oh JK, Kane GC, Seward JB, Tajik AJ, eds. *The Echo Manual*. 4th ed.  Wolters Kluwer; 2019:Chapter 8. ISBN 9781496312198.

**9.** Correct Answer: B. At the tips of the MV in the left ventricle

*Rationale:* The sample volume of PWD has to be positioned at the tips of the MV leaflets in the left ventricle. Doppler interrogation line should be aligned with the direction of inflow into the left ventricle during diastole. (See also **Figure 50.46**.)

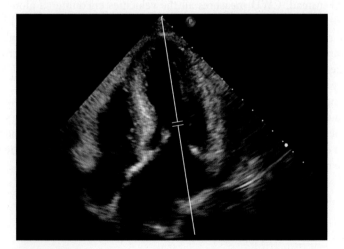

**Figure 50.46**

Selected Reference

1. Nagueh SF, Smiseth OA, Appleton CP, et al. Recommendations for the evaluation of left ventricular diastolic function by echocardiography: an update from the American Society of Echocardiography and the European Association of Cardiovascular Imaging. *J Am Soc Echocardiogr.* 2016 Apr;29(4):277-314. doi:10.1016/j.echo.2016.01.011.

**10.** Correct Answer: D. Coexisting aortic regurgitation (AR)

*Rationale:* Imperfect alignment of the Doppler interrogation line with the flow will result in *under*estimation of the velocity, not its overestimation. Doppler shift can only estimate the component of the velocity parallel to the insonation beam. Recall that the Doppler equation contains a correction factor cos*θ*.

Doppler equation: $$V = \frac{\Delta f \times c}{2 \times f\text{insonation} \times \cos\theta},$$

where *c* is the speed of sound in the tissue, $\Delta f$ is Doppler shift, $f_{\text{insonation}}$ is insonation frequency, and *θ* is the angle of insonation relative to the flow.

As the angle of insonation increases between 0 and 90°, the cosine of that angle decreases, and the estimated velocity will decrease. Consequently, assuming that the angle of insonation is zero (with its cosine being equal to 1) while in reality it is not, will *under*estimate the velocity.

Positioning Doppler sample volume in the LA is likely to underestimate the inflow velocities, because flow accelerates in the narrower tract.

Flow of MR and AS occurs in systole and will not affect measurements of diastolic mitral inflow. Both may result in high diastolic LV pressures, but that is a physiologic effect, not an error of measurement.

In contrast, flow of AR occurs in diastole, at the same time as normal mitral inflow. Because of the anatomic proximity of the LV in in- and outflow tracts, the jet of AR can be easily mixed with the mitral inflow, especially if the sample box is positioned too close to the LV outflow tract. Pressure gradient across a regurgitant aortic valve is much higher than across a normal open MV. From Bernoulli's equation, high pressure gradient corresponds to high flow velocities, and, therefore, mitral inflow velocities may be significantly overestimated.

Selected Reference

1. Kerut EK, McIlwain EF, Plotnick GD. *Handbook of Echo-Doppler Interpretation.* 2nd ed. Futura, an imprint of Blackwell Publishing; 2004. ISBN: 0-4051-1903-9.

**11.** Correct Answer: A. Continuous-wave Doppler (CWD) was used instead of PWD.

*Rationale:* Mitral inflow velocity tracing is obtained by PWD with the sample volume positioned at the tips of the MV leaflets within the left ventricle. PWD measures velocities of flow only within the space defined by the sample volume, usually denoted by two small parallel hatches on the interrogation line. PWD is thus the modality used to evaluate flow velocities at a particular point in space.

In this recording CWD was used instead. CWD measures all the velocities encountered along the interrogation line, and, therefore, does not have a sample volume. The fact that CWD rather than PWD is being used is indicated by a closed rhomboid shape on the interrogation line. Position of the rhomboid symbol along that line is of no relevance and does not change the fact that all points along the interrogation line are surveyed. To be sure, the rhombus is *not* a sample volume. (Note that the indicator of CWD modality may vary among devices by various manufacturers.)

There are two other ways to distinguish CWD from PWD. Because, as mentioned, all velocities along the interrogation line are detected, a wide spectrum of velocity values will be detected, and tracing's envelope will be filled. In contrast, if the flow is laminar, PWD samples a limited range of velocities and the envelope will have an outline, but an empty middle. Finally, CWD designation can be seen along the left margin of the screen, identifying the modality used.

A potential issue with using CWD is that any simultaneously present flow will be mixed-in with the mitral inflow signal. For example, significant AR is expected to affect the measurements.

Inflow velocities can be done in several different apical views, but A4 is a standard preferred view, which was used in this case, as can be seen in the accompanied B-mode image.

Tissue Doppler records velocity of moving myocardium, not the blood and is not used for detection of mitral inflow velocities. Tissue movement velocities are one to two orders of magnitude slower than velocity of blood flow. It was not used in this case.

### Selected Reference

1. Kerut EK, McIlwain EF, Plotnick GD. *Handbook of Echo-Doppler Interpretation.* 2nd ed. Futura, an imprint of Blackwell Publishing; 2004. ISBN: 0-4051-1903-9.

**12.** Correct Answer: C. Grade II diastolic dysfunction

*Rationale:* According to the 2016 ASE guidelines, the first step in evaluation of diastolic function is assessment for the presence of myocardial pathology. This patient has several risk factors for myocardial disease (age, HTN, and obesity), but normal LV systolic function. In the absence of known myocardial disease, qualitative presence of diastolic dysfunction is confirmed based on the presence of three of four criteria in the guidelines, which are:

- septal e' <7 cm/s, lateral e' <10 cm/s—present in this case
- average E/e' ratio >14 (lateral E/e' ratio >13 or a septal E/e' >15)—absent in this case
- LA maximum volume index >34 mL/m$^2$—present in this case
- peak TR velocity >2.8 m/s—present in this case

Note that presence or absence of myocardial disease should *not* be equated with the presence or absence of CHF. In fact, clinical history of coronary heart disease, hypertensive heart disease, or CHF is a sufficient ground to state that the patient has diastolic dysfunction. Presence of systolic dysfunction too is taken as evidence of coexisting diastolic dysfunction.

Other echo and Doppler parameters may indicate the presence of diastolic dysfunction, such as increased Ar-A duration, significant change in mitral inflow pattern with Valsalva maneuver, significant discrepancy between inflow patterns across mitral and tricuspid valves, and presence of L-wave on the spectral tracing of mitral inflow. These guidelines, among other things, were meant to increase specificity of assessment for diastolic dysfunction, at the expense of lower sensitivity. It remains to be seen how these changes in criteria play out clinically.

Once the presence of diastolic dysfunction has been ascertained (or at least its probability is thought to be high enough), the next step is quantification of diastolic dysfunction, with the main goal of identifying patients with increased, as opposed to normal, LV filling pressures.

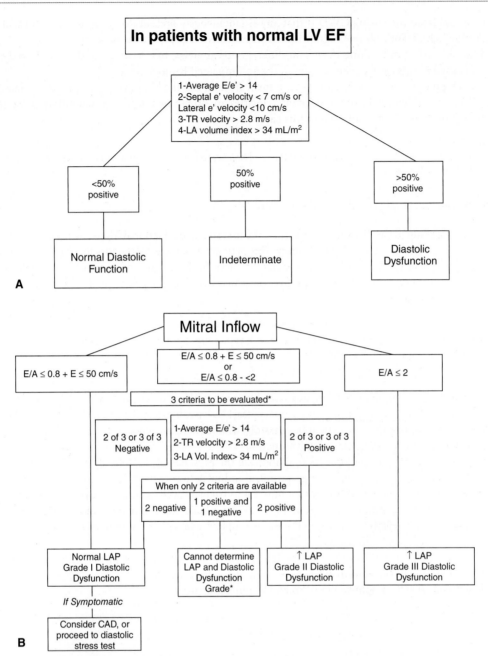

**Figure 50.47** Classification of diastolic function with known myocardial disease.

The classification scheme shown in **Figure 50.47** is based on the variability of diastolic mitral inflow velocity patterns shown in Figure 50.45 in **Answer 3**, but with some refinements:

1. The upper limit of normal E/A ratio is not 1 (E=A), but rather 0.8, meaning that E-wave does not have to be greater than A-wave, but still may not be less than A-wave by >20%.
2. A second criterion for normal inflow pattern is added: E-wave velocity cannot be too high (has to be ≤50 cm/s). Both the criteria must be met for the pattern to be normal (or pseudonormal).
3. Among patients with pseudonormal mitral inflow pattern, abnormal tissue Doppler velocity (E/e' >14) does not automatically classify a patient as having grade II diastolic dysfunction and at least one additional criterion is required: either a dilated LA or presence of pulmonary hypertension (PHTN). If abnormally high E/e' is the sole finding, the patient is classified as having grade I diastolic dysfunction. This distinction is important, because grade I implies normal LA pressure. In

fact, these three criteria (high E/e', large LA, PHTN) are treated as equally important. Diagnosis of grade II diastolic dysfunction requires presence of at least two of the three.

The flowchart provided in the ASE guidelines may be somewhat cumbersome to follow. A simplified flowchart of the same classification is given in **Figure 50.48**.

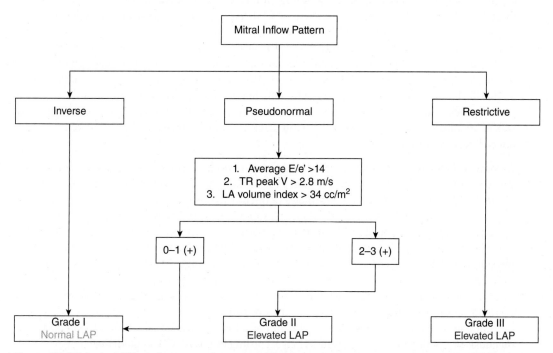

**Figure 50.48** A simplified diagram of the classification of diastolic dysfunction by 2016 American Society of Echocardiography (ASE) guidelines. Note that no supra-normal or normal inflow patterns feature in this diagram. This is because this classification algorithm is only applicable to patients with established myocardial disease. This flowchart is limited to the cases where all three criteria are available. Special provisions are made for cases when only two measures are available. For definitions of inflow patterns see Figure 50.45.

The patient in this question has E/A slightly over 0.8 (E/A = 0.83), which is characteristic of normal or, in the presence of myocardial disease, pseudonormal inflow pattern. His E/e' is low, but he does fulfill the other two criteria listed in Figure 50.47, namely, TR $V_{max}$ >2.8 m/s and LAVI >34 cc/m². Thus, this case would be classified as grade II diastolic dysfunction, with the implication that LA pressure is elevated. Note that the physiologic classification (Figure 50.45), which does not take LA size or PHTN into consideration, would yield a different result and classify this patient's diastolic dysfunction as grade I, which implies *normal* mean LA pressure.

Selected Reference

1. Nagueh SF, Smiseth OA, Appleton CP, et al. Recommendations for the evaluation of left ventricular diastolic function by echocardiography: an update from the American Society of Echocardiography and the European Association of Cardiovascular Imaging. *J Am Soc Echocardiogr.* 2016 Apr;29(4):277-314. doi:10.1016/j.echo.2016.01.011.

**13.** Correct Answer: D. LA volume index (LAVI)

*Rationale:* LA size does not decrease despite decrease in LAP with diuretic therapy.

Selected References

1. Greenstein YY, Mayo PH. Evaluation of left ventricular diastolic function by the intensivist. *Chest.* 2018 Mar;153(3):723-732. doi:10.1016/j.chest.2017.10.032. Epub 2017 Nov 4.
2. Oh JK, Miranda WR, Bird JG, Kane GC, Nagueh SF. The 2016 diastolic function guideline: is it already time to revisit or revise them? *JACC Cardiovasc Imaging.* 2020 Jan;13(1 Pt 2):327-335. doi:10.1016/j.jcmg.2019.12.004.

**14.** Correct Answer: B.

*Rationale:* Constrictive pericarditis is in the differential of severe diastolic dysfunction, that is, restrictive filling in a patient with a clinical picture consistent with CHF. Currently the most robust and validated diagnostic approach is that by the Mayo Clinic. It includes several parameters other than mitral annular diastolic velocity, such as clinical presence of CHF, plethoric IVC, abnormal respiratory septal movement (septal bounce), restrictive filling pattern, significant respiratory mitral inflow variation, and prominent hepatic vein expiratory diastolic flow reversals (expiratory end-diastolic reversal velocity/forward flow velocity $\geq 0.8$). Reversal of normal relationship of e' lateral > e' medial is termed *annulus reversus*. Among patients with clinical CHF and plethoric IVC, annulus reversus had LR($-$) of 0.3 and LR($+$) = 5. This likelihood ratio by itself would not be sufficient to rule out constrictive pericarditis if a reasonable pretest probability existed. The patient in this case has an extremely low suspicion for constriction and lack of annulus reversus effectively rules it out. Lack of septal bounce is the most useful variable in ruling out constriction with LR = 0.1.

**Answer A.** IVRT is a time interval between the closure of the aortic valve and opening of the MV. In the course of diastolic dysfunction progression IVRT follows a biphasic course analogous to E/A pattern. Normal IVRT is 70 to 90 ms. Trained athletes frequently have supra-normal filling and their IVRT would be shorter than normal. As the LV diastolic relaxation becomes impaired and delayed (grade I diastolic dysfunction), IVRT lengthens to >90 ms, and often >110 ms. As diastolic dysfunction progresses to grade II, marked by transition from normal to elevated LV filling pressures (and from the "pull" to "push" physiology), IVRT shortens and falls back into the normal range. In grade III, that is, restrictive filling, IVRT progressively shortens and falls below the lower end of normal 70 ms. It follows that IVRT of 52.8 ms could represent either a supra-normal LV filling in an athlete or stage IV diastolic dysfunction. It would certainly be inappropriate to discount a possibility of this symptomatic patient having diastolic dysfunction based solely on low IVRT value. Importantly, IVRT is not a part of the general algorithm for diagnosis or grading of diastolic dysfunction, according to the 2016 ASE guidelines.

**Answer B.** E-DT is a time from the peak of the E-wave velocity to zero velocity (or extrapolation to baseline). Like IVRT, E-DT follows a biphasic course with increasing severity of diastolic dysfunction. Normal E-DT is 160 to 200 ms, but in a vigorously relaxing athletic heart E-DT will be shorter. In grade I diastolic dysfunction, as the suctioning force of the left ventricle decreases and becomes delayed, E-DT lengthens (>200 ms). Beginning with grade II diastolic dysfunction, as physiology of LV filling switches from "pull" to "push," E-DT progressively shortens. A comparison to a car braking on sand, as compared to braking on ice, may be useful. On sand, the resistance is high and decrease in velocity is rapid. As the kinetic energy is rapidly dissipated, the car will come to a stop after only a short skidding distance. On the contrary, when driving on ice, the resistance is low, and the skidding distance will be long. Similarly, a compliant accommodating left ventricle will result in a slow decrease in inflow velocity, whereas hitting a "wall" of a stiff, highly noncompliant ventricle will result in a rapid drop in the velocity and short E-DT.

|        | Supra-normal | Normal     | Grade I   | Grade II   | Grade III |
| ------ | ------------ | ---------- | --------- | ---------- | --------- |
| **IVRT** | <70 ms     | 70-90 ms   | >90 ms    | 70-90 ms   | <70 ms    |
| **E-DT** | <160 ms    | 160-200 ms | >200 ms   | 160-200 ms | <160 ms   |

Note that it is not really the declaration time, but the rate of deceleration (slope) that has physiologic meaning. This is illustrated by the fact that in some cases of restrictive filling, when E-velocity is very high (>120 cm/s) it takes a long time for the atrium to empty and E-DT may be longer than 160 ms. The reason E-DT has been in use in cardiology, instead of the slope of deceleration, is largely historic: earlier machines lacked automatic tools to calculate slopes, whereas time intervals could be readily measured. It is thus clear that E-DT alone is insufficient to make diagnosis of diastolic dysfunction. E-DT is too not a part of the general algorithm for diagnosis or grading of diastolic dysfunction, according to the 2016 ASE guidelines.

**Answer C.** Peak velocity of tricuspid regurgitant flow (TR $V_{max}$) can be used to estimate systolic pulmonary arterial pressure (PAPs). According to the modified Bernoulli equation,

$\Delta P = 4 \times V^2$, where $\Delta P$ is peak systolic pressure gradient across the tricuspid valve and $V = TR\ V_{max}$, and

$$\Delta P = P_{RV} - P_{RA}$$

In the absence of pulmonic stenosis, $P_{RV}$ ø PAPs, and so

$$PAPs - P_{RA} = 4 \times V^2 \text{ and}$$

$$PAPs = 4 \times V^2 + P_{RA}$$

Note that because RAP estimates are very crude, they introduce a large error into the estimate. Consequently, TR velocity alone has been used as a surrogate for PAPs.

Normal peak tricuspid transvalvular pressure gradient is ≤30 mm Hg, which corresponds to peak velocity ≤2.8 m/s. In this case the TR $V_{max} = 2.1$, which is below the threshold (corresponding pressure gradient is 18 mm Hg, which is normal).

**Answer D.** In diastolic dysfunction E/e' is *increased* and e' is *decreased*, therefore answer D is incorrect.

### Selected References

1. Claessens PJ, Claessens CW, Claessens MM, Claessens MC, Claessens JE. Supernormal left ventricular diastolic function in tri-athletes. *Tex Heart Inst J.* 2001;28(2):102-110.
2. Reuss CS, Wilansky SM, Lester SJ, et al. Using mitral "annulus reversus" to diagnose constrictive pericarditis. *Eur J Echocardiogr.* 2009 May;10(3):372-375. doi:10.1093/ejechocard/jen258. Epub 2008 Oct 24.
3. Silbiger JJ. Pathophysiology and echocardiographic diagnosis of left ventricular diastolic dysfunction. *J Am Soc Echocardiogr.* 2019 Feb;32(2):216-232.e2. doi:10.1016/j.echo.2018.11.011.
4. Welch TD, Ling LH, Espinosa RE, et al. Echocardiographic diagnosis of constrictive pericarditis: Mayo Clinic criteria. *Circ Cardiovasc Imaging.* 2014 May;7(3):526-534. doi:10.1161/CIRCIMAGING.113.001613. Epub 2014 Mar 14.

---

**15.** Correct Answer: **A. Normal diastolic function**

*Rationale:* Recall that assessment of diastolic function starts with the clinical context and echocardiographic evaluation for the presence of overt myocardial disease, in essence an estimation of probability of diastolic dysfunction. This patient has no historical clues to any preexisting cardiac disease and her B-mode echo images reveal normal LV size, thickness, and systolic function. Further, the patient does not fulfill any of the four criteria listed in the 2016 ASE guidelines (**Figure 50.49**). This patient has a normal diastolic function and an alternative explanation to her dyspnea on exertion must be sought, such as, for example, deconditioning.

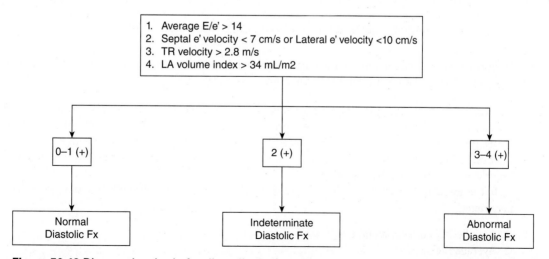

**Figure 50.49** Diagnostic criteria for diastolic dysfunction in patients without avert myocardial disease according to 2016 American Society of Echocardiography (ASE) guidelines. Note the criteria were meant to increase specificity of the diagnosis, and hence it is not sufficient to have abnormal tissue Doppler to be classified as having diastolic dysfunction.

**Selected References**

1. Nagueh SF, Smiseth OA, Appleton CP, et al. Recommendations for the evaluation of left ventricular diastolic function by echocardiography: an update from the American Society of Echocardiography and the European Association of Cardiovascular Imaging. *J Am Soc Echocardiogr.* 2016 Apr;29(4):277-314. doi:10.1016/j.echo.2016.01.011.
2. Oh JK, Kane GC, Seward JB, Tajik AJ, eds. *The Echo Manual.* 4th ed.  Wolters Kluwer; 2019.

**16.** Correct Answer: **D. None of the above**

*Rationale:* In standard notation blood flow spectral Doppler waves are labeled with Latin capital letters, such as E and A, as shown in **Figure 50.50A**. Tissue velocities are designated by addition of apostrophe to a (usually lower case) Latin letter, such as e', a', and s'. The waves of the MV movement are shown in **Figure 50.50B**. Note that both e'- and a'-wave are diastolic events. Systolic movement of the mitral (and tricuspid) annulus toward the apex is designated as s'.

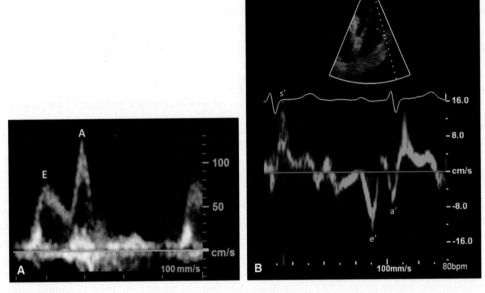

**Figure 50.50**

**Selected Reference**

1. Oh JK, Kane GC, Seward JB, Tajik AJ, eds. *The Echo Manual.* 4th ed.  Wolters Kluwer; 2019.

**17.** Correct Answer: **A. Evaluation for the presence of myocardial disease, such as decreased LV systolic function, LVH, and known diastolic dysfunction**

*Rationale:* The 2016 ASE guidelines separate assessment of diastolic function into two steps. The first is to determine whether myocardial disease is present. "Myocardial disease" is a broad notion here. Importantly, it is NOT limited to CHF with reduced LV systolic function (heart failure with reduced ejection fraction [HFrEF]), but includes conditions such as LVH, and hypertensive heart disease, as well as *qualitatively* present diastolic dysfunction.

In the absence of other myocardial disease, qualitative assessment of diastolic function is based on four parameters:

1. Septal e' <7 cm/s or lateral e' <10 cm/s
2. Average E/e' >14
3. TR velocity >2.8 m/s (equivalent to pressure gradient of >31.4 mm Hg)
4. LAVI >34 mL/m$^2$

If >50% of the criteria are fulfilled (3 or 4)—diastolic dysfunction is present.
If <50% of the criteria are fulfilled (0 or 1)—diastolic dysfunction is absent.

If exactly 50% of the criteria are fulfilled (2)—diastolic function is indeterminate.

*Severity* of diastolic dysfunction, which in practicality boils down to estimation of mean LAP, is reserved for the subsequent step in the evaluation.

Note that inflow pattern is not part of the first step in that algorithm (Figure 50.47), but is the basis of the classification in step 2.

### Selected Reference

1. Nagueh SF, Smiseth OA, Appleton CP, et al. Recommendations for the evaluation of left ventricular diastolic function by echocardiography: an update from the American Society of Echocardiography and the European Association of Cardiovascular Imaging. *J Am Soc Echocardiogr.* 2016 Apr;29(4):277-314. doi:10.1016/j.echo.2016.01.011.

**18.** Correct Answer: C. Grade II diastolic dysfunction

*Rationale:* In this case Doppler parameters are as follows:

E = 0.85 m/s
A = 1.3 m/s
E/A = 0.65
e' septal = 4.2 cm/s
e' lateral = 6.2 cm/s
E/e' septal = = 20.3
E/e' lateral = 13.7
E/e' mean = 17
TR $V_{max}$ = 2.3 m/s
Recall that LAVI = 35 mL/m$^2$

This patient has risk factors for diastolic dysfunction, such as HTN. Presence of hypertensive heart disease by itself (unless HTN is of very recent onset in a young person) can be taken as evidence of diastolic dysfunction. However, if no such historical clues were available, then according to the 2016 ASE guidelines one would start by assessing LV anatomy and systolic function, which in this case are all both normal. Next, in the absence of any myocardial disease, we would have to ascertain the presence of diastolic dysfunction based on four parameters:

1. septal e' <7 cm/s, lateral e' <10 cm/s
2. average E/e' ratio >14 (lateral E/e' ratio >13 or a septal E/e' >15)
3. LA maximum volume index >34 mL/m$^2$
4. peak TR velocity >2.8 m/s

This patient fulfills criteria #1-3, but not #4. He therefore has diastolic dysfunction.

The next step is grading of diastolic dysfunction, which is first done based on the inflow pattern and E/A ratio. In this case E/A = 0.65, which is below the cutoff of 0.8, that is, an A-dominant pattern is present. However, ASE guidelines identify a special subgroup of patients with A-dominant inflow pattern, those with very high E-wave velocity (>50 cm/s) and puts them together with those with "pseudonormal" filling (see Figure 50.47B).

This patient's E-velocity is 85 cm/s, and therefore, the next step requires consideration of additional three criteria:

1. Average E/e' >14
2. TR velocity >2.8 m/s
3. LAVI >34 mL/m$^2$

This patient satisfies criteria #1 and #3, but not #2. Two of three positive criteria classify this patient as having grade II diastolic dysfunction. Note that if LAVI was not available, the diastolic function would be classified as "indeterminate" and would require further assessment.

Grade II diastolic dysfunction implies elevated mean LAP.

### Selected Reference

1. Nagueh SF, Smiseth OA, Appleton CP, et al. Recommendations for the evaluation of left ventricular diastolic function by echocardiography: an update from the American Society of Echocardiography and the European Association of Cardiovascular Imaging. *J Am Soc Echocardiogr.* 2016 Apr;29(4):277-314. doi:10.1016/j.echo.2016.01.011.

**19.** Correct Answer: B. Grade I diastolic dysfunction with normal LV filling pressures

*Rationale:* Normal pattern of PV flow is such that S < D. (See also **Figure 50.51**.)

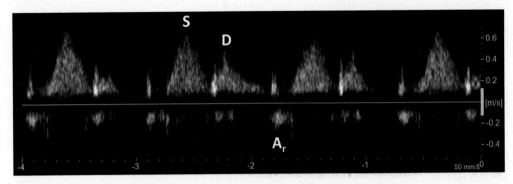

**Figure 50.51** Spectral Doppler of pulmonary venous (PV) flow obtained from the superior medial pulmonary vein with district waves labeled. Several parameters are used for assessment of diastolic function based on PV flow.

With advancing stages of diastolic dysfunction, like many other Doppler parameters, S/D undergoes a biphasic change. First, in grade I diastolic dysfunction, S becomes larger than D. However, as the severity of diastolic dysfunction progresses, S/D normalizes (pseudonormalizes) in stage II and then drops further in restrictive filling (stage III) with S<<D. Consequently, interpretation of S/D, just like interpretation of E/A, is not straightforward. In patients with impaired systolic function, in whom normal (and supra-normal) filling patterns are excluded by definition, S/D < 1 indicates elevated LAP. In patients with normal LV function, interpretation is more complex and depends on other parameters:

S/D

D-wave deceleration time (D-DT) (**Figure 50.52A**)
Duration of Ar-wave and particularly,

- Difference between duration of PV Ar (**Figure 50.52B**) and duration of mitral inflow A-wave (**Figure 50.53**), Ar-A duration.

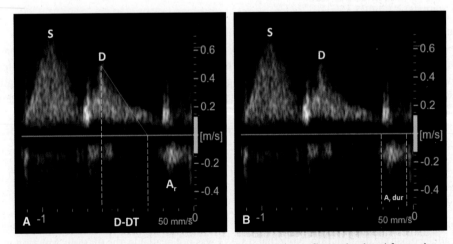

**Figure 50.52** A. Spectral Doppler of pulmonary venous flow obtained from the superior medial pulmonary vein with district waves labeled. D-DT is D-wave deceleration time. B. Spectral Doppler of pulmonary venous flow obtained from the superior medial pulmonary vein with district waves labeled. Ar-wave duration (Ar-dur) is labeled.

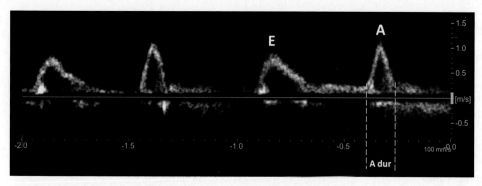

**Figure 50.53** Spectral Doppler of mitral inflow. A-wave duration (A dur) is labeled.

S/D ratio follows a biphasic course as severity of diastolic dysfunction progresses. In this case S>D, suggesting either a supra-normal filling or grade I diastolic dysfunction, both of which would be associated with normal LAP. Note that in this case presence of multiple risk factors and LVH should be taken as evidence of impaired diastolic function, thus excluding supra-normal pattern from the differential.

|  | Supra-normal | Normal | Grade I | Grade II | Grade III |
|---|---|---|---|---|---|
| **IVRT** | <70 ms | 70-90 ms | >90 ms | 70-90 ms | <70 ms |
| **E-DT** | <160 ms | 160-200 ms | >200 ms | 160-200 ms | <160 ms |
| **S/D** | S<<D | S<D | S>D | S<D | S<<D |

D-wave corresponds to the flow from the PV into the LA during rapid filling. In this phase of the cardiac cycle there is a continuous column of blood between the PV, LA, and left ventricle. Thus, in the absence of MS, recordings of flow from PV and MV inflow measure the flow of the same column of blood at two different locations. Consequently, changes in that flow will affect both measurements similarly. As a result, E-DT and D-DT have similar interpretation. Both E-DT and D-DT undergo biphasic changes as diastolic dysfunction progresses. In grade I it lengthens. As physiology switches from "pull" to "push" in grade II diastolic dysfunction, DT shortens again. DT becomes very short in grade III (restrictive filling). The reported cutoff for the DT in restrictive filling for the E-wave is <160 ms (if E-wave peak is <120 cm/s) and **<150 ms for the D-wave**. In this case E-DT can be estimated to be >200 ms, which is abnormally long (normal is 160-200 ms). D-DT in this case is also long at 300 ms.

Finally, Ar and A are registering flows generated by the contracting LA, albeit in the opposite direction. The duration of these waves will depend (among other factors) on compliance of the left ventricle and PV circuit, respectively. As LV filling pressure increases, duration of the A-wave decreases and Ar-A duration lengthens. The advantage of this parameter is that it does *not* follow a biphasic course with progression of diastolic dysfunction, and it appears that a long **Ar-A duration (>30 ms)** is associated with elevated LAP regardless of the systolic LV function. In this case, A duration is approximately 140 ms and Ar duration is approximately 150 ms, thus the difference between the two is not significant.

Of note, it has been suggested that among patients with normal grade I filling patterns based on mitral inflow velocities and mitral annular tissue Doppler parameters, there may exist a subgroup of patients (a so-called grade Ib) who may have elevated LAP. These patients are identified based on Ar-A duration being prolonged. This subclassification has not been included in the 2016 ASE guidelines.

In conclusion, this patient likely has grade I diastolic dysfunction with normal LAP. Her dyspnea is unlikely to be due to cardiac etiology and is likely solely due to acute viral pneumonia.

### Selected References

1. Nagueh SF, Smiseth OA, Appleton CP, et al. Recommendations for the evaluation of left ventricular diastolic function by echocardiography: an update from the American Society of Echocardiography and the European Association of Cardiovascular Imaging. *J Am Soc Echocardiogr.* 2016 Apr;29(4):277-314. doi:10.1016/j.echo.2016.01.011.
2. Silbiger JJ. Pathophysiology and echocardiographic diagnosis of left ventricular diastolic dysfunction. *J Am Soc Echocardiogr.* 2019 Feb;32(2):216-232.e2. doi:10.1016/j.echo.2018.11.011.
3. Tabata T, Thomas JD, Klein AL. Pulmonary venous flow by Doppler echocardiography: revisited 12 years later. *J Am Coll Cardiol.* 2003 Apr 16;41(8):1243-1250. doi: 10.1016/s0735-1097(03)00126-8.
4. Yamamoto K, Nishimura RA, Chaliki HP, Appleton CP, Holmes DR Jr, Redfield MM. Determination of left ventricular filling pressure by Doppler echocardiography in patients with coronary artery disease: critical role of left ventricular systolic function. *J Am Coll Cardiol.* 1997 Dec;30(7):1819-1826. doi:10.1016/s0735-1097(97)00390-2.

**20.** Correct Answer: D. Grade III diastolic dysfunction

*Rationale:* Doppler parameters in this case are as follows:

TR $V_{max}$ = 2.9 m/s
E = 118 cm/s
A = 35 cm/s
E/A = 3.4
e' septal = 8.1 cm/s
e' lat = 8.9 cm/s
E/e' septal = 14.5
E/e' lat = 13.3
E/e' mean = 13.9
LAVI is not available

This patient has a history of HTN and DM2, which are both risk factors for diastolic dysfunction. In addition, he has significant LVH on the echo, placing him in the category of having (or being at very high risk of having) diastolic dysfunction. The next step is assessment of the degree of diastolic dysfunction, which starts with assessment of E/A. This patient has a restrictive filling pattern with E/A > 2, which categorizes him as having grade III diastolic dysfunction. Restrictive filling pattern implies elevated LAP.

**21.** Correct Answer: C. Elevated LAP as estimated echocardiographically (e.g., by E/e') predicts failure to extubate.

*Rationale:* Despite initial enthusiasm about E/e' being linearly related to mean LAP, further research showed that the correlation is rather weak ($r^2$ = 0.3). Application of 2016 ASE guidelines leaves between 17% and 49% of patients with indeterminate diastolic function. In mechanically ventilated patients, sensitivity and specificity of the ASE algorithm were both 74%, with corresponding LR(+) of 2.8 and LR(−) of 0.35, hardly a spectacular performance. On the other hand, there is evidence that elevated LAP, as estimated by echocardiography, is associated with increased mortality in sepsis and with failure to extubate. In practical terms, it is critical to understand that positive end-expiratory pressure (PEEP) decreases both pre- and afterload on the left ventricle, and that removing PEEP has a potential to suddenly overload a noncompliant ventricle, resulting in flash pulmonary edema and failure to extubate.

### Selected References

1. Brault C, Marc J, Mercado P, et al. Estimation of pulmonary artery occlusion pressure using Doppler echocardiography in mechanically ventilated patients. *Crit Care Med.* 2020 Oct;48(10):e943-e950. doi:10.1097/CCM.0000000000004512.
2. Lancellotti P, Galderisi M, Edvardsen T, et al. Echo-Doppler estimation of left ventricular filling pressure: results of the multicentre EACVI Euro-Filling study. *Eur Heart J Cardiovasc Imaging.* 2017 Sep 1;18(9):961-968. doi:10.1093/ehjci/jex067.
3. Mourad M, Chow-Chine L, Faucher M, et al. Early diastolic dysfunction is associated with intensive care unit mortality in cancer patients presenting with septic shock. *Br J Anaesth.* 2014 Jan;112(1):102-109. doi:10.1093/bja/aet296. Epub 2013 Sep 17.
4. Nagueh SF, Middleton KJ, Kopelen HA, Zoghbi WA, Quiñones MA. Doppler tissue imaging: a noninvasive technique for evaluation of left ventricular relaxation and estimation of filling pressures. *J Am Coll Cardiol.* 1997 Nov 15;30(6):1527-1533. doi:10.1016/s0735-1097(97)00344-6.
5. Nauta JF, Hummel YM, van der Meer P, Lam CSP, Voors AA, van Melle JP. Correlation with invasive left ventricular filling pressures and prognostic relevance of the echocardiographic diastolic parameters used in the 2016 ESC heart failure guidelines and in the 2016 ASE/EACVI recommendations: a systematic review in patients with heart failure with preserved ejection fraction. *Eur J Heart Fail.* 2018 Sep;20(9):1303-1311. doi:10.1002/ejhf.1220. Epub 2018 Jun 7.
6. Sanfilippo F, Di Falco D, Noto A, et al. Association of weaning failure from mechanical ventilation with transthoracic echocardiography parameters: a systematic review and meta-analysis. *Br J Anaesth.* 2020. https://doi.org/10.1016/j.bja.2020.07.059.
7. Sturgess DJ, Marwick TH, Joyce C, et al. Prediction of hospital outcome in septic shock: a prospective comparison of tissue Doppler and cardiac biomarkers. *Crit Care.* 2010;14(2):R44. doi:10.1186/cc8931. Epub 2010 Mar 24.

**22.** Correct Answer: D. All of the above

*Rationale:* Assessment of diastolic function is complex, and the 2016 ASE algorithm leaves many patients in the indeterminate category. Many additional parameters have been proposed as indices of elevated LA pressure in certain clinical circumstances.

All the choices would be indicative of a restrictive filling pattern except for the listed PV flow parameters.

PV flow velocities on transthoracic echocardiography (TTE) are usually obtained from the right superior PV in the apical four-chamber view (**Figure 50.54**). Unfortunately, in many patients, the PV may not be visualized, limiting the utility of PV flow velocities.

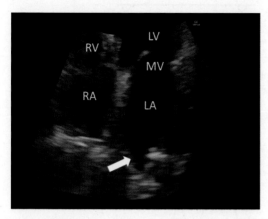

**Figure 50.54** Apical four-chamber view, zoomed-in on the left atrium. Right superior pulmonary vein is indicated with an *arrow*.

Normal PV flow pattern is shown in **Figure 50.55A**. Recorded from the apical four-chamber view, spectral PWD of the PV flow features three positive deflections (flow toward the heart) and one negative deflection (flow away from the heart). The systolic (positive) deflections are designated as S1 and S2, the diastolic positive flow as D, and negative deflection (also diastolic) as Ar (for atrial reversal). In most people S1 and S2 waves are fused together forming a single systolic S-wave, as shown in **Figure 50.55B**. Most of the S-wave is generated by the suctioning effect of the relaxing left ventricle, which draws blood from the LA into the left ventricle, and simultaneously from the PVs into the LA. In early diastole during rapid LV filling, blood flows through the open MV from the LA into the left ventricle. The passive emptying of the LA draws blood from the PVs into the LA, generating the D-wave. Finally, in late diastole, the LA contracts and pushes blood into the left ventricle, but simultaneously backward into the PVs. **Figure 50.55C** illustrates that, in healthy people, the PV D-wave corresponds to the same physiologic event as the mitral inflow E-wave. Consequently, both peak D-wave velocity and D-DT have interpretation similar to the corresponding parameters of the mitral E-wave.

In a normal heart, the PV S-wave is smaller than the D-wave. With progression of the degree of diastolic dysfunction, S/D ratio undergoes biphasic changes similar to E/A ratio, as shown in **Figure 50.55D-F**. In grade I diastolic dysfunction the S-wave becomes larger than the D-wave. In grade II, however, the ratio normalizes (a pseudonormal pattern) with S< D. In grade III (restrictive filling) the D-wave becomes much larger than S, a pattern that can also be seen in healthy young athletes (supra-normal pattern).

As can be expected based on the knowledge of E-DT, the pattern of D-DT also follows a biphasic course. In grade I diastolic dysfunction D-DT lengthens. Then, as the physiology of LV filling changes from "pull" to "push," in grade II diastolic dysfunction D-DT shortens again. D-DT becomes very short in grade III (restrictive filling). The reported cutoff for the D-DT in restrictive filling for the E-wave is <160 ms (if E-wave peak is <120 cm/s) and <150 ms for the D-wave.

The Ar-wave corresponds to the A-wave of the mitral inflow but is quite identical to it. As the LA contracts, the blood is ejected in two directions: into the left ventricle and back into the PVs. Difference in durations of Ar- and A-waves is meaningful and lengthens as compliance of the left ventricle decreases. In restrictive filling Ar-A is usually >30 ms. The peak of pulmonary wave Ar is also usually high in patients with elevated LVEDPs. Note that, just like the A-wave, Ar-wave is absent in patients with atrial fibrillation.

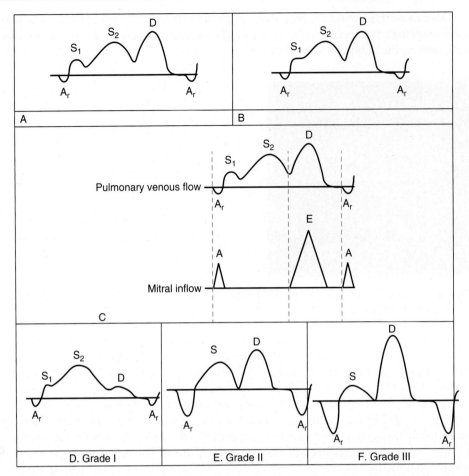

**Figure 50.55** A. On invasive monitoring, and occasionally on spectral Doppler, there are two systolic waves, labeled $S_1$ and $S_2$. These are followed by a diastolic wave (D). Finally, during atrial contraction, atrial reversal flow is seen (Ar-wave), which coincides with atrial contraction. B. Frequently $S_1$ and $S_2$ waves fuse together and the fusion is termed simply "S-wave." C. Timing of the D-wave of pulmonary venous flow corresponds to the E-wave of mitral inflow, while the Ar-wave (in normal individuals) starts simultaneously with the A-wave. D-F. Different patterns of pulmonary vein flow by the grade of diastolic dysfunction. (D: Grade I; E: Grade II, F: Grade III.)

## Selected References

1. Nagueh SF, Smiseth OA, Appleton CP, et al. Recommendations for the evaluation of left ventricular diastolic function by echocardiography: an update from the American Society of Echocardiography and the European Association of Cardiovascular Imaging. *J Am Soc Echocardiogr.* 2016 Apr;29(4):277-314. doi:10.1016/j.echo.2016.01.011.
2. Oh JK, Kane GC, Seward JB, Tajik AJ, eds. *The Echo Manual.* 4th ed. Wolters Kluwer; 2019.
3. Tabata T, Thomas JD, Klein AL. Pulmonary venous flow by Doppler echocardiography: revisited 12 years later. *J Am Coll Cardiol.* 2003 Apr 16;41(8):1243-1250. doi:10.1016/s0735-1097(03)00126-8.
4. Yingchoncharoen T, Wuttichaipradit C, Klein AL. Echo Doppler parameters of diastolic function. In: Lang RM, Goldstein SA, Kronzon I, Khandheria BK, Mor-Avi V, eds. *ASE's Comprehensive Echocardiography.* 2nd ed. Saunders, an imprint of Elsevier Inc.; 2016. ISBN: 978-0-323-26011-4

---

**23.** Correct Answer: D. Short E-DT is consistent with high LV filling pressures.

*Rationale:* This patient has moderately decreased LV systolic function and is in atrial fibrillation, as stated in the clinical vignette. (See also **Figures 50.56, 50.57,** and **50.58.**)

- LA size in patients with chronic atrial fibrillation does not correlate with LV filling pressures.
- Peak velocity and DT of mitral E-wave vary with the length of the cardiac cycle. Ideally, measurements from several cardiac cycles with relatively normal R-R intervals should be averaged.
- Absence of atrial contraction eliminates A-wave of mitral inflow and Ar-wave of PV flow.

- S-wave of PV flow consists of two components: S1 and S2. S1 is believed to reflect atrial relaxation (after atrial contraction in late diastole). In atrial fibrillation, the atrium does not contract in an organized manner and therefore there is no organized relaxation. Consequently, the S1 component and the composite S-wave are almost always diminished in atrial fibrillation.

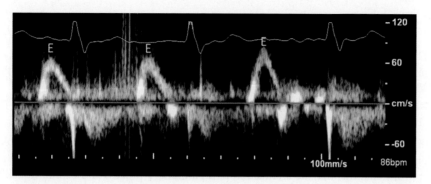

**Figure 50.56** Mitral inflow velocity spectral pulse-wave Doppler. The R-R intervals are varied and there are no P-waves present on the electrocardiogram. There is no A-wave present on the Doppler tracing. E-waves are labeled.

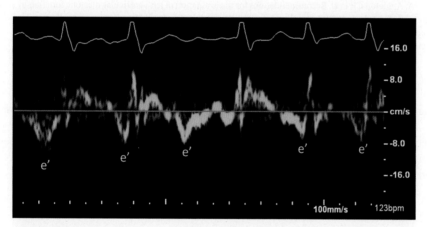

**Figure 50.57** Medial tissue Doppler imaging of the mitral annulus. e'-waves are labeled. Atrial fibrillation.

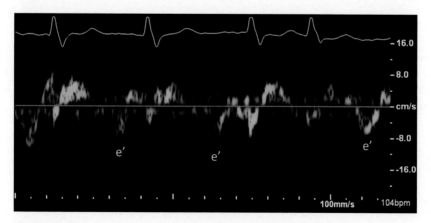

**Figure 50.58** Lateral tissue Doppler imaging of the mitral annulus. e'-waves are labeled. Atrial fibrillation.

Assessment of diastolic function in patients with atrial fibrillation is better studied in patients with depressed LV systolic function. Several parameters have been shown to correlate with LV filling pressures:

- E-DT ≤160 ms[#][*]
- IVRT ≤65 ms
- PV D-DT ≤220 ms
- E/mitral Vp (E/Vp) ≥1.4[^]
- E/e' ratio ≥11

# E-DT should be measured only in cycles in which E-wave terminates before the onset of QRS.

* E-DT is a particularly useful parameter for assessment of diastolic function in patients with decreased systolic LV function.

^ this parameter combines mitral inflow Doppler E-wave height with a CMM parameter—flow propagation velocity.

In this case, the patient's E-DT = 108 ms and E/e' = 94, which are both consistent with elevated LV filling pressure. High TR $V_{max}$ suggests elevated PAP. However, in a patient with chronic COPD and acute severe interstitial pneumonia, this may be a reflection of a pulmonary process and cannot be taken as evidence of elevated LA pressure.

### Selected References

1. Kotecha D, Mohamed M, Shantsila E, Popescu BA, Steeds RP. Is echocardiography valid and reproducible in patients with atrial fibrillation? A systematic review. *Europace*. 2017 Sep 1;19(9):1427-1438. doi:10.1093/europace/eux027.
2. Nagueh SF, Smiseth OA, Appleton CP, et al. Recommendations for the evaluation of left ventricular diastolic function by echocardiography: an update from the American Society of Echocardiography and the European Association of Cardiovascular Imaging. *J Am Soc Echocardiogr*. 2016 Apr;29(4):277-314. doi:10.1016/j.echo.2016.01.011.
3. Oh JK, Kane GC, Seward JB, Tajik AJ, eds. *The Echo Manual*. 4th ed. Wolters Kluwer; 2019.

**24.** Correct Answer: A. In patients with severe MAC E/e' is unreliable.

*Rationale:* In patients with MAC E-velocity tends to be falsely elevated because of the mild narrowing of the valve. E' tends to be lower, because of the restriction of the stiff calcified annulus, particularly in its lateral part. Consequently, E/e' ratio can be elevated solely because of the valve calcification. This does not mean that LV filling pressures in patients with severe MAC cannot be estimated.

From the provided data the measured Doppler parameters are as follows:

TR $V_{max}$ (m/s): 3.5
E' med = 3 cm/s
E' lat = 6 cm/s
E' mean = 4.5 cm/s
E= 180 cm/s
A = 80 cm/s
E/A = 2.25
E/e' mean = 40

An algorithm based on E/A appears to perform well in patients with moderate-severe MAC (**Figure 50.59**). According to this classification scheme, patients with E/A in excess of 1.8 are very likely to have elevated LV filling pressures, patients with E/A <0.8 are very unlikely to have elevated LV filling pressure, and those in the intermediate group can be further classified based on IVRT.

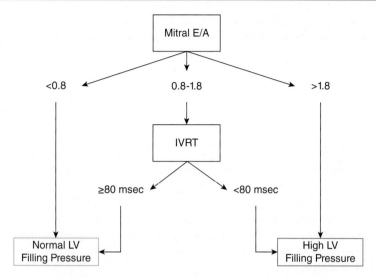

**Figure 50.59** Algorithm for estimation of left ventricular filling pressure in patients with moderate-severe mitral annular calcification.

Other reliable estimates of LV filling pressures are based on PV velocities and TR velocity.

This patient has significantly elevated E/A and high peak TR velocity, strongly suggesting elevated LA pressure.

### Selected References

1. Abudiab MM, Chebrolu LH, Schutt RC, Nagueh SF, Zoghbi WA. Doppler echocardiography for the estimation of LV filling pressure in patients with mitral annular calcification. *JACC Cardiovasc Imaging.* 2017 Dec;10(12):1411-1420. doi:10.1016/j.jcmg.2016.10.017. Epub 2017 Mar 15.
2. Oh JK, Kane GC, Seward JB, Tajik AJ, eds. *The Echo Manual.* 4th ed. Wolters Kluwer; 2019.

**25.** Correct Answer: A. The findings are suggestive of elevated LV filling pressures, and therefore diastolic CHF may be contributing to her symptoms.

*Rationale:* Mitral inflow spectral Doppler tracing (**Figure 50.60**) in this case shows the presence of an L-wave as well as a restrictive filling pattern in an elderly patient with arterial HTN.

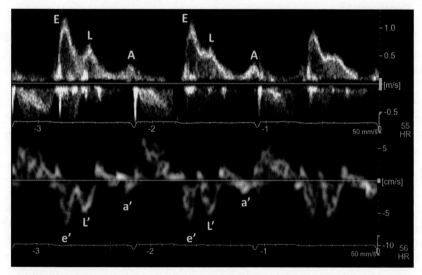

**Figure 50.60** Mitral inflow and tissue Doppler imaging of the lateral mitral annulus with waves labeled.

The L-wave in this case may be incorrectly identified as an A-wave, leading to completely wrong conclusions. In this case the measurements were as follows:

E = 1.1 m/s
A = 0.35 m/s
E/A = 3.54
E' lateral = 0.07 m/s
E/e' lat = 16

Mechanism of L-wave generation is controversial, but it seems to occur when the left ventricle is stiff and transmitral flow is high. In certain clinical scenarios, this can be taken as evidence of increased LV filling pressure. Other conditions, notably severe MR, can result in an L-wave. Importantly, normal bradycardic patients may exhibit this filling pattern as well. In this patient recorded HR is 55 bpm, which by itself may have produced an L-wave. Nonetheless, a combination of L-wave with a restrictive filling pattern (E/A >> 2) is highly suggestive of elevated LV filling pressures. When performed, tissue Doppler of the mitral annulus also showed an L'-wave, corresponding to the L-wave of mitral inflow. E/e' = 16 is also consistent with elevated LV filling pressures.

Selected Reference

1. Kerut EK. The mitral L-wave: a relatively common but ignored useful finding. *Echocardiography*. 2008 May;25(5):548-550. doi:10.1111/j.1540-8175.2007.00626.x. Epub 2008 Feb 12.

---

**26.** Correct Answer: D. None of the above

*Rationale:* The patient is certainly in normal sinus rhythm as evidenced by the ECG shown in Figure 50.37. Despite the presence of synchronized electrical atrial activity detected as a P-wave on ECG, it takes weeks after conversion to normal sinus rhythm for the atrium to recover its organized mechanical contractility. Consequently, diminished A-wave and false "restrictive filling pattern" are known to occur in these patients in the period immediately following cardioversion. PV flow Ar-wave is caused by the same atrial contraction as the A-wave of mitral inflow and is expected to be absent or greatly diminished in this patient.

Selected Reference

1. Manning WJ, Silverman DI, Katz SE, et al. Impaired left atrial mechanical function after cardioversion: relation to the duration of atrial fibrillation. *J Am Coll Cardiol*. 1994 Jun;23(7):1535-1540. doi:10.1016/0735-1097(94)90652-1.

---

**27.** Correct Answer: A. Significant AS

*Rationale:* Standard approach to assessment of LV diastolic function is valid in patients with significant AS.

The following conditions are specifically identified in the 2016 ASE guidelines as requiring deviation from the standard recommended approach to LV diastolic function assessment.

**Hypertrophic cardiomyopathy**

| | |
|---|---|
| Average E/e' >14<br>Ar-A duration ≥ 30 ms<br>TR $V_{max}$ >2.8 m/s<br>LAVI >34 mL/m² | < 2 criteria fulfilled—grade I + LAP wnl (within normal limits)<br>>2/4 criteria or >1/3 criteria fulfilled—grade II + high LAP<br>2/4 criteria fulfilled—inconclusive |
| Restrictive pattern (E/A > 2) Low mitral annular e' (septal <7 cm/s, lateral <10 cm/s) | If both criteria fulfilled—grade III + high LAP |

**Restrictive Cardiomyopathy (Figure 59.61)**

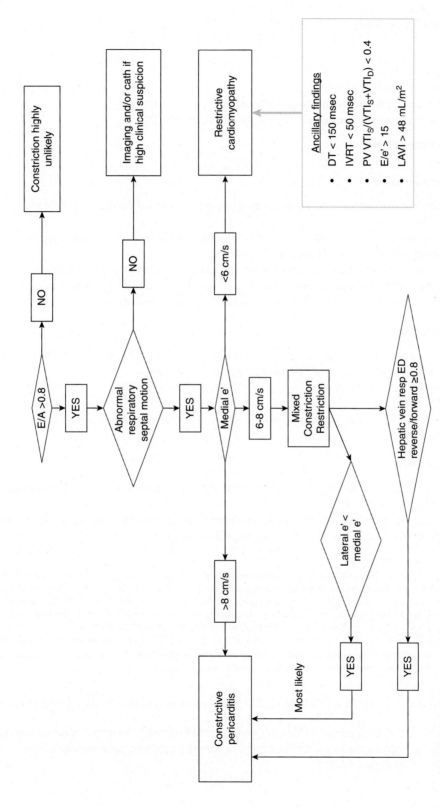

**Figure 50.61**

### MS

IVRT <60 ms—high specificity
IVRT/$T_{E-e'}$ <4.2
Mitral A velocity >1.5 m/s

### MR

Ar-A duration ≥ 30 ms
IVRT <60 ms—high specificity
IVRT/$T_{E-e'}$ <5.6 (if LV systolic function is normal)
Average E/e' >14 (may be considered in patients with depressed EF)

### MAC (see Figure 59.59)

### Heart Transplantation

- Depending on the surgical technique, LA may be partially excised during transplantation, altering mitral inflow pattern.
- Posttransplant, the heart is denervated and is frequently tachycardic at rest, resulting in E-A fusion and making analysis of mitral inflow impossible.
- Performance of standard parameters in heart transplant recipients is largely unknown.
- E/e' lateral > 22 had sensitivity 56%, spec 95%, LR(+) = 11, and LR(−) = 0.46 for detection of PCWP >12 mm Hg, indicating limited ability to r/o diastolic dysfunction.

### Atrial Fibrillation

- E-DT ≤ 160 ms. Note: DT should be measured only when E-velocity ends before the onset of QRS. Better parameter in patients with decreased systolic LV function.
- IVRT ≤65 ms
- PV D-DT ≤220 ms
- E/mitral Vp (E/Vp) ≥1.4—combination of Doppler E-wave and CMM parameters
- E/e' ratio ≥11

### Noncardiac PHTN

When cardiac etiology is present, lateral E/e' is >13, whereas in patients with PHTN due to a noncardiac etiology, lateral E/e' is <8.

Neither significant AS nor significant AR requires modification of the approach. Special care must be taken in significant AR to place Doppler sampling volume correctly.

Selected References
1. Badano LP, Miglioranza MH, Edvardsen T, et al. European Association of Cardiovascular Imaging/Cardiovascular Imaging Department of the Brazilian Society of Cardiology recommendations for the use of cardiac imaging to assess and follow patients after heart transplantation. *Eur Heart J Cardiovasc Imaging.* 2015 Sep;16(9):919-948. doi:10.1093/ehjci/jev139. Epub 2015 Jul 2.
2. Broch K, Al-Ani A, Gude E, Gullestad L, Aakhus S. Echocardiographic evaluation of left ventricular filling pressure in heart transplant recipients. *Scand Cardiovasc J.* 2014 Dec;48(6):349-356. doi:10.3109/14017431.2014.981579.
3. Nagueh SF, Smiseth OA, Appleton CP, et al. Recommendations for the evaluation of left ventricular diastolic function by echocardiography: an update from the American Society of Echocardiography and the European Association of Cardiovascular Imaging. *J Am Soc Echocardiogr.* 2016 Apr;29(4):277-314. doi:10.1016/j.echo.2016.01.011.

**28.** Correct Answer: **D. Color M-mode (CMM). Mitral inflow propagation velocity is being assessed.**

*Rationale:* As the name suggests, CMM combines M-mode with color Doppler. Unlike conventional color Doppler, CMM displays color-coded velocity of flow along a single interrogation line (aligned with inflow jet) over time. (See **Figure 50.62.**)

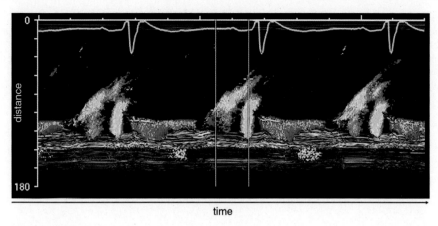

**Figure 50.62**

Recall that in M-mode display distance is plotted on the Y-axis and time on the X-axis.

Color Doppler for these purposes is obtained in the apical four-chamber view, with the M-mode interrogation line aligned with the mitral inflow.

The baseline of the color Doppler is shifted up to allow for more aliasing within the early diastolic jet tracing. All the points along the first aliasing interface (the border between the yellow and the blue) are moving with the same velocity (aliasing velocity) and form an isovelocity curve. In its initial segment the curve is usually a straight line, that is, isovelocity line. The other way to conceptualize isovelocity line is to think of it as a depiction of a particular velocity "moving" in space: propagating from the MV into the LV cavity over time. The slope of the isovelocity line is the velocity with which the flow front propagates, termed flow propagation velocity and labeled as Vp. Normal Vp <50 cm/s (0.5 m/s). An indexed value of E/Vp has been used for assessment of diastolic function with E/Vp ≥ 2.5 predicting LAP > 15.

**Selected Reference**

1. Oh JK. Assessment of diastolic function. *In*: Oh JK, Kane GC, Seward JB, Tajik AJ, eds. *The Echo Manual*. 4th ed. Wolters Kluwer; 2019.

---

**29. Correct Answer: A. It suggests that LV end-diastolic pressure (EDP) is elevated.**

*Rationale:* The finding, termed "A-dip," has been described in critically ill patients with elevated LVEDP. AR need not be severe, but acute AR is more likely than chronic to cause elevation in LVEDP. In this case AR was mild-moderate. A-dip disappeared with diuretic therapy and inotropic support.

**Selected References**

1. Giannakopoulos G, Rey F, Müller H. Pathophysiology of the aortic regurgitation Doppler signal end-diastolic notching: "a-dip insight." *Echocardiography*. 2020 Jul;37(7):1116-1119. doi:10.1111/echo.14774. Epub 2020 Jun 20.
2. Sethi JS, Shah A, Benenstein R, Rosenzweig BP, Tunick PA, Kronzon I. The a-dip of aortic regurgitation. *J Am Soc Echocardiogr*. 2003 Oct;16(10):1078-1079. doi:10.1016/S0894-7317(03)00473-5.

---

**30. Correct Answer: D. Diastolic MR**

*Rationale:* Downward deflection on the spectral graph is seen before the onset of QRS, timing it to diastole. All the choices listed are associated with elevated LVEDP. A-dip is a notch on the AR spectral Doppler tracing. B-bump is a late diastolic opening of the MV, usually seen in M-mode. L-wave is an "extra" mid-diastolic mitral inflow wave usually detected by PWD.

Diastolic MR is only possible when there is a positive pressure gradient between the left ventricle and the LA. This gradient can be achieved by either unusually low LA pressure or unusually high LV pressure. The former is the case in a variety of conditions in which there is a long time interval between atrial emptying and ventricular systole (atrioventricular block, long interval in atrial fibrillation). The latter is seen in cases of either systolic or diastolic heart failure. In published literature, the most common condition leading to elevated LVEDP is acute aortic insufficiency.

Selected References

1. Silbiger JJ. Pathophysiology and echocardiographic diagnosis of left ventricular diastolic dysfunction. *J Am Soc Echocardiogr.* 2019 Feb;32(2):216-232.e2. doi:10.1016/j.echo.2018.11.011.
2. Veyrat C, Sebaoun G, Fitoussi M, Abitbol G, Dumora P, Kalmanson D. Detection of diastolic mitral regurgitation using pulsed Doppler and its implications. *Eur Heart J.* 1987 Aug;8(8):878-887. doi:10.1093/oxfordjournals.eurheartj.a062352.

# 51 | ECHOCARDIOGRAPHY IN ASSESSMENT AND MANAGEMENT OF ACUTE AND CHRONIC RIGHT HEART FAILURE

Talal Dahhan and Fawaz Alenezi

1. Which of the following indicates the correct location for measurement of the inferior vena cava (IVC) diameter in this view (**Figure 51.1**)?

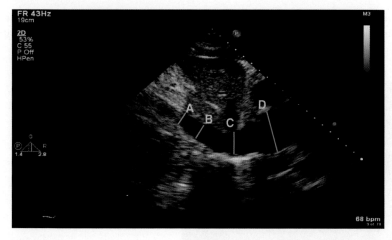

**Figure 51.1**

A. A
B. B
C. C
D. D

2. A 47-year-old woman with a diagnosis of massive acute pulmonary embolism is admitted to the intensive care unit (ICU). She is intubated and is receiving mechanical ventilation. Transthoracic echocardiography is performed. Based on the hepatic vein Doppler flow pattern (**Figure 51.2**), what is the estimate of the right atrial pressure (RAP)?

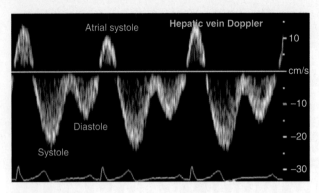

**Figure 51.2**

A. Normal RAP
B. Cannot be estimated
C. Low RAP
D. High RAP

3. Which of the following is the most sensitive and specific echocardiographic parameter for RAP assessment?

A. Tricuspid valve regurgitation severity
B. RA size
C. Tricuspid annular plane systolic excursion (TAPSE)
D. Hepatic vein systolic filling fraction

4. What is the estimated pulmonary artery pressure (PAP) in this patient if the tricuspid regurgitation (TR) peak velocity is 3.2 m/s (**Figure 51.3**) and the IVC diameter is 2.3 cm while collapsing 20% with inspiration?

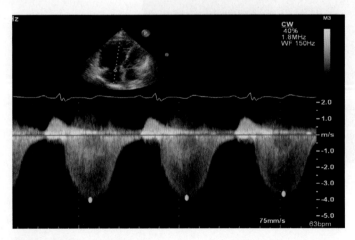

**Figure 51.3**

A. 30 to 39 mm Hg
B. 40 to 49 mm Hg
C. 50 to 59 mm Hg
D. 60 to 69 mm Hg

5. In **Figure 51.4**, which of the following is the correct location of the basal right ventricular (RV) dimension?

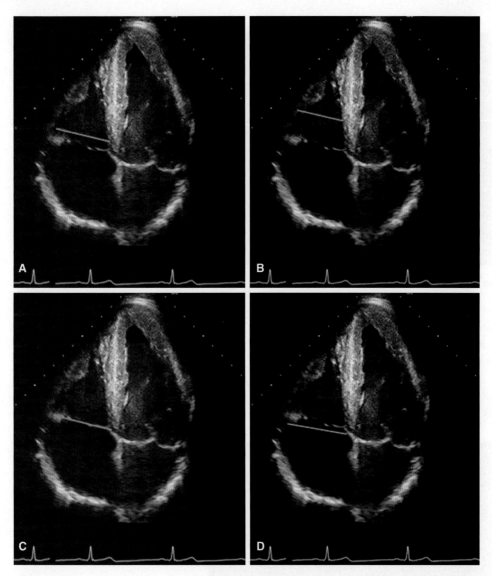

**Figure 51.4**

A. A
B. B
C. C
D. D

6. A 63-year-old man presents with shortness of breath, bilateral lower limb edema, and elevated jugular venous pressure. What is the possible diagnosis based on the views shown in **Figure 51.5** and ▶ **Video 51.1**?

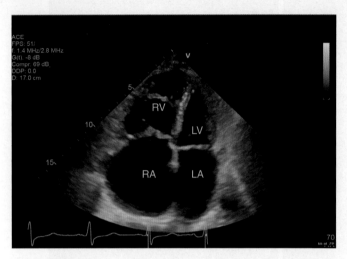

**Figure 51.5**

**A.** RV infarction
**B.** Pulmonary arterial hypertension
**C.** Acute pulmonary embolism
**D.** Carcinoid heart disease

7. Which of the following letters indicates the correct TAPSE M-mode cursor alignment from **Figure 51.6**?

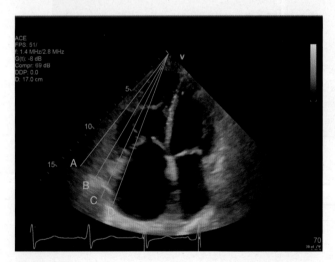

**Figure 51.6**

**A.** A
**B.** B
**C.** C
**D.** D

8. What is the estimated "degree of pulmonary hypertension" based on this tricuspid regurgitant Doppler (**Figure 51.7**) velocity?

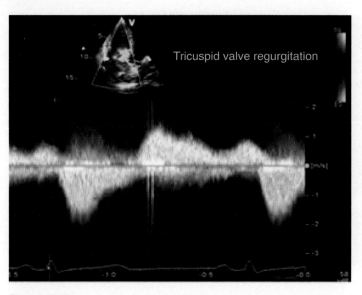

Tricuspid valve regurgitation

**Figure 51.7**

A. Mild pulmonary hypertension
B. Moderate pulmonary hypertension
C. Severe pulmonary hypertension
D. Cannot determine

9. In this short-axis transthoracic echocardiogram (▶ **Video 51.2** and **Figure 51.8**) of the left ventricle at the level of papillary muscle, what is the most probable diagnosis?

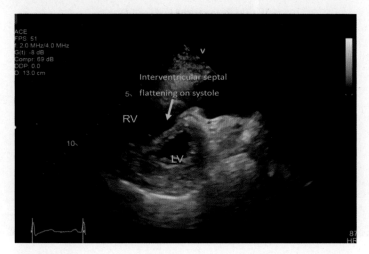

Interventricular septal flattening on systole

RV

LV

**Figure 51.8**

A. Normal RV pressure and volume
B. Low RV pressure
C. RV pressure overload
D. RV volume overload

**10.** In this short-axis transthoracic echocardiogram (▶ **Video 51.3** and **Figure 51.9**) of the left ventricle at the level of papillary muscle, what is the most probable diagnosis?

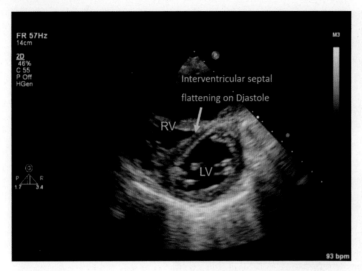

**Figure 51.9**

**A.** Significant tricuspid valve regurgitation
**B.** Significant pulmonary valve stenosis
**C.** Left ventricular volume overload
**D.** RV pressure overload

**11.** What is the estimated RAP based on the IVC diameter and collapse in **Figure 51.10** and ▶ **Video 51.4**?

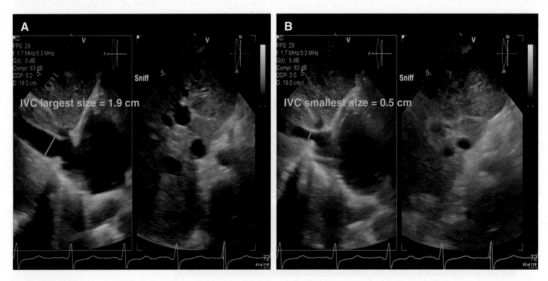

**Figure 51.10**

**A.** 3 to 5 mm Hg
**B.** 20 to 25 mm Hg
**C.** 10 to 15 mm Hg
**D.** 15 to 20 mm Hg

**12.** The pulsed-wave (PW) Doppler through the RV outflow tract (RVOT)/pulmonary valve shown in **Figure 51.11** is *most* commonly associated with which of the following diagnoses?

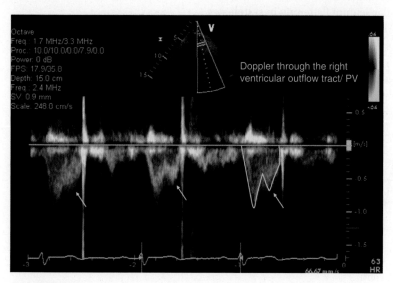

**Figure 51.11**

**A.** Normal RV pressure
**B.** Pulmonary valve stenosis
**C.** RV pressure overload
**D.** Sub-pulmonary valve stenosis

**13.** What is the estimated mean PAP in this patient (shown in **Figure 51.12**) with tricuspid valve regurgitation velocity of 3.2 m/s, pulmonary regurgitation (PR) peak diastolic pressure of 2.9 m/s, and RAP of 10 mm Hg?

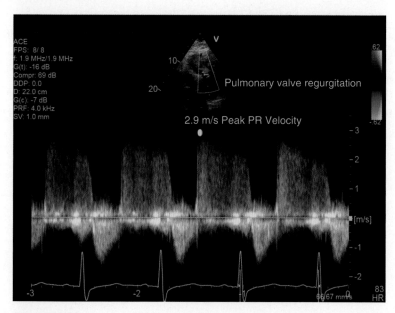

**Figure 51.12**

**A.** 57.6 mm Hg
**B.** 31.5 mm Hg
**C.** 43.6 mm Hg
**D.** 33.3 mm Hg

14. Which of the following is the least helpful echocardiographic sign of pulmonary arterial hypertension?

    **A.** Pulmonary artery acceleration time <80 ms
    **B.** D shape interventricular septum flattening in systole
    **C.** Midsystolic notching in PW Doppler of pulmonary valve
    **D.** TAPSE >1.9 cm

15. Which of the following statements is true about TAPSE (**Figure 51.13**)?

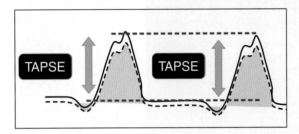

**Figure 51.13**

    **A.** Normal TAPSE is <1.7 cm.
    **B.** TAPSE represents the global longitudinal RV function.
    **C.** TAPSE measurement is accurate in patients after tricuspid valve surgery.
    **D.** TAPSE represents the regional longitudinal RV function.

16. Which phrase is wrong about classifying the degree of severity of pulmonary hypertension using transthoracic echocardiography?

    **A.** Mild pulmonary hypertension is suggested by systolic PAP between 40 and 50 mm Hg.
    **B.** Moderate pulmonary hypertension is suggested by systolic PAP between 50 and 69 mm Hg.
    **C.** Severe pulmonary hypertension is suggested by systolic PAP ≥ 70 mm Hg.
    **D.** All are incorrect.

17. Which of the following statements regarding the usefulness of echocardiography in the diagnosis of pulmonary hypertension is *most* correct?

    **A.** Echocardiography is not useful for the assessment of PAP.
    **B.** Echocardiography is the gold standard for assessment of the PAP.
    **C.** Echocardiography is not diagnostic but can help in the diagnosis and can be used as a screening test.
    **D.** None of the above.

18. A 47-year-old woman with newly diagnosed systemic sclerosis is admitted to the ICU with respiratory failure. Based on the echocardiographic images (**Figure 51.14A-C** and ▶ **Video 51.5**), what is the best description of her RV size and systolic function?

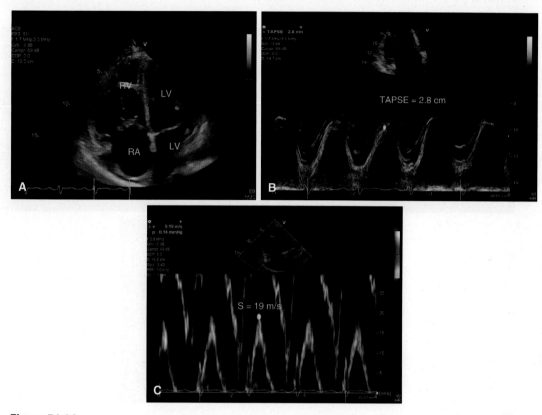

**Figure 51.14**

A. Normal RV size and systolic function
B. Abnormal RV size with normal systolic function
C. Normal RV size and abnormal systolic function
D. D. Abnormal RV size and systolic function

19. Which of the following is not a method for the assessment of RV function?

A. TAPSE
B. Tissue Doppler tricuspid annular systolic velocity
C. RV global longitudinal strain
D. Biplane Simpson's ejection fraction method

20. A 67-year-old woman is admitted to the ICU with acute shortness of breath and mild lower limb edema. The patient has a history of antiphospholipid syndrome and chronic obstructive pulmonary disease. Based on the echocardiographic images shown at end diastole in **Figure 51.15A-C** and ▶ **Video 51.6,** which of the following diagnoses is most correct?

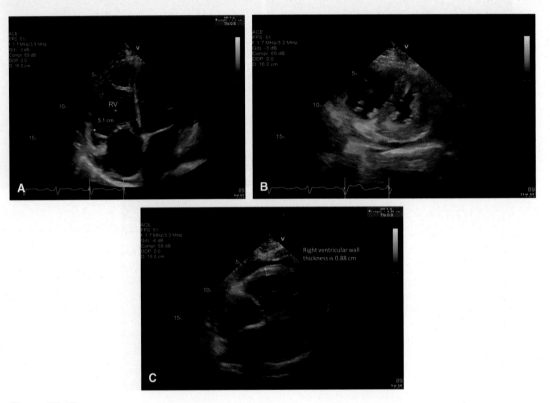

**Figure 51.15**

A. Acute pulmonary hypertension likely related to an acute pulmonary embolism
B. Chronic pulmonary hypertension likely related to chronic obstructive pulmonary disease
C. Normal right heart with hyperdynamic function
D. Acute left ventricular systolic dysfunction

**21.** Which of the following statements is not true about the RV global longitudinal strain in **Figure 51.16** and ▶ **Video 51.7**?

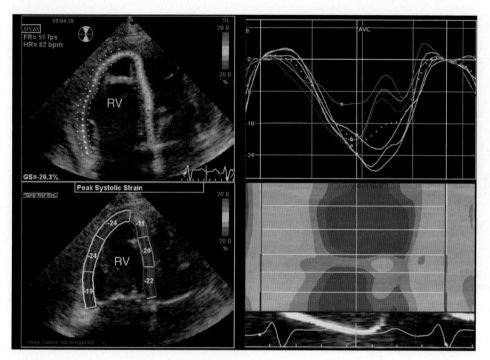

**Figure 51.16**

**A.** It is abnormal.
**B.** It is affected by volume status.
**C.** It is strongly correlated with prognosis.
**D.** It is normal.

**22.** What is the best estimation of the PAP in this image assuming a RAP of 10 mm Hg and PR (**Figure 51.17**) with an end-diastolic velocity of 2.2 m/s?

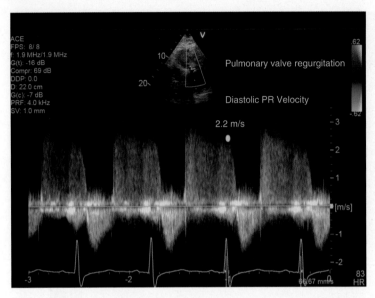

**Figure 51.17**

    **A.** Normal
    **B.** Moderate elevation
    **C.** Severe (systemic) elevation
    **D.** None of the above

**23.** The smallest regurgitant flow area immediately beyond the flow convergence region and before expansion of the turbulent regurgitant jet was measured to be 8 mm. Systolic flow reversal of hepatic vein flow is also present. The amount of TR in this patient is (▶ **Video 51.8A and B** and **Figure 51.18**):

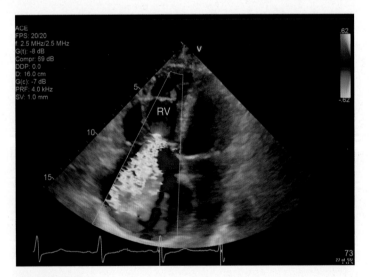

**Figure 51.18**

    **A.** Mild
    **B.** Moderate
    **C.** Severe
    **D.** Cannot quantify

**24.** The PR signal shown in **Figure 51.19** is suggestive of:

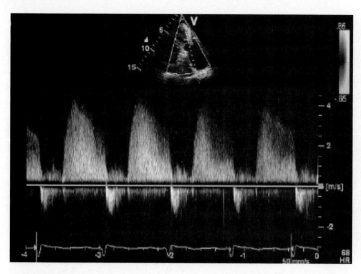

**Figure 51.19**

A. Severe pulmonary hypertension
B. Severe systemic hypertension
C. Mild pulmonary hypertension
D. Mild right heart failure

**25.** Which of the following findings is present in the M-mode image shown in **Figure 51.20**?

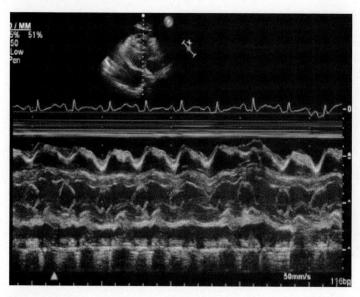

**Figure 51.20**

A. Normal M-mode through the heart
B. Diastolic collapse of the right ventricle
C. Pericardial thickening
D. Constrictive pericarditis

26. In this RV view (**Figure 51.21**) which of the tricuspid valve leaflets is indicated by (*A, arrow*)?

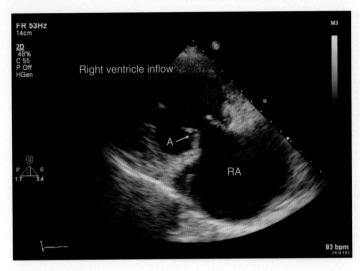

**Figure 51.21**

A. Anterior tricuspid valve leaflets
B. Septal tricuspid valve leaflets
C. Posterior tricuspid valve leaflets
D. Cannot be determined from this view only

27. In this RV view (**Figure 51.22**), what is the structure indicated by the *arrow*?

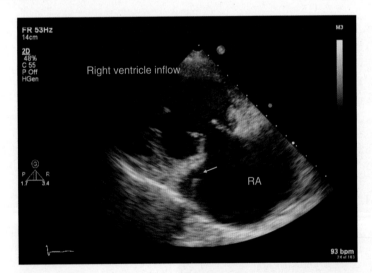

**Figure 51.22**

A. Inferior vena cava
B. Superior vena cava
C. Coronary sinus
D. Eustachian valve

28. Which of the following echocardiographic parameters is least likely to be used to assess RV function?

    **A.** Myocardial performance or Tei Index
    **B.** TAPSE
    **C.** Right ventricular fractional area of change (RVFAC)
    **D.** RV ejection fraction

29. A 39-year-old man presents to the Emergency Department with acute shortness of breath and chest pain. Blood pressure is 110/60 mm Hg, heart rate is 120 bpm, and respiratory rate is 32 breaths/min. Bedside echocardiography is performed, and ▶ **Video 51.9** represents an apical four chamber view window.

    Based on ▶ **Video 51.9**, which statement is *most* correct regarding the diagnosis of pulmonary embolism?
    **A.** Definitive diagnosis
    **B.** Possible diagnosis
    **C.** Can be excluded
    **D.** The video is insufficient to make any statement.

# Chapter 51 ▪ Answers

**1.** Correct Answer: C. C

*Rationale:* The diameter of the IVC should be measured in the subcostal long-axis view with the patient in the supine position at 1.0 to 2.0 cm from the junction with the right atrium. For accuracy, this measurement should be made perpendicular to the IVC long axis. The diameter of the IVC decreases in response to inspiration when negative intrathoracic pressure leads to an increase in RV filling from the systemic veins. The diameter of the IVC and the percentage decrease in the diameter during inspiration correlate with RAP.

Selected References
1. Ommen SR, Nishimura RA, Hurrell DG, Klarich KW. Assessment of right atrial pressure with 2-dimensional and Doppler echocardiography: a simultaneous catheterization and echocardiographic study. *Mayo Clin Proc.* 2000;75:24-29.
2. Rudski LG, Lai WW, Afilalo J, et al. Guidelines for the echocardiographic assessment of the right heart in adults: a report from the American Society of Echocardiography. *J Am Soc Echocardiogr.* 2010;23:685-713.
3. Weyman A. *Cross-Sectional Echocardiography.* Lea & Febiger; 1981.

**2.** Correct Answer: A. Normal RAP

*Rationale:* In Figure 51.2, the hepatic vein pattern is dominant in systole, which indicates a normal RAP. In ventilated patients, the IVC pattern might be useful to estimate the RAP. In the normal hepatic vein waveform, the S wave is larger than or equal to the D wave. This is expected, considering that the powerful systolic movement of the tricuspid annulus toward the cardiac apex causes a large antegrade rush of blood into the heart.

Selected References
1. Rudski LG, Lai WW, Afilalo J, et al. Guidelines for the echocardiographic assessment of the right heart in adults: a report from the American Society of Echocardiography. *J Am Soc Echocardiogr.* 2010;23:685-713.
2. Scheinfeld MH, Bilali A, Koenigsberg M. Understanding the spectral Doppler waveform of the hepatic veins in health and disease. *RadioGraphics.* 2009;29:2081-2098.

**3.** Correct Answer: D. Hepatic vein systolic filling fraction

*Rationale:* Among echocardiographic and Doppler parameters of RA and RV function, hepatic venous flow dynamics relate best to mean RAP. This information can be used clinically to estimate mean RAP. The higher the RAP, the lower the pressure gradient between the hepatic veins and the right atrium and thus the lower the forward systolic flow. This observation was described previously in patients with restrictive heart disease and elevated filling pressures. The hepatic vein systolic filling fraction is the ratio $V_s/(V_s+V_d)$ and a value $<55\%$ was found to be the most sensitive and specific sign of elevated RAP. Particularly systolic filling fraction, derived with either time-velocity integrals or maximal velocities, had the best relation to mean RAP and allowed a good estimation of atrial pressure in patients with a variety of underlying clinical conditions.

Selected Reference

1. Nagueh SF, Kopelen HA, Zoghbi WA. Relation of mean right atrial pressure to echocardiographic and Doppler parameters of right atrial and right ventricular function. *Circulation.* 1996;93:1160-1169.

**4.** Correct Answer: C. 50 to 59 mm Hg

*Rationale:* The pulmonary artery systolic pressure is given by $4V^2$ + RAP. The RAP is estimated by the diameter and change in diameter of the IVC with inspiration. IVC diameter $\leq 2.1$ cm that collapses $>50\%$ with a sniff suggests a normal RAP of 3 mm Hg (range, 0-5 mm Hg), whereas an IVC diameter $>2.1$ cm that collapses $<50\%$ with a sniff suggests a high right trial pressure of 15 mm Hg (range, 10-20 mm Hg). In indeterminate cases in which the IVC diameter and collapse do not fit this paradigm, an intermediate value of 8 mm Hg (range, 5-10 mm Hg) may be used or, preferably, secondary indices of elevated RAP should be integrated.
In this case, $4(3.2)^2 + 15 = 55.9$ mm Hg.

Selected References

1. Aduen JF, Castello R, Lozano MM, et al. An alternative echocardiographic method to estimate mean pulmonary artery pressure: diagnostic and clinical implications. *J Am Soc Echocardiogr.* 2009;22(7):814-819.
2. Rudski LG, Lai WW, Afilalo J, et al. Guidelines for the echocardiographic assessment of the right heart in adults: a report from the American Society of Echocardiography. *J Am Soc Echocardiogr.* 2010;23:685-713.

**5.** Correct Answer: A. A

*Rationale:* RV basal linear dimension is easily obtained on an apical four-chamber view at end diastole. RV end-diastolic basal diameter has been shown to be a predictor of survival in patients with chronic pulmonary artery disease. The basal diameter is generally defined as the maximal short-axis dimension in the basal one-third of the right ventricle seen on the four-chamber view. The upper reference limit for the RV basal dimension is 4.2 cm. Respiration influences the size of the right ventricle. During inspiration, it is slightly larger. It is important to take the patient's body surface area into account.

Selected References

1. Lang RM, Bierig M, Devereux RB, et al. Recommendations for chamber quantification: a report from the American Society of Echocardiography's Guidelines and Standards Committee and the Chamber Quantification Writing Group, developed in conjunction with the European Association of Echocardiography, a branch of the European Society of Cardiology. *J Am Soc Echocardiogr.* 2005;18:1440-1463.
2. Rudski LG, Lai WW, Afilalo J, et al. Guidelines for the echocardiographic assessment of the right heart in adults: a report from the American Society of Echocardiography. *J Am Soc Echocardiogr.* 2010;23:685-713.

**6.** Correct Answer: B. Pulmonary arterial hypertension

*Rationale:* In this case, the diagnosis is pulmonary arterial hypertension since it is most consistent with the clinical presentation of right heart failure with elevation of RAP. The degree of immobility of the free RV wall, the wall thickness observed, and the size of the RA make the process more likely to be chronic than acute. This makes carcinoid heart disease, acute pulmonary embolism, and RV infarction very less likely.

Selected References

1. Lang RM, Bierig M, Devereux RB, et al. Recommendations for chamber quantification: a report from the American Society of Echocardiography's Guidelines and Standards Committee and the Chamber Quantification Writing Group, developed in conjunction with the European Association of Echocardiography, a branch of the European Society of Cardiology. *J Am Soc Echocardiogr.* 2005;18:1440-1463.
2. Rudski LG, Lai WW, Afilalo J, et al. Guidelines for the echocardiographic assessment of the right heart in adults: a report from the American Society of Echocardiography. *J Am Soc Echocardiogr.* 2010;23:685-713.

## 7. Correct Answer: C. C

*Rationale:* The systolic movement of the base of the RV free wall provides one of the most visibly obvious movements on normal echocardiography. TAPSE is a method to measure the distance of systolic excursion of the RV annular segment along its longitudinal plane, from a standard apical four-chamber window at the level of lateral tricuspid valve annulus. TAPSE represents longitudinal function of the right ventricle in the same way as mitral annular plane systolic excursion by Doppler tissue imaging does with the left ventricle. It is inferred that the greater the descent of the base in systole, the better the RV systolic function. TAPSE is simple, less dependent on optimal image quality, and reproducible, and it does not require sophisticated equipment or prolonged image analysis. A TAPSE cutoff value <17 mm has high specificity, though low sensitivity to distinguish abnormal from normal subjects.

Selected Reference

1. Rudski LG, Lai WW, Afilalo J, et al. Guidelines for the echocardiographic assessment of the right heart in adults: a report from the American Society of Echocardiography. *J Am Soc Echocardiogr.* 2010;23:685-713.

## 8. Correct Answer: C. Severe pulmonary hypertension

*Rationale:* It is important to note that TR jet velocity is not related to the volume of regurgitant flow. In fact, very severe TR is often associated with a low jet velocity (2 m/s), with near equalization of RV and RA systolic pressures. A truncated, triangular jet contour with early peaking of the maximal velocity indicates elevated RAP and a prominent regurgitant pressure wave ("V wave") in the right atrium. It should be noted that this pattern may be present in patients with milder degrees of TR and severe elevation of RAP (reduced right atrial compliance). It usually reflects a high RAP. When we get severe TR and normal RV systolic pressure, the antegrade and retrograde continuous-wave flow signals across the valve can appear qualitatively very similar with a "sine wave" appearance, corresponding to the "to-and-fro" flow across the severely incompetent valve.

Selected References

1. Rudski LG, Lai WW, Afilalo J, et al. Guidelines for the echocardiographic assessment of the right heart in adults: a report from the American Society of Echocardiography. *J Am Soc Echocardiogr.* 2010;23:685-713.
2. Zoghbi WA, Adams D, Bonow RO, et al. Recommendations for noninvasive evaluation of native valvular regurgitation a report from the American Society of Echocardiography developed in collaboration with the Society for Cardiovascular Magnetic Resonance. *J Indian Acad Echocardiogr Cardiovasc Imaging.* 2020;4(1):58-121.

## 9. Correct Answer: C. RV pressure overload

*Rationale:* In ▶ **Video 51.2** and Figure 51.8, the interventricular septum is flattening in systole, which is suggestive of RV pressure overload. This is a systolic D-shaped left ventricle. When it is present during systole only, it is a sign of high RV pressure. Answers A, B, and D are incorrect.

Selected References

1. Lang RM, Badano LP, Mor-Avi V, et al. Recommendations for cardiac chamber quantification by echocardiography in adults: an update from the American Society of Echocardiography and the European Association of Cardiovascular Imaging. *Eur Heart J Cardiovasc Imaging.* 2015;16:233-271.
2. Rudski LG, Lai WW, Afilalo J, et al. Guidelines for the echocardiographic assessment of the right heart in adults: a report from the American Society of Echocardiography. *J Am Soc Echocardiogr.* 2010;23:685-713.

**10.** Correct Answer: A. Significant tricuspid valve regurgitation

*Rationale:* In ▶ **Video 51.3** and Figure 51.9, the interventricular septal is flattening in diastole, which is suggestive of RV volume overload, like from significant tricuspid valve regurgitation or significant pulmonary valve regurgitation. This is a diastolic D-shaped left ventricle. When it is present during diastole only, it is a sign of RV volume overload, such as tricuspid valve regurgitation.

Selected References
1. Lang RM, Badano LP, Mor-Avi V, et al. Recommendations for cardiac chamber quantification by echocardiography in adults: an update from the American Society of Echocardiography and the European Association of Cardiovascular Imaging. *Eur Heart J Cardiovasc Imaging.* 2015;16:233-271.
2. Rudski LG, Lai WW, Afilalo J, et al. Guidelines for the echocardiographic assessment of the right heart in adults: a report from the American Society of Echocardiography. *J Am Soc Echocardiogr.* 2010;23:685-713.

**11.** Correct Answer: A. 3 to 5 mm Hg

*Rationale:* The RAP can be estimated by looking at the dimension of the IVC diameter and its relative change in size during respiration. This method of assessing the RAP, although simple, might underestimate the true RAP, especially in cases of severe RV dysfunction or severe tricuspid valve regurgitation where the RAP can be much higher than 15 mm Hg (the maximal value obtained by this method). IVC diameter ≤2.1 cm that collapses >50% with a sniff suggests normal RAP of 3 mm Hg (range, 0-5 mm Hg), whereas IVC diameter >2.1 cm that collapses <50% with a sniff suggests high RAP of 15 mm Hg (range, 10-20 mm Hg). In scenarios in which IVC diameter and collapse do not fit this paradigm, an intermediate value of 8 mm Hg (range, 5-10 mm Hg) may be used or, preferably, other indices of RAP should be integrated to downgrade or upgrade to the normal or high values of RAP.

Selected References
1. Lang RM, Badano LP, Mor-Avi V, et al. Recommendations for cardiac chamber quantification by echocardiography in adults: an update from the American Society of Echocardiography and the European Association of Cardiovascular Imaging. *Eur Heart J Cardiovasc Imaging.* 2015;16:233-271.
2. Rudski LG, Lai WW, Afilalo J, et al. Guidelines for the echocardiographic assessment of the right heart in adults: a report from the American Society of Echocardiography. *J Am Soc Echocardiogr.* 2010;23:685-713.

**12.** Correct Answer: C. RV pressure overload

*Rationale:* Prominent midsystolic notching obtained by PW Doppler through the RVOT is suggestive of high RV pressure. The decrease in RV-pulmonary artery pressure gradient and forward flow accompanied by midsystolic partial closure occurs with earlier and higher prevailing pressure, suggesting forces opposing ejection with higher pressure. In pulmonary arterial hypertension (PAH), the notched profile of RVOT Doppler flow velocity envelope appears to integrate indicators of pulmonary vascular load and RV function and serves as a marker for adverse outcomes. Answers A, B, and D are incorrect.

Selected References
1. Tahara M, Tanaka H, Nakao S, et al. Hemodynamic determinants of pulmonary valve motion during systole in experimental pulmonary hypertension. *Circulation.* 1981;64:1249-1255.
2. Takahama H, McCully RB, Frantz RP, Kane GC. Unraveling the RV ejection Doppler envelope. Insight into pulmonary artery hemodynamics and disease severity. *JACC Cardiovasc Imaging.* 2017;10:1268-1277.
3. Weyman AE, Dillon JC, Feigenbaum H, Chang S. Echocardiographic patterns of pulmonic valve motion with pulmonary hypertension. *Circulation.* 1974;50:905-910.

**13.** Correct Answer: C. 43.6 mm Hg

*Rationale:* The diagnosis of pulmonary artery hypertension is made based on a mean PAP, as determined by right heart catheterization. There are several methods of estimating mean PAP by echo, several of them with excellent correlation with right heart catheterization. Estimation of mean PAP obtained through measurement of TR velocity is a technique similar to that used to obtain the mean gradient across the aortic valve. The complete TR jet envelope can be traced, giving TR TVI and yielding a mean RV-RA pressure gradient. Adding an estimated RAP as described yields an estimated mean PAP. This method has the attraction of being most physiologically sound. Estimation of mean PAP can be obtained through measurement of peak PR velocity: mPAP = 4 × Peak PR velocity$^2$ + RAP.

### Selected References

1. Aduen JF, Castello R, Lozano MM, et al. An alternative echocardiographic method to estimate mean pulmonary artery pressure: diagnostic and clinical implications. *J Am Soc Echocardiogr.* 2009;22(7):814-819.
2. Rudski LG, Lai WW, Afilalo J, et al. Guidelines for the echocardiographic assessment of the right heart in adults: a report from the American Society of Echocardiography. *J Am Soc Echocardiogr.* 2010;23:685-713.

---

**14.** Correct Answer: D. TAPSE >1.9 cm

*Rationale:* The systolic movement of the base of the RV free wall provides one of the most visibly obvious movements on normal echocardiography. TAPSE is a method to measure the distance of systolic excursion of the RV annular segment along its longitudinal plane, from a standard apical four-chamber window. It is inferred that the greater the descent of the base in systole, the better the RV systolic function. TAPSE is simple, less dependent on optimal image quality, and reproducible, and it does not require sophisticated equipment or prolonged image analysis. In a study of 750 patients with a variety of cardiac conditions, compared with 150 age-matched normal controls, a TAPSE cutoff value <17 mm yielded high specificity, though low sensitivity to distinguish abnormal from normal subjects. Answers A, B, and C are incorrect.

### Selected Reference

1. Rudski LG, Lai WW, Afilalo J, et al. Guidelines for the echocardiographic assessment of the right heart in adults: a report from the American Society of Echocardiography. *J Am Soc Echocardiogr.* 2010;23:685-713.

---

**15.** Correct Answer: D. TAPSE represents the regional longitudinal RV function.

*Rationale:* The systolic movement of the base of the RV free wall provides one of the most visibly obvious movements on normal echocardiography. TAPSE is a method to measure the distance of systolic excursion of the RV annular segment along its longitudinal plane, from a standard apical four-chamber window. It is inferred that the greater the descent of the base in systole, the better the RV systolic function. TAPSE is simple, less dependent on optimal image quality, and reproducible, and it does not require sophisticated equipment or prolonged image analysis. In a study of 750 patients with a variety of cardiac conditions, compared with 150 age-matched normal controls, a TAPSE cutoff value <17 mm yielded high specificity, though low sensitivity to distinguish abnormal from normal subjects. Having tricuspid valve surgery with a repair or replacement may change the angle of the annulus and make known standardized measurements less helpful. Answers A, B, and C are incorrect.

### Selected References

1. Brierre G, Blot-Souletie N, Degano B, Têtu L, Bongard V, Carrié D. New echocardiographic prognostic factors for mortality in pulmonary arterial hypertension. *Eur J Echocardiogr.* 2010;11:516-522.
2. Forfia PR, Fisher MR, Mathai SC, et al. Tricuspid annular displacement predicts survival in pulmonary hypertension. *Am J Respir Crit Care Med.* 2006;174:1034-1041.
3. Rudski LG, Lai WW, Afilalo J, et al. Guidelines for the echocardiographic assessment of the right heart in adults: a *report from the American* Society of Echocardiography. *J Am Soc Echocardiogr.* 2010;23:685-713.

---

**16.** Correct Answer: D. All are incorrect.

*Rationale:* One should always remember that systolic PAP is a function of stroke volume, *according to the* equation $P = Q \times R$, where $P$ is pressure, $Q$ *is* flow, and $R$ is resistance. As pulmonary hypertension becomes very severe and the RV decompensates, the PAP may actually fall due to the fall in stroke volume. Similarly, in cirrhosis (high cardiac output), the systolic PAP may be elevated despite normal resistance. Documenting the overall stroke volume (obtained by the continuity equation, measuring the cross-sectional area of the outflow tract and the velocity time integral through that outflow tract) might be helpful in the initial assessment when evaluating the etiology. Stroke volume or cardiac output may also be helpful during follow-up when mentioning the systolic PAP in the context of RV systolic function. Answers A, B, and C are incorrect.

Selected References
1. McQullian BM, Picard MH, Leavitt M, Weyman AE. Clinical correlates and reference intervals for pulmonary artery systolic pressure among echocardiographically normal subjects. *Circulation.* 2001;104:2797-2802.
2. Rudski LG, Lai WW, Afilalo J, et al. Guidelines for the echocardiographic assessment of the right heart in adults: a report from the American Society of Echocardiography. *J Am Soc Echocardiogr.* 2010;23:685-713.

**17.** Correct Answer: C. Echocardiography is not diagnostic but can help in the diagnosis and can be used as a screening test.

*Rationale:* Echocardiography remains an important starting point in screening for pulmonary hypertension and RV systolic function, but other investigations, such as right heart catheterization and cardiac magnetic resonance, are employed to make a definitive diagnosis. Cardiac magnetic resonance imaging (MRI) is the gold standard for RV assessment and right heart catheter is the gold standard for assessment of the right-sided pressure. Answers A, B, and D are incorrect.

Selected References
1. McQullian BM, Picard MH, Leavitt M, Weyman AE. Clinical correlates and reference intervals for pulmonary artery systolic pressure among echocardiographically normal subjects. *Circulation.* 2001;104:2797-2802.
2. Rudski LG, Lai WW, Afilalo J, et al. Guidelines for the echocardiographic assessment of the right heart in adults: a report from the American Society of Echocardiography. *J Am Soc Echocardiogr.* 2010;23:685-713.

**18.** Correct Answer: B. Abnormal RV size with normal systolic function

*Rationale:* This patient has an abnormal RV size and normal RV function. The basal diameter is generally defined as the maximal short-axis dimension in the basal one-third of the right ventricle seen on the four-chamber view (Figure 51.14.A). The upper reference limit for the RV basal dimension is 4.2 cm. In this patient, the basal RV diameter is 6.0 cm, which is dilated. However, the RV function does appear to be preserved at least based on the TAPSE (2.7 cm) and the systolic motion (S'), which is 19 m/s. Answers A, C, and D are incorrect.

Selected References
1. Lang RM, Badano LP, Mor-Avi V, et al. Recommendations for cardiac chamber quantification by echocardiography in adults: an update from the American Society of Echocardiography and the European Association of Cardiovascular Imaging. *Eur Heart J Cardiovasc Imaging.* 2015;16:233-271.
2. Rudski LG, Lai WW, Afilalo J, et al. Guidelines for the echocardiographic assessment of the right heart in adults: a report from the American Society of Echocardiography. *J Am Soc Echocardiogr.* 2010;23:685-713.

**19.** Correct Answer: D. Biplane Simpson's ejection fraction method

*Rationale:* Visual estimation using different imaging planes is still one of the most commonly used methods for RV assessment. RV TAPSE, tissue Doppler tricuspid annular systolic velocity, and RV global longitudinal strain are all used for RV assessment. However, unlike the left ventricle, there are no orthogonal views that allow measurement of biplane Simpson's ejection fraction and the RV has a more complex shape than the LV. Answers A, B, and C are incorrect.

Selected References
1. Lang RM, Badano LP, Mor-Avi V, et al. Recommendations for cardiac chamber quantification by echocardiography in adults: an update from the American Society of Echocardiography and the European Association of Cardiovascular Imaging. *Eur Heart J Cardiovasc Imaging.* 2015;16:233-271.
2. Rudski LG, Lai WW, Afilalo J, et al. Guidelines for the echocardiographic assessment of the right heart in adults: a report from the American Society of Echocardiography. *J Am Soc Echocardiogr.* 2010;23:685-713.

**20.** Correct Answer: B. Chronic pulmonary hypertension likely related to chronic obstructive pulmonary disease

*Rationale:* Echocardiography can be helpful in differentiating between pulmonary hypertension due to acute causes, for example, pulmonary embolism, or chronic causes, for example, chronic obstructive pulmonary disease. In acute pulmonary hypertension, the PAP may not be particularly high (often not more than about 50 mm Hg). The right ventricle is not hypertrophied, maybe not dilated, and the ventricle apical contraction is preserved. In more chronic pulmonary hypertension, the right ventricle will be hypertrophied and dilated. The RV pressure will be higher and the RV systolic dysfunction will be global. Answers A, C, and D are incorrect.

### Selected References
1. Fields JM, Davis J, Girson L, et al. Transthoracic echocardiography for diagnosing pulmonary embolism: a systematic review and meta-analysis. *J Am Soc Echocardiogr.* 2017;30:714-723.
2. Konstantinides SV, Torbicki A, Agnelli G, et al. 2014 ESC guidelines on the diagnosis and management of acute pulmonary embolism. *Eur Heart J.* 2014;35:997-1053.69a-69k.

**21.** Correct Answer: **A. It is abnormal.**

*Rationale:* Strain imaging is sensitive to early impairments in systolic function that may develop despite the presence of normal appearing contractility by 2D imaging. This makes strain potentially valuable for assessment of the right ventricle, including early disease. Longitudinal systolic strain measurement is also especially well-suited to assess RV function because RV contractility predominantly occurs in the longitudinal plane due to the principal orientation of myocardial fibers. Unlike TAPSE, strain is more global and has been demonstrated to be more accurate for global RV function assessment. Among patients with pulmonary hypertension, a moderate reduction in RV global longitudinal strain (absolute value <20%) is associated with worse outcomes. Answers B, C, and D are incorrect.

### Selected Reference
1. Fine NM, Chen L, Bastiansen PM, et al. Outcome prediction by quantitative right ventricular function assessment in 575 subjects evaluated for pulmonary hypertension. *Circ Cardiovasc Imaging.* 2013;6:711-721.

**22.** Correct Answer: **B. Moderate elevation**

*Rationale:* End-diastolic PR velocity is 2 m/s, consistent with a PA to RV end-diastolic gradient of 16 mm Hg ($4 \times 2 \times 2$) and assuming that the RV end-diastolic pressure is close to the mean RAP, the PA diastolic pressure will be 26 mm Hg. Answers A, C, and D are incorrect.

### Selected References
1. Aduen JF, Castello R, Lozano MM, et al. An alternative echocardiographic method to estimate mean pulmonary artery pressure: diagnostic and clinical implications. *J Am Soc Echocardiogr.* 2009;22(7):814-819.
2. Rudski LG, Lai WW, Afilalo J, et al. Guidelines for the echocardiographic assessment of the right heart in adults: a report from the American Society of Echocardiography. *J Am Soc Echocardiogr.* 2010;23:685-713.

**23.** Correct Answer: **C. Severe**

*Rationale:* This is severe given that the vena contracta that is defined as the smallest regurgitant flow area immediately beyond the flow convergence before expansion of the turbulent regurgitant jet is ≥ 7 mm and there is systolic flow reversal of hepatic vein flow. A vena contracta of <0.3 is consistent with mild TR. Of note, the two-dimensional image shows lack of tricuspid leaflet coaptation, leading to wide-open TR. The mechanism is tricuspid annular dilatation and hence is functional, probably secondary to previous pulmonary hypertension due to mitral valve disease resulting in RV and RA dilatation, thus stretching the tricuspid annulus. This is repairable with tricuspid annuloplasty. Also note the partly seen mitral prosthesis. TR quantification by using the three components of the jet is not well validated. Answers A, B, and D are incorrect.

### Selected References
1. Lang RM, Badano LP, Mor-Avi V, et al. Recommendations for cardiac chamber quantification by echocardiography in adults: an update from the American Society of Echocardiography and the European Association of Cardiovascular Imaging. *Eur Heart J Cardiovasc Imaging.* 2015;16:233-271.
2. Rudski LG, Lai WW, Afilalo J, et al. Guidelines for the echocardiographic assessment of the right heart in adults: a report from the American Society of Echocardiography. *J Am Soc Echocardiogr.* 2010;23:685-713.

**24.** Correct Answer: A. Severe pulmonary hypertension

*Rationale:* The PR pressure profile reflects a PA to RV diastolic pressure gradient. Hence, this patient's PA end-systolic pressure is four times the square of early diastolic PR velocity + RV diastolic pressure, which would be similar to the RAP ($4V^2 + RAP$). In this patient, this is calculated to be in the range of 80 mm Hg, which would also be similar to the mean PA pressure. The PR end-diastolic velocity is about 3 m/s. Hence, the PA diastolic pressure is 36 + RAP. This patient does not have significant pulmonary stenosis, as is shown by the accompanying systolic flow. In fact, a markedly reduced duration is indicative of low cardiac output as well, as a consequence of pulmonary hypertension. Answers B, C, and D are incorrect.

### Selected References
1. Lang RM, Badano LP, Mor-Avi V, et al. Recommendations for cardiac chamber quantification by echocardiography in adults: an update from the American Society of Echocardiography and the European Association of Cardiovascular Imaging. *Eur Heart J Cardiovasc Imaging.* 2015;16:233-271.
2. Rudski LG, Lai WW, Afilalo J, et al. Guidelines for the echocardiographic assessment of the right heart in adults: a report from the American Society of Echocardiography. *J Am Soc Echocardiogr.* 2010;23:685-713.

**25.** Correct Answer: B. Diastolic collapse of the right ventricle

*Rationale:* The M-mode image shows RV diastolic collapse resulting from a significant pericardial effusion. This is a sign of cardiac tamponade that might be clinically imminent and the need for urgent pericardiocentesis. Answers A, B, and C are incorrect.

### Selected References
1. Lang RM, Badano LP, Mor-Avi V, et al. Recommendations for cardiac chamber quantification by echocardiography in adults: an update from the American Society of Echocardiography and the European Association of Cardiovascular Imaging. *Eur Heart J Cardiovasc Imaging.* 2015;16:233-271.
2. Rudski LG, Lai WW, Afilalo J, et al. Guidelines for the echocardiographic assessment of the right heart in adults: a report from the American Society of Echocardiography. *J Am Soc Echocardiogr.* 2010;23:685-713.

**26.** Correct Answer: C. Posterior tricuspid valve leaflets

*Rationale:* Echocardiographic assessment of the tricuspid valve is challenging due to unfavorable retrosternal position of the valve and the inability to simultaneously visualize all three leaflets in standard transthoracic views. In the right ventricular inflow view (RVIF), the leaflet seen to the right of the 2D image (nearest the aortic valve) is always the anterior leaflet. When the RVIF view is acquired with the septum in view, the anterior-septal leaflet combination is seen. When the septum is not visualized, it was not possible to determine whether the septal or posterior leaflet is being imaged, because the 2D image with the anterior-septal leaflet combination and the image with the anterior-posterior combination look similar. Answers A, B, and D are incorrect.

### Selected References
1. Addetia K, Yamat M, Mediratta A, et al. Comprehensive two-dimensional interrogation of the tricuspid valve using knowledge derived from three-dimensional echocardiography. *J Am Soc Echocardiogr.* 2016;29:74-82.
2. Tricuspid and Pulmonary Valves. In: Armstrong WF, Ryan T. *Feigenbaum's Echocardiography.* 8th ed. Philadelphia, PA: Wolters Kluwer; 2019.
3. García-Fernández MA, Gomez de Diego JJ. Transthoracic echocardiography. In: Galuito L, ed. *The EAE Textbook of Echocardiography.* Oxford University Press; 2011:18-19.
4. Lancellotti P, Moura L, Pierard LA, et al. European Association of Echocardiography recommendations for the assessment of valvular regurgitation. Part 2: mitral and tricuspid regurgitation (native valve disease). *Eur J Echocardiogr.* 2010;11(4):307-332.

**27.** Correct Answer: C. Coronary sinus

*Rationale:* Figure 51.22 is the coronary sinus. It is a normal finding in occasional views of echocardiographic assessment of the right atrium. The location of this is less likely to be related to other anatomic structures such as the entry of superior vena cava and IVC, or the Eustachian valve. Answers A, B, and D are incorrect.

### Selected References

1. Lang RM, Badano LP, Mor-Avi V, et al. Recommendations for cardiac chamber quantification by echocardiography in adults: an update from the American Society of Echocardiography and the European Association of Cardiovascular Imaging. *Eur Heart J Cardiovasc Imaging.* 2015;16:233-271.
2. Rudski LG, Lai WW, Afilalo J, et al. Guidelines for the echocardiographic assessment of the right heart in adults: a report from the American Society of Echocardiography. *J Am Soc Echocardiogr.* 2010;23:685-713.

**28.** Correct Answer: **D. RV ejection fraction**

*Rationale:* Myocardial performance or Tei Index, TAPSE, RVFAC, global and free wall strains have been studied to assess RV function. RV ejection fraction is a cardiac MRI-related measurement and is not yet established or validated as echocardiographic techniques. Answers A, B, C are signs but incorrect to answer the question. See also **Figure 51.23**.

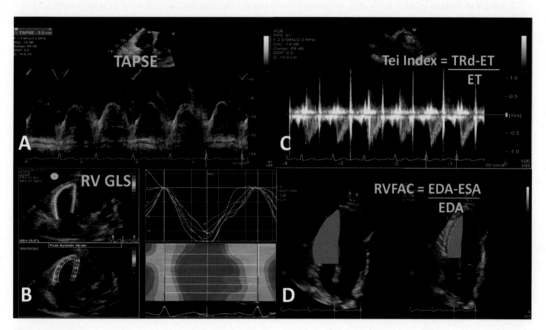

**Figure 51.23**

### Selected References

1. Lang RM, Badano LP, Mor-Avi V, et al. Recommendations for cardiac chamber quantification by echocardiography in adults: an update from the American Society of Echocardiography and the European Association of Cardiovascular Imaging. *Eur Heart J Cardiovasc Imaging.* 2015;16:233-271.
2. Rajagopal S, Forsha DE, Risum N, et al. Comprehensive assessment of right ventricular function in patients with pulmonary hypertension with global longitudinal peak systolic strain derived from multiple right ventricular views. *J Am Soc Echocardiogr.* 2014 Jun;27(6):657-665.

**29.** Correct Answer: **B. Possible diagnosis**

*Rationale:* ▶ **Video 51.9** provides one of the signs for determining severity of pulmonary embolism (PE) cases, but does not confirm the diagnosis. Acute pulmonary embolism is a disease that is diagnosed with a high sensitivity and specificity using CT pulmonary angiogram. An alternative would be ventilation and perfusion scan. Echocardiography may serve as a definitive diagnostic test if clots are visualized "in transit" from the right ventricle. McConnell's sign, where immobility and dilatation of the RV free wall is seen in the presence of apical mobility, is a sign of severity of RV dysfunction. Answers A, B, and D are incorrect.

### Selected References
1. Fields JM, Davis J, Girson L, et al. Transthoracic echocardiography for diagnosing pulmonary embolism: a systematic review and meta-analysis. *J Am Soc Echocardiogr.* 2017 Jul;30(7):714-723.
2. Lang RM, Badano LP, Mor-Avi V, et al. Recommendations for cardiac chamber quantification by echocardiography in adults: an update from the American Society of Echocardiography and the European Association of Cardiovascular Imaging. *Eur Heart J Cardiovasc Imaging.* 2015;16:233-271.

# 52 | PNEUMOTHORAX

Alberto Goffi, Gian Alfonso Cibinel, and Paolo Persona

1. A 35-year-old female patient has sustained a severe multisystem trauma as a result of a car accident. Upon arrival in the Emergency Department, her Glasgow Coma Scale is severely reduced (E1V1M2) and her systolic BP is approximately 90 mm Hg. Immediate endotracheal intubation is performed. Due to poor vascular access, you attempt a right subclavian vein cannulation, but it proves unsuccessful. Postattempt, you notice significant reduction in the air entry on the right side and worsening oxygenation. Lung ultrasound (LUS) is immediately performed. The two accompanying videos are acquired at the right (▶ **Video 52.1A**) and left (▶ **Video 52.1B**) third intercostal space between the parasternal and the midclavicular line. Based on the LUS findings, which answer is the most correct?

   **A.** Right pneumothorax (PTX)
   **B.** Left PTX
   **C.** Right bronchial obstruction
   **D.** Right lung contusion
   **E.** Right hemothorax

2. A 24-year-old male patient is transported to the Emergency Department after sustaining a chest trauma. He reports falling off his bicycle and hitting his left hemithorax on the ground. He complains of severe left-sided chest pain and shortness of breath. He is hemodynamically stable, tachypneic (respiratory rate 32 breaths/min), not hypoxemic (SpO$_2$ 98% room air). He does not report any significant past medical history. Based on the LUS findings, identified at the level of the left second intercostal space, medially to the midclavicular line (▶ **Video 52.2** and **Figure 52.1**) which condition can be immediately ruled out?

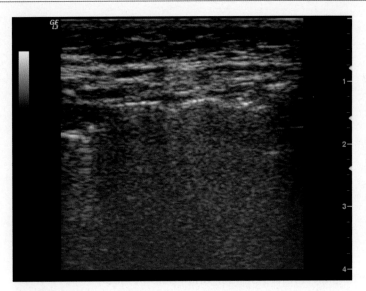

**Figure 52.1**

A. Pneumothorax
B. Lung contusion
C. Hemothorax
D. Endobronchial obstruction
E. None of the above

3. A 59-year-old man presents to the Emergency Department after being hit by a car while walking in a parking lot. His systolic BP is 88 mm Hg and HR 130 bpm after 2 L of Lactated Ringer's solution is infused. His abdomen is distended and tender, and abdominal ultrasound shows free fluid in the left upper quadrant and pelvis. A supine anteroposterior chest X-ray (CXR) is performed (**Figure 52.2**) to determine if a chest tube should be placed for PTX before laparotomy. Which of the following statements about the test characteristics of LUS for PTX is correct?

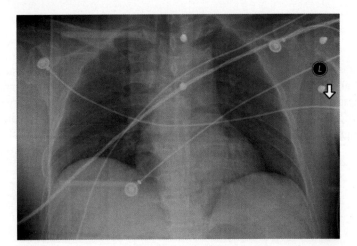

**Figure 52.2** Supine anteroposterior chest radiography performed in the Emergency Department.

A. LUS is more sensitive and less specific than CXR for detection of PTX
B. LUS is more sensitive but equally specific to CXR for detection of PTX
C. LUS is equally sensitive but more specific than CXR for detection of PTX
D. LUS is less sensitive but more specific than CXR for detection of PTX
E. None of the above

4. You are on call for the critical care rapid response team and you have just been called by the anesthesia team to help with a 64-year-old man who just underwent a right supraclavicular brachial plexus block in preparation for wrist surgery. Immediately following block insertion, the patient has developed shortness of breath, chest pain, and SpO₂ 85% on room air. He has a past medical history significant for emphysema. Distant breath sounds are auscultated on both sides. On the ultrasound, lung sliding, lung pulse, and vertical artifacts are all absent over the anterior right hemithorax. You slide the transducer more laterally and obtain two separate videos (▶ **Video 52.3A** and **B**). Which finding confirms the diagnosis of a right-sided PTX in this patient?

   A. ▶ **Video 52.3A** demonstrates a lung point, a highly specific finding for PTX
   B. ▶ **Video 52.3A** demonstrates a lung point, a highly sensitive finding for PTX
   C. ▶ **Video 52.3B** demonstrates a lung pulse, a highly specific finding for PTX
   D. ▶ **Video 52.3B** demonstrates a lung point, a highly sensitive finding for PTX
   E. None of the above

5. A 53-year-old male patient is transported to the Emergency Department after falling off a step-ladder while repairing a fence in his backyard. He reports left-sided chest trauma and moderate pain. He is hemodynamically stable, mildly tachycardic (115 bpm), tachypneic (respiratory rate 28 breaths/min) but not hypoxemic (SpO₂ 99% room air). Solely based on the LUS findings demonstrated in ▶ **Video 52.4**, diagnosis of PTX is:

   A. Unlikely, lung sliding is detected
   B. Unlikely, lung pulse is detected
   C. Unlikely, A-lines are detected
   D. Likely, neither lung sliding nor pulse is detected
   E. None of the above

6. A 45-year-old man is transported to the Emergency Department after a car accident. Paramedics report signs of head injury and chest trauma. His BP is 110/75 mm Hg, HR 120 bpm, respiratory rate 18 breaths/min, SpO₂ 95% on 2 L nasal cannula. You cannot clearly identify lung sliding or lung pulse on the right chest, and you decide to perform an M-mode examination (**Figure 52.3**) of the dubious area.

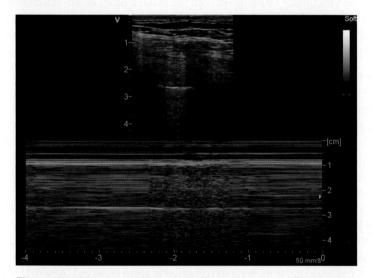

**Figure 52.3** M-mode ultrasound of the right chest of patient presented in Question 6.

The findings depicted in Figure 52.3 suggest:
A. Normal sliding
B. PTX
C. Lack of ventilation
D. Image acquisition pitfall
E. None of the above

7. A 75-year-old man with no previous respiratory history has been admitted after sustaining a syncopal episode in which he fell at home. Chest radiograph, electrocardiogram (ECG), and troponin levels are normal. The nurse calls you to assess him because of worsening dyspnea and desaturation. Based on the ultrasound findings identified in ▶ **Video 52.5** and **Figure 52.4**, which condition can be immediately diagnosed?

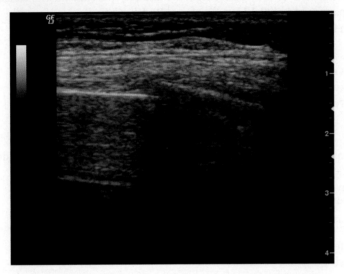

**Figure 52.4**

A. Pneumothorax
B. Rib fracture
C. Hemothorax
D. Diaphragmatic injury
E. None of the above

8. A 26-year-old man presents at the Emergency Department with the sudden onset of left-sided chest pain and shortness of breath. He reports that the symptoms started while exercising approximately 45 minutes prior and is exacerbated by deep breathing. LUS examination reveals the following image (▶ **Video 52.6**). What is the *most* appropriate medical decision based on this LUS finding?

A. Insert pleural drainage for PTX
B. Reassure patient that there is no PTX and discharge
C. Keep the patient for monitoring and repeat LUS examination
D. Computed tomography to rule out PTX
E. None of the above

9. A 68-year-old man was admitted to the intensive care unit (ICU) for severe respiratory failure secondary to bilateral pneumonia. He required endotracheal intubation and initiation of mechanical ventilation. Initially, he was ventilated in volume control ventilation (tidal volume = 6 mL/kg ideal body weight), respiratory rate of 28 breaths/min, and a positive end-expiratory pressure (PEEP) of 8 cmH$_2$O. LUS was performed, with ▶ **Videos 52.7** showing the right (▶ **Video 52.7A**) and left (▶ **Video 52.7B**) anterosuperior zones. Due to ongoing hypoxemia, PEEP was progressively increased, up to 14 cmH$_2$O. After an initial improvement in oxygenation, worsening oxygenation is again observed. A new LUS is performed in the same regions (▶ **Video 52.7C** and **D**). Which condition is *most* likely?

A. Pneumothorax
B. Atelectasis
C. Worsening interstitial syndrome
D. Lung overdistension
E. None of the above

# Chapter 52 ▪ Answers

*Rationale:* When suspecting a PTX, the three most useful findings to look for are: 1) lung sliding; 2) lung pulse; and 3) presence of vertical artifacts. In the case of a PTX, visceral and parietal pleura are separated by intrapleural air, causing complete reflection and attenuation of ultrasound waves at the level of the parietal pleura. Thus, when PTX is present, *all* three of the aforementioned pulmonary ultrasound findings are not detectable by surface ultrasound. Absence of lung sliding alone has very poor specificity for PTX, with a positive predictive value of only 22%. On the contrary, the identification of *even one* of these findings is sufficient to rule out PTX in the insonated area (**Figure 52.5**), making LUS an excellent technique to "rule out" but not necessarily "rule in" PTX.

In ▶ **Video 52.1B**, both lung sliding and pulse can be identified, immediately ruling out PTX on the left side. In ▶ **Video 52.1A**, lung sliding is absent, but lung pulse can still be identified, ruling out PTX also on the right side. Pleural effusion, defined as an anechoic collection between the parietal and visceral pleura, is not demonstrated in ▶ **Video 52.1A**; therefore, right hemothorax is not the correct answer, although we cannot exclude presence of hemothorax in this patient; such a determination would require the scanning of more dependent areas of the pleural cavity. Finally, lung contusion cannot be confirmed in these videos as neither B-lines nor lung consolidations are detected. The most likely correct answer in this case is therefore right bronchial obstruction. Lack of sliding in this case was caused by lack of ventilation related to left mainstem endobronchial intubation. Since the visceral and parietal pleura are still in physical contact, lung pulse (i.e., ultrasonographic detection of transmission of cardiac contraction through lung tissue) is still present.

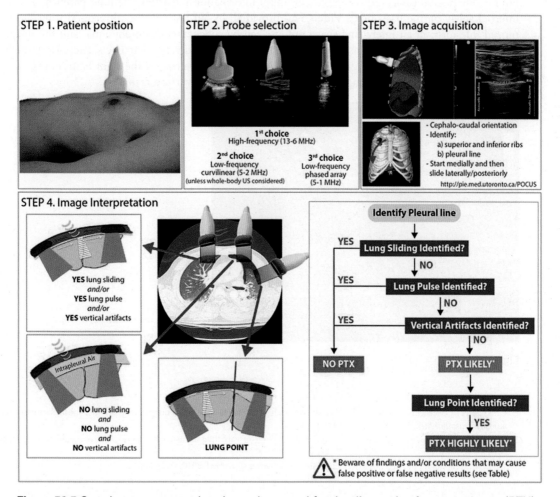

**Figure 52.5** Step-by-step approach to lung ultrasound for the diagnosis of pneumothorax (PTX).

**Selected References**

1. Goffi A, Kruisselbrink R, Volpicelli, G. The sound of air: point-of-care lung ultrasound in perioperative medicine. *Can J Anesth.* 2018;65(4):399-416.
2. Lichtenstein DA, Menu Y. A bedside ultrasound sign ruling out pneumothorax in the critically Ill: lung sliding. *Chest.* 1995;108(5):1345-1348.
3. Volpicelli G. Sonographic diagnosis of pneumothorax. *Intensive Care Med.* 2010;37(2):224-232.
4. Volpicelli G, Elbarbary M, Blaivas M, et al. International evidence-based recommendations for point-of-care lung ultrasound. *Intensive Care Med.* 2012;38(4):577-591.

**2.** Correct Answer: E. None of the above

*Rationale:* ▶ **Video 52.2** demonstrates the sonographic appearance of subcutaneous emphysema. The linear hyperechoic artifacts (*white arrow*, **Figure 52.6**) do not originate from the pleural line, but within the subcutaneous tissues, above the parietal pleura, as demonstrated by the *red arrows* in Figure 52.6, where costal cartilage and underlying pleural line can be observed. These artifacts are generated by the high acoustic impedance difference created by the interface between subcutaneous tissues and air bubbles. Sometimes, they can also produce vertical reverberation artifacts (also known as "E-lines") that can be mistakenly interpreted as B-lines. The key aspect in differentiating E-lines from B-lines is the fact that the first ones do not originate from the pleural line. A "false pleural sliding" can sometimes be observed, generated by the contraction of respiratory muscles during inspiration. Although PTX cannot be diagnosed with certainty, identification of subcutaneous emphysema in this specific context (chest trauma) is highly suspicious for presence of PTX.

Presence of subcutaneous emphysema can significantly affect LUS acquisition and performance; air in the subcutaneous tissues acts as a barrier for the ultrasounds and therefore the pleura cannot be reached. As the pleural line cannot be insonated at this level, no information can be provided on lung sliding and pulse, presence of vertical artifacts originating from the pleural line, and/or collection of fluid in the pleural cavity. For example, no useful information regarding the lung parenchyma can be inferred solely on the basis of ▶ **Video 52.2** provided. In our patient, the ultrasound transducer was moved inferiorly, in an intercostal space not affected by subcutaneous emphysema, and the image acquired (▶ **Video 52.8A**) demonstrated lack of sliding, pulse, and vertical artifacts, supporting the likely diagnosis of traumatic PTX (Figure 52.1). ▶ **Video 52.8B**, acquired on the right hemithorax, demonstrates normal lung findings (lung sliding, lung pulse, and short vertical artifacts).

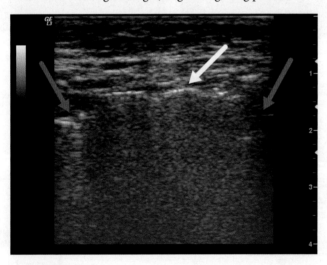

**Figure 52.6**

**Selected References**

1. Chiappetta M, Meacci E, Cesario A, et al. Postoperative chest ultrasound findings and effectiveness after thoracic surgery: a pilot study. *Ultrasound Med. Biol.* 2018;44(9):1960-1967.
2. Goffi A, Kruisselbrink R, Volpicelli, G. The sound of air: point-of-care lung ultrasound in perioperative medicine. *Can J Anesth.* 2018;65(4):399-416.
3. Volpicelli G. Sonographic diagnosis of pneumothorax. *Intensive Care Med.* 2010;37(2):224-232.

**3.** Correct Answer: B. LUS is more sensitive but equally specific to CXR for detection of PTX.

*Rationale:* In the hands of a trained operator and in patients with a high pretest probability (e.g., dyspnea or chest pain posttrauma or central line insertion), LUS is overall more accurate than CXR for the detection of a PTX. In particular, the sensitivity of LUS is higher than supine CXR (79%-91% versus 40%-52%, respectively) (Answers C and D are incorrect), whereas specificity is equally very high for both (98%-99% versus 99%-100%, respectively) (Answer A is incorrect, B is correct). However, as most studies on the diagnostic accuracy of LUS for PTX are in trauma or postprocedural patients, these numbers may overestimate LUS performance in other settings (e.g., nontrauma patients with preexisting conditions such as emphysema).

### Selected References

1. Alrajab S, Youssef A, Akkus N, Caldito G. Pleural ultrasonography versus chest radiography for the diagnosis of pneumothorax: review of the literature and meta-analysis. *Crit Care.* 2013;17(5):R208.
2. Alrajhi K, Woo MY, Vaillancourt C. Test characteristics of ultrasonography for the detection of pneumothorax: a systematic review and meta-analysis. *Chest.* 2012;141(3):703-708.
3. Ding W, Shen Y, Yang J, He X, Zhang M. Diagnosis of pneumothorax by radiography and ultrasonography: a meta-analysis. *Chest.* 2011;140(4):859-866.

**4.** Correct Answer: A. ▶ **Video 52.3A** demonstrates a lung point, a highly specific finding for PTX

*Rationale:* Although highly suspicious, the absence of lung sliding, lung pulse, and vertical artifacts is not sufficient to diagnose PTX with certainty. Certain lung conditions (e.g., severe chronic obstructive pulmonary disease, bullous disease, lung overdistension) can create a similar sonographic pattern. Observation of a "lung point," where the pleural layers meet adjacent to the edge of the PTX, confirms the presence of PTX (*red arrow*, **Figure 52.7**).

As observed in ▶ **Video 52.3A**, the respiratory (sliding) and oscillatory (pulse) patterns are visualized on the left side of the screen and intermittently replace the motionless pleura, representing a "lung point," a "positive" finding with a high specificity but low sensitivity (Answer A is correct, Answer B is incorrect). This "replacement movement" allows differentiation between a true lung point (i.e., confirmation of PTX) and the transition between ventilating and nonventilating areas as they can be observed in patients with pleural adhesions. The presence of a lung pulse excludes PTX. ▶ **Video 52.3B** does show a lung pulse, a finding not seen in PTX (Answers C, D are incorrect).

A lung point cannot be visualized in a larger PTX, where the pleural layers are separated completely, because the "edge" of the PTX is not in an area accessible by ultrasound. In other cases, the lung point may not be visible as it can be hidden behind osseous structures (ribs and scapula). In stable patients, the absence of a lung point does not allow definitive PTX diagnosis and should prompt further investigations (e.g., chest radiography or computed tomography). Finally, although precise quantification of PTX is not possible with LUS, the more laterally the lung point is detected, the greater is the extension of the PTX.

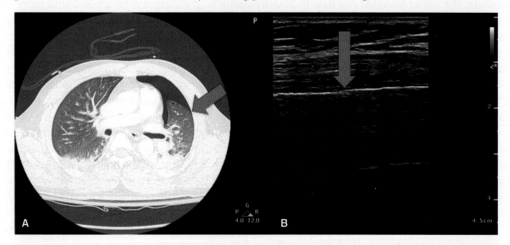

**Figure 52.7** A, Axial image from chest computed tomography (CT) demonstrating left pneumothorax. B, Lung ultrasound image demonstrating the transition point ("lung point") between intrapleural air (no sliding, no pulse, and no vertical artifacts) and a normally aerated area (sliding, pulse, and/or vertical artifacts). *Red arrows* indicate the transition areas.

Selected References
1. Goffi A, Kruisselbrink R, Volpicelli, G. The sound of air: point-of-care lung ultrasound in perioperative medicine. *Can J Anesth.* 2018;65(4):399-416.
2. Volpicelli G. A lung point that is not a lung point. *Intensive Care Med.* 2019;45(9):1326-1326.
3. Volpicelli G. Sonographic diagnosis of pneumothorax. *Intensive Care Med.* 2010;37(2):224-232.
4. Volpicelli G, Boero E, Sverzellati N, et al. Semi-quantification of pneumothorax volume by lung ultrasound. *Intensive Care Med.* 2014;40(10):1460-1467.
5. Volpicelli G, Elbarbary M, Blaivas M, et al. International evidence-based recommendations for point-of-care lung ultrasound. *Intensive Care Med.* 2012;38(4):577-591.

**5.** Correct Answer: D. Likely, neither lung sliding nor pulse is detected

*Rationale:* In ▶ **Video 52.4**, no sliding or vertical artifacts are seen originating from the pleural line. The "focal" pulsatility observed is generated by the arterial pulsation of the intercostal artery seen immediately about the parietal pleural and not by the transmission of cardiac contractions through the lung parenchyma. Therefore, this video is suspicious for the presence of PTX; in this patient, a lateral movement of the transducer identified a lung point confirming the diagnosis of traumatic PTX.

Several pitfalls have been described in acquisition and interpretation of LUS images in the context of possible PTX, leading to both false-positive and false-negative results. False-negative results can be caused by: 1) failure to insonate the least dependent zone of the chest (typically when scanning a patient in a sitting or semi-recumbent position); 2) misinterpretation of the absence of lung point as a sign of no PTX instead of complete PTX; 3) misinterpretation of vertical artifacts originating in the subcutaneous tissues (E-lines) as vertical artifacts originating from the pleural line (see question 2); 4) presence of loculated PTX; 5) small left PTX at the level of the paracardiac area; 6) misinterpretation of intercostal or internal thoracic artery pulsations as lung pulse; and/or 7) failure to identify lung pulse in the context of severe bradycardia and hypotension. On the contrary, false-positive results can be caused by: 1) absence of lung sliding (e.g., apnea, inflammatory adherences, over-inflation, severe bullous disease, decrease in lung compliance, pleural symphysis, endobronchial intubation); 2) absence of lung pulse in bullous disease and over-inflation/-distension; 3) position of transducer over a rib instead of the intercostal space; and/or 4) misinterpretation of pericardial movement (paracardiac area), diaphragm (supradiaphragmatic area), or transition point between normal lung and lung bullae or adhesions as lung point.

Selected References
1. Goffi A, Kruisselbrink R, Volpicelli, G. The sound of air: point-of-care lung ultrasound in perioperative medicine. *Can J Anesth.* 2018;65(4):399-416.
2. Soldati G, Testa A, Sher S, Pignataro G, La Sala M, Silveri NG. Occult traumatic pneumothorax: diagnostic accuracy of lung ultrasonography in the emergency department. *Chest.* 2008;133(1):204-211.

**6.** Correct Answer: D. Image acquisition pitfall

*Rationale:* The use of M-mode can help to identify subtle lung sliding and lung pulse with more confidence than B-mode. In a recent study, Avila et al. demonstrated that the addition of M-mode images to B-mode studies improves the accuracy of LUS for diagnosis of PTX, but only for providers who have performed less than 250 LUS studies. When M-mode is used to insonate normal lung, a series of hyperechoic continuous lines, generated by the relatively motionless subcutaneous tissues and muscles, can be identified above the pleural line. Below this line, the movement generated by lung sliding produces a "granular" appearance of the M-mode pattern that has been compared to the sand of a beach, with the straight continuous lines above the pleura looking like ocean waves, hence the "seashore" sign (**Figure 52.8A**).

In the presence of PTX, because of the lack of movement seen between pleural layers, the same motionless lines observed above the pleural line are observed below it, generating a typical pattern that resembles a "barcode" (or, as initially described by Lichtenstein, the "stratosphere," **Figure 52.8B**). On M-mode, lack of lung sliding but the presence of lung pulse (as seen in conditions causing lack of ventilation as apnea or bronchial obstruction) generates an alternating pattern where a barcode sign is rhythmically interrupted by short seashore signs (Figure 52.8A).

In Figure 52.3, a barcode sign is suddenly interrupted by a granular pattern that initially may be confused with a seashore sign. With more careful analysis, the granular pattern is noted to be present not only below the pleural line but also above it. This "full thickness" granular appearance of the M-mode signal is generated by an artifactual sudden motion of the transducer relative to the chest wall (Answer D is correct). Because it occurs both above and below the pleura, it is distinct from pleural movement (Answer A is incorrect). Because the motion artifact occupies much of the area of interest, it is not accurate to make an assessment about the presence or absence of ventilation (Answer C) or PTX (Answer B). By repeating the examination in the same area without artifactual movement, the presence of a PTX may be confirmed.

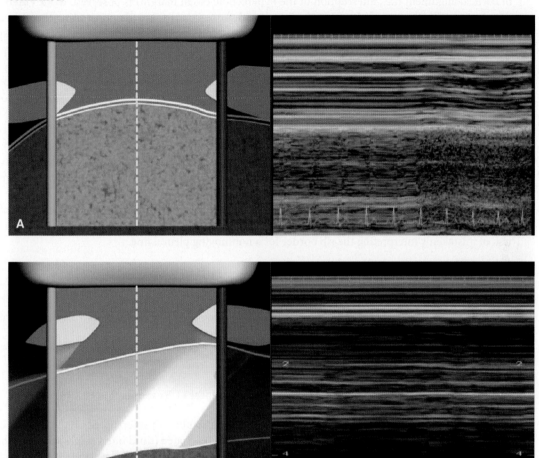

**Figure 52.8** A, M-mode ultrasound appearance of normally aerated lung in the absence of pneumothorax. A series of hyperechoic continuous lines, generated by the relatively motionless subcutaneous tissues and muscles, can be identified above the pleural line. Below this line, the movement generated by lung sliding produces a "granular" appearance of the M-mode pattern that has been compared to the sand of a beach, hence the "seashore" sign, with the straight continuous lines looking like ocean waves. Lack of lung sliding but presence of lung pulse (as seen in conditions causing lack of ventilation as apnea or bronchial obstruction) generates an alternating pattern where a barcode sign is rhythmically interrupted by short seashore signs. Images adapted with permission from http://pie.med.utoronto.ca/POCUS. B, M-mode ultrasound appearance of pneumothorax. Because of the lack of lung sliding and pulse, motionless lines above the pleural line are also observed below it, generating a typical pattern that resembles a "barcode" (or, as initially described by Lichtenstein, the "stratosphere").

### Selected References

1. Avila J, Smith B, Mead T, et al. Does the addition of M-mode to B-mode ultrasound increase the accuracy of identification of lung sliding in traumatic pneumothoraces? *J Ultrasound Med.* 2018;37(11):2681-2687.
2. Lichtenstein D, Mezière G, Biderman P, Gepner A. The "lung point": an ultrasound sign specific to pneumothorax. *Intensive Care Med.* 2000;26(10):1434-1440.
3. Prada G, Vieillard-Baron A, Martin AK, et al. Tracheal, lung, and diaphragmatic applications of M-mode ultrasonography in anesthesiology and critical care. *J Cardiothorac Vasc Anesth.* 2021;35(1):310-322 [Epub ahead of print].

**7.** Correct Answer: B. Rib fracture

*Rationale:* ▶ **Video 52.5** and Figure 52.4 demonstrate the sonographic appearance of a displaced rib fracture. The high-frequency linear transducer is placed parallel to the long axis of the rib and discontinuity of cortical alignment (i.e., interruption of the hyperechoic costal margin) is observed. In ▶ **Video 52.9**, the operator tilts the transducer from the intercostal to the costal space, demonstrating the differences between the two areas. In this video, a lung point is also observed at the level of the intercostal space, demonstrating the presence of a PTX that was missed during the initial CXR performed in the Emergency Department.

This case highlights two key concepts: 1) the utility of point-of-care ultrasound for the diagnosis of rib fractures; and 2) the importance of proper transducer positioning and image acquisition for correct interpretation.

Ultrasound has been shown to be more sensitive than chest radiography for the diagnosis of rib fractures in the Emergency Department (sensitivity of 80.3%-90% versus 15%-23.7%, respectively), although it may be time consuming. If the patient is able to collaborate, identification of the site of maximal tenderness may significantly shorten performance time and increase diagnostic accuracy. Sometimes, a hypoechoic hematoma can be seen at the fracture site.

We recommend to always begin lung insonation by placing the transducer in a cephalocaudal orientation to allow visualization of at least two ribs and the pleural line between. This approach lessens the risk of mistakenly interpreting the rib border for a nonmoving pleural line.

### Selected References

1. Chan SS-W. Emergency bedside ultrasound for the diagnosis of rib fractures. *Am J Emerg Med.* 2009;27(5):617-620.
2. Griffith JF, Rainer TH, Ching AS, Law KL, Cocks RA, Metreweli C. Sonography compared with radiography in revealing acute rib fracture. *Am J Roentgenol.* 1999;173(6):1603-1609.
3. Lalande É, Wylie K. Towards evidence-based emergency medicine: best BETs from the Manchester Royal Infirmary. BET 1: ultrasound in the diagnosis of rib fractures. *Emerg Med J.* 2014;31(2):169-170.
4. Rainer TH, Griffith JF, Lam E, Lam PKW, Metreweli C. Comparison of thoracic ultrasound, clinical acumen, and radiography in patients with minor chest injury. *J Trauma.* 2004;56(6):1211-1213.

**8.** Correct Answer: C. Keep the patient for monitoring and repeat LUS examination

*Rationale:* In ▶ **Video 52.6**, the lung sliding seems to be intermittently interrupted on the left side of the screen, raising concerns for a lung point. However, the area insonated (third intercostal space at the hemiclavicular line) suggests a cautious approach to a definitive diagnosis, as at this level pulmonary structures are in close relationship with mediastinal structures. In a study by Soldati et al., LUS incorrectly classified three patients undergoing computed tomography (CT) for suspicion of PTX (two false-negative results and one false-positive one). In all three cases, the LUS misinterpretation was in images obtained at the level of the left paracardiac region. Careful observation of ▶ **Video 52.8A** demonstrates that what may initially be interpreted as a lung point is instead the pleuro-pericardial interface, with pleural line shifting caused by cardiac contractions. In the study by Soldati et al., LUS was performed using a low-frequency transducer, which may have contributed to the three incorrect LUS interpretations; we recommend use of high-frequency transducers for the detection of PTX, when available.

In this patient, the combination of LUS findings, pain characteristics, and lack of significant risk factors allowed us to quickly rule out primary spontaneous PTX and also did not suggest high risk for pulmonary embolism. However, the presence of several B-lines raised concerns for an interstitial process. The patient underwent further investigations and later developed fever and respiratory symptoms consistent with an infectious process. LUS ultrasound performed a few days later demonstrated a lung consolidation with small parapneumonic pleural effusion.

### Selected References

1. Alrajab S, Youssef A, Akkus N, Caldito G. Pleural ultrasonography versus chest radiography for the diagnosis of pneumothorax: review of the literature and meta-analysis. *Crit Care.* 2013;17(5):R208.
2. Alrajhi K, Woo MY, Vaillancourt C. Test characteristics of ultrasonography for the detection of pneumothorax: a systematic review and meta-analysis. *Chest.* 2012;141(3):703-708.
3. Goffi A, Kruisselbrink R, Volpicelli, G. The sound of air: point-of-care lung ultrasound in perioperative medicine. *Can J Anesth.* 2018;65(4):399-416.
4. Soldati G, Testa A, Sher S, Pignataro G, La Sala M, Silveri NG. Occult traumatic pneumothorax: diagnostic accuracy of lung ultrasonography in the emergency department. *Chest.* 2008;133(1):204-211.

**9.** Correct Answer: D. Lung overdistension

*Rationale:* LUS has been proposed as a monitoring tool for mechanically ventilated patients. Assessment of real-time changes through LUS patterns (normal aeration, isolated B-lines, coalescent B-lines, and lung consolidation) allows for the detection of lung reaeration after interventions such as prone positioning, recruitment maneuvers, or changes in PEEP. However, one of the main limitations of LUS in the assessment of lung recruitability during mechanical ventilation is its inability to effectively quantify lung over-inflation. Once the lung is completely reaerated, further distension of the alveolar units does not significantly change the LUS pattern (A-lines with absent B-lines). Nevertheless, changes in lung sliding and/or lung pulse may suggest worsening inflation of normally aerated areas. In our case, at PEEP of 8 cmH$_2$O, both sliding and pulse were clearly identified in the least dependent zones of the chest (● **Video 52.7A** and **B**), whereas at PEEP of 14 cmH$_2$O, lung sliding was no longer evident in the same regions (● **Video 52.7C** and **D**), suggesting a reduction in regional ventilation consistent with overdistension (Answer D). The presence of a lung pulse immediately excludes PTX in this patient at both locations (Answer A is incorrect). Atelectasis and worsening interstitial syndrome are usually associated with the presence of B-lines, which are not observed (Answer B and C are incorrect).

### Selected References

1. Bouhemad B, Brisson H, Le-Guen M, Arbelot C, Lu Q, Rouby JJ. Bedside ultrasound assessment of positive end-expiratory pressure-induced lung recruitment. *Am J Respir Crit Care Med.* 2011;183:341-347.
2. Bouhemad B, Mongodi S, Via G, Rouquette I. Ultrasound for "lung monitoring" of ventilated patients. *Anesthesiology.* 2015;122:437-447.
3. Cereda M, Xin Y, Goffi A, et al. Imaging the injured lung: mechanisms of action and clinical use. *Anesthesiology.* 2019;131(3): 716-749.
4. Lichtenstein D. Novel approaches to ultrasonography of the lung and pleural space: where are we now? *Breathe.* 2017;13:100-111.

# 53 | CARDIOGENIC PULMONARY EDEMA, NONCARDIOGENIC PULMONARY EDEMA (ARDS), DIFFUSE PARENCHYMAL LUNG DISEASE (INTERSTITIAL PNEUMONITIS)

Christopher N. Parkhurst

1. A 75-year-old man with a medical history that includes heart failure with reduced ejection fraction and atrial fibrillation presents to the Emergency Department with 4 months of worsening shortness of breath with ambulation. He has a 45 pack-year smoking history and is a current every-day smoker. His atrial fibrillation is treated with amiodarone. Vital signs are notable for an SpO$_2$ of 85% at rest and are otherwise unremarkable. His physical examination is notable for moderate lower extremity edema with evidence of chronic venous stasis and fine rales in the lower and midlung fields. A focused lung ultrasound examination demonstrates the following finding in multiple fields in the anterior, posterior, and midaxillary lines (**Figure 53.1** and ▶ **Video 53.1**).

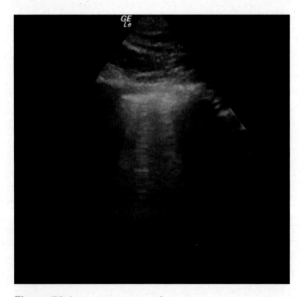

**Figure 53.1**

Given the above finding, the *least* likely etiology of this patient's shortness of breath is:

A. Chronic obstructive pulmonary disease (COPD)
B. Idiopathic pulmonary fibrosis (IPF)
C. Amiodarone toxicity
D. Decompensated heart failure

2. A 65-year-old man with a past medical history of heart failure with preserved ejection fraction is brought to the Emergency Department by ambulance with 3 days of worsening dyspnea. He is emergently intubated due to respiratory distress and brought to the intensive care unit (ICU). Over the next 24 hours, he develops worsening hypoxemia, and increasing inspiratory pressures are required to maintain an adequate minute ventilation. Nasopharyngeal polymerase chain reaction (PCR)-based testing is positive for influenza A virus. The estimated central venous pressure (CVP) derived from an internal jugular central venous catheter is normal. Bilateral breath sounds are heard on lung auscultation. The lung ultrasound findings that would be *most* consistent with the cause of this patient's worsening oxygenation and compliance are:

   A. Large unilateral pleural effusion
   B. Bilateral B-line profile
   C. Interspersed areas of B-lines and normal lung
   D. Absence of A-lines

3. The finding *most* specific for a diagnosis of interstitial lung disease (ILD) is:

   A. A thickened and fragmented pleural line
   B. Absence of lung sliding
   C. Diffuse bilateral B-lines
   D. Bilateral A-line profile

4. A 50-year-old woman with metastatic breast cancer is admitted to the hospital with approximately 1 week of worsening dyspnea on exertion and is found to have a large right-sided pleural effusion. Thoracentesis is performed using local anesthesia with 1% lidocaine, and 2.5 L of clear yellow fluid is removed without any obvious complication. Immediately after the procedure, the patient experiences relief of her dyspnea; however, over the next 2 hours, she becomes increasingly short of breath and develops respiratory distress. Focused ultrasound of the lungs is performed with the patient in the supine position and the following findings over the right anterior and lateral hemithorax are demonstrated in **Figure 53.2** and ▶ **Videos 53.2, 53.3, 53.4.**

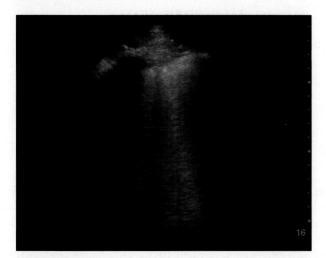

**Figure 53.2**

The most likely etiology of this patient's postprocedural dyspnea is:
A. Pneumothorax
B. Hemothorax
C. Lidocaine toxicity
D. Reexpansion pulmonary edema

5. A 70-year-old man is admitted to the ICU for the treatment of septic shock. He is intubated and mechanically ventilated, and is being treated with antibiotics, a vasopressor infusion, and crystalloid infusions due to persistent hypotension. On his third day in the ICU, it is noted that both his $FiO_2$ and inspiratory pressure requirements have increased to maintain adequate oxygenation and ventilation. A member of the ICU team suspects pulmonary edema due to iatrogenic volume overload and begins a focused lung ultrasound examination. Which of the following findings would *most* likely suggest that pulmonary edema is *not* the etiology for the patient's change in oxygenation and lung compliance?

     **A.** The absence of B-lines in the anterior lung fields
     **B.** The absence of a pleural effusion
     **C.** The absence of multiple B-lines in the posterior lung fields
     **D.** Normal bilateral lung sliding

6. The greatest number of B-line artifacts that may be seen within a single intercostal space in a healthy adult patient is:

     **A.** 1
     **B.** 2
     **C.** 3
     **D.** 5

7. A 65-year-old woman with a medical history of chronic hypersensitivity pneumonitis (cHP, a form of ILD) and heart failure with reduced ejection fraction is brought to the Emergency Department with several days of progressive dyspnea and worsening lower extremity edema. Her oxygen saturation by pulse oximetry on arrival is noted to be 83% on 6 L of supplemental oxygen (she does not normally use supplemental oxygen at home), and her breathing is mildly labored. Ultrasound examination of her lungs demonstrates a diffuse B-line pattern in all lung fields examined. The lung ultrasound findings observed in this patient indicate that her dyspnea and hypoxia are *most* likely due to which of the following?

     **A.** Exacerbation of congestive heart failure
     **B.** Exacerbation of cHP
     **C.** Pulmonary embolism
     **D.** The etiology cannot be determined from this data

8. Which of the following scenarios is the *least* likely to produce B-lines?

     **A.** Transfusion-related acute lung injury (TRALI)
     **B.** Asthma exacerbation
     **C.** Subarachnoid hemorrhage
     **D.** Endotracheal tube obstruction

9. A 67-year-old man with a long-standing history of poorly controlled hypertension is brought to the Emergency Department from home with several days of fever and increasing lethargy. He is found to be hypotensive and tachycardic and has a serum lactate level of 7 mmol/L. He is admitted to the ICU and treated with broad-spectrum antibiotics, crystalloid fluid resuscitation, and vasopressors. Despite this early therapy, his condition declines and he is intubated. Overnight, his oxygen requirements increase, and by the following day his P:F ratio is 150. He has received a total of 8 L of intravenous fluid since admission for ongoing hypotension. A portable chest X-ray is obtained and shows diffuse bilateral infiltrates and no evidence of a pneumothorax. Ultrasound is performed and shows numerous and diffuse B-lines bilaterally, in addition to the finding shown in ▶ **Video 53.5**. The most likely etiology for this patient's hypoxemia is:

     **A.** Cardiogenic pulmonary edema (CPE)
     **B.** Pneumothorax
     **C.** Acute respiratory distress syndrome (ARDS)
     **D.** Ventilator-associated pneumonia

**10.** A patient undergoes an ultrasound examination of the lung, which demonstrates a normal-appearing pleural line, normal lung sliding, no B-lines, and a loss of A-lines in all lung fields examined. What are these findings most consistent with?

 **A.** Idiopathic pulmonary fibrosis
 **B.** Pneumothorax
 **C.** Chronic obstructive lung disease
 **D.** Normal lung tissue with advanced age

**11.** A 65-year-old man is evaluated in the Emergency Department with several weeks of worsening dyspnea. He has no known history of pulmonary disease. He is noted to be hypoxemic with SpO$_2$ of 85% on room air. The pleural ultrasound images (**Figure 53.3, ▶ Video 53.6, ▶ Video 53.7**) are obtained in multiple lung regions bilaterally. Cardiac ultrasound examination demonstrates grossly normal left and right ventricular size and function, and Doppler ultrasonography indicates normal diastolic pressures within the left ventricle.

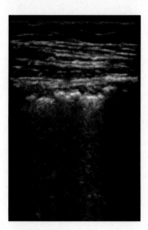

**Figure 53.3**

The *most* likely diagnosis is which of the following?
 **A.** Interstitial lung disease
 **B.** Pulmonary edema
 **C.** Pneumothorax
 **D.** Pneumonia

**12.** A 23-year-old woman is brought by ambulance to the trauma bay of the Emergency Department after she was found unconscious in a nearby park by bystanders. Upon arrival, emergency medical service practitioners found her unresponsive with sporadic shallow breaths and she was intubated. After arrival to the Emergency Department, it is noted that it is becoming increasingly difficult to ventilate through the endotracheal tube using a bag-valve device. Vital signs are temperature 34°C, BP 110/70 mm Hg, and HR 50 bpm. She is noted to have pinpoint pupils and the physical examination is otherwise unremarkable. While the secondary trauma survey is taking place, a Focused Assessment with Ultrasound for Trauma (FAST) examination is performed. The cardiac and abdominal portions of the examination are normal (except for bradycardia), and the pulmonary portion of the examination reveals a diffuse B-line pattern in a bilateral distribution. The most likely diagnosis in this patient is:

 **A.** Right mainstem bronchus intubation
 **B.** Pulmonary edema
 **C.** Pulmonary contusion
 **D.** Hemothorax

**13.** A 45-year-old man with human immunodeficiency virus (HIV)/acquired immunodeficiency syndrome (AIDS) is being treated for *Pneumocystis jiroveci* pneumonia in the ICU. A computed tomography (CT) scan on admission demonstrated severe parenchymal disease with diffuse ground-glass opacification (GGO) and multifocal pulmonary blebs. He was intubated several days ago for hypoxemic respiratory failure and has required increasing inspiratory pressure in order to provide an adequate tidal volume. The peak airway pressure alarm sounds, and it is noted that his peak airway pressure has increased dramatically. Focused ultrasound of the pleura demonstrates bilateral lung points consistent with bilateral pneumothorax, and chest tubes are emergently placed in each hemithorax with successful evacuation of air and a fall in the peak airway pressure. After this intervention, the patient undergoes repeat pleural ultrasonography of the anterior chest wall in the supine position and **Figure 53.4** and ▶ **Video 53.8** are obtained. This finding is *most* consistent with which of the following?

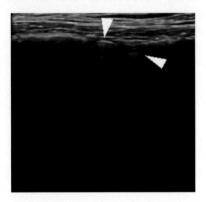

**Figure 53.4**

**A.** Residual pneumothorax
**B.** Atelectatic lung
**C.** Pulmonary edema
**D.** Subcutaneous emphysema

**14.** What do the features highlighted by the *arrowhead* in **Figure 53.5** represent? (See also ▶ **Video 53.9**.)

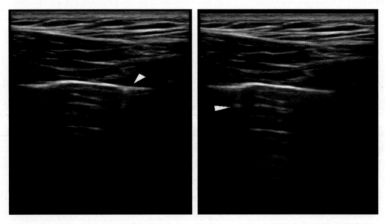

**Figure 53.5**

**A.** Normal lung tissue
**B.** Pulmonary edema
**C.** Idiopathic pulmonary fibrosis
**D.** Chronic obstructive pulmonary disease

15. **Figure 53.6** was obtained 1 minute apart from each other on the same patient in exactly the same thoracic imaging site.

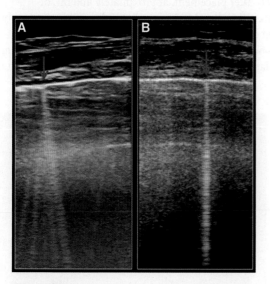

**Figure 53.6**

Between the acquisition of Figure 53.6A and Figure 53.6B, an adjustment is made to the ultrasound machine's software. This *most* likely adjustment is which of the following?
A. Near-field gain increased
B. Near-field gain decreased
C. Second harmonics turned on
D. Second harmonics turned off

16. A patient with suspected pulmonary edema undergoes lung ultrasound. Apparent B-lines are imaged in all lung regions, as in **Figure 53.7** and ▶ **Video 53.10**.

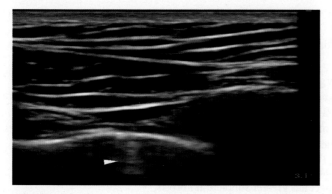

**Figure 53.7**

In order to confirm that the image does indeed contain B-lines, which of the following adjustments should be made to the ultrasound machine?
A. Beam focus depth increased
B. Beam focus depth decreased
C. Imaging depth increased
D. Imaging depth decreased

17. A 57-year-old woman is admitted to the hospital with a diagnosis of community-acquired pneumonia (CAP), complicated by pleural effusion. She undergoes placement of a "pigtail" pleural catheter for drainage of the pleural collection. Immediately after placement, approximately 400 mL of cloudy-appearing yellow fluid drains into the collection chamber, before the drainage spontaneously stops, after which no further material is collected over the next 24 hours. The patient continues to complain of shortness of breath, and an ultrasound examination of the lungs is performed, providing **Figure 53.8** and ▶ **Video 53.11** over the anterolateral chest wall (ipsilateral to the chest tube), with the patient in the supine position.

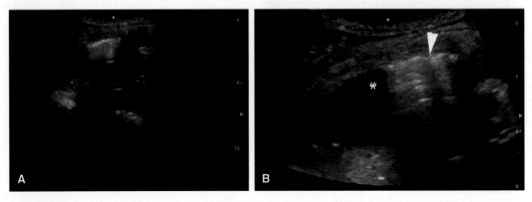

**Figure 53.8**

What do the findings *most* likely represent?
A. Reexpansion pulmonary edema
B. Atelectatic lung tissue
C. Hydropneumothorax
D. Cardiogenic pulmonary edema

18. Which of the following is *not* an absolute criterion for B-lines?

A. They arise from the pleural line.
B. They project to the bottom of the screen without fading.
C. They erase A-lines.
D. They move synchronously with lung sliding.

19. Two patients with known ILD undergo pleural ultrasound. The examinations of both patients are notable for diffuse B-line profiles in both lungs, as well as a fractured and irregular-appearing pleural line. It is noted that one patient has B-lines that are spaced 3 mm apart, while the other patient has B-lines that are 7 mm apart. Which of the following statements *best* describes the correlation of these ultrasound findings to CT scan of the chest in this patient population?

A. The patient with B-lines 3 mm apart has more advanced disease.
B. The patient with B-lines 7 mm apart has greater subpleural fibrosis.
C. The patient with B-lines 7 mm apart has greater subpleural GGO.
D. The distance between B-lines is not correlated with the CT lung examination.

**20.** A 76-year-old man with a medical history of well-controlled hypertension and type 2 diabetes presents from home with several days of productive cough and fatigue. His vital signs are remarkable for a fever of 38°C. A chest X-ray is performed and does not show any abnormality. A point-of-care cardiac and lung ultrasound examination is performed. The cardiac examination is unremarkable; however, the lung examination demonstrates a diffuse bilateral B-line profile in both lungs, and there are no pleural effusions or consolidated/atelectatic lung regions. Lung sliding is intact, and the pleural line appears normal in all regions examined. Based on this information, the *most* likely diagnosis is which of the following?

**A.** Idiopathic pulmonary fibrosis
**B.** Cardiogenic pulmonary edema
**C.** Lymphangitic carcinomatosis of the lung
**D.** Pneumonia

# Chapter 53 ▪ Answers

**1.** Correct Answer: **A. Chronic obstructive pulmonary disease (COPD)**

*Rationale:* The presence of B-lines is a nonspecific finding that signifies the presence of an interstitial syndrome. The pathologies that underlie this finding are numerous and include pulmonary edema (both cardiogenic and noncardiogenic), drug-induced lung injury, and tissue fibrosis. This older man with a significant smoking history (both risk factors for IPF), heart failure, amiodarone use (risk for pulmonary drug toxicity), and reduced left ventricular function has multiple possible etiologies for his breathlessness. The presence of B-lines does not rule out any of these processes except for COPD, which should demonstrate a normal A-line profile. Note that the B-line profile seen in this patient *does not* rule out the presence of underlying COPD, as it is possible to have pulmonary edema on top of obstructive lung disease.

Selected References
1. Hasan AA, Makhlouf HA. B-lines: transthoracic chest ultrasound signs useful in assessment of interstitial lung diseases. *Ann Thorac Med.* 2014;9(2):99-103. doi:10.4103/1817-1737.128856.
2. Soldati G, Copetti R, Sher S. Sonographic interstitial syndrome: the sound of lung water. *J Ultrasound Med.* 2009;28(2):163-174. doi:10.7863/jum.2009.28.2.163.

**2.** Correct Answer: **C. Interspersed areas of B-lines and normal lung**

*Rationale:* This case involves differentiating the cause of worsening hypoxia and lung compliance in a patient presenting with acute respiratory failure. Although his underlying cardiac dysfunction, specifically a stiff left ventricle, puts him at risk for cardiogenic pulmonary edema (CPE), the low CVP makes this a less likely etiology. Given the presence of an influenza viral infection, worsening oxygenation, and decreasing lung compliance, ARDS is the most likely diagnosis in the patient. Because the pattern of lung injury seen in ARDS is typically nonuniform, lung ultrasound often demonstrates a patchy distribution of B-lines alternating with areas of normal lung, whereas fulminant pulmonary edema more typically shows B-lines in multiple imaging fields.

Selected Reference
1. Copetti R, Soldati G, Copetti P. Chest sonography: a useful tool to differentiate acute cardiogenic pulmonary edema from acute respiratory distress syndrome. *Cardiovasc Ultrasound.* 2008;6:16. doi:10.1186/1476-7120-6-16.

**3.** Correct Answer: **A. A thickened and fragmented pleural line**

*Rationale:* The ILDs are a heterogeneous group of pulmonary diseases affecting the lung parenchyma that ultimately progress to lung fibrosis and include idiopathic pulmonary fibrosis, connective tissue disease–related ILD, and hypersensitivity pneumonitis. In a lung ultrasound study of patients with ILD, the most common finding present in ILD vs. healthy control patients was irregularity and thickening of the pleural line (see **Figure 53.9** for example images).

### Selected Reference
1. Reissig A, Kroegel C. Transthoracic sonography of diffuse parenchymal lung disease: the role of comet tail artifacts. *J Ultrasound Med.* 2003;22(2):173-180. doi:10.7863/jum.2003.22.2.173.

---

**4.** Correct Answer: D. Reexpansion pulmonary edema

*Rationale/Critique:* A number of complications are associated with common bedside pleural procedures. These include hemothorax from injury to intercostal vessels, pneumothorax due to inadvertent interruption of the pleura, and reexpansion pulmonary edema. This type of non-CPE (NCPE) occurs after the removal of air or pleural fluid from the pleural space, typically within several hours of the procedure. Here the presence of lung sliding and absence of fluid in the pleural space rule out pneumothorax and hemothorax, respectively. Although the mechanism is incompletely understood, reexpansion pulmonary edema appears as an interstitial syndrome with ultrasound, and therefore creates a diffuse B-line profile. Although these findings are typically seen ipsilateral to the procedure, it is important to note that in rare cases reexpansion pulmonary edema can occur in the lung contralateral to the procedure, and so—as with all lung ultrasound—both lungs should be examined.

### Selected References
1. Gomes R, Rocha B, Morais R, Araujo I. Acute non-cardiogenic pulmonary oedema due to contralateral pulmonary re-expansion after thoracentesis: an uncommon complication. *BMJ Case Rep.* 2018. doi:10.1136/bcr-2018-224903.
2. Mahfood S, Hix WR, Aaron BL, Blaes P, Watson DC. Reexpansion pulmonary edema. *Ann Thorac Surg.* 1988;45(3):340-345. doi: 10.1016/s0003-4975(10)62480-0.

---

**5.** Correct Answer: C. The absence of multiple B-lines in the posterior lung fields

*Rationale:* The patient in the scenario has a suspected interstitial syndrome due to iatrogenic volume overload, a commonly-encountered situation in the postresuscitation setting. The presence of multiple B-lines on lung ultrasound can help to confirm this diagnosis; however, it is important to remember that fluid accumulation is gravity-dependent. Unlike a patient with acute respiratory failure from flash pulmonary edema, B-lines may be most prominent in the lateral or posterior fields, and it is important to scan all lung fields. This is especially relevant in a typical ICU population, in which many patients may be lying in the supine position for extended periods of time due to sedation/ventilation requirements.

### Selected Reference
1. Lichtenstein D, Meziere G, Biderman P, Gepner A, Barre O. The comet-tail artifact. An ultrasound sign of alveolar-interstitial syndrome. *Am J Respir Crit Care Med.* 1997;156(5):1640-1646. doi:10.1164/ajrccm.156.5.96-07096.

---

**6.** Correct Answer: B. 2

*Rationale:* Although the presence of a B-line profile may indicate an interstitial syndrome, it is important to remember that up to two of these artifacts may be seen in a given intercostal space in a healthy adult patient and that isolated B-lines in the otherwise asymptomatic patient should not necessarily be considered a pathologic finding.

### Selected Reference
1. Chiesa AM, Ciccarese F, Gardelli G, et al. Sonography of the normal lung: comparison between young and elderly subjects. *J Clin Ultrasound.* 2015;43(4):230-234. doi:10.1002/jcu.22225.

---

**7.** Correct Answer: D. The etiology cannot be determined from this data.

*Rationale:* The patient in the vignette carries two diagnoses that may be contributing to her worsening respiratory status, one an intrinsic lung process (cHP) and the other cardiogenic (congestive heart failure [CHF]). Although it is tempting to use lung ultrasound to aid in differentiating between these two processes, the presence of an ILD makes interpretation of B-lines more challenging, if not impossible, given that diffuse B-lines are present in a significant percentage of ILD patients, regardless of the degree of extravascular lung water. In this patient, focused echocardiography may be of more utility in determining the etiology of her acute respiratory failure.

Selected Reference

1. Lichtenstein DA, Meziere GA, Lagoueyte JF, Biderman P, Goldstein I, Gepner A. A-lines and B-lines: lung ultrasound as a bedside tool for predicting pulmonary artery occlusion pressure in the critically ill. *Chest.* 2009;136(4):1014-1020. doi:10.1378/chest.09-0001.

## 8. Correct Answer: B. Asthma exacerbation

*Rationale:* B-lines are hyperechoic, streak-like artifacts that arise from and move with the pleural surface, projecting in a perpendicular manner to the deepest point in the image. They are the result of a reverberation artifact that occurs when the normally aerated subpleural alveoli are altered by the presence of fluid or fibrotic lung tissue. To correctly interpret the meaning of these artifacts, it is important to remember that B-lines represent an alveolar-interstitial syndrome. Any process that leads to this syndrome, rather than a single disease process, is therefore able to produce B-lines. TRALI is an acute inflammatory reaction within the lung due to allogenic blood products that result in leakage of plasma proteins into the alveolar space. Subarachnoid hemorrhage and other traumatic brain injuries can lead to non-cardiogenic pulmonary edema (NCPE) through neurovascular activation. Large negative pressure efforts made against a closed glottis or obstructed endotracheal tube can lead to negative pressure pulmonary edema. All three of these conditions can certainly lead to the presence of B-lines. Asthma, a disease that may involve a significant degree of air trapping, does not typically result in an interstitial syndrome and would not be expected to result in the formation of B-lines.

Selected Reference

1. Lichtenstein DA, Meziere GA. Relevance of lung ultrasound in the diagnosis of acute respiratory failure: the BLUE protocol. *Chest.* 2008;134(1):117-125. doi:10.1378/chest.07-2800.

## 9. Correct Answer: C. Acute respiratory distress syndrome (ARDS)

*Rationale/Critique:* Differentiating CPE from ARDS remains a significant challenge due to multiple shared diagnostic features. The patient in the above vignette typifies this challenge: he has received multiple liters of intravenous crystalloid fluids in the setting of sepsis and likely has an increased left ventricular end-diastolic pressure (LVEDP) due to long-standing uncontrolled hypertension, making CPE likely. However, his rapidly worsening P:F ratio in the setting of sepsis would also be consistent with ARDS. Although the total number of patients was low (58 total patients), Copetti, et al. found that 100% of patients with a final diagnosis of ARDS demonstrated reduced or absent lung sliding in at least one examined lung zone compared to 0% of patients with a final diagnosis of CPE. This finding is demonstrated in ▶ **Video 53.5** (the slight movement of the pleura is a lung pulse—the movement induced by the beat of the heart, not by pleural sliding during respiration). Of course, pneumothorax must also be considered in this patient population given the typically poor lung compliance and high inspiratory pressures required to maintain adequate ventilation, but the presence of the lung pulse excludes pneumothorax at this location. Additional findings from this study are summarized in **Table 53.1**.

### Table 53.1 Percentage of the Different Signs in the Two Groups

| Ultrasound Finding | ALI/ARDS (%) | Acute CPE (%) | p-Value |
|---|---|---|---|
| B-lines | 100 | 100 | ns |
| Pleural line abnormalities | 100 | 25 | <0.0001 |
| Reduced or absent lung sliding | 100 | 0 | <0.0001 |
| Spared areas | 100 | 0 | <0.0001 |
| Consolidations | 83 | 0 | <0.0001 |
| Pleural effusion | 66 | 95 | 0.004 |

Selected Reference

1. Copetti R, Soldati G, Copetti P. Chest sonography: a useful tool to differentiate acute cardiogenic pulmonary edema from acute respiratory distress syndrome. *Cardiovasc Ultrasound.* 2008;6:16. doi:10.1186/1476-7120-6-16.

**10.** Correct Answer: D. Normal lung tissue with advanced age

*Rationale:* Although A-lines are present in nearly 100% of healthy persons <65 years of age, they are often absent in the elderly population. Although the etiology of the loss of A-lines is unclear, it may be in part due to subtle subpleural fibrosis that frequently occurs in the senile lung. In a healthy patient, this finding should not be considered pathologic.

Selected References

1. Chiesa AM, Ciccarese F, Gardelli G, et al. Sonography of the normal lung: comparison between young and elderly subjects. *J Clin Ultrasound.* 2015;43(4):230-234. doi:10.1002/jcu.22225.
2. Copley SJ, Wells AU, Hawtin KE, et al. Lung morphology in the elderly: comparative CT study of subjects over 75 years old versus those under 55 years old. *Radiology.* 2009;251(2):566-573. doi:10.1148/radiol.2512081242.

**11.** Correct Answer: A. Interstitial lung disease

*Rationale:* Figure 53.3 demonstrates a diffuse bilateral B-line profile along with a thickened and "fractured" or "broken" pleural line (indicated by the *arrowheads* in Figure 53.9). The diffuse B-line profile simply indicates an interstitial syndrome, which has a wide differential diagnosis associated with it. However, the normal cardiac ultrasound examination including the normal left ventricular filling pressures argues against pulmonary edema as the etiology. The pleural imaging seen with the linear probe in the accompanying videos demonstrates lung sliding (excluding pneumothorax); however, the broken pleural line in the context of diffuse B-lines suggests either acute lung injury (ALI/ARDS, which is not listed as a choice) or ILD.

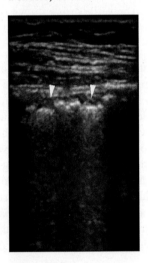

**Figure 53.9**

Selected Reference

1. Sekiguchi H, Schenck LA, Horie R, et al. Critical care ultrasonography differentiates ARDS, pulmonary edema, and other causes in the early course of acute hypoxemic respiratory failure. *Chest.* 2015;148(4):912-918. doi:10.1378/chest.15-0341.

**12.** Correct Answer: B. Pulmonary edema

*Rationale:* This patient is suffering from one of the many types of NCPE. In this example of a patient found unconscious with bradypnea, pinpoint pupils, normotension, and a grossly normal cardiac and abdominal ultrasound (FAST) examination, the pulmonary edema is likely secondary to an overdose of opioids. Although the incidence of opioid-related NCPE has decreased significantly over the past decades (possibly due to the greatly increased availability of naloxone), the overall incidence of opioid overdose has skyrocketed, reinforcing the continued need for familiarity with this condition. Right mainstem intubation is possible, but an ultrasound examination would likely show a lack of lung sliding and possibly atelectasis over the left hemithorax, whereas this patient has a diffuse bilateral B-line pattern. Pulmonary contusion and hemothorax are also important considerations in the undifferentiated trauma patient with increasing airway resistance; however, these etiologies are less likely in a patient with no signs of blunt force trauma and without pleural fluid. Other reported etiologies for NCPE include: ARDS, reexpansion pulmonary edema, high-altitude pulmonary edema (HAPE), neurogenic pulmonary edema, salicylate toxicity, pulmonary embolism, TRALI, and reperfusion pulmonary edema.

### Selected Reference

1. Sprung CL, Rackow EC, Fein IA, Jacob AI, Isikoff SK. The spectrum of pulmonary edema: differentiation of cardiogenic, intermediate, and noncardiogenic forms of pulmonary edema. *Am Rev Respir Dis.* 1981;124(6):718-722. doi: 10.1164/arrd.1981.124.6.718.

**13.** Correct Answer: **D. Subcutaneous emphysema**

*Rationale:* The finding highlighted by the arrowheads is known as an "E-line" or an "O-line" (referred to here as E/O-lines) and represents subcutaneous emphysema, a common finding after pneumothorax. It is important to differentiate between E/O-lines and B-lines, as they indicate very different underlying pathologic processes. The major difference in appearance is that while B-lines always arise from the pleural surface, E/O-lines appear to arise from *above* the pleural line, in the subcutaneous tissue.

### Selected Reference

1. Francisco MJ Neto, Rahal A, Vieira FA, Silva PS, Funari MB. Advances in lung ultrasound. *Einstein (Sao Paulo).* 2016;14(3): 443-448. doi:10.1590/S1679-45082016MD3557.

**14.** Correct Answer: **A. Normal lung tissue**

*Rationale:* The finding demonstrated in this image is known as a "Z-line" and is an artifact that may be seen in normal lung tissue due to normal pleural irregularities. They can be easily mistaken for B-lines; however, unlike true B-lines, Z-lines are typically ill-defined and vanish quickly after a few centimeters of depth, while B-lines extend to the edge of the image (Figure 53.5).

### Selected References

1. Lee FC. Lung ultrasound—a primary survey of the acutely dyspneic patient. *J Intensive Care.* 2016;4(1):57. doi:10.1186/s40560-016-0180-1.
2. Yue Lee FC, Jenssen C, Dietrich CF. A common misunderstanding in lung ultrasound: the comet tail artefact. *Med Ultrason.* 2018;20(3):379-384. doi:10.11152/mu-1573.

**15.** Correct Answer: **D. Second harmonics turned off**

*Rationale/Critique:* Modern ultrasound machines often include multiple hardware and software features that are designed to increase imaging sensitivity and decrease noise. Although these features can be beneficial in many circumstances, they can be detrimental when trying to detect and quantify the artifacts that are the hallmarks of lung ultrasound, including B-lines. In this example, in Figure 53.6A, a secondary harmonic feature is activated, which produces the appearance of multiple B-lines arising from the pleural surface. The careful observer will notice that these B-lines all appear to be originating from a single point on the pleural surface, a hint that they may be artificially generated. This is confirmed by turning off this feature, producing the image seen in Figure 53.6B. A second finding consistent with the use of a secondary harmonic feature is the appearance of a thicker pleural line in the image on the left. The use of secondary harmonic imaging often results in an artificial thickening of structures. While alterations in gain could enhance or diminish the appearance of B-lines, they cannot cause a single B-line to spread into multiple B-lines with the same origin as in the example in Figure 53.6.

With most modern ultrasound machines, lung ultrasound should be performed using either the abdominal or a dedicated lung imaging mode, with all harmonic and noise-reducing features turned off.

### Selected Reference

1. Mongodi S, Stella A, Orlando A, Mojoli F. B-lines visualization and lung aeration assessment: mind the ultrasound machine setting. *Anesthesiology.* 2019;130(3):444. doi:10.1097/ALN.0000000000002522.

**16.** Correct Answer: C. Imaging depth increased

*Rationale:* By definition, B-lines should be continuous and should not attenuate with increasing depth. The scale on the right of this image indicates that it is set to a maximum imaging depth of 3.1 cm. In order to ensure that the artifacts are in fact B-lines (and not Z-lines, which quickly diminish in intensity with increasing depth from the pleural line), the imaging depth must be increased.

Selected Reference

1. Lichtenstein DA, Meziere GA, Lagoueyte JF, Biderman P, Goldstein I, Gepner A. A-lines and B-lines: lung ultrasound as a bedside tool for predicting pulmonary artery occlusion pressure in the critically ill. *Chest.* 2009;136(4):1014-1020. doi:10.1378/chest.09-0001.

**17.** Correct Answer: C. Hydropneumothorax

*Rationale:* Figure 53.8 shows an A-line pattern (*arrowhead*) overlying a hyperechoic pleural effusion (*) with consolidated lung deeper in the imaging field (the left ventricle is also visible in the lower-left portion of the screen, momentarily). This pattern is a recently named artifact known as a "hydro point" and represents the convergence of air and fluid within the pleural space. It is analogous to the lung point seen in pneumothorax. It is common to entrain air during pleural procedures, including chest tube insertion. This typically resolves along with the drainage of fluid from the pleural space, but in this case, it is likely that the chest tube has kinked, clogged, or is otherwise blocked, which has trapped both air and fluid in the pleural space. As the comet tail artifacts present do not actually arise from the parietal pleura (which is trapped below the air-fluid collection in this case), these are not B-lines and do not represent pulmonary edema (cardio- or noncardiogenic).

Selected Reference

1. Volpicelli G, Boero E, Stefanone V, Storti E. Unusual new signs of pneumothorax at lung ultrasound. *Crit Ultrasound J.* 2013;5(1):10. doi:10.1186/2036-7902-5-10.

**18.** Correct Answer: C. They erase A-lines.

*Rationale:* The initial definition of a B-line included a total of seven criteria: (1) comet tail artifact, (2) arises from the pleural line, (3) moves in concert with lung sliding, (4) long and well-defined, (5) laser like, (6) hyperechoic, and (7) erasing A-lines. However, in the most recent version of the international evidence-based recommendations for point-of-care lung ultrasound, the requirement for B-lines to "erase" or "obliterate" A-lines has been removed, as these two artifacts may be seen simultaneously. The finding of simultaneous A- and B-lines does not alter the meaning of the B-line profile when other criteria are met.

Selected Reference

1. Volpicelli G, Elbarbary M, Blaivas M, et al. International evidence-based recommendations for point-of-care lung ultrasound. *Intensive Care Med.* 2012;38(4):577-591. doi:10.1007/s00134-012-2513-4.

**19.** Correct Answer: B. The patient with B-lines 7 mm apart has greater subpleural fibrosis.

*Rationale:* Patients with the various forms of ILD present a diagnostic dilemma with regard to lung ultrasound, as the presence of even subtle subpleural abnormalities results in the presence of diffuse B-lines, which are almost always seen in this patient population. However, in patients with an established ILD diagnosis, the presence of B-lines can actually help in determining the degree of lung fibrosis. When the subpleural abnormalities are in earlier stages of the fibrotic process and are represented by GGOs on CT, B-lines on pleural ultrasound are likely to be spaced at a distance of around 3 mm (also known as a "B3" pattern). When the underlying process has progressed to the level of fibrosis, the B-lines are more likely to be separated by a distance of around 7 mm ("B7" pattern). This increased distance between B-lines has a strong correlation with additional measures of lung function including forced vital capacity (FVC), total lung capacity (TLC), diffusing capacity for carbon monoxide (DLCO), and $PaO_2$. Differentiating between B3 and B7 patterns may also be useful in contexts other than pulmonary fibrosis. For example,

B3 patterns typically emerge in the context of intralobular selective flooding and partial alveolar collapse such as in pneumonia, while B7 patterns typically emerge during conditions resulting in thickened interlobular septa such as pulmonary edema.

### Selected References

1. Hasan AA, Makhlouf HA. B-lines: transthoracic chest ultrasound signs useful in assessment of interstitial lung diseases. *Ann Thorac Med.* 2014;9(2):99-103. doi:10.4103/1817-1737.128856.
2. Soldati G, Demi M, Inchingolo R, Smargiassi A, Demi L. On the physical basis of pulmonary sonographic interstitial syndrome. *J Ultrasound Med.* 2016;35(10):2075-2086. doi:10.7863/ultra.15.08023.

---

**20.** Correct Answer: D. Pneumonia

*Rationale:* Although all of the answers provided are capable of producing a bilateral B-line profile, the patient has a clinical history that is most compatible with pneumonia (cough, fatigue, and fever for several days). Although it may be tempting to assign another etiology for this patient's symptoms in the absence of findings on chest X-ray and a diffuse bilateral B-line pattern, this pattern is most compatible with a diagnosis of CAP. The performance of plain film chest radiography for ruling out pneumonia is imperfect. Furthermore, although less common than other ultrasound findings supportive of pneumonia (tissue-like lung echotexture, hepatization, pleural thickening, pleural effusion), a bilateral B-line profile in the correct clinical context is compatible with pneumonia. This is due to the fact that the above-mentioned changes to the lung parenchyma and pleura are only detectable by ultrasound if the consolidative process reaches the pleural surface.

### Selected References

1. Cortellaro F, Colombo S, Coen D, Duca PG. Lung ultrasound is an accurate diagnostic tool for the diagnosis of pneumonia in the emergency department. *Emerg Med J.* 2012;29(1):19-23. doi:10.1136/emj.2010.101584.
2. Upchurch CP, Grijalva CG, Wunderink RG, et al. Community-acquired pneumonia visualized on CT scans but not chest radiographs: pathogens, severity, and clinical outcomes. *Chest.* 2018;153(3):601-610. doi:10.1016/j.chest.2017.07.035.

Tanping Wong

1. An 82-year-old woman with a history of hypertension, atrial fibrillation, and heart failure with preserved ejection fraction presents with 1 week of shortness of breath, cough, 10-kg weight gain, and increasing lower extremity edema. Her admission chest X-ray shows bilateral pleural effusions and increased interstitial markings. She is treated with diuresis for respiratory failure secondary to decompensated heart failure in the setting of rhinovirus infection and improves over the course of the week. However, 1 week later, she develops worsening dyspnea and hypoxia. She is afebrile with a HR of 70 bpm and has crackles in bilateral lung fields, despite improved lower extremity edema. A repeat chest X-ray shows persistent central vascular congestion and increased bibasilar opacities. A point-of-care ultrasound is performed as shown in **Figure 54.1A** (▶ **Video 54.1A**) and **Figure 54.1B** (▶ **Video 54.1B**).

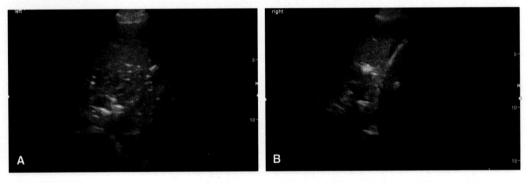

**Figure 54.1**

What is the *most* appropriate next step in management for this patient?
A. Start broad-spectrum antibiotics as the patient has developed pneumonia.
B. Continue diuresis given her improvement over the course of the past week.
C. Increase diuresis because the patient has worsening heart failure.
D. Perform thoracentesis given the change in clinical status of the patient and X-ray showing pleural effusion.

2. An 87-year-old woman with a history of pulmonary fibrosis, severe obstructive lung disease (FEV1 36% predicted), who is dependent on home oxygen (3 L nasal cannula), presents with 4 days of worsening cough and shortness of breath. She also has a history of heart failure and pulmonary hypertension with right ventricular dilation. In the Emergency Department, she is noted to be in respiratory distress, with a RR of 28/min, HR 120 bpm BP of 100/70 mm Hg, and SpO$_2$ is 95% on 3 L nasal cannula. She is afebrile. On physical examination, jugular venous distention, diffuse wheezing, and basilar crackles are noted. A portable chest X-ray shows diffuse increased interstitial markings and increased opacity of the right lower lung field. Her white blood cell count (WBC) is 13,000/mm$^3$ with 85% neutrophils. A point-of-care ultrasound is performed (**Figure 54.2** and ▶ **Video 54.2**).

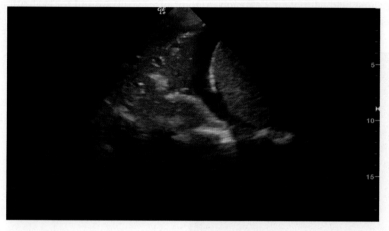

**Figure 54.2**

Which of the following conclusions is *most* accurate?
A. The patient likely has a viral infection leading to exacerbation of her obstructive lung disease.
B. The patient likely has pneumonia, given the consolidation seen on ultrasound.
C. The patient likely has an exacerbation of heart failure, given the pleural effusion seen on ultrasound.
D. The patient likely has progression of her underlying pulmonary fibrosis.

3. Which of the following findings (**Figure 54.3** and ▶ **Video 54.3**) on ultrasound does not support a diagnosis of pneumonia?

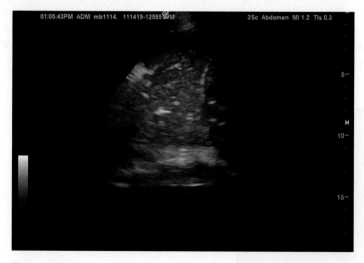

**Figure 54.3**

A. Hepatization of the lung parenchyma
B. Shred sign
C. A-lines
D. Dynamic air bronchograms

4. A 57-year-old previously healthy man presents with fever, cough, and fatigue. His symptoms began as nasal congestion and rhinorrhea 1 week prior, when his young children were also sick at home. He was treated with oral azithromycin for 5 days, with a worsening cough and new onset of fever. On presentation, his temperature is 39°C, with HR 100 bpm, BP 100/60 mm Hg, RR 22/min with SpO$_2$ 94% on 3 L of oxygen via nasal cannula. His leukocyte count is 3000 cells/mm$^3$. A portable chest X-ray shows opacity in the right lower lung field with pleural effusion. A point-of-care ultrasound for evaluation of the pleural effusion is performed (**Figure 54.4** and ▶ **Video 54.4**).

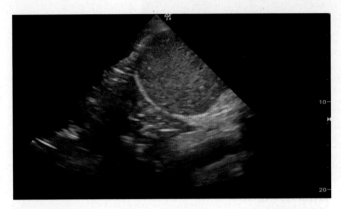

**Figure 54.4**

What is the *most* appropriate next step in his management?
A. Perform diagnostic thoracentesis to rule out the presence of empyema.
B. The ultrasound shows a complex loculated pleural effusion; call expert consultation for chest tube placement.
C. Start intravenous (IV) antibiotics for the treatment of community-acquired pneumonia.
D. Place a nasogastric tube to evacuate the stomach contents seen on ultrasound.

5. An 84-year-old woman who is a resident of a nursing home presents with fatigue and anorexia. She was noted to have low-grade fevers and suprapubic tenderness. She reports a chronic cough, but does not have shortness of breath or chest pain. Her temperature is 37°C, HR 84 bpm, BP 116/72 mm Hg, RR 12/min, and SpO$_2$ 95% on room air. Her portable chest X-ray is hazy at the lower lung fields bilaterally. A point-of-care ultrasound is performed for better visualization of her lung fields (**Figure 54.5** and ▶ **Video 54.5**).

**Figure 54.5**

Which of the following is seen on the ultrasound image?
A. Consolidation
B. Complex pleural effusion
C. Mirror artifact with curtain sign
D. Diffuse B-lines

6. A 27-year-old man was an unrestrained backseat passenger in a motor vehicle collision 1 week prior to presentation. He was seen in the Emergency Department at the time of the accident. A chest X-ray done at that time did not show pneumothorax or rib fractures. Since the accident, he's been experiencing pleuritic chest pain, and over the past 3 days, he has a cough and low-grade fever. A repeat chest X-ray is reported as normal. Ultrasound at the site of reproducible chest wall tenderness is shown (▶ **Video 54.6**).

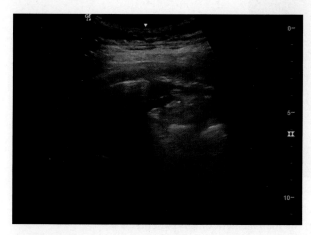

**Figure 54.6**

Based on **Figure 54.6**, which of the following is the *most* likely explanation for his symptoms?
A. A displaced rib fracture is seen.
B. The ultrasound shows subcutaneous emphysema, suggesting a pneumothorax.
C. The patient likely suffered lung contusion that developed into pneumonia.
D. Normal lung parenchyma is seen. The patient likely suffered a chest wall contusion.

7. A 25-year-old man with a past history of asthma presents with 1 week of fever, cough, right-sided pleuritic chest pain, and shortness of breath. On presentation to the Emergency Department, he has an RR of 32/min and $SpO_2$ 68% on room air. On auscultation, wheezing and bronchial breath sounds are noted on the right lower lung field. He is emergently intubated for respiratory distress. A point-of-care ultrasound is performed and shown in **Figure 54.7** and ▶ **Video 54.7**.

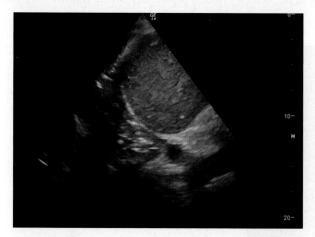

**Figure 54.7**

What is the *most* likely diagnosis of this patient's clinical presentation?

A. The patient is having a severe asthma exacerbation.

B. The patient presents with severe community-acquired lobar pneumonia.

C. The patient has a complex pleural effusion, likely empyema.

D. The patient likely suffered blunt trauma, as hemothorax is seen on ultrasound.

8. A 17-year-old college student presents with 1 week of nasal congestion, sore throat, myalgias, cough fatigue, and fever. Chest X-ray shows blunting of bilateral costophrenic angles, without clear consolidation. A point-of-care ultrasound is performed (**Figure 54.8** and ▶ **Video 54.8**).

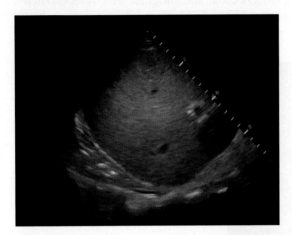

**Figure 54.8**

What is the *most* appropriate next step in the management of this patient?

A. It is not possible to determine from the image provided.

B. Supportive therapy for an upper respiratory infection given normal mirror artifact seen on ultrasound.

C. The patient has developed empyema as a complication of his pneumonia. Chest tube placement is indicated.

D. The patient has developed pneumonia as supported by visualization of a consolidation and the spine sign.

9. An 87-year-old man with a history of ischemic dilated cardiomyopathy with an ejection of 25%, atrial fibrillation, and stage II chronic kidney disease was admitted 1 week prior with dyspnea, hypoxia, edema, and chest X-ray findings of increased interstitial markings and a right-sided pleural effusion. He was treated for decompensated heart failure with diuresis, with improvement in symptoms. Currently, he is afebrile, breathing comfortably on 2 L nasal cannula, and has bilateral basilar crackles on lung examination. A point-of-care ultrasound is performed to assess pulmonary edema (**Figure 54.9** and ▶ **Video 54.9**).

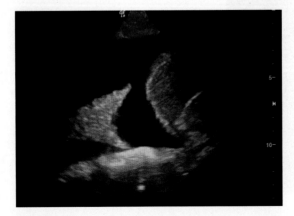

**Figure 54.9**

Which of the following is *least* likely to benefit this patient?

**A.** Start vancomycin and piperacillin/tazobactam for treatment of hospital-acquired pneumonia seen on bedside ultrasound.

**B.** Continue diuresis.

**C.** Diagnostic thoracentesis given persistent pleural effusion.

**D.** Encourage the use of incentive spirometer and mobilization.

**10.** A 57-year-old man presents with 2 weeks of fever and shortness of breath. On initial examination, his temperature is 38.6°C, HR 100 bpm, BP 90/60 mm Hg, RR 20/min, and SpO$_2$ 90% on room air. A parasternal short-axis view of the heart at the aortic valve level is shown (**Figure 54.10** and ▶ **Video 54.10**).

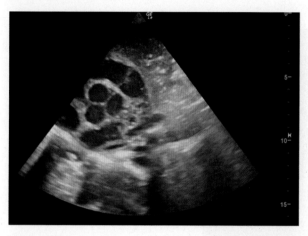

**Figure 54.10**

What is the *most* appropriate next step in the management of this patient?

**A.** Obtain echocardiogram to assess for cardiac tamponade.

**B.** Obtain computed tomography (CT) scan of the chest to better delineate this anterior mediastinal mass.

**C.** Perform thoracentesis and place a chest tube for this complex pleural effusion.

**D.** Start antibiotics for community-acquired pneumonia.

**11.** A 75-year-old man is admitted to the hospital with gallstone pancreatitis. He underwent successful endoscopic retrograde cholangiopancreatography (ERCP) on hospital day 1. Three days after ERCP, he develops fever, cough, and abdominal pain. A portal chest X-ray shows haziness of the left costophrenic angle. A coronal view with point-of-care ultrasound is performed at the left mid-axillary line at the level of the xiphoid (**Figure 54.11** and ▶ **Video 54.11**).

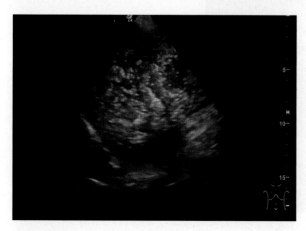

**Figure 54.11**

What is the *most* appropriate next step in the management of this patient?

A. Start broad-spectrum antibiotics for hospital-acquired pneumonia of the left lower lobe.

B. Place a chest tube for complex pleural effusion.

C. Place a nasogastric tube to decompress a distended stomach with gastric contents.

D. Perform paracentesis for complex ascites.

12. A 90-year-old man with dementia is admitted after a fall and is found to have a femoral neck fracture as well as a urinary tract infection. He is treated with ceftriaxone for the infection and subsequently undergoes surgical repair of his hip fracture. On hospital day 3, he abruptly becomes hypoxemic, with RR 28/min and SpO₂ 88% on room air. His chest X-ray shows increased interstitial markings and obscured diaphragmatic borders. A point-of-care ultrasound is performed and shown in **Figure 54.12** and ▶ **Video 54.12**.

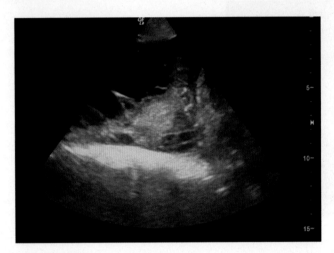

**Figure 54.12**

What is the *most* appropriate next step in his management?

A. Diuresis to improve pulmonary edema, likely exacerbated by IV fluids

B. Encourage the use of an incentive spirometer and physical therapy, as the patient likely has atelectasis

C. Start antibiotics for healthcare-associated pneumonia

D. Start antibiotics and place a chest tube for treatment of empyema

13. A 45-year-old man presents with 1 day of right-sided pleuritic chest pain. A chest X-ray is normal. A point-of-care ultrasound performed in a transverse plane in the right third intercostal space on the lateral chest wall is shown (**Figure 54.13** and ▶ **Video 54.13**).

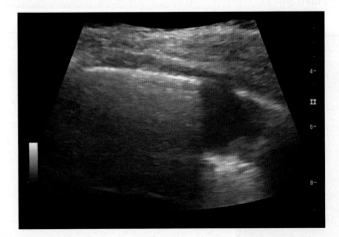

**Figure 54.13**

Based on the ultrasound findings, which of the following should be considered *most* likely in the differential diagnosis?

A. Pneumonia, pulmonary embolism, pulmonary edema
B. Pneumonia, pulmonary embolism, pulmonary contusion
C. Pneumonia, pulmonary contusion, pulmonary edema
D. Pulmonary edema, pulmonary embolism, pulmonary contusion

14. Which ultrasound feature of pneumonia is indicated by the *arrow* in **Figure 54.14**? (See also ▶ **Video 54.14**.)

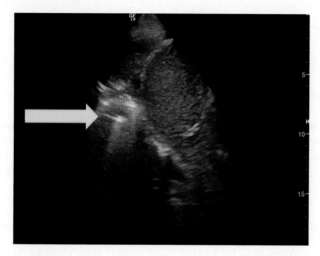

**Figure 54.14**

A. Plankton sign
B. B-Lines
C. Jellyfish sign
D. Shred sign

15. A 47-year-old man with a history of smoking and alcohol abuse presents with sudden-onset right-sided anterior chest pain. The pain is worse on inspiration and cough. There is no history of fall, trauma, or cancer. On presentation, there is no tachypnea, tachycardia, hypoxemia, or hypotension. Lung sounds are coarse.

A point-of-care lung ultrasound is performed with a linear array transducer at the spot identified by the patient as the most painful (**Figure 54.15A** and ▶ **Video 54.15A**). There are several additional areas with a similar appearance scattered throughout both lungs. The rest of the lungs showed an A-pattern bilaterally. An apical four-chamber view of the heart is shown (**Figure 54.15B** and ▶ **Video 54.15B**).

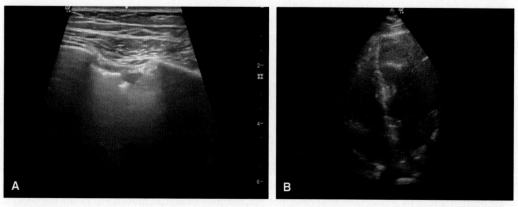

**Figure 54.15**

Based on the ultrasound findings, which of the following would be the *most* appropriate next step in his management?

**A.** The ultrasound findings are highly suggestive of pneumonia, and the patient should start antibiotics.

**B.** The ultrasound findings are pathognomonic for pulmonary infarction, suggesting the patient has a pulmonary embolism and should start anticoagulation and obtain confirmatory studies.

**C.** The differential diagnosis for the ultrasound findings is broad, and additional evaluation with lower extremity focused ultrasound is indicated.

**D.** The ultrasound findings suggest pneumothorax. A confirmatory chest X-ray should be performed.

# Chapter 54 ▪ Answers

**1.** Correct Answer: A. Start broad-spectrum antibiotics as the patient has developed pneumonia.

*Rationale:* Figure 5.1A, B and ▶ **Videos 54.1A, B** show bilateral consolidations in the lower lung fields without significant pleural effusion, likely representing pneumonia. The accuracy of lung ultrasound in the diagnosis of pneumonia has been shown to be superior to the accuracy of X-ray. The improved lower extremity edema, as well as the consolidations on ultrasound argue against worsening heart failure, and drainage of the effusions is not necessary at this time.

### Selected References
1. Alzahrani SA, Al-Salamah MA, Al-Madani WH, Elbarbary MA. Systematic review and meta-analysis for the use of ultrasound versus radiology in diagnosing of pneumonia. *Crit Ultrasound J.* 2017;9(1):6. doi:10.1186/s13089-017-0059-y.
2. Chavez MA, Shams N, Ellington LE, et al. Lung ultrasound for the diagnosis of pneumonia in adults: a systemic review and meta-analysis. *Respir Res.* 2014;15:50.

**2.** Correct Answer: B. The patient likely has pneumonia, given the consolidation seen on ultrasound.

*Rationale:* Possible etiologies for this patient's respiratory distress include progression of her pulmonary fibrosis, exacerbation of her obstructive lung disease, worsening heart failure, viral infection, and bacterial pneumonia. Ultrasound is useful in the evaluation of such patients, as they are often unstable for further imaging with a CT scan. The ultrasound shows dense consolidation in the right lower lung field (left side of Figure 54.2, above the curved diaphragm), with surrounding pleural effusion, suggesting pneumonia and parapneumonic effusion. A heart failure exacerbation, chronic obstructive pulmonary disease (COPD) exacerbation, or progression of pulmonary fibrosis would not be expected to produce this type of consolidation.

### Selected References
1. Ye X, Xiao H, Chen B, Zhang SY. Accuracy of lung ultrasonography versus chest radiography for the diagnosis of adult community-acquired pneumonia: review of the literature and meta-analysis. *PLoS One.* 2015;10(6):e0130066.
2. Zanobetti M, Scorpiniti M, Gigli C, et al. Point-of-care ultrasound for evaluation of acute dyspnea in the ED. *Chest.* 2017;151(6):1295-1301.

**3.** Correct Answer: C. A-lines

*Rationale:* Characteristics on ultrasound that are highly suggestive of pneumonia include hepatization, dynamic air bronchograms, and the shred sign. Hepatization refers to the hypoechoic appearance of the lung formed by pus-filled bronchi. The shred sign is a shredded deep border of the tissue-like image adjacent to the aerated lung. Air bronchograms are linear or punctiform hyperechoic features seen within the consolidation from regions of aerated airspaces. Mobile or dynamic air bronchograms are specific for the diagnosis of pneumonia. In this situation, the respiratory movement of gas bubbles within the bronchi indicates patency of the airway. This is in contrast to static air bronchograms, which are seen in atelectasis. Limitations of dynamic air bronchograms include being off-plane during examination (which will cause air bronchogram to transiently disappear, but not because of actual movement of air bubbles) and the development of atelectasis (with static air bronchograms) within pneumonia. The combined presence of hepatization, shred sign, and air bronchograms has a positive likelihood ratio of 12 and a negative likelihood ratio of 0.16 for the diagnosis of pneumonia. A-line represent a strong reflection from aerated lung tissue, and would not be expected in the presence of consolidated lung tissue.

### Selected References

1. Alzahrani SA, Al-Salamah MA, Al-Madani WH, Elbarbary MA. Systematic review and meta-analysis for the use of ultrasound versus radiology in diagnosing of pneumonia. *Crit Ultrasound J.* 2017;9(1):6. doi:10.1186/s13089-017-0059-y.
2. Reissig A, Copetti R, Mathis G, et al. Lung ultrasound in the diagnosis and follow-up of community-acquired pneumonia: a prospective, multicenter, diagnostic accuracy study. *Chest.* 2012;142(4):965-972. doi:10.1378/chest.12-0364.

**4.** Correct Answer: C. Start intravenous (IV) antibiotics for the treatment of community-acquired pneumonia

*Rationale*: This patient developed a right lower lobe pneumonia. His hypoxemia and fever after antibiotic therapy warrant additional treatment. There is no pleural effusion on the ultrasound, thus thoracentesis is not indicated. Although gastric content can appear as hyperechoic specks, the stomach is located under the diaphragm (to the right side of the image), and ultrasound typically shows a mix of hypo- and hyperechogenic content. The liver is visualized below the diaphragm of Figure 54.4. Ultrasound is useful in clarifying nonspecific opacities seen in the lower lung fields of chest X-rays.

The ultrasound shows consolidated lung above the diaphragm (left side of Figure 54.4), containing hyperechoic lines and dots that move with respiration. These are dynamic air bronchograms that represent trapped air within the small airways, with a sensitivity of 94% and specificity of 61% in the diagnosis of pneumonia.

### Selected References

1. Alzahrani SA, Al-Salamah MA, Al-Madani WH, Elbarbary MA. Systematic review and meta-analysis for the use of ultrasound versus radiology in diagnosing of pneumonia. *Crit Ultrasound J.* 2017;9(1):6. doi:10.1186/s13089-017-0059-y.
2. Lichtenstein D, Meziere G, Seitz J. The dynamic air bronchogram* a lung ultrasound sign of alveolar consolidation ruling out atelectasis. *Chest.* 2009;135:1421-1425.

**5.** Correct Answer: C. Mirror artifact with curtain sign

*Rationale*: Liver tissue is visible on the right of ▶ **Video 54.5**, as well as the hyperechoic diaphragm in the center. To the left of the diaphragm is a mirror artifact. The curtain sign is seen coming into view during respiration.

The mirror image artifact is seen when there is a highly reflective surface such as the diaphragm in the path of the primary beam, which is reflected back to the transducer. The reflection of the liver is seen beyond the diaphragm and may be confused for hepatized lung. This artifact can be distinguished from hepatization of the lung by the absence of the spine sign and the presence of the curtain sign (**Figure 54.16**).

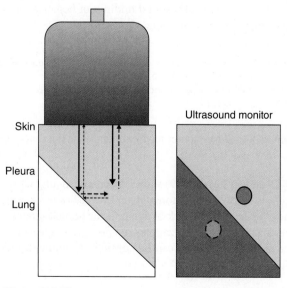

**Figure 54.16**

Selected Reference

1. Chichra A, Makaryus M, Chaudhri P, Narasimhan M. Ultrasound of the pulmonary consultant. *Clin Med Insights Circ Respir Pulm Med.* 2016;10:1-9.

## 6. Correct Answer: C. The patient likely suffered lung contusion that developed into pneumonia

*Rationale*: Lung contusion is common after blunt chest trauma and can be missed on an initial chest X-ray. On ultrasound, lung contusion can appear as hypoechoic subpleural peripheral parenchymal lesions. It can also appear as an alveolointerstitial syndrome with B-line artifacts. Complications like infection can develop from contusions. Pain control, improvement of respiratory mechanics, and secretion clearance are the main treatments. Antibiotics may be necessary if superinfection develops.

Selected References

1. Helmy S, Beshay B, Hady MA, Mansour A. Role of chest ultrasound in the diagnosis of lung contusion. *Egypt Soc Chest Dis Tuberc.* 2015;64:469-475. doi:10.1016/j.ejcdt.2014.11.021.
2. Soldati G, Testa A, Silva FR, Carbone L, Portale G, Silveri NG. Chest ultrasound in lung contusion. *Chest.* 2006;130(2):533-538.

## 7. Correct Answer: B. The patient presents with severe community-acquired lobar pneumonia

*Rationale*: The ultrasound (Figure 54.7 and ▶ **Video 54.7**) shows complete consolidation of the right lung with dynamic air bronchograms. This dense consolidation is often referred to as "hepatization," as it has a similar appearance to the sonographic appearance of the liver. It is formed by bronchi filled with pus and secretions that appear hypoechoic. The trapped air bubbles form linear or punctate hyperechoic structures referred to as air bronchograms. The spine is seen in the far-field, indicating the presence of lung transmitting the sound wave, which is abnormal. Normally aerated lung reflects ultrasound waves and the spine cannot be visualized through the pleura This patient's bronchoalveolar lavage culture subsequently grew *Streptococcus pneumoniae*.

Selected References

1. Lichtenstein D, Mezière G, Seitz J. The dynamic air bronchogram: a lung ultrasound sign of alveolar consolidation ruling out atelectasis. *Chest.* 2009;135(6):1421-1425. doi:10.1378/chest.08-2281.
2. Reissig A, Copetti R, Mathis G, et al. Lung ultrasound in the diagnosis and follow-up of community-acquired pneumonia: a prospective, multicenter, diagnostic accuracy study. *Chest.* 2012;142(4):965-972. doi:10.1378/chest.12-0364.

## 8. Correct Answer: D. The patient has developed pneumonia as supported by visualization of a consolidation and the spine sign.

*Rationale*: The spine sign is an ultrasound finding in which the thoracic spine is visualized extending above the diaphragm. In normally aerated lung tissue, air obscures the transmission of sound waves above the diaphragm, leading to an abrupt cutoff of the hyperechoic vertebral bodies above the diaphragm. The presence of fluid or consolidation allows for the transmission of ultrasound waves and thus visualization of the vertebral bodies above the diaphragm. Together with ultrasound findings of hepatization and air bronchograms, the spine sign is helpful in the diagnosis of pneumonia.

Selected References

1. Alzahrani SA, Al-Salamah MA, Al-Madani WH, Elbarbary MA. Systematic review and meta-analysis for the use of ultrasound versus radiology in diagnosing of pneumonia. *Crit Ultrasound J.* 2017;9(1):6. doi:10.1186/s13089-017-0059-y.
2. Dickman E, Terentiev V, Likourezos A, Derman A, Haines L. Extension of the thoracic spine sign. *J Ultrasound Med.* 2015;34:1555-1561. https://onlinelibrary.wiley.com/doi/pdf/10.7863/ultra.15.14.06013.

## 9. Correct Answer: A. Start vancomycin and piperacillin/tazobactam for treatment of hospital-acquired pneumonia seen on bedside ultrasound

*Rationale*: The bedside ultrasound (Figure 54.9 and ▶ **Video 54.9**) shows consolidated lung with pleural effusion. The findings likely represent atelectasis and not pneumonia given the lack of fever, worsening hypoxia, and cough. The large volume of the effusion and the lack of dynamic air bronchograms further support this as atelectasis. Continued diuresis as well as mobilization are appropriate measures. A diagnostic thoracentesis given the persistence of pleural effusion can be considered, although follow-up evaluation after resolution of heart failure is reasonable and less invasive. The patient lacks infectious symptoms and clinical deterioration to warrant initiation of broad-spectrum antibiotics.

### Selected References

1. Alzahrani SA, Al-Salamah MA, Al-Madani WH, Elbarbary MA. Systematic review and meta-analysis for the use of ultrasound versus radiology in diagnosing of pneumonia. *Crit Ultrasound J.* 2017;9(1):6. doi:10.1186/s13089-017-0059-y.
2. Lichtenstein DA, Lascols N, Meziere G, Gepner A. Ultrasound diagnosis of alveolar consolidation in the critically ill. *Intensive Care Med.* 2004; 30(2):276-281.

**10.** Correct Answer: D. Start antibiotics for community-acquired pneumonia

*Rationale*: On this parasternal short-axis view (Figure 54.10 and ▶ **Video 54.10**), there is tissue-like density anterior to the heart, which is a consolidated lung. One can see hyperechoic specks and tubes representing air in the bronchi. A shred sign is seen at the lateral edge of the consolidated lung on the right side of the screen, further supporting the presence of a left-sided pneumonia.

### Selected References

1. Lichtenstein D, Mezière G, Seitz J. The dynamic air bronchogram: a lung ultrasound sign of alveolar consolidation ruling out atelectasis. *Chest.* 2009;135(6):1421-1425. doi:10.1378/chest.08-2281.
2. Reissig A, Copetti R, Mathis G, et al. Lung ultrasound in the diagnosis and follow-up of community-acquired pneumonia: a prospective, multicenter, diagnostic accuracy study. *Chest.* 2012;142(4):965-972. doi:10.1378/chest.12-0364.

**11.** Correct Answer: C. Place a nasogastric tube to decompress a distended stomach with gastric contents

*Rationale*: ▶ **Video 54.11** shows a dilated stomach with gastric contents, which appears heterogeneous with hypoechoic food and fluid, along with hyperechoic specks of air. It is important to recognize the landmarks in lung ultrasound, as the stomach is seen below the diaphragm (shown as a thin partially visible crescent on the left side of ▶ **Video 54.11**).

### Selected References

1. Blanco P, Volpicelli G. Common pitfalls in point-of-care ultrasound: a practical guide for emergency and critical care physicians. *Crit Ultrasound J.* 2016;8(1):15.
2. Kruisselbrink R, Gharapetian A, Chaparro LE, et al. Diagnostic accuracy of point-of-care gastric ultrasound. *Anesth Analg.* 2019;128(1):89-95. doi:10.1213/ANE.0000000000003372.

**12.** Correct Answer: D. Start antibiotics and place a chest tube for treatment of empyema

*Rationale*: ▶ **Video 54.12** shows a consolidation with surrounding complex pleural effusion, as indicated by the septated strands seen in the hypoechoic pleural effusion. Visible septations and debris within a pleural effusion are strongly suggestive of empyema. Although the lung tissue does appear consolidated, consistent with pneumonia, the empyema warrants drainage in addition to antibiotics.

### Selected Reference

1. Koppurapu V, Meena N. A review of the management of complex para-pneumonic effusion in adults. *J Thorac Dis.* 2017. http:// jtd.amegroups.com/article/view/14711/11905.

**13.** Correct Answer: B. Pneumonia, pulmonary embolism, pulmonary contusion

*Rationale*: This ultrasound (Figure 54.13 and ▶ **Video 54.13**) is obtained in the intercostal space in a transverse plane, showing a large section of pleura horizontally across the image. There is a hypoechoic (dark) density, which is subpleural and round. Pulmonary infarcts can be seen as hypoechoic round or wedge-shaped lesions under the pleura. Early pulmonary contusions can have a similar appearance and can be considered if supported by the clinical history. Similarly, anterior subpleural consolidations caused by pneumonia can be considered in a patient with fever and cough. Pulmonary edema is seen as an interstitial pattern with bilateral B-lines, which are not present in this image, making significant pulmonary edema unlikely.

**Selected References**
1. Lichtenstein DA. Relevance of lung ultrasound in the diagnosis of acute respiratory failure: The BLUE Protocol. *Chest.* 2008;134(1):117-125. doi:10.1378/chest.07-2800.
2. Mathis G, Metzler J, Fussenegger D, Sutterlütti G, Feurstein M, Fritzsche H. Sonographic observation of pulmonary infarction and early infarctions by pulmonary embolus. *Eur Heart J.* 1993;14(6):8040808. doi:10.1093/eurheartj/14.6.804.
3. Reissig A, Heyne JP, Kroegel C. Sonography of lung and pleura in pulmonary embolism. *Chest.* 2001;120(6):1977-1983. doi:10.1378/chest.120.6.1977.

**14.** Correct Answer: D. Shred sign

*Rationale*: A shred sign is seen when the deeper border of the consolidated tissue makes contact with hyperechoic aerated lung. This irregular border is also sometimes referred to as the fractal line. It has high sensitivity and specificity for pneumonia but can be absent in large lobar consolidations without adjacent aerated lung tissue. Plankton and jellyfish signs are seen in pleural effusion, which is not seen in Figure 54.14.

**Selected References**
1. Chichra A, Makaryus M, Chaudhri P, Narasimhan M., Ultrasound for the pulmonary consultant. *Clin Med Insights Circ Respir Pulm Med.* 2016;10:1-9.
2. Lichtenstein DA. Lung ultrasound in the critically ill. *Ann Intensive Care.* 2014;4(1):1.

**15.** Correct Answer: C. The differential diagnosis for the ultrasound findings is broad, and additional evaluation with lower extremity focused ultrasound is indicated.

*Rationale*: The finding of a hypoechoic round nodule in a subpleural location may represent a variety of processes, including pneumonia and pulmonary infarct. Distinguishing between the two based on sonography alone is not feasible. Demonstration of a lower extremity venous clot would significantly increase the likelihood of pulmonary embolism, as this patient did indeed turn out to have (⊙ **Video 54.16**).

It is critical to understand the limitations of right ventricular strain to inform the likelihood of pulmonary embolism. Lack of right ventricular strain does suggest that shock in a patient is unlikely to be due to a pulmonary embolism, but does not exclude a smaller pulmonary embolism without hemodynamic compromise.

**Selected References**
1. Mathis G, Metzler J, Fussenegger D, Sutterlütti G, Feurstein M, Fritzsche H. Sonographic observation of pulmonary infarction and early infarctions by pulmonary embolus. *Eur Heart J.* 1993;14(6):8040808. doi:10.1093/eurheartj/14.6.804.
2. Volpicelli G, Frascisco M. Lung ultrasound in the evaluation of patients with pleuritic pain in the emergency department. *Ultrasound Emerg Med.* 2008;34(2):179-186. doi:10.1016/j.jemermed.2007.06.024.

# 55 | PLEURAL EFFUSIONS

Jina Bai

1. An 89-year-old woman with a past medical history of chronic obstructive pulmonary disease, diastolic heart failure, and hypothyroidism is admitted with urosepsis. She initially improves with intravenous (IV) antibiotics and fluid resuscitation. On day 3, she has new-onset dyspnea. Her vital signs show a temperature of 36.9°C, BP 165/75 mm Hg, HR 98 bpm, RR 28/min, and SpO$_2$ 74% on room air, which increases to 100% with a non-rebreather mask.

   Point-of-care lung ultrasound is performed with the probe at the midclavicular lines bilaterally (**Figure 55.1A**), as well as in the coronal plane at the right (**Figure 55.1B**) and left (**Figure 55.1C**) midaxillary lines.

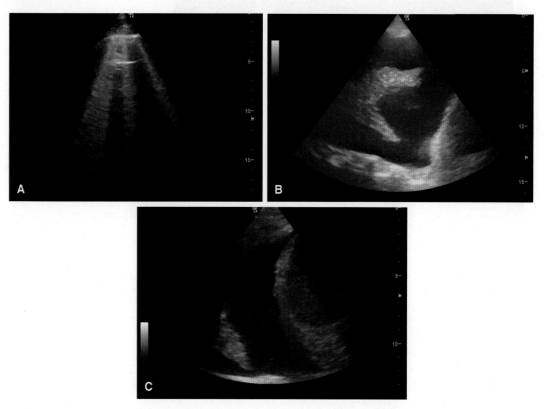

**Figure 55.1**

What is the *most* appropriate next step in her management?

A. Order computed tomography (CT) to rule out pulmonary angiogram and start heparin drip

B. Give IV furosemide and order echocardiogram

C. Broaden antibiotics

D. Perform diagnostic thoracentesis

2. A 48-year-old man is brought to the hospital after a motor vehicle collision with multiple injuries, including an open femur fracture. There was a prolonged extrication time, as the car had rolled down an embankment. Upon arrival, the patient is confused, BP 88/55 mm Hg, HR 124 bpm, RR 30/min, SpO$_2$ 68% on room air, and he is placed on a non-rebreather mask. Point-of-care cardiac ultrasound shows no pericardial effusion, a hyperdynamic left ventricle (LV), and a normal-sized right ventricle (RV) with increased contractility. Lung ultrasound is obtained in the left coronal plane at the midaxillary line (**Figure 55.2**).

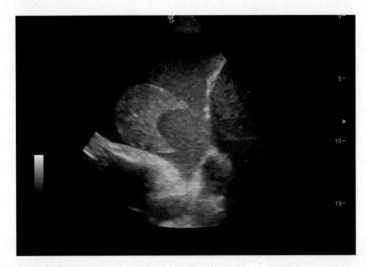

**Figure 55.2**

What is the *most likely* cause of the patient's hypoxemia?

A. Pneumothorax

B. Hemothorax

C. Fat embolism from open femur fracture

D. Empyema

3. A 92-year-old woman is admitted from a nursing home with left lower lobe pneumonia. Empiric treatment is started with piperacillin/tazobactam and vancomycin. On hospital day 3, she develops hypotension and a persistent fever. Lung ultrasound is obtained in the right coronal plane at the midaxillary line (**Figure 55.3**).

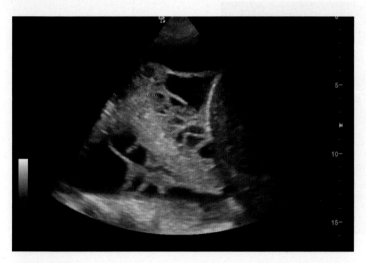

**Figure 55.3**

What is the *most appropriate* next step in her management?
A. Chest tube insertion, with consideration for VATS (video-assisted thoracoscopic surgery)
B. Diagnostic thoracentesis
C. Broaden antibiotic coverage
D. CT chest

4. A 76-year-old woman is admitted with progressively worsening dyspnea on exertion and cough over the past 3 months, culminating in a near-syncopal episode while climbing stairs. Chest X-ray shows a large left-sided pleural effusion. Lung ultrasound is performed, and **Figure 55.4** is acquired in the left coronal plane at the midaxillary line.

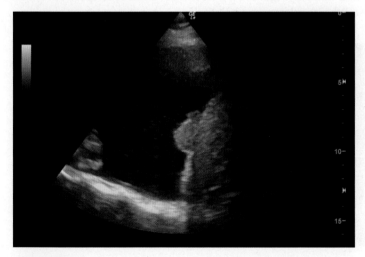

**Figure 55.4**

What is the *most likely* etiology of her symptoms?
A. Congestive heart failure (CHF)
B. Tuberculosis (TB)
C. Empyema
D. Malignant pleural effusion

5. A 63-year-old man presents with rapidly-progressive dyspnea and chest pain. He is not able to walk up to his bedroom on the second floor due to his symptoms and was brought to the hospital by his son. A point-of-care ultrasound is performed, and a selected image is shown in **Figure 55.5**.

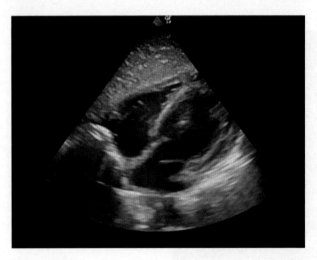

**Figure 55.5**

Which of the following *best* describes the findings in this image?
A. There is a pericardial effusion.
B. There is a right pleural effusion.
C. There is a left pleural effusion.
D. There is no apparent abnormality.

6. A 28-year-old man presents to the Emergency Department with a cough and fever for 3 days. He was recently diagnosed with human immunodeficiency virus (HIV) and TB, and started on antiretroviral treatment and treatment for TB 2 weeks prior to arrival. He has a temperature of 39°C, BP 85/45 mm Hg, HR 120 bpm, RR 30/min, and $SpO_2$ 88% on room air. Point-of-care cardiac ultrasound shows a hyperdynamic LV with a small pericardial effusion and a collapsible inferior vena cava (IVC). There is a moderate-sized right-sided pleural effusion (**Figure 55.6**). He is started on broad-spectrum antibiotics and given 30 mL/kg IV Lactated Ringer's solution as a bolus.

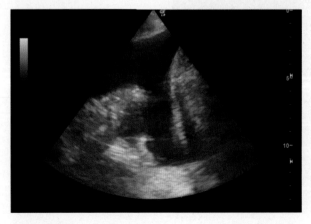

**Figure 55.6**

What is the *most appropriate* next step in his management?
A. Give diuretics to improve pleural effusion
B. Perform diagnostic thoracentesis, send adenosine deaminase (ADA)
C. Empirically start anticoagulation therapy and order a CT scan
D. Placement of an emergent chest tube and consideration for VATS

7. A 48-year-old man with a history of alcohol abuse and cirrhosis is admitted to the intensive care unit for alcohol withdrawal, and incidentally found to have a large right-sided pleural effusion. Point-of-care cardiac ultrasound shows no pericardial effusion and a hyperdynamic LV and RV. Lung ultrasound is obtained in the right coronal plane at the midaxillary line (**Figure 55.7**).

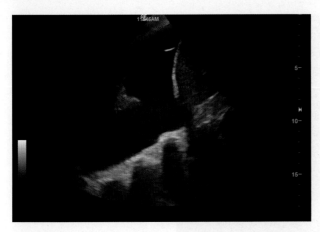

**Figure 55.7**

What is the most likely cause of this pleural effusion?
A. Empyema from aspiration pneumonia
B. Transudative effusion from CHF
C. Uncomplicated parapneumonic effusion from community-acquired pneumonia
D. Hepatic hydrothorax

8. An 81-year-old man with prostate cancer receiving chemotherapy presents to the Emergency Department with sudden-onset dyspnea and chest pain. His temperature is 37°C, BP 160/100 mm Hg, HR 108 bpm, RR 26/min, and SpO$_2$ 94% on room air. Electrocardiogram (ECG) shows sinus tachycardia, and is otherwise normal. Laboratory evaluation is significant for Troponin T 20 ng/L (mild elevation) and B-type natriuretic peptide (BNP) 380 pg/mL (moderate elevation).

Lung ultrasound obtained in the right coronal plane at the midaxillary line is shown in **Figure 55.8**.

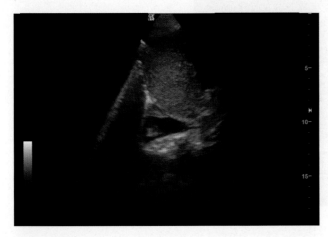

**Figure 55.8**

What is the *most appropriate* next step in his management?
A. Perform diagnostic thoracentesis and initiate antibiotic therapy
B. Order CT chest angiogram and initiate a heparin infusion
C. Perform echocardiography and initiate diuresis with furosemide
D. Call interventional cardiology for urgent coronary angiogram and administer aspirin

9. A 78-year-old man is admitted to the hospital with alcohol withdrawal. He is not able to give his medical history. He has a temperature of 37°C, BP 160/110 mm Hg, HR 110 bpm, and $SpO_2$ 94% on room air. His chest X-ray shows a left-sided pleural effusion. A point-of-care lung ultrasound is performed in the coronal plane at the left midaxillary line, as shown in **Figure 55.9**.

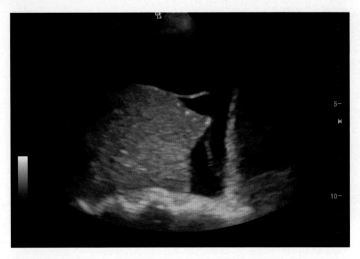

**Figure 55.9**

What is the most likely diagnosis of this pleural effusion?
**A.** Parapneumonic effusion from undiagnosed pneumonia
**B.** Malignant pleural effusion
**C.** Transudative pleural effusion from CHF
**D.** Hepatic hydrothorax from cirrhosis

10. Which answer choice names the structures A, B, and C correctly in **Figure 55.10**?

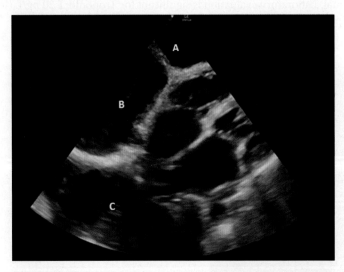

**Figure 55.10**

**A.** A = Ascites, B = Ascites, C = R pleural effusion
**B.** A = R pleural effusion, B = Ascites, C = L pleural effusion
**C.** A = Ascites, B = R pleural effusion, C = L pleural effusion
**D.** A = R pleural effusion, B = Ascites, C = Vertebral body

11. Your intern brings you a sonographic image of a patient who is admitted for evaluation of dyspnea. **Figure 55.11** was acquired in the coronal plane at the right midaxillary line.

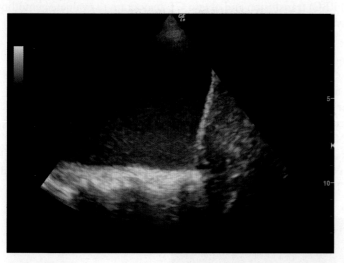

**Figure 55.11**

What is the *best* advice you can give your intern regarding this image?
A. The image is sufficient for the diagnosis of a large pleural effusion, advise them to perform a diagnostic and therapeutic thoracentesis.
B. The image is sufficient for the diagnosis of a large pleural effusion, advise them to place a chest tube.
C. Ask the intern to order a CT scan to confirm the diagnosis of right pleural effusion.
D. Ask the intern to obtain additional sonographic images, as you cannot diagnose pleural effusion based on the image shown.

12. A 78-year-old man with known CHF and cirrhosis secondary to hepatitis C is admitted for evaluation of dyspnea on exertion and a persistent right-sided pleural effusion.

A diagnostic and therapeutic thoracentesis is performed, with the removal of 1.5 L of yellow fluid. A follow-up chest X-ray after the procedure shows resolution of the right pleural effusion and no pneumothorax. Overnight, the patient complains of worsening dyspnea. His vital signs show a temperature of 37°C, BP 90/60 mm Hg, HR 120 bpm, RR 24/min, $SpO_2$ 90% on 6 L supplemental oxygen. Point-of-care lung ultrasound reveals **Figure 55.12** in the right coronal plane at the midaxillary line.

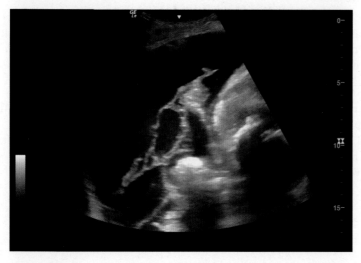

**Figure 55.12**

What is the *most appropriate* next step in his management?
A. Administer furosemide for reexpansion pulmonary edema
B. Obtain a surgical consult for diaphragmatic injury
C. Order packed red blood cell (PRBC) transfusion and obtain CT angiogram to evaluate hemothorax
D. Closely monitor as transient dyspnea is expected after thoracentesis

13. A 96-year-old man with a history of heart failure with a reduced ejection fraction (EF 19%) and atrial fibrillation on warfarin presents to the Emergency Department with weakness. His vital signs are temperature 35°C, BP 103/66 mm Hg, HR 108 bpm, RR 22/min, and $SpO_2$ 97% on 4 L supplemental oxygen. Laboratory evaluation reveals a white blood cell (WBC) of $12 \times 10^9$/L, hemoglobin (Hgb) 10.3 g/dL, electrolytes within normal limits, creatinine 1.4 mg/dL (baseline 1.1), international normalized ratio (INR) 5. Point-of-care cardiac ultrasound shows severely reduced systolic LV function, a dilated left atrium (LA), normal RV size and function, dilated right atrium (RA), significant tricuspid regurgitation (TR), and significant mitral regurgitation (MR). Lung ultrasound shows bilateral pleural effusions. The right pleural effusion is shown in **Figure 55.13**.

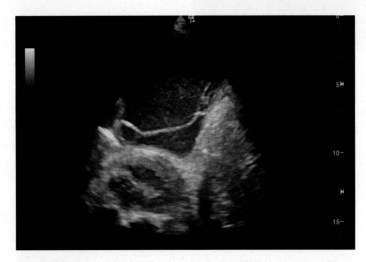

**Figure 55.13**

What is the most likely etiology of the patient's presentation?
A. Pneumonia with parapneumonic empyema
B. Exacerbation of CHF
C. Hemothorax from supratherapeutic INR
D. Cardiogenic shock from valve failure

14. Ultrasound is a simple noninvasive procedure that can detect pleural effusions with higher sensitivity than chest X-ray. Sonographic quantification of pleural effusion by antero-posterior depth has been reported to be correlated with drained pleural volume. Which of the following statements is *false* regarding the estimate of pleural effusion volume with ultrasound?

A. The PLD (pleura-lung distance) is defined by the distance between the posterior chest wall and the lung when the patient is supine and the probe is in a transverse plane.
B. A pleural effusion >800 mL is predicted by a PLD > 45 mm on the right or >50 mm on the left.
C. A pleural effusion of >500 mL is predicted by a PLD > 50 mm.
D. PLD overestimates pleural volume with a massive pleural effusion.

15. Ultrasound assessment of pleural effusion by posterior depth has been correlated with the drained pleural volume. Pleura-lung distance (PLD) is defined by the distance between the posterior chest wall and the lung when the patient is supine and the probe is placed in a transverse plane. Which part in **Figure 55.14** correctly measures PLD in estimating pleural effusion volume?

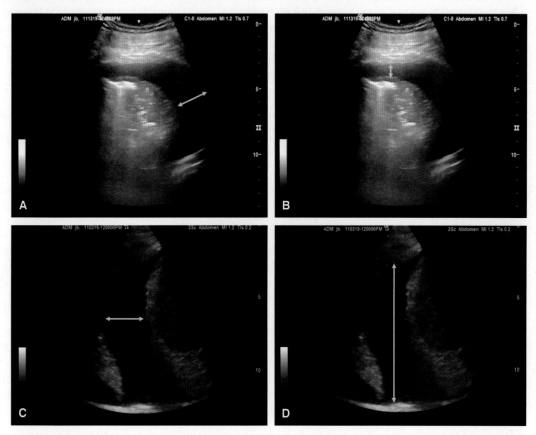

**Figure 55.14**

A. Figure 55.14A
B. Figure 55.14B
C. Figure 55.14C
D. Figure 55.14D

# Chapter 55 ▪ Answers

1. **Correct Answer: B. Give IV furosemide and order echocardiogram**

*Rationale:* Sonographic evidence of anechoic simple bilateral pleural effusions with diffuse bilateral B lines is suggestive of hydrostatic pulmonary edema (e.g., from congestive heart failure or volume overload). Homogeneously anechoic simple pleural effusions are suggestive of a transudative pleural effusion. If there is a strong suspicion of heart failure as a cause of the effusion and no competing reason for emergent thoracentesis (such as clinically suspected infection), then a trial of medical therapy for heart failure can be prescribed prior to consideration of thoracentesis. Pulmonary embolism and pneumonia are not suggested by the ultrasound imaging.

Selected Reference
1. Light R. Clinical practice pleural effusion. *N Engl J Med.* 2002 Jun;346(25):1971-1977.

**2.** Correct Answer: B. Hemothorax

*Rationale:* Pleural effusions that are diffusely echogenic are usually due to debris, which may be RBCs, WBCs, or even protein clumps. Most commonly, these are exudative effusions, such as hemothorax or empyema. It is difficult to differentiate hemothorax from empyema based on sonographic images alone, but the clinical history of recent trauma and rib fractures suggests hemothorax is most likely. It is important to note that even a small volume of blood within a transudative effusion can cause this appearance, as well as setting the 2D gain too high while obtaining images. Evaluation of the pleura would help identify pneumothorax, which is not apparent here. Fat embolism is an important cause of respiratory failure after orthopedic trauma or surgery, but the hemothorax is the most likely cause in this case.

Selected References
1. Ferreira AC, Filho FM, Braga T, Fanstone GD, Charbel I, Chodraui B. Radiologia Brasileira. *Radiol Bras.* 2006;39(2):1-9. doi:10.1590/S0100-39842006000200014.
2. Soni NJ, Franco R, Velez MI, et al. Ultrasound in the diagnosis and management of pleural effusions. *J Hosp Med.* 2015 Dec;10(12):811-816. doi:10.1002/jhm.2434.

**3.** Correct Answer: A. Chest tube insertion, with consideration for VATS (video-assisted thoracoscopic surgery)

*Rationale:* Figure 55.3 shows a multiloculated effusion with septations. Fibrin strands and septae are commonly seen in all exudates, including empyema, hemothorax, uremic and malignant pleural effusions. However, the clinical picture of sepsis is strongly suggestive of empyema, which requires drainage. A diagnostic thoracentesis is unnecessary because of the high suspicion for empyema, and it will only delay treatment. A multiloculated effusion with septation is a late stage of parapneumonic effusion, and it requires chest tube insertion with consideration for VATS. Intrapleural tissue plasminogen activator (tPA) and DNAse may facilitate drainage if it is inadequate. Common indications for VATS drainage include multiloculated empyema, empyema refractory to tube thoracostomy, and the presence of a pleural "rind." Increasing antibiotic coverage may be indicated if a resistant organism is suspected, but evacuation of the infected fluid is the preferred next step in management. CT may help classify additional lesions or evaluate response to drainage, but the ultrasound image is adequate to initiate treatment immediately with thoracostomy.

Selected References
1. Koppurapu V, Meena N. A review of the management of complex parapneumonic effusion in adults. *J Thorac Dis.* 2017;9(7):2135-2141. doi:10.21037/jtd.2017.06.21.
2. Yang PC, Luh KT, Chang DB, Wu HD, Yu CJ, Kuo SH. Value of sonography in determining the nature of pleural effusion: analysis of 320 cases. *Am J Roentgenol.* 1992;159(1):29-33. doi:10.2214/ajr.159.1.1609716.

**4.** Correct Answer: D. Malignant pleural effusion

*Rationale:* Sonographic evidence of a pleural nodule is a specific finding in patients with malignant effusion. In a paper by Gorg, et al., 210 patients with exudative pleural effusions were studied by ultrasound for sonographic signs of pleural carcinomatosis. Images were evaluated for echoes within the fluid, septations, sheet-like or nodular pleural masses, and associated lesions of the lung. The study concluded that sonographic findings of echogenic or septated fluid were not specific for malignancy. Only the evidence of pleural masses was characteristic of malignant effusion. CHF is an important cause of pleural effusion, but the visualized nodule is more suggestive of malignancy. Similarly, TB may cause pleural effusion, but is not the most likely cause in this case. Empyema is less likely given the indolent presentation and anechoic appearance of the fluid, but remains a possibility as well.

Selected References
1. Görg C, Restrepo I, Schwerk WB. Sonography of malignant pleural effusion. *Eur Radiol.* 1997;7(8):1195-1198. doi:10.1007/s003300050273.
2. Yang PC, Luh KT, Chang DB, Wu HD, Yu CJ, Kuo SH. Value of sonography in determining the nature of pleural effusion: Analysis of 320 cases. *Am J Roentgenol.* 1992;159(1):29-33. doi:10.2214/ajr.159.1.1609716.

**5.** Correct Answer: B. There is a right pleural effusion.

*Rationale/Critique:* Figure 55.5 is a subcostal four-chamber view of the heart, with the liver at the top of the image, adjacent to the RV (see also **Figure 55.15**). Deep to the heart on the right side of the image is the left pleura. The right pleural space is present on the left side of the image, with a large anechoic region, representing a pleural effusion. There is no evidence for pericardial effusion, which would typically be apparent between the liver and the RV, at the top of the image.

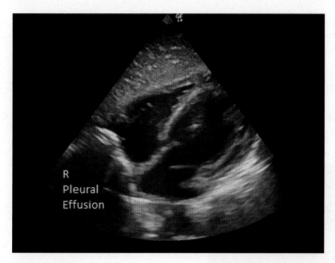

**Figure 55.15**

**6.** Correct Answer: B. Perform diagnostic thoracentesis, send adenosine deaminase (ADA)

*Rationale:* This is a case of TB and HIV-associated immune reconstitution inflammatory syndrome (IRIS). IRIS develops after antiretroviral therapy initiation. Clinically, it can present in a wide variety of ways, consistent with systemic inflammation. Even without concomitant HIV, TB can paradoxically worsen once anti-TB treatment is initiated because of immune system reconstitution, known as a "paradoxical response." This effect is more common and prominent with concomitant initiation of HIV treatment.

Figure 55.6 shows a tuberculous pleural effusion, which is usually small to moderate in size. Diagnostic thoracentesis should be performed and ADA and lactate dehydrogenase (LDH) levels should be sent. Demonstration of an elevated pleural fluid ADA level is useful in the diagnosis of TB pleural effusion. Patients with severe symptoms of IRIS should be started on glucocorticoids to suppress the inflammatory immune response. His hyperdynamic heart suggests that heart failure is not the cause of his pleural effusion, and with hypotension, he is unlikely to benefit from diuresis. While pulmonary embolism is an important cause of respiratory failure and hypotension, it is not suggested by the ultrasound findings, which should demonstrate abnormal RV function and a dilated IVC if it is causing this degree of hemodynamic insult.

Selected Reference

1. Naidoo K, Yende-Zuma N, Padayatchi N, et al. The immune reconstitution inflammatory syndrome after antiretroviral therapy initiation in patients with tuberculosis: findings from the SAPiT trial. *Ann Internal Med.* 2012;157(5):313-324. doi:10.7326/0003-4819-157-5-201209040-00004.

**7.** Correct Answer: D. Hepatic hydrothorax

*Rationale:* Hepatic hydrothorax is defined as the presence of pleural effusion in a patient with cirrhosis who does not have other reasons to have pleural effusion. Hepatic hydrothorax is a right-sided effusion in approximately 85% of cases. It is thought to be caused by the movement of ascites into the chest via diaphragmatic defects, driven by a pressure gradient from the peritoneal to the pleural space. The lack of infectious symptoms and hyperdynamic ventricles makes empyema, parapneumonic effusion, and CHF less likely.

**Selected Reference**
1. Garbuzenko DV, Arefyev NO. Hepatic hydrothorax: an update and review of the literature. *World J Hepatol.* 2017;9(31): 1197-1204. doi:10.4254/wjh.v9.i31.1197.

**8.** Correct Answer: B. Order CT chest angiogram and initiate a heparin infusion

*Rationale/Critique:* Figure 55.8 shows a trace or small right-sided pleural effusion, evidenced by the spine sign (**Figure 55.16**).

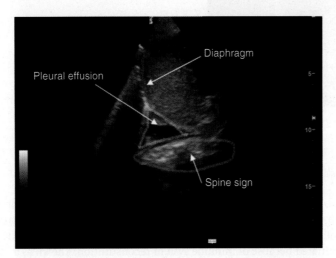

**Figure 55.16**

This presentation is concerning for acute pulmonary embolism, and it is appropriate to initiate therapy while awaiting confirmatory testing. The patient's cancer history is a risk factor, and the sudden-onset tachycardia, and combination of chest pain and dyspnea support this concern. The mildly elevated serum troponin and BNP levels are also consistent with acute pulmonary embolism (PE), and suggest myocardial strain, which may also be evident on ECG, but not reliably so. Ultrasound of the pleural space is never diagnostic for PE, but may still be helpful in excluding alternative causes. About 20%-50% of patients with pulmonary embolism have an associated pleural effusion, which is usually small and almost always exudative. One can consider diagnostic thoracentesis in the above case, but the effusion shown in the image is too small for bedside diagnostic thoracentesis and is certainly not responsible for the patient's symptoms. Parapneumonic pleural effusion is less likely, as the patient has no infectious symptoms. CHF is not a usual cause of pleuritic chest pain, and with such a small effusion, there would be no urgency in diuretic administration. Although coronary syndromes can present with normal ECG findings, there is no urgency in coronary angiography in this case.

**Selected Reference**
1. Porcel JM, Light RW. Pleural effusions due to pulmonary embolism. *Curr Opin Pulm Med.* 2008;14(4):337-342. doi:10.1097/MCP.0b013e3282fcea3c.

**9.** Correct Answer: B. Malignant pleural effusion

*Rationale:* Figure 55.9 is likely a complex effusion with fibrin strands. A malignant pleural effusion should be considered with a new left-sided exudative pleural effusion with fibrous strands in the absence of any infectious symptoms. Malignant pleural effusions are the second leading cause of exudative effusions, after parapneumonic effusions. Parapneumonic effusion is less likely in this case with a lack of infectious symptoms. The lack of apparent air bronchograms in this image also suggests compressive atelectasis as the cause of the lung density, rather than pneumonia. A unilateral effusion without a history of heart failure makes CHF a less likely cause. Hepatic hydrothorax would be expected on the right side of the chest.

Selected Reference

1. American Thoracic Society. Management of malignant pleural effusions. *Am J Respir Crit Care Med.* 2000;162(5):1987-2001. doi:10.1164/ajrccm.162.5.ats8-00.

**10.** Correct Answer: A. A = Ascites, B = Ascites, C = R pleural effusion

*Rationale/Critique:* Figure 55.10 is taken from a subcostal window in a patient with large ascites and a pleural effusion. Normally, the liver would be apparent at the top of the image, but it is displaced by the large volume of ascites. A subcostal (subxiphoid) four-chamber view of the heart is present on the right side of Figure 55.10 (see also **Figure 55.17**). There is a right-sided pleural effusion adjacent to the atria in the deep portion of the screen (C). The large volume of ascites makes the falciform ligament apparent, between (A) and (B).

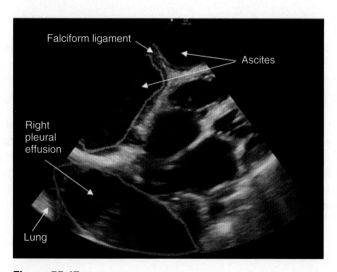

**Figure 55.17**

Selected Reference

1. Kerut E, Dearstine M, Hanawalt C. Utility of identification of the falciform ligament in the echocardiography laboratory. *Echocardiography.* 2007 Sep;24(8):887-888. doi:10.1111/j.1540-8175.2007.00481.x.

**11.** Correct Answer: D. Ask the intern to obtain additional sonographic images, as you cannot diagnose pleural effusion based on the image shown.

*Rationale:* The three criteria for the diagnosis of pleural effusion by bedside ultrasound are: (1) The presence of proper anatomic boundaries (chest wall, diaphragm, lung, and spine [or aorta]). (2) The presence of a hypo- or an anechoic space—the effusion—within the above boundaries. (3) The presence of respiratory-phasic lung movements—the so-called "swirling lung signs" (jellyfish sign and sinusoid sign). All three of these must be present to confidently diagnose pleural effusion. The image above does not show any lung tissue, and hence the upper boundary of the "effusion" is not seen. This may lead to erroneous identification of structures, for example, the collection may be intra-abdominal. In addition, a lack of visualized lung precludes one from identifying any dynamic lung signs. Consequently, a dense right lower lobe consolidation with hepatization of the lung can give a similar appearance to the image above.

#### Selected Reference

1. Doerschug KC, Schmidt GA. Intensive care ultrasound: III. Lung and pleural ultrasound for the intensivist. *Ann Am Thorac Soc.* 2013;10(6):708-712. doi:10.1513/AnnalsATS.201308-288OT.

**12.** Correct Answer: C. Order packed red blood cell (PRBC) transfusion and obtain CT angiogram to evaluate hemothorax

*Rationale:* **Figure 55.12** shows a complex pleural effusion with fibrin strands. Fibrin strands may be seen in exudates, including empyema, hemothorax, uremic and malignant pleural effusions. The etiology of the effusion cannot be determined from the sonographic images alone. Given the rapid accumulation of fluid, a hemothorax secondary to the recent procedure should be considered at the top of the differential diagnosis. Other than getting STAT labs and giving a transfusion if indicated, a CT angiogram or diagnostic thoracentesis may confirm the diagnosis of hemothorax, and placement of a chest tube is usually indicated for initial treatment. Surgical intervention or endovascular embolization is occasionally necessary for persistent large-volume hemorrhage. Reexpansion pulmonary edema is a complication of thoracentesis, but the pleural effusion image shown in the question is not consistent with reexpansion edema. A parapneumonic effusion from healthcare-acquired pneumonia is not impossible, but it is not the most likely scenario, and it is unusual to accumulate a large pleural effusion with fibrin strands within hours, especially in a patient without any infectious symptoms.

#### Selected References

1. Ault MJ, Rosen BT, Scher J, Feinglass J, Barsuk JH. Thoracentesis outcomes: a 12-year experience. *Thorax.* 2015;70(2):127-132. doi:10.1136/thoraxjnl-2014-206114.
2. Cantey EP, Walter JM, Corbridge T, Barsuk JH. Complications of thoracentesis: Incidence, risk factors, and strategies for prevention. *Curr Opin Pulm Med.* 2016;22(4):378-185. doi:10.1097/MCP.0000000000000285.

**13.** Correct Answer: A. Pneumonia with parapneumonic empyema

*Rationale:* The patient has a history of CHF and point-of-care cardiac ultrasound showing reduced systolic function and valvular abnormalities. However, the pleural ultrasound shows a complex effusion (presence of fibrin strands), making the diagnosis of an exudate virtually certain. In addition, hypothermia would not be readily accounted for by a CHF exacerbation or valvular abnormalities. A hemothorax from a supratherapeutic INR can also be considered for a pleural effusion with fibrin strands, but it is less likely in this patient with infectious symptoms.

#### Selected Reference

1. Yang PC, Luh KT, Chang DB, Wu HD, Yu CJ, Kuo SH. Value of sonography in determining the nature of pleural effusion: analysis of 320 cases. *Am J Roentgenol.*1992;159(1):29-33. doi:10.2214/ajr.159.1.1609716.

**14.** Correct Answer: D. PLD overestimates pleural volume with a massive pleural effusion.

*Rationale:* Ultrasound assessment of pleural effusion volume by measuring its posterior depth has been reported in several studies. In a study by Vignon, et al., a pleural effusion >800 mL was predicted when this distance was > 45 mm (right) or >50 mm (left). In another study by Roch, et al., it was found that an effusion width of 5 cm predicted an effusion volume of 500 mL. However, the volume assessment with PLD underestimates the volume in a massive pleural effusion because the lung also collapses superiorly, and PLD does not account for the fluid accumulation in the lung base.

#### Selected References

1. Balik M, Plasil P, Waldauf P, et al. Ultrasound estimation of volume of pleural fluid in mechanically ventilated patients. *Intensive Care Med.* 2006;32(2):318-321. doi:10.1007/s00134-005-0024-2.
2. Roch A, Bojan M, Michelet P, et al. Usefulness of ultrasonography in predicting pleural effusions> 500 mL in patients receiving mechanical ventilation. *Chest.* 2005;127(1):224-232. doi:10.1378/chest.127.1.224.
3. Vignon P, Chastagner C, Berkane V, et al. Quantitative assessment of pleural effusion in critically ill patients by means of ultrasonography. *Crit Care Med.* 2005;33(8):1757-1763. doi:10.1097/01.CCM.0000171532.02639.08

**15.** Correct Answer: A. Figure 55.14A

*Rationale:* PLD is the distance between the posterior chest wall and the lung when the patient is supine and the probe is placed in a transverse plane at the posterior axillary line. The probe is placed in a coronal plane in Figure 55.14C and 55.14D. PLD is measured by the maximal posterior distance between parietal and visceral pleura in the transverse plane, which corresponds to Choice A, Figure 55.15A. Figure 55.15B measures pleural distance from the lateral chest wall. There are alternative techniques to quantify the pleural effusion, and not one method is validated among the others. Another technique is a multiplane ultrasound approach, suggested by Remerand, et al., where the height of the pleural effusion is measured, multiplied by the area of the effusion (in transverse plane) in the midpoint of the height.

### Selected References

1. Balik M, Plasil P, Waldauf P, et al. Ultrasound estimation of volume of pleural fluid in mechanically ventilated patients. *Intensive Care Med.* 2006;32(2):318-321. doi:10.1007/s00134-005-0024-2.
2. Remerand F, Dellamonica J, Mao Z, et al. Multiplane ultrasound approach to quantify pleural effusion at the bedside. *Intensive Care Med.* 2010;36(4):656-664.
3. Roch A, Bojan M, Michelet P, et al. Usefulness of ultrasonography in predicting pleural effusions> 500 mL in patients receiving mechanical ventilation. *Chest.* 2005;127(1):224-232. doi:10.1378/chest.127.1.224.
4. Usta E, Mustafi M, Ziemer G. Ultrasound estimation of volume of postoperative pleural effusion in cardiac surgery patients. *Interact Cardiovasc Thorac Surg.* 2010;10(2):204-207.

# 56 | DIFFERENTIATING PULMONARY EDEMA, PNEUMONIA, COPD/ASTHMA, BRONCHIOLITIS, ARDS, PULMONARY EMBOLISM

Kevin M. Swiatek and Sammy Pedram

1. A 56-year-old man develops acute respiratory failure and is mechanically ventilated. Point-of-care ultrasound is used to evaluate the etiology of his respiratory failure. His anterior chest shows the pattern with lung ultrasound in **Figure 56.1**.

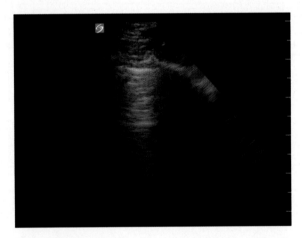

**Figure 56.1**

Which of the following *most* accurately describes this pattern?
A. A horizontal reverberation artifact that represents air-pleura interface
B. Horizontal artifacts that repeat the distance from the probe to the nearest blood vessels
C. A vertical reverberation artifact that represents fully inflated lung
D. Vertical artifacts indicating an underlying interstitial syndrome

2. Based on the case presented in **Question 1** and Figure 56.1, which of the following is *most* true regarding this pattern of lung ultrasound findings?

A. This pattern is commonly seen in patients with edematous interlobular septae.
B. This pattern is commonly seen in patients with dry interlobular septae.
C. This pattern excludes pneumothorax at this location.
D. This pattern suggests an interstitial syndrome as the cause of respiratory failure.

3. Based on the case presented in **Question 1** and Figure 56.1, which of the following techniques can help better visualize this pattern on lung ultrasound?

   A. Low gain, probe at an oblique axis to the surface of the skin
   B. Low gain, probe at a perpendicular axis to the surface of the skin
   C. High gain, probe at an oblique axis to the surface of the skin
   D. High gain, probe at a perpendicular axis to the surface of the skin

4. A 76-year-old man with a history of coronary artery disease presents complaining of shortness of breath and wheezing. He notes a 7 lb weight gain over the past 2 weeks. He has orthopnea and dyspnea on exertion, as well as lower extremity edema. Chest ultrasound is used to evaluate his complaint and reveals **Figure 56.2** and ▶ **Video 56.1**.

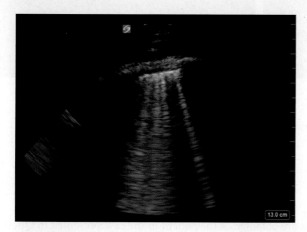

**Figure 56.2**

Which of the following best describes the characteristics seen in Figure 56.2 and ▶ Video 56.1?
A. Profuse B-lines are present and consistent with an interstitial syndrome.
B. An A-line predominant pattern is present and consistent with pneumonia.
C. Few B-lines are present, consistent with dry interlobular septa.
D. A C-profile pattern is seen, consistent with heart failure.

5. Based on the case presented in **Question 4**, Figure 56.2, and ▶ Video 56.1, which of the following are mandatory characteristics of this finding?

   I. Comet-tail artifact
   II. Makes A-lines more prominent
   III. Arises from the pleural line
   IV. Moves in concert with lung sliding

   A. I, II, and III
   B. I, II, and IV
   C. II, III, and IV
   D. I, III, and IV

6. On auscultation, the patient from **Question 4** is found to have a blowing systolic murmur and bilateral rales. Point-of-care cardiac ultrasound demonstrates the finding seen in ▶ Video 56.2. Putting all of these findings together, which of the following is the *most likely* diagnosis?

   A. Pneumonia
   B. Pulmonary embolism
   C. Heart failure exacerbation
   D. Pneumothorax

7. A 74-year-old man presents to the Emergency Department (ED) with a 1-day history of shortness of breath and cough productive of purulent sputum. His temperature is 38.5°C, BP 115/60 mm Hg, HR 110 bpm, RR 20/min, and $SpO_2$ 90% on room air. His chest is examined with lung ultrasound, which reveals **Figure 56.3**.

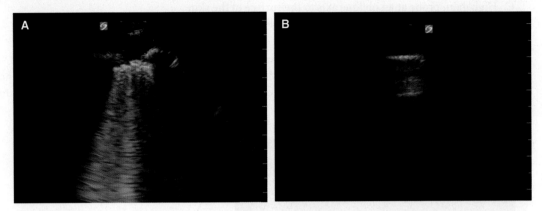

**Figure 56.3**

Which of the following patterns is *most* consistent with the ultrasound findings?
A. Diffuse B-lines
B. A-lines
C. A/B pattern
D. Consolidation

8. Additional images of the right hemithorax are obtained of the patient in the case presented in **Question 7**. Which of the following signs is seen in **Figure 56.4**?

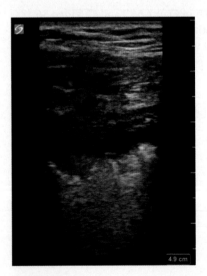

**Figure 56.4**

A. Shred sign
B. Sinusoid sign
C. Stratosphere sign
D. Bat sign

9. The patient's symptoms (**Questions 7** and **8**) and ultrasound findings (Figures 56.3 and 56.4) are *most* consistent with which clinical diagnosis?

    **A.** Community-acquired pneumonia
    **B.** Acute respiratory distress syndrome (ARDS)
    **C.** Congestive heart failure exacerbation
    **D.** Chronic obstructive pulmonary disease (COPD) exacerbation

10. A patient is mechanically ventilated for acute respiratory failure. Lung ultrasound is performed as shown in **Figure 56.5** and ▶ **Videos 56.3A** and **B**. Lung sliding is present, but reduced in a scattered distribution.

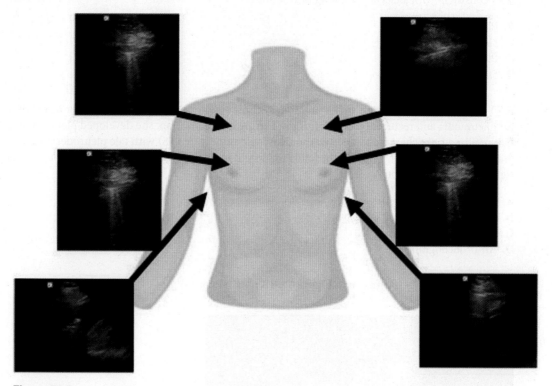

**Figure 56.5**

What is the *most* likely diagnosis?
**A.** Acute respiratory distress syndrome
**B.** Pulmonary edema
**C.** Pulmonary embolism with infarct
**D.** Asthma exacerbation

11. Over the next 6 hours, the patient from **Question 10** develops hemodynamic decline. The physician performs reassessment with lung ultrasound and notes the same findings as before. Which of the following is *most* true regarding this patient's lung ultrasound findings?

    **A.** The presence of B-lines rules out pneumothorax.
    **B.** An A-line predominant pattern is consistent with ARDS.
    **C.** The number of B-lines does not predict mortality in ARDS.
    **D.** The patient should receive diuretics for pulmonary edema.

12. A 56-year-old woman presents to the outpatient office to establish and receive care for her pulmonary fibrosis. Clinically, she has advanced disease requiring chronic supplemental oxygen therapy, and a forced vital capacity (FVC) that is 45% of predicted. Which pattern is *most* likely to be seen at the bases of her lungs on lung ultrasound?

   A. Few B-lines, wide separation between B-lines
   B. Few B-lines, narrow separation between B-lines
   C. Diffuse B-lines, wide separation between B-lines
   D. Diffuse A-lines, narrow separation between B-lines

13. A consolidation pattern (C-profile) can be seen with atelectasis or pneumonia. Which of the following is *most* consistent with atelectasis on lung ultrasound?

   A. Plankton sign
   B. Hepatization of lung
   C. Pleural effusion
   D. Static air bronchograms

14. A 70-year-old woman presents to her pulmonary clinic appointment for follow-up after hospitalization for pneumonia and recurrent pleural effusion. During hospitalization, she developed pleural adhesions that required right chest video-assisted thoracoscopic surgery (VATS) with talc pleurodesis. Once the pneumonia has resolved, which of the following would *most* likely be seen on lung ultrasound of the right chest of this patient?

   A. Profuse B-lines with lung sliding
   B. Absent lung sliding
   C. Consolidation pattern
   D. Air bronchograms

15. Lung ultrasound is performed, and **Figure 56.6** is obtained.

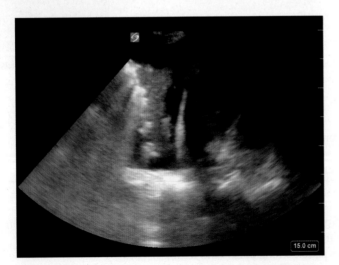

**Figure 56.6**

Which of the following *best* describes Figure 56.6?
A. Complex pleural effusion with compressive atelectasis
B. Ascites with air bronchograms
C. Pleural effusion with air bronchograms
D. Pleural effusion, ascites, compressive atelectasis

16. A patient presents with several days of cough and fever consistent with pneumonia. A urine legionella antigen test is positive. A chest X-ray is obtained and shown in **Figure 56.7A**.

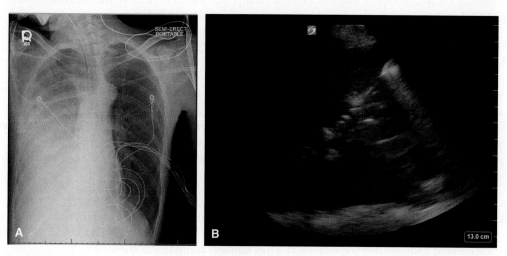

**Figure 56.7**

Lung ultrasound is performed (**Figure 56.7B** and ▶ **Video 56.4**) is performed and demonstrates which of the following?
A. Diffuse B-lines
B. Absence of lung sliding with a B-line pattern
C. Shred sign with lung rockets
D. Consolidation pattern with dynamic air bronchograms

17. A 17-year-old man is seen in the ED after sudden-onset shortness of breath and wheezing while mowing the lawn. A lung ultrasound is performed, which shows an A-line pattern symmetrically, with bilateral lung sliding present. The posterolateral aspects of both lungs appear normal on ultrasound. Both lower extremities are negative for deep vein thrombosis (DVT). Which of the following is the *most* likely diagnosis?

A. Pulmonary embolism
B. Asthma
C. Pneumonia
D. ARDS

18. A 71-year-old man is referred to an outpatient pulmonary clinic for evaluation of his severe bullous emphysema associated with stable COPD. He has no new symptoms and is on 2 L of supplemental nasal cannula oxygen at home. In patients with COPD and bullous emphysema, which of the following is *most* likely to be seen on chest ultrasound?

A. A-line profile without lung sliding
B. B-line predominant pattern
C. B-lines in the apex with A-lines in the remaining lung
D. Increased diaphragm movement with inspiration

19. A woman presents to the ED with 1 week of worsening cough and copious sputum production. She has a history of COPD and endorses similar symptoms with previous exacerbations. She denies fever and laboratory evaluation reveals white blood cells (WBC) $9.0 \times 10^9$/L. Which of the following would be *most* likely to be seen with ultrasound in the posterolateral lung zones?

    A. Absent lung sliding
    B. A-lines
    C. B-lines with decreased lung sliding
    D. Subpleural consolidations

20. A 2-year-old child is seen by her pediatrician for cough and wheezing. The parents have also noticed a fever and decreased appetite. A lung ultrasound is performed with the hope of avoiding ionizing radiation exposure from a chest X-ray. Which of the following statements about lung ultrasound in this population is *most* accurate?

    A. In contrast to adults, hilar pathology is well seen on lung ultrasound of children.
    B. X-ray is superior to ultrasound in the diagnosis of bronchiolitis in children under the age of 24 months.
    C. Ultrasound findings correlate with chest X-ray findings accurately in children.
    D. The use of lung ultrasound delays the diagnosis of bronchiolitis in infants.

21. Infants and young children are among the patients at greatest risk of being hospitalized for acute respiratory illness. Guidelines do not currently support the routine use of X-ray in the diagnostic evaluation of these patients (except in those that are critically ill). Which of the following is *most* true regarding the use of lung ultrasound in this population?

    A. Ultrasound can be helpful to predict the trajectory of acute respiratory illness in children.
    B. X-ray accurately predicts the progression to respiratory failure.
    C. X-ray is more accurate than ultrasound at determining the severity of disease.
    D. Lung ultrasound can be used to distinguish pneumonia from acute bronchiolitis .

22. A 65-year-old man presents to the ED with worsening respiratory distress. He is found to have COVID-19 infection. Over the next 24 hours, he develops worsening hypoxemia and is intubated and placed on mechanical ventilation. Chest X-ray reveals diffuse patchy bilateral infiltrates. Which of the following will *most* likely be seen on chest ultrasound?

    A. A-line profile
    B. Normal lung sliding
    C. Lung point
    D. Lung pulse

23. A 61-year-old man is admitted to the medical intensive care unit (ICU) for respiratory failure. He has a history of heart failure, but also had fever, malaise, and cough prior to presentation. B-lines are seen on lung ultrasound. Which of the following findings would be *most* consistent with ARDS on lung ultrasound?

    A. Profuse B-lines
    B. Scattered/patchy B-lines
    C. Subpulmonic effusion
    D. Normal lung sliding

24. A young woman is seen in the ED after a transcontinental flight, during which she acutely developed dyspnea. A lung ultrasound is performed to identify the cause of her dyspnea, and is shown in **Figure 56.8**.

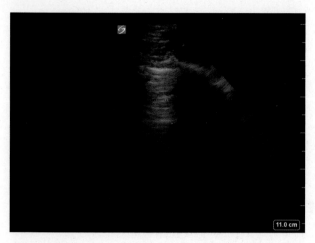

**Figure 56.8**

In addition to abnormal lower extremity venous compression ultrasound, which of the following ultrasound findings is the *most* consistent with this presentation?
   A. Normal lung sliding, A-lines
   B. Absent or decreased lung sliding, A-lines
   C. Normal lung sliding, B-lines
   D. Absent or decreased lung sliding, B-lines

25. A 65-year-old man presents with acute onset of right-sided chest pain and dyspnea on exertion. A point-of-care ultrasound examination of the heart reveals an enlarged right ventricle in the parasternal short-axis and apical four-chamber views, with septal bowing into the left ventricle during systole. Lung ultrasound demonstrates multiple 1 cm subpleural consolidations in the right lower lung field. Lung sliding and A-lines are seen throughout the remainder of the chest. Based on this information, what test is *most* likely to confirm the diagnosis?

   A. Sputum culture
   B. Troponin and B-natriuretic peptide (BNP)
   C. Chest X-ray
   D. Lower extremity ultrasound

26. A 22-year-old woman with no past medical history who is 37 weeks pregnant presents to the ED for acute onset of shortness of breath and "racing heart." Lung ultrasound shows bilateral lung sliding with A-lines. Which of the following is the *most* appropriate next step?

   A. D-dimer and computed tomography (CT) pulmonary angiogram
   B. Chest X-ray and repeat lung ultrasound in 30 minutes
   C. Cardiac and lower extremity ultrasound
   D. Serial electrocardiogram (ECG) and troponin evaluation, and admit for observation

27. A 35-year-old woman with a history of systemic lupus erythematosus presents with right-sided chest pain for 3 days. She has a history of pulmonary embolism and ran out of her medications last month. Which of the following items below are *most* likely to be seen on lung ultrasound?

   **I.** Subpleural consolidation(s)
   **II.** Absent lung sliding
   **III.** Pleural effusion
   **IV.** B-line pattern

   **A.** I, II, III
   **B.** I, III
   **C.** II, III, IV
   **D.** III, IV

# Chapter 56 ▪ Answers

**1.** Correct Answer: A. A horizontal reverberation artifact that represents air-pleura interface

*Rationale:* A-lines are horizontal reverberation artifacts that represent a strong reflection from the air-pleura interface. The presence of A-lines is not itself pathologic. The distance between A-lines is equal to the distance from the probe to the air-pleura interface.

Selected References

1. Doerschug KC, Schmidt GA. Intensive care ultrasound: III. Lung and pleural ultrasound for the intensivist. *Ann Am Thorac Soc.* 2013;10(6):708-712. doi:10.1513/annalsats.201308-288ot.
2. Lichtenstein DA. BLUE-protocol and FALLS-protocol. *Chest.* 2015;147(6):1659-1670. doi:10.1378/chest.14-1313.

**2.** Correct Answer: B. This pattern is commonly seen in patients with dry interlobular septae

*Rationale:* An A-line predominant pattern, as shown in Figure 56.1, indicates that the interlobular septae are characteristically dry. The A-line reverberation artifact is an apparent "second" pleural reflection, deep to the pleura, twice the distance of the original pleural reflection. It represents a strong reflection from the aeration just below the pleural line, which is consistent with aerated lung, but can also be present with pneumothorax. The presence of B-lines would suggest an interstitial syndrome or edematous interlobular septae (pulmonary edema), which are not seen here. Additionally, in an ICU population of mechanically ventilated patients, an A-line pattern has a 93% specificity, 50% sensitivity, and 97% positive predictive value for a pulmonary artery occlusion pressure (PAOP) ≤18 mm Hg. However, in a later study, lung ultrasound was shown to be of limited usefulness for predicting PAOP.

Selected References

1. Lichtenstein DA. BLUE-protocol and FALLS-protocol. *Chest.* 2015;147(6):1659-1670. doi:10.1378/chest.14-1313.
2. Lichtenstein DA, Mezière GA, Lagoueyte J-F, Biderman P, Goldstein I, Gepner A. A-lines and B-lines: lung ultrasound as a bedside tool for predicting pulmonary artery occlusion pressure in the critically ill. *Chest.* 2009;136(4):1014-1020, ISSN 0012-3692, doi:10.1378/chest.09-0001.
3. Volpicelli G, Skurzak S, Boero E, et al. Lung ultrasound predicts well extravascular lung water but is of limited usefulness in the prediction of wedge pressure. Anesthesiology. 2014;121(2):320-327.

**3.** Correct Answer: B. Low gain, probe at a perpendicular axis to the surface of the skin

*Rationale:* A-lines and lung sliding are best visualized with the linear or phased array transducers, but the phased array probe may be needed to achieve the depth adequate to visualize A-lines. The linear transducer allows for high-frequency detailed visualization of the pleural line. Proper positioning of the probe perpendicular to the skin with a low gain setting will optimize these artifacts.

### Selected Reference

1. Doerschug KC, Schmidt GA. Intensive care ultrasound: III. Lung and pleural ultrasound for the intensivist. *Ann Am Thorac Soc.* 2013;10(6):708-712. doi:10.1513/annalsats.201308-288ot.

**4.** Correct Answer: A. Profuse B-lines are present and consistent with an interstitial syndrome.

*Rationale:* B-lines are vertical reverberation artifacts commonly seen in patients with interstitial syndromes. In this case, the patient appears to have signs and symptoms consistent with heart failure. On ultrasound, an occasional B-line may be a normal finding between rib spaces, but this patients has many B-lines (more than three) in a single image, which is abnormal. A thin pleural line and profuse B-lines in a symmetric distribution are highly suggestive of an interstitial syndrome (e.g., pulmonary edema). Evidence also suggests that if many B-lines are detected in a bilateral, symmetric distribution in all lung zones, this is associated with increased left ventricular filling pressure.

### Selected References

1. Hubert A, Girerd N, Breton HL, et al. Diagnostic accuracy of lung ultrasound for identification of elevated left ventricular filling pressure. *Arch Cardiovasc Dis.* 2019;11(1):53. doi:10.1016/j.acvdsp.2018.10.115.
2. Lichtenstein DA. BLUE-protocol and FALLS-protocol. *Chest.* 2015;147(6):1659-1670. doi:10.1378/chest.14-1313.
3. Muniz RT, Mesquita ET, Souza Junior CV, Martins WA. Pulmonary ultrasound in patients with heart failure—systematic review. *Arq Bras Cardiol.* 2018;110(6):577-584. doi:10.5935/abc.20180097.

**5.** Correct Answer: D. I, III, and IV

*Rationale:* Lichtenstein describes three mandatory criteria used to identify B-lines: a comet-tail (reverberation) artifact, arising from the pleural line, which moves in concert with lung sliding when present. Four other criteria are often seen with B-lines: extend from pleural line to the distal edge of the image, well-defined, erases A-lines, hyperechoic. These criteria help to distinguish B-lines from other comet-tail artifacts.

### Selected References

1. Lichtenstein D. Novel approaches to ultrasonography of the lung and pleural space: where are we now? *Breathe.* 2017;13(2):100-111. doi:10.1183/20734735.004717.
2. Miller A. Practical approach to lung ultrasound. *BJA Educ.* 2016;16(2):39-45. doi:10.1093/bjaceaccp/mkv012.

**6.** Correct Answer: C. Heart failure exacerbation

*Rationale:* Pulmonary edema can develop rapidly in patients with mitral regurgitation from a myocardial infarction or acute heart failure. In this instance, B-lines help to confirm the diagnosis of pulmonary edema as the cause for impending respiratory failure. A systematic review and meta-analysis of ED patients with acute heart failure suggests that point-of-care lung ultrasound can be used accurately and reliably as an adjunct to other diagnostic modalities.

### Selected References

1. Lichtenstein DA. BLUE-protocol and FALLS-protocol. *Chest.* 2015;147(6):1659-1670. doi:10.1378/chest.14-1313.
2. Mcgivery K, Atkinson P, Lewis D, et al. Emergency department ultrasound for the detection of B-lines in the early diagnosis of acute decompensated heart failure: a systematic review and meta-analysis. *CJEM.* 2018;20(3):343-352. doi:10.1017/cem.2018.27.

**7.** Correct Answer: C. A/B Pattern

*Rationale:* In this scenario, the patient presents with the clinical syndrome of pneumonia associated with focal B-lines on lung ultrasound. Figure 56.3A demonstrates B-lines and the pleura appears somewhat irregular, which is consistent with an inflammatory interstitial syndrome. In contrast, Figure 56.3B demonstrates normal pleura with an A-line pattern. An A/B pattern describes an A-profile (normal appearance) in one hemithorax and a B-profile (B-lines) in the other. This suggests a heterogeneous distribution of the inflammatory process, as may be seen with pneumonia, in contrast to a diffuse pattern, which would be expected with cardiogenic pulmonary edema.

**Selected References**

1. Bhatt H, Patel C, Parikh S, Jhaveri B, Puranik J. Bedside lung ultrasound in emergency protocol as a diagnostic tool in patients of acute respiratory distress presenting to emergency department. *J Emerg Trauma Shock.* 2018;11(2):125. doi:10.4103/jets.jets_21_17.
2. Lichtenstein DA, Mezière GA. Relevance of lung ultrasound in the diagnosis of acute respiratory failure*: the BLUE protocol. *Chest.* 2008;134(1):117-125. doi:10.1378/chest.07-2800.

**8.** Correct Answer: A. Shred sign

*Rationale:* Figure 56.4 demonstrates a shred sign. The shred sign artifact is seen when there is subpleural consolidation of lung tissue, in which a portion of consolidated lung is visualized adjacent to the reflection from a deeper, aerated portion of lung. The irregular interface between the consolidated and aerated lung tissues gives a "shredded" appearance. The shred sign is nonspecific, but can help to define lung pathology in a clinical context. For example, in the case presented in **Questions 7** and **8**, this likely represents ultrasound evidence of pneumonia. It should be noted that the shred sign can also be seen with pulmonary infarct, subpleural lung abscess, and lung cancer.

**Selected References**

1. Biswas A, Lascano JE, Mehta HJ, Faruqi I. The utility of the "shred sign" in the diagnosis of acute respiratory distress syndrome resulting from multifocal pneumonia. *Am J Respir Crit Care Med,* 2017;195(2). doi:10.1164/rccm.201608-1671im.
2. Mojoli F, Bouhemad B, Mongodi S, Lichtenstein D. Lung ultrasound for critically ill patients. *Am J Respir Crit Care Med.* 2019;199(6):701-714. doi:10.1164/rccm.201802-0236ci.
3. Rinaldi L, Milione S, Fascione MC, et al. Relevance of lung ultrasound in the diagnostic algorithm of respiratory diseases in a real-life setting: a multicentre prospective study. *Respirology.* 2019. doi:10.1111/resp.13659.

**9.** Correct Answer: A. Community-acquired pneumonia

*Rationale/Critique:* The case presented in **Questions 7, 8,** and **9** and chest ultrasound findings (Figures 56.3 and 56.4) suggest a focal inflammatory or infectious process, such as community-acquired pneumonia. ARDS would demonstrate a patchy pattern of B-lines with hypoxia, which would be bilateral. Hydrostatic pulmonary edema from a heart failure exacerbation would show a thickened pleural line with many B-lines bilaterally. Chest ultrasound examination of those with COPD and asthma can be normal (A-line pattern) and would also be expected to appear symmetric.

**Selected Reference**

1. Lichtenstein DA. BLUE-protocol and FALLS-protocol. *Chest.* 2015;147(6):1659-1670. doi:10.1378/chest.14-1313.

**10.** Correct Answer: A. Acute respiratory distress syndrome

*Rationale:* Figure 56.5 and ▶ **Videos 56.3A** and **B** demonstrate a bilateral heterogeneous distribution of B-lines. In the figure, the left upper lobe is spared. The left lower lobe, right upper lobe, and right lower lobe with B-lines are shown. The right posterolateral aspect has a pleural effusion and left appears normal. This distribution is consistent with ARDS. Pulmonary edema is a profuse pattern of B-lines with intact lung sliding. Pulmonary embolism with infarct would demonstrate A-line pattern, with or without shred sign, and pleural effusion. Asthma exacerbation would also demonstrate an A-line predominant pattern.

**Selected References**

1. Copetti R, Soldati G, Copetti P. Chest sonography: a useful tool to differentiate acute cardiogenic pulmonary edema from acute respiratory distress syndrome. *Cardiovasc Ultrasound.* 2008;6(1). doi:10.1186/1476-7120-6-16.
2. Doerschug KC, Schmidt GA. Intensive care ultrasound: III. Lung and Pleural ultrasound for the intensivist. *Ann Am Thorac Soc.* 2013;10(6):708-712. doi:10.1513/annalsats.201308-288ot.

**11.** Correct Answer: A. The presence of B-lines rules out pneumothorax.

*Rationale:* ARDS is a heterogeneous disease process that can produce a B-line predominant pattern in a heterogeneous distribution. With high-pressure ventilation, pneumothorax can develop. However, the presence of B-lines rules out pneumothorax with 100% sensitivity and 100% negative predictive value, because two opposing layers of pleura must be present to create this artifact. In addition, the number of B-lines may have a prognostic impact on ARDS mortality and the likelihood of successfully weaning from a ventilator. The asymmetric heterogeneous B-line pattern argues against cardiogenic pulmonary edema.

### Selected References

1. Mojoli F, Bouhemad B, Mongodi S, Lichtenstein D. Lung ultrasound for critically ill patients. *Am J Respir Crit Care Med.* 2019;199(6):701-714. doi:10.1164/rccm.201802-0236ci.
2. Soummer A, Perbet S, Brisson H, et al. Ultrasound assessment of lung aeration loss during a successful weaning trial predicts postextubation distress. *Crit Care Med.* 2012;40(7):2064-2072. doi:10.1097/ccm.0b013e31824e68ae.

**12.** Correct Answer: C. Diffuse B-lines, wide separation between B-lines

*Rationale:* Diffuse B-lines are the predominant finding on lung ultrasound in cases of pulmonary fibrosis. The distance between two B-lines is thought to correlate with the severity of the disease, and is inversely related to the DLCO, $PaO_2$, FVC %, and TLC %. While these findings are seen on lung ultrasound, they should not be used in isolation to make an initial diagnosis, and other clinical and diagnostic testing would be needed.

### Selected References

1. Makhlouf H, Hasan A. B-lines: transthoracic chest ultrasound signs useful in assessment of interstitial lung diseases. *Ann Thorac Med.* 2014;9(2):99. doi:10.4103/1817-1737.128856.
2. Manolescu D, Davidescu L, Traila D, Oancea C, Tudorache V. The reliability of lung ultrasound in assessment of idiopathic pulmonary fibrosis. *Clin Interv Aging.* 2018;13:437-449. doi:10.2147/cia.s156615.

**13.** Correct Answer: D. Static air bronchograms

*Rationale:* Both atelectasis and pneumonia can demonstrate consolidation patterns on lung ultrasound. Commonly, clinical factors are enough to differentiate the two entities. Dynamic air bronchograms appear and disappear with ventilation and help to exclude bronchial obstruction, suggesting pneumonia as the diagnosis. Static air bronchograms are more consistent with atelectasis and are demonstrated in **Figure 56.9**, as well as a pleural effusion. The presence of hepatization is associated with pneumonia, and the plankton sign describes swirling debris within a complex pleural effusion.

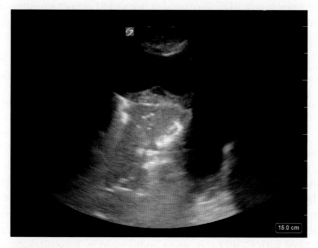

**Figure 56.9**

### Selected References

1. Lichtenstein D, Mezière G, Seitz J. The dynamic air bronchogram. A lung ultrasound sign of alveolar consolidation ruling out atelectasis. *Chest.* 2009;135(6):1421-1425. doi:10.1378/chest.08-2281.
2. Miller A. Practical approach to lung ultrasound. *BJA Educ.* 2016;16(2):39-45. doi:10.1093/bjaceaccp/mkv012.

**14.** Correct Answer: B. Absent lung sliding

*Rationale:* Pleurodesis will result in apposition and scarring of the visceral and parietal pleura. For lung sliding to be present, there must be free movement of visceral and parietal pleura.

Selected Reference

1. Ahmed Abd El Megied El Hadidy, Kamel KM, Amany Atf Al Kareem Abo Zaid, Kamal E, Fayiad, H. E. Role of chest ultrasound in detecting successful pleurodesis. *Egyptian J Chest Dis Tuberc.* 2017;66(2):279-283. doi:10.1016/j.ejcdt.2016.11.009.

**15.** Correct Answer: D. Pleural effusion, ascites, compressive atelectasis

*Rationale:* In Figure 56.6, there are anechoic fluid collections both above (to the left of the image) and below the diaphragm (to the right of the image), representing pleural effusion and ascites, respectively. There are associated static air bronchograms in the posterolateral aspect of the lower lobe, which is consistent with atelectasis (left side of the image). In Figure 56.6, there is no evidence to suggest a complex fluid collection.

Selected Reference

1. Miller A. Practical approach to lung ultrasound. *BJA Educ.* 2016;16(2):39-45. doi:10.1093/bjaceaccp/mkv012.

**16.** Correct Answer: D. Consolidation pattern with dynamic air bronchograms

*Rationale/Critique:* Figure 56.7 and ▶ **Video 56.4** demonstrate a densely consolidated right lower lobe with dynamic air bronchograms. Dense consolidation can obscure lung sliding, which is not seen in this clip. In addition, B-lines are also not appreciated here, but are commonly seen with typical and atypical pneumonia patterns. A shred sign is not apparent, because there is no delineation visible between consolidated and aerated lung.

Selected References

1. Lichtenstein DA, Mezière GA. Relevance of lung ultrasound in the diagnosis of acute respiratory failure*: the BLUE protocol. *Chest.* 2008;134(1):117-125. doi:10.1378/chest.07-2800.
2. Lichtenstein D, Mezière G, Seitz J. The dynamic air bronchogram. A lung ultrasound sign of alveolar consolidation ruling out atelectasis. *Chest.* 2009;135(6):1421-1425. doi:10.1378/chest.08-2281.

**17.** Correct Answer: B. Asthma

*Rationale:* The Basic Lung Ultrasound Examination (BLUE) protocol helps to better define the cause of shortness of breath in this patient. If pulmonary embolism were present, we would be more likely to find a DVT in the lower extremity veins. If pneumonia or ARDS were present, we would expect a posterolateral alveolar or pleural syndrome, B', or C-profiles, as well as infectious symptoms, and likely a more indolent onset. Of the options provided, asthma is the most likely diagnosis.

Selected References

1. Lichtenstein D. Novel approaches to ultrasonography of the lung and pleural space: where are we now? *Breathe.* 2017;13(2):100-111. doi:10.1183/20734735.004717.
2. Lichtenstein DA, Mezière GA. Relevance of lung ultrasound in the diagnosis of acute respiratory failure: the BLUE protocol. *Chest.* 2008;134(1):117-125. doi:10.1378/chest.07-2800.

**18.** Correct Answer: A. A-line profile without lung sliding

*Rationale:* A-lines are the predominant feature of COPD and asthma on lung ultrasound. In cases of bullous emphysema, lung sliding may be absent in the apex because of the abnormal pleural movement from aeration of large blebs adjacent to the pleura. B-lines are associated with interstitial processes like pulmonary edema, although occasional B-lines are a normal finding. Decreased diaphragmatic motion and decreased muscle thickness is associated with COPD and can be appreciated by lung ultrasound.

Selected References

1. Lichtenstein DA, Mezière GA. Relevance of lung ultrasound in the diagnosis of acute respiratory failure*: the BLUE protocol. *Chest.* 2008;134(1):117-125. doi:10.1378/chest.07-2800.
2. Nair G, Jain S, Nuchin A, Uppe A. Study of the diaphragm in chronic obstructive pulmonary disease using ultrasonography. *Lung India.* 2019;36(4):299. doi:10.4103/lungindia.lungindia_466_18.

**19.** Correct Answer: B. A-lines

*Rationale:* The question stem is describing a patient with an acute exacerbation of COPD. Using the BLUE protocol as a guide, she would likely demonstrate an A-line predominate pattern showing normal aeration of the peripheral lung tissue. In patients with a COPD exacerbation without pneumonia, the posterolateral lung zones would be expected to appear normal as well, including the costophrenic angle, which may display intermittent aeration with inspiration (curtain sign). Absent lung sliding would be expected with pneumothorax, although decreased lung sliding may be apparent in regions with heavy bullous disease. B-lines would be expected with an interstitial process, like pulmonary edema or pneumonia, and would favor pneumonia in the presence of decreased lung sliding. Visualization of subpleural consolidations (C-profile) would suggest pneumonia, which is less likely in the absence of fever or leukocytosis.

Selected References

1. Lichtenstein DA, Mezière GA. Relevance of lung ultrasound in the diagnosis of acute respiratory failure*: the BLUE protocol. *Chest.* 2008;134(1):117-125. doi:10.1378/chest.07-2800.
2. Staub LJ, Biscaro RR, Kaszubowski E, Maurici R. Lung ultrasound for the emergency diagnosis of pneumonia, acute heart failure, and exacerbations of chronic obstructive pulmonary disease/asthma in adults: a systematic review and meta-analysis. *J Emerg Med.* 2019;56(1):53-69. doi:10.1016/j.jemermed.2018.09.009.

**20.** Correct Answer: C. Ultrasound findings correlate with chest X-ray findings accurately in children.

*Rationale:* Bronchiolitis remains the most common cause of hospitalization of children in the first year of life. Multiple studies have looked at alternatives to chest radiograph for the diagnosis of bronchiolitis. Bronchiolitis can present with multiple findings on lung ultrasound including B-lines and subpleural consolidations. Transthoracic lung ultrasound can effectively evaluate the lung parenchyma without using ionizing radiation when compared to chest X-ray.

Selected References

1. Jaszczołt S, Polewczyk T, Dołęga-Kozierowska M, Woźniak M, Doniec Z. Comparison of lung ultrasound and chest X-ray findings in children with bronchiolitis. *J Ultrason.* 2018;18(74):193-197. doi:10.15557/jou.2018.0029.
2. Özkaya AK, Yilmaz HL, Kendir ÖT, Gökay SS, Eyüboğlu I. Lung ultrasound findings and bronchiolitis ultrasound score for predicting hospital admission in children with acute bronchiolitis. *Pediatr Emerg Care.* 2018;1. doi:10.1097/pec.0000000000001705.

**21.** Correct Answer: A. Ultrasound can be helpful to predict the trajectory of acute respiratory illness in children.

*Rationale:* The routine use of chest X-ray is not recommended as a screening or prognostication tool in children. However, point-of-care lung ultrasound has demonstrated utility in clinically generating a lung ultrasound score (LUS), which is useful to predict risk of hospitalization, severity of disease, and the need for invasive and noninvasive ventilation in pediatric patients with acute bronchiolitis.

Selected References

1. Özkaya AK, Yilmaz HL, Kendir ÖT, Gökay SS, Eyüboğlu I. Lung ultrasound findings and bronchiolitis ultrasound score for predicting hospital admission in children with acute bronchiolitis. *Pediatr Emerg Care.* 2018;1. doi:10.1097/pec.0000000000001705.
2. Supino MC, Buonsenso D, Scateni S, et al. Point-of-care lung ultrasound in infants with bronchiolitis in the pediatric emergency department: a prospective study. *Eur J Pediatr.* 2019;178(5):623-632. doi:10.1007/s00431-019-03335-6.

**22.** Correct Answer: D. Lung pulse

*Rationale:* Lung sliding represents physiologic apposition of the visceral and parietal pleural surfaces. In a normal examination, the pleural surfaces freely move past each other with respiration, which creates a shimmering pleural artifact. In any pulmonary disease process that greatly reduces air movement throughout the lung, such as ARDS, lung sliding will be reduced or absent. Absent lung sliding can also be seen with mainstem bronchial intubation, mucus plugging, severe pneumonia, and apnea. A lung pulse can be a helpful way to differentiate absent lung sliding from pneumothorax versus other causes of decreased lung movement. The movement of the heart during the cardiac cycle is normally transmitted through the lung and demonstrated as subtle movement between the pleural layers at regular intervals, even when lung movement from ventilation is absent. The absence of a lung pulse suggests that the two pleural layers are not contiguous, that is, a pneumothorax is present. A lung point describes visualization of the edge of a pneumothorax, which is not suggested in this case.

Selected References

1. Levitov A, Mayo PH, Slonim AD. *Critical Care Ultrasonography*. McGraw-Hill Education Medical; 2014.
2. Lichtenstein DA. Lung ultrasound in the critically ill. *Ann Intensive Care*. 2014;4(1):1. doi:10.1186/2110-5820-4-1.

---

**23.** Correct Answer: B. Scattered/patchy B-lines

*Rationale:* ARDS is a heterogeneous disease process, with regions of the lung that are commonly spared, leading to inconsistent presence of B-lines. It also involves abnormalities of the pleura, which is reflected by reduced or absent lung sliding, pleural thickening, or coarse pleural irregularities. Pleural effusions can definitely exist in the setting of ARDS, but are not the most consistent finding.

Selected References

1. Copetti R, Soldati G, Copetti P. Chest sonography: a useful tool to differentiate acute cardiogenic pulmonary edema from acute respiratory distress syndrome. *Cardiovasc Ultrasound*. 2008;6(1). doi:10.1186/1476-7120-6-16.
2. Doerschug KC, Schmidt GA. Intensive care ultrasound: III. Lung and pleural ultrasound for the intensivist. *Ann Am Thorac Soc*. 2013;10(6):708-712. doi:10.1513/annalsats.201308-288ot.

---

**24.** Correct Answer: A. Normal lung sliding, A-lines

*Rationale:* This patient likely has an acute pulmonary embolism as the cause of her dyspnea, supported by the abnormal lower extremity compression ultrasound suggesting DVT. Lung sliding will normally be preserved in the setting of pulmonary embolism, in contrast to pneumothorax or pneumonia, which may display absent or decreased lung sliding. A-lines are expected as well, as the peripheral lung tissue should remain well-aerated, in contrast to interstitial processes like pulmonary edema or pneumonia, which would be expected to produce B-lines.

Selected Reference

1. Lichtenstein DA. BLUE-protocol and FALLS-protocol. *Chest*. 2015;147(6):1659-1670. doi:10.1378/chest.14-1313.

---

**25.** Correct Answer: D. Lower extremity ultrasound

*Rationale:* The patient has signs and symptoms consistent with a submassive pulmonary embolism, with right heart strain. Mathis, *et al.* demonstrated that in high-risk patients, the presence of two or more subpleural consolidations (0.5-3 cm in size) or one subpleural consolidation in the presence of a pleural effusion has a high sensitivity of 74% and specificity of 95% for the diagnosis of pulmonary embolism. In addition, the majority of the emboli were found in the lower lobes. An A-line pattern with normal lung sliding can also be seen with pulmonary embolism. A lower extremity ultrasound compression test would be helpful to increase the accurate diagnosis of DVT and pulmonary embolism. Troponin and BNP evaluation may help stratify the degree of right heart strain, but do not help differentiate the cause of the patient's symptoms. Sputum culture to evaluate for pneumonia and chest X-ray are less likely to help diagnose the suspected diagnosis of pulmonary embolism.

Selected References

1. Lichtenstein DA, Mezière GA. Relevance of lung ultrasound in the diagnosis of acute respiratory failure*: the BLUE protocol. *Chest*. 2008;134(1):117-125. doi:10.1378/chest.07-2800.
2. Mathis G, Blank W, Reißig A, et al. Thoracic ultrasound for diagnosing pulmonary embolism. *Chest*. 2005;128(3):1531-1538. doi:10.1378/chest.128.3.1531.

---

**26.** Correct Answer: C. Cardiac and lower extremity ultrasound

*Rationale:* In this example, the pretest probability for pulmonary embolism is high and a normal lung ultrasound does not rule out pulmonary pathology. If she is hemodynamically stable, the best next step would include cardiac echocardiography looking for right heart strain and lower extremity ultrasound examination for DVT assessment. This may also help evaluate for alternative causes of her symptoms, like peripartum cardiomyopathy, but findings of pulmonary edema (B-lines) would be expected if this was the cause of her dyspnea. If ultrasound testing is not diagnostic and the clinical suspicion for pulmonary embolism remains high, definitive testing (e.g., CT pulmonary angiogram) should be considered.

### Selected Reference

1. Lichtenstein D, Malbrain ML. Critical care ultrasound in cardiac arrest. Technological requirements for performing the SESAME-protocol—a holistic approach. *Anesthesiol Intensive Ther.* 2015;47(5):471-481. doi:10.5603/ait.a2015.0072.

---

**27.** Correct Answer: B. I, III

*Rationale:* The patient likely has an acute pulmonary embolism, which may include areas of pulmonary infarction. A typical ultrasound finding consistent with pulmonary infarct would include two or more "typical" lesions, 0.5-3 cm subpleural consolidations. Pleural effusions can also be seen in addition to subpleural consolidations. Absent lung sliding or a B-line pattern should prompt the operator to consider an alternative diagnosis.

### Selected References

1. Mathis G, Blank W, Reißig A, et al. Thoracic ultrasound for diagnosing pulmonary embolism. *Chest.* 2005;128(3):1531-1538. doi:10.1378/chest.128.3.1531.
2. Nazerian P, Vanni S, Volpicelli G, et al. Accuracy of point-of-care multiorgan ultrasonography for the diagnosis of pulmonary embolism. *Chest.* 2014;145(5):950-957. doi:10.1378/chest.13-1087.

# 57 | ESOPHAGEAL VERSUS ENDOTRACHEAL INTUBATION

Alberto Goffi and Paolo Persona

1. A 65-year-old man with a history of locally advanced oropharyngeal squamous cell carcinoma and previous treatment with chemotherapy and localized radiation therapy presents to the Emergency Department with stridor and upper airway obstruction. On physical examination, the patient has trismus and significant lymphadenopathy on the right neck, and you cannot palpate the trachea. In agreement with the otolaryngologist, you decide to transfer the patient to the operating room and attempt awake fiberoptic intubation. The backup plan is to perform a tracheostomy, and the surgeon asks you to help with ultrasound identification of the cricothyroid membrane and the trachea. Using a transverse orientation, you find the trachea significantly deviated to the left side. By rotating the transducer longitudinally, you identify the cricoid and tracheal cartilages. Which of the structures labeled in **Figure 57.1** corresponds to the first tracheal ring?

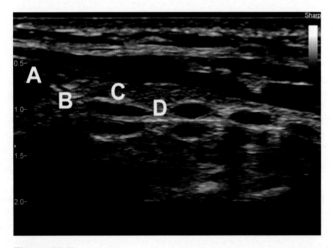

**Figure 57.1**

**A.** A
**B.** B
**C.** C
**D.** D

2. A 58-year-old woman with a past medical history of poorly controlled hypertension is brought to the Emergency Department with a decreased level of consciousness. She is comatose (Glasgow Coma Scale E1V1M2) and severely hypertensive (215/115 mm Hg). You decide to let your resident perform emergency endotracheal intubation for head computed tomography, and you monitor the procedure with ultrasound. Based on the ultrasound loop provided (▶ **Video 57.1** and **Figure 57.2**), what should be done next?

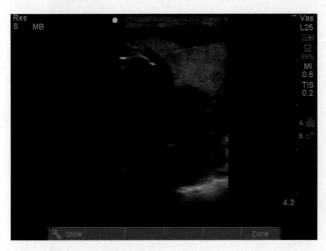

**Figure 57.2**

A. Initiation of mechanical ventilation
B. Advance the endotracheal tube 2 cm
C. Retract the endotracheal tube 2 cm
D. Remove the endotracheal tube from esophagus

# Chapter 57 ▪ Answers

1. Correct Answer: C

*Rationale:* When performing sonographic assessment of the airway, it is extremely important to follow a systematic step-by-step approach. Two techniques have been described for identification of the crico-thyroid membrane: (a) the longitudinal "String of Pearls" (SOP) and (b) the transverse "Thyroid-Airline-Cricoid-Airline" (TACA). The SOP technique is the most commonly used and it also allows identification of the interspaces between tracheal cartilages. The transverse TACA technique can be very useful in patients with short neck or severe neck flexion limitation. In the SOP technique, the first step requires identification of the trachea in a transverse approach at the level of the suprasternal notch (**Figure 57.3A,** *top row*). At this point, the transducer is slid to the patient's right side until only half of the tracheal carti-lage is displayed on the screen (**Figure 57.3B,** *second row*). Then, the transducer is rotated 90° clockwise, carefully maintaining it over the tracheal midline; this rotation allows visualization of the trachea in a longitudinal plane, with several hypoechoic rounded structures (cricoid and tracheal cartilages) aligned anteriorly to a hyperechoic line (air-mucosa interface), similar to a "string of pearls" (**Figure 57.3C**, *third row*). The cricoid cartilage appears as a larger and more anterior structure compared to the tracheal rings, with the first ring usually appearing as the longest one (Figure 57.1, *structure C*). The distal part of the thyroid cartilage is then seen cephalad to the cricoid cartilage. The cricothyroid membrane can be identified between the cricoid and thyroid cartilages (**Figure 57.3D**, *last row*).

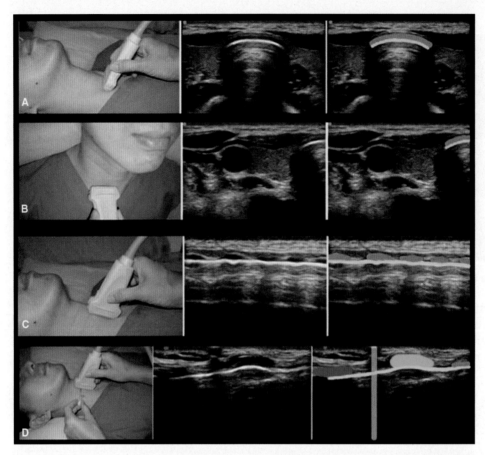

**Figure 57.3** The longitudinal "String of Pearls" (SOP) technique for the identification of the cricothyroid membrane and the interspaces between tracheal rings. Orange-red = tracheal ring; light blue = the tissue-air border; green = the cricoid cartilage; purple = the distal end of the thyroid cartilage; yellow = the shadow from the needle slid in between the transducer and the skin. www.airwaymanagement.dk

For the transverse TACA technique, the first step requires identification of thyroid cartilage (seen as a triangular structure) (**Figure 57.4A**, *top row*), followed by a caudal movement of the transducer until the cricothyroid membrane can be identified (**Figure 57.4B**, *second row*). Further caudal movement will reveal the cricoid cartilage, appearing as a hypoechoic horse-shoe structure (**Figure 57.4C**, *third row*). The final step is a cranial movement of the transducer, aimed at reidentification of the cricothyroid membrane (**Figure 57.4D**, *last row*) and marking of the skin for possible cricothyroidotomy.

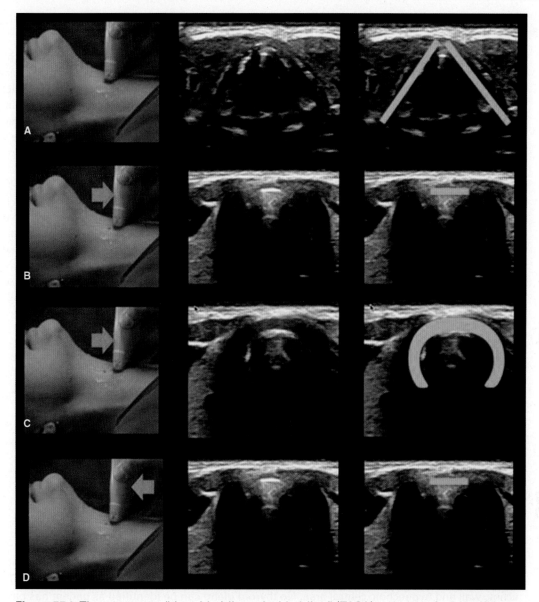

**Figure 57.4** The transverse "thyroid-airline-cricoid-airline" (TACA) technique for identifying the cricothyroid membrane. Blue triangle = thyroid cartilage; blue horizontal line = the "airline" = the cricothyroid membrane; blue "lying C" = the anterior part of the cricoid cartilage. www.airwaymanagement.dk.

## Selected References

1. Kristensen MS. Ultrasonography in the management of the airway. *Acta Anaesthesiol Scand.* 2011;55(10):1155-1173.
2. Kristensen MS, Teoh WH, Rudolph SS, Hesselfeldt R, Børglum J, Tvede MF. A randomised cross-over comparison of the transverse and longitudinal techniques for ultrasound-guided identification of the cricothyroid membrane in morbidly obese subjects. *Anaesthesia.* 2016;71(6):675-683.
3. Osman A, Meng Sum K. In: Diaz-Gomez J, Nikravan S, Conlon S, eds. Airway management in "Comprehensive Critical Care Ultrasound". 2nd ed. Society of Critical Care Medicine; 2020:325-333.
4. You-Ten KE, Siddiqui N, Teoh WH, Kristensen MS. Point-of-care ultrasound (POCUS) of the upper airway. *Can J Anesth.* 2018;65(4):473-484.

**2.** Correct answer: D. Remove the endotracheal tube from esophagus

*Rationale:* ▶ **Video 57.1** demonstrates a transverse plane of the neck at the level of the thyroid isthmus and left thyroid lobe. A tracheal cartilage with the air-mucosa interface can be observed on the left side of the screen, while the cervical esophagus runs posteriorly to the thyroid gland and laterally to the trachea. This ultrasound was performed in real time as the person performing the intubation was attempting to pass the endotracheal tube through the vocal cords. The sudden appearance, posterolateral to the trachea (in correspondence of the anatomic location of the esophagus), of a second hyperechoic structure with posterior acoustic shadowing ("double tract sign") is consistent with esophageal intubation and therefore immediate retraction of the tube is recommended.

Correct placement of the tube endotracheally will not reveal the appearance of the second air-filled structure. When performing tracheal/esophageal ultrasound for real-time confirmation of tracheal intubation, it is important to preidentify the esophagus. Although at the cervical level the esophagus is usually located to the left of the trachea, in some patients it can be identified on the right side, whereas in others it is not seen on ultrasound because it is located posterior to the trachea. In this latter circumstance, ultrasound is not able to correctly identify esophageal intubation as the tracheal air will impede proper visualization. **Figure 57.5** and ▶ **Video 57.2** demonstrate the same cervical plane and identify the esophagus, seen as an oval structure with a hyperechoic wall and hypoechoic central area. In ▶ **Video 57.2**, the patient swallows and a small amount of water and esophageal peristalsis can be appreciated.

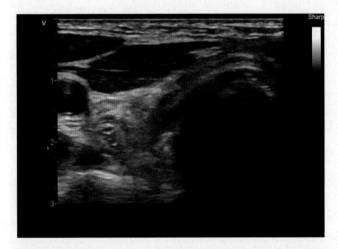

**Figure 57.5** Transverse plane of the neck. Esophagus is seen as an oval structure with a hyperechoic wall and hypoechoic central area. No thyroid gland can be identified as patient has past medical history of thyroidectomy.

In a recent systematic review and meta-analysis, Gottlieb et al. identified 17 studies (n = 1595 patients) exploring the accuracy of transtracheal ultrasound for identification of endotracheal tube position and demonstrated a pooled sensitivity of 98.7% (95% confidence interval [CI] 97.8%-99.2%) and specificity of 97.1% (95% CI 92.4%-99%), with a mean time to confirmation of only 13 seconds.

Selected References

1. Arya R, Schrift D, Choe C, Al-Jaghbeer M. Real-time tracheal ultrasound for the confirmation of endotracheal intubations in the intensive care unit: an observational study. *J Ultrasound Med.* 2019;38(2):491-497.
2. Gottlieb M, Holladay D, Peksa GD. Ultrasonography for the confirmation of endotracheal tube intubation: a systematic review and meta-analysis. *Ann Emerg Med.* 2018;72:627-636.
3. Ma G, Davis DP, Schmitt J, Vilke GM, Chan TC, Hayden SR. The sensitivity and specificity of transcricothyroid ultrason*ography to co*nfirm endotracheal tube placement in a cadaver model. *J Emerg Med.* 2007;32(4):405-407.
4. You-Ten KE, Siddiqui N, Teoh WH, Kristensen MS. Point-of-care ultrasound (POCUS) of the upper airway. *Can J Anesth.* 2018;65(4):473-484.

# 58 | OPTIMIZATION AND FACILITATION OF WEANING FROM THE VENTILATOR

Vinca W. Chow

1. A 72-year-old man with severe chronic obstructive pulmonary disease and lung cancer is recovering from a right upper lobectomy, and his ventilator has been transitioned to pressure support. **Figure 58.1A** and **B** are representative images obtained at end-inspiration and end-expiration, respectively, from the midclavicular subcostal view in the supine position.

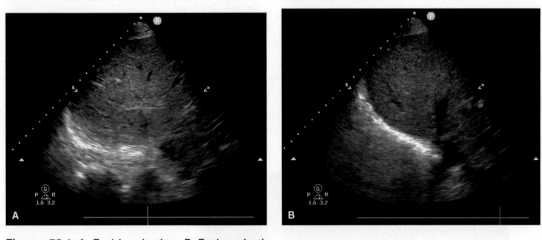

**Figures 58.1** A: End-inspiration. B: End-expiration.

Which statement is the *most* accurate description of these images?
**A.** Normal pleural sliding
**B.** Pleural thickening with impaired sliding
**C.** Normal diaphragmatic movement
**D.** Paradoxical diaphragmatic movement

2. A 46-year-old woman with rib fractures and blunt abdominal trauma after a motor vehicle collision has been intubated for 4 days. In consideration of extubation, an ultrasound image (**Figure 58.2**) is obtained in the anterolateral subcostal position during a spontaneous breathing trial (SBT). Which is the *most* appropriate course of action based on Figure 58.2?

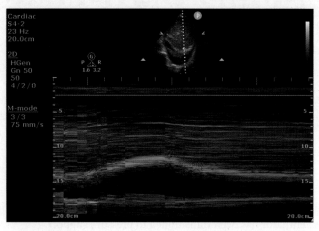

**Figures 58.2**

A. Ventilator weaning should proceed based on the degree of diaphragmatic excursion.
B. A chest tube for drainage of the large pleural effusion should be placed prior to attempts at extubation.
C. A chest tube should be placed urgently as the barcode pattern in M-mode is indicative of a pneumothorax.
D. Recruitment maneuvers should be performed given the "hepatization" of the lung in the near field.

3. A 65-year-old man has been intubated for 3 days after an exploratory laparotomy for bowel perforation. An ultrasound image (**Figure 58.3**) is obtained below the ninth rib in the anterior axillary line during an SBT.

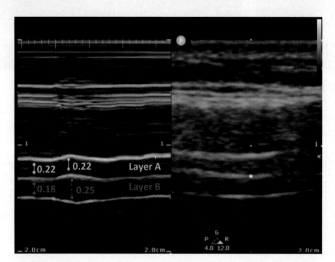

**Figures 58.3**

Which statement is the *most* accurate regarding his ventilator weaning?
A. The absence of intercostal muscle thickening in layer A predicts weaning failure.
B. The absence of diaphragmatic thickening in layer A predicts weaning failure.
C. The degree of intercostal thickening in layer B predicts weaning success.
D. The degree of diaphragmatic thickening in layer B predicts weaning success.

4. A 22-year-old woman was intubated for an asthma exacerbation 1 day ago. An ultrasound is performed below the eighth rib in the anterior axillary line. Which statement is best supported by **Figure 58.4**?

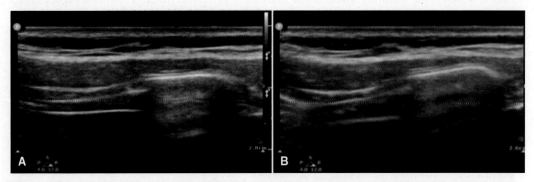

**Figures 58.4** A: Expiration. B: Inspiration.

A. There is a lung point concerning for pneumothorax
B. There is appropriate diaphragmatic excursion
C. There is appropriate diaphragmatic thickening
D. There is appropriate intercostal muscle thickening

5. A 28-year-old woman with acute respiratory distress syndrome (ARDS) and acute myocarditis secondary to influenza is weaned to pressure support after 2 days of induced paralysis and stress-dose steroids. The representative images seen in **Figure 58.5** were obtained during tidal breathing in the anterior axillary line.

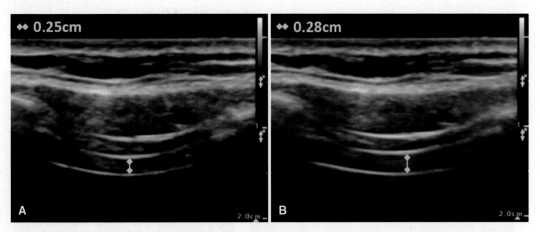

**Figures 58.5** A: End-expiration. B: End-inspiration.

Which of the following most accurately describes the diaphragmatic thickening fraction?
A. DT = (0.28 − 0.25)/0.28 = 0.11, indicating normal DT
B. DT = (0.28 − 0.25)/0.28 = 0.11, indicating impaired DT
C. DT = (0.28 − 0.25)/0.25 = 0.12, indicating normal DT
D. DT = (0.28 − 0.25)/0.25 = 0.12, indicating impaired DT

6. A 60-year-old man with a history of a coronary artery bypass graft and a left ventricular ejection fraction of 25% was intubated 4 days ago for respiratory failure in the setting of urosepsis. An ultrasound is performed to assess his respiratory function at the end of a spontaneous breathing trial (SBT). Which of the following would be the most likely additional findings based on **Figure 58.6**?

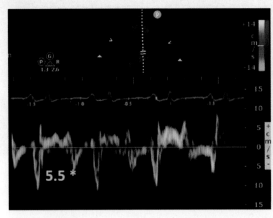 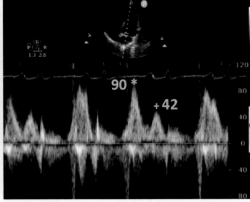

**Figures 58.6**

A. Bilateral diffuse B-lines with left ventricular end-diastolic pressure (LVEDP) of 10 mm Hg
B. Focal B-lines in the right lower lobe with LVEDP of 10 mm Hg
C. Bilateral diffuse B-lines with LVEDP of 20 mm Hg
D. Focal B-lines in the right lower lobe with LVEDP of 20 mm Hg

7. A 66-year-old man with a left ventricular ejection fraction of 35% was intubated 3 days ago for a chronic obstructive pulmonary disease exacerbation. His vital signs during an SBT are notable for HR 92 bpm, BP 171/99 mm Hg, and SpO$_2$ 88% on 40% O$_2$. Which is the most appropriate intervention to facilitate extubation based on **Figure 58.7**?

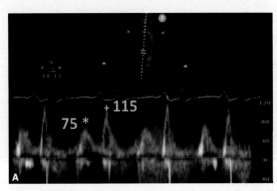 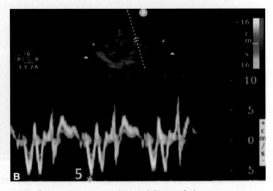

**Figures 58.7** A: During pressure support. B: At the end of spontaneous breathing trial.

A. Administer a fluid bolus
B. Administer an inotrope
C. Administer a vasodilator
D. Administer a bronchodilator

8. An 88-year-old woman with a history of hypertension, congestive heart failure with a left ventricular ejection fraction of 30%, and chronic kidney disease was intubated for septic shock 5 days ago. Her vital signs during an SBT are notable for HR 95 bpm, BP 175/105 mm Hg, respiratory rate (RR) 42/min, and SpO$_2$ 82% on 30% O$_2$. Which intervention is the *least* appropriate based on **Figure 58.8**?

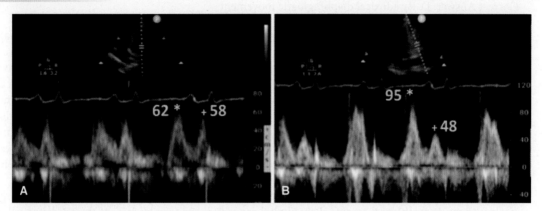

**Figures 58.8** A: During pressure support. B: At the end of spontaneous breathing trial.

A. Administer inhaled nitric oxide
B. Administer diuretic
C. Administer afterload reduction
D. Initiate noninvasive pressure support ventilation after extubation

9. In a patient with a left ventricular ejection fraction of 18% and currently in atrial fibrillation, the decision to administer a diuretic to facilitate ventilator weaning is best supported by which of the following change in echocardiographic findings after transitioning from pressure support ventilation to an SBT?

A. A change in *E/A* ratio from 14 to 16
B. A change in *E/A* ratio from 16 to 14
C. A change in E-wave deceleration time (DTE) from 120 ms to 140 ms
D. A change in DTE from 140 to 120 ms

10. A 45-year-old woman with hypertension was intubated 1 day ago after a motor vehicle collision causing multiple rib fractures and sternal fracture. During attempts to wean the ventilator, she becomes tachycardic, hypertensive, tachypneic, and hypoxic. Based on **Figure 58.9** of the parasternal long-axis view, which is the most appropriate next step in her management?

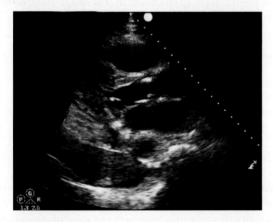

**Figure 58.9**

A. Transesophageal echocardiogram to assess for dissection flap in the descending aorta
B. Chest computed tomography angiogram to assess for injury to the descending aorta
C. Emergent pericardiocentesis
D. Chest tube placement or thoracentesis to drain pleural effusion

# Chapter 58 ▪ Answers

**1.** Correct Answer: D. Paradoxical diaphragmatic movement

*Rationale:* The craniocaudal excursion of the posterior third of the diaphragm can be assessed by imaging the subcostal region between the midclavicular and anterior axillary lines, with the transducer directed medially, cranially, and posteriorly. The diaphragm is the echogenic curvilinear structure located between the liver in the near field and lung in the far field. Diaphragm dysfunction can be detected with a high degree of specificity. There is better correlation between the inspired volume and diaphragmatic movement in the supine position compared to sitting or standing. Paradoxical movement is more pronounced in the supine position as compensatory expiration by the abdominal wall is reduced. In diaphragmatic dysfunction, compensatory contraction from the inspiratory muscles of the rib cage and neck causes the weakened diaphragm to move in a cephalad direction, as illustrated in these images with the movement of the diaphragm away from the transducer during inspiration (Figure 58.1A).

Diaphragm dysfunction arising from phrenic nerve injury could occur during cardiothoracic surgery, neck surgery, or mechanical trauma. Forced vital capacity is reduced by 30% of the predicted value in unilateral hemidiaphragmatic paralysis, and further reduced by 75% in bilateral paralysis.

## Selected References

1. Houston JG, Morris AD, Howie CA, Reid JL, McMillan N. Technical report: quantitative assessment of diaphragmatic movement--a reproducible method using ultrasound. *Clin Radiol.* 1992;46(6):405-407.
2. Kokatnur L, Rudrappa M. Diaphragmatic palsy. *Diseases.* 2018;6:E16.
3. McCool FD, Manzoor K, Minami T. Disorders of the diaphragm. *Clin Chest Med.* 2018;39(2):345-360.
4. Sarwal A, Walker FO, Cartwright MS. Neuromuscular ultrasound for evaluation of the diaphragm. *Muscle Nerve.* 2013;47(3):319-329.
5. Umbrello M, Formenti P. Ultrasonographic assessment of diaphragm function in critically ill subjects. *Respir Care.* 2016;61(4):542-555.

**2.** Correct Answer: A. Ventilator weaning should proceed based on the degree of diaphragmatic excursion.

*Rationale:* The right and left hemidiaphragms can be imaged through the liver and spleen windows, respectively, to assess the degree of craniocaudal excursion. This M-mode image illustrates an excursion of nearly 3 cm. Normal diaphragmatic excursion in adults has been reported to range from 1.9 to 9 cm, with various correction factors for age, sex, weight, and height proposed by different studies. Although currently there are no uniform guidelines for defining diaphragmatic dysfunction and adjusting for baseline characteristics, an excursion of less than 1 cm is widely agreed upon as indicative of diaphragm dysfunction.

This image shows a pleural effusion with atelectasis and an additional assessment of the size of the effusion should be considered. However, the narrow pleural separation shown in this image alone does not reveal an effusion of significant size to support proceeding immediately to a chest tube.

## Selected References

1. Boussuges A, Gole Y, Blanc P. Diaphragmatic motion studied by m-mode ultrasonography: methods, reproducibility, and normal values. *Chest.* 2009;135(2):391-400.
2. Sarwal A, Walker FO, Cartwright MS. Neuromuscular ultrasound for evaluation of the diaphragm. *Muscle Nerve.* 2013;47(3):319-329.
3. Weerakkody Y, Reddy U, et al. Diaphragmatic paralysis. *Radiopaedia.* Accessed September 5, 2019. https://radiopaedia.org/articles/diaphragmatic-paralysis-1?lang=us.

**3.** Correct Answer: D. The degree of diaphragmatic thickening in layer B predicts weaning success.

*Rationale:* When weaning from mechanical ventilation, ultrasound assessment of the diaphragm has been applied to help predict extubation failure. A linear array transducer placed along the anterior axillary line at the intercostal spaces between the seventh and ninth ribs provides images at the zone of apposition to enable assessment of diaphragm thickness and echogenicity. Diaphragm thickness varies with inspiratory effort and level of contraction. The diaphragm (Layer B) is visualized as the hypoechoic layer of muscle in-between two hyperechoic connective tissue layers (the parietal pleura and peritoneum), deep to the intercostal muscles (Layer A). M-mode echocardiography in this image shows a dynamic increase in diaphragm thickness from 0.18 to 0.25 cm during inspiration, giving a thickening fraction of 39%. A thickening fraction above 30% is indicative of normal diaphragm contractility and has been found to predict extubation success with 71% specificity.

While various studies have identified different thresholds for thickening fraction in predicting ventilator weaning failure, a thickening fraction of less than 20% is widely agreed upon as indicative of diaphragm weakness. The absence of thickening correlates well with invasive measurements of transdiaphragmatic pressure and enables the diagnosis of diaphragm paralysis with high sensitivity and specificity.

**Selected References**
1. Harper CJ, Shahgholi L, Cieslak K, Hellyer NJ, Strommen JA, Boon AJ. Variability in diaphragm motion during normal breathing, assessed with B-mode ultrasound. *J Orthop Sports Phys Ther.* 2013;43:927-931.
2. Matamis D, Soilemezi E, Tsagourias M, et al. Sonographic evaluation of the diaphragm in critically ill patients. Technique and clinical applications. *Intensive Care Med.* 2013;39(5):801-810.
3. Sarwal A, Walker FO, Cartwright MS. Neuromuscular ultrasound for evaluation of the diaphragm. *Muscle Nerve.* 2013;47(3):319-329.
4. Summerhill EM, El-Sameed YA, Glidden TJ, McCool FD. Monitoring recovery from diaphragm paralysis with ultrasound. *Chest.* 2008;133(3):737-743.

**4.** Correct Answer: C. There is appropriate diaphragmatic thickening

*Rationale:* These B-mode images illustrate diaphragm thickening at the intercostal space along the anterior axillary line at the zone of apposition, where the diaphragm contacts the rib cage. In these images, the rib is on the right (**Figure 58.10,** *marked by* *). During inspiration, the diaphragm is seen "peeling away" from the chest wall as it increases in thickness (option C). While there is insufficient evidence to support routine evaluation of the intercostal muscles in assessing respiratory function, an intercostal thickening fraction of greater than 8% is suggestive of a pathologic respiratory pattern.

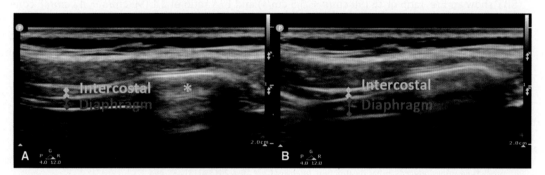

**Figure 58.10** A: Expiration. B: Inspiration.

**Selected Reference**
1. Matamis D, Soilemezi E, Tsagourias M, et al. Sonographic evaluation of the diaphragm in critically ill patients. Technique and clinical applications. *Intensive Care Med.* 2013;39(5):801-810.

**5.** Correct Answer: D. DT = (0.28 − 0.25)/0.25 = 0.12, indicating impaired DT

*Rationale:* Identification of diaphragm dysfunction with ultrasonography has been found to be predictive of extubation failure. Diaphragm atrophy and weakness develop in the first few days of mechanical ventilation and critical illness, and are exacerbated by the use of paralytic agents and steroids. Diaphragm thickness has been correlated with the strength of the diaphragm and muscle shortening, but not with endurance or fatigability. Good association has been found between the thickening fraction and transdiaphragmatic pressure measurements. The thickening fraction is defined as:

(End-Inspiratory Thickness – End-Expiratory Thickness) ÷ End-Expiratory Thickness

Thresholds for predicting extubation failure vary between studies. However, the consensus is that a thickening fraction of less than 0.2 indicates diaphragm dysfunction.

**Selected References**
1. Gottesman E, McCool FD. Ultrasound evaluation of the paralyzed diaphragm. *Am J Respir Crit Care Med.* 1997;155(5):1570-1574.
2. Matamis D, Soilemezi E, Tsagourias M, et al. Sonographic evaluation of the diaphragm in critically ill patients. Technique and clinical applications. *Intensive Care Med.* 2013;39(5):801-810.

**6.** Correct Answer: C. Bilateral diffuse B-lines with LVEDP of 20 mm Hg

*Rationale:* Weaning-induced cardiac dysfunction is an important contributor to ventilator weaning failure. The transition from positive-pressure ventilation to spontaneous breathing generates negative inspiratory intrathoracic pressure that leads to an increase in both left ventricular preload and afterload. Patients with decompensated heart failure can experience significant hemodynamic impact from even small changes in intrathoracic pressure, leading to pulmonary edema. In one series, Caille et al. determined that cardiac dysfunction accounted for 87% of 23 patients who failed ventilator weaning. Furthermore, compared to those who were successfully weaned, patients who failed had a significantly lower left ventricular ejection fraction and higher filling pressures prior to the start of the SBT.

Patients with weaning-induced pulmonary edema, defined by Dres et al. as "weaning intolerance associated with an increase in pulmonary arterial occlusion pressure (PAOP) above 18 mm Hg at the end of the SBT," were found by transpulmonary thermodilution to have increased extravascular lung water in conjunction with acute blood volume contraction. In a series of 100 ventilated patients, B-type natriuretic peptide (BNP) significantly increased in patients who had heart failure–associated SBT failure, and basal BNP was found to be higher in patients with post-extubation distress compared to those who extubated successfully. The identification of B-lines on pulmonary ultrasound has been validated as a sensitive measure of extravascular lung water. Bilateral diffuse B-lines would be more consistent with cardiogenic pulmonary edema, whereas focal B-lines are nonspecific findings of consolidation that could represent pneumonia, atelectasis, contusion, hemorrhage, pulmonary infarction, neoplasia, and so on.

This patient with a history of congestive heart failure is at high risk of cardiogenic interstitial edema during ventilator weaning secondary to volume overload and left ventricular decompensation in the setting of acute kidney injury, sepsis, and fluid resuscitation. The spectral images obtained at the end of the SBT show an E/e′ ratio of 16 (90 cm/s ÷ 5.5 cm/s) and E/A ratio of 2.1 (90 cm/s ÷ 42 cm/s), consistent with at least Grade 3 diastolic dysfunction. Lamia, et al. found that an E/e′ ratio above 8.5 and E/A ratio above 0.95 at the end of an SBT predicted a PAOP higher than 18 mm Hg with 82% sensitivity and 91% specificity. As such, it would be expected that this patient has an elevated LVEDP greater than 18 mm Hg and bilateral B-lines.

**Selected References**
1. Caille V, Amiel JB, Charron C, Belliard G, Vieillard-Baron A, Vignon P. Echocardiography: a help in the weaning process. *Crit Care.* 2010;14:R120.
2. Dres M, Teboul JL, Anguel N, Guerin L, Richard C, Monnet X. Extravascular lung water, B-type natriuretic peptide, and blood volume contraction enable diagnosis of weaning-induced pulmonary edema. *Crit Care Med.* 2014;42(8):1882-1889.
3. Dres M, Teboul JL, Anguel N, Guerin L, Richard C, Monnet X. Passive leg raising performed before a spontaneous breathing trial predicts weaning-induced cardiac dysfunction. *Intensive Care Med.* 2015;41(3):487-494.
4. Lamia B, Maizel J, Ochagavia A, et al. Echocardiographic diagnosis of pulmonary artery occlusion pressure elevation during weaning from mechanical ventilation. *Crit Care Med.* 2009;37:1696-1701.
5. Teboul JL. Weaning-induced cardiac dysfunction: where are we today? *Intensive Care Med.* 2014;40(8):1069-1079.
6. Teboul JL, Monnet X, Richard C. Weaning failure of cardiac origin: recent advances. *Crit Care.* 2010;14(2):211.
7. Tobin MJ. Extubation and the myth of "minimal ventilator settings". *Am J Respir Crit Care Med.* 2012;185(4):349-350.
8. Zapata L, Vera P, Roglan A, Gich I, Ordonez-Llanos J, Betbesé AJ. B-type natriuretic peptides for prediction and diagnosis of weaning failure from cardiac origin. *Intensive Care Med.* 2011;37:477-485.

**7.** Correct Answer: C. Administer a vasodilator

*Rationale:* Patients with decompensated heart failure can experience significant hemodynamic impact from even small changes in intrathoracic pressure. The negative inspiratory pressure during spontaneous ventilation increases left ventricular preload and afterload, elevating the risk of cardiogenic pulmonary edema. Zapata, et al. found that BNP significantly increased in patients with heart failure–associated SBT failure, and that basal BNP was higher in patients with post-extubation distress compared to those extubated successfully. Additionally, the combination of increased work of breathing and left ventricular afterload during SBT intensifies the workload on the heart, predisposing the patient to cardiac ischemia and worsening ventricular function.

This patient with E/e′ ratio of 15 (75 ÷ 5) and E/A ratio of 0.65 (115 cm/s ÷ 75 cm/s) demonstrates impaired relaxation with Grade 1 diastolic dysfunction. The combination of diastolic dysfunction and hypertension during the SBT places the patient at risk of developing cardiogenic pulmonary edema. Administering a vasodilator would reduce preload in a noncompliant ventricle, as well as alleviate afterload to promote forward flow. Although administering an inotrope could enhance left ventricular contractility, in a patient who is already hypertensive, the increase in cardiac workload could potentiate cardiac ischemia and further impair function.

### Selected References
1. Tobin MJ. Extubation and the myth of "minimal ventilator settings". *Am J Respir Crit Care Med.* 2012;185(4):349-350.
2. Zapata L, Vera P, Roglan A, Gich I, Ordonez-Llanos J, Betbesé AJ. B-type natriuretic peptides for prediction and diagnosis of weaning failure from cardiac origin. *Intensive Care Med.* 2011;37:477-485.

### 8. Correct Answer: A. Administer inhaled nitric oxide

*Rationale:* These images demonstrate an increase in E/A ratio after an SBT, indicating worsened diastolic dysfunction with increased filling pressure. In patients with left ventricular dysfunction who failed a ventilator wean, a statistically significant increase in E/A ratio and shortening of the DTE were observed during SBT compared to pressure support. Furthermore, a systolic blood pressure above 180 mm Hg or an increase of greater than 20% during SBT has been found to be indicators of weaning failure.

Diuresis would decrease preload and filling pressures (option B). Afterload reduction would promote forward flow and alleviate cardiac workload (option C). In patients with baseline cardiac dysfunction, noninvasive ventilation (NIV) has been found to augment extubation success by lessening the work of breathing, as well as improve hemodynamics by reducing preload and afterload. For patients at high risk of extubation failure, which includes those with congestive heart failure, the American Thoracic Society and the American College of Chest Physicians recommend the immediate application of preventive NIV to enhance extubation success (option D). As this patient has no history of pulmonary hypertension or right ventricular dysfunction, inhaled nitric oxide would not be an appropriate intervention.

### Selected References
1. Boles JM, Bion J, Connors A, et al. Weaning from mechanical ventilation. *Eur Respir J.* 2007;29:1033-1056.
2. Caille V, Amiel JB, Charron C, Belliard G, Vieillard-Baron A, Vignon P. Echocardiography: a help in the weaning process. *Crit Care.* 2010;14:R120.
3. Lemaire F, Teboul JL, Cinotti L, et al. Acute left ventricular dysfunction during unsuccessful weaning from mechanical ventilation. *Anesthesiology.* 1988;69:171-179.
4. Nava S, Gregoretti C, Fanfulla F, et al. Noninvasive ventilation to prevent respiratory failure after extubation in high-risk patients. *Crit Care Med.* 2005;33:2465-2470.
5. Schmidt GA, Girard TD, Kress JP, et al. Official executive summary of an American Thoracic Society/American College of Chest Physicians clinical practice guideline: liberation from mechanical ventilation in critically ill adults. *Am J Respir Crit Care Med.* 2017;195:115-119.

### 9. Correct Answer: D. A change in DTE from 140 to 120 ms

*Rationale:* Patients with left ventricular dysfunction have been found to demonstrate a statistically significant increase in E/A ratio and shortening of DTE during SBT. E/A ratio cannot be assessed in patients in atrial fibrillation due to the absence of atrial contraction. DTE is affected by atrioventricular compliance and mitral valve area, and correlates with filling pressures in patients with depressed ejection fraction. As such, a decrease in DTE is reflective of rising filling pressures, which in turn has been found to be associated with increased extravascular lung water. A patient with depressed systolic function and a shortening DTE (option D) during SBT would likely benefit from diuresis.

### Selected References
1. Caille V, Amiel JB, Charron C, Belliard G, Vieillard-Baron A, Vignon P. Echocardiography: a help in the weaning process. *Crit Care.* 2010;14:R120.
2. Dres M, Teboul JL, Anguel N, Guerin L, Richard C, Monnet X. Extravascular lung water, B-type natriuretic peptide, and blood volume contraction enable diagnosis of weaning-induced pulmonary edema. *Crit Care Med.* 2014;42(8):1882-1889.
3. Lemaire F, Teboul JL, Cinotti L, et al. Acute left ventricular dysfunction during unsuccessful weaning from mechanical ventilation. *Anesthesiology.* 1988;69:171-179.
4. Symanski JD, Nishimura RA, Hurrell DG. Doppler parameters of left ventricular filling are poor predictors of diastolic performance in patients with hypertrophic cardiomyopathy. *Circulation.* 1995;92(suppl I):269.

**10.** Correct Answer: D. Chest tube placement or thoracentesis to drain pleural effusion

*Rationale:* In the parasternal long-axis view, the descending thoracic aorta is used to differentiate between a pericardial and pleural effusion. A pericardial effusion is confined anteriorly to the aorta, whereas a pleural effusion extends posteriorly. This image shows a fluid collection posterior to the descending aorta (DA), indicative of a pleural effusion (PEff). As such, further evaluation or drainage of her pleural effusion would be the next appropriate step to optimize ventilator weaning.

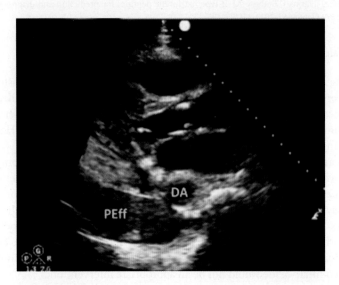

**Figure 58.11**

The descending aorta is visible in short axis on the parasternal long-axis view. **Figure 58.11** shows no evidence of dissection or aneurysm.

Selected Reference

1. "Pericardial effusion and pleural effusion." *Critical Care Sonography.* September 14, 2016. Accessed September 28, 2019. https://www.criticalcare-sonography.com/2016/09/14/pericardial-effusion-and-pleural-effusion/

Hassan Mashbari, Ahmed Al Hazmi, Osaid Alser, Matthew Mueller, and Christopher R. Tainter

1. A 75-year-old woman with a history of chronic obstructive pulmonary disease (COPD) and recent viral upper respiratory tract infection presents to the Emergency Department (ED) with shortness of breath. She reports that her breathing has become more labored over the last 24 hours and she is using her inhaler more frequently than usual. Her vital signs are significant for HR 120 bpm, BP 150/85 mm Hg, RR 24/min, $SpO_2$ 90% on 4 L/min by nasal cannula, and a temperature of 38.3°C. On examination, breath sounds are diminished over the left lower lobe and diffuse expiratory wheezes are appreciated. Point-of-care ultrasound is performed and demonstrates **Figure 59.1** (relevant structures marked by the white arrows) from her left lateral chest wall.

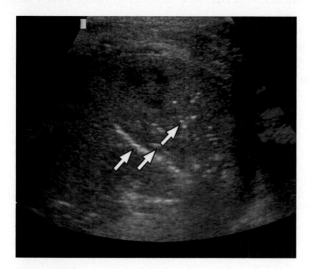

**Figure 59.1**

What is the most likely diagnosis?
A. Pleural effusion
B. Community-acquired pneumonia
C. Pulmonary edema
D. Pneumothorax

2. A 32-year-old woman with an elevated body mass index (BMI) presents to the ED with shortness of breath, hemoptysis, and calf pain 1 day after returning home from international travel. On presentation, her vital signs are significant for HR 115 bpm, BP 90/55 mm Hg, RR 22/min, SpO$_2$ 92% on room air, and temperature 37.9°C. On examination, she is tachypneic, her lungs are clear to auscultation bilaterally, and her right lower extremity is tender, erythematous, and has 2+ pitting edema. A point-of-care echocardiogram is performed (**Figure 59.2**).

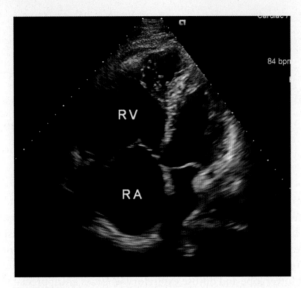

**Figure 59.2**

Given the most likely etiology of her presentation, what additional ultrasound finding is likely to be present?
A. Tricuspid annular plane systolic excursion (TAPSE) 1.5 cm
B. Septal motion toward the right ventricle during diastole
C. Right ventricular (RV):left ventricular (LV) ratio 0.6
D. RV apical hypokinesis, sparing the base

3. A 65-year-old man with a history of hypertension, hyperlipidemia, and insulin-dependent diabetes presents to the ED with chest pain and shortness of breath that awoke him from sleep. On presentation, his vital signs are significant for HR 115 bpm, BP 190/105 mm Hg in his right arm and 160/90 in his left arm, RR 18/min, temperature 37.2°C, and SpO$_2$ 88% on 5 L by nasal cannula. Physical examination demonstrates an anxious, pale, and diaphoretic man with asymmetric radial pulses. A point-of-care echocardiogram demonstrates the finding shown in **Figure 59.3**.

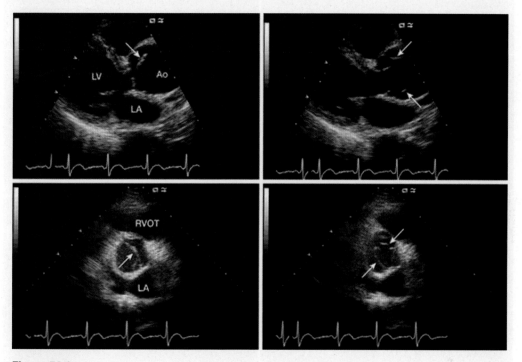

**Figure 59.3**

The acute, severe valvulopathy associated with this condition can be diagnosed by which of the following criteria?
A. Peak velocity > 4 m/s
B. Vena contracta width > 5 mm
C. Central jet ≥65% of the LV outflow tract (LVOT)
D. Mean pressure gradient >50 mm Hg

4. You are called to evaluate a 27-year-old man with a history of intravenous (IV) drug abuse for worsening dyspnea. He presented to the ED the prior day with chest pain and shortness of breath. He was diagnosed with infective endocarditis, started on broad-spectrum antibiotics, and admitted to the hospital, although he eloped overnight. On evaluation, the patient is in respiratory distress and has audible crackles. A point-of-care echocardiogram is performed demonstrating **Figure 59.4**.

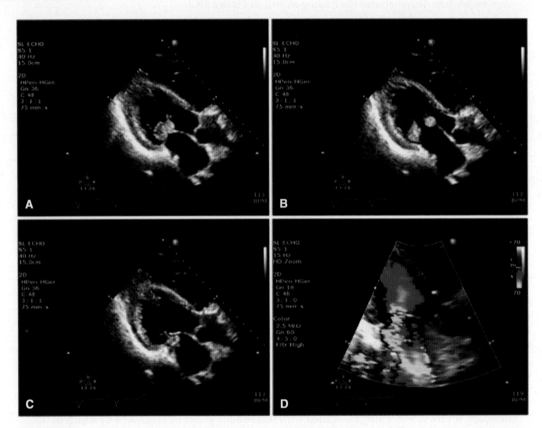

**Figure 59.4**

Which of the following structures is the most likely to be impacted?
A. Chordae tendineae
B. Pectinate muscles
C. Moderator band
D. Trabeculae carneae

5. A 34-year-old man with a history of IV drug use and bioprosthetic tricuspid valve presents to the ED with shortness of breath and fatigue. His vital signs are significant for HR 105 bpm, BP 105/55 mm Hg, RR 22/min, temperature 38.2°C, and SpO$_2$ 87% on room air. A point-of-care echocardiogram is shown in **Figure 59.5**.

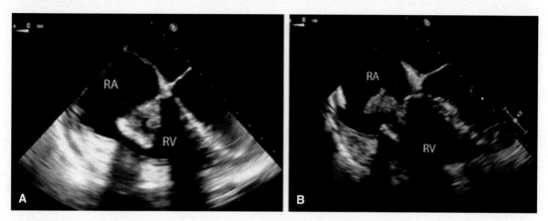

**Figure 59.5**

Which of the following is the *most* likely additional ultrasonographic finding?
A. Mitral valve mean gradient >10 mm Hg
B. LV end-diastolic pressure >25 mm Hg
C. Pulmonary artery pressure 60 mm Hg
D. Hepatic vein flow reversal

6. A 72-year-old man with a history of COPD and group 3 pulmonary hypertension is admitted to the intensive care unit (ICU) for respiratory failure and hypotension. The patient is started on nebulized bronchodilators and noninvasive positive pressure ventilation. Point-of-care echocardiography is performed and demonstrates **Figure 59.6**.

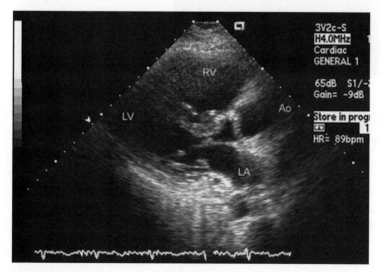

**Figure 59.6**

Which of the following is *most* consistent with right heart failure?
A. Pulsed-wave Doppler S-wave >9.5 cm/s
B. TAPSE < 17 mm
C. RV fractional area change <45%
D. RV myocardial performance index (MPI) 0.8

7. A 70-year-old woman with COPD and a 50 pack-year smoking history presents to the ED with shortness of breath. She reports that her dyspnea is worsened on exertion, her cough is newly productive of green sputum, and she is using inhaled bronchodilators every hour with minimal relief. On presentation, she is tachypneic, has audible wheezes, and breath sounds are diminished at the right lung base. Nebulized bronchodilators and oral glucocorticoids are administered for presumed COPD exacerbation. Point-of-care ultrasound is performed to further evaluate the etiology of the auscultatory finding. What is the smallest volume of pleural fluid that can be visualized on thoracic ultrasound?

   A. 5 mL
   B. 50 mL
   C. 150 mL
   D. 200 mL

8. A 25-year-old woman with a past medical history of severe persistent asthma presents to the ED with sudden-onset shortness of breath and wheezing. On presentation, she is in respiratory distress and is brought to the resuscitation bay for immediate evaluation. Vital signs are significant for HR 130 bpm, RR 30/min, BP 80/50 mm Hg, temperature 38.0°C, and SpO$_2$ 88% on 15 L via non-rebreather mask. Point-of-care ultrasound demonstrates **Figure 59.7**.

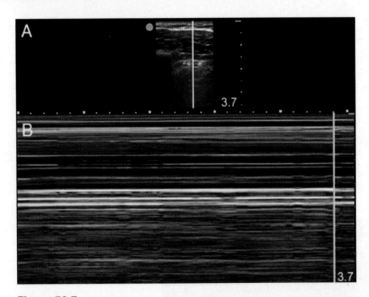

**Figure 59.7**

What is the next best step?
A. Administer inhaled bronchodilators
B. Intubate
C. Tube thoracostomy
D. Administer 30 mL/kg crystalloid bolus

9. What ultrasonographic finding has the *highest* specificity for a pneumothorax?

   A. Seashore sign
   B. Barcode sign
   C. Lung point
   D. Lung pulse

10. A 50-year-old 6-foot-tall man with acute respiratory distress syndrome (ARDS) has been intubated in the ICU for 12 days and has now been on pressure support ventilation for 4 hours. He is receiving a driving pressure of 5 cmH$_2$O and positive end-expiratory pressure of 5 cmH$_2$O, and he is capable of generating 1000 mL tidal volume breaths. The patient's RR is 14/min, SpO$_2$ is 99% on 30% FiO$_2$, and PaO$_2$ is 100 mm Hg. Point-of-care ultrasound is performed (**Figure 59.8**).

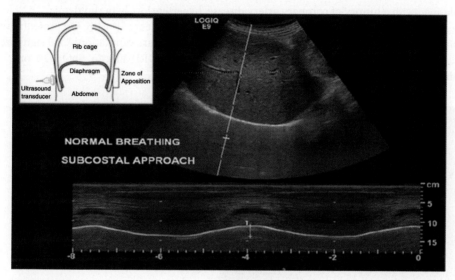

**Figure 59.8**

Which of the following diaphragmatic findings would suggest that the patient is at low risk for reintubation?
A. Diaphragmatic excursion <20 mm
B. Diaphragmatic excursion >20 mm
C. Upward diaphragmatic movement during inspiration
D. Diaphragm thickness 0.1 cm

11. A 50-year-old woman with a recent history of surgical repair for a midshaft femur fracture presents to the ED for chest pain. Immediately upon arrival, the patient has a cardiac arrest and cardiopulmonary resuscitation (CPR) is initiated. During the first rhythm check, there is no palpable pulse and point-of-care ultrasound is performed demonstrating **Figure 59.9**.

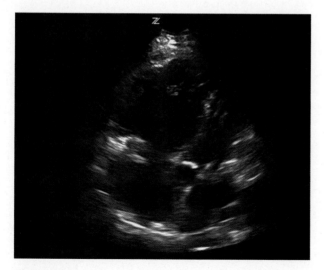

**Figure 59.9**

What is the most appropriate next step in her management?
A. Proceed to emergent coronary angiography.
B. Perform a resuscitative thoracotomy.
C. Administer IV thrombolytics (IV tissue plasminogen activator [tPA]).
D. Stop resuscitation attempts due to futility.

12. A 70-year-old man with a history of coronary artery disease, hypertension, hyperlipidemia, insulin-dependent diabetes, and COPD presents to the ED with shortness of breath. On presentation, he is in respiratory distress and is placed on noninvasive positive pressure ventilation. Vital signs are significant for a temperature of 37°C, HR 110 bpm, BP 110/65 mm Hg, RR 30/min, SpO$_2$ 92% on 0.4 FiO$_2$. Point-of-care ultrasound is performed (**Figure 59.10**).

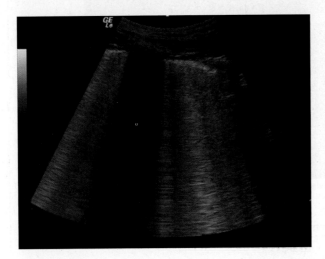

**Figure 59.10**

What is the next best step?
A. Administer furosemide.
B. Perform tube thoracostomy.
C. Administer ceftriaxone and azithromycin.
D. Administer albuterol and methylprednisolone.

13. What is the maximum number of B-lines that is considered normal in older patients?

A. One
B. Two
C. Three
D. Four

**14.** A 32-year-old woman who is postpartum day 3 following an uncomplicated cesarean section develops shortness of breath while in the hospital. You are called to evaluate the patient and on your arrival you find a young woman who is in moderate distress. Vital signs are notable for a HR 125 bpm, RR 22/min, BP 102/70 mm Hg, T 37.9°C, and SpO$_2$ 90% on room air. Based on the ultrasound shown in **Figure 59.11**, what is the next best step?

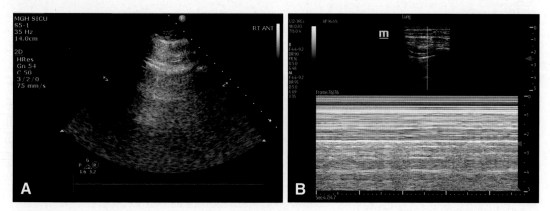

**Figure 59.11**

**A.** Start broad-spectrum antibiotics
**B.** Computed tomography (CT) pulmonary angiography
**C.** Tube thoracostomy
**D.** Bronchoscopy

# Chapter 59 ▪ Answers

**1.** Correct Answer: **B.** Community-acquired pneumonia

*Rationale/Critique:* Older patients and those with underlying lung disease, such as COPD, are at an increased risk for developing community-acquired pneumonia. Pneumonia may not be present on chest radiography early in its course, but can be visualized by ultrasound with >95% sensitivity and >90% specificity. Areas of focal consolidation appear as a hypoechoic disruption of the pleural line. Fluid-filled consolidated lung causes a heterogeneous appearance on ultrasound, similar to liver tissue, which is termed "hepatization." Air bronchograms (white arrows in Figure 59.1) can also be seen (as in the image above), which are scattered small hyperechoic structures caused by focal areas of aeration reflecting the ultrasound waves.

A pleural effusion (**Answer A**) will appear as a hypoechoic region in dependent lung regions. The presence of B-lines suggests pulmonary edema (**Answer C**). The absence of lung sliding or the presence of a lung point suggests a pneumothorax.

### Selected References
1. Chavez MA, Shams N, Ellington LE, et al. Lung ultrasound for the diagnosis of pneumonia in adults: a systematic review and meta-analysis. *Respir Res.* 2014;15(1):50. doi:10.1186/1465-9921-15-50.
2. Ellington LE, Gilman RH, Chavez MA, et al. Lung ultrasound as a diagnostic tool for radiographically-confirmed pneumonia in low resource settings. *Respir Med.* 2017;128:57-64. doi:10.1016/j.rmed.2017.05.007.

**2.** Correct Answer: **A.** Tricuspid annular plane systolic excursion (TAPSE) 1.5 cm

*Rationale:* Point-of-care ultrasound can support the diagnosis of pulmonary embolism (PE) in a patient with a high pretest probability, such as this patient. Sonographic findings suggestive of PE include:

- RV dilatation
- End-diastolic RV:LV ratio ≥1 visualized in the apical four- or five-chamber view

- McConnell sign: RV free wall akinesis/hypokinesis sparing the apex, suggesting acute regional ventricular dysfunction
- D-sign: interventricular septal flattening can be visualized on the parasternal short-axis view of the heart.
- Paradoxical motion of the interventricular septum
- RV hypokinesis: TAPSE <1.6 cm

### Selected Reference

1. Dudzinski DM, Hariharan P, Parry BA, Chang Y, Kabrhel C. Assessment of right ventricular strain by computed tomography versus echocardiography in acute pulmonary embolism. *Acad Emerg Med.* 2017;24(3):337-343. doi:10.1111/acem.13108.

---

**3.** Correct Answer: C. Central jet ≥ 65% of the LV outflow tract (LVOT)

*Rationale:* According to the Stanford classification of aortic dissection, a Type A dissection involves the ascending aorta and may also involve the descending aorta, while a Type B dissection includes only the descending aorta. Type A dissections can cause acute, severe aortic insufficiency, which can be diagnosed by measuring the central jet as ≥65% of the LVOT (**Answer C**). Other findings include:

- Vena contracta >6 mm
- Regurgitant volume >60 mL/beat
- Regurgitant fraction >50%
- Effective regurgitant orifice area ≥0.30 cm$^2$

Peak velocity and mean gradient are typically used to evaluate stenotic lesions.

### Selected References

1. Orde S. Valvulopathy quantification. In: Slama M, eds. *Echocardiography in ICU.* Springer; 2020. https://doi.org/10.1007/978-3-030-32219-9_22.
2. Sobczyk D, Nycz K. Feasibility and accuracy of bedside transthoracic echocardiography in diagnosis of acute proximal aortic dissection. *Cardiovasc Ultrasound.* 2015;13:15. doi:10.1186/s12947-015-0008-5.
3. von Homeyer P, Oxorn DC. Aortic regurgitation: echocardiographic diagnosis. *Anesth Analg.* 2016;122(1):37-42. doi:10.1213/ANE.0000000000001013.

---

**4.** Correct Answer: A. Chordae tendineae

*Rationale:* Acute mitral regurgitation can occur as a result of rupture of the chordae tendineae (**Answer A**) or papillary muscles and can be a result of infective endocarditis, acute myocardial infarction, cardiac disease (eg, rheumatic heart disease), or may occur spontaneously. Acute mitral regurgitation can result in the rapid progression of pulmonary edema secondary to cardiogenic shock. Echocardiographic findings consistent with severe mitral regurgitation are:

- Jet area: >8 cm$^2$
- Jet area: left atrial area: >40%
- Vena contracta: >7 mm
- Estimated orifice area: >0.4 cm$^2$

### Selected References

1. Grigioni F, Russo A, Pasquale F, et al. Clinical use of Doppler echocardiography in organic mitral regurgitation: from diagnosis to patients' management. *J Cardiovasc Ultrasound.* 2015;23(3):121-133. doi:10.4250/jcu.2015.23.3.121.
2. Orde S. Valvulopathy quantification. In: Slama M, eds. *Echocardiography in ICU.* Springer; 2020. https://doi.org/10.1007/978-3-030-32219-9_22.

---

**5.** Correct Answer: D. Hepatic vein flow reversal

*Rationale:* IV drug use can lead to tricuspid endocarditis and subsequently to tricuspid regurgitation. Valvular vegetations appear as echogenic masses that may be loose and mobile throughout the cardiac cycle. Ultrasonographic findings consistent with severe tricuspid regurgitation are:

- Regurgitant jet area: >10 cm$^2$
- Vena contracta: >7 mm
- Regurgitant volume: >45 mL

- Tricuspid inflow E-wave velocity: >1 m/s
- Hepatic vein systolic flow reversal

Of the answer choices listed, tricuspid regurgitation would only lead to hepatic vein flow reversal.

Selected References

1. Badano LP, Muraru D, Enriquez-Sarano M. Assessment of functional tricuspid regurgitation. *Eur Heart J*. 2013;34(25): 1875-1885. doi:10.1093/eurheartj/ehs474.
2. Yuan XC, Liu M, Hu J, Zeng X, Zhou AY, Chen L. Diagnosis of infective endocarditis using echocardiography. *Medicine (Baltimore)*. 2019;98(38):e17141. doi:10.1097/MD.0000000000017141.

---

**6.** Correct Answer: B. TAPSE < 17 mm

*Rationale:* COPD and PE are common causes of cor pulmonale, which is defined as enlargement of the right ventricle with resultant RV failure. Echocardiogram demonstrates RV hypertrophy or dilatation, and right atrial enlargement, and in most cases pulmonary hypertension and tricuspid regurgitation can be seen. RV dysfunction can be diagnosed on echocardiography by measuring TAPSE on an apical four-chamber view (**Answer B**). Findings consistent with RV dysfunction include:

- TAPSE <17 mm
- Pulsed-wave Doppler S-wave <9.5 cm/s
- Tissue Doppler S-wave <6 cm/s
- RV fractional area change <35%
- RV ejection fraction <45%
- Pulsed-wave Doppler MPI >0.43
- Tissue Doppler MPI >0.54
- E-wave deceleration time <119 or >242 msec
- E/A <0.8 or >2.0
- e'/a' <0.52
- e' <7.8
- E/e' >6.0

Selected References

1. Lang RM, Badano LP, Mor-Avi V, et al. Recommendations for cardiac chamber quantification by echocardiography in adults: an update from the American Society of Echocardiography and the European Association of Cardiovascular Imaging [published correction appears in Eur Heart J Cardiovasc Imaging. 2016;17(4):412 [published correction appears in *Eur Heart J Cardiovasc Imaging*. 2016;17 (9):969]. *Eur Heart J Cardiovasc Imaging*. 2015;16(3):233-270. doi:10.1093/ehjci/jev014
2. Vieillard-Baron A, Prin S, Chergui K, Dubourg O, Jardin F. Echo-Doppler demonstration of acute cor pulmonale at the bedside in the medical intensive care unit. *Am J Respir Crit Care Med*. 2002;166(10):1310-1319. doi:10.1164/rccm.200202-146CC.

---

**7.** Correct Answer: A. 5 mL

*Rationale:* Thoracic ultrasound can detect as little as 5 mL of pleural fluid (**Answer A**), but sensitivity and specificity are improved when ≥ 20 mL is present. Posteroanterior radiographs require 200 mL of pleural fluid to be detected, while lateral views can detect effusions when at least 50 mL of pleural fluid is present.

Selected References

1. Brogi E, Gargani L, Bignami E, et al. Thoracic ultrasound for pleural effusion in the intensive care unit: a narrative review from diagnosis to treatment. *Crit Care*. 2017;21(1):325. doi:10.1186/s13054-017-1897-5
2. Miles MJ, Islam S. Point of care ultrasound in thoracic malignancy. *Ann Transl Med*. 2019;7(15):350. doi:10.21037/atm.2019.05.53.
3. Soni NJ, Franco R, Velez MI, et al. Ultrasound in the diagnosis and management of pleural effusions. *J Hosp Med*. 2015;10(12):811-816. doi:10.1002/jhm.2434.

---

**8.** Correct Answer: C. Tube thoracostomy

*Rationale:* This patient has a tension pneumothorax and immediate chest tube placement is necessary (**Answer C**). Pneumothorax can be diagnosed via ultrasound with high sensitivity and specificity, 90% and 100% respectively. Findings include:

- Absent lung sliding
- "Barcode" or "Stratosphere" sign on M-mode (as seen in this image)

- Lung point: junction between the sliding lung and absent lung sliding
- Absent lung pulse (transmitted cardiac motion observed at the pleural line)

The patient is likely experiencing an asthma exacerbation as evidenced by wheezing, which can lead to increased alveolar pressure and spontaneous pneumothorax. A simple pneumothorax can develop into a tension pneumothorax and requires prompt intervention. Inhaled bronchodilators (**Answer A**) are an important treatment option for an asthma exacerbation, but the first priority is resolution of the tension physiology to prevent cardiopulmonary arrest. Viral infections and pneumonias are often implicated as the etiology of an asthma exacerbation. While the patient is febrile, hypotensive, and may have an underlying infection, the tension pneumothorax is the likely cause of this patient's hypotension, rather than septic shock. Following placement of a chest tube and further management of the patient's asthma, intubation may be considered if she exhibits a persistent respiratory acidosis or if she can no longer compensate for a respiratory acidosis due to fatigue.

### Selected References

1. Doerschug KC, Schmidt GA. Intensive care ultrasound: III. Lung and pleural ultrasound for the intensivist. *Ann Am Thorac Soc.* 2013;10(6):708-712. doi:10.1513/AnnalsATS.201308-288OT.
2. Sekiguchi H, Schenck LA, Horie R, et al. Critical care ultrasonography differentiates ARDS, pulmonary edema, and other causes in the early course of acute hypoxemic respiratory failure. *Chest.* 2015;148(4):912-918. doi:10.1378/chest.15-0341.
3. Volpicelli G, Elbarbary M, Blaivas M, et al. International evidence-based recommendations for point-of-care lung ultrasound. *Intensive Care Med.* 2012;38(4):577-591. doi:10.1007/s00134-012-2513-4.
4. From Karthika M, Wong D, Nair SG, Pillai LV, Mathew CS. Lung Ultrasound: The Emerging Role of Respiratory Therapists. *Respir Care.* 2019;64(2):217-229. Figure 9.

**9.** Correct Answer: C. Lung point

*Rationale:* The lung point has near 100% specificity for diagnosing pneumothorax (**Answer C**). The lung point is the junction where the visceral pleura begins to separate from the parietal pleura at the edge of the pneumothorax. Pneumothorax can be diagnosed via ultrasound with high sensitivity and specificity, 90% and 100% respectively. The seashore sign (**Answer B**) is a term used to describe the appearance of normal pleural sliding in M-mode, in contrast to the barcode (stratosphere) (**Answer D**), which suggests pneumothorax, but with less specificity. A lung pulse is the rhythmic beating of the pleura as a result of transmitted cardiac motion, which excludes pneumothorax.

### Selected References

1. Sekiguchi H, Schenck LA, Horie R, et al. Critical care ultrasonography differentiates ARDS, pulmonary edema, and other causes in the early course of acute hypoxemic respiratory failure. *Chest.* 2015;148(4):912-918. doi:10.1378/chest.15-0341.
2. Volpicelli G, Elbarbary M, Blaivas M, et al. International evidence-based recommendations for point-of-care lung ultrasound. *Intensive Care Med.* 2012;38(4):577-591. doi:10.1007/s00134-012-2513-4.

**10.** Correct Answer: B. Diaphragmatic excursion > 20 mm

*Rationale:* Diaphragmatic excursion is a useful tool to evaluate diaphragmatic weakness. A low-frequency ultrasound probe is placed at the anterior axillary line with the diaphragm centered in the field of view, and the diaphragm can be seen contracting toward the probe. M-mode allows for quantitative measurement of diaphragmatic excursion, and values <10 mm identify patients who are at high risk for reintubation or for difficulty weaning from mechanical ventilation (**Answer A**). Normal diaphragmatic excursion is ≥18 mm in men and ≥16 mm in women during quiet breathing (**Answer B**). Paradoxical upward movement during inspiration (**Answer C**) or thinning of the diaphragm <0.2 cm suggests diaphragmatic paralysis (**Answer D**).

### Selected References

1. Boussuges A, Gole Y, Blanc P. Diaphragmatic motion studied by m-mode ultrasonography: methods, reproducibility, and normal values. *Chest.* 2009;135(2):391-400. doi:10.1378/chest.08-1541.
2. Doerschug KC, Schmidt GA. Intensive care ultrasound: III. Lung and pleural ultrasound for the intensivist. *Ann Am Thorac Soc.* 2013;10(6):708-712. doi:10.1513/AnnalsATS.201308-288OT.
3. Sarwal A, Walker FO, Cartwright MS. Neuromuscular ultrasound for evaluation of the diaphragm. *Muscle Nerve.* 2013;47(3):319-329. doi:10.1002/mus.23671.

**11.** Correct Answer: C. Administer IV thrombolytics (IV tissue plasminogen activator [tPA])

*Rationale/Critique:* Figure 59.9 demonstrates a massively dilated right ventricle with septal flattening, which suggests a massive PE as the cause of the patient's cardiac arrest. The American Heart Association recommends thrombolysis in patients in cardiac arrest and with known or suspected PE. Echocardiographic findings suggestive of PE include:

- RV dilatation.
- End-diastolic RV:LV ratio ≥ 1 visualized in the apical four- or five-chamber view
- McConnell sign: RV free wall akinesis/hypokinesis sparing the apex, suggesting acute regional ventricular dysfunction
- D-sign: interventricular septal flattening can be visualized on the parasternal short-axis view of the heart.
- Paradoxical motion of the interventricular septum
- RV hypokinesis: TAPSE <1.6 cm

The patient may benefit from urgent cardiac catheterization (**Answer A**) after return of spontaneous circulation (ROSC) is obtained, but this is not the best next step. A resuscitative thoracotomy (**Answer B**) is recommended following penetrating thoracic injury and subsequent traumatic cardiac arrest, which does not apply to this situation. Since a potentially reversible cause is identified, further resuscitation attempts should not be considered futile.

### Selected References

1. Logan JK, Pantle H, Huiras P, Bessman E, Bright L. Evidence-based diagnosis and thrombolytic treatment of cardiac arrest or periarrest due to suspected pulmonary embolism. *Am J Emerg Med.* 2014;32(7):789-796. doi:10.1016/j.ajem.2014.04.032.
2. Panchal AR, Bartos JA, Cabañas JG, et al. Part 3: Adult basic and advanced life support: 2020 American Heart Association Guidelines for cardiopulmonary resuscitation and emergency cardiovascular care. *Circulation.* 2020;142(16_suppl_2):S366-S468. doi:10.1161/CIR.0000000000000916.

---

**12.** Correct Answer: A. Administer furosemide

*Rationale:* This patient is presenting in respiratory distress likely secondary to pulmonary edema and would likely benefit from diuresis in addition to positive pressure ventilation (**Answer A**). The ultrasound image demonstrates B-lines, also known as comet tails, and is suggestive of pulmonary edema. B-lines may be a normal finding in older adults, but are pathologic when more than two B-lines are observed, as in this image.

Tube thoracostomy (**Answer B**) would be warranted if the patient had a pneumothorax or large pleural effusion, which are not evident in this image. Antibiotics (**Answer C**) would be appropriate for the treatment of pneumonia, which is also not demonstrated by this image. Albuterol and methylprednisolone (**Answer D**) may be appropriate given his history of COPD, but do not appear to address the immediate cause of his shortness of breath.

### Selected References

1. Dietrich CF, Mathis G, Blaivas M, et al. Lung B-line artefacts and their use. *J Thorac Dis.* 2016;8(6):1356-1365. doi:10.21037/jtd.2016.04.55.
2. Mayo PH, Copetti R, Feller-Kopman D, et al. Thoracic ultrasonography: a narrative review. *Intensive Care Med.* 2019;45(9):1200-1211. doi:10.1007/s00134-019-05725-8.
3. Sekiguchi H, Schenck LA, Horie R, et al. Critical care ultrasonography differentiates ARDS, pulmonary edema, and other causes in the early course of acute hypoxemic respiratory failure. *Chest.* 2015;148(4):912-918. doi:10.1378/chest.15-0341.
4. Volpicelli G, Elbarbary M, Blaivas M, et al. International evidence-based recommendations for point-of-care lung ultrasound. *Intensive Care Med.* 2012;38(4):577-591. doi:10.1007/s00134-012-2513-4.

---

**13.** Correct Answer: B. Two

*Rationale:* B-lines are discrete hyperechoic reverberation artifacts that arise from the pleura and suggest the presence of an interstitial syndrome. They have been described as "comet tails" in some references, and fewer than three B-lines (**Answer C**) per field is considered normal in older patients. In fact, B-lines may be seen in almost 40% of elderly patients.

### Selected References

1. Dietrich CF, Mathis G, Blaivas M, et al. Lung B-line artefacts and their use. *J Thorac Dis.* 2016;8(6):1356-1365. doi:10.21037/jtd.2016.04.55.
2. Sekiguchi H, Schenck LA, Horie R, et al. Critical care ultrasonography differentiates ARDS, pulmonary edema, and other causes in the early course of acute hypoxemic respiratory failure. *Chest.* 2015;148(4):912-918. doi:10.1378/chest.15-0341.
3. Volpicelli G, Elbarbary M, Blaivas M, et al. International evidence-based recommendations for point-of-care lung ultrasound. *Intensive Care Med.* 2012;38(4):577-591. doi:10.1007/s00134-012-2513-4.

**14.** Correct Answer: B. Computed tomography (CT) pulmonary angiography

*Rationale:* The lung ultrasound (Figure 59.11) in this patient shows an A-line profile and "seashore sign." Based on bedside lung ultrasound in emergency (BLUE) protocol for lung ultrasonography, presence of A-line profile in a patient with respiratory distress points toward COPD/asthma exacerbation or pneumothorax. The absence of B-lines makes pneumonia and pulmonary edema less likely. The presence of seashore sign on lung ultrasound rules out pneumothorax. Seashore sign is seen in the absence of pneumothorax when the normal movement of lung parenchyma with respiration is captured on M-mode.

In the context of this patient's clinical presentation, and given that no lung pathology is identified on ultrasound, obtaining a CT pulmonary angiography is the best answer (**Answer B**). While the patient is also at risk for developing pneumonia following surgery, the ultrasound image does not depict a consolidation that would suggest pneumonia (**Answer A**). A tube thoracostomy (**Answer C**) is warranted for patients with a clinically significant pneumothorax or pleural effusion, neither of which this patient has. A bronchoscopy can assist in visualization of airway epithelium; however, this patient does not have an immediate indication for bronchoscopy (**Answer D**).

In this case, although lung ultrasound is not diagnostic for PE, it provides supportive evidence to rule out other important causes of shortness of breath and hypoxia.

### Selected References

1. Lichtenstein DA. Lung ultrasound in the critically ill. *Ann Intensive Care.* 2014 9;4(1):1. doi: 10.1186/2110-5820-4-1.
2. Nazerian P, Vanni S, Volpicelli G, et al. Accuracy of point-of-care multiorgan ultrasonography for the diagnosis of pulmonary embolism. *Chest.* 2014;145(5):950-957. doi: 10.1378/chest.13-1087.

# SECTION XII | TRAUMA ULTRASOUND AND E-FAST EXAM

# 60 | TRAUMA ULTRASOUND AND E-FAST EXAMINATION

Morgan J. Crigger and Vicki Sein

1. A 25-year-old man presents after a high-speed motorcycle crash. His BP is 85/50 mm Hg, HR 120 bpm, and SpO$_2$ 90% on a non-rebreather mask. To prioritize operative versus diagnostic procedures, a Focused Assessment with Sonography in Trauma (FAST) examination is performed. Which of the following views/windows are included in this examination?

   A. Hepatorenal, splenorenal, anterior left chest, anterior right chest
   B. Hepatorenal, parasternal, splenorenal, subxiphoid
   C. Hepatorenal, splenorenal, suprapubic, subxiphoid
   D. Hepatorenal, anterior left chest, anterior right chest, subxiphoid

2. A 55-year-old man is brought to the Emergency Department after being struck by a car while crossing a residential street. His BP is 90/55 mm Hg, HR 105 bpm, respiratory rate (RR) 18/min, and SpO$_2$ 95% on 2 L nasal cannula. A FAST examination reveals hypoechoic fluid in the pelvis, and his BP improves and stabilizes after 1 L intravenous (IV) lactated Ringer's solution. What is the *minimum* volume needed in the peritoneal cavity to result in a positive FAST examination?

   A. 100 mL
   B. 200 mL
   C. 500 mL
   D. 1000 mL

3. A 45-year-old man is brought to the Emergency Department after falling about 10 feet from a roof and striking a concrete driveway. The paramedics report that they initially had clear breath sounds bilaterally. Focused ultrasound of the lung is performed to evaluate for pneumothorax, and the following M-mode image is seen in **Figure 60.1**.

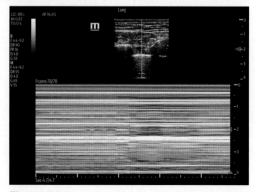

**Figure 60.1**

Which of the following is the *most* appropriate probe position to assess for pneumothorax?

A. Second-third intercostal space, midclavicular line
B. Fourth-fifth intercostal space, midclavicular line
C. Second-third intercostal space, midaxillary line
D. Fourth-fifth intercostal space, midaxillary line

4. After Figure 60.1 is obtained, the trauma surgeon questions the diagnosis and requests that a chest x-ray be performed. What is the sensitivity of the extended FAST (eFAST) examination for diagnosing pneumothorax?

A. 0% to 25%
B. 26% to 50%
C. 50% to 85%
D. 86% to 100%

5. A patient presents to the Emergency Department after sustaining a gunshot wound to the chest. An eFAST examination is performed, demonstrating hypoechoic fluid in the pleural space. A chest tube is placed, and 300 mL of blood is drained. What is the approximate sensitivity of the eFAST examination for diagnosing hemothorax?

A. 25%
B. 50%
C. 75%
D. >90%

6. A 45-year-old woman presents to the Emergency Department after a motor vehicle collision (MVC). Her BP is 120/65 mm Hg, HR 90 bpm, RR 14/min, and SpO$_2$ 99% on room air. An eFAST examination is performed and is noted to be positive in the right upper quadrant and in the pelvis. What is the sensitivity of eFAST for diagnosing hemoperitoneum in a patient without a hemodynamically significant amount of blood loss?

A. 15% to 20%
B. 30% to 40%
C. 60% to 70%
D. 90% to 100%

7. In which of the following scenarios is the use of eFAST most appropriate?

A. A 95-year-old man with BP 110/65 mm Hg after an MVC
B. A 45-year-old woman with BP 85/50 mm Hg after an MVC
C. A 35-year-old man with BP 120/65 mm Hg after a gunshot wound to the abdomen
D. A 25-year-old woman with BP 80/40 mm Hg after a gunshot wound to the abdomen

8. What is the most appropriate transducer to use for the abdominal portion of the eFAST examination?

A. 2 to 5 MHz curvilinear probe
B. 1 to 5 MHz phased array probe
C. 5 to 12 MHz linear probe
D. 8 to 13 MHz intracavitary probe

9. A 35-year-old woman presents to the Emergency Department after an MVC. Her BP is 110/60 mm Hg, HR 90 bpm, RR 22/min, and SpO$_2$ 90% on room air. An eFAST examination is performed. Which of the following images is *most* consistent with a pneumothorax?

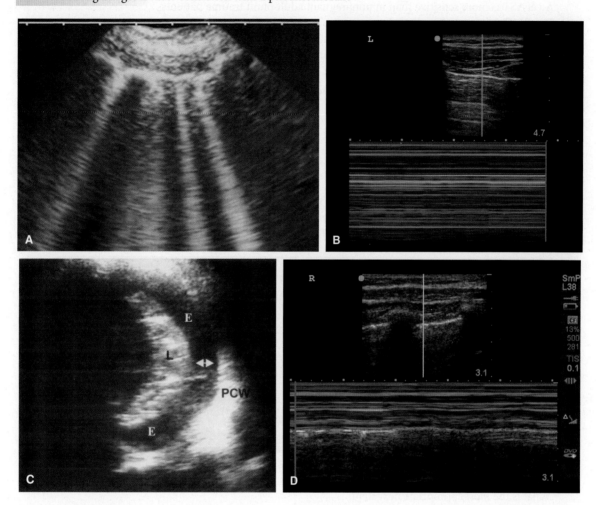

**A.** Figure 60.2A
**B.** Figure 60.2B
**C.** Figure 60.2C
**D.** Figure 60.2D

10. A 45-year-old man with a history of hepatitis C cirrhosis arrives in the Emergency Department after an MVC. His BP is 90/55 mm Hg, HR 102 bpm, RR 18/min, and SpO$_2$ 95% on room air. Which of the following is true regarding the eFAST examination in a patient with ascites?

**A.** Blood appears more dense or with visible cells compared to ascites
**B.** The peritoneal fluid echogenicity can be compared to the pleural fluid echogenicity to distinguish blood from ascites
**C.** The eFAST examination has little diagnostic value for hemoperitoneum in this setting
**D.** Only the thoracic views of the eFAST should be performed in a patient with known ascites

11. A 32-year-old woman who is 26 weeks pregnant is brought to the Emergency Department following a high-speed MVC. Which of the following is true regarding eFAST examination of her abdomen?

    A. eFAST is more sensitive than in nonpregnant adult blunt trauma patients
    B. eFAST is less sensitive than in nonpregnant adult blunt trauma patients
    C. eFAST has similar sensitivity to nonpregnant adult blunt trauma patients
    D. eFAST is not reliable in assessing pregnant adult blunt trauma patients

12. Which of the following factors is *most* likely to cause a false-negative eFAST examination in blunt abdominal trauma patients?

    A. Clotted intra-abdominal blood
    B. Presence of ascites
    C. Injury Severity Score (ISS) < 25
    D. Trendelenburg positioning

13. A 3-year-old boy presents to the Emergency Department with abdominal pain after a fall from approximately 5 feet. His BP is 100/50 mm Hg, HR 95 bpm, RR 18/min. His FAST examination is shown in **Figure 60.3**.

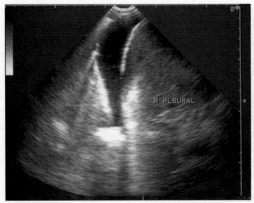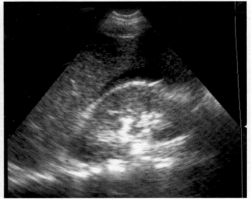

R PLEURAL

**Figure 60.3**

What is the *most* appropriate next step?

A. Computed tomography (CT) scan of the abdomen/pelvis with IV contrast
B. Monitor with serial abdominal examinations
C. Take to the operation room (OR) for emergent operation
D. Repeat FAST examination

14. A patient is brought to the trauma room after sustaining a stab wound to the chest, just to the left of the sternum, at the fifth intercostal space. An eFAST is performed and the following result is obtained from the subxiphoid view and shown in **Figure 60.4**.

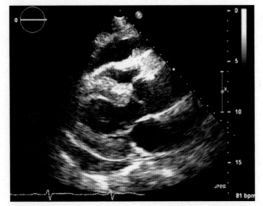

81 bpm

**Figure 60.4**

What is the minimal amount of blood that is required to produce this finding?

A. 10 mL
B. 20 mL
C. 50 mL
D. 200 mL

15. An 86-year-old man presents to the Emergency Department with point tenderness on the left chest after a fall. Which of the following represents a rib fracture on the eFAST examination?

A. Seashore sign
B. Spine sign
C. Anterior echogenic margin
D. Lighthouse phenomenon

16. A 37-year-old woman presents to the Emergency Department after a high-speed MVC with prolonged extrication. She has a temperature of 35°C, BP 80/55 mm Hg, HR 125 bpm, RR 22/min, SpO$_2$ 95% on facemask with 15 L/min of O$_2$. She has mobility of the pelvis when compressed. Which of the following statements is correct regarding the use of the FAST examination in this unstable patient with a suspected pelvic fracture?

A. There is high sensitivity and specificity for detecting intra-abdominal hemorrhage
B. The specificity is good, but the sensitivity is low to detect intra-abdominal hemorrhage
C. The sensitivity is good, but the specificity is too low to assess for intra-abdominal hemorrhage
D. Both the sensitivity and specificity are inadequate to assess for intra-abdominal hemorrhage in this patient

17. A 45-year-old man is admitted to the intensive care unit following an MVC. His BP has decreased from 110/65 mm Hg on initial presentation to 90/55 mm Hg now. A repeat eFAST examination is negative for pneumothorax, pleural fluid, and intraperitoneal fluid. What is the lower limit of a normal inferior vena cava (IVC) diameter?

A. 3.5 cm
B. 2.5 cm
C. 1.5 cm
D. 0.5 cm

18. A 47-year-old woman presents to the Emergency Department after a high-speed MVC. She has abdominal pain and a belt-shaped contusion across her abdomen. Which of the following is true regarding the eFAST examination in the assessment of hollow organ injury?

A. It has high sensitivity and high specificity
B. It has low sensitivity and low specificity
C. It has high sensitivity and low specificity
D. It has low sensitivity and high specificity

19. A 42-year-old man is brought to the Emergency Department after he crashed his motorcycle into a barrier. His temperature is 36°C, BP 92/50 mm Hg, HR 120 bpm, RR 28/min, and SpO$_2$ 92% on a non-rebreather facemask. Which among these injuries would be *least* likely to be identified on an eFAST examination?

A. Grade 2 liver laceration
B. Retroperitoneal hematoma
C. Grade 2 splenic laceration
D. Intraperitoneal bladder rupture

**20.** Performance of how many FAST examinations are recommended for a trainee to develop a level of proficiency with performing the examination?

**A.** 50
**B.** 100
**C.** 150
**D.** 20

# Chapter 60 ▪ Answers

**1.** Correct Answer: C. Hepatorenal, splenorenal, suprapubic, subxiphoid

*Rationale:* The FAST examination is indicated in patients who are hemodynamically unstable following blunt trauma. The examination allows for rapid assessment for hemoperitoneum and hemopericardium as the cause of hypotension. In addition, solid organ injury may be identified, but the sensitivity is inadequate to exclude these injuries on the basis of ultrasound alone. The FAST examination includes views of the pericardium from the subxiphoid window and the abdomen from the right upper quadrant (hepatorenal), left upper quadrant (splenorenal), and suprapubic (pelvic) windows. Views of the left and right chest are obtained in the eFAST examination to evaluate for pneumothorax and hemothorax. Additional views can be pursued for additional information (e.g., parasternal), but are not part of the traditional FAST examination.

Selected Reference
1. Rozyck GS, Oschner MG, Schmidt JA, et al. A prospective study of surgeon performed ultrasound as the primary adjuvant modality for the injured patient assessment. *J Trauma.* 1995;39(3):492-498.

**2.** Correct Answer: B. 200 mL

*Rationale:* It takes approximately 200 mL of free fluid to be reliably detected on ultrasound. A volume smaller than this may be occasionally visible, but is unlikely to be the cause of hemodynamic instability. That said, one should repeat the FAST examination if ongoing bleeding is suspected, as an initial examination may be negative because of a small fluid volume. Also, a positive FAST does not necessarily mean that a patient needs an intervention, since many injuries can be managed nonoperatively.

Selected Reference
1. Branney SW, Wolfe RE, Moore EE, et al. Quantitative sensitivity of ultrasound in detecting free intraperitoneal fluid. *J Trauma.* 1995;39:375-380.

**3.** Correct Answer: A. Second-third intercostal space, midclavicular line

*Rationale:* Pneumothoraces tend to be "antidependent," because the lung tissue is heavier than the pleural airspace. Therefore, evaluation for pneumothorax generally starts anteriorly and apically, at approximately the second or third intercostal space, in the midclavicular line, where a small pneumothorax is most likely to be detected. However, localized pleural disease is possible, so a more thorough examination of the chest is warranted if clinical suspicion is high.

Selected Reference
1. Kirkpatrick AW, Sirois M, Laupland K, et al. Hand-held thoracic sonography for detecting post-traumatic pneumothoraces: the extended focused assessment with sonography for trauma (EFAST). *J Trauma Inj Infect Crit Care.* 2004;57(2):288-295.

**4.** Correct Answer: D. 86% to 100%

*Rationale:* The eFAST is composed of the traditional FAST examination with added views of the chest to identify and diagnose pneumothorax and hemothorax. The sensitivity for pneumothorax with this examination approaches 86% to 100%, in contrast with chest x-ray, which has a sensitivity 30% to 80%.

**Selected Reference**

1. Schellenberg M, Inaba K, Bardes JM, et al. The combined utility of extended focused assessment with sonography for trauma and chest x-ray in blunt thoracic trauma. *J Trauma Acute Care Surg.* 2018;85(1):113-117.

## 5. Correct Answer: D. >90%

*Rationale:* Ultrasound is an excellent tool for detecting hemothorax in the trauma patient with blunt and penetrating chest injury. Multiple studies have assessed the utility of ultrasound to detect clinically significant hemothorax and they have shown 100% sensitivity and specificity with no false-negative or false-positive findings.

**Selected Reference**

1. Governatori NJ, Saul T, Siadecki SD, Lewis RE. Ultrasound in the evaluation of penetrating thoraco-abdominal trauma: a review of the literature. *Med Ultrason.* 2015;17(4):528-534.

## 6. Correct Answer: C. 60% to 70%

*Rationale:* An eFAST examination can be used to detect intra-abdominal injury in the blunt and penetrating trauma patient, but the sensitivity for solid organ injury and small-volume hemoperitoneum is significantly less than that for CT scan. With a small volume of fluid (<200 mL), the sensitivity is 60% to 70%, which has been shown over multiple trials. Fortunately, the sensitivity increases with increasing blood volume and is excellent when a hemodynamically significant amount of blood is present in the peritoneum. For this reason, serial reassessment is important if ongoing bleeding is suspected.

The moderate sensitivity may argue against performing eFAST in a hemodynamically stable patient. But, it is important to note that even though the sensitivity is low, the specificity of a positive eFAST is quite high (>90%) in most studies. Hence, a positive eFAST after an abdominal trauma identifies at-risk patients, though it cannot rule out solid organ injury.

**Selected References**

1. Branney SW, Wolfe RE, Moore EE, et al. Quantitative sensitivity of ultrasound in detecting free intraperitoneal fluid. *J Trauma Inj Infect Crit Care.* 1995;39(2):375-380.
2. Dolich MO, McKenney MG, Varela JE, et al. 2,576 Ultrasounds for blunt abdominal trauma. *J Trauma Inj Infect Crit Care.* 2001; 50(1):108-112.
3. Natarajan B, Gupta PK, Cemaj S, Sorensen M, Hatzoudis GI, Forse RA. FAST scan: is it worth doing in hemodynamically stable blunt trauma patients? *Surgery.* 2010;148(4):695-701.

## 7. Correct Answer: B. A 45-year-old woman with BP 85/50 mm Hg after an MVC

*Rationale:* The FAST and eFAST examinations are noninvasive tests that can be performed concomitantly with resuscitation. The use of ultrasound evaluation is most indicated in a blunt trauma patient who is not stable to transport to CT, to evaluate for intraperitoneal fluid and determine the need for immediate operative intervention. CT is the preferred method of imaging for a stable patient and may provide information about other organ injuries as well. Penetrating trauma patients would be expected to have some degree of fluid in the chest or abdomen (depending on the site of injury), and a negative eFAST examination would not provide adequate reassurance; thus, it would not help clinical decision-making.

**Selected Reference**

1. EAST Practice Management Guidelines Work Group. *J Trauma.* 2002;53(3):602-615.

## 8. Correct Answer: A. 2 to 5 MHz curvilinear probe

*Rationale:* Ultrasound probes penetrate tissue levels according to the frequency (MHz) of the transducer. Higher frequency probes have less penetration, but greater resolution at shallow depths. Lower frequency probes have greater penetration and allow for visualization of deeper structures. The 2 to 5 MHz curvilinear or convex array probe is best used to evaluate deep abdominal structures for injury. The 1 to 5 MHz phased array probe has a smaller footprint and allows for more advanced manipulation of the ultrasound beam, which is best used for pediatric examinations and echocardiography, although it would be a reasonable alternative if the curvilinear array probe was unavailable. The 5 to 12 MHz linear transducer probe is best used for superficial structures and vascular access, as well as evaluation of pneumothorax. The 8 to

13 MHz intracavitary probe is best used for transvaginal and oral evaluations due to its high-resolution images and the shape, which allows it to image from within a body cavity.

### Selected Reference

1. Enriquez JL, Wu TS. An introduction to ultrasound equipment and knobology. *Crit Care Clin*. 2014;30(1):25-45.

---

**9.** Correct Answer: B. Figure 60.2B

*Rationale:* In addition to lung sliding seen on real-time B-mode ultrasound, M-mode can be used to detect motion. In normal lung ultrasound, a "seashore sign" is seen, indicating motion of the pleural layers below the chest wall, as seen in Figure 60.2D. The "barcode" or "stratosphere" sign indicates no motion of the pleura or lung, as seen in Figure 60.2B, and is indicative of pneumothorax. B-lines are seen with pulmonary interstitial fluid (Figure 60.2A), and their presence excludes pneumothorax at that location. A dark stripe around the lung can be seen with a pleural effusion or hemothorax (Figure 60.2C).

### Selected Reference

1. Lichtenstein DA. Lung ultrasound in the critically ill. *Ann Intensive Care*. 2014;4(1). doi:10.1186/2110-5820-4-1.

---

**10.** Correct Answer: C. The eFAST examination has little diagnostic value for hemoperitoneum in this setting

*Rationale:* The eFAST will detect intra-abdominal or intrathoracic fluid, but is unable to reliably differentiate between types of fluid. Although a hematocrit level may be apparent after blood cells have settled, in the acute setting, blood cannot be reliably differentiated from other fluids. Because of this, the abdominal and posterior thoracic views of the examination may be confounding, and additional clinical information may be necessary to guide management.

### Selected Reference

1. Maitra S, Jarman R, Halford N, Richards S. When FAST is a FAFF: is FAST scanning useful in non-trauma patients? *Ultrasound*. 2008;16(3):165-168.

---

**11.** Correct Answer: C. eFAST has similar sensitivity to nonpregnant adult blunt trauma patients

*Rationale:* The sensitivity of the FAST examination in pregnancy is 83%, which is similar to the nonpregnant patient sensitivity of 79% to 98%, even during the third trimester.

### Selected Reference

1. Goodwin H, Holmes JF, Wisner DH. Abdominal ultrasound examination in pregnant blunt trauma patients. *J Trauma*. 2001;50(4):689-693; discussion 694.

---

**12.** Correct Answer: A. Clotted intra-abdominal blood

*Rationale:* False-negative findings can occur with the eFAST examination. Patients with old hemorrhage that is now clotted show a mixed echogenicity instead of the anechoic look of fresh blood. The presence of ascites will lead to an increased false-positive rate. An ISS > 25 is associated with a higher false-negative rate. Trendelenburg positioning may increase sensitivity for peritoneal fluid in the upper abdomen. Serial FAST examinations improve the sensitivity of the study.

### Selected Reference

1. Savatmongkorngul S, Wongwaisayawan S, Kaewlai R. Focused assessment with sonography for trauma: current perspectives. *Open Access Emerg Med*. 2017;9:57-62.

---

**13.** Correct Answer: A. CT scan of the abdomen/pelvis with IV contrast

*Rationale:* In children, the eFAST examination has a reported sensitivity of 80%. In the pediatric population with a positive eFAST examination in a hemodynamically stable patient, a CT scan should be the next step in the evaluation of a patient with a high suspicion for intra-abdominal injuries. Monitoring the patient with serial abdominal examinations could delay the diagnosis of an intra-abdominal injury requiring intervention. Taking the patient to the OR for an emergent operation while hemodynamically stable would not be appropriate as the false-negative rate for laparotomy is too high to justify this action. Repeating the FAST examination would not help as there is already a positive finding.

Selected Reference

1. Holmes JF, Gladman A, Chang CH. Performance of abdominal ultrasonography in pediatric blunt trauma patients: a meta-analysis. *J Pediatr Surg.* 2007;42(9):1588-1594.

**14.** Correct Answer: B. 20 mL

*Rationale:* **Figure 60.5** shows a pericardial effusion, presumed to be hemorrhage in the setting of penetrating trauma to the area. Approximately 20 mL is the smallest volume of fluid in the pericardium that can be reliably seen on ultrasound. Although smaller volumes may be visualized by experienced sonographers, these small-volume effusions are probably clinically insignificant. Patients with chronic pericardial effusions may have very large volumes but may not have the hemodynamic issues seen when a small-volume effusion occurs acutely because the pericardium can expand over time.

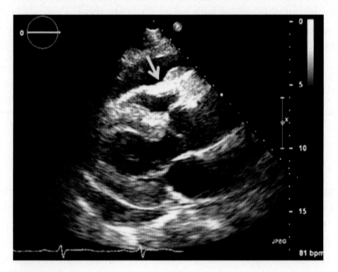

**Figure 60.5**

Selected Reference

1. Governatori NJ, Saul T, Siadecki SD, Lewis RE. Ultrasound in the evaluation of penetrating thoraco-abdominal trauma: a review of the literature. *Med Ultrason.* 2015;17(4):528-534.

**15.** Correct Answer: D. Lighthouse phenomenon

*Rationale:* Rib fractures can be detectable with ultrasound by noting the lighthouse phenomenon—an acoustic shadow seen deep to the posterior rib border (like the beam from a lighthouse) , as seen in **Figure 60.6**. The seashore sign (Figure 60.2D) is the M-mode appearance of normal lung tissue moving the pleural layers, creating a sand-like appearance against the chest wall. The spine sign is seen when fluid is in the pleural space. An intact anterior echogenic margin is seen with a normal rib.

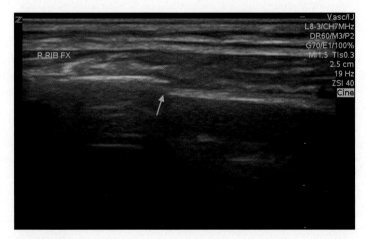

**Figure 60.6**

Selected References
1. Ahmed AA, Martin JA, Saul T, Lewiss RE. The thoracic spine sign in bedside ultrasound. Three cases report. *Med Ultrason.* 2014;16(2):179-181.
2. Smereczynski A, Kolaczyk K, Bernatowicz E. Chest wall—underappreciated structure in sonography. Part II: non-cancerous lesions. *J Ultrason.* 2017;17(71):275-280.
3. Turk F, Kurt AB, Saglam S. Evaluation by ultrasound of traumatic rib fractures missed by radiography. *Emerg Radiol.* 2010;17(6):473-477.

**16.** Correct Answer: A. There is high sensitivity and specificity for detecting intra-abdominal hemorrhage

*Rationale:* The eFAST examination can reliably detect intra-abdominal hemorrhage in unstable blunt trauma patients with or without life-threatening pelvic fractures with high specificity and sensitivity, approaching 96% for each. Once 200 to 250 mL of intra-abdominal blood has accumulated, it can be easily seen with the eFAST examination. In the unstable patient with pelvic fractures, this is a valuable tool to assess for bleeding and determine if operative intervention for an intra-abdominal pathology is necessary in addition to pelvic fixation. Of note, it is critical to reassess with a repeat eFAST examination if the clinical picture changes.

Selected Reference
1. Christian NT, Burlew CC, Moore EE, et al. The focused abdominal sonography for trauma examination can reliably identify patients with significant intra-abdominal hemorrhage in life-threatening pelvic fractures. *J Trauma Acute Care Surg.* 2018;84(6):924-928.

**17.** Correct Answer: C. 1.5 cm

*Rationale:* A decreased IVC diameter may be a manifestation of hypovolemia. The average diameter of the IVC is normally 1.5 to 2.5 cm in a euvolemic patient. It is important to perform this examination on expiration as the IVC collapses 50% of its normal size on physiologic inspiration.

Selected Reference
1. Richards JR, McGahan JP. Focused Assessment with Sonography in Trauma (FAST) in 2017: what radiologists can learn. *Radiology.* 2017;283(1):30-48.

**18.** Correct Answer: B. It has low sensitivity and low specificity

*Rationale:* The FAST examination has a low sensitivity and specificity for detection of a hollow organ injury. The sensitivity for gastrointestinal injury was reported to be >40% for detection within the first 12 hours. Of note, this increases to above 80% when greater than 12 to 24 hours. It is important to use eFAST only as an adjunct when assessing for hollow organ injury. Other forms of imaging, like CT or serial abdominal examinations, in conjunction with clinical judgment are a more appropriate strategy for assessment of hollow organ injury.

Selected Reference
1. Savatmongkorngul S, Wongwaisayawan S, Kaewlai R. Focused assessment with sonography for trauma: current perspectives. *Open Access Emerg Med.* 2017;9:57-62.

**19.** Correct Answer: B. Retroperitoneal hematoma

*Rationale:* An eFAST examination is directed at the identification of intra-abdominal blood, hemothorax, or pneumothorax. However, solid organ injuries may be identified as well, including liver lacerations, splenic lacerations, and kidney lacerations. It is not typically able to detect retroperitoneal hematomas or intestinal injury.

Selected References
1. Bloom BA, Gibbons RC. Focused Assessment with Sonography for Trauma (FAST). *StatPearls. Treasure Island (FL).* 2019.
2. Savatmongkorngul S, Wongwaisayawan S, Kaewlai R. Focused assessment with sonography for trauma: current perspectives. *Open Access Emerg Med.* 2017;9:57-62.

**20.** Correct Answer: A. 50

*Rationale:* Medical providers who are learning the FAST examination experience false-negative rates early in their training. During the first FAST consensus conference, it was noted that 200 supervised examinations are needed to be considered **experienced**, and a level of proficiency was achieved by 50 examinations. Most errors occur during the first 10 FAST examinations, with accuracy improving with each examination.

### Selected References

1. Scalea TM, Rodriguez A, Chiu WC, et al. Focused assessment with sonography for trauma (fast): results from an international consensus conference. *J Trauma Inj Infect Crit Care.* 1999;46(3):466-472.
2. Shackford SR, Rogers FB, Osler TM, Trabulsy ME, Clauss DW, Vane DW. Focused abdominal sonogram for trauma: the learning curve of nonradiologist clinicians in detecting hemoperitoneum. *J Trauma Inj Infect Crit Care.* 1999;46(4):553-564.

# 61 | LIVER AND GALLBLADDER

George Kasotakis, Meredith L. Whitacre, Suresh "Mitu" Agarwal, and Katherine Albutt

1. What is the optimal ultrasound (US) probe to be used for hepatobiliary evaluation?

   A. A phased array probe with high frequency (5-13 MHz)
   B. A curvilinear probe with a low frequency (3.5-5.0 MHz)
   C. A phased array probe with a low frequency (2-8 MHz)
   D. A curvilinear probe with a high frequency (8-13 MHz)

2. You are performing an abdominal US on an adult patient with right upper quadrant pain. You wish to differentiate the common bile duct (CBD) from the portal vein and hepatic artery. Which of the following adjustments will be the *most* effective in making this distinction?

   A. Decrease the depth.
   B. Move the focal zone over the area of interest.
   C. Add color flow Doppler.
   D. Increase the gain.

3. A 24-year-old woman is admitted to the intensive care unit (ICU) in blastic crisis and has right upper abdominal pain. You are attempting to visualize the gallbladder with a curvilinear probe in the subcostal area, but the images are limited because of her elevated body mass index (BMI). Which of the following would be *most* likely to improve imaging of the gallbladder?

   A. Change to a linear array probe with high frequency (5-13 MHz).
   B. Change to a phased array probe (frequency 2-8 MHz).
   C. Increase the imaging depth.
   D. Move the probe to another location.

4. What is described by the "Mickey Mouse sign" with respect to liver US?

   A. The normal appearance of the CBD, portal vein, and hepatic artery seen on their short axis
   B. The appearance of the three hepatic veins as they enter the inferior vena cava (IVC)
   C. The appearance of the gallbladder adjacent to the IVC and fluid-filled duodenum
   D. The appearance of a trilobar septated abscess in the liver

5. What is the sonographic Murphy's sign?

   A. Tenderness in the right upper quadrant during a physical examination by the ultrasonographer
   B. Tenderness in the right upper quadrant when pressure is applied while the US probe is over the gallbladder
   C. Tenderness in the left upper quadrant when pressure is applied while the US probe is over the gallbladder
   D. The classic US triad of cholecystitis: cholelithiasis, gallbladder wall thickening, and pericholecystic fluid

6. A 54-year-old woman with an elevated BMI is admitted to the hospital with an asthma exacerbation. On day 2, she complains of right upper quadrant and epigastric abdominal discomfort after eating a fatty meal. Her pain resolves within the hour. The obtained US is shown in **Figure 61.1**.

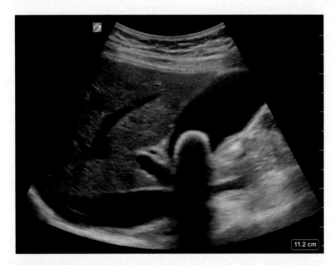

**Figure 61.1**

What is the *most* likely diagnosis?
A. Symptomatic cholelithiasis
B. Acute cholecystitis
C. Acalculous cholecystitis
D. Gallstone ileus

7. An 81-year-old man has been in the surgical ICU for over 2 weeks following multiple small bowel resections for acute mesenteric ischemia. He is receiving total parenteral nutrition (TPN) due to delayed return of bowel function. His laboratory evaluation is significant for leukocytosis, normal liver function tests (LFTs), and US **Figure 61.2** is obtained.

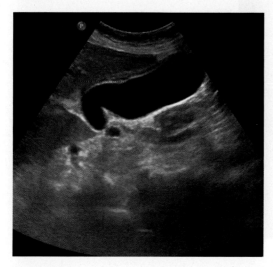

**Figure 61.2**

What is the *most* likely diagnosis?
A. Symptomatic cholelithiasis
B. Acute cholecystitis
C. Acalculous cholecystitis
D. Choledocholithiasis

8. A 55-year-old woman is admitted to the hospital after a complicated abdominal hysterectomy and bilateral salpingo-oophorectomy. After improving for several days, she starts complaining of unrelenting right upper quadrant pain after her first regular meal. She has a positive Murphy's sign, white blood cell count (WBC) 15,000/mm$^3$/L, and a temperature of 38.1°C. **Figure 61.3** US is obtained.

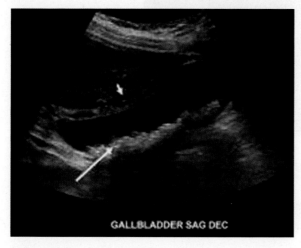

**Figure 61.3**

Which of the following is the *most* likely diagnosis?
A. Symptomatic cholelithiasis
B. Acute cholecystitis
C. Acute acalculous cholecystitis
D. Choledocholithiasis

9. A 60-year-old woman is admitted to the ICU with hemorrhagic shock from lower gastrointestinal bleeding. Point-of-care US is performed to assess volume status and cardiac function, and **Figure 61.4** of the gallbladder is obtained.

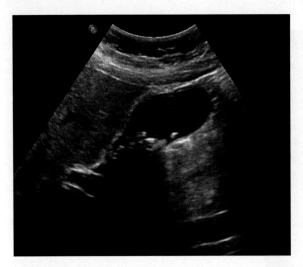

**Figure 61.4**

The patient declines any relevant right upper quadrant or epigastric symptomatology, and laboratory evaluation reveals normal LFTs.

What is the *most* likely diagnosis?
A. Symptomatic cholelithiasis
B. Acute cholecystitis
C. Acute acalculous cholecystitis
D. Chronic cholecystitis

10. An obviously malnourished, frail 90-year-old woman with uncontrolled diabetes is admitted to the ICU with sepsis and right upper quadrant abdominal pain. US is shown in **Figure 61.5**.

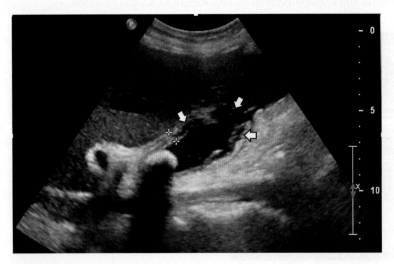

**Figure 61.5**

What is the *most* likely diagnosis?
A. Acute cholecystitis
B. Emphysematous cholecystitis
C. Acute acalculous cholecystitis
D. Chronic cholecystitis

11. A 50-year-old man with a history of bilateral lung transplant now presents with sepsis and right upper quadrant abdominal pain. A point-of-care US demonstrates **Figure 61.6**.

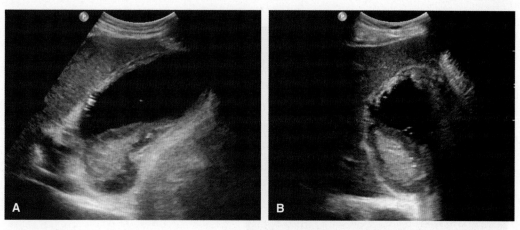

**Figure 61.6**

What is the *most likely* diagnosis?
A. Gangrenous cholecystitis
B. Choledocholithiasis
C. Acute acalculous cholecystitis
D. Chronic cholecystitis

12. A 67-year-old woman is admitted to the ICU with sepsis, fever, leukocytosis, jaundice, and right upper quadrant pain. **Figure 61.7** is obtained with point-of-care US.

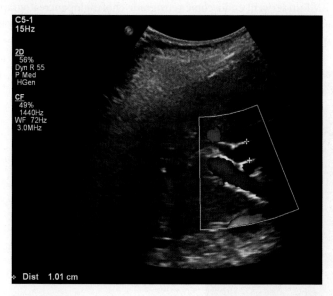

**Figure 61.7**

Which of the following is the *most likely* diagnosis?
A. Acute cholecystitis
B. Cholelithiasis without cholecystitis
C. Cholangitis
D. Chronic cholecystitis

13. A 78-year-old man with a history of coronary artery disease and peripheral vascular disease is admitted to the ICU with severe abdominal pain and sepsis. A point-of-care US of the liver is shown in **Figure 61.8**.

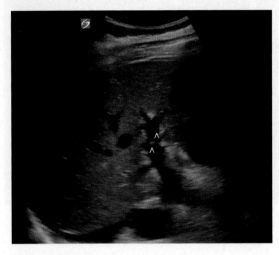

**Figure 61.8**

What *abnormal* finding is represented in Figure 61.8?
A. Acute hepatitis
B. Pneumobilia
C. Portal venous gas
D. Cirrhosis

14. A 44-year-old woman with elevated BMI underwent endoscopic retrograde cholangiopancreatography (ERCP) for complicated gallstone pancreatitis yesterday and now complains of worsening right upper quadrant discomfort. A right upper quadrant US is shown in **Figure 61.9**.

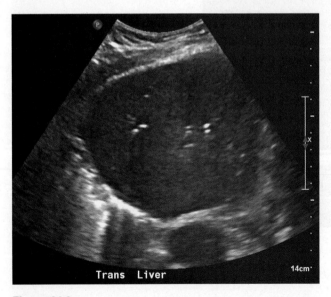

**Figure 61.9**

What *abnormal* finding is represented in this image?
A. Acute hepatitis
B. Pneumobilia
C. Portal venous gas
D. Cirrhosis

15. A 77-year-old man with a long-standing history of smoking, coronary artery disease, and congestive heart failure is admitted to the ICU for a heart failure exacerbation. He complains of abdominal distention and early satiety, but denies any fever, vomiting, or diarrhea. A point-of-care US of the liver demonstrates an enlarged liver (19 cm at the midclavicular line) and is shown in **Figure 61.10**.

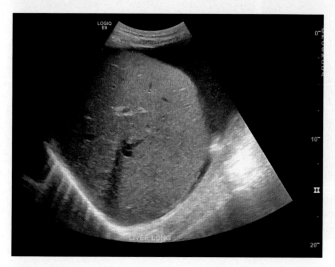

**Figure 61.10**

What is the *most* likely diagnosis?
A. Acute viral hepatitis
B. Acute cholecystitis
C. Hepatomegaly without hepatitis
D. Cirrhosis

16. A 66-year-old man with a long-standing history of alcoholism is admitted to the ICU with hematemesis. A point-of-care liver US reveals **Figure 61.11**.

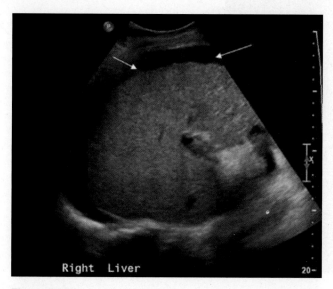

**Figure 61.11**

Which of the following is suggested by the US shown in Figure 61.11?
A. Choledocholithiasis
B. Elevated right atrial pressure
C. Acalculous cholecystitis
D. Cirrhosis

17. A 56-year-old man with a long-standing history of hepatitis C is admitted with pancytopenia and splenomegaly. An image from his liver US is shown in **Figure 61.12**.

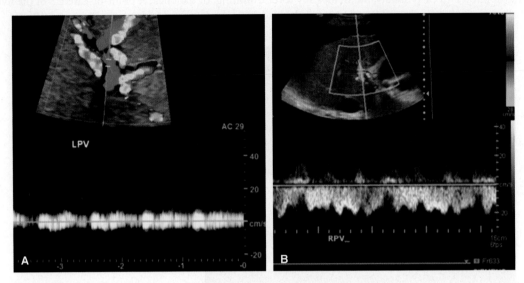

**Figure 61.12**

What is the *most* likely diagnosis?
A. Choledocholithiasis
B. Elevated right atrial pressure
C. Portal hypertension
D. Budd-Chiari syndrome

18. A 40-year-old female with a history of Factor V Leiden presents with acute abdominal pain, ascites, and right upper quadrant discomfort. An image from her liver US is shown in **Figure 61.13**.

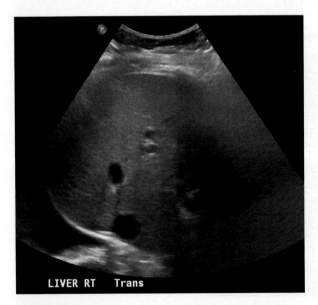

**Figure 61.13**

Which of the following is the *most* likely diagnosis?
A. Acute viral hepatitis
B. Choledocholithiasis
C. Portal venous thrombosis
D. Budd-Chiari syndrome

19. A 55-year-old man underwent a pancreaticoduodenectomy (Whipple procedure) for pancreatic adenocarcinoma 3 days ago. Today, he developed acute epigastric pain. An US image from his right upper quadrant is shown in **Figure 61.14**.

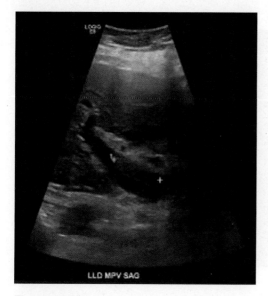

**Figure 61.14**

What is the *most* likely diagnosis?
A. Pancreatic leak
B. Portal vein thrombosis
C. Biliary stricture
D. Budd-Chiari syndrome

20. A 24-year-old is admitted to the ICU with malaise, high fevers, and right upper quadrant pain after recently moving to the United States from Mexico. Laboratory evaluation reveals leukocytosis and mild alkaline phosphatase elevation. A right upper quadrant US is shown in **Figure 61.15**.

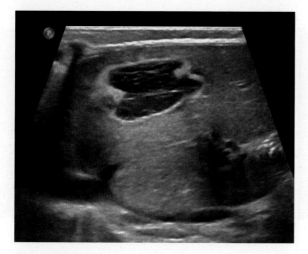

**Figure 61.15**

What is the *most* likely diagnosis?
A. Simple hepatic cyst
B. Acute cholecystitis
C. Liver abscess
D. Hepatocellular carcinoma

21. A 33-year-old woman was an unrestrained passenger in a motor vehicle collision and was admitted to the ICU. She has several right-sided rib fractures and a grade III liver laceration. After starting a clear liquid diet this morning, she developed acute right upper quadrant pain. A point-of-care US image is displayed in **Figure 61.16**.

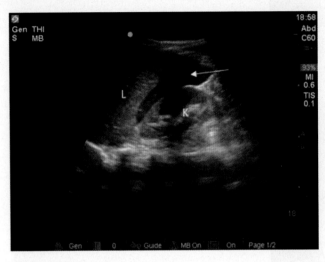

**Figure 61.16**

What is the *most* likely diagnosis?
A. Acute cholecystitis
B. Hemoperitoneum
C. Vena cava injury
D. Gastric perforation

22. A 40-year-old female who is 2 months postpartum underwent a laparoscopic cholecystectomy for recurrent cholecystitis. Her gallbladder was noted to be gangrenous and the dissection was tedious. Two weeks postoperatively, she presents to the office with jaundice and vague abdominal pain. An US is obtained followed by a hepatobiliary iminodiacetic acid (HIDA) scan. Based on **Figure 61.17**, what is the *most* likely diagnosis?

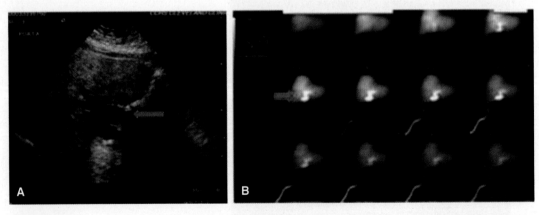

**Figure 61.17**

A. Biloma and CBD injury
B. Biloma secondary to traumatic injury
C. Postoperative liver abscess
D. Postoperative hematoma

**23.** A 38-year-old woman is in the ICU with acute respiratory failure from pneumonia. She has a right upper quadrant US that reveals **Figure 61.18**.

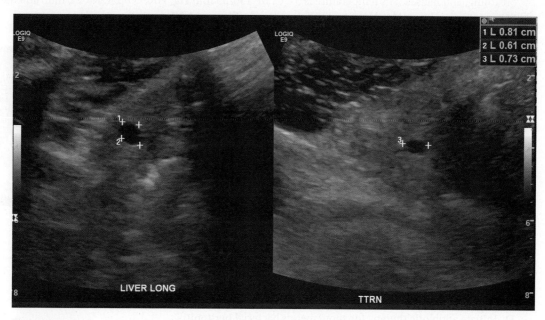

**Figure 61.18**

Which of the following is the *most* likely diagnosis?
**A.** Simple hepatic cyst
**B.** Hepatic abscess
**C.** Hypovolemia from diuresis
**D.** Acute cholecystitis

**24.** A 70-year-old man is in the ICU after a complicated right hemicolectomy for cancer. He complains of right upper quadrant pain with the initiation of his diet. Selected images from his right upper quadrant US are displayed in **Figure 61.19**.

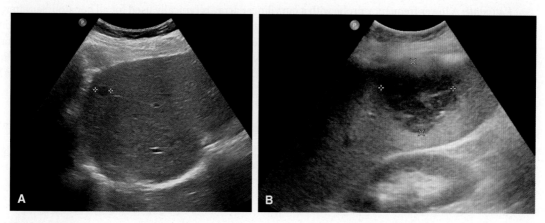

**Figure 61.19**

What is the *most* likely diagnosis?
**A.** Hepatic abscess
**B.** Simple hepatic cyst
**C.** Metastatic liver disease
**D.** Hepatocellular carcinoma

**25.** A 66-year-old man with chronic hepatitis C complicated by cirrhosis is admitted to the ICU. He has noticed progressively worsening abdominal pain and distention over the last several weeks, difficulty breathing, and nausea. His temperature is 37°C, BP 130/55 mm Hg, HR 95 bpm, RR 22/min, and SpO$_2$ 98% on 2 L nasal cannula. Abdominal US is shown in **Figure 61.20**.

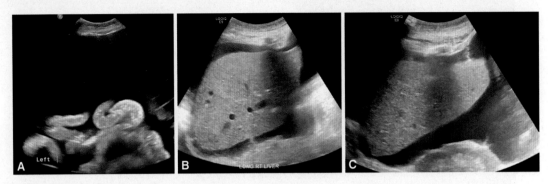

**Figure 61.20**

What is the *most* appropriate next step in his treatment?
**A.** Surgical consult for hemoperitoneum
**B.** Paracentesis to relieve abdominal distention
**C.** Nasogastric lavage to evaluate for variceal bleeding
**D.** Initiate antibiotic therapy for spontaneous bacterial peritonitis

# Chapter 61 ▪ Answers

**1.** Correct Answer: B. A curvilinear probe with low frequency (3.5-5.0 MHz)

*Rationale:* A lower frequency probe with a curvilinear array is typically used for all hepatobiliary imaging. The curvilinear alignment of the crystals allows a fanning out of the beam, which allows visualization of a much wider area than the probe's footprint. The low frequency also allows better tissue penetration, which may be necessary for obese patients, in whom gallstone disease is typically more common. Phased array probes offer a variety of imaging options, but generally contain fewer crystals, thus fewer scan lines and less spatial resolution.

**Selected References**
1. Fentress M. Does the patient have cholelithiasis or cholecystitis?. In: Bornemann P, ed. *Ultrasound for Primary Care.* Wolters Kluwer; 2021:151-157.
2. Izadifar Z, Izadifar Z, Chapman D, Babyn P. An introduction to high intensity focused ultrasound: systematic review on principles, devices, and clinical applications. *J Clin Med.* 2020 Feb;9(2):pii: E460.

**2.** Correct Answer: C. Add color flow Doppler

*Rationale/Critique:* The addition of color flow Doppler allows identification of vascular structures, as blood flow will display flow velocity within the portal vein and hepatic arteries, but not in the CBD. The CBD also typically lies anterior and to the right of the portal vein, while the hepatic artery commonly lies anterior to the portal vein and toward the midline (left). Adjusting the depth, focal zone, and gain may all help improve visualization of the CBD, but are less helpful for its identification. (See also **Figure 61.21**.)

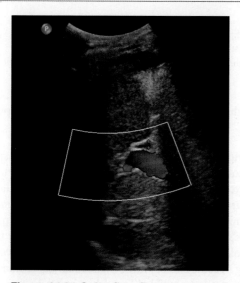

**Figure 61.21** Color flow Doppler overlying the portal triad. The common bile duct is marked with calipers.

Selected Reference

1. Gubernick JA, Rosenberg HK, Ilaslan H, Kessler A. US approach to jaundice in infants and children. *Radiographics.* 2000 Jan-Feb;20(1):173-195.

**3.** Correct Answer: **D. Move the probe to another location**

*Rationale:* The gallbladder is best visualized using a curvilinear probe in the right subcostal area. This should be done in both a longitudinal and transverse axis, to fully study the organ. When excess bowel gas obscures the gallbladder, or in obese patients with high riding livers, imaging through the rib spaces may be beneficial. Rib shadowing may obscure visualization, which can be improved by aligning the imaging plane with the intercostal space. The probe can be angled obliquely or slid anteriorly or laterally until the gallbladder is fully seen. Increasing the depth or using a higher frequency or phased array probe would not improve attenuation of the US signal or the quality of the image.

Selected Reference

1. Lee JM, Boll DT. Disease of the gallbladder and biliary tree. In: Hodler J, Kubik-Huch RA, von Schulthess GK, eds. *Diseases of the Abdomen and Pelvis 2018-2021: Diagnostic Imaging - IDKD Book [Internet].* Springer; 2018:Chapter 5.

**4.** Correct Answer: **A. The normal appearance of the CBD, portal vein, and hepatic artery seen on their short axis**

*Rationale/Critique:* Viewing the porta hepatis in its short axis demonstrates the three structures in a "Mickey Mouse" head configuration, with the portal vein representing the head, the CBD the right ear, and hepatic artery the left. (See **Figure 61.22**.)

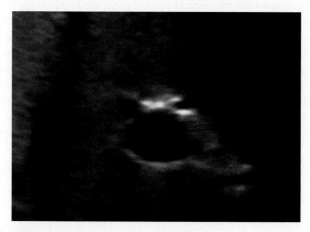

**Figure 61.22** The "Mickey Mouse" sign.

Selected References

1. Izadifar Z, Izadifar Z, Chapman D, Babyn P. An introduction to high intensity focused ultrasound: systematic review on principles, devices, and clinical applications. *J Clin Med.* 2020 Feb 7;9(2):pii: E460.

2. Xiang H, Han J, Ridley WE, Ridley LJ. Mickey mouse signs. *J Med Imaging Radiat Oncol.* 2018 Oct;62 suppl 1:92. doi:10.1111/1754-9485.39_12784.

## 5. Correct Answer: B. Tenderness in the right upper quadrant when pressure is applied while the US probe is over the gallbladder

*Rationale:* Murphy's sign refers to tenderness of the right upper quadrant on palpation during inspiration. The pain is severe enough to arrest deep inspiration. A "sonographic Murphy's sign" is similar to the Murphy's sign elicited during abdominal palpation, except that the positive response is observed during palpation with the US transducer. This is more accurate than hand palpation because it can confirm that it is indeed the gallbladder that is being pressed by the imaging transducer. Sonographic findings of cholecystitis include gallstones, sonographic Murphy's sign, gallbladder distension, pericholecystic fluid, and gallbladder wall thickening. The presence of cholelithiasis combined with a positive sonographic Murphy's sign is the most specific sonographic finding in acute cholecystitis. Gallbladder distension (>4 cm transverse and 10 cm in length) and an impacted stone in the gallbladder neck or cystic duct are suggestive findings. Gallbladder wall thickening measuring >3 mm and pericholecystic fluid are additional findings that can be seen; however, they are less specific than the signs previously described.

Selected References

1. Oppenheimer DC, Rubens DJ. Sonography of acute cholecystitis and its mimics. *Radiol Clin North Am.* 2019 May;57(3):535-548. doi:10.1016/j.rcl.2019.01.002. Epub 2019 Feb 10.

2. Ralls PW, Colletti PM, Lapin SA, et al. Real-time sonography in suspected acute cholecystitis. Prospective evaluation of primary and secondary signs. *Radiology.* 1985 Jun;155(3):767-771. doi:10.1148/radiology.155.3.3890007.

3. Simeone JF, Brink JA, Mueller PR, et al. The sonographic diagnosis of acute gangrenous cholecystitis: importance of the Murphy sign. *AJR Am J Roentgenol.* 1989 Feb;152(2):289-290.

## 6. Correct Answer: A. Symptomatic cholelithiasis

*Rationale:* The US (Figure 61.1) demonstrates a large dependent stone in the gallbladder neck with posterior shadowing, suggestive of cholelithiasis. The gallbladder wall does not appear thickened or distended, and there is no pericholecystic edema, making cholecystitis unlikely. While pain unrelated to her gallbladder remains possible, the US findings, onset with fatty food, and quick resolution suggest that symptomatic cholelithiasis without cholecystitis is the most likely explanation.

Selected References

1. Murphy MC, Gibney B, Gillespie C, Hynes J, Bolster F. Gallstones top to toe: what the radiologist needs to know. *Insights Imaging.* 2020 Feb;11(1):13. doi:10.1186/s13244-019-0825-4.

2. Ross M, Brown M, McLaughlin K, et al. Emergency physician-performed ultrasound to diagnose cholelithiasis: a systematic review. *Acad Emerg Med.* 2011 Mar;18(3):227-235.

## 7. Correct Answer: C. Acalculous cholecystitis

*Rationale/Critique:* The US (Figure 61.2) demonstrates a thickened, distended gallbladder with pericholecystic fluid but no stones. These findings, along with the clinical presentation, are highly suggestive of acalculous cholecystitis. This is a fairly common condition in the ICU. Prolonged fasting, TPN, prolonged mechanical ventilation, polytrauma, sepsis, shock, extensive burns, multiple transfusions, and medications (sedatives, vasopressors, opiates) have all been identified as risk factors for the development of acalculous cholecystitis, although the condition is not uncommon in the outpatient population. Common sonographic findings include a typically thickened gallbladder wall (>3.5 mm), distended gallbladder, and pericholecystic fluid (hypoechoic halo). Given the typically high acuity of ICU patients with acalculous cholecystitis, management revolves around minimally invasive (percutaneous) drainage of the gallbladder. When the patient recovers from critical illness, an elective cholecystectomy can be considered.

Selected Reference

1. Yokoe M, Hata J, Takada T, et al. Tokyo guidelines 2018: diagnostic criteria and severity grading of acute cholecystitis. *J Hepatobiliary Pancreat Sci.* 2018 Jan;25(1):41-54.

**8.** Correct Answer: B. Acute cholecystitis

*Rationale/Critique:* The US (Figure 61.3) demonstrates a thickened gallbladder with stones and pericholecystic edema. These findings, along with the clinical presentation, are suggestive of acute calculous cholecystitis. US findings are the same as in acalculous cholecystitis (see the previous vignette), with the presence of obvious stones (hyperechoic masses inside the gallbladder that create acoustic shadowing). The normal LFTs suggest that there is no biliary tract obstruction, and the pathology is isolated distal to the cystic duct. Depending on the patient's overall clinical condition, this may be addressed with cholecystectomy or percutaneous cholecystostomy.

Selected Reference

1. Oppenheimer DC, Rubens DJ. Sonography of acute cholecystitis and its mimics. *Radiol Clin North Am.* 2019 May;57(3):535-548.

**9.** Correct Answer: D. Chronic cholecystitis

*Rationale:* The US (Figure 61.4) demonstrates a thickened gallbladder with dependent stones present, but no pericholecystic edema. This, along with the clinical presentation, is suggestive of chronic cholecystitis, likely the result of multiple subclinical episodes of biliary colic and chronic low-grade inflammation, secondary to chronic gallstone disease. The normal LFTs argue against obstructive biliary disease. Chronic cholecystitis that is an incidental imaging finding may be addressed on an outpatient basis.

Selected Reference

1. Oppenheimer DC, Rubens DJ. Sonography of acute cholecystitis and its mimics. *Radiol Clin North Am.* 2019 May;57(3):535-548.

**10.** Correct Answer: B. Emphysematous cholecystitis

*Rationale/Critique:* Emphysematous cholecystitis is a rare subtype of acute cholecystitis caused by gas-forming bacteria. It typically presents in elderly, debilitated patients and poorly controlled diabetes is a common risk factor. The diagnosis is suggested by the presence of bright gas locules in the gallbladder wall, ring-down artifacts, and mobile gaseous echoes within the gallbladder lumen. Figure 61.5 demonstrates such gaseous locules within the gallbladder wall. (See **Figure 61.23.**)

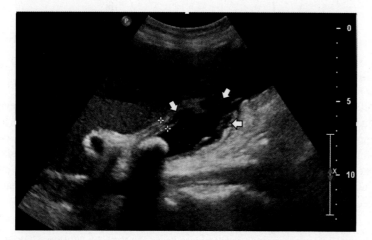

**Figure 61.23**

In **Figure 61.24**, the US demonstrates the "champagne sign" or "effervescent gallbladder." This is a term used to describe the hyperechoic appearance of air bubbles secondary to gas formation in the gallbladder lumen. On US, the air in the gallbladder lumen appears highly echogenic with low-level posterior shadowing and reverberation artifacts due to the gas within the lumen of the gallbladder. A less common appearance consists of tiny hyperechoic foci within the lumen released from gas-producing bacteria. These hyperechoic foci are reminiscent of champagne bubbles rising inside a flute of champagne.

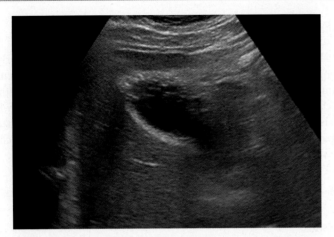

**Figure 61.24** The "Champagne sign."

Selected References
1. Minault Q, Gaiddon C, Veillon F, Venkatasamy A. The champagne sign. *Abdom Radiol (NY)*. 2018 Oct;43(10):2888-2889. doi:10.1007/s00261-018-1544-x.
2. Oppenheimer DC, Rubens DJ. Sonography of acute cholecystitis and its mimics. *Radiol Clin North Am*. 2019 May;57(3):535-548.

**11.** Correct Answer: A. Gangrenous cholecystitis

*Rationale:* Gangrenous cholecystitis is a severe, highly morbid complication of acute cholecystitis, in which portions of the gallbladder wall have become ischemic and necrosed. This is manifested sonographically by sloughed mucosal membranes (sometimes visualized as small hyperechoic foci in the gallbladder lumen—as in Figure 61.6), focal wall bulge, ulceration, and disruption of the gallbladder wall (as shown in Figure 61.6). When perforation has occurred, a pericholecystic abscess may be noted, as is seen in the above images. Immunosuppression is a common risk factor, as minimally perceived pain enables the infection to progress before medical attention is sought. Free fluid may or may not be adjacent to the gallbladder, depending on whether the perforation took place on the hepatic or peritoneal surface of the gallbladder.

Selected Reference
1. Oppenheimer DC, Rubens DJ. Sonography of acute cholecystitis and its mimics. *Radiol Clin North Am*. 2019 May;57(3):535-548.

**12.** Correct Answer: C. Cholangitis

*Rationale:* The patient presents with the typical Charcot's triad of leukocytosis, jaundice (or elevated bilirubin), and right upper quadrant pain, which suggests ascending cholangitis. The US (Figure 61.7) demonstrates a dilated common bile duct (CBD). This is suggestive of distal biliary obstruction, commonly from a stone at the sphincter of Oddi, which can lead to a potentially lethal infection. The size of the CBD ranges by patient size and weight, but as a rule of thumb, its size increases by 1 mm for every decade of life over the age of 60. In younger patients, it is approximately 4 to 5 mm, but may increase to 10 mm in diameter after cholecystectomy.

Selected Reference
1. Oppenheimer DC, Rubens DJ. Sonography of acute cholecystitis and its mimics. *Radiol Clin North Am*. 2019 May;57(3):535-548.

**13.** Correct Answer: C. Portal venous gas

*Rationale:* The US (Figure 61.8) demonstrates discrete hyperechoic foci that move with blood flow, consistent with gas in the portal vein. In smaller, more peripheral branches of the portal venous system, these may extend into the hepatic parenchyma toward the periphery and be confused with parenchymal pathology. Doppler may demonstrate disruption of the monophasic flow of the portal vein. Portal venous gas should be distinguished from pneumobilia, in which the hyperechoic foci that represent gas are typically seen within the liver parenchyma, entirely outside the vascular system. Common causes of portal venous gas include intestinal ischemia, pneumatosis coli, abdominal sepsis, and severe abdominal inflammation (e.g., complicated diverticulitis). Findings suggestive of acute hepatitis include hepatomegaly (most sensitive sign), gallbladder wall thickening, accentuated brightness of portal vein radicle walls, and overall decreased echodensity. Cirrhosis generally appears with surface nodularity or an overall coarse and heterogeneous echotexture, reduced size, or signs of portal hypertension. (See also **Figure 61.25**.)

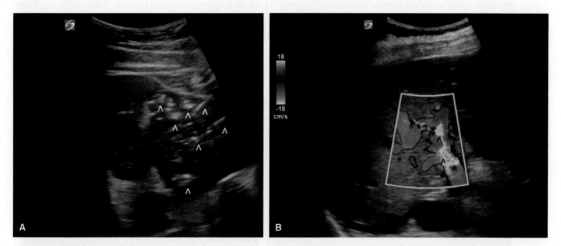

**Figure 61.25** A, Hyperechoic foci within the more peripheral branches of the portal venous system. B, Disruption of the monophasic flow of the portal vein.

### Selected References

1. Connor-Schuler R, Binz S, Clark C. Portal venous gas on point-of-care ultrasound in a case of cecal ischemia. *J Emerg Med*. 2020 Mar;58(3):e117-e120. doi:10.1016/j.jemermed.2019.10.033. Epub 2019 Dec 13.
2. Liang KW, Huang HH, Tyan YS, Tsao TF. Hepatic portal venous gas: review of ultrasonographic findings and the use of the "meteor shower" sign to diagnose it. *Ultrasound Q*. 2018 Dec;34(4):268-271.

---

**14.** Correct Answer: B. Pneumobilia

*Rationale:* Pneumobilia is commonly seen after instrumentation of the sphincter of Oddi, or hepatobiliary bypass procedures. Less commonly, it is seen in cases of bilioenteric fistulas, emphysematous cholecystitis, and perforated duodenal ulcers. The US shown in Figure 61.9 demonstrates hyperechoic foci in more central large-caliber ducts and these foci are not seen to be mobile or inside the portal circulation. Additionally, acute hepatitis may demonstrate abnormal overall density or size, or accentuated brightness of portal vein walls (not seen in Figure 61.9). Cirrhosis generally appears with surface nodularity or an overall coarse and heterogeneous echotexture, reduced size, or signs of portal hypertension.

### Selected Reference

1. Huang J, Stone MB. Ultrasound identification of traumatic pneumobilia. *Am J Emerg Med*. 2010 Feb 28(2):255.e5-e6.

---

**15.** Correct Answer: C. Hepatomegaly without hepatitis

*Rationale/Critique:* This liver is enlarged (75% of patients have a liver that measures <15 cm in the midclavicular line) and has a "starry night" appearance, in which multiple hyperechoic dots (enhancing portal venous walls) appear within a hypoechoic parenchyma (Figure 61.10). Ascites is present due to portal hypertension and enlarged hepatic veins can be seen. In the absence of inflammatory symptoms like fever, these changes most likely represent hepatomegaly from chronic right heart failure. Cholecystitis may be challenging to diagnose in the setting of portal hypertension, as pericholecystic fluid or edema may be present at baseline, but the gallbladder is not visualized here, and the lack of inflammatory symptoms is reassuring. Cirrhosis would be expected to demonstrate a smaller liver with irregular texture.

### Selected Reference

1. Kratzer W, Fritz V, Mason RA, Haenle MM, Kaechele V, Roemerstein Study Group. Factors affecting liver size: a sonographic survey of 2080 subjects. *J Ultrasound Med*. 2003;22(11):1155.

**16.** Correct Answer: D. Cirrhosis

*Rationale:* Although cirrhosis causes hepatomegaly in its initial stages, over time the liver shrinks and obtains a coarse, irregular surface with nodular parenchymal appearance. The loss of normal, homogeneous liver architecture is also seen. Figure 61.11 is suggestive of cirrhosis. Although the CBD is not identified, there is no intrahepatic biliary dilatation to suggest choledocholithiasis. A dilated IVC is not apparent to suggest elevated right atrial pressure. The gallbladder wall appears to have normal thickness without pericholecystic fluid, which does not support the diagnosis of acalculous cholecystitis. (See also **Figure 61.26.**)

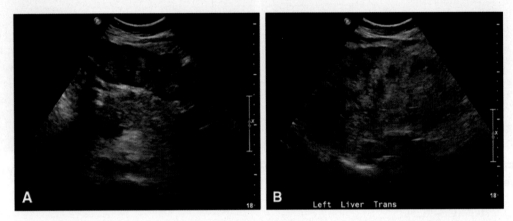

**Figure 61.26** Cirrhotic liver with loss of normal homogeneous liver architecture.

Selected References
1. Aubé C, Bazeries P, Lebigot J, Cartier V, Boursier J. Liver fibrosis, cirrhosis, and cirrhosis-related nodules: Imaging diagnosis and surveillance. *Diagn Interv Imaging.* 2017 Jun;98(6):455-468.
2. Irshad A, Anis M, Ackerman SJ. Current role of ultrasound in chronic liver disease: surveillance, diagnosis and management of hepatic neoplasms. *Curr Probl Diagn Radiol.* 2012 Mar-Apr;41(2):43-51. doi:10.1067/j.cpradiol.2011.07.003.

**17.** Correct Answer: C. Portal hypertension

*Rationale:* In this patient with cirrhosis, evidence of portal hypertension is seen. As portal hypertension worsens, portal flow is altered. Doppler measurements within the portal vein will show monophasic, biphasic (Figure 61.12A), and eventually hepatofugal flow (Figure 61.12B). Additional findings on US may include an enlarged diameter of the portal vein (**Figure 61.27**), a decrease in respiratory variation (<20% variation of the portal vein diameter), and changes in blood flow as described earlier. Dilatation of the biliary system is not apparent to suggest choledocolithiasis. The IVC is not prominent to suggest elevated right atrial pressure. The hepatic veins are not well-visualized to suggest Budd-Chiari syndrome.

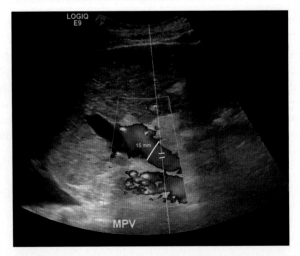

**Figure 61.27** Enlarged diameter of the main portal vein.

Selected References

1. Hammoud GM, Ibdah JA. Utility of endoscopic ultrasound in patients with portal hypertension. *World J Gastroenterol*. 2014 Oct 21;20(39):14230-14236.
2. Siegel MJ, Masand PM. Liver. In: Siegel MJ, ed. *Pediatric Sonography*. 5th ed. Wolters Kluwer; 2019:211-272.

**18.** Correct Answer: D. Budd-Chiari syndrome

*Rationale:* In this hypercoagulable patient, thrombosis of the hepatic veins has occurred (Budd-Chiari syndrome). The veins appear dilated due to the lack of blood flow and presence of thrombus. Doppler mode sonography shows decreased or absent blood flow, depending on the severity of thrombosis. Distinguishing portal veins from hepatic veins within the liver parenchyma may be challenging. The distinction can be made by the echogenicity of the vessel walls—portal veins typically have hyperechoic walls (as they are invested by Glisson capsule), and thus appear bright, while hepatic veins typically do not have reflective walls. The distinct composition of the hepatic vein wall renders it a specular reflector, which is hyperechoic only when the angle between the US beam and the vessel wall is close to 90°, whereas the composition of the portal vein wall enables it to appear hyperechoic at a wide range of beam-vessel angles. Acute viral hepatitis would be expected to show an enlarged liver with decreased echogenicity. There is no biliary dilatation to suggest choledocolithiasis. The portal veins do not appear dilated to suggest portal hypertension, although Doppler evaluation would be more sensitive. (See also **Figure 61.28**.)

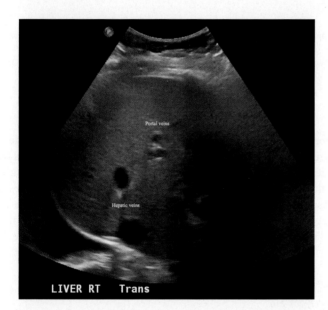

**Figure 61.28** Distinguishing portal veins from hepatic veins within the liver parenchyma.

Selected Reference

1. Hammoud GM, Ibdah JA. Utility of endoscopic ultrasound in patients with portal hypertension. *World J Gastroenterol*. 2014 Oct;20(39):14230-14236.

**19.** Correct Answer: B. Portal vein thrombosis

*Rationale/Critique:* The portal vein appears dilated (Figure 61.14) and has an endoluminal thrombus (immobile luminal defect). Portal vein thrombi range in echogenicity from anechoic or hypoechoic to hyperechoic. The degree of dilatation of the portal vein is dependent on the severity and chronicity of the thrombosis. Doppler mode ultrasonography demonstrates a lack of blood flow in the area occupied by the thrombus. Identifying an area of absent intraluminal flow in the portal vein on color Doppler is particularly useful when the thrombus is isoechoic to the adjacent normal portal vein. Sepsis, trauma, neoplasms, hypercoagulable states, and severe acute dehydration may lead to portal venous thrombosis. (See also **Figure 61.29**.)

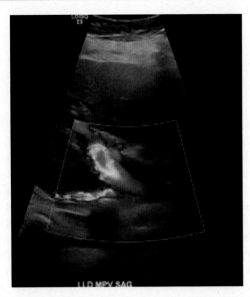

**Figure 61.29** Portal venous clot with lack of Doppler flow in the area of thrombus.

Selected References
1. Hammoud GM, Ibdah JA. Utility of endoscopic ultrasound in patients with portal hypertension. *World J Gastroenterol.* 2014 Oct;20(39):14230-14236.
2. Oppenheimer DC, Rubens DJ. Sonography of acute cholecystitis and its mimics. *Radiol Clin North Am.* 2019 May;57(3):535-548. doi:10.1016/j.rcl.2019.01.002. Epub 2019 Feb 10.

**20.** Correct Answer: C. Liver abscess

*Rationale:* The US (Figure 61.15) demonstrates a hypoechoic lesion with a hyperechoic wall, suggestive of a liver abscess. Pyogenic hepatic abscesses have a variable sonographic appearance, which ranges from complex fluid collections with heterogeneous echogenicity, thick-walled cystic lesions with or without septations, or cystic lesions with fluid-fluid levels. The history of travel from an endemic area raises suspicion for an *Entamoeba histolytica* abscess. A simple hepatic cyst is usually asymptomatic, has a thin, smooth wall, and should not display septations. Malignant tumors may have irregular shapes and thickness, and areas of vascular flow. The gallbladder is not visualized in this image and is usually on the inferior border of the liver.

Selected Reference
1. Mavilia MG, Pakala T, Molina M, Wu GY. Differentiating cystic liver lesions: a review of imaging modalities, diagnosis and management. *J Clin Transl Hepatol.* 2018 Jun;6(2):208-216.

**21.** Correct Answer: B. Hemoperitoneum

*Rationale/Critique:* Figure 61.16 reveals a hypoechoic fluid collection in the right upper quadrant over the liver and in the hepatorenal recess. This is highly suggestive of free fluid in the peritoneal cavity, which in the vast majority of cases represents blood (succus is a far less common source of free intraperitoneal fluid) after trauma. This is further suggested by the known liver injury, for which the patient was being monitored in the ICU. The gallbladder is not visualized in this image. Enteral contents (from a gastric perforation) may include debris and air (causing acoustic shadowing) and likely result in a small volume of peritoneal fluid, which may not be present on US.

Selected References
1. Corvino A, Catalano O, Corvino F, Sandomenico F, Petrillo A. Diagnostic performance and confidence of contrast-enhanced ultrasound in the differential diagnosis of cystic and cystic like liver lesions. *AJR Am J Roentgenol.* 2017 Sep;209(3):W119-W127.
2. Pace J, Arntfield R. Focused assessment with sonography in trauma: a review of concepts and considerations for anesthesiology. *Can J Anaesth.* 2018 Apr;65(4):360-370. English. doi:10.1007/s12630-017-1030-x. Epub 2017 Dec 4.

**22.** Correct Answer: A. Biloma and CBD injury

*Rationale:* Figure 61.17 demonstrates CBD injury and biloma formation after laparoscopic cholecystectomy for gangrenous cholecystitis. A biloma is a well-demarcated collection of bile outside the biliary tree. Traumatic and iatrogenic injuries, most commonly secondary to cholecystectomy, are the usual causes. In the context of a previous laparoscopic cholecystectomy and the presence of a fluid collection, it is imperative to have a high clinical suspicion for biloma. The reasons for biliary leaks after cholecystectomy include iatrogenic injury to the CBD, cystic duct stump leak, or anatomic variants, including the accessory ducts of Luschka. The US demonstrates an ill-defined anechoic collection with posterior acoustic enhancement within the porta hepatis and the HIDA demonstrates prompt tracer uptake by the liver and accumulation of tracer in the porta hepatis. CBD injury is a feared complication of cholecystectomy, with an incidence of 0.1% to 0.6%. US may visualize an extrahepatic fluid collection consistent with a biloma. It also allows for accurate assessment of CBD diameter, which is enlarged in distal occlusive injuries. The addition of Doppler imaging can aid in the diagnosis of concomitant vascular injury.

Selected References

1. Cohen JT, Charpentier KP, Beard RE. An update on iatrogenic biliary injuries: identification, classification, and management. *Surg Clin North Am.* 2019 Apr;99(2):283-299. doi:10.1016/j.suc.2018.11.006. Epub 2019 Feb 10.
2. Copelan A, Bahoura L, Tardy F, Kirsch M, Sokhandon F, Kapoor B. Etiology, diagnosis, and management of bilomas: a current update. *Tech Vasc Interv Radiol.* 2015 Dec;18(4):236-243. doi:10.1053/j.tvir.2015.07.007. Epub 2015 Jul 15.

**23.** Correct Answer: A. Simple hepatic cyst

*Rationale:* The US (Figure 61.18) demonstrates a round, well-marginated anechoic lesion, with a very thin wall. This is consistent with a simple hepatic cyst, likely of minimal clinical significance. Simple hepatic cysts may be round or ovoid and may demonstrate acoustic shadowing, depending on the size and echogenicity of their wall, which is typically thin. A few minor septae may be present, and there is no internal vascularity on color Doppler. Abscesses may be more complex, with multiple septations and thicker walls. Because the lesion is imaged from two axes, we can see that it is not cylindrical (like the IVC) or pouch-shaped (like the gallbladder).

Selected Reference

1. Corvino A, Catalano O, Corvino F, Sandomenico F, Petrillo A. Diagnostic performance and confidence of contrast-enhanced ultrasound in the differential diagnosis of cystic and cysticlike liver lesions. *AJR Am J Roentgenol.* 2017 Sep;209(3):W119-W127.

**24.** Correct Answer: C. Metastatic liver disease

*Rationale/Critique:* The US (Figure 61.19) demonstrates several round, well-defined, hypoechoic masses, some of which appear to exert a mass effect on adjacent vascular structures. These are concerning for metastatic disease. Malignant tumors may also display a hypoechoic halo, which is due to compression of the adjacent liver parenchyma. Because of the known colon cancer and the appearance of multiple lesions, metastases are the most likely diagnosis. Cystic, calcified, and diffuse infiltrative hyperechoic structures may also represent malignancy, depending on the chronicity and originating organ.

Selected Reference

1. Corvino A, Catalano O, Corvino F, Sandomenico F, Petrillo A. Diagnostic performance and confidence of contrast-enhanced ultrasound in the differential diagnosis of cystic and cystic like liver lesions. *AJR Am J Roentgenol.* 2017 Sep;209(3):W119-W127.

**25.** Correct Answer: B. Paracentesis to relieve abdominal distention

*Rationale/Critique:* The patient is a known cirrhotic who presents with free intraperitoneal fluid (large hypoechoic fluid on US) and abdominal distention. As he is hemodynamically normal, this likely represents ascites, a known complication of long-standing uncompensated cirrhosis. It is significant enough to cause shortness of breath, which warrants a paracentesis, in most cases. Without hypotension, tachycardia, or a history of trauma or bleeding, hemoperitoneum or bleeding esophageal varices are unlikely. Although spontaneous bacterial peritonitis remains a possibility, it is not the most likely diagnosis given this scenario and empiric antibiotic therapy would not be indicated.

Selected Reference

1. Narasimhan M, Koenig SJ, Mayo PH. A whole-body approach to point of care ultrasound. *Chest.* 2016 Oct;150(4):772-776.

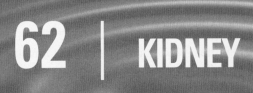

# 62 | KIDNEY

Etienne J. Couture, William Beaubien-Souligny, and Andre Y. Denault

1. A 60-year-old man presents with acute renal failure in the context of septic shock from community-acquired pneumonia. What is the best interpretation of his kidney size, as measured by the ultrasound shown in **Figure 62.1**?

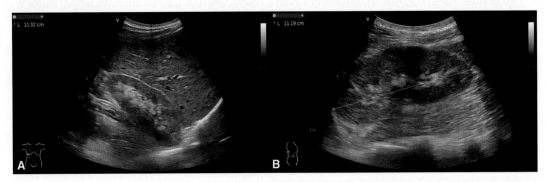

**Figure 62.1** Kidney size. 2D ultrasound evaluation of the kidney. An **(A)** Anterior or **(B)** lateral longitudinal view of the kidney can be used to measure kidney length. The length of the imaged kidney is 11 cm.

A. The size of the kidney is normal.
B. The kidney shows atrophy due to chronic kidney disease.
C. The kidney shows atrophy related to age.
D. The kidney is hypertrophied due to undiagnosed infiltrative disease.

2. When assessing renal blood flow using point-of-care ultrasound, what is the direction of the venous and arterial blood flow of the kidney with the probe held as a reference point?

A. Venous: toward, arterial: toward
B. Venous: away, arterial: toward
C. Venous: away, arterial: away
D. Venous: toward, arterial: away

3. How is the arterial renal resistive index (RRI) calculated?

   A. (peak systolic velocity − end-diastolic velocity)/peak systolic velocity
   B. (peak systolic velocity − end-diastolic velocity)/mean velocity
   C. (peak systolic velocity − end-diastolic velocity)/end-diastolic velocity
   D. (peak systolic velocity − mean velocity)/end-diastolic velocity

4. Which of the following is associated with an increase in arterial RRI?

   A. Hypernatremia
   B. Aortic insufficiency
   C. Aortic stenosis
   D. Renal artery stenosis

5. Which of the following clinical situations will be associated with an increased arterial RRI but normal splenic and hepatic arterial resistive indices?

   A. Right ventricular failure
   B. Acute tubular necrosis
   C. Abdominal compartment syndrome
   D. Advanced age

6. What is the expected effect on the RRI with an increase in mean arterial pressure using norepinephrine in the context of septic shock?

   A. A linear increase of RRI
   B. An exponential increase of RRI
   C. No change in RRI
   D. A decrease in RRI

7. What renal venous flow pattern progression is seen when heart function progresses from normal to failure?

   1. *Biphasic with an interruption between systole and diastole*
   2. *Continuous systolic-diastolic uninterrupted venous flow*
   3. *Monophasic with venous flow restricted to diastole*
   4. *Continuous systolic-diastolic flow with a brief interruption during atrial contraction*

   A. 2-4-1-3
   B. 2-3-4-1
   C. 3-2-4-1
   D. 3-4-1-2

8. How is the venous flow impedance index calculated?

   A. (Peak maximal venous flow velocity − nadir flow velocity)/nadir flow velocity
   B. (Peak maximal venous flow velocity − nadir flow velocity)/peak maximal venous flow velocity
   C. (Peak maximal venous flow velocity − nadir flow velocity)/mean venous flow velocity
   D. (Peak maximal venous flow velocity − mean flow velocity)/nadir flow velocity

9. What change to the renal blood flow pattern would be expected when an intravenous fluid bolus is given to a euvolemic patient with heart failure (with or without reduced ejection fraction), compared to normal subjects?

   A. Increase of renal venous impedance index and unchanged arterial resistance index
   B. Increase of renal venous impedance index and increase of arterial resistance index
   C. Decrease of renal venous impedance index and unchanged arterial resistance index
   D. Decrease of renal venous impedance index and increase of arterial resistance index

10. How does the renal venous flow impedance index predict diuresis in response to diuretic administration?

    A. A low venous impedance index will predict a low response to diuretics.
    B. A low venous impedance index will predict absent response to diuretics.
    C. A high venous impedance index will predict a low response to diuretics.
    D. Response to diuretics administration is not correlated with venous impedance index.

11. The renal venous stasis index (RVSI) was originally created to better characterize renal congestion. Which of the following has been associated with an increase in the RVSI?

    A. Increase in serum B-type natriuretic peptide (BNP) level
    B. Decrease in arterial RRI
    C. Decrease in intra-abdominal pressure
    D. Increase in tricuspid annular plane systolic excursion

12. What renal Doppler flow pattern would be expected after aggressive intravascular fluid resuscitation in a patient with marked right ventricular failure?

    A. Decrease in arterial renal resistance index
    B. Discontinuous monophasic renal venous flow
    C. Pulsatile renal venous flow
    D. Renal venous impedance index close to 0

13. Which of the following has the most impact on intrarenal vein flow patterns?

    A. Arterial renal blood flow
    B. Systolic blood pressure
    C. Diameter of the abdominal aorta
    D. Right heart function

14. Which of the following would be most consistent with an uninterrupted venous flow at Doppler evaluation?

    A. Reduction in right ventricular fractional area change
    B. Moderate to severe tricuspid regurgitation
    C. Lower hepatic systolic to diastolic velocity ratio (hepatic vein S/D < 0.55)
    D. High systolic velocity of the lateral portion of the tricuspid annular plane

15. Which of the following is *not* a sign of increased intra-abdominal pressure?

    A. Increased arterial resistive index
    B. Decreased arterial diastolic flow velocity
    C. Blunted renal venous flow
    D. Increased venous flow velocity

16. Which of the following should be the first step in the ultrasound evaluation of a patient who suddenly stopped making urine upon intensive care unit (ICU) admission after cardiac surgery?

    A. Calculation of arterial resistive index
    B. Evaluation of bladder volume
    C. Calculation of venous impedance index
    D. Inferior vena cava (IVC) diameter and cardiac output

# Chapter 62 ▪ Answers

**1.** Correct Answer: A. The size of the kidney is normal.

*Rationale:* The maximal longitudinal length of the kidney is generally measured between 9 and 12 cm in an average-sized adult, and depends on age and body size. A kidney length smaller than 10 cm before 60 years of age, or smaller than 9 cm at any age, is uncommon and highly suggestive of renal atrophy. The maximal kidney length is generally reached around 18 years of age, followed by a very small reduction during adulthood. Due to loss of parenchyma, the size of the kidney tends to decrease after 50 years of age. Renal atrophy is highly suggestive of underlying chronic kidney disease. However, diabetic nephropathy can present with normal kidney size, even in the presence of significant chronic kidney disease. A hypertrophied kidney can be due to infiltrative disease, polycystic disease, pyelonephritis, or multiple myeloma.

### Selected References

1. Beaubien-Souligny W, Denault A, Robillard P, Desjardins G. The role of point-of-care ultrasound monitoring in cardiac surgical patients with acute kidney injury. *J Cardiothorac Vasc Anesth.* 2019;33(10):2781-2796.
2. O'Neill WC. Sonographic evaluation of renal failure. *Am J Kidney Dis.* 2000;35(6):1021-1038.

**2.** Correct Answer: B. Venous: away, arterial: toward

*Rationale:* Assessment of the kidney is accomplished with a curvilinear or a phased array probe. A large curvilinear abdominal ultrasound probe (2-5 MHz) is preferred, due to improved tissue penetration of a wider field of view, allowing for a complete view of the kidney for measurements. A phased array probe (2-10 MHz), commonly used for echocardiography, can also be used for abdominal ultrasound. Its smaller footprint compared to the curvilinear abdominal ultrasound probe makes it easier to obtain images from smaller acoustic windows, such as within an intercostal space.

In order to interrogate renal blood flow, a probe should be positioned in the posterior axillary line to obtain a longitudinal view of the kidney. Pulsed-wave Doppler is used, after the interlobar vessels are localized (usually with color Doppler, using a reduced Nyquist limit [10-25 cm/s]). It is important to adjust the sample volume, to use the low-velocity filter in order to avoid low-velocity signals, and to use a low pulse repetition frequency of 1 to 1.5 kHz to avoid aliasing. Using pulsed-wave Doppler interrogation, renal arterial flow will be displayed in the positive velocity range, directed toward the renal cortex and toward the ultrasound probe, whereas renal venous flow will be displayed in the negative velocity range, directed away from the renal cortex and away from the ultrasound probe (**Figure 62.2**).

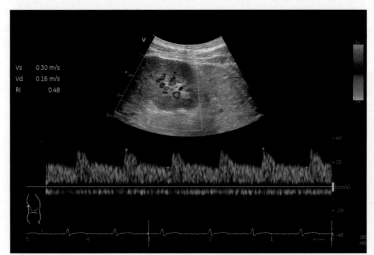

**Figure 62.2** Arterial and venous Doppler flow evaluation in the kidney. A longitudinal view of the kidney is obtained using 2D ultrasound imaging. Color flow Doppler is then used to visualize the vascular structures. In this case, red represents flow coming toward the ultrasound probe,

and blue represents blood flow going away from the ultrasound probe. Then, using pulsed-wave Doppler, sampling of the interlobar vessels can be obtained. Positive velocities represent arterial flow and negative velocities represent venous flow. A renal resistive index (RRI) can be calculated from the peak systolic (PS) and the end-diastolic (ED) velocities.

### Selected References

1. Beaubien-Souligny W, Benkreira A, Robillard P, et al. Alterations in portal vein flow and intrarenal venous flow are associated with acute kidney injury after cardiac surgery: a prospective Observational Cohort Study. *J Am Heart Assoc.* 2018;7(19):e009961.
2. Beaubien-Souligny W, Denault A, Robillard P, Desjardins G. The role of point-of-care ultrasound monitoring in cardiac surgical patients with acute kidney injury. *J Cardiothorac Vasc Anesth.* 2019;33(10):2781-2796.

---

**3.** Correct Answer: A. (peak systolic velocity – end-diastolic velocity)/peak systolic velocity

*Rationale:* The RRI, or Pourcelot index, can be calculated from the maximal velocity (Vmax) occurring during systole and the minimal velocity (Vmin) occurring during diastole. An RRI between 0.50 and 0.70 is considered normal.

The RRI increases in clinical situations characterized by renal vasoconstriction or increased intracapsular pressure such as acute tubular necrosis, hepatorenal syndrome, intra-abdominal compartment syndrome, venous congestion, acute rejection in a renal transplant, or urinary obstruction. A high RRI ($> 0.7$) is an early marker of acute kidney injury and predicts progression toward severe stages of severe acute injury.

### Selected References

1. Beaubien-Souligny W, Denault A, Robillard P, Desjardins G. The role of point-of-care ultrasound monitoring in cardiac surgical patients with acute kidney injury. *J Cardiothorac Vasc Anesth.* 2019;33(10):2781-2796.
2. Granata A, Zanoli L, Clementi S, Fatuzzo P, Di Nicolo P, Fiorini F. Resistive intrarenal index: myth or reality? *Br J Radiol.* 2014;87(1038):20140004.
3. Tang WH, Kitai T. Intrarenal venous flow: a window into the congestive kidney failure phenotype of heart failure? *JACC Heart Fail.* 2016;4(8):683-686.

---

**4.** Correct Answer: B. Aortic insufficiency

*Rationale:* The RRI is calculated as the ratio of renal end-systolic (ES) minus end-diastolic (ED) velocities over end-systolic velocity (ES) (**Figure 62.3**). Hemodynamic alterations that increase arterial RRI occur with either an increase in systolic velocity or a decrease in the diastolic velocity, which therefore increases the renal pulse pressure. Thus, renal artery stenosis is associated with a decreased RRI, generally $< 0.6$, as a result of lower pulse pressure because of the reduced peak systolic velocity distal to the stenosis. Under normal conditions, bradycardia and aortic insufficiency should increase stroke volume, pulse pressure, and systolic velocities, and therefore increase the RRI. It is important to remember that the RRI is measured at the level of the intrarenal arteries (segmental or interlobar). Any condition associated with reduced diastolic arterial pressure can also increase the resistance index. If two completely different arterial Doppler sites (hepatic artery, splenic artery, or middle cerebral artery for instance) have similar resistance index, it is unlikely that there is a renal problem but a more global one, such as aortic insufficiency.

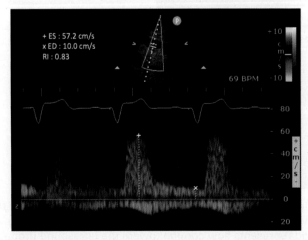

**Figure 62.3** Renal resistive index (RRI). The RRI is calculated as the ratio of renal systolic (ES) minus diastolic (ED) velocities over systolic velocity (ES).

Selected Reference

1. Granata A, Zanoli L, Clementi S, Fatuzzo P, Di Nicolo P, Fiorini F. Resistive intrarenal index: myth or reality? *Br J Radiol.* 2014;87(1038):20140004.

**5.** Correct Answer: **B. Acute tubular necrosis**

*Rationale:* An isolated increase in the RRI, concomitantly with normal systemic resistive indices, signifies an intrarenal etiology. Decompensated right heart failure, venous congestion, or advanced age, for example, tend to increase resistive indices in multiple different organs (liver, spleen, kidney). In acute tubular necrosis, renal flow dynamics will be altered without alteration in other organs. It is therefore important to not interpret any abnormal arterial Doppler signal in isolation.

Selected Reference

1. Beaubien-Souligny W, Denault A, Robillard P, Desjardins G. The role of point-of-care ultrasound monitoring in cardiac surgical patients with acute kidney injury. *J Cardiothorac Vasc Anesth.* 2019;33(10):2781-2796.

**6.** Correct Answer: **D. A decrease in RRI**

*Rationale:* The RRI has been shown to decrease by increasing the mean arterial pressure with norepinephrine from 65 to 75 mm Hg in patients with septic shock. This decrease in the RRI was also associated with an increase in urine output. A decrease in the RRI might result from a proportionally larger increase in diastolic flow velocity; however, increasing mean arterial pressure from 75 to 85 mm Hg did not result in any additional decrease in the RRI. Individual optimization of mean arterial pressure with norepinephrine using end-organ perfusion indices such as the RRI might be useful to obtain optimal end-organ blood flow. This approach could be useful in patients with cardiovascular disease or long-term hypertension that might have shifted their autoregulatory curves.

Selected Reference

1. Deruddre S, Cheisson G, Mazoit JX, Vicaut E, Benhamou D, Duranteau J. Renal arterial resistance in septic shock: effects of increasing mean arterial pressure with norepinephrine on the renal resistive index assessed with Doppler ultrasonography. *Intensive Care Med.* 2007;33(9):1557-1562.

**7.** Correct Answer: **A. 2-4-1-3**

*Rationale:* Stages of renal venous congestion can be defined by different intrarenal venous flow patterns. The absence of congestion will present as a continuous venous flow without any restriction of venous drainage. The first stage of congestion will present as a brief interruption of venous flow during atrial contraction. The second stage will present with biphasic venous flow with interruption between systole and diastole, and finally, the third stage of renal venous congestion will appear as a monophasic venous flow restricted to diastole. Congestion from elevated right atrial pressure will distend the venous system, creating a rigid liquid column between the right atrium and intrarenal venous system. Central venous oscillation will be transmitted to end-organ individual venous systems.

It is also important to mention that left renal vein phasicity may be attenuated due to its anatomic location and possible entrapment between the abdominal aorta and superior mesenteric artery (Nutcracker syndrome). Lastly, the left ovarian or left testicular veins drain into the left renal vein and may, in rare circumstances of ovarian or testicular varicosis, affect renal venous flow (**Figure 62.4**).

Selected References

1. Beaubien-Souligny W, Denault AY. Real-time assessment of renal venous flow by transesophageal echography during cardiac surgery. *A A Pract.* 2019;12(1):30-32.
2. Husain-Syed F, Birk HW, Ronco C, et al. Doppler-derived renal venous stasis index in the prognosis of right heart failure. *J Am Heart Assoc.* 2019;8(21):e013584.

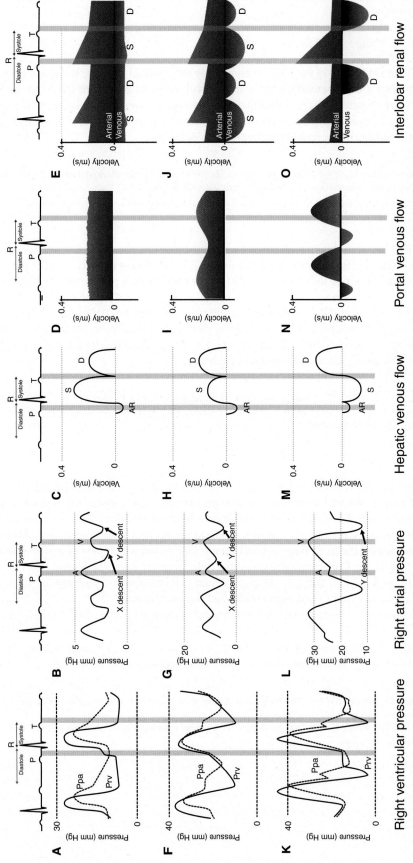

Right ventricular pressure   Right atrial pressure   Hepatic venous flow   Portal venous flow   Interlobar renal flow

**Figure 62.4** Correlation between right ventricular pressure waveform, right atrial pressure waveform, hepatic venous flow (HVF), portal venous flow, and interlobar renal flow. Right ventricular pressure (Prv), right atrial pressure, HVF, portal venous flow, and interlobar arterial and venous renal flow in normal patients (A, B, C, D, E) and typical patterns commonly observed in patients with mild (F, G, H, I, J) and severe (K, L, M, N, O) right ventricular dysfunction. AR, atrial reversal HVF velocity; D, diastolic HVF Doppler velocity; Ppa, pulmonary artery pressure; S, systolic HVF velocity. (Adapted from Raymond M, Gronlykke L, Couture EJ, et al. Perioperative Right Ventricular Pressure Monitoring in Cardiac Surgery. *J Cardiothorac Vasc Anesth.* 2019;33(4):1090-104.)

**8.** Correct Answer: B. (Peak maximal venous flow velocity − nadir flow velocity)/peak maximal venous flow velocity

*Rationale:* Renal venous flow impedance can be calculated from the maximal venous flow velocity (Vmax) and the minimal venous flow velocity (Vmin) occurring during the cardiac cycle.

Classification of renal venous flow using different categories may miss important distinctions within categories. In order to better define renal congestion, renal venous flow impedance has been proposed as an index to evaluate renal congestion using a continuum based on Doppler measurement of renal venous flow. A normal renal venous flow impedance should be near 0, as renal venous flow should be continuous throughout the cardiac cycle. The presence of renal congestion will appear as increasing values of venous flow impedance since systolic venous flow and, eventually, diastolic venous flow will reduce in duration.

**Selected References**

1. Damman K, Voors AA. The fastest way to the failing heart is through the kidneys. *JACC Heart Fail.* 2017;5(9):682-683.
2. Husain-Syed F, Birk HW, Ronco C, et al. Doppler-derived renal venous stasis index in the prognosis of right heart failure. *J Am Heart Assoc.* 2019;8(21):e013584.
3. Nijst P, Martens P, Dupont M, Tang WHW, Mullens W. Intrarenal flow alterations during transition from euvolemia to intravascular volume expansion in heart failure patients. *JACC Heart Fail.* 2017;5(9):672-681.

**9.** Correct Answer: A. Increase of renal venous impedance index and unchanged arterial resistance index

*Rationale:* A recent study by Nijst, et al. showed that intravascular volume expansion with 0.6 L led to unchanged renal arterial resistance indices in patients with or without heart failure. Conversely, a significant blunting of venous flow in heart failure patients following a fluid bolus could be demonstrated. In addition, blunting of renal venous flow during intravascular volume expansion was related to a lower diuretic response in heart failure patients with and without reduced ejection fraction, independent of the underlying renal function.

**Selected Reference**

1. Nijst P, Martens P, Dupont M, Tang WHW, Mullens W. Intrarenal flow alterations during transition from euvolemia to intravascular volume expansion in heart failure patients. *JACC Heart Fail.* 2017;5(9):672-681.

**10.** Correct Answer: C. A high venous impedance index will predict a low response to diuretics.

*Rationale:* Nijst, et al. showed that in heart failure patients, the highest venous impedance index during intravascular volume expansion demonstrated a lower diuretic response after 3 and 24 hours. Importantly, the relation between venous impedance index and renal response remained significant after correction for the underlying glomerular filtration rate.

**Selected Reference**

1. Nijst P, Martens P, Dupont M, Tang WHW, Mullens W. Intrarenal flow alterations during transition from euvolemia to intravascular volume expansion in heart failure patients. *JACC Heart Fail.* 2017;5(9):672-681.

**11.** Correct Answer: A. Increase in serum BNP level

*Rationale:* The RVSI has been proposed to characterize the full continuum of renal congestion (**Figure 62.5**). It indicates the proportion of the cardiac cycle during which there is no renal venous outlet flow and is calculated as follows:

(cardiac cycle duration − venous flow duration)/cardiac cycle duration

In nonpathologic conditions, the index is zero due to the presence of continuous renal venous flow. Progression of venous congestion decreases free venous flow, and a time interval appears where there is an absence of venous flow. This leads to a decrease in total venous flow duration, hence an increase in the RVSI. It has been shown that the RVSI might be superior to individual intrarenal venous flow patterns in predicting outcome, probably due to the fact that the former is a continuum that might have the ability to catch changes that discrete classification might have missed. Clinical parameters of right heart dysfunction and hypervolemia (e.g., BNP elevation) are associated with an increase in the RVSI.

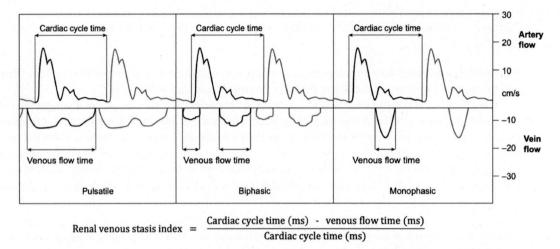

$$\text{Renal venous stasis index} = \frac{\text{Cardiac cycle time (ms)} - \text{venous flow time (ms)}}{\text{Cardiac cycle time (ms)}}$$

**Figure 62.5** Renal venous stasis index (RVSI). Pulsed-wave Doppler samples of renal congestion patterns in the interlobar renal vessel. Cardiac cycle length is based on electrocardiogram or intrarenal arterial flow, whereas venous flow time is used to evaluate congestion or stasis. Under physiologic conditions, venous drainage is continuous and uninterrupted, hence RVSI is zero, and it increases with rising severity of congestion. The figure illustrates the method of measurement of RVSI in different stages of congestion. ms indicates milliseconds.

**Selected Reference**

1. Husain-Syed F, Birk HW, Ronco C, et al. Doppler-derived renal venous stasis index in the prognosis of right heart failure. *J Am Heart Assoc.* 2019;8(21):e013584.

---

**12.** Correct Answer: **B. Discontinuous monophasic renal venous flow**

*Rationale:* Overzealous fluid resuscitation in a patient with right ventricular failure will lead to an increase in central venous pressure that will be transmitted to end-organ venous systems. The resultant increase in mean venous systemic pressures will be perceived as the last stage of renal venous congestion, which is a discontinuous monophasic renal venous flow pattern. Venous impedance will approach 1, and a venous stasis index will be greater than 0.5. The arterial RRI will tend to increase as diastolic flow will be decreased due to an increase in intra-abdominal and intracapsular renal pressure as a consequence of the accumulation of extravascular fluid.

**Selected Reference**

1. Beaubien-Souligny W, Denault AY. Real-time assessment of renal venous flow by transesophageal echography during cardiac surgery. *A A Pract.* 2019;12(1):30-32.

---

**13.** Correct Answer: **D. Right heart function**

*Rationale:* The recognized main determinants of renal venous flow patterns are central venous pressure, abdominal pressure and right heart function. Phasic variations of renal venous flow are associated with respiration and right heart function. As mentioned earlier, venous flow phasicity of the left kidney might be blunted due to entrapment of the left renal vein between the abdominal aorta and the superior mesenteric artery (Nutcracker syndrome). As veins are high-capacitance vessels with minimal resistance, pulsatile venous flow patterns emerge from surrounding tissue compliance. Besides the association with tissue characteristics, renal venous flow is strictly dependent on right heart function. During end-diastole, any increase in central venous pressures can be transmitted to renal veins, especially in patients with congestion in the IVC. This clinical portrait of venous congestion will impede normal venous drainage from the kidneys and can result in reversal of renal venous flow.

**Selected Reference**

1. Grande D, Terlizzese P, Iacoviello M. Role of imaging in the evaluation of renal dysfunction in heart failure patients. *World J Nephrol.* 2017;6(3):123-131.

**14. Correct Answer: D. High systolic velocity of the lateral portion of the tricuspid annular plane**

*Rationale:* The presence of renal venous congestion, as evidenced by a discontinuous monophasic venous flow, is usually due to reduced right heart function and elevated central venous pressure. Any marker of reduced right ventricular function (reduction in right ventricular fractional area change, moderate to severe tricuspid regurgitation, lower hepatic systolic to diastolic velocity ratio [hepatic vein S/D <0.55], and high right atrial pressure) could be found in a patient with discontinuous monophasic venous flow with renal Doppler evaluation. High systolic velocity of the lateral portion of the tricuspid annular plane suggests good right ventricular function.

### Selected References

1. Iida N, Seo Y, Sai S, et al. Clinical implications of intrarenal hemodynamic evaluation by doppler ultrasonography in heart failure. *JACC Heart Fail.* 2016;4(8):674-682.
2. Tang WH, Kitai T. Intrarenal venous flow: a window into the congestive kidney failure phenotype of heart failure? *JACC Heart Fail.* 2016;4(8):683-686.

**15. Correct Answer: D. Increased venous flow velocity**

*Rationale:* Normal intra-abdominal pressure is in the range of 5 to 7 mm Hg in critically ill patients. Intra-abdominal hypertension is defined by sustained or repeated pathologic elevation of intra-abdominal pressure >12 mm Hg. Acute compartment syndrome is defined as a sustained intra-abdominal pressure of >20 mm Hg (with or without an abdominal perfusion pressure < 60 mm Hg) that is associated with new organ dysfunction or failure.

An increase in intra-abdominal pressure is associated with decreased venous flow from intra-abdominal organs due to a loss of the venous gradient between the organ and the right atrium. A decrease in arterial diastolic flow velocity is also seen in intra-abdominal hypertension, which results in an increase in the arterial resistive index and lowers the venous flow velocity.

### Selected Reference

1. Kirkpatrick AW, Roberts DJ, De Waele J, et al. Intra-abdominal hypertension and the abdominal compartment syndrome: updated consensus definitions and clinical practice guidelines from the World Society of the Abdominal Compartment Syndrome. *Intensive Care Med.* 2013;39(7):1190-1206.

**16. Correct Answer: B. Evaluation of bladder volume**

*Rationale:* The first and perhaps the easiest thing to exclude is a dislodged or obstructed Foley catheter, which will present with a dilated bladder. Once a malfunctioning Foley is excluded (or other cause of bladder outlet obstruction), more sophisticated ultrasound techniques can be used to identify the etiology of an acute kidney injury.

### Selected References

1. Beaubien-Souligny W, Denault A, Robillard P, Desjardins G. The role of point-of-care ultrasound monitoring in cardiac surgical patients with acute kidney injury. *J Cardiothorac Vasc Anesth.* 2019;33(10):2781-2796.
2. Denault A, Canty D, Azzam M, Amir A, Gebhard CE. Whole body ultrasound in the operating room and intensive care unit. *Korean J Anesthesiol.* 2019;72(5):413-428.

# 63 | DETECTION OF FREE FLUID AND AIR

Samir Sethi, Sana Na Javeed, and Rohan K. Panchamia

1. Which of the following ultrasound findings during a focused assessment with sonography in trauma (FAST) examination is concerning for intra-abdominal free fluid?

   A. Anechoic area between the liver and right kidney
   B. Hyperechoic area between the diaphragm and spleen
   C. Edge-shaped hypoechoic area in Morison's pouch that is bounded on both sides by echogenic lines
   D. A mirror image of the liver seen above the diaphragm

2. Regarding the FAST examination, which of the following statements is *most* true?

   A. FAST is more sensitive in patients with higher body mass index (BMI).
   B. FAST is able to identify free intra-abdominal and/or pericardial fluid in the trauma patient.
   C. FAST is sensitive for intra-abdominal organ injury.
   D. FAST is able to reliably identify retroperitoneal hemorrhages.

3. Which of the following is the *most* sensitive window for detecting intra-abdominal free fluid?

   A. Right upper quadrant (RUQ) view
   B. Left upper quadrant (LUQ) view
   C. Subxiphoid view
   D. Suprapubic view

4. Which of the following statements is most accurate in regard to a LUQ examination?

   A. It is the most easily visualized of the four FAST views.
   B. It is typically found more caudad and anterior when compared to the RUQ view.
   C. The phrenicocolic ligament restricts the flow of free fluid to the LUQ.
   D. Free fluid preferentially flows between the left paracolic gutter and the LUQ.

5. The landmarks used to obtain the RUQ window during the FAST exam are best described by:

The intersection of the horizontal subxiphoid line with the midaxillary line

   A. The intersection of the horizontal subxiphoid line with the posterior axillary line
   B. Inferior to the xiphoid process
   C. Midline and just superior to the pubic symphysis

6. A 45-year-old woman presents to the Emergency Department after a motor vehicle collision. She is awake and alert, complaining of abdominal pain. Her BP is 110/55 mm Hg, and HR is 95 bpm. She has an abrasion across her abdomen consistent with the shape of a seat belt. A FAST examination is performed, and a hyperechoic density is noted circumferentially around the right kidney. What is the *most* likely etiology of this finding?

   A. Subcapsular renal hematoma
   B. Hemoperitoneum with liquid blood
   C. Hemoperitoneum with clotted blood
   D. A normal appearance of perinephric fat

7. Which of the following findings is shown in **Figure 63.1?**

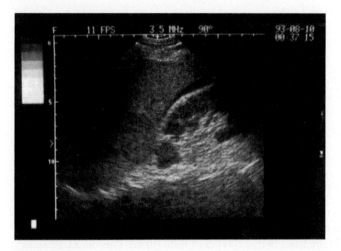

**Figure 63.1**

   A. Free fluid in Morison's pouch
   B. Free fluid in the pelvis
   C. Pleural effusion
   D. Pericardial effusion

8. Which finding is identified by the *red arrow* in **Figure 63.2**?

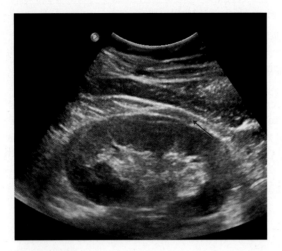

**Figure 63.2**

A. Spine sign
B. Mirror artifact
C. Intra-abdominal free fluid
D. Double line sign

9. Which structure would be *least* likely to cause a false-positive FAST result?

A. Gallbladder
B. Stomach contents
C. Perinephric fat in the RUQ
D. Full bladder

10. Which of the following is *not* a limitation of the FAST examination?

A. A negative examination does not rule out intra-abdominal injuries.
B. Clotted blood does not appear as anechoic fluid.
C. The FAST examination cannot differentiate between types of fluid (urine, bile, blood, or ascites).
D. The FAST examination is only able to reliably detect more than 500 mL of free fluid.

11. Which sign (*red arrow*) is depicted in the RUQ of **Figure 63.3**?

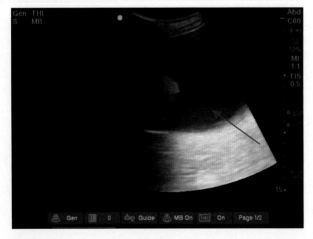

**Figure 63.3**

A. Plankton sign
B. Hematocrit sign
C. Double line sign
D. Spine sign

12. Which ultrasound artifact is represented by the *red arrow* in the RUQ image shown in **Figure 63.4**?

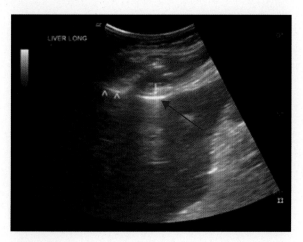

**Figure 63.4**

A. Mirror image
B. Acoustic enhancement
C. Enhanced peritoneal stripe
D. Rib shadow

13. In the supine patient, what is the best initial location to look for a pneumoperitoneum with ultrasound?

A. Right lumbar region
B. Suprapubic region
C. Left hypochondrium region (LUQ)
D. Right hypochondrium region (RUQ)

14. What maneuver can be performed to enhance the detection of intraperitoneal air with ultrasound?

A. Applying and then releasing slight pressure to an ultrasound transducer
B. Positioning the patient in the right lateral decubitus position
C. Asking the patient to take a deep breath
D. Placing the patient in Trendelenburg position

15. What is highlighted by the white arrow in the RUQ ultrasound shown in **Figure 63.5**?

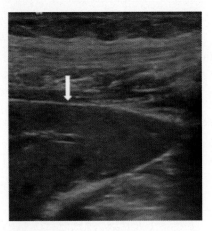

**Figure 63.5**

A. Pneumoperitoneum
B. Intraluminal free air
C. Pseudopneumoperitoneum
D. Normal peritoneum

16. In **Figure 63.6A-D,** which figure is *not* appropriately matched to the clinical scenario?

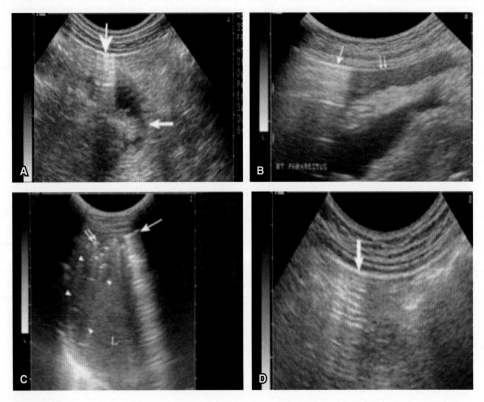

**Figure 63.6**

A. Figure 63.6A, a 30-year-old man with an ileal perforation
B. Figure 63.6B, a 35-year-old man with no acute medical pathology
C. Figure 63.6C, a 50-year-old male with perforation of a duodenal ulcer
D. Figure 63.6D, a 41-year-old woman who underwent laparoscopy 2 hours previously

# Chapter 63 ▪ Answers

**1.** Correct Answer: A. Anechoic area between the liver and right kidney

*Rationale:* Intra-abdominal free fluid normally appears anechoic on ultrasound, unless clotted blood is present, in which case the image can appear hyperechoic, hypoechoic, or have mixed echogenicity. RUQ abdominal ultrasound views obtained to look for fluid include Morison's pouch (hepatorenal recess), right paracolic gutter, and suprahepatic areas; the LUQ views evaluate the splenorenal recess, left paracolic gutter, and suprasplenic spaces in identifying free fluid. Perinephric fat is often confused for intra-abdominal fluid since both can appear as hypoechoic images; however, perinephric fat is bounded on both sides by echogenic lines, clearly distinguishing it from free fluid. The mirror image of the liver seen above the diaphragm, which is a strong reflector of ultrasound waves, is a normal artifact that essentially excludes the presence of a pleural effusion. See also **Figure 63.7.**

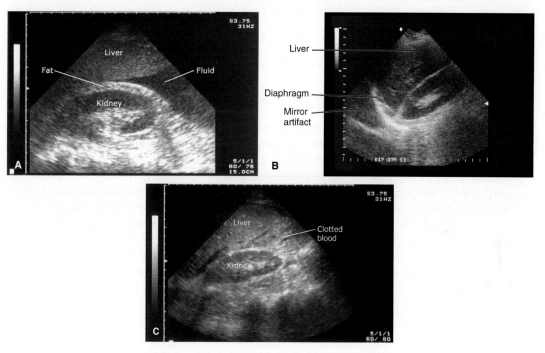

**Figure 63.7**

Selected References

1. Kelley K, Rose JS, Bair AE. Fundamentals of ultrasound. In: Cosby KS, Kendall JL, eds. *Practical Guide to Emergency Ultrasound.* 2nd ed. Wolters Kluwer; 2014:10-20.
2. Laselle BT, Kendall JL. Trauma. In: Cosby KS, Kendall JL, eds. *Practical Guide to Emergency Ultrasound.* 2nd ed. Wolters Kluwer; 2014:21-53.
3. Mohammad A, Hefny AF, Abu-Zidan FM. Focused assessment sonography for trauma (FAST) training: a systematic review. *World J Surg.* 2014;38(5):1009-1018.
4. Rozycki GS, Ochsner MG, Jaffin JH, Champion HR. Prospective evaluation of surgeons' use of ultrasound in the evaluation of trauma patients. *J Trauma.* 1993;34(4):516-526.

2. **Correct Answer: B.** FAST is able to identify free intra-abdominal and/or pericardial fluid in the trauma patient.

*Rationale:* FAST is a rapid ultrasonographic examination performed to determine the presence of fluid—blood in the trauma patient—within the peritoneum, pericardium, and/or thorax. It interrogates four different areas: subxiphoid, suprapubic, RUQ, and LUQ. One downside to the examination is that a significant volume of fluid is necessary to be reliably visualized sonographically (generally >100-200 mL). For this reason, serial examinations are encouraged if ongoing bleeding is suspected. Another limitation is the examination's inability to image the retroperitoneum due to overlying abdominal gas and viscera and suboptimal patient positioning. FAST has a lower sensitivity for the detection of solid organ injuries since they may not result in detectable free fluid, and has a very low sensitivity for hollow organ injuries. Obesity can severely limit the assessment of the peritoneal cavity and make the examination less useful.

Selected References
1. Abu-Zidan FM, Zayat I, Sheikh M, Mousa I, Behbehani A. Role of ultrasonography in blunt abdominal trauma: a prospective study. *Eur J Surg.* 1996;162:361-365.
2. Brahee D, Ogedegbe C, Hassler C, et al. Body mass index and abdominal ultrasound image quality: a pilot survey of sonographers. *J Diagn Med Sonogr.* 2013;29(2):66-72.
3. Richards JR, McGahan JP. Focused assessment with sonography in trauma (FAST) in 2017: what radiologists can learn. *Radiology.* 2017;283(1):30-48.
4. Rozycki GS, Root HD. The diagnosis of intraabdominal visceral injury. *J Trauma.* 2010;68(5):1019-1023.

3. **Correct Answer: A.** Right upper quadrant (RUQ) view

*Rationale:* In the supine patient, the RUQ window is the most sensitive view for identifying free peritoneal fluid. As fluid accumulates, it settles in dependent areas of the peritoneal cavity, primarily the RUQ and suprapubic regions. Changing the patient's position can increase the sensitivity in a specific area (e.g., Trendelenburg positioning will increase sensitivity in upper abdominal views, while reverse Trendelenburg may improve sensitivity from the suprapubic view). The space between the caudal liver edge and the inferior pole of the right kidney has recently been suggested to be a more sensitive indicator for free fluid than Morison's pouch. Although the suprapubic region is a dependent area of the peritoneal cavity, free fluid could be missed if the bladder is empty or if there is attenuation from bowel gas. The spleen's reduced size compared to the liver makes the LUQ window more challenging to view free fluid. The subxiphoid view would be helpful in determining the presence of pericardial effusion, not intraperitoneal free fluid. See also **Figure 63.8.**

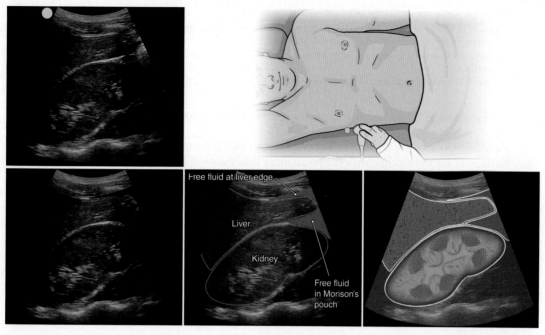

**Figure 63.8** Positive RUQ FAST view showing free fluid between caudal liver edge and inferior pole of the right kidney.

### Selected References

1. Focused Assessment with Sonography for Trauma (FAST). In: Loukas M, Burns D, eds. *Essential Ultrasound Anatomy*. 1st ed. Wolters Kluwer; 2020:246-258.
2. Lobo V, Hunter-Behrend M, Cullnan E, et al. Caudal edge of the liver in the right upper quadrant (RUQ) view is the most sensitive area for free fluid on the FAST Exam. *West J Emerg Med.* 2017;18(2):270-280.

4. **Correct Answer: C.** The phrenicocolic ligament restricts the flow of free fluid to the LUQ.

*Rationale/Critique:* Morison's pouch and the space between the caudal liver edge and inferior kidney pole are the most dependent areas in the supine patient. On the left, the phrenicocolic ligaments restrict the flow of fluid from the left paracolic gutter to the splenorenal recess; therefore, intra-abdominal free fluid tends to cross midline and move into RUQ spaces. The phrenicocolic ligaments also explain why LUQ fluid is more likely to collect in the subphrenic/suprasplenic space before accumulating in the splenorenal recess. The LUQ view is typically found more cephalad and posterior compared to the RUQ view. Due to the more posterior location and smaller size of the spleen when compared to the liver, free fluid in the LUQ is often more difficult to visualize on ultrasound. See also **Figure 63.9.**

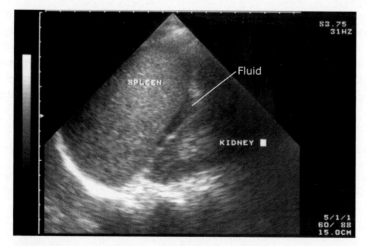

**Figure 63.9** Left upper quadrant FAST view, demonstrating the spleen, left kidney, and a hypoechoic region of free fluid between them.

Selected References

1. Bahner D, Blaivas M, Cohen HL, et al. AIUM practice guideline for the performance of the focused assessment with sonography for trauma (FAST) examination. *J Ultrasound Med*. 2008;27(2):313-318.
2. Laselle BT, Kendall JL. Trauma. In: Cosby KS, Kendall JL, eds. *Practical Guide to Emergency Ultrasound*. 2nd ed. Wolters Kluwer; 2014:21-53.
3. Rose JS. Ultrasound in abdominal trauma. *Emerg Med Clin North Am*. 2004;22:581-599.

---

**5. Correct Answer: A.** The intersection of the horizontal subxiphoid line with the midaxillary line

*Rationale/Critique:* RUQ structures are viewed by placing the ultrasound probe at the intersection of the horizontal subxiphoid line with the midaxillary line, between the 8th and 11th rib spaces. After identifying the hepatorenal recess, one should scan cephalad to look at the right subphrenic space, as well as caudally to assess the space between the caudal liver edge and inferior kidney pole. In the LUQ view, the spleen can often be technically more difficult to image due to its posterior location and smaller size. To obtain a window, place the probe at the intersection of the horizontal subxiphoid line with the posterior axillary line at the level of the 8th rib (generally about two rib spaces superior to the RUQ view, and more posterior). A probe is placed inferior to the xiphoid process to evaluate for pericardial fluid. Positioning the probe midline and just superior to the pubic symphysis is the approach taken to image the pelvis. See **Figure 63.10**.

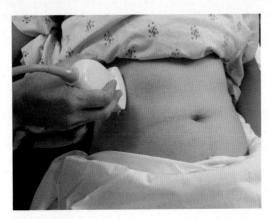

**Figure 63.10**

Selected Reference

1. Rozycki GS, Ochsner MG, Feliciano DV, et al. Early detection of hemoperitoneum by ultrasound examination of the right upper quadrant: a multicenter study. *J Trauma*. 1998;45(5):878-883.

---

**6. Correct Answer: D.** A normal appearance of perinephric fat

*Rationale/Critique:* Perinephric fat can be confused for clotted blood or free fluid in Morison's pouch. It is usually of even thickness, hypoechoic with sharp borders, and does not shift with movement. In contrast, free fluid tends to appear anechoic and can accumulate more in the RUQ with changes in positioning. In this case, her presentation immediately after injury makes clotted blood less likely, and a hypoechoic region of liquid blood is not described in the stem. A subcapsular renal hematoma would be expected to have a hypoechoic appearance initially, like free fluid, although after a clot develops, it may appear hyperechoic.

Selected References

1. Salen PN, Melanson SW, Heller MB. The focused abdominal sonography for trauma (FAST) examination: considerations and recommendations for training physicians in the use of a new clinical tool. *Acad Emerg Med*. 2000;7(2):162-168.
2. Sierzenski PR, Schofer JM, Bauman MJ. The double-line sign: a false positive finding on the focused assessment with sonography for trauma (FAST) examination. *J Emerg Med*. 2011;40(2):188-189.

**7.** Correct Answer: A. Free fluid in Morison's pouch

*Rationale:* This RUQ image (Figure 63.1) demonstrates free fluid in Morison's pouch: an anechoic stripe in the potential space between the liver and right kidney. An ultrasonographic fluid collection in the pelvis would appear in the rectovesical pouch (space between the bladder and prostate) in males and in the pouch of Douglas (posterior to the uterus) in females. A pleural effusion is found above the diaphragm in the RUQ or LUQ view, and a pericardial effusion is seen best on a subxiphoid view.

### Selected References

1. Branney SW, Wolfe RE, Moore EE, et al. Quantitative sensitivity of ultrasound in detecting free intraperitoneal fluid. *J Trauma Acute Care Surg.* 1995;39(2):375-380.
2. Pearl WS, Todd KH. Ultrasonography for the initial evaluation of blunt abdominal trauma: a review of prospective trials. *Ann Emerg Med.* 1996;27(3):353-361.

**8.** Correct Answer: D. Double line sign

*Rationale:* Figure 63.2 demonstrates the double line sign, which is often mistaken for intra-abdominal clotted blood or free fluid in Morison's pouch on the RUQ examination. The red arrow highlights two hyperechoic fascial edges (the double line sign) outlining the perinephric fat that surrounds the kidney. Clotted blood in Morison's pouch would not have these two hyperechoic lines surrounding it. A mirror image of the liver parenchyma above the diaphragm is a normal artifact and excludes the presence of a significant pleural effusion. The spine sign is abnormal visualization of thoracic vertebral bodies above the diaphragm, which signals the presence of a pleural effusion.

### Selected References

1. Auckland AK. Unexplained hematocrit drop. In: Sanders RC, ed. *Clinical Sonography: A Practical Guide.* 5th ed. Wolters Kluwer; 2016:588-595.
2. Patwa AS, Cipot S, Lomibao A. Prevalence of the "double-line" sign when performing focused assessment with sonography in trauma (FAST) examinations. *Intern Emerg Med.* 2015;10(6):721-724.

**9.** Correct Answer: D. Full bladder

*Rationale/Critique:* Inexperienced ultrasonographers may misinterpret normal abdominal structures for free fluid. On abdominal ultrasound, free fluid has sharp edges, dives between structures, and shifts with movement or respiration, features that help distinguish it from normal fluid-filled structures. Gastric contents typically present as a mix of hypoechoic and hyperechoic densities, and again commonly have rounded edges. Perinephric fat located near Morison's pouch is identified by the double line sign and has a higher echodensity than fresh blood. In the suprapubic region, acoustic enhancement produced by urine in the bladder can obscure posteriorly positioned free fluid, generating a false-negative examination. Therefore, it is important to scan in both transverse and sagittal planes to completely assess for free fluid in the pelvis. See also **Figure 63.11**.

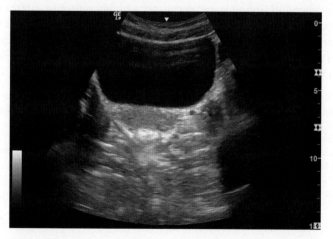

**Figure 63.11** An axial view of the pelvis, demonstrating a hypoechoic full bladder, with posterior acoustic enhancement.

Selected Reference
1. Jang T, Kryder G, Sineff S, Naunheim R, Aubin C, Kaji AH. The technical errors of physicians learning to perform focused assessment with sonography in trauma. *Acad Emerg Med.* 2012;19(1):98-101.

**10.** Correct Answer: D. The FAST examination is only able to reliably detect more than 500 mL of free fluid.

*Rationale:* While ultrasound is a very useful tool to detect intra-abdominal free fluid, it is crucial to understand its limitations. A negative examination does not rule out a solid organ injury, and if one is suspected, further testing including a computed tomography (CT) scan should be done. It has particularly poor sensitivity for hollow organ injuries. FAST examinations performed in patients with a delayed presentation may show clotted blood, which tends to appear hypoechoic and not anechoic, on ultrasound. While ultrasound can help detect fluid collections in the abdomen, it fails to distinguish blood from other fluid types like ascites, urine, or bile. Ultrasound has been shown to be sensitive in detecting anywhere from 150 to 500 mL of intraperitoneal free fluid, depending on the experience of the ultrasonographer.

Selected Reference
1. Kornezos I, Chatziioannou A, Kokkonouzis I, et al. Findings and limitations of focused ultrasound as a possible screening test in stable adult patients with blunt abdominal trauma: a Greek study. *Eur Radiol.* 2010;20(1):234-238.

**11.** Correct Answer: B. Hematocrit sign

*Rationale:* Figure 63.3 shows a large amount of free fluid in the RUQ. Occasionally, as in this image, cellular components settle in a layering effect called the hematocrit sign. The plankton sign is the observation of swirling debris within an anechoic pleural effusion, which cannot easily be demonstrated on a still image. The double line sign (as described previously) is indicative of perinephric fat, which is often confused with free fluid. The spine sign is the ability to visualize the thoracic vertebral bodies through the pleural spaces, as a consequence of a pleural effusion.

Selected Reference
1. Bolliger CT, Herth FJF, Mayo PH, Miyazawa T, Beamis JF. eds. Clinical chest ultrasound: from the ICU to the bronchoscopy suite. *Prog Respir Res.* Basel, Karger. 2009;37:I-IX.

**12.** Correct Answer: C. Enhanced peritoneal stripe

*Rationale:* The enhanced peritoneal stripe sign describes a highly echogenic and thickened peritoneal line associated with a pneumoperitoneum. Under normal conditions, ultrasound waves pass through the anterior abdominal wall and contact peritoneal fluid and solid organs, resulting in a smooth, thin peritoneal line. However, the accumulation of air in the abdomen produces a significant acoustic impedance mismatch at the peritoneum-gas interface, creating a bright reflection with the sonographic appearance of peritoneal enhancement and thickening. If large quantities of air are present, different types of reverberation artifacts, including a comet tail artifact (fleeting, echogenic vertical artifact) can be seen. A mirror image artifact is seen when ultrasound waves encounter a highly reflective surface (e.g., diaphragm), generating multiple beam reflections and a mirror image of an object above the reflector. Fluid-filled structures increase transmission of the ultrasound beam and can enhance the appearance of deeper structures, an artifact known as acoustic enhancement. A rib shadow would occur shallow to the peritoneal line, as a bright reflection with a hypoechoic "shadow" extending deep to it.

Selected References
1. Asrani A. Sonographic diagnosis of pneumoperitoneum using the 'enhancement of the peritoneal stripe sign.' A prospective study. *Emerg Radiol.* 2007 Apr;14(1):29-39.
2. Goudie A. Detection of intraperitoneal free gas by ultrasound. *Australas J Ultrasound Med.* 2013 May;16(2):56-61.
3. Prabhu SJ, Kanal K, Bhargava P, Vaidya S, Dighe MK. Ultrasound artifacts: classification, applied physics with illustrations, and imaging appearances. *Ultrasound Q.* 2014 Jun;30(2):145-157.

**13.** Correct Answer: D. Right hypochondrium region (RUQ)

*Rationale:* Due to its low density, air will rise to the highest point in the peritoneal cavity. In the supine patient, this location is anterior or superficial to the liver. A practical approach to visualizing free air is scanning over the epigastric area with a curved array transducer, then moving to the right hypochondrium. Repositioning the patient in the left lateral decubitus position could further displace free air over the region. Once over a region of interest, the sonographer can switch to a linear high-frequency transducer to increase the sensitivity of detecting free air.

Selected References
1. Asrani A. Sonographic diagnosis of pneumoperitoneum using the 'enhancement of the peritoneal stripe sign.' A prospective study. *Emerg Radiol.* 2007 Apr;14(1):29-39.
2. Kricun BJ, Horrow MM. Pneumoperitoneum. *Ultrasound Q.* 2012 Jun;28(2):137-138.

**14.** Correct Answer: A. Applying and then releasing slight pressure to an ultrasound transducer

*Rationale/Critique:* Shifting a patient from supine to a left lateral decubitus position can move free air from the anterior liver to the lateral aspect of the liver, confirming its free movement and enhancing the operator's ability to detect its presence. Nevertheless, clinical circumstances may render repositioning unsafe, in which case the "scissors" maneuver can be applied to replicate shifting positions. This technique involves orienting a linear-array transducer parasagittally over the liver to see if the enhanced peritoneal stripe and acoustic reverberations, sonographic findings suggestive of pneumoperitoneum, are present. If free air is suspected, the operator can then apply gentle pressure to the caudal aspect of the transducer, shifting air away from the anterior liver to other parts of the peritoneal cavity, attenuating the appearance of the peritoneal stripe. Upon the release of probe pressure, free air should relocate to the anterior liver and positive intraperitoneal sonographic findings should become more prominent.

Selected References
1. Goudie A. Detection of intraperitoneal free gas by ultrasound. *Australas J Ultrasound Med.* 2013 May;16(2):56-61.
2. Karahan OI, Kurt A, Yikilmaz A, Kahriman G. New method for the detection of intraperitoneal free air by sonography: scissors maneuver. *J Clin Ultrasound.* 2004 Oct;32(8):381-385.

**15.** Correct Answer: D. Normal peritoneum

*Rationale:* The structure is a normal peritoneal stripe seen at the interface between the anterior abdominal wall and liver. It is described as a discrete, thin line that is echogenic to surrounding tissue, wedged between abdominal wall musculature and underlying intra-abdominal fluid or solid organs. With the introduction of pathologic air, the peritoneal stripe becomes enhanced, highlighting the soft tissue-gas interface, and appears as a thickened bright line—known as the enhanced peritoneal stripe (sign). Large quantities of air can yield shadowing, comet-tail, and/or reverberation artifacts, in addition to the enhanced peritoneal stripe. Intraluminal air (physiologic air) can be confused for pathologic air since both produce similar ultrasound artifacts. Nevertheless, there are several features that distinguish intraluminal air from intra-abdominal air: (1) an association with a normal overlying peritoneal line; (2) intraluminal air will move with bowel peristalsis; and (3) gas within bowel will be near the peritoneal line, but separated from it by bowel wall (hypoechoic line). Pseudoperitoneum refers to Chilaiditi syndrome, a condition where the bowel is sandwiched between the liver and diaphragm, mimicking free air under the diaphragm. Shifting the patient's position should show that there isn't mobile pathologic air in the peritoneum. See **Figure 63.12**, with the enhanced peritoneal stripe (*downward arrow*) juxtaposed with normal peritoneal stripe (*upward arrow*).

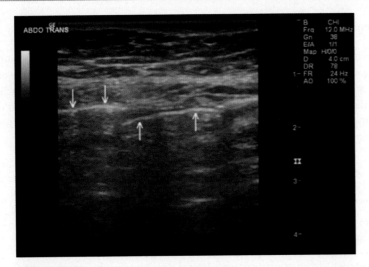

**Figure 63.12**

**Selected References**

1. Asrani A. Sonographic diagnosis of pneumoperitoneum using the 'enhancement of the peritoneal stripe sign.' A prospective study. *Emerg Radiol.* 2007 Apr;14(1):29-39.
2. Goudie A. Detection of intraperitoneal free gas by ultrasound. *Australas J Ultrasound Med.* 2013 May;16(2):56-61.
3. Hoffmann B, Nürnberg D, Westergaard MC. Focus on abnormal air: diagnostic ultrasonography for the acute abdomen. *Eur J Emerg Med.* 2012 Oct;19(5):284-291.
4. Indiran V, Vinoth Kumar R, Jefferson B. Enhanced peritoneal stripe sign. *Abdom Radiol (NY).* 2018 Dec;43(12):3518-3519.
5. Kricun BJ, Horrow MM. Pneumoperitoneum. *Ultrasound Q.* 2012 Jun;28(2):137-138.

**16.** Correct Answer: B. Figure 63.6B, a 35-year-old man with no acute medical pathology

*Rationale:* Figure 63.6A-D depicts focal thickening and increased echogenicity of the peritoneal stripes, with concern for intraperitoneal free air. Of note, A-line reverberation artifacts are pictured; this is due to the ultrasound wave bouncing back and forth between the probe and soft tissue-gas interface, creating bright horizontal lines at uniform intervals. A healthy individual without known intra-abdominal pathology would be expected to have a discrete, smooth, slightly echogenic peritoneal stripe, certainly lacking any associated imaging artifacts, like shadowing or reverberations. See also **Figure 63.13.**

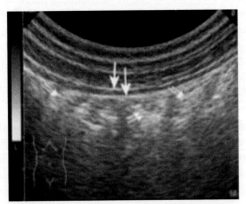

**Figure 63.13** Normal peritoneal stripe (*large arrows*) in a healthy male.

**Selected References**

1. Asrani A. Sonographic diagnosis of pneumoperitoneum using the 'enhancement of the peritoneal stripe sign.' A prospective study. *Emerg Radiol.* 2007 Apr;14(1):29-39.
2. Prabhu SJ, Kanal K, Bhargava P, Vaidya S, Dighe MK. Ultrasound artifacts: classification, applied physics with illustrations, and imaging appearances. *Ultrasound Q.* 2014 Jun;30(2):145-157.

# 64 | SMALL BOWEL OBSTRUCTION, PERFORATION, AND OTHER BOWEL PATHOLOGY

Gunter Michael Krauthamer and John T. Moeller

1. An 87-year-old man is admitted to the intensive care unit (ICU) for ascending cholangitis. Two days after admission, he complains of worsening abdominal pain, nausea, and vomiting. His nurse notes that he hasn't had a bowel movement in 48 hours. Point-of-care ultrasound of his abdomen reveals **Figure 64.1**.

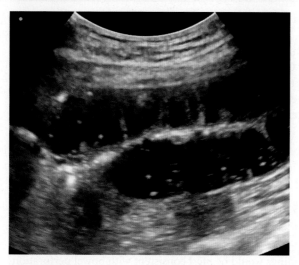

**Figure 64.1**

Which is the *most* appropriate next step in management?
A. Obtain a right upper quadrant ultrasound to evaluate for worsening biliary disease.
B. Obtain a surgical consult for bowel perforation.
C. Obtain a computed tomography (CT) scan to evaluate for gallstone ileus.
D. Obtain an abdominal X-ray to evaluate for pneumoperitoneum.

2. A 70-year-old man with diabetes is admitted to the hospital for septic shock, attributed to severe cellulitis of his left upper extremity. He begins treatment with intravenous (IV) clindamycin. Three days after admission, the patient begins to complain of profuse, watery diarrhea. On examination, he is diffusely tender, and his abdomen is tense. His vital signs are: temperature 39.0°C, BP 80/50 mm Hg, HR 125 bpm, and SpO$_2$ 90% on room air. Abdominal ultrasound reveals **Figure 64.2A** and **B.**

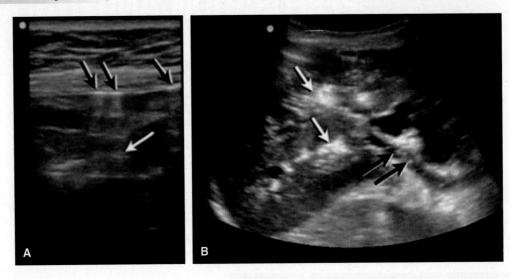

**Figure 64.2**

What is the *most* appropriate next step in his management?
A. Broaden antibiotic coverage to include *Clostridium difficile.*
B. Obtain a CT angiogram to evaluate for mesenteric ischemia.
C. Obtain an upright abdominal X-ray to evaluate for intraperitoneal free air.
D. Begin IV fluid resuscitation and emergently consult general surgery.

3. Which of the following is *most* closely associated with an ultrasonographic diagnosis of appendicitis?

A. Compressibility
B. Intraluminal air
C. Anterior to posterior measurement of 5 mm
D. Appendicolith

4. What combination of ultrasonographic findings would be *most* consistent with bowel perforation?

A. Enhanced echogenicity of the peritoneal stripe and thickened bowel loops
B. Target sign and surrounding localized free fluid
C. Dilated loops of bowel with keyboard sign
D. Thin peritoneal strip and dirty shadowing

5. A 46-year-old man sustained deep partial-thickness burns to his back and legs. He has a prolonged ICU course complicated by sepsis. Three weeks after admission, he abruptly develops epigastric abdominal pain and dyspnea. His abdomen is not distended, but is exquisitely tender. Ultrasound of his abdomen reveals **Figure 64.3**.

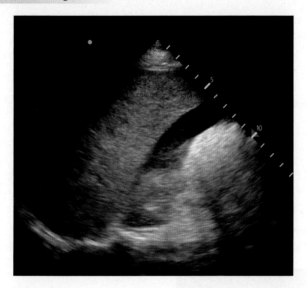

**Figure 64.3**

What is the *most* appropriate next step in his management?
A. Start stool softeners and encourage physical activity
B. Obtain a right upper quadrant ultrasound to evaluate for cholecystitis
C. Obtain a chest CT to further evaluate the pleural effusion
D. Begin resuscitation and get an emergent surgery consult

6. While working in a rural hospital, a nurse informs you that your patient is complaining of severe abdominal pain, nausea, and vomiting. On physical examination, the patient's abdomen is tense and diffusely tender. You are concerned about small bowel obstruction (SBO) and start evaluating the patient's abdomen with ultrasound. The patient's nurse asks if it would be better to obtain an acute abdominal series. You explain that ultrasound is preferable because:

A. While an acute abdominal series may have a higher sensitivity for diagnosing SBO, ultrasound has a higher specificity.
B. While an acute abdominal series may have a higher specificity for diagnosing SBO, ultrasound has a higher sensitivity.
C. X-ray and ultrasound have comparable sensitivity and specificity for diagnosing SBO, but ultrasound does not expose the patient to ionizing radiation.
D. Ultrasound is both more sensitive and specific for diagnosing SBO compared to an acute abdominal series.

7. A 78-year-old woman is admitted to the ICU with cardiogenic shock requiring norepinephrine and dopamine. Two days after admission, she complains of cramping abdominal pain, diarrhea, and blood in her stool. Laboratory evaluation reveals a white blood cell (WBC) count of 13,000/mm³. Ultrasound of her abdomen reveals a thickened colonic wall. What other finding would you *most* likely see on ultrasound of her colon?

A. Decreased Doppler signal
B. Spine sign
C. Kerckring folds
D. McConnell sign

8. An 82-year-old man admitted to your service begins to complain of severe abdominal pain, nausea, and vomiting. He has a 6 cm mass palpable at the umbilicus with overlying skin erythema. You decide to ultrasound the area in question. What would be the *most* likely ultrasonographic findings associated with this pathology?

   A. Multiconcentric rings when viewed in cross section
   B. Loops of thickened bowel with anechoic free fluid
   C. Extensive dirty shadowing and peristalsis
   D. A noncompressible, blind-end pouch

9. Which of the following ultrasound findings is *most* concerning for a high-grade SBO?

   A. Tanga sign
   B. Keyboard sign
   C. Twinkle sign
   D. Mickey Mouse sign

10. You admit a delirious patient with diabetic ketoacidosis to the ICU. The patient continues to have profuse vomiting despite treatment and complains of abdominal pain. She is tender over her periumbilical area but has no definite mass. An ultrasound image of the area is shown in **Figure 64.4**.

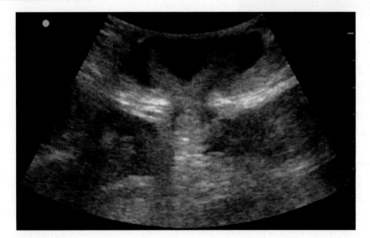

**Figure 64.4**

Based on the ultrasound appearance, what is the *most* appropriate next step in management?
A. Consult obstetrics and gynecology
B. Initiate antibiotic therapy for the cellulitis
C. Perform a bedside incision and drainage of the abscess
D. Consult general surgery

11. A 50-year-old man complains of 12 hours of midepigastric abdominal pain radiating to his right lower quadrant. Ultrasound of his lower abdomen reveals **Figure 64.5A-C**.

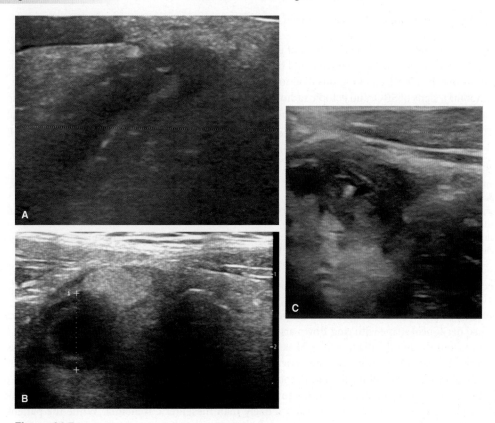

**Figure 64.5**

Figure 64.5A-C is most consistent with what disease process?
A. Appendicitis
B. Cholecystitis
C. Small bowel obstruction
D. Bowel perforation

12. The ultrasound in **Figure 64.6** is *most* concerning for which of the following?

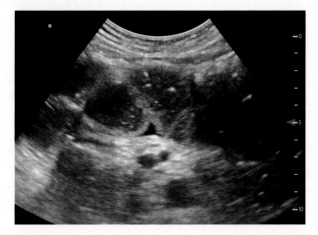

**Figure 64.6**

A. Small bowel obstruction
B. Large bowel obstruction
C. Ileus
D. Diverticulitis

# Chapter 64 ▪ Answers

**1.** Correct Answer: C. Obtain a CT scan to evaluate for gallstone ileus.

*Rationale:* Figure 64.1 shows dilated loops of small bowel with plicae circulares. These findings are concerning for a bowel obstruction, which could be due to gallstone ileus in the setting of his biliary disease. Plain films may be used in making this diagnosis, classically showing Rigler's triad: air in the biliary tree (pneumobilia), signs of SBO, and ectopic radiopaque gallstones, but CT has improved sensitivity and may show alternative pathology. There is no evidence of bowel perforation on this image, which may manifest as peritoneal air or fluid. While medical management may be appropriate for functional ileus or adhesive bowel obstruction, gallstone ileus typically requires surgical treatment.

### Selected References
1. Chang L, Chang M, Chang HM, Chang AI, Chang F. Clinical and radiological diagnosis of gallstone ileus: a mini review. *Emerg Radiol.* 2018;25(2):189-196.
2. Chuah PS, Curtis J, Misra N, Hikmat D, Chawla S. Pictorial review: the pearls and pitfalls of the radiological manifestations of gallstone ileus. *Abdom Radiol.* 2016;42(4):1169-1175.
3. Nuño-Guzmán CM, Marín-Contreras ME, Figueroa-Sánchez M, Corona JL. Gallstone ileus, clinical presentation, diagnostic and treatment approach. *World J Gastrointest Surg.* 2016;8(1):65-76.

**2.** Correct Answer: D. Begin IV fluid resuscitation and emergently consult general surgery.

*Rationale:* The patient has evidence of intraperitoneal free air on ultrasound (Figure 64.2) including a thickened peritoneal stripe with ring-down artifact. Portal venous gas is also noted (*white arrows in liver*). While ultrasound is not the diagnostic gold standard for intraperitoneal free air, it is a reasonable bedside test to evaluate patients who have acute-onset abdominal pain and hypotension. The ultrasonographic findings of free air in this clinical context should raise suspicion for toxic megacolon leading to colon perforation. The history of diarrhea and acute abdominal pain in the setting of recent antibiotic use makes sequela from *C. difficile* infection more likely than mesenteric ischemia. While the patient may need additional antibiotic coverage, intestinal perforation is typically an indication for emergent surgery. While radiographs may be useful to further evaluate for free air, resuscitation and surgical consult should not be delayed for additional imaging.

### Selected References
1. Coppolino F, Gatta G, Di Grezia G, et al. Gastrointestinal perforation: ultrasonographic diagnosis. *Crit Ultrasound J.* 2013;5(suppl 1):S4. doi:10.1186/2036-7902-5-S1-S4.
2. Hefny AF, Abu-Zidan FM. Sonographic diagnosis of intraperitoneal free air. *J Emerg Trauma Shock.* 2011;4(4):511-513. doi:10.4103/0974-2700.86649.
3. Hoffmann B, Nürnberg D, Westergaard M. Focus on abnormal air. *Eur J Emerg Med.* 2012;19(5):284-291. doi:10.1097/mej.0b013e3283543cd3.
4. Ma O. *Ma and Mateer's Emergency Ultrasound.* McGraw-Hill Education Medical; 2014.

**3.** Correct Answer: D. Appendicolith

*Rationale:* Noncompressibility, a visualized appendicolith, and an anterior-posterior measurement >7 mm are all findings consistent with appendicitis. Intraluminal air is typically a normal finding, although the presence of air does not *exclude* the diagnosis of appendicitis.

### Selected References
1. Jeffrey RB, Jain KA, Nghiem HV. Sonographic diagnosis of acute appendicitis: interpretive pitfalls. *Am J Roentgenol.* 1994;162(1):55-59.
2. Ma O. *Ma and Mateer's Emergency Ultrasound.* McGraw-Hill Education Medical; 2014.
3. Mostbeck G, Adam EJ, Nielsen MB, et al. How to diagnose acute appendicitis: ultrasound first. *Insights Imaging.* 2016;7(2):255-263. doi:10.1007/s13244-016-0469-6.

**4.** Correct Answer: A. Enhanced echogenicity of the peritoneal stripe and thickened bowel loops

*Rationale:* Enhanced echogenicity of the peritoneal stripe and thickened bowel loops would be most consistent with bowel perforation. These findings are primary and secondary findings of bowel perforation, respectively. Scattering of sound waves at the interface of soft tissue and air causes a reverberation artifact that enhances the echogenicity of the peritoneal stripe and causes the appearance of A-lines. Thickened bowel loops suggest bowel edema, which often accompanies underlying bowel pathology leading to perforation. A target sign with surrounding free fluid would be more consistent with appendicitis. A thin peritoneal stripe and dirty shadowing are normal ultrasonographic findings.

Selected References

1. Coppolino F, Gatta G, Di Grezia G, et al. Gastrointestinal perforation: ultrasonographic diagnosis. *Crit Ultrasound J.* 2013;5(suppl 1):S4. doi:10.1186/2036-7902-5-S1-S4.
2. Hefny AF, Abu-Zidan FM. Sonographic diagnosis of intraperitoneal free air. *J Emerg Trauma Shock.* 2011;4(4):511-513. doi:10.4103/0974-2700.86649.
3. Hoffmann B, Nürnberg D, Westergaard M. Focus on abnormal air. *Eur J Emerg Med.* 2012;19(5):284-291. doi:10.1097/mej.0b013e3283543cd3.
4. Ma O. *Ma and Mateer's Emergency Ultrasound.* McGraw-Hill Education Medical; 2014.

5. Correct Answer: D. Begin resuscitation and get an emergent surgery consult

*Rationale:* While current recommendations advocate against the use of ulcer prophylaxis in all hospitalized patients, this patient has multiple risk factors for stress ulcers including burns and sepsis requiring a prolonged ICU stay. His ultrasound (Figure 64.3) demonstrates free fluid in Morison's pouch, which raises suspicion for a stress ulcer with perforation, and an emergent surgery consult would be the preferred next step in management. Cholecystitis is not apparent on this image and the gallbladder is not visualized. This fluid is not a pleural effusion and a chest CT is unnecessary.

Selected References

1. Fashner J, Gitu AC. Diagnosis and treatment of peptic ulcer disease and *H. pylori* infection. *Am Fam Physician.* 2015;91(4):236-242.
2. Ma O. *Ma and Mateer's Emergency Ultrasound.* McGraw-Hill Education Medical; 2014.
3. Pruitt BA, Goodwin CW. Stress ulcer disease in the burned patient. *World J Surg.* 1981;5:209-220. doi:10.1007/BF01658293.

6. Correct Answer: D. Ultrasound is both more sensitive and specific for diagnosing SBO compared to an acute abdominal series.

*Rationale/Critique:* While CT imaging remains the gold standard for diagnosing SBO, multiple studies have demonstrated the superiority of ultrasound compared to radiographs as an early, rapid diagnostic modality for diagnosing SBO, particularly in situations where CT is not available or delayed. Compared to radiographs, ultrasound is both more sensitive and specific for diagnosing SBO. Findings consistent with SBO include dilated loops of bowel >25 mm, abnormal peristalsis, bowel wall edema (normal bowel wall is typically <3 mm), and plicae circulares, also known as "keyboard sign" (see **Figure 64.7**).

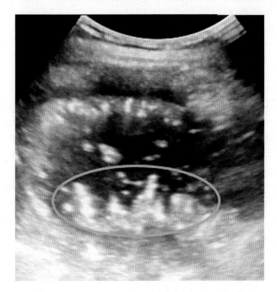

**Figure 64.7**

**Selected References**

1. Becker BA, Lahham S, Gonzales MA, et al. A prospective, multicenter evaluation of point-of-care ultrasound for small-bowel obstruction in the emergency department. *Acad Emerg Med.* 2019;26(8):921-930.
2. Gottlieb M, Peksa GD, Pandurangadu AV, Nakitende D, Takhar S, Seethala RR. Utilization of ultrasound for the evaluation of small bowel obstruction: a systematic review and meta-analysis. *Am J Emerg Med.* 2018;36(2):234-242.
3. Pourmand A, Dimbil U, Drake A, Shokoohi H. The accuracy of point-of-care ultrasound in detecting small bowel obstruction in emergency department. *Emerg Med Int.* 2018;2018:3684081.

**7.** Correct Answer: A. Decreased Doppler signal

*Rationale:* While ultrasound is not the ideal diagnostic modality for ischemic colitis, it can be useful for rapidly evaluating undifferentiated abdominal pathology at the bedside. Ultrasonographic findings consistent with ischemic colitis include bowel wall thickening and decreased blood flow to the affected bowel, reflected as decreased or absent Doppler signal on ultrasound. In the clinical scenario provided, this patient has multiple risk factors and findings concerning for ischemic colitis. The spine sign is a finding associated with pleural effusions/hemothorax. Kerckring folds refer to the plicae circulares that are sometimes visualized on ultrasound in patients with SBO. McConnell sign is an echocardiographic finding associated with right heart strain.

**Selected References**

1. Granat N, Gabrieli S, Alpert EA. Point-of-care ultrasound to diagnose colitis in the emergency department: a case series and review of the literature. *J Emerg Med.* 2019. doi:10.1016/j.jemermed.2019.08.035.
2. Ma O. *Ma and Mateer's Emergency Ultrasound.* McGraw-Hill Education Medical; 2014.
3. Ripollés T, Simó L, Martínez-Pérez MJ, Pastor MR, Igual A, López A. Sonographic findings in ischemic colitis in 58 patients. *Am J Roentgenol.* 2005;184(3):777-785. doi:10.2214/ajr.184.3.01840777.
4. Taourel P, Aufort S, Merigeaud S, Doyon FC, Hoquet MD, Delabrousse E. Imaging of ischemic colitis. *Radiol Clin North Am.* 2008;46:909-924.

**8.** Correct Answer: B. Loops of thickened bowel with anechoic free fluid

*Rationale:* The patient's findings are concerning for a strangulated umbilical hernia. On ultrasound, one would expect to see bowel wall edema with surrounding free fluid due to inflammation and bowel ischemia. Multiconcentric intestinal rings are an ultrasonographic finding consistent with intussusception. A noncompressible, blind-end pouch is an ultrasonographic finding suggestive of appendicitis. Non-pathologic abdominal ultrasound often shows "dirty shadowing," which is a term to describe the artifacts caused by bowel gas which makes visualizing normal bowel challenging.

**Selected References**

1. Arend CF. Static and dynamic sonography for diagnosis of abdominal wall hernias. *J Ultrasound Med.* 2013;32(7):1251-1259.
2. Ma O. *Ma and Mateer's Emergency Ultrasound.* McGraw-Hill Education Medical; 2014.
3. Young J, Gilbert AI, Graham MF. The use of ultrasound in the diagnosis of abdominal wall hernias. *Hernia.* 2007;11:347.

**9.** Correct Answer: A. Tanga sign

*Rationale:* The tanga sign is the name given to free fluid interspersed between dilated loops of small bowel and is indicative of a high-grade bowel obstruction as intraluminal pressure exceeds capillary pressure. It is named after a style of bikini bottom, reflecting the shape of the anechoic fluid between the rounded loops of bowel. Presence of the tanga sign should raise concern for impending bowel ischemia and warrants immediate surgical consultation. The keyboard sign is also associated with SBO, but is not associated with high-grade SBO, per se. The twinkle sign refers to the rapid flickering of Doppler color when placed over a stationary echogenic object such as a kidney stone. The Mickey Mouse sign describes the ultrasonographic appearance of the portal triad when viewed in short axis.

**Selected References**

1. Grassi R, Romano S, D'Amario F, et al. The relevance of free fluid between intestinal loops detected by sonography in the clinical assessment of small bowel obstruction in adults. *Eur J Radiol.* 2004;50(1):5-14.
2. Jones J. Small bowel obstruction: radiology reference article. Radiopaedia Blog RSS. Accessed November 14, 2019. https://radiopaedia.org/articles/small-bowel-obstruction?lang=us.
3. Ma O. *Ma and Mateer's Emergency Ultrasound.* McGraw-Hill Education Medical; 2014.

**10.** Correct Answer: D. Consult general surgery

*Rationale:* This patient has history and findings concerning for a strangulated hernia. The ultrasound image (Figure 64.4) reveals a dilated loop of bowel protruding through the peritoneum, with surrounding free fluid. These findings warrant an emergent surgical consult. While this patient may ultimately get a CT scan, given the specificity of the ultrasound findings and overall clinical picture, early consultation with a surgeon for definitive management is important. The ultrasound does not reflect gynecologic pathology. The erythema is likely secondary to the strangulated hernia and does not represent cellulitis. The ultrasound shows a loop of bowel, not an abscess, and thus incision and drainage would not be appropriate.

Selected References
1. Arend CF. Static and dynamic sonography for diagnosis of abdominal wall hernias. *J Ultrasound Med.* 2013;32(7):1251-1259.
2. Ma O. *Ma and Mateer's Emergency Ultrasound.* McGraw-Hill Education Medical; 2014.
3. Young J, Gilbert AI, Graham MF. The use of ultrasound in the diagnosis of abdominal wall hernias. *Hernia.* 2007;11:347.

**11.** Correct Answer: A. Appendicitis

*Rationale/Critique:* Figure 64.5 ultrasound(s) show a blind-ended pouch with a thickened, dilated wall and appendicolith. Given the overall clinical picture, this finding is most consistent with acute appendicitis. Ultrasonographic findings classically associated with appendicitis include: a noncompressible appendix, dilated to >7 mm (the diameter of the appendix in the presented case is ~2.5cm), and a visible appendicolith. The image does not show cholecystitis. Ultrasonographic findings of SBO include dilated bowel (>2.5-3 cm) abnormal peristalsis, and visible plicae circulares (keyboard sign). Ultrasonographic findings of bowel perforation include a thickened peritoneal stripe and reverberation artifact.

Selected References
1. Jeffrey RB, Jain KA, Nghiem HV. Sonographic diagnosis of acute appendicitis: interpretive pitfalls. *Am J Roentgenol.* 1994;162(1):55-59.
2. Ma O. *Ma and Mateer's Emergency Ultrasound.* McGraw-Hill Education Medical; 2014.
3. Mostbeck G, Adam EJ, Nielsen MB, et al. How to diagnose acute appendicitis: ultrasound first. *Insights Imaging.* 2016;7(2):255-263. doi:10.1007/s13244-016-0469-6.

**12.** Correct Answer: A. Small bowel obstruction

*Rationale/Critique:* The ultrasound image (Figure 64.6) shows findings consistent with a SBO, including dilated loops of bowel >2.5 cm in diameter and areas of surrounding free fluid referred to as the tanga sign. Large bowel obstruction is often difficult to visualize on ultrasound due to overlying bowel gas, but is typically delineated by an area of bowel dilation (>5 cm) with feculent material and dense spot echoes within the lumen of the bowel, or wide gas echoes along the edges of the abdomen. Ileus would be unlikely to result in bowel edema and transudative edema. Diverticulitis would be suggested by hypoechoic wall thickening, typically in the left lower quadrant and may also show a hyperechoic fecalith.

Selected References
1. Becker BA, Lahham S, Gonzales MA, et al. A prospective, multicenter evaluation of point-of-care ultrasound for small-bowel obstruction in the emergency department. *Acad Emerg Med.* 2019;26(8):921-930.
2. Gottlieb M, Peksa GD, Pandurangadu AV, Nakitende D, Takhar S, Seethala RR. Utilization of ultrasound for the evaluation of small bowel obstruction: a systematic review and meta-analysis. *Am J Emerg Med.* 2018;36(2):234-242.
3. Ma O. *Ma and Mateer's Emergency Ultrasound.* McGraw-Hill Education Medical; 2014.
4. Pourmand A, Dimbil U, Drake A, Shokoohi H. The accuracy of point-of-care ultrasound in detecting small bowel obstruction in emergency department. *Emerg Med Int.* 2018;2018:3684081.

# 65 | BLADDER ULTRASOUND

Tanping Wong

1. A 68-year-old man with a history of benign prostatic hypertrophy, who underwent transurethral resection of the prostate (TURP) 7 years prior, presents with 6 weeks of dyspepsia, anorexia, and weight loss. He is noted to have a creatinine of 10 mg/dL (normal when checked 2 years prior). Transverse (**Figure 65.1A,** ▶ **Video 65.1A**) and sagittal (**Figure 65.1B,** ▶ **Video 65.1B**) ultrasound views are obtained at the level of the umbilicus.

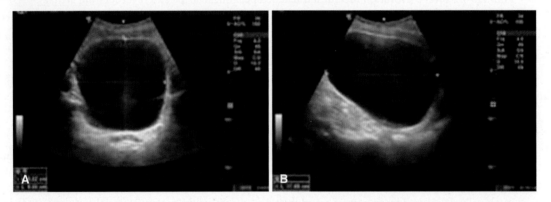

**Figure 65.1**

What is the *most appropriate* next step in his management?
A. Computed tomography (CT) scan for further evaluation of abdominal mass
B. Emergent surgery/urology consult for bladder rupture
C. Nephrology consult to initiate emergent hemodialysis
D. Place a Foley catheter for obstructive uropathy

2. A 68-year-old man with a history of benign prostatic hypertrophy presents with 4 weeks of abdominal pain, anorexia, weight loss, and decreased urine output. On physical examination, the bladder is palpable at the level of the umbilicus, and point-of-care ultrasound shows a distended bladder with bilateral hydronephrosis. A Foley catheter is placed and 400 mL of urine output is noted. Repeat ultrasound of the bladder is shown in **Figure 65.2** and ▶ **Video 65.2**.

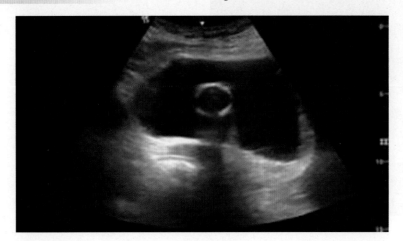

**Figure 65.2**

What is the *most appropriate* next step in the management of this patient's renal failure?
**A.** Initiate intravenous (IV) hydration.
**B.** Measure urine sodium and urine creatinine.
**C.** Reposition or replace the Foley catheter.
**D.** Perform a CT to evaluate for obstructing malignancy.

3. An 80-year-old man with a history of emphysema was admitted to the medical intensive care unit (ICU) for the treatment of a chronic obstructive pulmonary disease (COPD) exacerbation. On hospital day 6, he was noted to be delirious. His vitals are normal, his neurologic examination is nonfocal, and he has abdominal tenderness. Point-of-care ultrasound is shown in **Figure 65.3A** (▶ **Video 65.3A**) and **Figure 65.3B** (▶ **Video 65.3**).

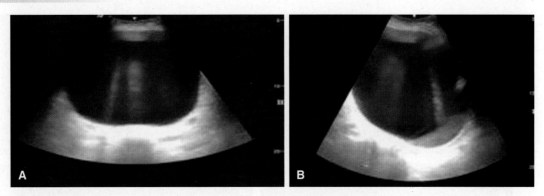

**Figure 65.3**

What is the *most appropriate* next step in the management of this patient's delirium?
**A.** Nonpharmacologic management including circadian rhythm reorientation
**B.** Start broad-spectrum antibiotics
**C.** Place a Foley catheter
**D.** Perform an emergent CT scan of his head

4. A 68-year-old man with a history of cirrhosis is admitted to the medical ICU with decompensated cirrhosis. He improves over the course of 5 days and his Foley catheter is removed. Six hours later, you are told by his nurse that the patient's bladder scan volume is 1500 mL. You perform an ultrasound of the bladder (**Figure 65.4** and ▶ **Video 65.4**).

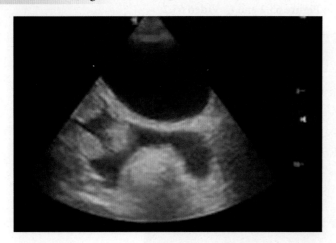

**Figure 65.4**

What is the *most appropriate* next course of action?
A. A Foley catheter should be reinserted
B. Perform a CT to evaluate for bladder obstruction
C. Perform a paracentesis to drain the ascites
D. Reassure the nurse, as the bladder volume is estimated to be approximately 300 mL

5. An 82-year-old man presents with 3 days of fever and dysuria. On presentation, he has a temperature of 38.5°C, HR 110 bpm, BP 90/60 mm Hg, RR 22/min, and SpO$_2$ 95% on room air. His physical examination is normal but laboratory evaluation is notable for white blood cells (WBC) 14 × 10$^9$/L, creatinine 2.0 mg/dL (baseline 1.0), and hemoglobin 9 g/dL. His urinalysis shows 100 red blood cells (RBC) and 50 WBC/high-power field (HPF). Point-of-care ultrasound is performed and shown in **Figure 65.5A** (▶ **Video 65.5A**) and **Figure 65.5B** (▶ **Video 65.5B**).

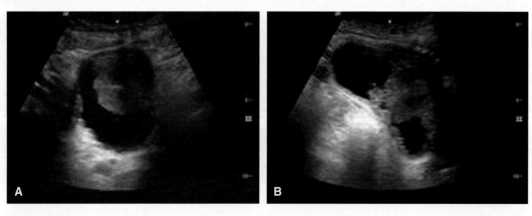

**Figure 65.5**

In addition to antibiotics and admission, what is the *most appropriate* management of this patient?
A. Send urine for cytology and order CT of the abdomen and pelvis
B. Start treatment for benign prostatic hyperplasia and refer the patient to Urology
C. Start antifungal treatment for a fungal urinary tract infection
D. Place a Foley catheter for acute urinary retention

6. A 56-year-old man was recently diagnosed with a liver abscess. He was treated with percutaneous drainage and antibiotics. He was discharged home but presents to the Emergency Department (ED) with difficulty urinating, pelvic pain, and fevers. His physical examination is notable only for a temperature of 38.6°C and suprapubic tenderness. Laboratory evaluation shows serum creatinine 0.9 mg/dL, WBC 20 × 10$^9$/L, and urinalysis shows three WBC/HPF. A point-of-care ultrasound is shown in **Figure 65.6A** (▶ **Video 65.6A**) and **Figure 65.6B** (▶ **Video 65.6B**).

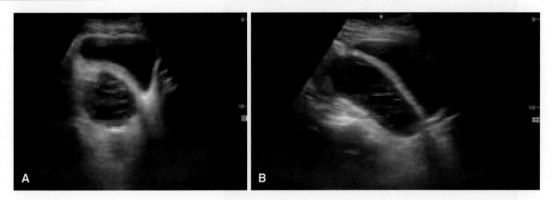

**Figure 65.6**

What does this ultrasound demonstrate?
A. Enlarged prostate causing urinary retention
B. Urinary sediment consistent with acute cystitis
C. A bladder mass suspicious for bladder carcinoma
D. Fluid collection posterior to bladder concerning for rectal abscess

7. An 84-year-old woman with metastatic pancreatic cancer presents with worsening back pain, weakness, and poor oral intake. Her admission evaluation reveals acute renal failure and she was subsequently admitted. Abdominal ultrasound shows a distended bladder with bilateral hydronephrosis. A Foley catheter is placed and 100 mL of urine is drained. A repeat ultrasound of the bladder is displayed in **Figure 65.7** and ▶ **Video 65.7**.

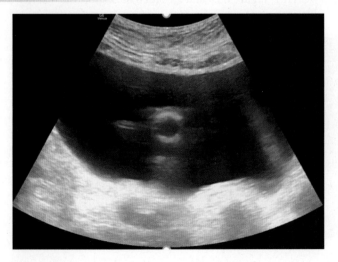

**Figure 65.7**

What is the *most appropriate* next step in the management of this patient?
A. Place bilateral percutaneous nephrostomy tubes
B. Give IV fluids
C. Continue the current management plan
D. Flush or adjust the Foley catheter

8. A 58-year-old man with a history of benign prostatic hyperplasia and recurrent urinary tract infections presents with dysuria, suprapubic pain, and difficulty urinating. He is afebrile, but suprapubic tenderness and fullness are noted on physical examination. The urinalysis from a voided specimen shows 50 RBC/HPF and 3 WBC/HPF. A point-of-care ultrasound image of the bladder is shown in **Figure 65.8** and ▸ **Video 65.8**.

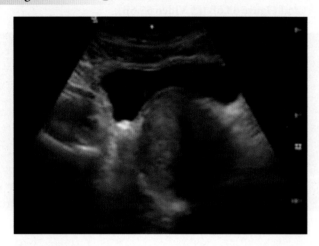

**Figure 65.8**

After Foley catheter placement, what is the *best* strategy to prevent recurrence of his urinary symptoms?
A. Urology consult for surgical evaluation
B. Obtain abdominal and pelvic CT for workup of bladder cancer
C. Start antibiotics for recurrent prostatitis
D. Aggressive treatment for constipation

9. A 42-year-old woman with a history of urinary tract infections presents with abdominal pain and dysuria. She is afebrile with normal vital signs but has lower abdominal tenderness on physical examination. Laboratory evaluation reveals WBC $11 \times 10^9$/L, serum creatinine 1.2 mg/dL, and urinalysis with 25 RBC/HPF and 10 WBC/HPF. **Figure 65.9** and ▸ **Video 65.9** show the bladder ultrasound.

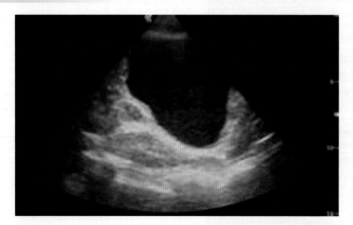

**Figure 65.9**

What is the *most appropriate* next step in her management?
A. This image shows complex ascites. Perform a diagnostic paracentesis.
B. This image shows debris in the bladder. Start antibiotics for a urinary tract infection.
C. This image shows urinary retention. Place a Foley catheter.
D. This image is uninterpretable. Adjust the gain and repeat the ultrasound.

10. A 58-year-old man with a history of non-Hodgkin lymphoma presents with 2 weeks of bilateral lower extremity edema, intermittent fevers, and difficulty urinating. Bulky inguinal lymphadenopathy is noted on physical examination. Laboratory evaluation reveals a serum creatinine 6.1 mg/dL (increased from 2.0 one week prior) and elevated calcium and uric acid. He is admitted for acute renal failure secondary to calcium and urate uropathy. A point-of-care ultrasound is shown in **Figure 65.10A** (▶ **Video 65.10A**) and **Figure 65.10B** (▶ **Video 65.10B**).

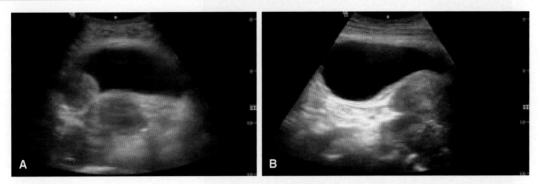

**Figure 65.10**

In addition to hypercalcemia and hyperuricemia, what is *most likely* contributing to this patient's acute renal failure?
A. The patient is hypovolemic and has a prerenal cause of his acute renal failure.
B. The patient has lymphoma infiltration of his bladder causing bladder outlet obstruction.
C. The patient has malignant ascites causing intravascular volume depletion.
D. The patient has lymphadenopathy causing bladder outlet obstruction.

11. A 70-year-old man presents with fatigue and is found to have acute renal failure with a serum creatinine of 4.2 mg/dL. A mass is palpated in the right lower quadrant of his abdomen. Point-of-care ultrasound shows moderate bilateral hydronephrosis and a distended bladder. A Foley catheter is placed and 100 mL of turbid urine is drained. A repeat bladder ultrasound is shown in **Figure 65.11** and ▶ **Video 65.11.**

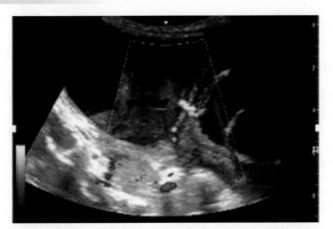

**Figure 65.11**

What do these ultrasounds demonstrate?
A. Perforated bladder
B. Colovesicular fistula
C. Bladder diverticulum
D. Ascites

**12.** A 35-year-old man without past medical history presents to the ED for sudden onset of intermittent severe left flank pain, associated with mild nausea. He denies hematuria, dysuria, or fever. His vitals are normal and he has no tenderness or masses on examination. Ultrasound of the kidneys shows moderate left hydronephrosis. An ultrasound image of the bladder in a transverse plane is shown in **Figure 65.12**

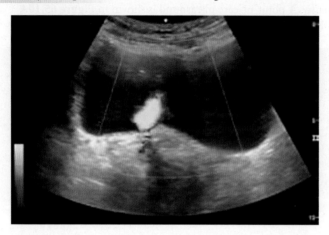

**Figure 65.12**

What is the next most appropriate action?
**A.** Start antibiotics for pyelonephritis pending urinalysis and urine culture
**B.** Obtain CT abdomen and pelvis to evaluate for appendicitis
**C.** Send urine for toxicology screen given suspicion of narcotic-seeking behavior
**D.** Start hydration and analgesics for renal colic

# Chapter 65 ■ Answers

**1.** Correct Answer: D. Place a Foley catheter for obstructive uropathy

*Rationale:* Detection of a distended bladder at the level of the umbilicus is highly suggestive of urinary retention. This patient had bilateral hydronephrosis and a Foley catheter was placed with 1000 mL of urine output. His creatinine eventually decreased to normal in the subsequent week. The etiology of his urinary retention is likely secondary to the recurrence of benign prostatic hypertrophy.

Point-of-care ultrasound is indicated to rapidly evaluate bladder volume with suspected obstruction. Bladder volume can be calculated using the formula (0.75 × width × length × height). CT scan may be indicated for further evaluation if an obstructing mass is suspected (unlikely in this scenario), but emergent bladder decompression is the most appropriate next step. There is no evidence of bladder rupture and free intraperitoneal fluid would not have the "rounded" appearance of the bladder, as seen here. Relief of the obstruction is the first step in the treatment of this patient's renal failure even if emergent dialysis is indicated.

Selected References
1. Boniface KS, Calabrese KY. Intensive care ultrasound: IV. *Abdominal ultrasound in critical care. Ann Am Thorac Soc.* 2013;10(6):713-724.
2. Chan H. Noninvasive bladder volume measurement. *J Neurosci Nurs.* 1993;25:309-312.
3. Kelly CE. Evaluation of voiding dysfunction and measurement of bladder volume. *Rev Urol.* 2004;6(suppl 1):S32-S37.

**2.** Correct Answer: C. Reposition or replace the Foley catheter

*Rationale:* An adequately positioned Foley catheter should completely drain the bladder. ▶ **Video 65.2** shows a distended bladder with the Foley catheter in place, suggesting that it is likely obstructed. Flushing, replacing, or repositioning the catheter would be the most appropriate action. Placement within the prostatic urethra is another common cause of catheter malfunction, which should prompt repositioning or replacement as well. Relief of the bladder obstruction should be performed prior to any further evaluation or treatment for additional causes of renal failure.

Selected References

1. Boniface KS, Calabrese KY. Intensive care ultrasound: IV. *Abdominal ultrasound in critical care. Ann Am Thorac Soc.* 2013;10(6):713-724.
2. Subramanian V. The risk of intra-urethral Foley catheter balloon inflation in spinal cord-injured patients: lessons learned from a retrospective case series. *Patient Saf Surg.* 2016:10(14):14.

**3.** Correct Answer: C. Place a Foley catheter

*Rationale:* Figure 65.3A, B shows a distended bladder, suggesting that acute urinary retention is the most likely cause of the patient's delirium. Risk factors for acute urinary retention are older age, history of benign prostatic hyperplasia, neurologic impairment, anticholinergic and sympathomimetic drugs, infection, bed-bound state, and constipation. Although being in the ICU is a risk factor for delirium, this is less likely as the patient has been improving, and specific treatments are limited. Infection is another common cause of delirium, but does not appear to be the most likely cause in this case. CT scan of the head is warranted in delirious patients with focal neurologic deficits, which are not present in this case, but may be considered for further evaluation if relief of the urinary obstruction is not therapeutic. ▶ **Video 65.3A** and **B** shows distended enlarged bladder in transverse and sagittal views.

Selected References

1. Chan H. Noninvasive bladder volume measurement. *J Neurosci Nurs.* 1993;25:309-312.
2. Waardenberg IE. Delirium caused by urinary retention in elderly people: a case report and literature review on the "cystocerebral syndrome". *J Am Geriatr Soc.* 2008;56(12):2371-2372. https://onlinelibrary.wiley.com/doi/abs/10.1111/j.1532-5415.2008.02035.x.

**4.** Correct Answer: D. Reassure the nurse, as the bladder volume is estimated to be approximately 300 mL

*Rationale:* ▶ **Video 65.4** shows a bladder with estimated volume of 300 mL (volume = 0.75 × width × length × height). ▶ **Video 65.4** also shows ascites inferior to the nondistended bladder. The patient should void and have his bladder volume monitored.

Early removal of catheters reduces the risk of catheter-associated urinary tract infection. Accuracy of postvoid bladder volume assessment avoids unnecessary bladder reinsertion, but bladder scans are often inaccurate in patients with obesity, anasarca, and ascites. Point-of-care ultrasound is more accurate in the assessment of bladder volume and can distinguish between bladder volume and ascites. CT imaging is not necessary to evaluate for bladder obstruction. Paracentesis is not indicated for the ultrasound findings in the absence of other concerns.

Selected References

1. Chan H. Noninvasive bladder volume measurement. *J Neurosci Nurs.* 1993;25:309-312.
2. Park YH, Ku JH, Oh S-J. Accuracy of post-void residual volume measurement using a portable ultrasound bladder scanner with real-time pre-scan imaging. *Neurourol Urodyn.* 2011;30:335-338. doi:10.1002/nau.20977.
3. Prentice DM, Sona C, Wessman BT, et al. Discrepancies in measuring bladder volumes with bedside ultrasound and bladder scanning in the intensive care unit: a pilot study. *J Intensive Care Soc.* 2018;19(2):122-126. https://www.ncbi.nlm.nih.gov/pubmed/29796068.

**5.** Correct Answer: A. Send urine for cytology and order CT of the abdomen and pelvis

*Rationale:* The ultrasound (Figure 65.5) shows a bladder mass that is highly suggestive of bladder cancer. Patients with bladder cancer present with hematuria, urinary symptoms, and constitutional symptoms. Further workup for carcinoma with urine cytology and CT scan is warranted. Ultrasound plays an important role in the detection of bladder lesions and the early diagnosis of bladder carcinoma. There is no evidence to suggest urinary retention or benign prostatic hyperplasia in this case, and fungal bladder infection is unlikely to cause a mass like this.

### Selected References

1. Gharibvand MM. The role of ultrasound in diagnosis and evaluation of bladder tumors. *J Fam Med Prim Care*. 2017;6(4):840-843. doi:10.4103/jfmpc.jfmpc_186_17.
2. Smereczynski A. Sonography of tumors and tumor-like lesions that mimic carcinoma of the urinary bladder. *J Ultrason*. 2014;14(56):36-48. doi:10.15557%2FJoU.2014.0004.

**6.** Correct Answer: D. Fluid collection posterior to bladder concerning for rectal abscess

*Rationale:* The bladder in transverse (Figure 65.6A) and sagittal (Figure 65.6B) views shows a hypoechoic septated mass posterior and external to the bladder. The distended bladder serves as an excellent acoustic window for ultrasound to image adjacent structures. The differential diagnosis of a fluid-filled heterogeneous mass posterior to the bladder in a male includes a distended rectum, abscess, and enlarged prostate. The septated fluid-filled mass is most suspicious for rectal abscess, which is the most likely cause of his recurrence of fever and leukocytosis. An enlarged prostate would appear more echodense. Sediment is not apparent in the bladder in Figure 65.6, and the mass appears outside of the bladder, in contrast to a bladder carcinoma.

### Selected References

1. Bor R, Fabian A, Szepes Z. Role of ultrasound in colorectal disease. *World J Gastroenterol*. 2016;22(43):9477-9487. doi:10.3748%2F-wjg.v22.i43.9477.
2. Hollerbach S, Geissler A, Schiegl H, et al. The accuracy of abdominal ultrasound in the assessment of bowel disorders. *Scand J Gastroenterol*. 1998;33(11):1201-1208. doi:10.1080/00365529850172575.

**7.** Correct Answer: D. Flush or adjust the Foley catheter

*Rationale:* A decompressed bladder should be visualized when it is adequately drained after Foley placement. The presence of a distended bladder indicates a malfunctioning Foley catheter. After adjustment of the Foley position, 1000 mL of urine returned and the patient had subsequent resolution of her renal failure. Bilateral hydronephrosis and bladder distention suggest obstruction distal to the bladder, and if bladder decompression is possible, this is preferable to nephrostomy tubes. IV fluids are unlikely to resolve her condition. While the Foley catheter does appear to be in the correct position within the bladder, it does need to be adjusted or replaced, as it is not functioning properly.

### Selected Reference

1. Boniface KS, Calabrese KY. Intensive care ultrasound: IV. Abdominal ultrasound in critical care. *Ann Am Thorac Soc*. 2013;10(6):713-724.

**8.** Correct Answer: A. Urology consult for surgical evaluation

*Rationale:* The ultrasound (Figure 64.8) shows an echogenic focus with posterior acoustic shadowing, consistent with a bladder stone, as well as a significantly enlarged prostate. Bladder calculi are a common complication of benign prostatic hyperplasia secondary to urinary stasis. They can lead to bladder outlet obstruction and an increased risk of recurrent urinary tract infections. A urology consultation for removal of the bladder stone is most likely to prevent recurrence of the bladder outlet obstruction. There is no mass observed within the bladder to suggest bladder cancer. Although his prostate is enlarged, no fever and a low WBC count from a voided specimen argue against prostatitis. While antibiotic treatment may still be considered, there is no clear role for prophylactic antibiotics. Constipation is also a common cause for bladder outlet obstruction/urinary retention, but the history and alternative pathology suggest that is not the most likely cause for this patient.

### Selected References

1. Huang W, Cao JJ, Cao M, et al. Risk factors for bladder calculi in patients with benign prostatic hyperplasia. *Medicine*. 2017;96(32):e7728. doi:10.1097%2FMD.0000000000007728.
2. Rosenfield AT, Taylor KJ, Weiss RM. Ultrasound evaluation of bladder calculi. *J Urol*. 1979;121(1):119-120. doi:10.1016/s0022-5347(17)56687-2.
3. Tahtali IN, Karatas T. Giant bladder stone: a case report and review of the literature. *Turk J Urol*. 2014;40(3):189-191.

**9.** Correct Answer: D. This image is uninterpretable. Adjust the gain and repeat the ultrasound

*Rationale:* ▶ **Video 65.9** shows the triangular-shaped sagittal view of the bladder. Adjacent bowel and uterus are visualized. In addition to posterior acoustic enhancement, Figure 65.9 is over-gained, which can lead to the appearance of sediment in the bladder that may not be present. Over-gained images also lead to inadequate visualization of the pouch of Douglas because of posterior acoustic enhancement. There is no ascites visible in this image. Although debris in the bladder would be concerning for an infection, the material apparent within the bladder is more likely an artifact. The bladder volume suggested by the single image, without knowing whether the patient has attempted to void, does not suggest urinary retention.

### Selected References
1. Abu-Zidan FM, Hefny AF, Corr P. Clinical ultrasound physics. *J Emerg Trauma Shock*. 2011;4(4):501-503. https://www.ncbi.nlm.nih.gov/pubmed/22090745.
2. Shriki J. Ultrasound physics. *Crit Care Clin*. 2014;30(1):1-24. doi:10.1016/j.ccc.2013.08.004.

**10.** Correct Answer: D. The patient has lymphadenopathy causing bladder outlet obstruction

*Rationale:* Bladder ultrasound may be helpful in differentiating causes for renal failure in patients presenting with multiple potential etiologies. In this patient, bulky lymphadenopathy is seen posterior and inferior to the bladder, potentially causing obstruction. Hydronephrosis would support this finding as well. Improvement in renal function after decompression (Foley catheter placement) will confirm the role of obstruction in this patient's acute renal failure. While dehydration may contribute, potential bladder outlet obstruction is likely and must be treated immediately. The masses observed on the ultrasound image are outside of the bladder and do not suggest infiltration into the bladder. There is no ascites visible on the ultrasound image (Figure 65.10).

### Selected Reference
1. Khalil MAM, Latif H, Rehman A, et al. Acute kidney injury in lymphoma: a single centre experience. *Int J Nephrol*. 2014;2014:272961. doi:10.1155/2014/272961.

**11.** Correct Answer: C. Bladder diverticulum

*Critique/Rationale:* Figure 65.11 shows the Foley catheter within the distended bladder. Color Doppler shows the communication between the bladder and the adjacent fluid-filled structure, which is a bladder diverticulum.

Diverticula of the bladder are seen in patients with chronically elevated bladder pressure. Its appearance can be confused with pelvic cystic structures and ascites. Demonstration of the point of communication aids in the diagnosis of bladder diverticula. Color Doppler can rapidly and easily demonstrate this communication (**Figure 65.13**).

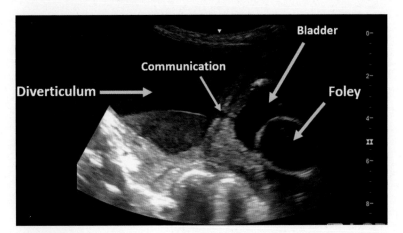

**Figure 65.13**

### Selected References
1. Levine D. Using color doppler jets to differentiate a pelvic cyst from a bladder diverticulum. *Am J Ultrasound Med*. 1994;13:575-577.
2. Maynor CH. Urinary bladder diverticula: sonographic diagnosis and interpretive pitfalls. *Am Inst Ultrasound Med*. 1996;16:189-194.

**12.** Correct Answer: D. Start hydration and analgesics for renal colic

*Rationale:* Ultrasound is useful in the detection of renal stones and hydronephrosis and can readily be done by physicians at the point of care. Early identification of a ureteral stone allows for the initiation of therapy with hydration and analgesics. The asymmetric ureteral jet here is suggestive of unilateral ureteral obstruction, likely secondary to a stone, which fits with the clinical suspicion for renal colic. CT scans have higher sensitivity and specificity for the detection of stones and should be used if more detailed information is needed. A lack of infectious symptoms puts pyelonephritis and appendicitis lower on the differential diagnosis. Drug-seeking behavior should be considered only after acute pathology has been evaluated. "Confirmation" with urine toxicology is usually not necessary and may provide both false positives and false negatives.

Selected References

1. Burge HJ, Middleton WD, McClennan BL, Hildebolt CF. Ureteral jets in healthy subjects and in patients with unilateral ureteral calculi: comparison with color Doppler US. *Radiology.* 1991;180(2):437. doi:10.1148/radiology.180.2.2068307.
2. Jandaghi AB, Falahatkar S, Alizadeh A, et al. Assessment of ureterovesical jet dynamics in obstructed ureter by urinary stone with color Doppler and duplex Doppler examinations. *Urolithiasis.* 2013;41:159-163.

# 66 | OBSTETRICS AND GYNECOLOGY

Benjamin S. Levin, Arielle Butterly, and William J. Sauer

1. Which best describes left ventricular (LV) function in a 36-week pregnant woman, when compared to a nonpregnant patient?

   **A.** Cardiac output unchanged, ejection fraction (EF) unchanged, LV size unchanged
   **B.** Cardiac output increased, EF increased, LV size unchanged
   **C.** Cardiac output increased, EF unchanged, LV size increased
   **D.** Cardiac output unchanged, EF decreased, LV size increased

2. A 28-year-old $G_3P_2$ woman who is 38 weeks pregnant underwent a transthoracic echocardiogram (TTE) for shortness of breath, and **Figure 66.1, Figure 66.2,** ▶ **Video 66.1,** and ▶ **Video 66.2** are obtained.

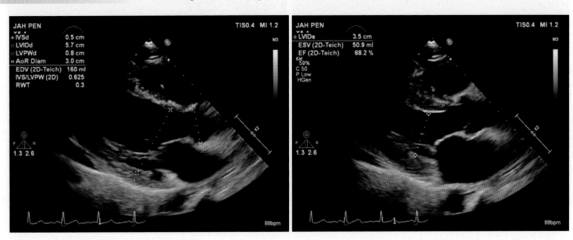

**Figures 66.1 and 66.2**

How would you best characterize this image from that echocardiogram?
**A.** Normal end-diastolic diameter, normal LV stroke volume
**B.** Normal end-diastolic diameter, increased LV stroke volume
**C.** Increased end-diastolic diameter, increased LV stroke volume
**D.** Normal end-diastolic diameter, decreased LV stroke volume

3. A 24-year-old $G_1P_0$ woman who is 38 weeks pregnant is admitted to the intensive care unit (ICU) with hypoxic respiratory failure. You are asked to perform a point-of-care echocardiogram to evaluate her dyspnea. Which of the following characteristics best supports the diagnosis of peripartum cardiomyopathy?

   **A.** Enlarged LV end-diastolic diameter, LVEF estimated at 30 to 35%
   **B.** Enlarged LV end-diastolic diameter, LVEF estimated at 60% to 65%
   **C.** Normal size LV end-diastolic diameter, LVEF estimated at 40% to 45%
   **D.** Normal LV end-diastolic diameter, LVEF estimated at 60% to 65%

4. A previously healthy 22-year-old woman at 38 weeks gestation is admitted to the ICU with an increasing oxygen requirement. **Figure 66.3** is obtained at the time of admission. Figure 66.3A and C are taken at end-diastole, and Figure 66.3B and D are taken at end-systole (see also ▶ **Video 66.3**).

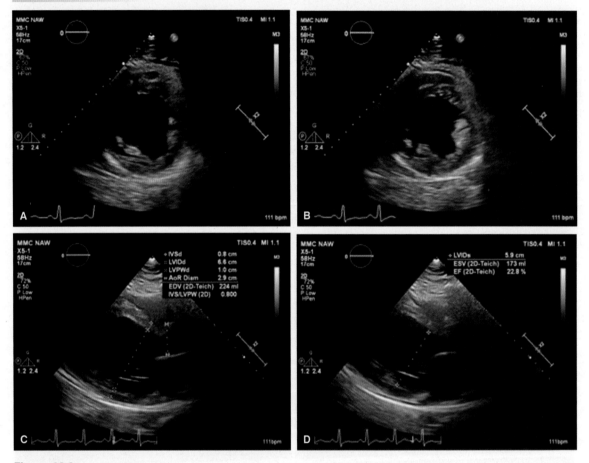

**Figure 66.3**

Which statement *most* accurately describes the findings?

   **A.** Normal LV size with normal systolic function
   **B.** Dilated LV with reduced systolic function
   **C.** Dilated LV with normal systolic function
   **D.** Normal LV size with reduced systolic function

5. A 39-year-old $G_1P_0$ woman is diagnosed with preeclampsia. A TTE is performed. Which of the following is most consistent with a diagnosis of hypertensive cardiomyopathy seen with preeclampsia?

   A. Reduced E/A ratio with normal E/e′
   B. Cardiac output is increased, with reduced E/A ratio
   C. Increased LV mass, elevated E/e′
   D. Normal LV stroke volume, increased LV mass

6. Following delivery at 38 weeks, a 28-year-old $G_2P_2$ woman became hypotensive after the obstetrician manually evacuated the uterus. The hypotension persisted despite ongoing resuscitation. You perform a transesophageal echo and obtain **Figures 66.4** and **66.5** (see also ▶ **Video 66.4**).

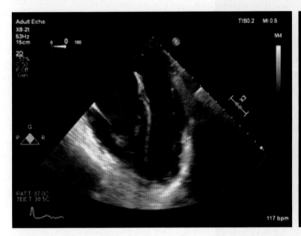 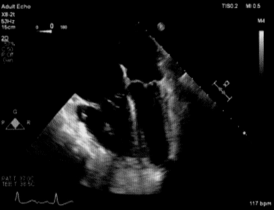

**Figures 66.4 and 66.5**

   Which of the following findings would likely *not* be present?

   A. Severe tricuspid regurgitation (TR)
   B. Leftward septal shift during systole
   C. Hypokinesis of the free wall of the right ventricle
   D. Collapsible inferior vena cava (IVC) with respiratory variation

7. A 34-year-old $G_3P_2$ woman has acute-onset dyspnea following a cesarean section. She has a persistently low oxygen saturation and is mildly hypotensive. The obstetric team is concerned for an amniotic fluid embolism (AFE). Which of these findings would *not* support that diagnosis?

   A. Dilated right ventricle (RV) with leftward shift of the intraventricular septum
   B. Tricuspid annular plane systolic excursion (TAPSE) of 12 mm with preserved LV systolic function
   C. D-shaped LV with reduced LV systolic function
   D. Dilated LV with systolic and diastolic impairment

8. A 30-year-old woman 35 weeks pregnant is hypotensive and complaining of chest pain. You perform a transesophageal echocardiogram (TEE) and obtain **Figure 66.6, Figure 66.7,** ▶ **Video 66.5,** and ▶ **Video 66.6.**

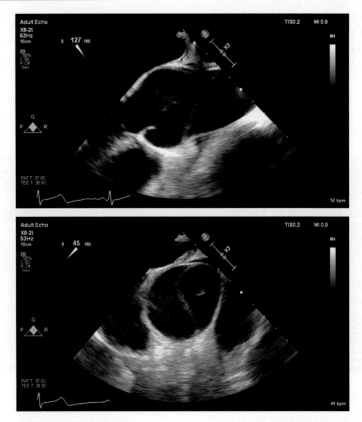

**Figures 66.6 and 66.7**

Which of the following statements is *most* accurate?

A. This is a Stanford Type B dissection
B. This is a DeBakey Type III dissection
C. This is a Stanford Type A dissection
D. This is artifact and does not represent a pathologic state

9. A 24-year-old $G_3P_2$ woman who is 34 weeks pregnant is short of breath, tachypneic, and hypoxemic. The resident who examined the patient is concerned that a previous murmur they heard is now louder. You perform a TTE exam and obtain the following images. Which of the following best describes the findings in **Figure 66.8**?

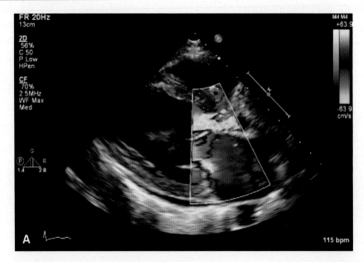

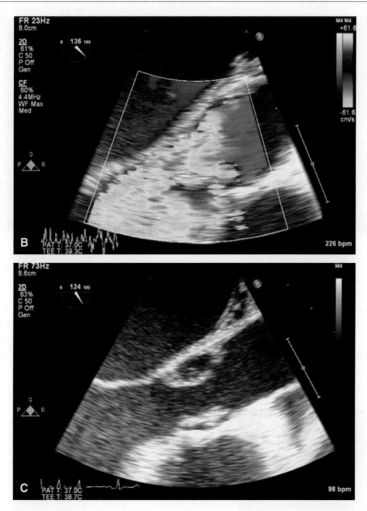

**Figure 66.8**

A. Trace aortic insufficiency from physiologic aortic root dilation
B. Acute aortic insufficiency from aortic dissection
C. Acute aortic insufficiency from aortic valve endocarditis
D. Pulmonic insufficiency from previously repaired tetralogy of Fallot

**10.** A 32-year-old G$_4$P$_4$ woman is admitted to the ICU following urgent C-section. Despite resuscitation with blood products, she remains hypotensive and requires vasopressor support. You perform a TTE, which yields **Figure 66.9**, ▶ **Video 66.7**, and ▶ **Video 66.8**. What is the *most* appropriate interpretation of Figure 66.9?

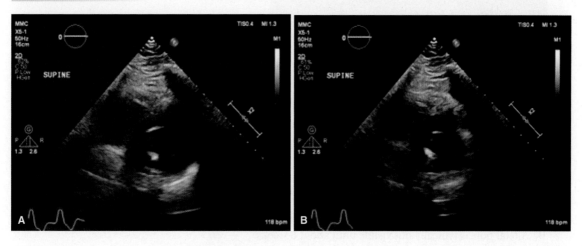

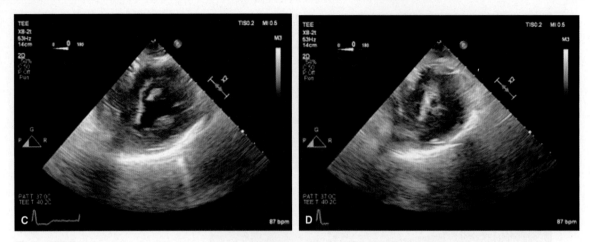

**Figure 66.9**

    **A.** Normal LV volume and reduced LVEF concerning for cardiogenic shock

    **B.** Normal LV volume and increased LVEF concerning for septic shock

    **C.** Low LV volume and increased LVEF concerning for hemorrhagic shock

    **D.** Low LV volume and reduced LVEF due to obstructive shock

**11.** You are performing a transvaginal ultrasound on a young woman for abdominal pain following a positive pregnancy test at home. Her last menstrual period was 5 weeks ago, and her betahuman chorionic gonadotropin (β-hCG) level is 1,500 mIU/mL. You obtain **Figure 66.10.**

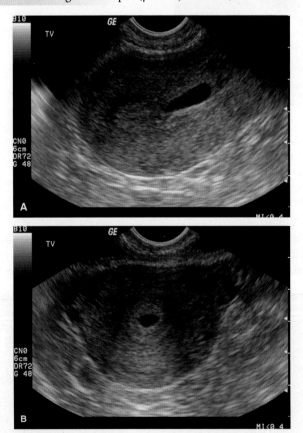

**Figure 66.10**

Which of the following statements is *most* correct?

    **A.** The serum β-hCG level should be <1,000 mIU/mL for this image to represent a normal pregnancy

    **B.** A fetal pole is typically not visible until about 8 weeks

    **C.** The presence of a double decidual sac sign (DDSS) indicates the presence of an intrauterine pregnancy (IUP)

    **D.** An IUP cannot be confirmed

**12.** A 32-year-old woman presents with left pelvic pain after a positive home pregnancy test. Her β-hCG level is 2,500 mIU/mL. You perform a transabdominal ultrasound and obtain **Figure 66.11** in the region of her left ovary.

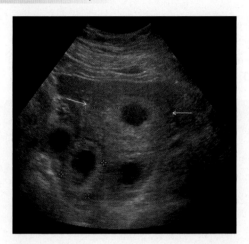

**Figure 66.11**

Which of the following statements is *most* correct?

**A.** This is most likely an ovarian cyst
**B.** Abdominal ultrasound is the preferred imaging modality for this diagnosis
**C.** This represents a possible ectopic pregnancy
**D.** A small amount of free fluid in the pelvis is physiologic

**13.** A 28-year-old woman is having vaginal bleeding and abdominal pain. You obtain the following images from transvaginal ultrasound (**Figure 66.12**).

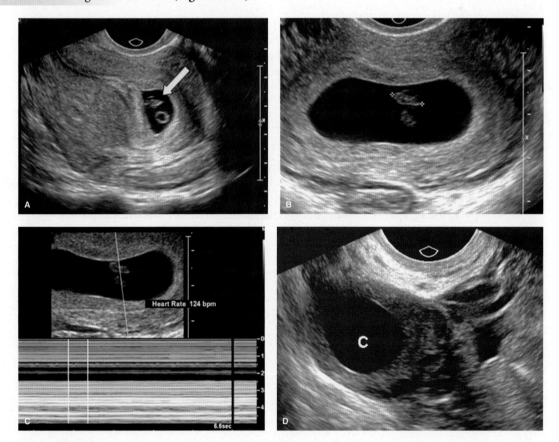

**Figure 66.12**

Which statement is *most* correct?

**A.** It is not possible to confirm if this is an IUP
**B.** The fetal heart rate (FHR) is 124 and is within normal range
**C.** The presence of a FHR confirms an IUP
**D.** Vaginal bleeding at this gestational age is likely to represent a spontaneous abortion

14. An 18-year-old woman reports severe abdominal pain for the last 8 hours. You perform an abdominal and transvaginal ultrasound and obtain **Figure 66.13**.

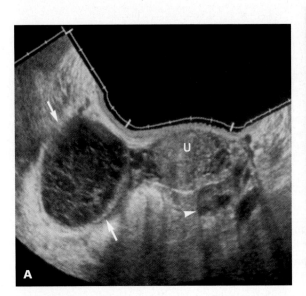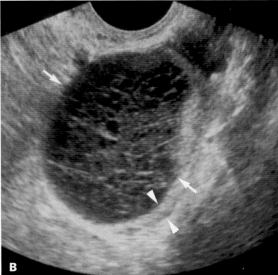

**Figure 66.13**

Which of the following is *most* correct?

**A.** This is a simple ovarian cyst and unlikely to be the cause of her pain
**B.** This is a complex ovarian cyst and is likely the cause of her pain
**C.** Simple ovarian cysts are premalignant and require gynecologic workup
**D.** The absence of teeth or a fluid level suggests a simple ovarian cyst

15. A 64-year-old woman is evaluated with ultrasound for a pelvic mass felt on examination. Which statement is *most* correct?

**A.** Transvaginal ultrasound has a low positive predictive value for malignancy.
**B.** Ovarian masses identified with ultrasound should be followed up with magnetic resonance imaging (MRI).
**C.** Abdominal ultrasound is considered the first-line screening modality for malignancy.
**D.** Computed tomography (CT) scan improves diagnostic certainty for pelvic malignancy.

**16.** A 32-year-old woman presents with lower abdominal pain. A urinary pregnancy test is negative. You obtain the transabdominal ultrasound shown in **Figure 66.14**.

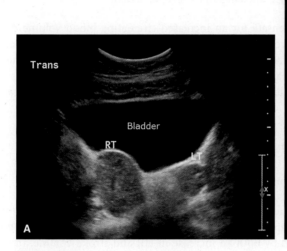
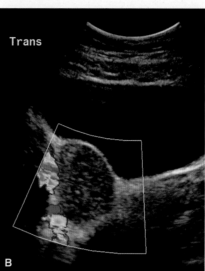

**Figure 66.14**

Which statement is *most* correct?

**A.** The presence of arterial Doppler flow rules out ovarian torsion.
**B.** Asymmetric enlargement of ovaries is normal during the menstrual cycle.
**C.** The presence of cysts on an ovary confirms the diagnosis of ovarian torsion.
**D.** A coiled vascular pedicle visualized on color flow suggests ovarian torsion.

**17.** A 42-year-old woman presents with pelvic pain and fever. Her temperature is 39 °C, BP 110/55 mm Hg, HR 110 bpm. She has left lower quadrant tenderness, and left adnexal fullness and tenderness. **Figure 66.15** shows the transvaginal ultrasound images obtained.

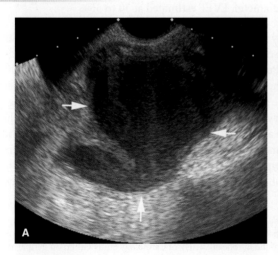
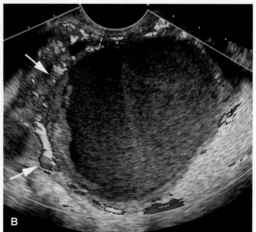

**Figure 66.15**

Which statement is *most* correct?

**A.** This is a complex ovarian cyst and warrants surgical drainage.
**B.** The high degree of vascularity surrounding the rim suggests an abscess.
**C.** A Fallopian tube size less than 10 mm is considered normal.
**D.** The lack of central color Doppler flow suggests ovarian torsion.

# Chapter 66 ▪ Answers

**1.** Correct Answer: **C. Cardiac output increased, EF unchanged, LV size increased**

*Rationale:* Cardiac output increases to compensate for an increased circulating blood volume during pregnancy. By the time a parturient is at 36 weeks, echocardiographic changes of LV size and function should be evident. In order to increase cardiac output, LV stroke volume increases, accomplished by increasing LV size, as measured by LV end-diastolic diameter. This increased diastolic size allows for a larger stroke volume but an unchanged EF. Elevation in resting HR also contributes to the increase in cardiac output during pregnancy.

**Selected Reference**
1. Liu, S, Elkayam U, Naqvi T. Echocardiography in pregnancy: part 1. *Curr Cardiol Rep.* 2016;18(9):92.

**2.** Correct Answer: **C. Increased end-diastolic diameter, increased LV stroke volume**

*Rationale:* During the course of pregnancy, cardiac output undergoes a gradual increase. By the time of delivery, cardiac output has increased by approximately 50% and can increase even more immediately following delivery. This is accomplished by both an increase in HR and stroke volume. In order to increase stroke volume, the LV end-diastolic diameter is increased, resulting in an increased stroke volume but unchanged EF. The images demonstrate an enlarged end-diastolic diameter of 57 mm compared to normal adult females who should have an end-diastolic diameter between 40 and 50 mm. The EF of 68% is not elevated but the stroke volume of 110 mL is also elevated compared to a normal value of 95 mL ± 10 mL. There is also physiologic LV hypertrophy as a result of the increased circulating blood volume. The hemodynamic and echocardiographic changes in pregnancy often resolve within 2 weeks postpartum. The supplemental videos demonstrate increased LV stroke volume and increased end-diastolic diameter.

**Selected Reference**
1. Liu, S, Elkayam U, Naqvi T. Echocardiography in pregnancy: part 1. *Curr Cardiol Rep.* 2016;18(9):92.

**3.** Correct Answer: **A. Enlarged LV end-diastolic diameter, LVEF estimated at 30 to 35%**

*Rationale:* The European Society of Cardiology working group defines peripartum cardiomyopathy as an idiopathic, dilated cardiomyopathy that presents during the last month of pregnancy or immediately postpartum, with symptoms of heart failure. Peripartum cardiomyopathy affects between 1:1,000 and 1:4,000 live births in the United States. While the underlying cause of peripartum cardiomyopathy is unknown, hypertension during pregnancy may be a risk factor. Peripartum cardiomyopathy is a diagnosis of exclusion, and hypertensive disease, coronary artery disease, and valvular disease must be excluded. Patients with peripartum cardiomyopathy have a reduced LVEF and abnormal contractility. An echocardiogram will reveal an LVEF of less than 45% and both the end-diastolic and end-systolic diameters will be increased. RV function is also affected in peripartum cardiomyopathy, and the TAPSE has been found to be significantly less in peripartum patients when compared to idiopathic dilated cardiomyopathy.

**Selected References**
1. Arany Z, Elkayam U. Peripartum cardiomyopathy. *Circulation.* 2016, 133:1397-1409.
2. Bauersachs J, König T, van der Meer P, et al. Pathophysiology, diagnosis and management of peripartum cardiomyopathy: a position statement from the Heart Failure Association of the European Society of Cardiology Study Group on peripartum cardiomyopathy. *Eur J Heart Fail.* 2019;21:827-843.
3. Liu, S, Elkayam U, Naqvi T. Echocardiography in pregnancy: part 1. *Curr Cardiol Rep.* 2016;18(9):92.

**4.** Correct Answer: **B. Dilated LV with reduced systolic function**

*Rationale:* Peripartum cardiomyopathy is characterized by a dilated left ventricle with a reduction in systolic function. One of the defining characteristics is the onset of heart failure symptoms within the last four weeks of the pregnancy or immediately postpartum. The LV end diastolic diameter increases in size during pregnancy and should measure between 50 and 60 mm in healthy parturients. The images show an increased end-diastolic diameter measuring 66 mm (Figure 66.3B). The increased end-diastolic diameter is accompanied by a calculated end-diastolic volume of 224 mL. The calculated EF seen in Figure 66.3D is 22%, which is below the diagnostic cutoff of 45%.

Selected References

1. Arany Z, Elkayam U. Peripartum cardiomyopathy. *Circulation*. 2016;133:1397-1409.
2. Bauersachs J, König T, van der Meer P, et al. Pathophysiology, diagnosis and management of peripartum cardiomyopathy: a position statement from the Heart Failure Association of the European Society of Cardiology Study Group on peripartum cardiomyopathy. *Eur J Heart Fail*. 2019;21:827-843.
3. Liu, S, Elkayam U, Naqvi T. Echocardiography in pregnancy: part 1. *Curr Cardiol Rep*. 2016;18(9):92.

**5.** Correct Answer: **C. Increased LV mass, elevated E/e′**

*Rationale:* The most common cause of nonobstetric death in pregnancy is cardiovascular disease. As discussed in previous questions, there are significant cardiovascular changes that occur during pregnancy. Patients with preeclampsia and gestational hypertension have increased vascular resistance and abnormal LV function. As the pregnancy progresses, cardiac output can fall, which leads to a higher vascular resistance to maintain placental perfusion pressure.

A compensatory response to the increased vascular resistance is for LV hypertrophy to develop. This increase in LV mass results in diminished diastolic relaxation, as evidenced by a decrease in the E/A ratio, and is seen in both preeclampsia and gestational hypertension. E/e′ can be used to differentiate hypertensive cardiomyopathy of preeclampsia from the effects of gestational hypertension. In preeclampsia, elevated LV end-diastolic pressure (LVEDP) is seen as a compensatory mechanism, and E/e′ will be elevated. These changes in diastolic dysfunction are more pronounced in patients that develop early preeclampsia and can often be seen before the clinical diagnosis of preeclampsia is made.

Echocardiographic findings in gestational hypertension include normal LV function and myocardial performance index, and an increase in LV mass resulting from concentric hypertrophy. The LV and LA diameters also increase. The E/A ratio is decreased further than in pregnant patients without hypertension.

Answers A, B and D are all changes found in normal pregnancy.

Selected Reference

1. Castleman JS, Ganapathy R, Taki R, Lip GYH, Steeds RP, Kotecha D. Echocardiographic structure and function in hypertensive disorders of pregnancy: a systematic review. *Circ Cardiovasc Imaging*. 2016;9:e004888.

**6.** Correct Answer: **D. Collapsible IVC with respiratory variation**

*Rationale:* Figures 66.4 and 66.5 show a distended right ventricle that has septal displacement into the left ventricle, which is more pronounced during systole. This finding is caused by both RV pressure and volume overload, in this case as a possible result of an amniotic fluid embolus. In acute volume overload, the right ventricle will cause a leftward septal shift that is most prominent at end diastole because that is when RV volume is the highest and RV end-diastolic pressure exceeds LVEDP. In acute RV pressure overload, the right ventricle contracts against a higher afterload, resulting in high RV systolic pressure and leftward septal shift during systole. The first signs of RV pressure overload will be a loss of septal motion and a flattening of the septum, resulting in a D-shaped left ventricle. As RV pressure rises, a leftward septal shift during systole is seen. Elevated RV pressures prolong RV systole, which also accounts for some of the septal shift. New severe TR is also a sign of RV dilation. With the dilation of the RV and the severe TR that accompanies it, the IVC will become distended and have minimal respiratory variation. Pulsed-wave Doppler of the hepatic vein flow will show systolic flow reversal.

Selected References

1. McDonnell, NJ, Percival V, Paech MJ. Amniotic fluid embolism: a leading cause of maternal death yet still a medical conundrum. *Int J Obstet Anesth*. 2013;22:329-336.
2. Sidebotham D. *Practical Perioperative Transoesophageal Echocardiography*. 3rd ed. Oxford University Press: 2018:209,211,285-288.

**7.** Correct Answer: D. Dilated LV with systolic and diastolic impairment

*Rationale:* AFE is a rare but potentially fatal event that can occur in the peripartum period. The incidence ranges between 1:12,000 in the United States and 1:50,000 in the UK. The sentinel event is disruption of the barrier between maternal and placental circulation and the entry of placental, amniotic, or fetal components into maternal circulation via the uterine veins. One theory is that an AFE causes a mechanical obstruction in the pulmonary artery leading to reduced cardiac output. A more recent theory suggests that AFE is an immune-mediated response. Amniotic fluid contains cytokines, vasoactive peptides, and procoagulant factors, which can trigger the immune response that results in pulmonary hypertension. The effect of either mechanical obstruction or pulmonary hypertension is acute RV pressure overload.

The first echo findings seen in AFE is acute RV failure from RV pressure overload. Septal shift can also decrease LV end-diastolic volume and affect LV function. TAPSE is likely to be decreased (<18 mm) with significant RV dysfunction. After the resolution of pulmonary hypertension, LV systolic dysfunction can still be seen; this may be due to ischemia from hypotension or direct myocardial depression from inflammatory mediators. There are also case reports of visualizing transient masses in the RV or pulmonary arteries. It is unclear if these masses are from development of disseminated intravascular coagulation (DIC), amniotic products, or thromboemboli.

AFE does not result in a dilated left ventricle and reduced systolic function, this would be more consistent with peripartum cardiomyopathy.

### Selected References

1. James CF, Feinglass NG, Menke DM, Grinton SF, Papadimo TJ. Massive amniotic fluid embolism: diagnosis aided by emergency transesophageal echocardiography. *Int J Obstet Anesth.* 2004; 13:279-283.
2. Katz J, Shear TD, Murphy GS, et al. Cardiovascular collapse in the pregnant patient, rescue transesophageal echocardiography and open heart surgery. *J Cardiothorac Vasc Anesth.* 2017;31:203-206.
3. McDonnell, NJ, Percival V, Paech MJ. Amniotic fluid embolism: a leading cause of maternal death yet still a medical conundrum. *Int J Obstet Anesth.* 2013;22:329-336.
4. Shamshursaz AA, Clark SL. Amniotic fluid embolism. *Obstet Gynecol Clin North Am.* 2016;43:779-790.

**8.** Correct Answer: C. This is a Stanford Type A dissection

*Critique/Rationale:* Half of aortic dissections that occur in patients under the age of 40 occur in a peripartum setting and are less commonly associated with hypertension as compared to non-parturients. In pregnancy, there are hormonal changes that lead to a weakening of aortic tissue and, when combined with an increase in shear stress due to an expansion in blood volume during the third trimester, aortic dissection can occur. Patients at a higher risk for peripartum aortic dissection are those with connective tissue disorders like Marfan syndrome, Ehlers-Danlos syndrome, and Loeys-Dietz syndrome. Management of an acute Type A aortic dissection would include emergent delivery of the fetus and surgical repair.

The diagnosis of aortic dissection can be made with CT angiography or echocardiography. CT angiography has a sensitivity of 100% and a specificity of 98%, and TEE has high sensitivity and specificity for detecting Stanford Type A dissection approaching 100%, as well. In pregnant patients, TEE has the benefit of not requiring ionizing radiation. TEE can also be useful to look for extension of the dissection into the aortic root and, according to one study, up to 79% of patients had severe acute aortic insufficiency.

Differentiating between the true and false lumen is important for surgical repair. This can be done by looking for systolic expansion of the true lumen and more turbulent higher velocity flow based on color flow Doppler within the true lumen. If the origin of the dissection flap is found, color flow can be used to visualize flow directly into the false lumen.

Hypertension is a risk factor for both Type A and Type B aortic dissections. A Stanford Type B dissection originates distal to the left subclavian artery and is often managed medically, while a Type A dissection originates anywhere more proximal and is managed surgically. Traumatic aortic dissections are most commonly seen in the descending thoracic aorta, and most originate where the ligamentum arteriosum tethers the aorta to the chest. TEE can be helpful in diagnosing and determining the origin of Type B dissections; it is also used for guidance during open and endovascular repair.

### Selected References

1. Borhart J, Palmer J. Cardiovascular emergencies in pregnancy. *Emerg Med Clin North Am.* 2019;37:339-350.
2. Sidebotham D. *Practical Perioperative Transoesophageal Echocardiography.* 3rd ed. Oxford University Press: 2018: 182-184.
3. Zhu JM, Ma WG, Peters S, et al. Aortic dissection in pregnancy: management strategy and outcomes. *Ann Thorac Surg.* 2017;103:1199-1206.

**9.** Correct Answer: C. Acute aortic insufficiency from aortic valve endocarditis

*Rationale:* Infective endocarditis during pregnancy is a rare but potentially catastrophic occurrence. The prevalence of infective endocarditis during pregnancy is estimated at 0.006%, but as high as 1.2% for patients with preexisting cardiac disease (prosthetic valve or surgically corrected congenital disease). The biggest risk factor for patients without preexisting cardiac disease is IV drug use. Maternal mortality from heart failure or embolic events is 33% and fetal mortality is 29%. Surgery, while high risk, may be required during pregnancy for heart failure symptoms from acute valvulopathy.

Chronic aortic insufficiency results in chronic LV volume overload, which can be well-tolerated because the LV can compensate with hypertrophy and by increasing in size. Acute aortic insufficiency causes rapid LV volume and pressure overload, which can result in an abrupt rise in left atrial and pulmonary pressures, resulting in acute pulmonary edema. The high regurgitant fraction seen with severe aortic insufficiency can result in reduced forward flow leading to cardiogenic shock. The increase in circulating blood volume during pregnancy can exacerbate or unmask underlying aortic insufficiency.

The images above are from a patient who developed sudden severe aortic insufficiency as a result of aortic valve endocarditis.

Selected References

1. Habib G, Lancellotti P, Antunes MJ, et al. 2015 ECS guidelines for the management of infective endocarditis. *Eur Heart J.* 2015;36:3075-3123.
2. Sidebotham D. *Practical Perioperative Transoesophageal Echocardiography.* 3rd ed. Oxford University Press: 2018:155-157.

**10.** Correct Answer: C. Low LV volume and increased LVEF concerning for hemorrhagic shock

*Rationale:* One of the most common causes of hypotension following cesarean delivery is hemorrhagic shock. These patients often receive massive transfusion and may be admitted to ICU for monitoring or further resuscitation. This patient has multiple risk factors for uterine atony and subsequent postpartum hemorrhage.

Hypovolemia and low afterload have similar echocardiographic appearances and must be often differentiated based on the clinical scenario. Characteristic echo findings of hypovolemia include reduced LV end-diastolic volume and an increased LVEF. When the LVEF is >70%, it is termed hyperdynamic. When examining the LV in a short-axis view, the LV volume will be reduced and at end systole it can appear that the papillary muscles are almost touching (the kissing papillary sign). In the case of hypovolemia, RV size is also decreased.

Low afterload states (e.g., sepsis, neuraxial anesthesia) will also have a hyperdynamic LV, but LV end-diastolic volume will be closer to normal. RV size may be normal or slightly decreased. Doppler measurement of cardiac output will reveal a reduced cardiac output in a hypovolemic state while low afterload often results in a high output state.

Selected Reference

1. Sidebotham D. *Practical Perioperative Transoesophageal Echocardiography.* 3rd ed. Oxford University Press: 2018:283-284.

**11.** Correct Answer: D. An IUP cannot be confirmed

*Rationale:* A DDSS is often seen with an IUP, but its presence alone does not confirm an IUP. A DDSS is two concentric rings filled with anechoic fluid with myometrium surrounding, as seen in the cross-sectional view in the second panel of the image. The DDSS is often the first sign of an IUP, but until the yolk sac is seen, an IUP cannot be confirmed. After the yolk sac is present, the fetal pole will develop in the yolk sac and a fetal heartbeat should be identifiable. A DDSS can be mistaken for a pseudo-gestational sac, which is a thin-walled anechoic sac filled with fluid that represents an intrauterine fluid collection, which is often seen with ectopic pregnancy.

The fetal pole would indicate that the patient has an IUP and can start to be seen around 6 weeks. Serum β-hCG levels strongly correlate with ultrasound findings in early normal pregnancy; however, a missed abortion or ectopic pregnancy may have lower-than-expected β-hCG levels. An important developmental milestone to remember is that a β-hCG level of about 2,500 mIU/mL correlates with the first appearance of a yolk sac in most cases, but findings can be variable between 1,000 and 2,000 mIU/mL. The fetal pole is usually visible at about 5,000 mIU/mL, and the fetal heartbeat at about 7,000 mIU/mL.

**Table 66.1 Developmental Milestones**

| Ultrasound | Weeks from LMP | β-hCG (mIU/mL) |
|---|:---:|:---:|
| Gestational sac (2-5 mm) | 5 | 1,000 |
| Discriminatory zone | 5-6 | 1,000-2,000 |
| Yolk sac | 6 | 2,500 |
| Fetal pole | 7 | 5,000 |
| Fetal heart motion | 6-7 | 7,000 |

LMP, last menstrual period.

Because of the variability of these ranges (**Table 66.1**), a single examination is often not sufficient to exclude or confirm IUP and should be repeated serially if uncertainty remains.

Selected Reference
1. Conolly AM, Ryan DH, Stuebe AM, Wolfe HM. Reevaluation of discriminatory and threshold levels for serum B-HCG in early pregnancy. *Obstetrics and Gynecology*. 2013;121(1):65-70.
2. Scibetta EW, Han CS. Ultrasound in early pregnancy. *Obstet Gynecol Clin N AM*. 2019;46:783-795.
3. Sohoni A, Bosley J, Miss JC. Bedside ultrasound for obstetric and gynecologic emergencies. *Crit Care Clin*. 2014;30:207-226.
4. Walls RM. Rosen's Emergency Medicine. 9th ed., Ch 178. Elsevier: 2018.

**12.** Correct Answer: C. This represents a possible ectopic pregnancy

*Rationale:* **Figure 66.16** shows a tubal ectopic pregnancy (EP) adjacent to the patient's left ovary (LO). The empty intrauterine gestational sac (I) can also be seen within the uterus, which does not confirm an IUP. In a patient with a positive pregnancy test, an extrauterine mass should be considered an ectopic pregnancy and can represent an obstetric emergency.

A β-hCG of 2,500 mIU/mL is usually not sufficient to see a fetal pole. Transvaginal ultrasound would be the preferred mode of imaging for this case, unless a definitive diagnosis is established with transabdominal ultrasound, which is usually performed first. Transvaginal ultrasound can detect a yolk sac representing an IUP at a β-hCG level as low as 2,000 mIU/mL, but this is typically not visible by abdominal ultrasound until around 6,000 mIU/mL. In a patient with free fluid in the pelvis, a positive pregnancy test and ovarian mass is suspicious for ruptured ectopic pregnancy and should be further evaluated.

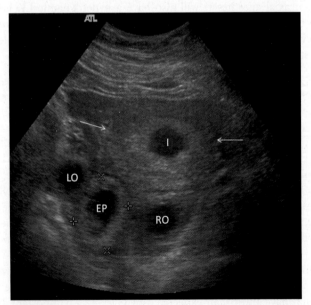

**Figure 66.16**

Selected Reference
1. Sohoni A, Bosley J, Miss JC. Bedside ultrasound for obstetric and gynecologic emergencies. *Crit Care Clin*. 2014;30:207-226.

**13.** Correct Answer: B. The fetal heart rate (FHR) is 124 and is within normal range

*Critique/Rationale:* The images represent an IUP. The gestational sac is visualized within the uterus and the fetal heart measures 124 (Figure 66.12, *Panel C*), which is within the normal range for a crown-rump length (CRL) (Figure 66.12, *Panel B*) of 7.5 mm. CRL is one of the methods of determining gestational age and, during early gestation, correlates with expected FHR. **Table 66.2** shows the CRL to FHR relationship. Fetal bradycardia increases the chance of miscarriage.

**Table 66.2 CRL and FHR Relationship**

| CRL (mm) | Est. Gest. Age (weeks) | Expected FHR (bpm) | <5% Expected FHR (bpm) |
|---|---|---|---|
| <5 | 6 | 100-120 | <100 |
| 5-9 | 6-7 | 120-140 | 100-120 |
| 10-15 | 7-8 | 140-160 | 120-140 |

Measurement of FHR is performed using M-mode across the fetal heart, one wavelength represents one heartbeat and FHR can be calculated that way. This calculation can also be done automatically by the ultrasound machine.

FHR can be present in ectopic pregnancies depending on gestational age. Vaginal bleeding in early pregnancy can be a symptom of pregnancy loss, and the patient should be counseled on this. However, pregnancy loss occurs in a minority (~10%) of these cases.

Selected References

1. Papaioannou GI, Syngelaki A, Poon LC, Ross JA, Nicolaides KH. Normal ranges of embryonic length, embryonic heart rate, gestational sac diameter and yolk sac diameter at 6–10 weeks. *Fetal Diagn Ther.* 2010;28(4):212-214.
2. Sohoni A, Bosley J, Miss JC. Bedside ultrasound for obstetric and gynecologic emergencies. *Crit Care Clin.* 2014;30: 207-226.
3. Varelas FK, Prapas NM, Liang RI, Prapas IM, Makedos GA. Yolk sac size and embryonic heart rate as prognostic factors of first trimester pregnancy outcome. *Eur J Obstet Gynecol Reprod Biol.* 2008;138(1):11.

**14.** Correct Answer: B. This is a complex ovarian cyst and is likely the cause of her pain

*Rationale:* Ovarian cysts can be a cause of acute abdominal pain in women. The densities within this cyst suggest that it is not a simple cyst. Simple ovarian cysts can vary in size from 2 to 8 cm, are thin-walled, and are filled with anechoic fluid without septations. If cysts are larger than 3 cm, they should have a follow-up ultrasound to ensure resolution.

Hemorrhagic cysts occur when a hemorrhage develops into an existing cyst, which can be painful and often leads patients to seek medical evaluation. The image above shows a hemorrhagic cyst of the left ovary (note the arrowheads in panel B are pointing to the thickened cyst wall). The internal structure of the cyst can have septations, a sponge-like appearance, or a more solid appearance.

Dermoid ovarian cysts, also called mature cystic teratomas, are germ cell tumors that can be premalignant and require urgent gynecologic follow-up. Dermoid cysts often have a fluid level and will have teeth visible on ultrasound. Even though the images do not show dermoid cyst characteristics, this cyst should have further gynecologic evaluation.

Selected References

1. Abbas AM, Amin MT, Tolba SM, Ali MK. Hemorrhagic ovarian cysts: clinical and sonographic correlation with the management options. *Middle East Fertil Soc J.* 2016;21:41-45.
2. Eskander R, Berman M, Keder L. ACOG practice bulletin: evaluation and management of adnexal masses, number 174. *Obstet Gynecol.* 2016;128(5):e210-e226.
3. Sohoni A, Bosley J, Miss JC. Bedside ultrasound for obstetric and gynecologic emergencies. *Crit Care Clin.* 2014;30:207-226.

**15.** Correct Answer: A. Transvaginal ultrasound has a low positive predictive value for malignancy.

*Rationale:* According to the American College of Obstetrics and Gynecology (ACOG) Practice guidelines on the evaluation of adnexal masses, transvaginal ultrasound is the preferred screening and initial diagnostic imaging modality. Transvaginal ultrasound is preferred because of its low cost, widespread use, and ability to provide anatomic information. However, transvaginal ultrasound has a low positive predictive value for malignancy due to difficulty differentiating between benign and malignant masses. The addition of color or spectral Doppler can increase the specificity for malignancy with transvaginal ultrasound.

Abdominal ultrasound is reasonable when pelvic masses distort the anatomy, but it is not considered first line for imaging or screening. CT imaging does not improve diagnostic certainty, but does help with staging by allowing for imaging of the other abdominal organs and looking for mesenteric or peritoneal implants. MRI is an imaging modality used for gynecologic evaluation, but based on ACOG recommendations is helpful mostly for identifying the origin of nonovarian masses.

Selected Reference

1. Eskander R, Berman M, Keder L. ACOG practice bulletin: evaluation and management of adnexal masses, number 174. *Obstet Gynecol*. 2016;128(5):e210-e226.

**16.** Correct Answer: D. A coiled vascular pedicle visualized on color flow suggests ovarian torsion.

*Rationale:* Transabdominal ultrasound is the preferred imaging method for patients with a concern for ovarian torsion, with sensitivity of approximately 92%. However, intervention should not be delayed for imaging if the diagnosis is apparent. The ultrasound findings that are most suggestive of ovarian torsion are unilateral enlargement of an ovary, ovarian edema (a hyperechoic ovary), peripherally displaced follicles, free pelvic fluid, and a coiled vascular pedicle ("whirlpool sign").

Reassuring findings that help exclude an ovarian torsion include symmetric ovarian size and location. A torsed ovary can be up to 12 times as large as its counterpart. Coexistence of ovarian cysts and torsion is high, but the presence of cysts does not confirm the diagnosis of torsion. Due to collateral arterial flow to the ovary, the presence of normal arterial Doppler flow does not rule out torsion and may be present in up to 60% of cases.

Selected References

1. Abraham M, Keyser EA. ACOG committee opinion on adnexal torsion in adolescents. *Obstet Gynecol*. 2019; 134(2):e56-e63.
2. Sohoni A, Bosley J, Miss JC. Bedside ultrasound for obstetric and gynecologic emergencies. *Crit Care Clin*. 2014;30:207-226.

**17.** Correct Answer: B. The high degree of vascularity surrounding the rim suggests an abscess.

*Rationale:* Figure 66.15 represents an enlarged Fallopian tube and tubo-ovarian abscess (TOA). On ultrasound, a TOA appears as an enlarged Fallopian tube filled with heterogeneous-appearing fluid. The use of color flow Doppler is helpful to demonstrate the hypervascularity seen in the wall of the abscess and suggests the presence of acute inflammation. A fluid-filled Fallopian tube that measures greater than 5 mm in diameter is classified as a hydrosalpinx. Systemic illness, tenderness to palpation, cervical motion tenderness, and the heterogeneous nature of the fluid suggest TOA, a more severe manifestation of pyosalpinx. Antibiotics are the initial treatment for a TOA and surgery (or drainage) is considered only if the patient fails to respond to medical management.

Selected References

1. Eskander R, Berman M, Keder L. ACOG practice bulletin: evaluation and management of adnexal masses, Number 174. *Obstetrics and Gynecology*. 2016;128(5):e210-e226.
2. Sohoni A, Bosley J, Miss JC. Bedside ultrasound for obstetric and gynecologic emergencies. *Crit Care Clin*. 2014;30:207-226.

Elaine Y. Gee

1. A 92-year-old man has a known 4.5 cm infrarenal abdominal aortic aneurysm. You decide to practice your abdominal vascular ultrasound and obtain the following image (**Figure 67.1** and ▶ **Video 67.1**).

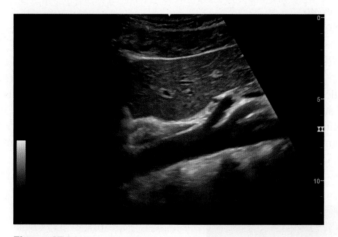

**Figure 67.1**

Which would *least* likely account for the discrepancy between your bedside imaging and the patient's history?
A. The aneurysm is saccular
B. The aneurysm has been repaired
C. The longitudinal image is along a parasagittal plane
D. The image does not extend distally enough

2. A 72-year-old woman with a past medical history of coronary artery disease, hypertension, and an AAA presents with recurrent abdominal pain after eating fatty foods. She is currently asymptomatic. While doing an abdominal ultrasound to evaluate her gallbladder, you obtain **Figure 67.2** and ▶ **Video 67.2** of the aorta.

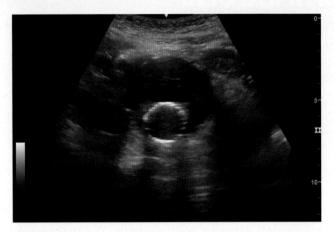

**Figure 67.2**

What is the *most* appropriate next step in her management regarding this finding?
A. Outpatient vascular surgery follow-up
B. Urgent inpatient vascular surgery consultation
C. Immediate anticoagulation
D. Urgent computed tomography angiography (CTA) of the abdomen and pelvis

3. A 95-year-old man with a past medical history of end-stage Alzheimer's dementia presents from his nursing facility with altered mental status. He is unable to provide any history, but is complaining of abdominal pain. His vital signs show a temperature of 38.5°C, HR 110 bpm, RR 16/min, and BP 170/70 mm Hg. His physical examination is notable for abdominal distension and lower abdominal tenderness, but no peritoneal signs. Distal pulses are intact. A point-of-care ultrasound (POCUS) reveals **Figure 67.3** and ▶ **Video 67.3**.

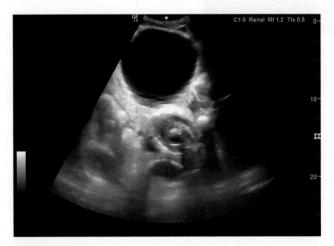

**Figure 67.3**

What is the *most* appropriate next step for the management of the abnormality noted within the aorta?
A. Outpatient follow-up with vascular surgery
B. Emergent vascular surgery consult
C. Start a beta-blocker
D. Emergent CTA of the abdomen and pelvis

4. Identify the structure indicated by the *arrow* in **Figure 67.4**. (See also ▶ **Video 67.4**.)

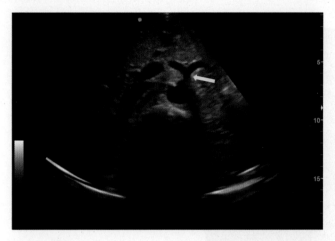

**Figure 67.4**

   **A.** Descending aorta
   **B.** Celiac trunk
   **C.** Superior mesenteric artery (SMA)
   **D.** Left renal artery

5. Identify the structure indicated by the *arrow* in **Figure 67.5**. (See also ▶ **Video 67.5**.)

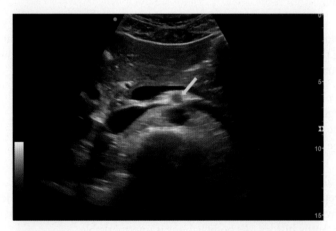

**Figure 67.5**

   **A.** Aorta
   **B.** Celiac trunk
   **C.** Superior mesenteric artery
   **D.** Inferior mesenteric artery

6. You perform a POCUS examination of the abdominal aorta for a patient with abdominal pain and obtain **Figure 67.6**.

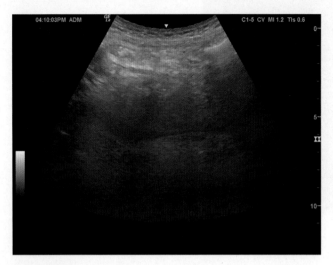

**Figure 67.6**

Which of the following maneuvers is *least* likely to improve visualization of the aorta?
A. Gentle continuous probe pressure
B. Right coronal scanning approach
C. Left lateral decubitus positioning
D. Deep inspiration with breath-hold

7. You are asked to ultrasound the abdominal aorta of a patient with a midline incision extending from the xiphoid to the umbilicus, rendering the standard imaging windows inaccessible. Which of the following would be the *least* appropriate alternative imaging approach?

A. Lateral to the wound with the probe angled toward midline
B. Coronal plane from either the right or left mid-axillary line, just below the costal margin
C. From the midline, with the probe below the umbilicus and angled cephalad
D. From the midline, with the probe above the xiphoid process and angled caudad

8. A 22-year-old man is serving as an ultrasound model for a teaching course. While scanning his abdominal aorta ( ▶ **Video 67.6**), you see the abnormality indicated by the *arrow* in **Figure 67.7**. He denies any past medical history of hypertension, symptoms of back or abdominal pain, or recent trauma or procedures. He is unaware of his family history. His body habitus is unremarkable.

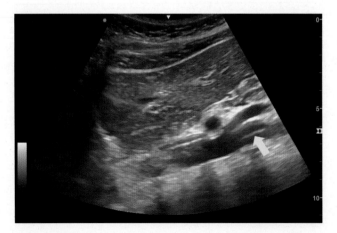

**Figure 67.7**

Which of the following would be *least* likely to exclude the presence of aortic dissection?
A. Scanning from the coronal plane
B. Scanning in the short axis in the standard transverse plane
C. Scanning in the long axis in an oblique plane
D. Evaluating with alternate imaging modality (CT or magnetic resonance imaging [MRI])

9. A 75-year-old man with a past medical history of hypertension, hyperlipidemia, and a 50-pack-year smoking history presents with acute-onset back and abdominal pain. The patient is alert, but his BP is 82/40 mm Hg and his HR is 140 bpm.

His abdominal examination is remarkable for diffuse tenderness, but no rebound or guarding. A point-of-care abdominal ultrasound shows **Figure 67.8** and ▶ **Videos 67.7A** and **B.**

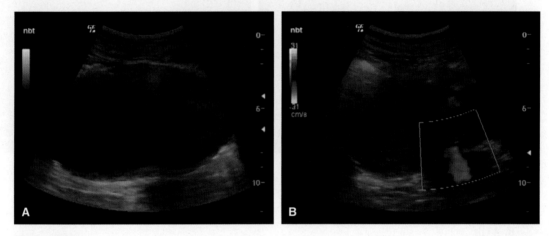

**Figure 67.8**

What is the *best* next step in his management?
A. Consult vascular surgery emergently
B. Order a STAT CTA abdomen and pelvis
C. Bolus 2 L of crystalloid
D. Perform STAT transesophageal echocardiogram (TEE)

10. A 75-year-old man with a known aortic aneurysm presents with vomiting and diarrhea. A POCUS of his aorta is performed and is shown in **Figure 67.9** and ▶ **Video 67.8.**

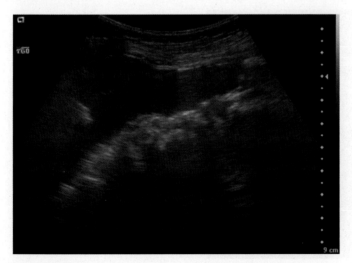

**Figure 67.9**

What is the maximum aortic diameter?

**A.** 3 cm

**B.** 4 cm

**C.** 6 cm

**D.** Cannot be determined

---

11. An 82-year-old woman with a past medical history of hypertension, hyperlipidemia, and hypothyroidism presents with abdominal pain. An abdominal ultrasound is performed and **Figure 67.10** and ▶ **Videos 67.9A** and **B** are obtained.

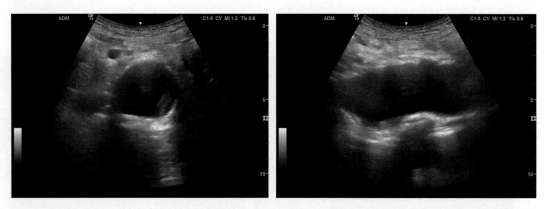

**Figure 67.10**

What is the diameter of the aorta at this point?

**A.** 3 cm

**B.** 4 cm

**C.** 5 cm

**D.** >9 cm

---

12. An 80-year-old man with a past medical history of hypertension and tobacco use presents with fever and lower abdominal pain. Upon arrival, his vital signs show a temperature of 38.6°C, HR 90 bpm, RR 16/min, and BP 120/70 mm Hg. His abdomen is soft, but he has mild right lower quadrant tenderness over a pulsatile mass. There are no peritoneal signs. Both lower extremities are warm and well-perfused, with no edema.

A POCUS of the kidneys reveals moderate right-sided hydronephrosis. Ultrasound of the abdomen shows **Figure 67.11**.

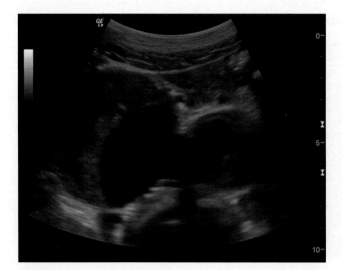

**Figure 67.11**

What is the *most appropriate* next step in the management of the patient?
A. CTA abdomen and pelvis
B. Bilateral lower extremity venous Doppler
C. Anticoagulation
D. Emergent vascular surgery consultation

13. An 81-year-old man with a past medical history of Alzheimer's dementia and a known AAA was brought in from his nursing home after an episode of syncope. The patient is currently lethargic and complaining of abdominal pain. His vital signs show a temperature of 37°C, BP 70/40 mm Hg, HR 140 bpm, RR 30/min, and SpO$_2$ 94% on room air. He has diffuse abdominal tenderness. An abdominal ultrasound shows no free peritoneal fluid, and **Figure 67.12** and ▶ **Videos 67.10A** and **B** are obtained.

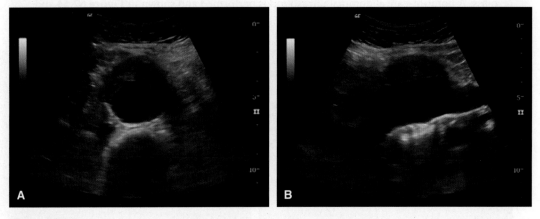

**Figure 67.12**

What is the *best* next step in his management?
A. Call vascular surgery emergently
B. Repeat the ultrasound in 15 minutes to see if fluid accumulates
C. Order a STAT CTA of the abdomen and pelvis
D. Perform point-of-care echocardiography to exclude other sources of shock

14. A 71-year-old woman with a past medical history of hypertension and atrial fibrillation presents from her nursing facility with a complaint of acute-onset abdominal pain. She is tachycardic to 140 bpm and has a BP of 70/40 mm Hg. Her abdomen is diffusely tender, but there is no rebound or guarding. There is no evidence of trauma. No free fluid is noted on ultrasound of her abdomen, and **Figure 67.13** and ▶ **Videos 67.11A** and **B** are obtained.

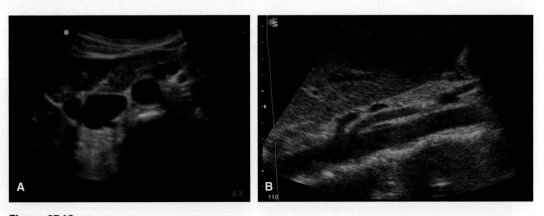

**Figure 67.13**

What is the *most* likely cause of her symptoms, and what is the *best* next step in her management?
A. This is an aortic rupture until otherwise proven. Call vascular surgery emergently.
B. This is a possible aortic rupture. Repeat the ultrasound in 15 minutes to see if fluid accumulates.
C. This is a possible aortic rupture. Since there is no evidence of free fluid, order a CTA of the abdomen and pelvis.
D. This is unlikely to be an aortic rupture. Look for another source of shock.

15. A 79-year-old man with a past medical history of hypertension, peripheral vascular disease, and a 60-pack-year smoking history presents with persistent dull abdominal pain for 3 days.

His vital signs show a temperature of 37.5°C, BP 110/60 mm Hg, HR 80 bpm, RR 14/min, and SpO$_2$ 96% on room air. His physical examination is remarkable for periumbilical tenderness and a pulsatile mass. A point-of-care abdominal ultrasound is performed and shown in **Figure 67.14** and ▶ **Videos 67.12A** and **B.**

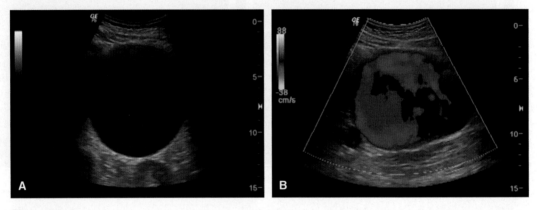

**Figure 67.14**

What is the *most* appropriate next step in his management?
A. Outpatient vascular surgery follow-up and routine surveillance imaging
B. Obtain a CTA abdomen and pelvis and consult vascular surgery
C. Defer further imaging and obtain an emergent vascular surgery consultation
D. Initiate an intravenous (IV) beta-blocker to lower the HR and BP

16. A 62-year-old man with a past medical history of coronary artery disease, hypertension, and hyperlipidemia presents with acute-onset upper back and abdominal pain. His vitals signs show a temperature of 37.2°C, BP 140/70 mm Hg right arm, 118/60 mm Hg left arm, HR 120 bpm, RR 18/min, and SpO$_2$ 94% on room air. His physical examination is remarkable for tachycardia, with a regular rhythm and a decrescendo diastolic murmur. The lungs are clear and the abdomen is diffusely tender, without rebound or guarding. Weak pedal pulses are noted bilaterally. A point-of-care abdominal ultrasound is performed and shows **Figure 67.15** and ▶ **Videos 67.13A** and **B.**

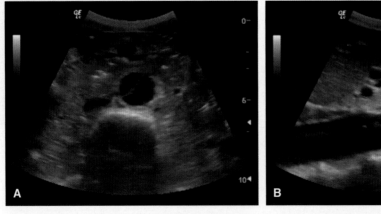

**Figure 67.15**

Which subsequent study would be the *least* helpful?
A. Transesophageal echocardiogram
B. Point-of-care cardiac ultrasound
C. CTA chest/abdomen/pelvis
D. Ankle-brachial index (ABI)

# Chapter 67 ▪ Answers

**1.** Correct Answer: B. The aneurysm has been repaired

*Rationale:* This is an image of a native aorta. An open or endovascular repair would appear as an echogenic foreign body within an aneurysm sac.

This case illustrates the importance of imaging the entirety of the abdominal aorta from the proximal aspect to the bifurcation, in both the transverse and longitudinal planes.

Saccular aneurysms (Choice A) expand asymmetrically from the aortic wall and are best seen in the transverse plane as it gives a circumferential view of the aorta. Even with fusiform aneurysms, which expand symmetrically, longitudinal views are prone to error due to the cylinder tangent effect (**Figure 67.16**). In this axis, the widest diameter is the true diameter. It is possible to underestimate the diameter of the aorta if the imaging plane is not midline, but parasagittal (Choice C). In the transverse axis, the smallest diameter is the true diameter, and it is possible to overestimate the true diameter if the angle of insonation is not exactly perpendicular. This is especially true when measuring a tortuous aorta.

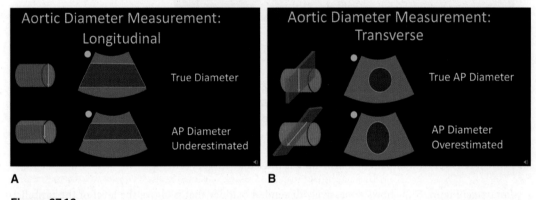

**Figure 67.16**

Choice D is possible because in this view, the distal aorta is not completely visualized. A complete abdominal aorta exam begins proximally at the xiphoid process and extends distally to the bifurcation of the aorta into the iliac arteries. While this image includes the more proximal part of the infrarenal aorta, it does not include the entire segment down to the bifurcation. Complete imaging of the abdominal aorta is important since 95% of abdominal aortic aneurysms are infrarenal.

Selected References
1. Dean AJ. Abdominal aorta. In: Cosby KS, Kendall JL, eds. *Practical Guide to Emergency Ultrasound.* 2nd ed. Wolters Kluwer Health; 2014:156-171.
2. Guideline developed in collaboration with the American College of Radiology; Society of Radiologists in Ultrasound. AIUM practice guideline for the performance of diagnostic and screening ultrasound examinations of the abdominal aorta in adults. *J Ultrasound Med.* 2015;34(8):1-6. doi:10.7863/ultra.34.8.15.13.0003.
3. Noble VE, Nelson BP, eds. Abdominal aorta ultrasound. In: *Manual of Emergency and Critical Care Ultrasound.* 2nd ed. Cambridge University Press; 2011:115-131.
4. Tainter CR. Abdominal aorta. In: Soni NJ, Arntfield R, Kory P, eds. *Point-of-Care Ultrasound.* 1st ed. Elsevier; 2015:167-173.

2. Correct Answer: A. Outpatient vascular surgery follow-up

*Rationale:* Figure 67.2 shows an AAA with a stent-graft in place following an endovascular aortic aneurysm repair (EVAR). The hyperechoic ring represents the walls of the stent-graft, which lies within the lumen of the aneurysmal aorta. The aneurysm sac is notable for the presence of extensive mural thrombus. The walls of the stent-graft could be mistaken for a calcified, non-aneurysmal aortic wall if care is not taken to identify the true aortic wall.

Urgent inpatient vascular surgery consultation (Choice B) or CTA of the abdomen and pelvis (Choice D) is unnecessary because the patient has no signs or symptoms of post-EVAR complications. She requires only routine outpatient vascular surgery follow-up and surveillance with CTA or ultrasound. Although there is evidence of mural thrombus in the aneurysm sac, there is no role for anticoagulation (Choice C) in this setting. See also **Figure 67.17**.

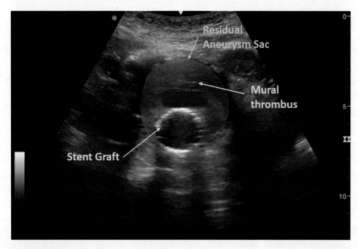

**Figure 67.17**

### Selected References

1. Chaikof EL, Dalman RL, Eskandari MK, et al. The Society for Vascular Surgery practice guidelines on the care of patients with an abdominal aortic aneurysm. *J Vasc Surg.* 2018;67(1):2-77.e2. doi:10.1016/j.jvs.2017.10.044.
2. Dean AJ. Abdominal aorta. In: Cosby KS, Kendall JL, eds. *Practical Guide to Emergency Ultrasound.* 2nd ed. Wolters Kluwer Health; 2014:156-171.

3. Correct Answer: A. Outpatient follow-up with vascular surgery

*Rationale:* Figure 67.3 shows a massively distended bladder that is above the level of the umbilicus. The fluid-filled bladder allows for excellent imaging of the aneurysmal aorta posterior. The aorta is remarkable for the presence of an endovascular stent-graft.

The patient's symptoms can be attributed to urinary retention and a possible urinary tract infection. A Foley catheter was placed and >1 L of urine was drained, with immediate resolution of his abdominal distension and pain. As the patient is asymptomatic from his previously repaired AAA, visible deep to the distended bladder (see image below), only routine follow-up with his vascular surgeon and surveillance imaging is required (Choice A). Emergent vascular surgery consult (Choice B) or CTA of the abdomen and pelvis (Choice D) is not warranted. Beta-blockers (Choice C) have not been shown to limit aneurysm sac expansion or increase regression post-EVAR.

This image demonstrates the importance of identifying the vertebral shadow as a key landmark for locating the aorta, which lies directly above it. This is particularly important when normal anatomy may be altered by previous surgery or acute issues, such as massive bladder distension (in this case). One could easily mistake the distended bladder for a massive 9 cm AAA and assume the aorta behind it to be the vertebral body. Through the bladder, posterior acoustic enhancement makes the anterior wall of the aorta much brighter than usual, similar to the appearance of the anterior surface of the vertebra. Additionally, the presence of the endovascular stent-graft and mural thrombus in the residual aneurysm sac significantly alter the usual anechoic appearance of the aorta. See also **Figure 67.18**.

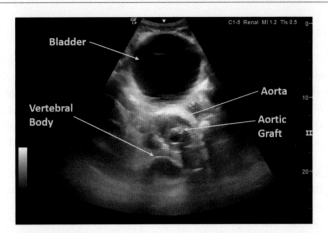

**Figure 67.18**

**Selected References**

1. Chaikof EL, Dalman RL, Eskandari MK, et al. The Society for Vascular Surgery practice guidelines on the care of patients with an abdominal aortic aneurysm. *J Vasc Surg.* 2018;67(1):2-77.e2. doi:10.1016/j.jvs.2017.10.044.
2. Kim W, Gandhi RT, Peña CS, et al. Effect of β-blocker on aneurysm sac behavior after endovascular abdominal aortic repair. *J Vasc Surg.* 2017;65(2):337-345. doi:10.1016/j.jvs.2016.06.111.

4. Correct Answer: B. Celiac trunk

*Rationale:* The celiac trunk is the first major branch of the abdominal aorta. It arises from the anterior aspect of the aorta, at the T12 vertebral level, and branches into the splenic artery to the left (right of the image) and the common hepatic artery to the right (left of the image), forming the characteristic "seagull sign," seen in Figure 67.4. See also **Figure 67.19**. The third branch of the trunk, the left gastric artery, often cannot be visualized on ultrasound.

The descending aorta (Choice A) is the round hypoechoic structure lying directly above the vertebral body. In this image, the left lateral wall of the aorta is obscured by an edge artifact. The SMA (Choice C) is the second major branch of the abdominal aorta. It arises from the anterior aspect of the aorta approximately 1 cm distal to the origin of the celiac trunk, at the L1 vertebral level, and does not have the characteristic bifurcation seen here. The bilateral renal arteries (Choice D) arise from the lateral aspects of the aorta, just distal to the origin of the SMA. They are often poorly visualized on ultrasound.

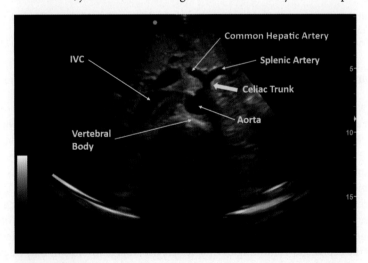

**Figure 67.19**

**Selected References**

1. Dean AJ. Abdominal aorta. In: Cosby KS, Kendall JL, eds. *Practical Guide to Emergency Ultrasound.* 2nd ed. Wolters Kluwer Health; 2014:156-171.
2. Noble VE, Nelson BP, eds. Abdominal aorta ultrasound. In: *Manual of Emergency and Critical Care Ultrasound.* 2nd ed. Cambridge University Press; 2011:115-131.
3. Tainter CR. Abdominal aorta. In: Soni NJ, Arntfield R, Kory P, eds. *Point-of-Care Ultrasound.* 1st ed. Elsevier; 2015:167-173.

**5.** Correct Answer: **C. Superior mesenteric artery**

*Rationale:* The SMA is the second major branch of the abdominal aorta. It arises from the anterior aspect of the aorta approximately 1 cm distal to the origin of the celiac trunk, at the L1 vertebral level. The SMA has a surrounding hyperechoic fat layer that forms the characteristic "mantle clock sign." Other important landmarks in this view include the splenic vein and the left renal vein (see **Figure 67.20**). The splenic vein can be seen coursing anteriorly to the SMA on its way to join the superior mesenteric vein (SMV) at the portal confluence. The left renal vein courses between the SMA and the aorta to empty into the inferior vena cava (IVC).

The aorta (Choice A) is the round hypoechoic structure lying directly above the vertebral body.

The celiac trunk (Choice B) is the first major branch of the abdominal aorta and will have branched off approximately 1 cm proximal to the origin of the SMA. The inferior mesenteric artery (Choice D) arises from the anterior aspect of the aorta at the L3 vertebral level. It is not well-visualized on the standard POCUS examination.

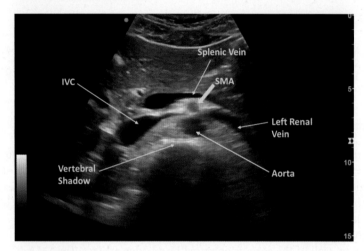

**Figure 67.20**

Selected References
1. Dean AJ. Abdominal aorta. In: Cosby KS, Kendall JL, eds. *Practical Guide to Emergency Ultrasound*. 2nd ed. Wolters Kluwer Health; 2014:156-171.
2. Noble VE, Nelson BP, eds. Abdominal aorta ultrasound. In: *Manual of Emergency and Critical Care Ultrasound*. 2nd ed. Cambridge University Press; 2011:115-131.
3. Tainter CR. Abdominal aorta. In: Soni NJ, Arntfield R, Kory P, eds. *Point-of-Care Ultrasound*. 1st ed. Elsevier; 2015:167-173.

**6.** Correct Answer: **D. Deep inspiration with breath-hold**

*Rationale:* Figure 67.6 shows overlying bowel gas.

A deep breath will displace the abdominal organs downward, improving imaging of the gallbladder or the heart in a subcostal approach. However, it is unlikely to displace bowel gas sufficiently to allow imaging of the abdominal aorta.

Gentle continuous pressure, often with a slight jiggling of the probe, encourages peristalsis and movement of bowel gas. A demonstration of this technique can be seen in ▶ **Video 67.14**.

The right coronal approach (from the mid-axillary line just below the diaphragm) uses the liver as an acoustic window to avoid bowel gas. The left coronal approach can also be used, though the spleen offers a smaller acoustic window. There are several key limitations to consider. The distal aorta will often be incompletely evaluated due to the cephalad positioning of the probe. Also, image resolution may be poor as the aorta will be further from the probe compared to the standard midline views. Left lateral decubitus positioning is often used in conjunction with the right coronal approach to further improve imaging. In this position, gravity encourages the bowel to fall away from the abdominal aorta. Similarly, right lateral decubitus positioning can be used with the left coronal approach.

Selected References

1. Dean AJ. Abdominal aorta. In: Cosby KS, Kendall JL, eds. *Practical Guide to Emergency Ultrasound.* 2nd ed. Wolters Kluwer Health; 2014:156-171.
2. Noble VE, Nelson BP, eds. Abdominal aorta ultrasound. In: *Manual of Emergency and Critical Care Ultrasound.* 2nd ed. Cambridge University Press; 2011:115-131.
3. Tainter CR. Abdominal aorta. In: Soni NJ, Arntfield R, Kory P, eds. *Point-of-Care Ultrasound.* 1st ed. Elsevier; 2015:167-173.

7. Correct Answer: D. From the midline, with the probe above the xiphoid process and angled caudad

*Rationale:* Alternative views are often necessary for a complete evaluation of the aorta. Each approach has its advantages and limitations.

The advantage of scanning lateral to the midline (Choice A) is that the probe can be moved from proximal to distal to evaluate the entire length of the abdominal aorta. Additionally, when in long axis, this oblique scan plane allows you to visualize the aortic bifurcation into the bilateral iliac arteries, although this approach may be limited by the presence of bowel gas.

Imaging from the right or left coronal plane (Choice B) uses the liver or spleen as an acoustic window, but views of the distal aorta are limited and the resolution may be poor due to the increased distance of the aorta from the probe.

The approach from below the umbilicus (Choice C) is often used to image the distal aorta when obscured by overlying bowel gas. The disadvantage of this technique is that it often offers no view of the more proximal aspects of the abdominal aorta and can be obscured by bowel gas as well.

With the probe above the xiphoid process (Choice D), the presence of bone and air would preclude imaging of the abdominal vessels, making this choice the least effective strategy.

Selected References

1. Dean AJ. Abdominal aorta. In: Cosby KS, Kendall JL, eds. *Practical Guide to Emergency Ultrasound.* 2nd ed. Wolters Kluwer Health; 2014:156-171.
2. Noble VE, Nelson BP, eds. Abdominal aorta ultrasound. In: *Manual of Emergency and Critical Care Ultrasound.* 2nd ed. Cambridge University Press; 2011:115-131.
3. Tainter CR. Abdominal aorta. In: Soni NJ, Arntfield R, Kory P, eds. *Point-of-Care Ultrasound.* 1st ed. Elsevier; 2015:167-173.

8. Correct Answer: B. Scanning in the short axis in the standard transverse plane

*Rationale:* The hyperechoic line indicated by the arrow is a reverberation artifact from the overlying SMA. It is formed by the reflection of ultrasound waves between the anterior and posterior walls of the SMA due to the hyperechoic fat layer surrounding the vessel. This hyperechoic fat gives the SMA its characteristic "mantle clock" appearance in transverse imaging. The reverberation artifact often appears as a hyperechoic mass (known as a "pseudo-mass") or, in this case, a bright stripe mimicking a dissection flap.

This artifact can be eliminated by imaging in such a way that the ultrasound beam does not pass directly through the SMA, such as through a coronal (Choice A) or oblique (Choice C) plane. Scanning in the standard transverse plane may not eliminate this artifact, as the ultrasound beam still passes through the anechoic SMA with hyperechoic edges, which creates the reverberation artifact. If the object remains despite changes in the scanning approach, the ultrasound finding should be confirmed with alternative imaging such as CT or MRI (Choice D).

Selected References

1. Kokhanovsky N, Nachtigal A, Reindorp N, Zeina AR. Superior mesenteric artery-related aortic pseudomass as a form of reverberation artifact in a 10-year-old boy. *J Clin Imaging Sci.* 2014;4:73. doi:10.4103/2156-7514.148268.
2. Mann GS, Robinson AJ, LeBlanc JG, Heran MK. Abdominal aortic pseudomass in a child: a diagnostic red herring. *J Ultrasound Med.* 2008;27(2):307-310. doi:10.7863/jum.2008.27.2.307.
3. Rubin JM, Gao J, Hetel K, Min R. Duplication images in vascular sonography. *J Ultrasound Med.* 2010;29(10):1385-1390. doi:10.7863/jum.2010.29.10.1385.

9. Correct Answer: A. Consult vascular surgery emergently

*Rationale:* This is a case of a ruptured aortic aneurysm. The longitudinal (sagittal) image in Figure 67.8A shows a markedly dilated aortic aneurysm with a maximum anteroposterior diameter of 8 cm and a posterior para-aortic hypoechoic area that is concerning for a hematoma. In the transverse (axial) image (Figure 67.8B), color Doppler confirms the flow of blood out of the aorta into the hypoechoic area.

Evidence of rupture is often not apparent on ultrasound, and the clinical triad of back and/or abdominal pain, hypotension, and AAA is sufficient to warrant emergent vascular surgery consultation (Choice A) with a goal door-to-intervention time of 90 minutes. Further confirmation with CT abdomen/pelvis (Choice B) is not necessary prior to consultation and should not delay evaluation of this hemodynamically unstable patient.

Further fluid boluses should be deferred to allow for permissive hypotension (or hypotensive hemostasis) with a target systolic BP of 70 to 90 mm Hg, as long as perfusion is adequate, pending definitive treatment.

Ultrasound findings suggestive of aortic rupture include:
- Para-aortic hypoechoic focus
- Inhomogeneous layered luminal thrombus
- Internal interruption of luminal thrombus
- Floating thrombus layer
- Focal wall interruption
- Retroperitoneal hematoma
- Hemoperitoneum

### Selected References

1. Catalano O, Siani A. Ruptured abdominal aortic aneurysm: categorization of sonographic findings and report of 3 new signs. *J Ultrasound Med.* 2005;24(8):1077-1083. doi:10.7863/jum.2005.24.8.1077.
2. Chaikof EL, Dalman RL, Eskandari MK, et al. The Society for Vascular Surgery practice guidelines on the care of patients with an abdominal aortic aneurysm. *J Vasc Surg.* 2018;67(1):2-77.e2. doi:10.1016/j.jvs.2017.10.044.
3. Dean AJ. Abdominal aorta. In: Cosby KS, Kendall JL, eds. *Practical Guide to Emergency Ultrasound.* 2nd ed. Wolters Kluwer Health; 2014:156-171.

**10.** Correct Answer: D. Cannot be determined

*Rationale:* Aneurysms are measured from outer wall to outer wall, and care must be taken to include any mural thrombus to avoid underestimation of the aneurysmal size. The aortic diameter needs to be measured in both the transverse and longitudinal planes. This is especially important in the case of a saccular aneurysm, like the one shown in Figure 67.9. Saccular aneurysms expand asymmetrically, making the determination of the maximal diameter inaccurate in the longitudinal axis, even if the scan plane is truly mid-sagittal. The transverse plane allows better evaluation of these aneurysms since it affords a view of the entire aortic circumference.

### Selected References

1. Dean AJ. Abdominal aorta. In: Cosby KS, Kendall JL, eds. *Practical Guide to Emergency Ultrasound.* 2nd ed. Wolters Kluwer Health; 2014:156-171.
2. Guideline developed in collaboration with the American College of Radiology; Society of Radiologists in Ultrasound. AIUM practice guideline for the performance of diagnostic and screening ultrasound examinations of the abdominal aorta in adults. *J Ultrasound Med.* 2015;34(8):1-6. doi:10.7863/ultra.34.8.15.13.0003.
3. Noble VE, Nelson BP, eds. Abdominal aorta ultrasound. In: *Manual of Emergency and Critical Care Ultrasound.* 2nd ed. Cambridge University Press; 2011:115-131.
4. Tainter CR. Abdominal aorta. In: Soni NJ, Arntfield R, Kory P, eds. *Point-of-Care Ultrasound.* 1st ed. Elsevier; 2015:167-173.

**11.** Correct Answer: C. 5 cm

*Rationale:* The abdominal aorta should be imaged in both transverse and longitudinal axes to best detect the presence of aneurysms. Transverse imaging allows the best determination of the aortic diameter because the entire circumference can be seen, and cannot be underestimated by a cylinder tangent effect (although it may be overestimated if the axis is not perpendicular, see explanation for **Question 1**). The largest transverse diameter is used, whether it is anterior-posterior, transverse, or oblique. Anterior-posterior measurements are often easiest because the walls will be well-defined as they are perpendicular to the angle of insonation. The transverse (medial-lateral) measurements can be complicated by a loss of wall definition due to edge artifact or the loss of lateral resolution, particularly with increasing depth of insonation. The aorta should be measured from outer wall to outer wall, and care must be taken to avoid underestimating the diameter by mistaking the surface of a mural thrombus for the vessel wall.

In the transverse plane, the anterior-posterior diameter is 4 cm (Choice B) and the transverse diameter is 5 cm, as illustrated in the figure. A mural thrombus is also seen at the 5 o'clock position. If this thrombus was not recognized and mistaken for the wall, a measurement of 3 cm (Choice A) would be obtained. (See also **Figure 67.21**.)

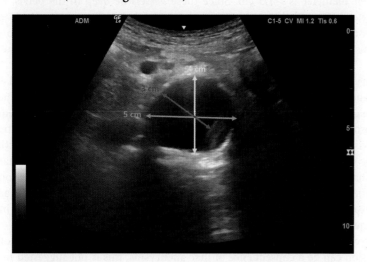

**Figure 67.21**

This is further illustrated in **Figure 67.22**, where a significant circumferential mural thrombus can give the appearance of a relatively normal aortic diameter and mask the presence of a large aneurysm.

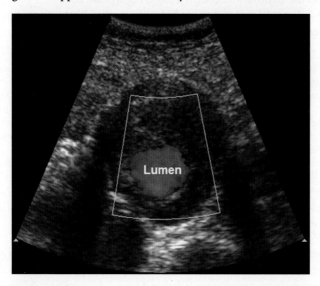

**Figure 67.22**

In the longitudinal image in the question stem, the anterior-posterior diameter is 4 cm. Measurement in this axis is inaccurate because the maximum diameter is not in the imaging plane. Longitudinal imaging is good for determining the length of dilatation, which in this case appears to be >9 cm (Choice D).

### Selected References

1. Dean AJ. Abdominal aorta. In: Cosby KS, Kendall JL, eds. *Practical Guide to Emergency Ultrasound.* 2nd ed. Wolters Kluwer Health; 2014:156-171.
2. Guideline developed in collaboration with the American College of Radiology; Society of Radiologists in Ultrasound. AIUM practice guideline for the performance of diagnostic and screening ultrasound examinations of the abdominal aorta in adults. *J Ultrasound Med.* 2015;34(8):1-6. doi:10.7863/ultra.34.8.15.13.0003.
3. Hannon KM. Vascular structures. In: Kawamura D, Lunsford B, eds. *Abdomen and Superficial Structures.* 3rd ed. Wolters Kluwer; 2013:57-100.
4. Noble VE, Nelson BP, eds. Abdominal aorta ultrasound. In: *Manual of Emergency and Critical Care Ultrasound.* 2nd ed. Cambridge University Press; 2011:115-131.
5. Tainter CR. Abdominal aorta. In: Soni NJ, Arntfield R, Kory P, eds. *Point-of-Care Ultrasound.* 1st ed. Elsevier; 2015:167-173.

**12.** Correct Answer: **A. CTA abdomen and pelvis**

*Rationale:* Figure 67.11 shows aneurysms of bilateral common iliac arteries. The iliac arteries are considered aneurysmal when their diameter is >1.5 cm. Since these vessels lie deep in the pelvis, these aneurysms are usually asymptomatic until they are quite large (>6 cm). Common presenting symptoms include the sequela of compression of adjacent structures (ureters, colon, lumbar plexus), thromboembolism, or rupture. In this case, compression of the right ureter led to hydronephrosis and resultant pyelonephritis.

Isolated iliac artery aneurysms are uncommon (<2% of all intra-abdominal aneurysms), and evaluation for other abdominal aneurysms is necessary. Ultrasound imaging of the abdominal and pelvic arteries may be limited by the depth and tortuosity of these vessels and overlying bowel gas. If adequate images can be obtained, ultrasound is the preferred modality for surveillance of asymptomatic patients. CTA of the abdomen and pelvis is preferred if other structures need evaluation (e.g., bowel obstruction), for those being considered for intervention (like this patient), or if adequate images cannot be obtained by ultrasound. Magnetic resonance angiography (MRA) can be utilized if there are contraindications to CTA. Indications for intervention include symptomatic or ruptured aneurysms, and asymptomatic aneurysms >3 cm, or with rapid expansion. Iliac aneurysms not meeting these criteria may be repaired in the setting of other aneurysms requiring intervention.

Bilateral lower extremity venous Doppler (Choice B) is incorrect because these vessels are not venous. While venous compression can be a consequence of iliac aneurysms, this is not suggested in this case. Veins can be distinguished from arteries by the fact they are more ovoid and larger than their corresponding artery, have thinner walls, exhibit respirophasic variability, and are compressible. Arteries are rounder with thicker, echogenic walls and exhibit pulsatility. The IVC may appear pulsatile due to transmission of pulsations from the aorta and the right ventricle, or tricuspid regurgitation.

Anticoagulation (Choice C) is not indicated for mural thrombi in aneurysms. The patient is hemodynamically stable, which makes emergent consultation (Choice D) unnecessary.

### Selected References

1. Chaikof EL, Dalman RL, Eskandari MK, et al. The Society for Vascular Surgery practice guidelines on the care of patients with an abdominal aortic aneurysm. *J Vasc Surg.* 2018;67(1):2-77.e2. doi:10.1016/j.jvs.2017.10.044.
2. Dean AJ. Abdominal aorta. In: Cosby KS, Kendall JL, eds. *Practical Guide to Emergency Ultrasound.* 2nd ed. Wolters Kluwer Health; 2014:156-171.
3. Guideline developed in collaboration with the American College of Radiology; Society of Radiologists in Ultrasound. AIUM practice guideline for the performance of diagnostic and screening ultrasound examinations of the abdominal aorta in adults. *J Ultrasound Med.* 2015;34(8):1-6. doi:10.7863/ultra.34.8.15.13.0003.
4. Krupski WC, Selzman CH, Floridia R, Strecker PK, Nehler MR, Whitehill TA. Contemporary management of isolated iliac aneurysms. *J Vasc Surg.* 1998;28(1):1-13. doi:10.1016/s0741-5214(98)70194-6.
5. Richardson JW, Greenfield LJ. Natural history and management of iliac aneurysms. *J Vasc Surg.* 1988;8(2):165-171.

**13.** Correct Answer: **A. Call vascular surgery emergently**

*Rationale:* Figure 67.12 is a ruptured aortic aneurysm until proven otherwise. Evidence of rupture is often not apparent on ultrasound, and the clinical triad of back and/or abdominal pain, hypotension, and AAA is sufficient to warrant emergent vascular surgery consultation (Choice A).

Repeating the focused assessment with sonography in trauma (FAST) examination (Choice B) to look for accumulation of free fluid is inappropriate because it will delay intervention and aortic aneurysms tend to bleed into the retroperitoneal space rather than cause hemoperitoneum. Other ultrasound findings suggestive of aortic rupture include a para-aortic hypoechoic focus, inhomogeneous layered luminal thrombus, internal interruption of luminal thrombus, floating thrombus layer, and focal wall interruption.

Confirmation with CT abdomen and pelvis (Choice C) is not necessary prior to consultation and should not delay evaluation of this hemodynamically unstable patient. Though this AAA is <5.5 cm, making the annual risk of rupture low, it does not preclude rupture in the appropriate clinical scenario. Looking for an alternative source of shock (Choice D) may be appropriate once emergent vascular surgery consultation has been initiated.

Selected References
1. Catalano O, Siani A. Ruptured abdominal aortic aneurysm: categorization of sonographic findings and report of 3 new signs. *J Ultrasound Med.* 2005;24(8):1077-1083. doi:10.7863/jum.2005.24.8.1077.
2. Chaikof EL, Dalman RL, Eskandari MK, et al. The Society for Vascular Surgery practice guidelines on the care of patients with an abdominal aortic aneurysm. *J Vasc Surg.* 2018;67(1):2-77.e2. doi:10.1016/j.jvs.2017.10.044.
3. Dean AJ. Abdominal aorta. In: Cosby KS, Kendall JL, eds. *Practical Guide to Emergency Ultrasound.* 2nd ed. Wolters Kluwer Health; 2014:156-171.

**14.** Correct Answer: D. This is unlikely to be an aortic rupture. Look for another source of shock.

*Rationale:* This aorta is not aneurysmal, making rupture an unlikely cause of her hypotension. Aneurysms are defined as diameter >3 cm in the abdominal aorta and >1.5 cm in the iliac arteries.

Non-aneurysmal aortic rupture can occur, especially in the setting of blunt trauma (often acceleration/deceleration injury in motor vehicle accidents) or with crush injuries, but this is also unlikely based on the clinical scenario. Other sources of shock should be evaluated first.

In the transverse view, it is important to not mistake the teardrop-shaped IVC, which is a little over 3.5 cm in greatest diameter, for an aneurysmal aorta. Identification of the vertebral body as the landmark for finding the aorta is helpful to prevent this error. Furthermore, the aorta is noncompressible, pulsatile, and the celiac (large arrow) and superior mesenteric (small arrows) arteries may be seen arising from its anterior aspect (**Figure 67.23**).

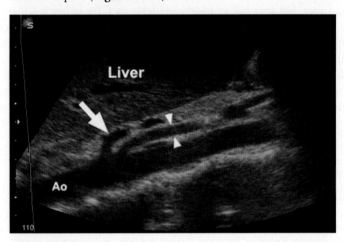

**Figure 67.23**

Selected References
1. Dean AJ. Abdominal aorta. In: Cosby KS, Kendall JL, eds. *Practical Guide to Emergency Ultrasound.* 2nd ed. Wolters Kluwer Health; 2014:156-171.
2. Noble VE, Nelson BP, eds. Abdominal aorta ultrasound. In: *Manual of Emergency and Critical Care Ultrasound.* 2nd ed. Cambridge University Press; 2011:115-131.
3. Tainter CR. Abdominal aorta. In: Soni NJ, Arntfield R, Kory P, eds. *Point-of-Care Ultrasound.* 1st ed. Elsevier; 2015:167-173.

**15.** Correct Answer: B. Obtain a CTA abdomen and pelvis and consult vascular surgery

*Rationale:* Figure 67.14 is a massive symptomatic AAA. As the risk of rupture is high, urgent intervention is warranted, beginning with a CTA abdomen/pelvis (to rule out rupture and for presurgical planning). Vascular surgery consultation is also essential and should be obtained while the patient is admitted. Outpatient vascular surgery follow-up (Choice A) is inappropriate for this high-risk condition. Emergent consultation (Choice C) is unnecessary because the patient is hemodynamically normal and there is no evidence of rupture. Beta-blockers (Choice D) have not been shown to decrease the rate of aneurysm growth or risk of rupture, which would be moot at this point since the patient already warrants repair.

This aorta is so markedly aneurysmal, it could be mistaken for the bladder or a large cyst/fluid collection. Identification of the vertebral body distal to the aorta and the presence of flow on color Doppler (as seen in the second image) confirms that this is the aorta.

Selected References

1. Chaikof EL, Dalman RL, Eskandari MK, et al. The Society for Vascular Surgery practice guidelines on the care of patients with an abdominal aortic aneurysm. *J Vasc Surg*. 2018;67(1):2-77.e2. doi:10.1016/j.jvs.2017.10.044.
2. Chaikof EL, Brewster DC, Dalman RL, et al. The care of patients with an abdominal aortic aneurysm: the Society for Vascular Surgery practice guidelines. *J Vasc Surg*. 2009;50(4 suppl):S2-S49. doi:10.1016/j.jvs.2009.07.002.
3. Dean AJ. Abdominal aorta. In: Cosby KS, Kendall JL, eds. *Practical Guide to Emergency Ultrasound*. 2nd ed. Wolters Kluwer Health; 2014:156-171.

**16.** Correct Answer: D. Ankle-brachial index (ABI)

*Rationale:* This is a case of aortic dissection. As nearly all dissections originate in the thoracic aorta, subsequent imaging of this area is warranted. Isolated abdominal aortic dissections are rare, accounting for only 1% to 4% of all cases.

In this clinical scenario, imaging of the thoracic aorta should occur emergently because the patient has symptoms concerning for ascending thoracic aorta involvement, including upper extremity BP differences and a murmur concerning for aortic insufficiency.

While the ABI will likely be abnormal, it does not provide any useful information about the ascending thoracic aorta.

The choice of imaging modality often depends on hemodynamic stability and local availability. When available, TEE (Choice A) is preferred in the hemodynamically unstable patient, as it can be done quickly at the bedside or in the operating room, but it is not as widely available as CTA (Choice C), is more operator-dependent, and requires sedation. Transthoracic cardiac ultrasound (Choice B) is significantly less sensitive and specific than other modalities (TEE, CTA, and MRA) in identifying aortic dissections, because only the proximal ascending aorta can be well-visualized. However, TTE may be useful in identifying cardiac complications of dissection, such as aortic insufficiency and hemopericardium, and thus is a reasonable study to perform while awaiting more definitive imaging. CTA is the preferred imaging modality in hemodynamically stable patients without evidence of ascending aorta involvement, or when TEE is unavailable.

Selected References

1. Farber A, Wagner WH, Cossman DV, et al. Isolated dissection of the abdominal aorta: clinical presentation and therapeutic options. *J Vasc Surg*. 2002;36(2):205-210. doi:10.1067/mva.2002.125028.
2. Hiratzka LF, Bakris GL, Beckman JA, et al. 2010 ACCF/AHA/AATS/ACR/ASA/SCA/SCAI/SIR/STS/SVM guidelines for the diagnosis and management of patients with Thoracic Aortic Disease: a report of the American College of Cardiology Foundation/American Heart Association Task Force on Practice Guidelines, American Association for Thoracic Surgery, American College of Radiology, American Stroke Association, Society of Cardiovascular Anesthesiologists, Society for Cardiovascular Angiography and Interventions, Society of Interventional Radiology, Society of Thoracic Surgeons, and Society for Vascular Medicine [published correction appears in Circulation. 2010 Jul 27;122(4):e410]. *Circulation*. 2010;121(13):e266-e369. doi:10.1161/CIR.0b013e3181d4739e.

# 68 | GASTRIC ULTRASOUND

Amanda Xi

**1.** Which is the correct identification of structures in **Figure 68.1?**

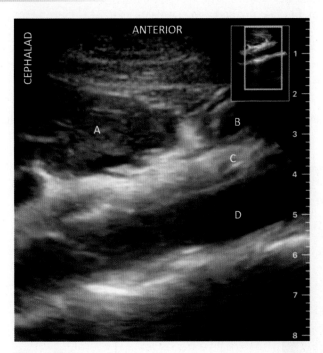

**Figure 68.1**

**A.** A: liver, B: superior mesenteric artery, C: gastric antrum, D: aorta
**B.** A: liver, B: gastric antrum, C: pancreas, D: aorta
**C.** A: liver, B: superior mesenteric artery, C: gastric antrum, D: inferior vena cava
**D.** A: liver, B: gastric antrum, C: pancreas, D: inferior vena cava

2. An obtunded patient is transferred to the intensive care unit. Due to mental status, the decision is made to prepare to intubate. Prior to induction, a gastric ultrasound is performed (**Figure 68.2**):

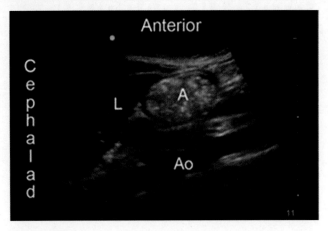

**Figure 68.2**

Based on Figure 68.2, what is the patient's *most likely* recent oral intake?
A. Recent ingestion of solid food
B. Recent ingestion of water
C. No recent ingestion
D. Unable to discern from this image

3. How can you optimize your probe/patient position to obtain a sagittal view of the gastric antrum shown in **Figure 68.3**?

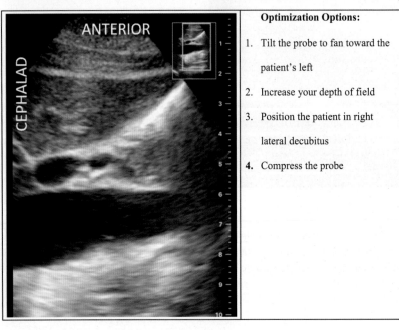

**Optimization Options:**

1. Tilt the probe to fan toward the patient's left

2. Increase your depth of field

3. Position the patient in right lateral decubitus

4. Compress the probe

**Figure 68.3**

A. Perform 1, 2, 3
B. Perform 1, 3
C. Perform 1, 3, 4
D. Perform all of the above

# Chapter 68 ▪ Answers

---

**1.** Correct Answer: B. A: liver, B: gastric antrum, C: pancreas, D: aorta

*Rationale:* In Figure 68.1, a low-frequency curvilinear probe was utilized to obtain this sagittal plane image. Utilizing familiar surrounding structures such as the aorta (*D*) and liver (*A*) can be helpful in identification of the gastric antrum (*B*) when learning gastric ultrasound. The pancreas (*C*) frequently appears as an echogenic structure deeper to the gastric antrum. The superior mesenteric artery is frequently captured when obtaining gastric ultrasound images; however, it does not appear in this particular image.

Selected References

1. El-Boghdadly K, Kruisselbrink R, Chan VWS, Perlas A. Images in anesthesiology: gastric ultrasound. *Anesthesiology.* 2016;125(3):595. doi:10.1097/ALN.0000000000001043.
2. Van de putte P, Perlas A. Ultrasound assessment of gastric content and volume. *Br J Anaesth.* 2014;113(1):12-22.

---

**2.** Correct Answer: A. Recent ingestion of solid food

*Rationale:* The gastric antrum shows hyperechoic, heterogeneous material, which is consistent with recent ingestion of thick or solid food. Liquids appear anechoic or hypoechoic, and if the patient has been without oral intake for several hours, the gastric antrum should be empty. Gastric ultrasonography has been utilized by gastroenterologists to assess gastric motility and emptying. With the increasing use of bedside ultrasound, gastric ultrasonography may be used as a tool to individualize aspiration risk.

Selected References

1. El-Boghdadly K, Kruisselbrink R, Chan VWS, Perlas A. Images in anesthesiology: gastric ultrasound. *Anesthesiology.* 2016;125(3):595. doi:10.1097/ALN.0000000000001043.
2. Van de putte P, Perlas A. Ultrasound assessment of gastric content and volume. *Br J Anaesth.* 2014;113(1):12-22.

---

**3.** Correct Answer: B. Perform 1, 3

*Rationale:* It is important to understand ways to optimize a gastric ultrasound image. In the image presented, the only obvious structure is the liver. From the indicators, it can be ascertained that this is a sagittal view. Familiar structures are helpful in identifying the gastric antrum; relative to the liver, the stomach is toward the patient's left. Thus, action 1, tilting/fanning the probe to the patient's left, may help bring the target into view. In this image, the scale on the right indicates that the depth of field is already at 10 cm. On average, obese patients' gastric antrum is at 7 cm, thus 10 cm is more than enough depth of field and action 2 is incorrect. Literature describing the use of gastric ultrasound recommends positioning the patient in the right lateral decubitus position, as this allows for a larger proportion of the stomach's content to flow to the more dependent distal antrum (action 3 is also correct). The current image has no view of the gastric antrum nor any of the usual structural landmarks (such as the aorta, pancreas); thus, compression will not optimize the image (action 4 is incorrect).

Selected References

1. El-Boghdadly K, Kruisselbrink R, Chan VWS, Perlas A. Images in anesthesiology: gastric ultrasound. *Anesthesiology.* 2016;125(3):595. doi:10.1097/ALN.0000000000001043.
2. Perlas A, Arzola C, Van de Putte P. Point-of-care gastric ultrasound and aspiration risk assessment: a narrative review. *Can J Anesth.* 2018;65:437-448.
3. Van de putte P, Perlas A. Ultrasound assessment of gastric content and volume. *Br J Anaesth.* 2014;113(1):12-22.

# 69 | ABDOMINAL EMERGENCIES

Hassan Mashbari, Ahmed Al Hazmi, Brittany K. Bankhead-Kendall, and Christopher R. Tainter

1. A 45-year-old woman presents complaining of acute-onset right upper quadrant (RUQ) abdominal pain associated with fever and vomiting. Her vital signs show a temperature of 38.6°C, HR 115 bpm, and her examination reveals tenderness in the RUQ. Based on **Figure 69.1**, which of the following additional sonographic findings would be *most* consistent with the suspected diagnosis?

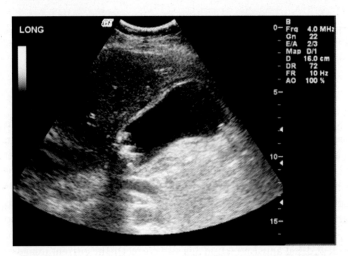

**Figure 69.1**

A. Gallbladder wall diameter is 3 mm
B. Contracted gallbladder
C. Pericholecystic fluid
D. Sludge visualized in the gallbladder

2. A 65-year-old man who presents for evaluation of flank pain and hematuria suddenly becomes hypotensive. His past medical history is significant for hypertension and a 30-pack-year smoking history. His initial BP was 160/90 mm Hg with a HR of 65 bpm. Repeat vital signs now show a BP of 85/45 mm Hg and HR 130 bpm. Which of the following ultrasound findings *best* correlates with this scenario and **Figure 69.2**?

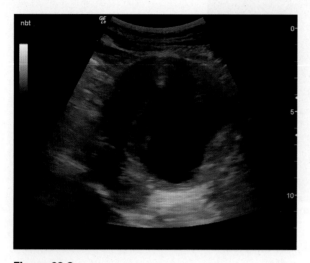

**Figure 69.2**

**A.** Calcifications of proximal abdominal aorta
**B.** Distal aorta diameter 6.5 cm
**C.** Dilated bowel with "target sign"
**D.** Bilateral grade 4 hydronephrosis

3. A 25-year-old man is brought to the Emergency Department (ED) after being involved in a high-speed motor vehicle collision. His initial vital signs showed a BP of 85/50 mm Hg and HR of 125 bpm after 2 L Lactated Ringer's fluid resuscitation. He has generalized abdominal tenderness. A Focused Assessment with Sonography in Trauma (FAST) examination is performed and is shown in **Figure 69.3**.

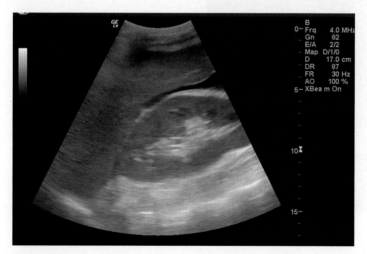

**Figure 69.3**

Which of the following is the *most* appropriate next step in his management?
**A.** Immediate operative intervention
**B.** Computed tomography (CT) to evaluate for intraperitoneal bleeding
**C.** Additional volume resuscitation for inferior vena cava (IVC) diameter <1.5 cm
**D.** Diagnostic peritoneal lavage

4. A 21-year-old woman presents to the ED with 2 days of periumbilical abdominal pain and nausea. The pain has migrated to the right lower quadrant (RLQ) and is now associated with fever and vomiting. Her physical examination demonstrates RLQ tenderness. A point-of-care ultrasound (POCUS) is performed, and a representative image is displayed in **Figure 69.4**.

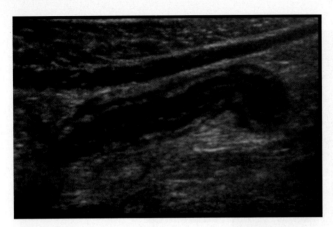

**Figure 69.4**

Which of the following findings would be *most* expected?
A. Free fluid visualized in the pouch of Douglas
B. Dilated loops of small bowel
C. Collapsed lumen of the colon
D. Target sign in the RLQ

5. A 62-year-old woman presents with abdominal pain and fever for the last 4 days. Her vital signs are notable for a temperature of 39°C, HR 122 bpm, BP 115/90 mm Hg, RR 16/min, and SpO$_2$ 95% on room air. Her physical examination reveals RUQ tenderness and jaundice. A POCUS reveals **Figure 69.5**.

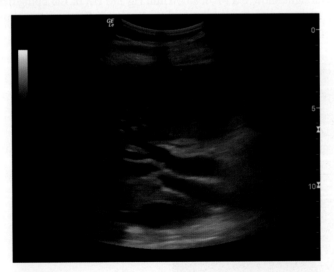

**Figure 69.5**

Which of the following ultrasound findings is *most* supportive of the diagnosis?
A. Gallbladder wall diameter > 3 mm
B. IVC diameter > 2.5 cm
C. Common bile duct diameter > 8 mm
D. Gallstones visualized within the gallbladder

6. A 45-year-old man presents to the ED with right flank pain. The pain is episodic and is associated with nausea and vomiting. His past medical history is significant for Crohn's disease. His vital signs are normal except for HR 100 bpm, and his physical examination is only remarkable for left flank tenderness. Which of the following sonographic findings is *most* consistent with the tentative diagnosis and **Figure 69.6**?

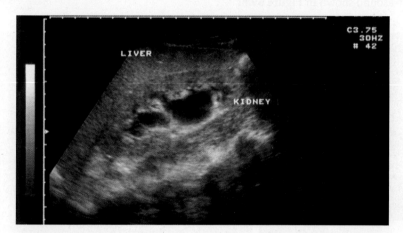

**Figure 69.6**

A. Increased echogenicity of the liver
B. Hyperechoic pancreatic tissue
C. Increased echodensity of the renal parenchyma
D. Dilatation of urinary collecting ducts

7. A 67-year-old man presents with diffuse abdominal pain, abdominal distention, and vomiting. His past medical history is significant for hypertension and previous abdominal surgery after a gunshot wound. His vital signs show HR 127 bpm and BP 110/80 mm Hg, and he has diffuse abdominal tenderness on physical examination. An image from a point-of care ultrasound is shown in **Figure 69.7**.

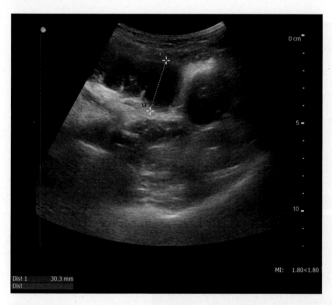

**Figure 69.7**

Which of the following ultrasound findings is *most* consistent with the presumptive diagnosis?
A. Free fluid in the peritoneum
B. Multiple hyperechogenic structures in the epigastrium
C. Bowel loop diameter 3.1 cm
D. Gallbladder diameter 3.1 cm

8. A 39-year-old woman presents with a 3-day history of fever, malaise, and right-sided back pain. She has been on antibiotics for a urinary tract infection (UTI) since last week. Her vital signs show a temperature of 39.1°C, HR 125 bpm, BP 110/70 mm Hg, RR 18/min, and SpO$_2$ 97% on room air. Her physical examination is notable only for right costovertebral angle (CVA) tenderness. What finding is demonstrated in her ultrasound shown in **Figure 69.8**?

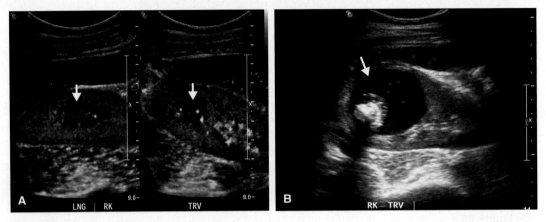

**Figure 69.8**

A. A complex renal abscess
B. Grade 3 hydronephrosis with an obstructing stone
C. Multiple gallstones within a thickened gallbladder wall
D. A hepatic mass medial to the gallbladder

9. A 35-year-old man is admitted to the intensive care unit (ICU) because of a fever and new-onset hypotension. He had a splenectomy 4 days ago following a motor vehicle collision. On examination, he has tenderness in the RUQ. Which of the following sonographic findings is demonstrated in **Figure 69.9**?

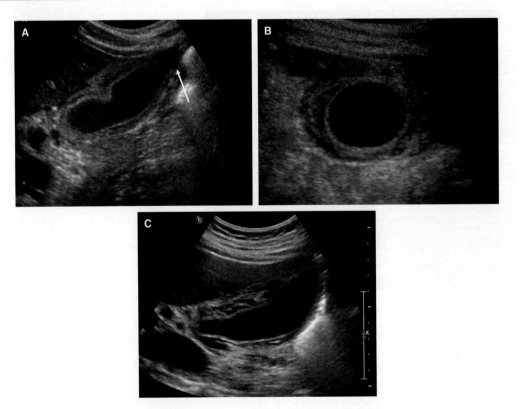

**Figure 69.9**

A. Hydronephrosis of the right kidney
B. Dilated loop of bowel
C. Distended gallbladder without gallstones
D. Intraparenchymal liver hematoma

10. A 72-year-old man presents to the ED with 2 days of fever, mental status changes, and RUQ abdominal pain. His temperature is 35°C, HR 130 bpm, BP 95/60 mm Hg, RR 20/min, and SpO$_2$ 89% on room air. His white blood cell (WBC) count is 17,000/mm$^3$, his alanine aminotransferase (ALT) is 350 U/L (10-55 U/L), and total bilirubin is 0.7 mg/dL (0.0-1.0 mg/dL). A POCUS is performed and reveals **Figure 69.10**.

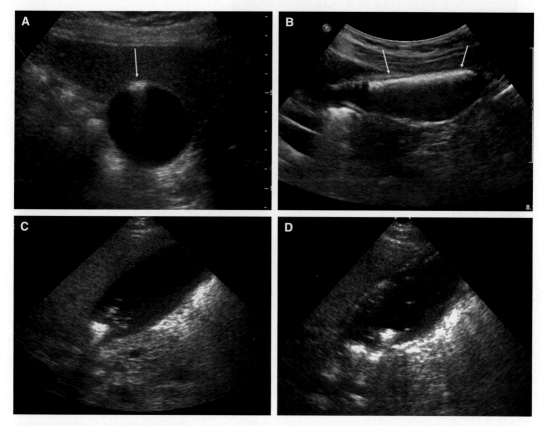

**Figure 69.10**

What is the *most* likely diagnosis?
A. Air within the gallbladder
B. Hypoechoic hepatic mass medial to the gallbladder
C. An obstructing gallstone in the common bile duct
D. Calcifications with the gallbladder wall

11. A 53-year-old man is brought to the ED following a motor vehicle collision. His HR is 125 bpm, BP is 98/55 mm Hg, and he has bruises over the left upper abdomen. Which of the following statements is *most* true about the FAST examination?

A. An empty bladder does not affect the ability to detect free fluid.
B. Up to 10% of FAST examinations may be indeterminate.
C. Peritoneal blood is hyperechoic when compared to ascites or urine.
D. A FAST examination is not indicated in this patient.

12. An 85-year-old man with a past medical history of hypertension and a 65-pack-year smoking history presents to the ED with epigastric pain. His temperature is 37°C, HR 81 bpm, BP 167/85 mm Hg, RR 14/min, and SpO$_2$ 95% on room air. His abdominal examination reveals a pulsatile, nontender abdominal mass but no other significant findings. Which of the following is *most* correct regarding the ultrasound shown in **Figure 69.11**?

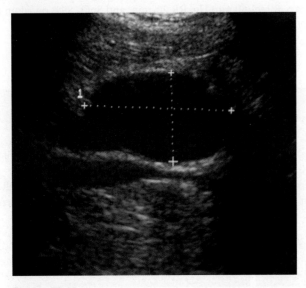

**Figure 69.11**

A. The calipers provide an accurate measurement of the aortic diameter.
B. The presence of abdominal gas helps with the ultrasound identification of an abdominal aortic aneurysm (AAA).
C. The cylinder-tangent effect may overestimate the size of an AAA.
D. The measured diameter of the aorta should include the outer walls.

13. A 21-year-old woman presents to the ED with sudden-onset RLQ abdominal pain and vomiting. She is sexually active and does not recall her last menstrual cycle. Her physical examination reveals mild tachycardia, focal tenderness in the RLQ, and right adnexal tenderness but no cervical discharge. Her urine beta human chorionic gonadotropin (BhCG) is positive. Which of the following is demonstrated in **Figure 69.12**?

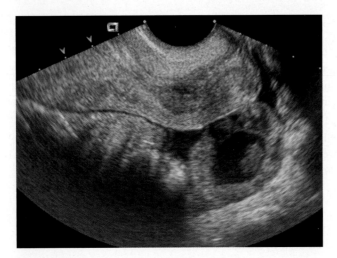

**Figure 69.12**

    **A.** Free fluid in Morrison's pouch
    **B.** A hypoechoic stripe in the pouch of Douglas
    **C.** An intrauterine pregnancy
    **D.** A double decidual sac

14. A 25-year-old man is being evaluated following a high-speed motor vehicle collision. He has equal bilateral breath sounds and diffuse abdominal tenderness. His BP is 95/45 mm Hg and HR is 140 bpm. Which of the following is true about the use of ultrasound in the evaluation of this patient?

    **A.** The extended FAST (eFAST) examination is an appropriate examination in a hemodynamically stable patient.
    **B.** The eFAST examination has a high sensitivity in penetrating trauma.
    **C.** The eFAST examination has a low sensitivity for pericardial injury.
    **D.** An eFAST examination is a reliable evaluation for intra-abdominal free fluid and hemopericardium.

15. A 42-year-old woman presents to the ED with sudden onset of periumbilical pain. Her past medical history is significant for hypertension and alcohol abuse. Her temperature is 37°C, HR 90 bpm, BP 105/60 mm Hg, RR 20/min, and SpO$_2$ 99% on room air. Her physical examination shows periumbilical tenderness without rebound, guarding, or distention. Which of the following statements is *most* correct regarding abdominal ultrasound?

    **A.** Free fluid in Morison's pouch can be distinguished from the gallbladder by its angular appearance.
    **B.** Identifying signs of chronic liver disease does not help distinguish ascites from hemoperitoneum.
    **C.** Injecting air through a nasogastric tube under ultrasound guidance will not help differentiate the stomach from free fluid.
    **D.** Ultrasound may miss up to 55% of traumatic injuries involving the bowel and up to 80% of solid organ injuries.

16. A 55-year-old man presents to the ED with 3 hours of epigastric pain. His past medical history is significant for hypertension, smoking, and alcohol abuse. His vitals are normal but he has epigastric tenderness without rebound or guarding. An ultrasound examination is performed and is displayed in **Figure 69.13**.

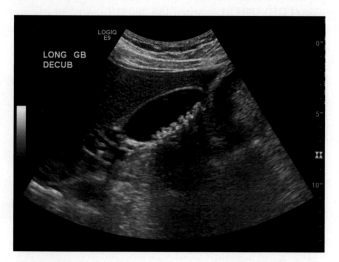

**Figure 69.13**

Which of the following is the *most* appropriate next step in his management?
    **A.** Obtain a surgical consult for acute cholecystitis.
    **B.** Treat his pain and reassess.
    **C.** Continue to evaluate for other causes of his pain.
    **D.** Give a proton pump inhibitor (PPI) and start antibiotic therapy.

**17.** An 80-year-old man presents with several days of increasing abdominal pain and constipation. He denies any past medical or surgical history, but admits that he does not seek care routinely. His temperature is 37°C, HR 110 bpm, BP 120/95 mm Hg, RR 22/min, and SpO$_2$ 95% on room air. His physical examination is remarkable for generalized abdominal tenderness and distension. Which of the following is *most* likely represented by **Figure 69.14**?

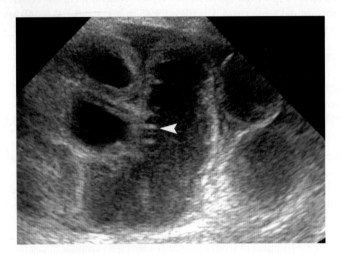

**Figure 69.14**

**A.** Dilated renal pelvis and renal collecting system due to bladder outlet obstruction
**B.** Free fluid from a perforated gastric ulcer
**C.** A dilated fluid-filled jejunal segment due to small bowel obstruction (SBO)
**D.** A distended gallbladder with pericholecystic fluid due to cholecystitis

**18.** A 55-year-old man with a history of chronic myelofibrosis presents to the ED with nontraumatic left-sided abdominal pain, nausea, and fever. He is not on anticoagulation. His temperature is 38°C, HR 105 bpm, BP 130/75 mm Hg, RR 20/min, and SpO$_2$ 96% on room air. He has left-sided abdominal tenderness, but an otherwise normal physical examination. Laboratory evaluation reveals a WBC count of 12,000/mm$^3$ and lactate dehydrogenase (LDH) 500 U/L (normal 140-280 U/L). A point-of-care abdominal ultrasound is performed and shown in **Figures 69.15A** and **C**. In addition, Doppler images are shown in **Figure 69.15B**.

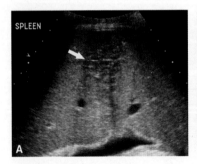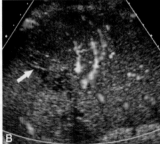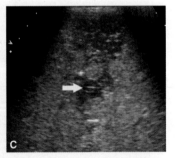

**Figure 69.15**

What is the *most* appropriate next step in his management?
**A.** Urgent splenectomy
**B.** Catheter-guided thrombolysis
**C.** Percutaneous drain placement by interventional radiology (IR)
**D.** Symptom management with pain medication

19. A 68-year-old man presents to the ED for evaluation of massive ascites causing severe abdominal distension, nausea, shortness of breath, bloating, and weight gain (36 lb in 9 months). He has a history of cirrhosis from hepatitis C and is on the liver transplant waiting list. His Model for End-stage Liver Disease (MELD) score is 22. Which of the following is *most* accurate about the ultrasound-guided procedure shown in **Figure 69.16**?

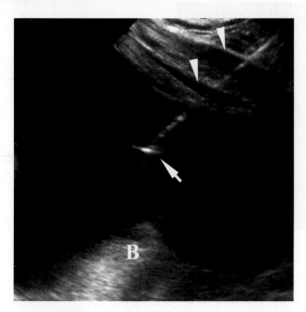

**Figure 69.16**

   A. Therapeutic paracentesis is a technique that removes a large volume of ascites (typically 100-1000 mL).
   B. The general area of the puncture site is localized 2 to 3 cm medial and 2 to 3 cm cephalad to the anterior superior iliac spine in the left lower quadrant.
   C. The success rate of ultrasound-guided paracentesis is the same as when using a traditional approach.
   D. Patients undergoing ultrasound-guided paracentesis have a higher risk of infection, but a lower rate of bleeding.

20. A 37-year-old man presents to the ED with severe umbilical pain, which occurred abruptly while he was helping his parents move furniture. On physical examination, there is an umbilical mass that is tender on palpation and has overlying skin erythema. The patient reports that he has noticed the mass intermittently for the last 6 months every time he coughs, but that it usually goes away on its own. His temperature is 38°C, HR 115 bpm, BP 140/75 mm Hg, RR 22/min, and SpO$_2$ 99% on room air. Which of the following is the *most* correct regarding ultrasound in the diagnosis of this condition?

   A. Ultrasound allows dynamic evaluation for a hernia during a Valsalva maneuver.
   B. Ultrasound can accurately identify the exact size of the fascial defects.
   C. Doppler cannot reliably identify compromised blood flow to a herniated bowel segment.
   D. Ultrasound cannot evaluate for postoperative seroma or hematoma formation

**21.** A 32-year-old woman presents to the ED with 1 day of suprapubic pain and hematuria. Her past medical history is significant for recurrent UTIs. Her vitals are normal and physical examination is remarkable only for suprapubic tenderness. Urinalysis is still pending. Which of the following is *not* an advantage to performing a pelvic ultrasound (**Figure 69.17**) with a full bladder?

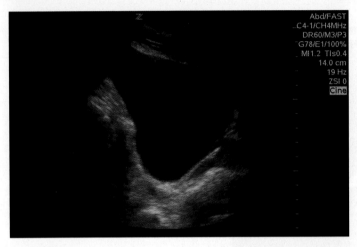

**Figure 69.17**

  **A.** To improve transvaginal imaging
  **B.** To improve the acoustic window
  **C.** To lower acoustic impedance
  **D.** To allow for better propagation of ultrasound waves

**22.** A 30-year-old man who was involved in a high-speed motor vehicle collision has just been brought to the ED. An eFAST examination was performed that showed **Figure 69.18**.

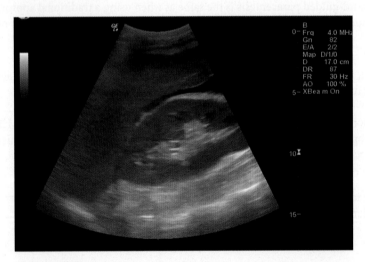

**Figure 69.18**

Which of the following is considered a limitation of eFAST?
  **A.** The examination is not able to evaluate for intrathoracic causes of hypotension.
  **B.** The examination cannot reliably identify pancreatic injuries.
  **C.** One cannot repeat the eFAST if there are any changes in the patient hemodynamics.
  **D.** Serial ultrasound examinations may delay CT evaluation.

23. A 22-year-old woman presents to the ED with 7 days of RUQ abdominal pain, nausea, and vomiting. Her temperature is 37°C, BP 110/60 mm Hg, HR 85 bpm, RR 14/min, and SpO$_2$ 100% on room air. Her physical examination is remarkable for hepatomegaly without abdominal tenderness. Laboratory evaluation reveals hemoglobin (Hb) 12 g/dL, WBC 8.4 × 10$^{-9}$/L, with 80% neutrophils and 8% eosinophils, total bilirubin 1.7 mg/dL (normal <1.2 mg/dL), aspartate transaminase (AST) 74 U/L (normal 0-32 U/L), ALT 58 U/L (normal 0-33 U/L), and alkaline phosphatase (ALP) of 18 U/L (normal 35-140 U/L). She reported a history of traveling to the Mediterranean for an internship recently. Ultrasound evaluation shows **Figure 69.19**.

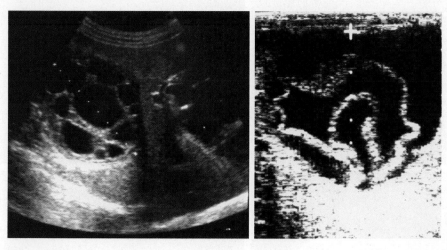

**Figure 69.19**

What is the *best* next step in management?
A. Test the patient by the echinococcosis indirect hemagglutination (IHA) test and/or enzyme-linked immunosorbent assay (ELISA).
B. Send the patient for an ultrasound-guided biopsy to r/o malignancy.
C. Send the patient to interventional radiology for hepatic abscess drain placement.
D. Consult surgery for a partial liver resection.

24. A 55-year-old man with a history of hypertension, hyperlipidemia (HLD), coronary artery disease, hepatitis B, and cirrhosis (MELD 29) presents to the ED with a history of abdominal pain, fever, and chills for several days. His temperature is 38.6°C, BP 100/50 mm Hg, HR 85 bpm, RR 18/min, and SpO$_2$ 92% on room air. Laboratory evaluation is remarkable for WBC of 21,000/mm$^3$. A CT shows large ascites but no other acute pathology. Peritoneal fluid sampling is requested. POCUS shows **Figure 69.20**.

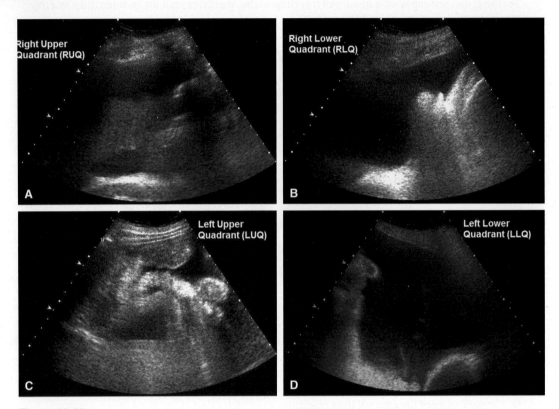

**Figure 69.20**

Which of the following statements about this procedure is *most* accurate?
A. There is no difference in the success of fluid aspiration with and without ultrasound.
B. Complications are similar with and without ultrasound.
C. Color-flow Doppler can help identify the inferior epigastric arteries.
D. A "Z-tract" technique is not recommended when performing this procedure under ultrasound.

25. A 27-year-old woman with no significant past medical history presents to the ED with sudden onset of severe right-sided lower abdominal pain that worsened over many hours. Her temperature is 37°C, BP 140/75 mm Hg, HR 105 bpm, RR 16/min, and SpO$_2$ 100% on room air. She has RLQ tenderness on examination. A POCUS of the ovaries is shown in **Figure 69.21** (Figure 69.21A is the right ovary, Figure 69.21B is the left).

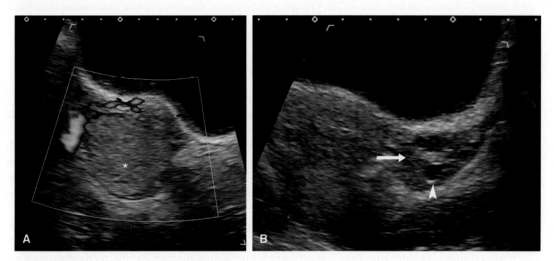

**Figure 69.21**

What is the *best* next step in her management?
A. Oral antibiotics and outpatient follow-up
B. Pain control and a comprehensive pelvic ultrasound
C. Admit for observation and serial abdominal examinations
D. Emergent consult for surgical exploration

# Chapter 69 ▪ Answers

1. Correct Answer: C. Pericholecystic fluid

*Rationale:* Acute calculous cholecystitis is inflammation of the gallbladder wall caused by a gallstone obstructing the cystic duct. RUQ ultrasound is the diagnostic test of choice due to its wide availability, portability, and efficiency. The overall sensitivity of ultrasound for acute cholecystitis is 90% to 95%, although the specificity is 78% to 80%. The sonographic findings of acute cholecystitis are well-described and include: the presence of gallstones (often seen at the gallbladder neck or cystic duct), gallbladder wall thickening (>3 mm), pericholecystic fluid, and a positive sonographic Murphy's sign. The presence of two of these is diagnostic, although each has its own sensitivity and specificity (see **Table 69.1**).

**Table 69.1 Screening Performance Characteristics of Emergency Department Bedside Sonography for Four Sonographic Findings of Acute Cholecystitis**

| Characteristics | Gallstone | Wall Edema | Fluid | Wall Thickness |
|---|---|---|---|---|
| Sensitivity | 92.7 (82.3-97.3) | 40.0 (13.6-72.6) | 68.2 (45.1-85.3) | 75.0 (59.4-86.3) |
| Specificity | 97.1 (94.1-98.6) | 97.5 (95.1-98.9) | 97.8 (95.3-99.0) | 97.3 (94.6-98.7) |
| Positive predictive value | 88.8 (78.7-94.7) | 33.3 (11.3-64.6) | 98.1 (45.1-85.3) | 80.5 (64.6-90.6) |
| Negative predictive value | 98.1 (95.5-99.3) | 98.2 (95.9-99.3) | 97.8 (95.3-99.0) | 96.3 (93.4-98.1) |

### Selected References

1. Bennett GL, Balthazar EJ. Ultrasound and CT evaluation of emergent gallbladder pathology. *Radiol Clin North Am.* 2003; 41(6):1203-1216. doi:10.1016/S0033-8389(03)00097-6.
2. Cosby KS, Kendall JL. Right upper quadrant: liver, gallbladder, and biliary tree. In: Cosby KS, Kendall JL, eds. *Practical Guide to Emergency Ultrasound.* 2nd ed. Wolters Kluwer; 2014:133-155.
3. Kiewiet JJS, Leeuwenburgh MMN, Bipat S, Bossuyt PMM, Stoker J, Boermeester MA. A systematic review and meta-analysis of diagnostic performance of imaging in acute cholecystitis. *Radiology.* 2012;264(3):708-720. doi:10.1148/radiol.12111561.
4. Shekarchi B, Rafsanjani SZH, Fomani NSR, Chahardoli M. Emergency department bedside ultrasonography for diagnosis of acute cholecystitis; a diagnostic accuracy study. *Emerg (Tehran).* 2018;6(1):e11.
5. Strasberg SM. Acute calculous cholecystitis. *N Engl J Med.* 2008;358(26):2804-2811. doi:10.1056/NEJMcp0800929.

**2.** Correct Answer: B. Distal aorta diameter 6.5 cm

*Rationale*: This presentation is concerning for a ruptured AAA. The classic presentation of AAA is the triad of abdominal or flank pain, palpable abdominal mass, and hypotension. Most aneurysms are asymptomatic and are usually found incidentally, but the diagnosis must be considered in any patient with risk factors (family history, hypertension, peripheral vascular disease, and history of tobacco use). The size of the AAA portends the risk of rupture, which carries a mortality rate of ~70%. A normal abdominal aortic diameter is < 3 cm on the transverse view. An aneurysm <5 cm in size does not require immediate operative repair unless it is symptomatic, but aneurysms >5 cm are usually repaired even in asymptomatic patients.

POCUS can rapidly identify AAA and both the sensitivity and specificity are nearly 100% for the detection of AAAs. The presence of a dilated aorta or a periaortic fluid collection or hematoma on ultrasound should prompt emergent management for presumed rupture. Aortic calcification may warrant additional evaluation in the proper scenario, but does not itself raise concern for AAA rupture. A dilated bowel with a "target sign" is suggestive of intussusception, which is less likely in this case. Hydronephrosis due to ureteral obstruction from an aneurysm may occur, but this is not the most likely scenario in this case.

### Selected References

1. Dean AJ. Abdominal Aorta. In: Cosby KS, Kendall JL, eds. *Practical Guide to Emergency Ultrasound.* 2nd ed. Wolters Kluwer; 2014:156-171.
2. Lech C, Swaminathan A. Abdominal aortic emergencies. *Emerg Med Clin North Am.* 2017;35(4):847-867. doi:10.1016/j.emc .2017.07.003.
3. Mellnick VM, Heiken JP. The acute abdominal aorta. *Radiol Clin North Am.* 2015;53(6):1209-1224. doi:10.1016/j.rcl.2015.06.007.

**3.** Correct Answer: A. Immediate operative intervention

*Rationale*: A hypoechoic stripe visualized in the hepatorenal recess (Morison's pouch) represents hemoperitoneum in this scenario. Given the hemodynamic instability, the most appropriate intervention is to proceed directly to exploratory laparotomy. Going to the CT scanner may be unsafe and would delay a necessary operative intervention. The IVC is not visualized in this image. Diagnostic peritoneal lavage may be considered if there is diagnostic uncertainty, if unable to obtain adequate views, or if there is an alternative explanation for the intra-abdominal fluid such as ascites (not the case in this scenario).

### Selected References

1. Bailitz J. A problem-based approach to resuscitation of acute illness or injury. In: Cosby KS, Kendall JL, eds. *Practical Guide to Emergency Ultrasound.* 2nd ed. Wolters Kluwer; 2014:96-107.
2. Lobo V, Hunter-Behrend M, Cullnan E, et al. Caudal edge of the liver in the right upper quadrant (RUQ) view is the most sensitive area for free fluid on the FAST exam. *West J Emerg Med.* 2017;18(2):270-280. doi:10.5811/westjem.2016.11.30435.
3. Richards JR, McGahan JP. Focused assessment with sonography in trauma (FAST) in 2017: what radiologists can learn. *Radiology.* 2017;283(1):30-48. doi:10.1148/radiol.2017160107.
4. Richards JR, McGahan JP, Pali MJ, Bohnen PA. Sonographic detection of blunt hepatic trauma: hemoperitoneum and parenchymal patterns of injury. *J Trauma Inj Infect Crit Care.* 1999;47(6):1092. doi:10.1097/00005373-199912000-00019.

4. Correct Answer: D. Target sign in the RLQ

*Rationale*: Abdominal pain is one of the most common complaints in the ED and there is a concern for the overuse of ionizing radiation with CT scans. For this reason, the American College of Emergency Physicians and American College of Radiology recommend ultrasonography (US) as the initial radiologic modality for evaluation of acute appendicitis (AA), especially in the pediatric population. Ultrasound is less sensitive than CT (~86%), but the specificity is high (~95%).

The diagnosis of AA can be achieved by direct visualization of the appendix or indirectly by observing signs of local inflammation. Direct signs include noncompressibility of the appendix (except in the case of perforation), a diameter >6 mm, wall thickness ≥3 mm, visualized appendicolith (hyperechoic structure with posterior shadowing), enhanced vascularity (seen in early stages of AA) or decreased/absent vascularity (seen with abscess and necrosis), or the presence of a "target sign." The target sign is described as a hypoechoic fluid-filled center surrounded by hyperechoic mucosa/submucosa, surrounded by a hypoechoic muscularis ring. Indirect signs of AA are free fluid surrounding the appendix, local abscess formation, increased echogenicity of adjacent mesenteric fat, enlarged mesenteric lymph nodes, thickening or hyperechogenicity of the peritoneum, and signs of secondary SBO.

Selected References

1. Benabbas R, Hanna M, Shah J, Sinert R. Diagnostic accuracy of history, physical examination, laboratory tests, and point-of-care ultrasound for pediatric acute appendicitis in the emergency department: a systematic review and meta-analysis. *Acad Emerg Med.* 2017;24(5):523-551. doi:10.1111/acem.13181.
2. Mostbeck G, Adam EJ, Nielsen MB, et al. How to diagnose acute appendicitis: ultrasound first. *Insights Imaging.* 2016;7(2): 255-263. doi:10.1007/s13244-016-0469-6.
3. Noguchi T, Yoshimitsu K, Yoshida M. Periappendiceal hyperechoic structure on sonography. *J Ultrasound Med.* 2005;24(3): 323-327. doi:10.7863/jum.2005.24.3.323.
4. Quigley AJ, Stafrace S. Ultrasound assessment of acute appendicitis in paediatric patients: methodology and pictorial overview of findings seen. *Insights Imaging.* 2013;4(6):741-751. doi:10.1007/s13244-013-0275-3.
5. Smith EA, Smith WL. Pediatric imaging. In: Farrell TA, ed. *Radiology 101.* Wolters Kluwer; 2020:144-174.

5. Correct Answer: C. Common bile duct diameter >8 mm

*Rationale*: Acute cholangitis is a potentially fatal biliary infection caused by obstruction of the common bile duct, usually by a gallstone. The sonographic findings of acute ascending cholangitis include bile duct wall thickening and intraductal debris, often with associated biliary ductal dilatation >7 mm. While gallbladder wall thickness >3 mm and the presence of gallstones support the diagnosis of cholecystitis, this is not the most likely diagnosis in this case. A dilated IVC may suggest elevated central venous pressure, which may contribute to hepatic dysfunction, but again, this is not the most likely diagnosis.

Selected References

1. Cosby KS, Kendall JL. Right upper quadrant: liver, gallbladder, and biliary tree. In: Cosby KS, Kendall JL, eds. *Practical Guide to Emergency Ultrasound.* 2nd ed. Wolters Kluwer; 2014:133-155.
2. Oppenheimer DC, Rubens DJ. Sonography of acute cholecystitis and its mimics. *Radiol Clin North Am.* 2019;57(3):535-548. doi:10.1016/j.rcl.2019.01.002.
3. Parulekar SG. Ultrasound evaluation of common bile duct size. *Radiology.* 1979;133(3):703-707. doi:10.1148/133.3.703.
4. Sokal A, Sauvanet A, Fantin B, de Lastours V. Acute cholangitis: diagnosis and management. *J Visc Surg.* June 2019. Article in press. doi:10.1016/j.jviscsurg.2019.05.007.

6. Correct Answer: D. Dilatation of urinary collecting ducts

*Rationale*: The presentation and imaging shown in Figure 69.6 are most consistent with ureteral obstruction by a kidney stone. Nephrolithiasis can occasionally be visualized with POCUS but typically the only evidence supporting the clinical suspicion is the presence of hydronephrosis. Hydronephrosis can be identified as dilatation of the renal collecting ducts, which appears as a hypoechoic structure within the renal parenchyma (severity is graded by its sonographic appearance). If urolithiasis can be identified, it will appear as a hyperechoic structure within the ureter or renal pelvis.

Selected References

1. Favus MJ, Feingold KR. Kidney stone emergencies. 2018 Sep 13. In: Feingold KR, Anawalt B, Boyce A, et al., eds. *Endotext [Internet].* MDText.com, Inc.; 2000. https://www.ncbi.nlm.nih.gov/books/NBK278956/.
2. Graham A, Luber S, Wolfson AB. Urolithiasis in the emergency department. *Emerg Med Clin North Am.* 2011;29(3):519-538. doi:10.1016/j.emc.2011.04.007.
3. Jendeberg J, Geijer H, Alshamari M, Cierzniak B, Lidén M. Size matters: the width and location of a ureteral stone accurately predict the chance of spontaneous passage. *Eur Radiol.* 2017;27(11):4775-4785. doi:10.1007/s00330-017-4852-6.
4. Laselle BT, Kendall JL. Trauma. In: Cosby KS, Kendall JL, eds. *Practical Guide to Emergency Ultrasound.* 2nd ed. Wolters Kluwer; 2014:21-25.
5. Ma OJ, Mateer JR, Reardon RF, Joing SA. *Emergency Ultrasound.* 3rd ed. McGraw-Hill Education; 2014.

## 7. Correct Answer: C. Bowel loop diameter 3.1 cm

*Rationale:* Figure 69.7 shows dilated loops of fluid-filled bowel, suggesting a small bowel obstruction (SBO). The most common cause for SBO is previous surgery resulting in adhesions. POCUS for SBO has a sensitivity over 97% and specificity of approximately 93%. Ultrasound findings of SBO include:

1. Bowel diameter >25 mm in three or more bowel loops
2. Bowel wall thickness >2 mm (caused by bowel wall edema)
3. Swirling motion of bowel content within the loops
4. Increased (to and from) or decreased peristaltic movements
5. Visible valvulae conniventes (plicae circulares) >2 mm (keyboard sign)
6. Noncompressible bowel close to collapsed, compressible small bowel (represents a transition point)

The presence of two or more of these findings in a critically ill patient is diagnostic for SBO and should prompt aggressive resuscitation, decompression of the bowel, and surgical evaluation.

Selected References

1. Abu-Zidan FM, Cevik AA. Diagnostic point-of-care ultrasound (POCUS) for gastrointestinal pathology: state of the art from basics to advanced. *World J Emerg Surg.* 2018;13(1):1-14. doi:10.1186/s13017-018-0209-y.
2. Frasure S. Accuracy of abdominal ultrasound for the diagnosis of small bowel obstruction in the emergency department. *World J Emerg Med.* 2018;9(4):267. doi:10.5847/wjem.j.1920-8642.2018.04.005.
3. Hefny AF, Corr P, Abu-Zidan FM. The role of ultrasound in the management of intestinal obstruction. *J Emerg Trauma Shock.* 2012;5(1):84-86. doi:10.4103/0974-2700.93109.
4. Schmutz GR, Benko A, Fournier L, Peron JM, Morel E, Chiche L. Small bowel obstruction: role and contribution of sonography. *Eur Radiol.* 1997;7(7):1054-1058. doi:10.1007/s003300050251.
5. Tayal VS, Lewis MR. Does the patient have a bowel obstruction? In: Bornemann P, ed. *Ultrasound for Primary Care.* Wolters Kluwer; 2021:158-16.
6. Ünlüer EE, Yavaşi Ö, Eroğlu O, Yilmaz C, Akarca FK. Ultrasonography by emergency medicine and radiology residents for the diagnosis of small bowel obstruction. *Eur J Emerg Med.* 2010;17(5):260-264. doi:10.1097/MEJ.0b013e328336c736.

## 8. Correct Answer: A. A complex renal abscess

*Rationale:* Perinephric and renal abscesses are rare complications of untreated UTIs, but the mortality rate approaches 50%. Due to the vague presentation and insidious onset, it can be difficult to make this diagnosis by examination alone. Symptoms can easily be mistaken for pyelonephritis. POCUS can help identify a perinephric or renal abscess as a fluid-filled mass with mixed echogenicity extending from the renal cortex into the perinephric fat. The presence of complicating factors includes prior stenting, urolithiasis, nephrolithiasis, and external compression.

Figure 69.8 shows a dual-image sonogram depicting a sagittal and transverse views of a complex renal abscess (*arrows*). Small air bubbles are seen as an echogenic focus.

Selected References

1. Bogler DM. Possible renal mass. In Sanders RC, eds. *Clinical Sonography: A Practical Guide.* 5th ed. Wolters Kluwer; 2015: 575-587.
2. Coelho RF, Schneider-Monteiro ED, Mesquita JLB, Mazzucchi E, Marmo Lucon A, Srougi M. Renal and perinephric abscesses: analysis of 65 consecutive cases. *World J Surg.* 2007;31(2):431-436. doi:10.1007/s00268-006-0162-x.
3. Gardiner RA, Gwynne RA, Roberts SA. Perinephric abscess. *BJU Int.* 2011;107(Suppl. 3):20-23. doi:10.1111/j.1464-410X.2011.10050.x.
4. Liu X-Q. Renal and perinephric abscesses in West China Hospital: 10-year retrospective-descriptive study. *World J Nephrol.* 2016;5(1):108. doi:10.5527/wjn.v5.i1.108.
5. Shu T, Green JM, Orihuela E. Renal and perirenal abscesses in patients with otherwise anatomically normal urinary tracts. *J Urol.* 2004;172(1):148-150. doi:10.1097/01.ju.0000132140.48587.b8.

### 9. Correct Answer: C. Distended gallbladder without gallstones

*Rationale*: Figure 69.9 shows a thickened gallbladder wall, sludge, and pericholecystic fluid (*arrow*) suggesting acute acalculous cholecystitis. Acute acalculous cholecystitis results from bile stasis within the gallbladder and remains an elusive diagnosis due to the complex clinical setting in which it occurs.

Ultrasound is the diagnostic test of choice given its availability, portability, and diagnostic accuracy. Ultrasound findings consistent with acalculous cholecystitis include gallbladder wall thickening >3 mm, pericholecystic fluid, sludge within the gallbladder, distention of the gallbladder, pneumobilia (intramural gas), and the absence of gallstones.

#### Selected References

1. Balmadrid B. Recent advances in management of acalculous cholecystitis. *F1000Research.* 2018;7:1-8. doi:10.12688/f1000research.14886.1.
2. Bieker TM. The gallbladder and biliary system. In: Kawamura D, Nolan T, eds. *Abdomen and Superficial Structures.* 4th ed. Wolters Kluwer; 2018:171-211.
3. Huffman JL, Schenker S. Acute acalculous cholecystitis: a review. *Clin Gastroenterol Hepatol.* 2010;8(1):15-22. doi:10.1016/j.cgh.2009.08.034.
4. Tana M, Tana C, Cocco G, Iannetti G, Romano M, Schiavone C. Acute acalculous cholecystitis and cardiovascular disease: a land of confusion. *J Ultrasound.* 2015;18(4):317-320. doi:10.1007/s40477-015-0176-z.

### 10. Correct Answer: A. Air within the gallbladder

*Rationale/Critique:* Figure 69.10 shows a highly echogenic reflection within the gallbladder wall, with posterior shadowing and reverberation artifact, representing intraluminal air (*arrows*). Emphysematous cholecystitis is a rare but rapidly progressing and life-threatening form of cholecystitis, with a mortality rate of up to 15%. Ultrasound will show signs of cholecystitis with a thickened gallbladder wall, pericholecystic fluid, and sonographic Murphy's sign. Gas within the lumen causes a sonographic reverberation artifact, which can be seen in any portion of the gallbladder. In some cases, there may be small echogenic foci floating within the gallbladder lumen.

#### Selected References

1. Aherne A, Ozaki R, Tobey N, Secko M. Diagnosis of emphysematous cholecystitis with bedside ultrasound in a septic elderly female with no source of infection. *J Emerg Trauma Shock.* 2017;10(2):85-86. doi:10.4103/JETS.JETS_75_16.
2. Bieker TM. The gallbladder and biliary system. In: Kawamura D, Nolan T, eds. *Abdomen and Superficial Structures.* 4th ed. Wolters Kluwer; 2018:171-211.
3. Bloom RA, Libson E, Lebensart PD, et al. The ultrasound spectrum of emphysematous cholecystitis. *J Clin Ultrasound.* 1989;17(4):251-256. doi:10.1002/jcu.1870170404.
4. Oyedeji FO, Voci S. Emphysematous cholecystitis. *Ultrasound Q.* 2014;30(3):246-248. doi:10.1097/RUQ.0000000000000101.
5. Parulekar SG. Sonographic findings in acute emphysematous cholecystitis. *Radiology.* 1982;145(1):117-119. doi:10.1148/radiology.145.1.7122865.
6. Wexler BB, Panebianco NL. The effervescent gallbladder: an emergency medicine bedside ultrasound diagnosis of emphysematous cholecystitis. *Cureus.* 2017;7(7):5-9. doi:10.7759/cureus.1520.

### 11. Correct Answer: B. Up to 10% of FAST examinations may be indeterminate

*Rationale*: The FAST examination has been established as a reliable method to rapidly evaluate for intra-abdominal blood in a trauma patient. However, its test characteristics are operator-dependent, and even in the hands of an experienced sonographer, up to 10% of scans can have a false negative. Small-volume hemorrhage can be missed and the presence of clot may be misinterpreted. Repeating the examination over time (or with a worsening clinical situation) can improve the sensitivity of the examination. An empty bladder decreases the acoustic window available for imaging the pelvis, which may decrease the sensitivity to a small blood volume. Fresh blood generally appears anechoic and is difficult to distinguish from urine or ascites. Because this patient shows signs of hemodynamic instability and has a suspected intra-abdominal injury, a FAST examination would be appropriate in his evaluation.

#### Selected Reference

1. Panebianco N. Ultrasound in acute trauma. In: Carmody KA, Moore CL, Feller-Kopman D, eds. *Handbook of Critical Care and Emergency Ultrasound.* McGraw-Hill; 2011: Chapter 24. Accessed November 13, 2019. http://accessanesthesiology.mhmedical.com/content.aspx?bookid=517&sectionid=41066810.

**12.** Correct Answer: D. The measured diameter of the aorta should include the outer walls.

*Rationale*: The correct measurement of a AAA includes the outer walls. Measurement of the interior hypoechoic portion underestimates the size of the aneurysm, as does the cylinder-tangent effect, which can be mitigated by measuring in two planes. The use of ultrasonography in the ED to detect an AAA has a pooled sensitivity of 99% (95% confidence interval [CI] 96%-100%) and specificity of 98% (95% CI 97%-99%). The presence of abdominal gas may impair the ability to visualize the aorta.

### Selected References

1. Carmody K, Moore CL. *Ultrasound of the aorta*. In: Carmody KA, Moore CL, Feller-Kopman D, *eds. Handbook of Critical Care and Emergency Ultrasound*. McGraw-Hill; 2011: Chapter 5. Accessed November 13, 2019. http://accessanesthesiology.mhmedical.com/content.aspx?bookid=517&sectionid=41066791.
2. Daffner RH, Hartman M. Abdominal radiographs. In: Daffner RH, Hartman M, eds. *Clinical Radiology*. 4th ed. Wolters Kluwer; 2014:215-251.

**13.** Correct Answer: B. A hypoechoic stripe in the pouch of Douglas

*Rationale/Critique*: Figure 69.12 shows an 8-week living ectopic pregnancy (with cardiac activity, not visualized in this image) in the cul-de-sac with an empty uterus and free pelvic fluid in the pouch of Douglas. POCUS can help diagnose an ectopic pregnancy using either the transabdominal or transvaginal approach, but the transabdominal approach should be attempted initially. A full bladder may facilitate visualization but is not required.

A definitive extrauterine pregnancy is diagnosed when a gestational sac with a yolk sac or fetal pole is seen outside the uterus. Findings suggestive of ectopic pregnancy include an empty uterus, pelvic free fluid (typically in the pouch of Douglas), an adnexal mass, or tubal rings.

### Selected References

1. Hsu S, Euerle BD. Ultrasound in pregnancy. *Emerg Med Clin North Am*. 2012;30(4):849-867. doi:10.1016/j.emc.2012.08.001.
2. Mukul LV, Teal SB. Current management of ectopic pregnancy. *Obstet Gynecol Clin North Am*. 2007;34(3):403-419. doi:10.1016/j.ogc.2007.07.001.
3. Murakami ME, Cernigliaro JG. Imaging in gynecologic emergencies. In: Benrubi GI, ed. *Handbook of Obstetric and Gynecologic Emergencies*. 4th ed. Wolters Kluwer; 2011:354-378.
4. Pontius E, Vieth JT. Complications in early pregnancy. *Emerg Med Clin North Am*. 2019;37(2):219-237. doi:10.1016/j.emc.2019.01.004.

**14.** Correct Answer: D. An eFAST examination is a reliable evaluation for intra-abdominal free fluid and hemopericardium.

*Rationale*: The eFAST examination is a noninvasive, rapid, widely available diagnostic imaging modality that is particularly useful in the evaluation of hemodynamically unstable patients. The eFAST has a sensitivity of only 28% to 48% in penetrating abdominal trauma, but does have a high specificity. Conversely, the sensitivity and specificity of the eFAST for pericardial injury are >99%. Ultrasound has very poor sensitivity and should not be used in isolation for early identification of hollow viscus injuries.

### Selected References

1. Biffl WL, Kaups KL, Cothren CC, et al. Management of patients with anterior abdominal stab wounds: A Western Trauma Association multicenter trial. *J Trauma*. 2009;66(5):1294-1301.
2. Hamada SR, Delhaye N, Kerever S, Harrois A, Duranteau J. Integrating eFAST in the initial management of stable trauma patients: the end of plain film radiography. *Ann Intensive Care*. 2016;6(1):62.
3. Soffer D, McKenney MG, Cohn S, et al. A prospective evaluation of ultrasonography for the diagnosis of penetrating torso injury. *J Trauma*. 2004;56(5):953-995.

**15.** Correct Answer: A. Free fluid in Morison's pouch can be distinguished from the gallbladder by its angular appearance.

*Rationale*: It is important to remember that ultrasound may miss a significant number of traumatic injuries involving the bowel or mesentery and up to 58% of solid organ injuries that have no associated hemoperitoneum. Small amounts of free fluid, especially < 400 mL, can easily be missed on ultrasound, highlighting the importance of repeat examinations when there is high clinical suspicion. Physiologic fluid-filled spaces (e.g., gallbladder, urinary bladder) tend to have rounded corners, while nonphysiologic spaces (e.g., peritoneum) tend to have "sharp" corners, as fluid collects between rounded structures like the bowel. One of the methods to differentiate the stomach from free fluid is to inject air or saline through a nasogastric tube under ultrasound guidance (and observe air entering the stomach). Identifying signs of chronic liver disease such as nodular cirrhosis, gallbladder wall thickening, hepatosplenomegaly, and portal vein enlargement should raise one's concern that ascites is the source of free fluid on ultrasound.

### Selected References

1. Catalano O, Aiani L, Barozzi L, et al. CEUS in abdominal trauma: multicenter study. *Abdon Imaging*. 2009;34(2):225-234.
2. Rose J. Ultrasound in abdominal trauma. *Emerg Med Clin North Am*. 2004;22(3):581-599.
3. Rozycki GS, Ochsner MG, Jaffin JH, Champion HR. Prospective evaluation of surgeons' use of ultrasound in the evaluation of trauma patients. *J Trauma*. 1993;34(4):516-526; discussion 26-27.

**16.** Correct Answer: C. Continue to evaluate for other causes of his pain

*Rationale:* In this scenario, the patient had cholelithiasis that resulted in acute pancreatitis. The majority of patients with gallstone pancreatitis have mild self-limited disease; however, approximately 20% of those patients will become critically ill. The presence of gallstones or biliary sludge in the setting of acute pancreatitis is insufficient to make the diagnosis of gallstone pancreatitis, and further evaluation is indicated.

There is no evidence of acute cholecystitis on Figure 69.13. Pain control and outpatient follow-up may be appropriate for symptomatic cholelithiasis, but without additional information (e.g., lipase) alternative pathologies have not been excluded. Similarly, a presumptive diagnosis of peptic ulcer disease may be premature without further evaluation. (See also **Figure 69.22**.)

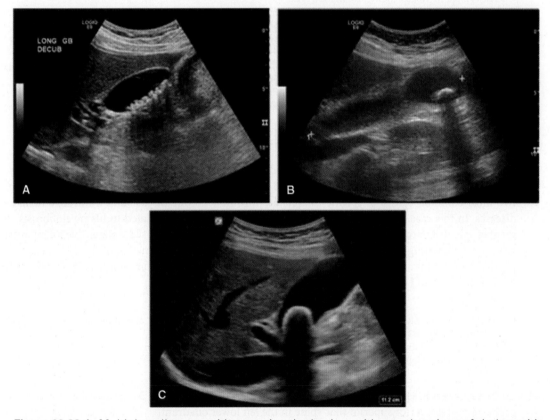

**Figure 69.22** A, Multiple gallstones with posterior shadowing, without other signs of cholecystitis. B, A large gallstone with posterior shadowing and gallbladder wall thickening in acute cholecystitis. C, A gallstone in the neck of a gallbladder.

### Selected References

1. Cucher D, Kulvatunyou N, Green DJ, Jie T, Ong ES. Gallstone pancreatitis. A review. *Surg Clin North Am*. 2014;94(2):257-280. doi:10.1016/j.suc.2014.01.006.
2. Fentress M. Does the patient have cholelithiasis or cholecystitis?. *In:* Bornemann P, *ed. Ultrasound for Primary Care*. Wolters Kluwer; 2021:151-157.
3. Shaffer EA. Epidemiology and risk factors for gallstone disease: has the paradigm changed in the 21st century? *Curr Gastroenterol Rep*. 2005;7(2):132-140. doi:10.1007/s11894-005-0051-8.

**17.** Correct Answer: C. A dilated fluid-filled jejunal segment due to small bowel obstruction (SBO)

*Rationale*: Figure 69.14 shows multiple dilated loops of fluid-filled bowel with visible plicae circularis (*arrow*) suggestive of an SBO. A CT of the abdomen and pelvis with contrast remains the gold standard to diagnose SBO, but it is not always available and may lead to a delay in diagnosis. POCUS is a useful tool in the hands of a trained practitioner, with a sensitivity over 97% and specificity of approximately 93%. Ultrasound findings of SBO include:

1. Loop dimensions of the jejunum >25 mm or ileum >15 mm, present in three or more bowel loops
2. Bowel wall thickness >2 mm (caused by bowel wall edema)
3. Swirling motion of bowel content within the loops
4. Increased (to and from) or decreased peristaltic movements
5. Visible valvular conniventes (plicae circulares) >2 mm (keyboard sign)
6. Noncompressible bowel close to collapsed compressible small bowel (represents a transition point)

The presence of two or more of these findings in a critically ill patient is diagnostic of SBO.

**Selected References**
1. Abu-Zidan FM, Cevik AA. Diagnostic point-of-care ultrasound (POCUS) for gastrointestinal pathology: state of the art from basics to advanced. *World J Emerg Surg*. 2018;13(1):1-14. doi:10.1186/s13017-018-0209-y.
2. Brant W. Abdomen Ultrasound. In: Klein J, Vinson EN, Brant WE, Helms CA, eds. *Brant and Helms' Fundamentals of Diagnostic Radiology*. 5th ed. Wolters Kluwer; 2019:1156-1191.
3. Frasure S. Accuracy of abdominal ultrasound for the diagnosis of small bowel obstruction in the emergency department. *World J Emerg Med*. 2018;9(4):267. doi:10.5847/wjem.j.1920-8642.2018.04.005.
4. Hefny AF, Corr P, Abu-Zidan FM. The role of ultrasound in the management of intestinal obstruction. *J Emerg Trauma Shock*. 2012;5(1):84-86. doi:10.4103/0974-2700.93109.
5. Schmutz GR, Benko A, Fournier L, Peron JM, Morel E, Chiche L. Small bowel obstruction: role and contribution of sonography. *Eur Radiol*. 1997;7(7):1054-1058. doi:10.1007/s003300050251.
6. Ünlüer EE, Yavaşi Ö, Eroğlu O, Yilmaz C, Akarca FK. Ultrasonography by emergency medicine and radiology residents for the diagnosis of small bowel obstruction. *Eur J Emerg Med*. 2010;17(5):260-264. doi:10.1097/MEJ.0b013e328336c736.

**18.** Correct Answer: D. Symptom management with pain medication

*Rationale*: Splenic infarction occurs when blood flow to the spleen is compromised, causing tissue ischemia and eventual necrosis. Splenic infarction may be the result of arterial or venous occlusion. The two most common causes of splenic infarcts are thromboembolic disease and infiltrative hematologic diseases. In this case, the interruption of splenic blood flow is likely related to his myelofibrosis. Treatment of splenic infarcts is based primarily on the underlying causative disease state. Splenic infarct in the noninfectious setting may be treated with analgesics, hydration, antiemetics, and other means of supportive care. Abdominal pain due to uncomplicated cases of splenic infarction usually resolves without intervention in 7 to 14 days.

**Selected References**
1. Llewellyn ME, Jeffrey RB, DiMaio MA, Olcott EW. The sonographic "bright band sign" of splenic infarction. *J Ultrasound Med*. 2014 Jun;33(6):929-938.
2. Wand O, Tayer-Shifman OE, Khoury S, Hershko AY. A practical approach to infarction of the spleen as a rare manifestation of multiple common diseases. *Ann Med*. 2018 Sep;50(6):494-500.

**19.** Correct Answer: B. The general area of the puncture site is localized 2 to 3 cm medial and 2 to 3 cm cephalad to the anterior superior iliac spine in the left lower quadrant.

*Rationale*: Ultrasound guidance for paracentesis results in greater success rates when compared to traditional techniques, 95% versus 61%, respectively. Patients undergoing ultrasound-guided paracentesis also have a decreased risk of bleeding, 0.27% versus 1.25% (without ultrasound), decreased hospital length of stay, and costs. There is no evidence to suggest that ultrasound guidance causes a higher infection rate.

Ultrasound guidance has several advantages over the landmark technique, including:

1. Reduced risk of serious complications (most commonly bleeding)
2. Identifies patients with insufficient volume of intraperitoneal free fluid
3. Improved success rates of the overall procedure

4. Helps identify a needle insertion site based on the size of the fluid collection, thickness of the abdominal wall, and proximity to abdominal organs
5. The needle insertion site can be evaluated using color-flow Doppler ultrasound to identify and avoid abdominal wall blood vessels along the anticipated needle trajectory.

### Selected References

1. Invasive procedures and surgical asepsis. In: Penny SM, ed. *Introduction to Sonography and Patient Care*. 2nd ed. Wolters Kluwer; 2021:387-409.
2. Mercaldi CJ, Lanes SF. Ultrasound guidance decreases complications and improves the cost of care among patients undergoing thoracentesis and paracentesis. *Chest*. 2013;143:532.
3. Nazeer SR, Dewbre H, Miller AH. Ultrasound-assisted paracentesis performed by emergency physicians vs the traditional technique: a prospective, randomized study. *Am J Emerg Med*. 2005;23:363-367.

20. Correct Answer: A. Ultrasound allows dynamic evaluation for a hernia during a Valsalva maneuver.

*Rationale*: As a real-time examination, ultrasound allows for data acquisition during Valsalva and other maneuvers that elicit hernia symptoms and can also detect peristalsis in herniated bowel. Ultrasound also has the ability to determine reducibility, as well as tenderness of the hernia with compression during the examination. In addition, Doppler flow can help evaluate perfusion to the herniated bowel segment. Two drawbacks are that fascial defects can be difficult to identify, and visualization of mesenteric or omental fat is often nonspecific. (See also **Figure 69.23**.)

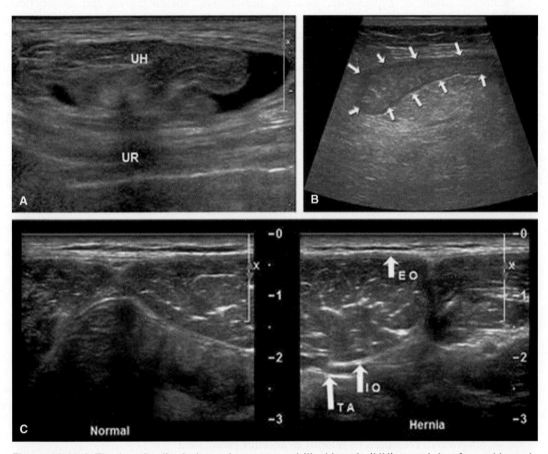

**Figure 69.23** A, The longitudinal plane shows an umbilical hernia (UH) containing fat and bowel that passed through a dilated umbilical ring (UR). B, On a different patient, the transverse plane shows a paraumbilical hernia (*arrows*) containing fat. C, The contiguous muscle can be seen on the normal abdominal wall on the left. On the left, the sonogram demonstrates a small Spigelian hernia (dotted outline) as it herniated through both the torn transversus abdominis (TA) and the internal oblique (IO) muscles. The external oblique (EO) muscle is intact. On this obese patient, there is a large amount of fat seen between IO and EO muscles. A mushroom-shaped or anvil-shaped hernia correlates with the inability to reduce and increased risk of strangulation.

Selected Reference

1. Bradley M, Morgan D, Pentlow B, Roe A. The groin hernia—an ultrasound diagnosis? *Ann R Coll Surg Engl.* 2003;85(3):178-180.

---

**21.** Correct Answer: A. To improve transvaginal imaging

*Rationale/Critique*: The acoustic "window" is the path through which the transducer "looks" at the deeper structures. A good acoustic window provides less impedance, scattering, and attenuation of the ultrasound beam. As the bladder is stretched, the folds of the bladder do not provide any impedance or irregular reflections. A full bladder may make transvaginal imaging more challenging by creating side-lobe artifacts from the same phenomenon (increased wave propagation) outside of the intended imaging plane.

Selected References

1. AIUM Practice parameter for the performance of an ultrasound examination of the female pelvis. *J Ultrasound Med.* 2020;39:E17.
2. AIUM Practice parameter for ultrasound examinations in reproductive medicine and infertility. https://www.aium.org/resources/guidelines/reproductiveMed.pdf.
3. Laselle BT, Kendall JL. Trauma. In: Cosby KS, Kendall JL, eds. *Practical Guide to Emergency Ultrasound.* 2nd ed. Wolters Kluwer; 2014:21-54.

---

**22.** Correct Answer: B. The examination cannot reliably identify pancreatic injuries.

*Rationale*: The extended FAST (eFAST) examination is able to reliably evaluate for some causes of intrathoracic causes of hypotension, including hemothorax, pneumothorax, and hemopericardium. Unfortunately, the FAST exam has poor sensitivity for hollow viscus injuries, diaphragmatic injuries, retroperitoneal injuries, or intra-abdominal injuries that do not produce a significant volume of hemorrhage. The FAST exam can detect volumes as small as 100 mL, though with decreased sensitivity relative to larger volumes of hemoperitoneum. In most studies, the overall sensitivity of the FAST examination for intraperitoneal hemorrhage ranges from 63% to 100%. Serial examination greatly improves the sensitivity, and ongoing bleeding that was initially not apparent may be more easily identified. If a significant injury is suspected and the eFAST examination is negative, the **hemodynamically stable** patient may require further evaluation (usually CT or serial clinical examinations). If there are any changes in the patient's hemodynamics, the eFAST examination should be repeated.

Selected References

1. Dolich MO, McKenney MG, Varela JE, Compton RP, McKenney KL, Cohn SM. 2,576 ultrasounds for blunt abdominal trauma. *J Trauma.* 2001;50:108.
2. Lingawi SS, Buckley AR. Focused abdominal US in patients with trauma. *Radiology.* 2000;217:426.
3. McGahan JP, Rose J, Coates TL, Wisner DH, Newberry P. Use of ultrasonography in the patient with acute abdominal trauma. *J Ultrasound Med.* 1997;16:653.
4. McGahan JP, Wang L, Richards JR. From the RSNA refresher courses: focused abdominal US for trauma. *Radiographics.* 2001;21 Spec No:S191.
5. Shanmuganathan K, Mirvis SE, Sherbourne CD, Chiu WC, Rodriguez A. Hemoperitoneum as the sole indicator of abdominal visceral injuries: a potential limitation of screening abdominal US for trauma. *Radiology.* 1999;212:423.

---

**23.** Correct Answer: A. Test the patient by the echinococcosis indirect hemagglutination (IHA) test and/or enzyme-linked immunosorbent assay (ELISA)

*Rationale*: The patient's presentation is consistent with hydatid liver disease, a severe, potentially lethal disease caused by Echinococcus granulosus larvae. Figure 69.19 shows the classic appearance of a cyst containing multiple daughter cysts. Several reports describe the sonographic features of hepatic hydatid disease. Lewall and McCorkell proposed the following four groups for hydatid cysts:

- Simple cysts containing no internal architecture except sand
- Cysts with detached endocyst secondary to rupture
- Cysts with daughter cyst matrix (echogenic material between daughter cysts)
- Densely calcified masses

Answer Choice options B and C are incorrect because performing a biopsy would put the patient at risk of anaphylactic shock from the spillage of the daughter cyst matrix. Answer Choice option D is incorrect because medical treatment alone is appropriate for most smaller cysts (<5 cm). While surgery may be necessary in certain situations, establishing the diagnosis of hydatid disease is essential for appropriate planning.

Selected References

1. Beggs I. The radiology of hydatid disease. *AJR Am J Roentgenol.* 1985;145(3):639-648.
2. Gharbi HA, Hassine W, Brauner MW, Dupuch K. Ultrasound examination of the hydatic liver. *Radiology.* 1981;139(2):459-463.
3. Lewall DB, McCorkell SJ. Hepatic echinococcal cysts: sonographic appearance and classification. *Radiology.* 1985;155(3):773-775.
4. Lightowlers MW. Vaccines against cysticercosis and hydatidosis: foundations in taeniid cestode immunology. *Parasitol Int.* 2006;55:S39-S43.
5. Milicevic MN. Echinococcal cyst—open and laparoscopic approach. In: Fischer J, ed. *Fischer's Mastery of Surgery.* 7th ed. Wolters Kluwer; 2019:1294-1314.
6. Polat P, Kantarci M, Alper F, et al. Hydatid disease from head to toe. *Radiographics.* 2003 Mar-Apr;23(2):475-494.
7. Yagci G, Ustunsoz B, Kaymakcioglu N, et al. Results of surgical, laparoscopic, and percutaneous treatment for hydatid disease of the liver: 10 years experience with 355 patients. *World J Surg.* 2005;29:1670.

---

**24.** Correct Answer: **C. Color-flow Doppler can help identify the inferior epigastric arteries**

*Rationale:* Paracentesis is an important diagnostic procedure for patients with new-onset ascites, as well as those patients with preexisting ascites who may have developed a new process, such as bacterial peritonitis. Ultrasound has been shown to significantly increase the success rate of paracentesis in the ED. In a prospective randomized study comparing traditional versus ultrasound-guided technique, Nazeer reported that 95% (40/42) of patients were successfully aspirated in the ultrasound group compared to only 61% (27/44) of those in the nonultrasound group.

If access sites in the lower quadrants are selected, it is important to avoid the inferior epigastric arteries. These vessels arise from the external iliac, immediately before they pass through the inguinal canal, so their origins can be identified by the femoral pulse in the groin. They course medially and superiorly, running up the anterior abdominal wall, analogous to the internal mammaries in the chest, about 5 cm on either side from the midline. Their location can usually be mapped using color-flow Doppler with appropriately adjusted (low-velocity) scale, depth, and gain settings. The probe should be angled as far as possible from perpendicular to the abdominal wall to maximize the Doppler signal from these small vessels.

Needle insertion along a "Z-tract" through the soft tissues may help decrease peritoneal leaking after needle/catheter removal.

Selected References

1. American College of Emergency Physicians. Emergency ultrasound guidelines. *Ann Emerg Med.* 2009;53:566.
2. Nazeer SR, Dewbre H, Miller AH. Ultrasound-assisted paracentesis performed by emergency physicians vs. the traditional technique: a prospective, randomized study. *Am J Emerg Med.* 2005;23:363.
3. Paracentesis: Multimedia. eMedicine. [Online]. Accessed December 28, 2010. http://emedicine.medscape.com/article/80944-media.
4. Rybyinski A. Sonography-guided interventional procedures. In: Kawamura D, Nolan T, eds. *Abdomen and Superficial Structures.* 4th ed. Wolters Kluwer; 2018:795-811.

---

**25.** Correct Answer: **D. Emergent consult for surgical exploration**

*Rationale:* Ovarian torsion is a surgical emergency. The goal of the surgical evaluation is to relieve the torsion and assess ovarian viability. A torsed ovary should be considered potentially viable as ovarian necrosis is rare; the vast majority of torsed ovaries can and should be salvaged (unless malignancy is suspected).

Figure 69.21A shows a color power Doppler image of the right ovary, which is enlarged and uniformly hyperechoic, with no visible normal ovarian follicles (*asterisk*). There is no detectable blood flow in the ovary. Figure 69.21B is a grayscale image of the normal left ovary (*arrow*), which appears to be normal in size and echotexture, with normal-appearing ovarian follicles (*arrowhead*).

Selected References

1. Beaunoyer M, Chapdelaine J, Bouchard S, Ouimet A. Asynchronous bilateral ovarian torsion. *J Pediatr Surg.* 2004;39:746.
2. Huchon C, Fauconnier A. Adnexal torsion: a literature review. *Eur J Obstet Gynecol Reprod Biol.* 2010;150:8.
3. Smith EA, Trout AT. Abdomen. In: Klein J, Vinson EN, Brant WE, Helms CA, eds. *Brant and Helms' Fundamentals of Diagnostic Radiology.* 5th ed. Wolters Kluwer; 2019:1495-1530.
4. Snfilippo JS, Rock JA. Surgery for benign disease of the ovary. In: Jones HW, Rock JA, eds. *TeLinde's Operative Gynecology.* 11th ed. Wolters Kluwer; 2015.

# 70 | DEEP VEIN THROMBOSIS

Todd A. Jaffe and Jarone Lee

1. A 47-year-old man presents to the Emergency Department with a 1-day history of right leg swelling. He was in a motor vehicle collision 2 weeks prior and underwent emergent orthopedic surgery for bilateral tibia fractures. Physical examination is notable for 2+ pitting edema of the entire right leg. Pulses are normal. Compression ultrasound at the level of the common femoral vessels (*A, B*) and popliteal vessels (*C, D*) as well as pulsed-wave Doppler at the level of the common femoral vessels (*E*) are shown in **Figure 70.1**:

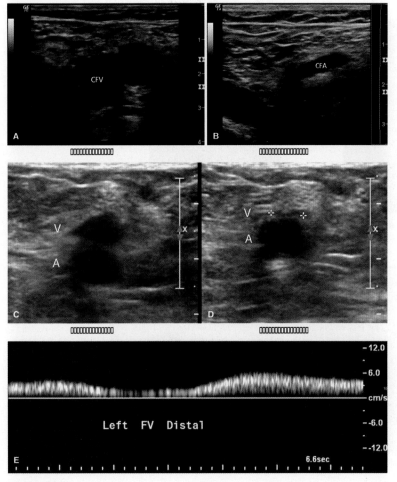

**Figure 70.1**

Which of the following describes the findings and recommended management?
**A.** Ultrasound with popliteal deep vein thrombosis (DVT); start therapeutic anticoagulation
**B.** Ultrasound with common femoral DVT; start therapeutic anticoagulation
**C.** Ultrasound without evidence of DVT; start lower extremity compression for postoperative edema
**D.** Ultrasound without evidence of DVT; obtain abdominal (iliocaval) imaging to assess for proximal occlusion

2. Which of the following is the correct pairing of a lower extremity DVT ultrasound modality and its description?

**A.** Two-region compression: compression of the upper leg from the common femoral to popliteal vein, and compression of the lower leg from the popliteal vein to the ankle
**B.** Extended compression: compression ultrasound of the femoral veins 1 to 2 cm above and below the saphenofemoral junction and the popliteal veins up to the calf veins confluence
**C.** Complete compression: compression from common femoral vein through the popliteal vein up to the calf veins confluence
**D.** Complete duplex: compression from the common femoral vein to the ankle, including color and spectral Doppler

3. A 67-year-old man with a history of metastatic prostate cancer is admitted to the intensive care unit (ICU) at a rural hospital with urosepsis. He develops acute onset left lower extremity swelling and pain. The facility does not have full ultrasound capabilities so you perform a point-of-care ultrasound to evaluate his leg. A two-region compression ultrasound with images at the level of the femoral vessels (*A, B*) and popliteal vessels (*C, D*) is shown in **Figure 70.2**.

**Femoral**

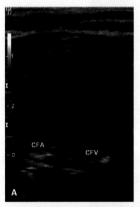 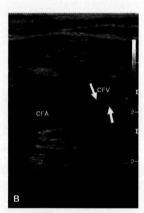

No compression                With compression

**Popliteal**

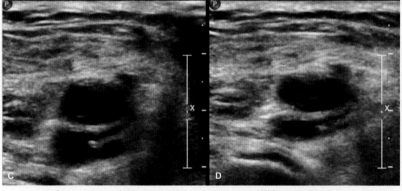

No compression                With compression

**Figure 70.2**

Which of the following best describes the findings?
A. DVT including the deep femoral and popliteal veins
B. Isolated deep femoral vein thrombus
C. Isolated popliteal vein thrombus
D. No evidence of DVT

4. A 48-year-old woman with a history of factor V Leiden presents with 2 days of chest pain and shortness of breath. Her vital signs on presentation include HR 102 bpm, BP 130/80 mm Hg, and SpO$_2$ 94% on 2 L nasal cannula. Point-of-care echocardiogram parasternal long- and short-axis views are shown in **Figure 70.3**.

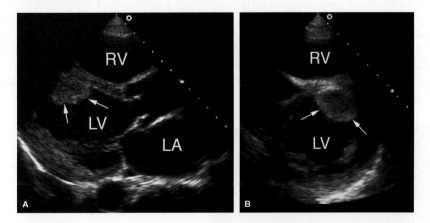

**Figure 70.3**

While in the Emergency Department, she endorses the acute onset of significant right lower extremity pain. Left foot dorsalis pedis pulse is 2+; however, pulses are not palpable in the right foot. An ultrasound of the right lower extremity at the level of the common femoral artery is shown in **Figure 70.4**.

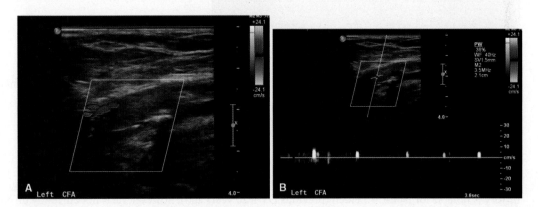

**Figure 70.4**

What is the *best* next step in the management of this patient?
A. Surgical consultation for arterial thrombectomy
B. Systemic thrombolytics
C. Broad-spectrum antibiotics
D. Systemic anticoagulation for DVT

5. A 72-year-old man with a history of lower extremity DVT is admitted to the ICU for pneumonia. While in the hospital, he develops worsening asymmetric lower extremity edema. You perform a point-of-care DVT evaluation and notice some venous abnormalities. Which of the following findings on ultrasound is more suggestive of residual venous thrombosis/scarring rather than acute DVT?

   A. Thrombus firmly adherent to vessel wall
   B. Vein dilation
   C. Smooth intraluminal material
   D. Intraluminal material that is deformable during compression

6. A 42-year-old woman presents to the Emergency Department with a 2-day history of right arm swelling. Her medical history is significant for a recent ICU admission for urosepsis the previous week. She appears uncomfortable, endorsing significant right arm pain. She has a temperature of 37.0°C, HR 104 bpm, BP 104/68 mm Hg, and SpO$_2$ 98% on room air. Physical examination is notable for 2+ edema from the right axilla to the right hand. Pulses in this arm are difficult to palpate but Doppler signals are present. Ultrasound of the R internal jugular vein and R carotid artery with and without compression is shown in **Figure 70.5**.

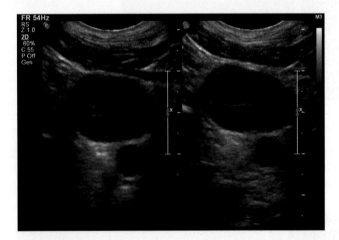

**Figure 70.5**

In addition to anticoagulation, which of the following is the *most* appropriate next step in management?
   A. Systemic thrombolytics
   B. Antibiotics, elevation and compression of the extremity
   C. Vascular surgery consultation for catheter-directed thrombolysis and/or thrombectomy
   D. Aspirin and Plavix

7. A 52-year-old man presents to the Emergency Department with a 2-day history of left arm swelling. His history is notable for factor V Leiden (previous DVT 20 years ago); however, he is not currently on any anticoagulation. Physical examination is notable for 1+ edema of the upper left arm and tenderness to palpation in the anterior left chest just below his clavicle. Which of the following is the *best* initial imaging study for this patient?

   A. Chest x-ray
   B. Duplex ultrasound of the upper extremities and chest
   C. Echocardiography
   D. V/Q scan

8. A 68-year-old man with history of a lower extremity DVT presents with 2 days of left arm swelling. Compression ultrasound of the left subclavian vein is shown in **Figure 70.6**.

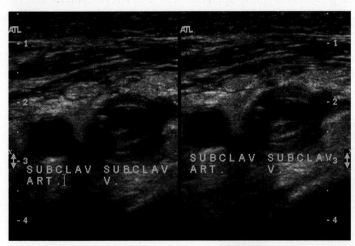

Without compression          With compression

**Figure 70.6**

The incidence of which complication is higher in this patient, compared to someone with the same pathology in the lower extremity?
A. Postthrombotic syndrome
B. 90-day mortality
C. Infection
D. Symptomatic pulmonary embolism (PE)

9. A 64-year-old man is admitted to the ICU for pneumonia. On day 3 of his hospital admission, he develops progressively increased pain and redness in his left arm. Compression ultrasound of the medial aspect of his proximal left upper extremity is shown in **Figure 70.7**.

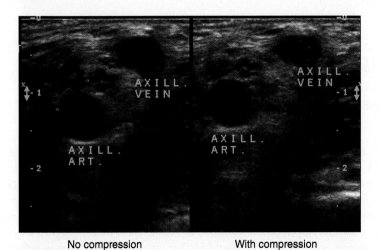

No compression          With compression

**Figure 70.7**

What are the ultrasound findings and recommended next steps?
A. Normal ultrasound, no additional workup is indicated
B. Normal ultrasound, empiric treatment for cellulitis
C. Upper extremity DVT, initiate anticoagulation
D. Upper extremity DVT, perform venogram for confirmatory study

10. A 58-year-old man presents to the Emergency Department with 2 days of right lower extremity swelling and pain. He reports that 3 days ago he flew from Japan to New York City, and shortly after returning he noticed the pain and swelling. On presentation, his temperature is 37.0°C, HR 86 bpm, BP 108/72 mm Hg, and SpO$_2$ 96% on room air. Physical examination is notable for 2+ edema of the entire right leg. A lower extremity ultrasound of the right leg demonstrates acute DVT of the femoral vein.

After the ultrasound examination, he develops chest pain. Repeat vital signs demonstrate a HR of 110 bpm, BP 88/68 mm Hg, and SpO$_2$ 78% on room air. **Figure 70.8** shows a parasternal short-axis view of the heart.

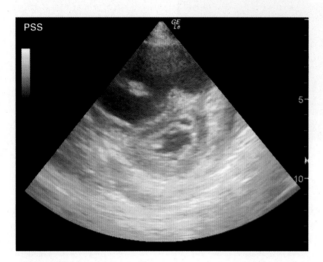

**Figure 70.8**

Which of the following ultrasonographic findings would be expected for this patient?
**A.** Right ventricular (RV)/left ventricular (LV) ratio less than 1
**B.** Tricuspid annular plane systolic excursion (TAPSE) <17 mm
**C.** Collapsible inferior vena cava (IVC) with respiratory variation
**D.** Hyperkinetic right ventricle

# Chapter 70 ▪ Answers

1. Correct Answer: D. Ultrasound without evidence of DVT; obtain abdominal (iliocaval) imaging to assess for proximal occlusion

*Rationale:* The patient in this question has evidence of significant asymmetric lower extremity edema and is at high risk for a DVT given his recent trauma and operations. The ultrasound provided does not demonstrate any evidence of DVT, as both the common femoral and popliteal veins are compressible. Swelling of the whole leg with a normal compression ultrasound raises concern for more proximal obstruction. Pulsed-wave Doppler interrogation of the femoral venous flow also gives additional information. Image E shows a loss of normal respirophasic variation in venous flow, which suggests there is a proximal occlusion. In these patients, guidelines recommend further investigation, including pelvic and abdominal imaging to further assess the vasculature.[1]

Selected References
1. Brant WE, Helms CA. Chapter 39, Vascular Ultrasound. In: *Fundamentals of Diagnostic Radiology*, 4th ed. Lippincott, Williams & Wilkins; 2012.
2. Cosby KS, Kendall JL. Chapter 17, Lower Extremity Venous Studies. In: *Practical Guide to Emergency Ultrasound*. Wolters Kluwer; 2013. ProQuest Ebook Central.
3. Needleman L, Cronan JJ, Lilly MP, et al. Ultrasound for lower extremity deep venous thrombosis: multidisciplinary recommendations from the society of radiologists in ultrasound consensus conference. *Circulation.* 2018;137:1505-1515.

**2.** Correct Answer: D. Complete duplex: compression from the common femoral vein to the ankle, including color and spectral Doppler

*Rationale:* Multiple modalities for assessment of DVT have been studied with varying efficacy. Most of these modalities include compression, Doppler flow, or both. Complete duplex ultrasound of the lower extremity includes compression from the common femoral vein to the ankle, also including color and spectral Doppler (**Figure 70.9**).

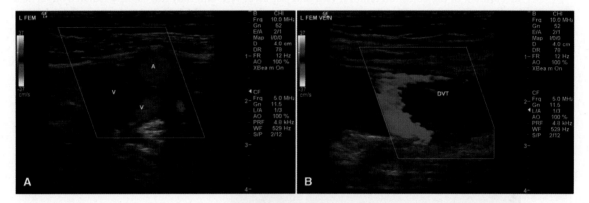

**Figure 70.9** Deep vein thrombosis with Doppler. **A.** Transverse orientation. **B.** Longitudinal orientation.

Deciding on the appropriate study for patients may depend on both operator comfort and available resources. Studies have demonstrated relatively similar failure rates for two-region compression and extended compression ultrasound, yet these studies are limited by the heterogeneity of patient population and operators. Further studies have shown that duplex ultrasound has the greatest sensitivity of the modalities at detecting DVT with a sensitivity of 96.5% for proximal DVTs and >70% for distal DVTs. **Table 70.1** summarizes the other commonly utilized modalities for DVT assessment and their description.

**Table 70.1. Lower Extremity Ultrasound Modalities**

| Lower extremity ultrasound modality | Description |
| --- | --- |
| *Two-region compression ultrasound (2-CUS)* | Compression ultrasound including the femoral veins 1-2 cm above and below the saphenofemoral junction and the popliteal veins up to the calf veins confluence |
| *Extended Compression Ultrasound (ECUS)* | Compression ultrasound from common femoral vein through the popliteal vein up to the calf veins confluence |
| *Complete Compression Ultrasound (CCUS)* | Compression ultrasound from common femoral vein to the ankle |
| *Complete Duplex Ultrasound (CDUS)* | Compression ultrasound from the common femoral vein to the ankle, color and spectral Doppler of the common femoral (or iliac veins) on both sides, color and spectral Doppler of the popliteal vein on the symptomatic side |

Selected References

1. Cosby KS, Kendall JL. Chapter 17, Lower extremity venous studies. In: *Practical Guide to Emergency Ultrasound*. Wolters Kluwer; 2013. ProQuest Ebook Central.
2. Kraaijpoel N, Carrier M, Le Gal G, et al. Diagnostic accuracy of three ultrasonography strategies for deep vein thrombosis of the lower extremity: a systematic review and meta-analysis. *PLoS One*. 2020;15:e0228788.
3. Goodacre S, Sampson F, Thomas S, van Beek E, Sutton A. Systematic review and meta-analysis of the diagnostic accuracy of ultrasonography for deep vein thrombosis. *BMC Med Imaging*. 2005;5:6.
4. Needleman L, Cronan JJ, Lilly MP, et al. Ultrasound for lower extremity deep venous thrombosis: multidisciplinary recommendations from the society of radiologists in ultrasound consensus conference. *Circulation*. 2018;137:1505-1515.

3. Correct Answer: C. Isolated popliteal vein thrombus

*Rationale:* The patient has signs and symptoms of acute DVT at a hospital with limited resources. The gold standard test for assessment of lower extremity DVT is complete duplex ultrasound; however, skilled ultrasonographers and necessary equipment may not be available in low-resource settings. Two- or three-region compression ultrasound, as well as extended compression ultrasound may be alternatives if complete duplex ultrasound capabilities are not available.[1] Two-region compression ultrasound includes assessment of the common femoral vein and popliteal vein and may not capture isolated superficial femoral vein thromboses. Three-region compression ultrasound, which includes the superficial femoral vein, has greater sensitivity for diagnosis of lower extremity DVT when compared with two-region compression. Both techniques include evaluation of the popliteal vein. In this question, the femoral vein is compressible while the popliteal vein is not. This finding is indicative of an isolated popliteal vein thrombus as shown in **Figure 70.10**.

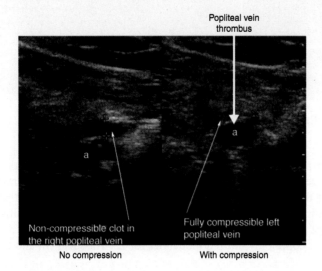

**Figure 70.10**

Selected References

1. Burnside PR, Brown MD, Kline JA. Systematic review of emergency physician-performed ultrasonography for lower-extremity deep vein thrombosis. *Acad Emerg Med.* 2008;15:493-498.
2. Kline JA, O'Malley PM, Tayal VS, Snead GR, Mitchell AM. Emergency clinician-performed compression ultrasonography for deep venous thrombosis of the lower extremity. *Ann Emerg Med.* 2008;52:437-445.
3. Zuker-Herman R, Ayalon Dangur I, Berant R, et al. Comparison between two-point and three-point compression ultrasound for the diagnosis of deep vein thrombosis. *J Thromb Thrombolysis.* 2018;45:99-105.
4. Hamper UM, DeJong MR, Scoutt LM. Ultrasound evaluation of the lower extremity veins. *Radiol Clin North Am.* 2007;45:525-47, ix.
5. Talbot SR, Oliver M. Duplex imaging of the lower extremity venous system. In: Kupinski AM, ed. *LWW Sonography: The Vascular System.* Wolters Kluwer; 2013:209-229. Figure 14.23.
6. Fox JC, Vandordaklou N. Lower extremity venous studies. In: Cosby KS, Kendall JL, eds. *Practical Guide to Emergency Ultrasound.* 2nd ed. Wolters Kluwer; 2014: 254-263.

4. Correct Answer: A. Surgical consultation for arterial thrombectomy

*Rationale:* This patient is hypercoagulable given her history of factor V Leiden, prompting a high suspicion for thromboembolic disease. The echocardiogram images demonstrate concern for a large thrombus in the left ventricle, but there is no flattening of the septum to suggest a PE. With the acute onset of severe lower extremity pain and asymmetric pulses, an arterial thromboembolic event is likely. The color Doppler ultrasound is included in **Figure 70.11.**

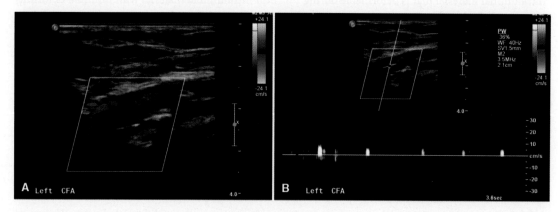

**Figure 70.11** Lower extremity Doppler with lack of arterial flow.

Color Doppler ultrasound may be adequate for identifying arterial stenosis and occlusions. Studies have found no difference in surgical outcomes and survival for patients with acute arterial emboli preoperatively assessed with ultrasound compared with those assessed with computed tomography angiography (CTA).

Urgent surgical consultation is indicated as the next step in management. Although thrombolysis may be considered for limb-threatening ischemia if surgical or radiological interventions are not available, it is not the preferred treatment. There is no indication for antibiotics in this scenario, and while systemic anticoagulation is appropriate, there is no evidence of venous thrombosis in Figures 70.3 or 70.4.

### Selected References

1. Crawford JD, Perrone KH, Jung E, Mitchell EL, Landry GJ, Moneta GL. Arterial duplex for diagnosis of *peripheral art*erial emboli. *J Vasc Surg.* 2016;64:1351-1356.
2. Hwang JY. Doppler ultrasonography of the lower extremity arteries: anatomy and scanning guidelines. *Ultrasonography.* 2017;36:111-119.
3. Armstrong WF, Ryan T. Masses, tumors, and source of embolus. *Feigenbaum's Echocardiography.* 8th ed. Wolters Kluwer; 2019:651-691.
4. Moneta GL, Zaccardi MJ. Duplex evaluation of lower extremity arterial occlusive disease. In: Zierler R, Dawson D, eds. *Strandness's Duplex Scanning in Vascular Disorders.* 5th ed. Wolters Kluwer; 2016:151-163.

**5.** Correct Answer: A. Thrombus firmly adherent to vessel wall

*Rationale:* In critically ill patients with a history of DVT, it may be difficult to differentiate between acute DVT and chronic venous scarring on ultrasound. Multiple findings are suggestive of acute venous thrombosis: (1) intraluminal material that is deformable during compression, (2) dilation of the vein, (3) smooth intraluminal material, (4) a free tail floating proximally from the attachment of the clot on the vein wall.[1] Over time, acute DVTs may evolve and demonstrate ultrasonographic signs of chronic scarring. These findings are largely dependent on the evolution of the thrombus, including lysis, thrombectomy, or embolic phenomena.[2] Residual thromboses may form chronic scars and are more likely to be firmly adherent to the vein wall. Acute DVTs are more likely to be free-floating with small attachment sites to the vessel wall. A list of ultrasonographic findings to differentiate acute DVT and chronic scarring is included in **Table 70.2.**

**Table 70.2 Ultrasound Findings of Acute DVT and Chronic Scarring**

| Acute deep vein thrombosis | Chronic scarring |
|---|---|
| Intraluminal material that is deformable during compression | Stiff intraluminal material with minimal deformity with compression |
| Vein dilation | Normal vein size or smaller in caliber |
| Smooth intraluminal material | Typically includes webs, bands, and vessel wall thickening |
| Free tail floating proximally from the attachment of the clot on the vein wall | Thrombus firmly adherent to the vessel wall |

Selected References
1. Murphy TP, Cronan JJ. Evolution of deep venous thrombosis: a prospective evaluation with US. *Radiology.* 1990;177:543-548.
2. Needleman L. Update on the lower extremity venous ultrasonography examination. *Radiol Clin North Am.* 2014;52:1359-1374.

**6. Correct Answer: C.** Vascular surgery consultation for catheter-directed thrombolysis and/or thrombectomy

*Rationale:* The patient in this question has significant arm pain, edema throughout the entire arm, and diminished pulses, which are all concerning for extensive thrombus. While not shown, the DVT appears to extend from the subclavian vein and into the internal jugular vein. Given the severe symptoms and extent of the thrombus, consideration of catheter-directed lysis and/or thrombectomy is the most appropriate management for this patient. A 2016 review in CHEST found that catheter-directed therapy should be considered when there are severe symptoms, extension from the subclavian to axillary vein, duration of symptoms <14 days, low risk of bleeding, and life expectancy >1 year. Systemic thrombolytics may be appropriate if the patient develops a life-threatening PE; however, treatment with systemic thrombolytics has significant greater risk of bleeding compared with catheter-directed treatment and is not recommended for upper extremity DVT without PE. Antibiotics and extremity compression/elevation would be appropriate for treatment of cellulitis or an infected thrombosis; however, this patient's presentation is more consistent with thrombosis without infection. Aspirin and Plavix may be appropriate for prophylaxis after stent placement; however, currently they are not included in the management of acute DVT.

Selected References
1. Caps MT, Mraz BA. Upper extremity venous thrombosis. In: Zierler R, Dawson D, eds. *Strandness's Duplex Scanning in Vascular Disorders.* 5th ed. Wolters Kluwer; 2016:250-273.
2. Feinberg J, Nielsen EE, Jakobsen JC. Thrombolysis for acute upper extremity deep vein thrombosis. *Cochrane Database Syst Rev.* 2017;12:CD012175.
3. Kearon C, Akl EA, Ornelas J, et al. Antithrombotic therapy for VTE disease: CHEST guideline and expert panel report. *Chest.* 2016;149:315-352.
4. Murphy E, Lababidi A, Reddy R, Mendha T, Lebowitz D. The role of thrombolytic therapy for patients with a submassive pulmonary embolism. *Cureus.* 2018;10:e2814.
5. Pillus D, Bruno E, Farcy D, Vilke GM, Childers R. Systematic review: the role of thrombolysis in intermediate-risk pulmonary embolism. *J Emerg Med.* 2019.

**7. Correct Answer: B.** Duplex ultrasound of the upper extremities and chest

*Rationale:* The patient in this question presents with left-sided chest discomfort as well as left upper arm pain. The differential diagnosis includes acute coronary syndrome (ACS), upper extremity DVT, pulmonary embolism (PE), and musculoskeletal pain. The physical examination and history are concerning for an upper extremity DVT given his arm edema and hypercoagulability. Duplex ultrasound of the upper extremities and chest is both sensitive and specific for the diagnosis of proximal upper extremity DVT. Although direct visualization of the proximal subclavian vein can be difficult with ultrasound, spectral analysis may show reduced or absent respiratory phasicity, which suggests a proximal obstruction. CT venography would be another method of diagnosis, but is not offered as a choice. A chest x-ray may be helpful for the diagnosis of pneumonia or congestive heart failure (CHF); however, it is not helpful in the diagnosis of venous thrombosis. Echocardiography may be obtained to evaluate for ACS or PE; however, the patient has no evidence of hemodynamic compromise or hypoxia. V/Q scan may be helpful in the diagnosis of a PE but the study is time-consuming and does not include imaging of the peripheral veins.

### Selected References

1. Baarslag HJ, van Beek EJ, Koopman MM, Reekers JA. Prospective study of color duplex ultrasonography compared with contrast venography in patients suspected of having deep venous thrombosis of the upper extremities. *Ann Intern Med.* 2002;136:865-872.
2. Di Nisio M, Van Sluis GL, Bossuyt PM, Buller HR, Porreca E, Rutjes AW. Accuracy of diagnostic tests for clinically suspected upper extremity deep vein thrombosis: a systematic review. *J Thromb Haemost.* 2010;8:684-692.
3. Knudson GJ, Wiedmeyer DA, Erickson SJ, et al. Color Doppler sonographic imaging in the assessment of upper-extremity deep venous thrombosis. *AJR Am J Roentgenol.* 1990;154:399-403.

## 8. Correct Answer: B. 90-day mortality

*Rationale:* The patient in this question has signs and symptoms concerning for an upper extremity DVT. Both upper extremity and lower extremity DVTs can be diagnosed with ultrasonography as demonstrated in the question. When compared to lower extremity thrombosis, upper extremity thrombosis is more rare, less likely to recur, and less likely to cause postthrombotic syndrome or symptomatic PE. It is, however, associated with a higher 3-month mortality, which may be due to the fact that upper extremity DVTs are more frequently identified in patients with malignancies. There is no evidence to suggest that upper extremity DVT has a higher rate of infection.

### Selected References

1. Engelberger RP, Kucher N. Management of deep vein thrombosis of the upper extremity. *Circulation.* 2012;126:768-773.
2. Munoz FJ, Mismetti P, Poggio R, et al. Clinical outcome of patients with upper-extremity deep vein thrombosis: results from the RIETE Registry. *Chest.* 2008;133:143-148.
3. Peripheral venous systems. In: Arger PH, Iyoob SD, eds. *Complete Guide to Vascular Ultrasound.* Wolters Kluwer; 2005:55-74.

## 9. Correct Answer: C. Upper extremity DVT, initiate anticoagulation

*Rationale:* The ultrasound findings indicate evidence of poor compressibility, concerning for an upper extremity DVT. The location of the ultrasound likely demonstrates DVT of the axillary vein, which, in addition to the brachial and subclavian veins, constitutes a deep vein of the upper extremity. Thromboses here are often associated with indwelling catheters, particularly central venous catheters. For proximal upper extremity DVTs (those proximal to the elbow), guidelines recommend initiation of anticoagulation for 3 months after diagnosis. Therapy may include heparin, low-molecular-weight heparin, vitamin K antagonists, or direct-acting oral anticoagulants such as rivaroxaban or apixaban. For a more distal idiopathic upper extremity DVT, the utility of anticoagulation is debated, but currently there is no consensus regarding the necessity of treatment. A CT or magnetic resonance (MR) venogram may be helpful when there is a high index of suspicion for DVT and an indeterminate or negative ultrasound study. In this example, the ultrasound clearly demonstrates a DVT and confirmatory testing is not indicated.

### Selected References

1. Ageno W, Haas S, Weitz JI, et al. Upper extremity DVT versus lower extremity DVT: perspectives from the GARFIELD-VTE Registry. *Thromb Haemost.* 2019;119:1365-1372.
2. Goodacre S, Sampson F, Thomas S, van Beek E, Sutton A. Systematic review and meta-analysis of the diagnostic accuracy of ultrasonography for deep vein thrombosis. *BMC Med Imaging.* 2005;5:6.
3. Kearon C, Akl EA, Comerota AJ, et al. Antithrombotic therapy for VTE disease: antithrombotic therapy and prevention of thrombosis, 9th ed. American College of Chest Physicians Evidence-Based Clinical Practice Guidelines. *Chest.* 2012;141:e419S-e496S.
4. Peripheral venous systems. In: Arger PH, Iyoob SD, eds. *Complete Guide to Vascular Ultrasound.* Wolters Kluwer; 2005:55-74.

## 10. Correct Answer: B. Tricuspid annular plane systolic excursion (TAPSE) <17 mm

*Rationale:* The echocardiogram image displays bowing of the interventricular septum into the left ventricle, resulting from acute RV volume or pressure overload in the setting of a PE. There is also a pericardial effusion present, but this is an incidental finding.

Additional evidence of right heart strain would include: increased RV/LV ratio (>1), dilated IVC without respiratory variation, and hypokinesis of the right ventricle. Measurement of the TAPSE has been studied as a method to assess right heart strain. TAPSE is typically assessed in M-mode by placing the cursor at the lateral tricuspid annulus. The maximum displacement during systole is then measured. Typically, a TAPSE <15 to 17 mm is quoted as associated with right ventricular impairment. An example of a normal image of the TAPSE (~26 mm) in M-mode is shown in **Figure 70.12**.

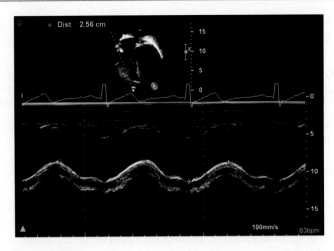

**Figure 70.12**

### Selected References

1. Bailitz J. A problem-based approach to resuscitation of acute illness or injury. In: Cosby KS, Kendall JL, eds. *Practical Guide to Emergency Ultrasound.* 2nd ed. Wolters Kluwer; 2014:96-107.

2. Carroll BJ, Heidinger BH, Dabreo DC, et al. Multimodality Assessment of Right Ventricular Strain in Patients With Acute Pulmonary Embolism. *Am J Cardiol* 2018;122:175-81.

3. Dwyer KH, Rempell JS, Stone MB. Diagnosing centrally located pulmonary embolisms in the emergency department using point-of-care ultrasound. *Am J Emerg Med.* 2018;36:1145-1150.

4. Eidem BW, O'Leary PW. Quantitative methods in echocardiography—basic techniques. In: Eidem BW, Cetta F, Johnson J, Lopez L, eds. *Echocardiography in Pediatric and Adult Congenital Heart Disease.* 3rd ed. Wolters Kluwer; 2021:42-66.

5. Lahham S, Fox JC, Thompson M, et al. Tricuspid annular plane of systolic excursion to prognosticate acute pulmonary symptomatic embolism (TAPSEPAPSE study). *J Ultrasound Med.* 2019;38:695-702.

# 71 | PSEUDOANEURYSM

Trent Lee Wei and Alejandro Pino

1. A pseudoaneurysm is a collection of blood that forms in which of the following areas?

   A. Between the adventitia and vasa vasorum
   B. Bound by the intima, media, and adventitia
   C. Between the media and adventitia
   D. Outside of the arterial wall

2. Which of the following is *most* likely to represent a recently formed femoral pseudoaneurysm on ultrasound?

   A. A homogeneous, predominantly hyperechoic area
   B. A heterogeneous, predominantly hyperechoic area
   C. A homogeneous, predominantly hypoechoic area
   D. A heterogeneous, predominantly hypoechoic area

3. Which best describes the "yin-yang sign" associated with a pseudoaneurysm?

   A. Alternating unidirectional, turbulent blood flow through the pseudoaneurysm
   B. Systolic and diastolic blood flow traversing longitudinally to the pseudoaneurysm
   C. Unidirectional, laminar blood flow through only one side of the pseudoaneurysm
   D. Bidirectional turbulent, swirling blood flow through the pseudoaneurysm

4. A 65-year-old woman receives a coronary angiogram following an abnormal stress test. The following day, an area of swelling is noted at the arterial puncture site that is evaluated with ultrasound (**Figure 71.1**).

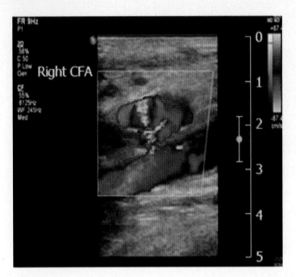

**Figure 71.1**

What is the preferred treatment of the pictured pseudoaneurysm?
A. Observation
B. Ultrasound-guided manual compression
C. Ultrasound-guided thrombin injection (UGTI)
D. Urgent surgical intervention

5. After femoral arterial catheterization, the ultrasound shown in **Figure 71.2** is obtained.

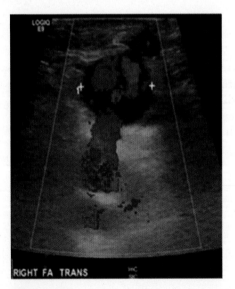

**Figure 71.2**

The defect has persisted after ultrasound-guided manual compression. Which of the following is a relative contraindication to UGTI?
A. History of stroke
B. Anticoagulation with heparin
C. Anticoagulation with apixaban
D. Large pseudoaneurysm neck diameter that is incompressible

6. A 75-year-old woman with type 2 diabetes and hypertension presents with acute myocardial infarction. She undergoes a cardiac catheterization via the right femoral artery. Four hours later, she develops a painful swelling at the access site in her right groin. She appears well and in no acute distress. Her vital signs reveal HR 80 bpm, BP 135/70 mm Hg, and RR 14/min. Point-of-care ultrasound with color Doppler of the right femoral artery shows **Figure 71.3**.

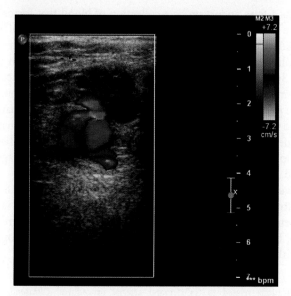

**Figure 71.3** A transverse color Doppler sonogram of the right groin in the region of the visible catheterization puncture site.

What is the *most appropriate* next step in the management of this patient?
A. Urgent surgical consultation
B. Local thrombin injection
C. Ultrasound-guided manual compression
D. Reevaluation in 1 hour

7. A 58-year-old man is in the cardiac intensive care unit following an acute anterior wall myocardial infarction. Two days prior, he underwent percutaneous coronary intervention via the right radial artery, and two drug-eluting stents (DES) were deployed. A palpable mass is noted on his forearm, and an ultrasound shows a 4.5 cm × 3.0 cm × 1.8 cm lesion arising from the origin of the right radial artery at the brachial artery.

What is the *most appropriate* next step in the management of this patient?
A. Urgent surgical consultation
B. Platelet transfusion
C. Local thrombin injection
D. Ultrasound-guided manual compression

# Chapter 71 ▪ Answers

**1. Correct Answer: C. Between the media and adventitia**

*Rationale:* A pseudoaneurysm, also known as a false aneurysm, is a collection of blood that forms between two of the layers of an artery, whereas a true aneurysm involves all three layers of the arterial wall. They typically form between the media and adventitia following trauma to the vessel. Pseudoaneurysms most commonly involve the femoral artery following angiography. The presentation may vary from clinically silent to life-threatening emergencies. Symptoms depend on the size and location of the pseudoaneurysm. Pain is common and occurs from increased pressure from swelling or nerve compression. On clinical examination, a pulsatile mass may be palpable, associated with a thrill or murmur. Pseudoaneurysms may cause significant morbidity due to an increased risk of rupture, thromboembolism, extrinsic compression of nearby neurovascular structures, or necrosis of overlying skin and subcutaneous tissue. Risk factors for pseudoaneurysms include a lower femoral puncture site, larger sheath size, anticoagulation or antifibrinolytic therapy, older age, and arterial hypertension.

Ultrasound of pseudoaneurysms can reveal a pulsatile anechoic saccular lesion with variable echogenicity, depending on the presence of an intraluminal thrombus. When there is no thrombus, it is anechoic; when the pseudoaneurysm is completely thrombosed, it may be difficult to differentiate from a hematoma. Images can also reveal swirling or fluid-fluid levels within a pseudoaneurysm. Color Doppler imaging shows a bidirectional, turbulent, swirling blood-flow pattern known as the yin-yang sign.

### Selected Reference

1. Chun EJ. Ultrasonographic evaluation of complications related to transfemoral arterial procedures. *Ultrasonography.* 2018;37(2):164-173.

**2. Correct Answer: D. A heterogeneous, predominantly hypoechoic area**

*Rationale:* The ultrasound appearance of pseudoaneurysms is expected to be heterogeneous. The variable echogenicity represents fluctuations of bleeding and rebleeding from the arterial wall lesion (**Figure 71.4**). Prior to thrombus formation, pseudoaneurysms are hypoechoic because they are predominantly anechoic liquid blood. Color flow Doppler may reveal a pulsatile, turbulent flow. The pathognomonic sign for pseudoaneurysm is a to-and-fro waveform within the arterial lesion on spectral or color Doppler imaging, often referred to as the yin-yang sign.

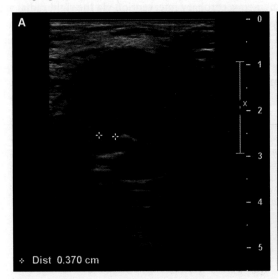 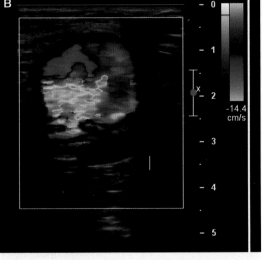

**Figure 71.4** Pseudoaneurysm. A, A transverse sonogram on a patient following postcardiac catheterization demonstrates a pseudoaneurysm in the common femoral artery. The neck is marked by calipers. B, The color Doppler sonogram demonstrates turbulent flow.

Selected References

1. Alerhand S, Apakama D, Nevel A, Nelson BP. Radial artery pseudoaneurysm diagnosed by point-of-care ultrasound five days after transradial catheterization: a case report. *World J Emerg Med.* 2018;9(3):223-226.
2. Rybyinski A. Sonography-guided interventional procedures. In: Kawamura D, Nolan T, eds. *Abdomen and Superficial Structures.* 4th ed. Wolters Kluwer; 2018:795-811.

3. Correct Answer: **D. Bidirectional turbulent, swirling blood flow through the pseudoaneurysm**

*Rationale:* The yin-yang sign seen with color Doppler ultrasound is a bidirectional, turbulent swirling, or fluid-fluid level within a pseudoaneurysm. This sign is commonly noted on large pseudoaneurysms that will partially thrombose, and blood may fill only part of the lesion.

The sign is created when blood on one side of an aneurysm or pseudoaneurysm travels toward the probe, and blood on the other side travels away from the probe in a turbulent pattern (**Figure 71.5**). Although this sign is helpful in differentiating aneurysms or pseudoaneurysms from hematomas, cysts, or solid masses, it is not solely associated with vascular abnormalities. Some neoplasms, such as solid and papillary epithelial neoplasms, may also demonstrate the "yin-yang sign." Furthermore, the absence of this sign does not rule out a pseudoaneurysm.

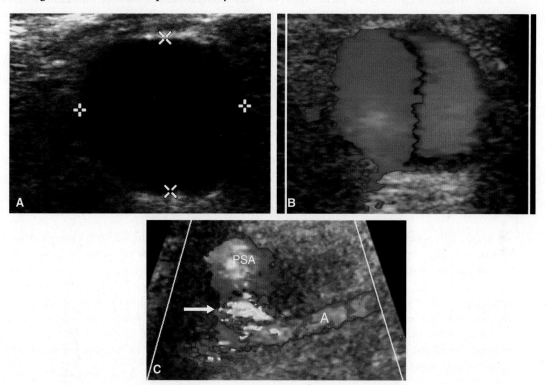

**Figure 71.5** Pseudoaneurysm. A, An echolucent mass with thrombus. B, Color Doppler image shows a swirling flow pattern, yin-yang sign, in the lumen of the pseudoaneurysm. C, Longitudinal color Doppler image demonstrates the broad neck (arrow) of the pseudoaneurysm (PSA), arising from the common femoral artery (A).

Selected References

1. Chun EJ. Ultrasonographic evaluation of complications related to transfemoral arterial procedures. *Ultrasonography.* 2018;37(2):164-173.
2. Helms WE. Vascular ultrasound. In: Klein J, Vinson EN, Brant WE, Helms CA, eds. *Brant and Helms' Fundamentals of Diagnostic Radiology.* 5th ed. Wolters Kluwer; 2019:1252-1276.
3. Lupattelli T. The yin-yang sign. *Radiology.* 2006;238:1070-1071.

4. Correct Answer: **A. Observation**

*Rationale:* Observation can be used as the treatment plan as long as the pseudoaneurysm is 2 cm or smaller, the lesion is stable for 24 hours, and the patient is asymptomatic. Patients with progressive hemorrhage, rapid expansion of the pseudoaneurysm, femoral neuralgia, or distal ischemia are not candidates for observation. The downsides of observation include increased time to resolution, the need for follow-up, unpredictability of thrombosis, and rupture potential. Resolution of postcatheterization pseudoaneurysms can take up to 8 weeks in some patients. Ultrasound can be used to guide compression of the tract connecting the native arterial lumen and the pseudoaneurysmal sac in patients who have a small pseudoaneurysm (usually <3.5 cm in diameter).

### Selected References
1. Chun EJ. Ultrasonographic evaluation of complications related to transfemoral arterial procedures. *Ultrasonography*. 2018;37(2):164-173.
2. Franklin JA, Brigham D, Bogey WM, Powell CS. Treatment of iatrogenic false aneurysms. *J Am Coll Surg*. 2003;197:293-301.
3. Mahmoud MZ, Al-Saadi M, Abuderman A, et al. "To-and-fro" waveform in the diagnosis of arterial pseudoaneurysms. *World J Radiol*. 2015;7(5):89-99. doi:10.4329/wjr.v7.i5.89.

**5.** Correct Answer: D. Large pseudoaneurysm neck diameter that is incompressible

*Rationale:* Pseudoaneurysms that are refractory to observation and ultrasound-guided manual compression will require percutaneous intervention. UGTI involves the administration of topical thrombin into the soft tissues comprising the pseudoaneurysm sac. Complications following thrombin injection are infrequent. The most serious complications, which are rare, include allergic reactions, arterial thrombosis, or distal embolization. For those in whom thrombin is not initially successful, repeat UGTI can be attempted.

A large neck diameter can theoretically increase the risk of distal embolization. Another contraindication is a pseudoaneurysm neck that is incompressible (unable to be compressed) due to concurrent compression of the native artery. Anticoagulation is not a contraindication to thrombin injection.

### Selected References
1. Loh EJ, Allen R. Endovascular treatment of refractory iatrogenic femoral artery pseudoaneurysm using Amplatzer vascular plugs following unsuccessful retrograde Angio-Seal deployment. *Indian J Radiol Imaging*. 2019;29(2):211-214.
2. Stone PA, Campbell JR II. Duplex evaluation and management of post-catheterization femoral pseudoaneurysms. In: AbuRahma AF, Bandyk DF, eds. *Noninvasive Vascular Diagnosis*. 3rd ed. London; 2013.

**6.** Correct Answer: C. Ultrasound-guided manual compression

*Rationale:* This patient has a symptomatic femoral artery pseudoaneurysm, which is a complication of the approach to percutaneous coronary intervention (PCI). Risk factors for pseudoaneurysms include advanced age, preexisting vascular disease, large sheath sizes, systemic anticoagulation, history of multiple catheter exchanges, and vascular site infection. This patient is hemodynamically stable with a relatively small pseudoaneurysm. While observation may be reasonable, it may allow for propagation of the pseudoaneurysm. The best initial management is compression and pressure, which may be done manually or by using a pneumatic device (i.e., inflated hemostatic band, sphygmomanometer). Thrombin injection may be considered if compression fails, and surgical consultation may be necessary if other treatment options fail or if she develops more severe symptoms.

### Selected Reference
1. Haystead C, Bowie JD, Kliewer MA, Hertzberg BS, Knutson TM, Carroll BA. Ultrasound. In: Provenzale JM, Nelson RC, Vinson EN, eds. *Duke Radiology Case Review*. 2nd ed. Wolters Kluwer; 2012:487-537.

**7.** Correct Answer: A. Urgent surgical consultation

*Rationale:* This case describes a pseudoaneurysm originating from the proximal radial artery. Due to the location and size of the pseudoaneurysm, neither manual compression nor thrombin injection would be considered given its proximity to the brachial artery. The patient will require surgery for repair of the pseudoaneurysm. Reversal of his antiplatelet therapy with a platelet transfusion would risk thrombosis of his new coronary stents.

### Selected Reference
1. Shah KJ, Halaharvi DR, Franz RW, Jenkins J. Treatment of iatrogenic pseudoaneurysms using ultrasound-guided thrombin injection over a 5-year period. *Int J Angiol*. 2011 Dec;20(4):235-242.

# 72 | ANEURYSM

Trent Lee Wei and Alejandro Pino

1. For which of the following patients is ultrasound screening recommended for abdominal aortic aneurysm (AAA)?

   A. A 75-year-old man with a 30 pack-year smoking history
   B. A 60-year-old woman with a 30 pack-year smoking history
   C. A 65-year-old man with a 30 pack-year smoking history
   D. A 60-year-old Hispanic man with diabetes

2. When analyzing AAAs with ultrasound in the transverse plane, which two landmarks should be identified to ensure complete visualization of the entire aorta?

   A. Superior mesenteric artery and inferior mesenteric artery
   B. Celiac trunk and the iliac bifurcation
   C. Celiac trunk and the inferior mesenteric artery
   D. The renal arteries and the iliac bifurcation

3. Which of the following helps differentiate the aorta from the inferior vena cava (IVC)?

   A. The aorta is on the patient's left, is noncompressible, and has no respiratory variation.
   B. The aorta is on the patient's right, is noncompressible, and has no respiratory variation.
   C. The aorta is on the patient's left, is compressible, and has respiratory variation.
   D. The aorta is on the patient's right, is compressible, and has respiratory variation.

4. Which of the following is *most* likely to obscure ultrasound visualization of the aorta?

   A. Hepatomegaly
   B. Splenomegaly
   C. Dilated loops of bowel with gas
   D. Ascites

5. Which of the following is *most* likely to cause underestimation of the size of an AAA?

   A. Measuring during inspiration
   B. Body positioning
   C. Intraluminal thrombus
   D. Perpendicular imaging plane

6. Which aortic landmark is pictured in **Figure 72.1**?

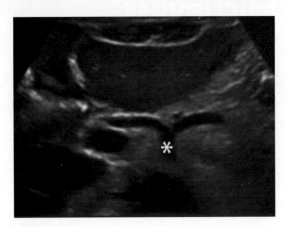

**Figure 72.1**

A. The celiac trunk bifurcating into the common hepatic artery and splenic artery
B. Bifurcation of the superior mesenteric artery into the right colic artery and middle colic artery
C. The common portal vein bifurcating into left and right portal vein
D. Bifurcation of the aorta into the right common iliac artery and the left common iliac artery

7. A 67-year-old man with a long smoking history presents to the Emergency Department with nontraumatic back pain for 1 day. An ultrasound of the abdominal aorta is shown in **Figure 72.2**.

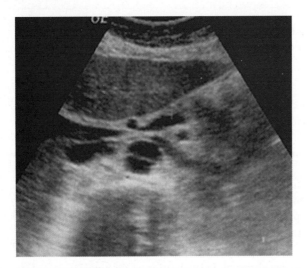

**Figure 72.2**

What is the *most* likely diagnosis based on the ultrasound findings?
A. Aortic dissection
B. Intramural thrombus
C. Aortic aneurysm
D. Atheromatous plaque

# Chapter 72 ▪ Answers

**1.** Correct Answer: C. A 65-year-old man with a 30 pack-year smoking history

*Rationale:* AAA is an abdominal aortic dilation of 3.0 cm or greater. The prevalence of AAA increases with age and is uncommon in persons younger than 50 years. The U.S. Preventive Services Task Force (USPSTF) updated guidelines recommend one-time screening with ultrasonography for men 65 to 75 years of age with a history of smoking, defined as at least 100 cigarettes over the individual's lifetime. Risk factors associated with a higher likelihood of AAA include first-degree relatives with AAA, history of other aneurysms, coronary artery disease, cerebrovascular disease, atherosclerosis, hypercholesterolemia, obesity, and hypertension. Factors associated with a decreased risk of AAA include black race, Hispanic ethnicity, and diabetes. The Society for Vascular Surgery recommends screening in all men and women 65 to 75 years of age.

### Selected References

1. Chaikof EL, Dalman RL, Eskandari MK, et al. The Society for Vascular Surgery practice guidelines on the care of patients with an abdominal aortic aneurysm. *J Vasc Surg.* 2018;67:2-77.e2.
2. U.S. Preventive Services Task Force. Screening for abdominal aortic aneurysm: recommendation statement. *Ann Intern Med.* 2014;161(4):281-290.

**2.** Correct Answer: B. Celiac trunk and the iliac bifurcation

*Rationale:* To fully evaluate the aorta, one must visualize the vessel in the transverse plane from the celiac trunk to the iliac bifurcation. The celiac trunk is the first major vessel to arise from the aorta immediately below the diaphragm. When visualized in the transverse plane, the celiac artery will appear as a "wide Y." At the level of the umbilicus the aorta will bifurcate into the iliac arteries, which can also be evaluated for aneurysmal disease if warranted.

In unstable patients, a right upper quadrant ultrasound or a focused assessment with sonography for trauma (FAST) to evaluate for pathologic fluid should be included. While the majority of AAAs rupture in the retroperitoneum, free rupture into the abdomen is rapidly fatal unless identified immediately. Lastly, assessing for the occurrence of an undulating intimal flap is important as this pathognomonic finding is 99%-100% specific for aortic dissections.

### Selected References

1. Fojtik JP, Costantino TG, Dean AJ. The diagnosis of aortic dissection by emergency medicine ultrasound. *J Emerg Med.* 2007;32:191-196.
2. Penny, SM. *Examination Review for Ultrasound: Abdomen and Obstetrics & Gynecology.* 1st ed. LWW; 2010.
3. Zucker EJ, Prabhakar AM. Abdominal aortic aneurysm screening: concepts and controversies. *Cardiovasc Diagn Ther.* 2018;8(suppl 1):S108-S117.

**3.** Correct Answer: A. The aorta is on the patient's left, is noncompressible, and has no respiratory variation.

*Rationale:* The aorta passes through the diaphragm at the level of the 12th thoracic vertebral body. It lies slightly to the left of the midline and bifurcates at the level of the 4th lumbar vertebral body. The anatomic landmark corresponding to the entry of the aorta through the diaphragm is the xiphoid process, and the landmark corresponding to the iliac bifurcation is the umbilicus. The aorta is to the left of the IVC, noncompressible, and lacks respiratory variation due to its thick arterial wall.

**4.** Correct Answer: C. Dilated loops of bowel with gas

*Rationale:* Ultrasound waves do not propagate well through gas, which appears as a bright reflective surface with shadowing that obscures the underlying anatomy. The interface with gas/air often causes long-path reverberation artifacts (for large gas collections) or short-path "ringdown" artifacts (for small gas collections). A gas-filled transverse colon often obscures visualization of the aorta. To remedy the situation, move the probe until an adequate sonographic window is visualized between loops of bowel or provide continuous compression with the probe until the gas moves out of the field of view.

Selected References

1. Hermsen K, Chong WK. Ultrasound evaluation of abdominal aortic and iliac aneurysms and mesenteric ischemia. *Radiol Clin North Am.* 2004;42:365-381.
2. Kuhn M, Bonnin RL, Davey MJ, Rowland JL, Langlois SL. Emergency department ultrasound scanning for abdominal aortic aneurysm: accessible, accurate, and advantageous. *Ann Emerg Med.* 2000;36(3):219-223.

5. Correct Answer: C. Intraluminal thrombus

*Rationale:* Measurement of AAA should be performed from outer wall to outer wall. Some AAAs contain intraluminal thrombus, and operators can confuse the thrombus with the arterial wall if the inner border is used. Doppler may be helpful in assessing the flow surrounding the thrombus. Other causes of inaccurate measurements of the aorta include oblique or angled planes, which can exaggerate the true aortic diameter, and sagittal sections of the aorta, which can lead to the appearance of a smaller diameter (the cylinder-tangent effect).

Selected References

1. Hermsen K, Chong WK. Ultrasound evaluation of abdominal aortic and iliac aneurysms and mesenteric ischemia. *Radiol Clin North Am.* 2004;42:365-381.
2. Kuhn M, Bonnin RL, Davey MJ, Rowland JL, Langlois SL. Emergency department ultrasound scanning for abdominal aortic aneurysm: accessible, accurate, and advantageous. *Ann Emerg Med.* 2000;36(3):219-223.

6. Correct Answer: A. The celiac trunk bifurcating into the common hepatic artery and splenic artery

*Rationale:* The celiac artery is an important landmark when assessing for an AAA. The division of the celiac artery into the splenic artery on the patient's left and hepatic artery on the patient's right forms the "seagull sign." The celiac artery forms the body of the seagull, and the splenic artery and hepatic artery form the wings. The splenic artery travels along the upper border of the pancreas, and the common hepatic artery travels toward the liver. This has also been called a "whale's tail sign," see **Figure 72.3**.

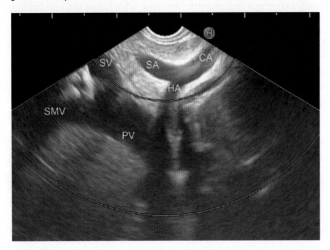

**Figure 72.3** Whale's tail sign visualized in long axis via transesophageal echocardiography. CA, celiac artery; HA, hepatic artery; PV, portal vein; SA, splenic artery; SMV, superior mesenteric vein; SV, splenic vein.

Selected References

1. Kupinski AM. *Diagnostic Medical Sonography: The Vascular System.* 2nd ed. Wolters Kluwer; 2018.
2. Pathak A, Shoukat A, Thomas NS, Mehta D, Sharma M. Seagulls of endoscopic ultrasound. *Endosc Ultrasound.* 2017;6(4):231-234.
3. Xiang H, Han J, Ridley WE, Ridley LJ. Seagull appearance: vascular anatomy on ultrasound. *J Med Imaging Radiat Oncol.* 2018;62(suppl 1):104.

7. Correct Answer: A. Aortic dissection

*Rationale:* Aortic dissections form when shearing intravascular forces separate the layers of the aortic wall. If untreated, patients with proximal aortic involvement have a 2-week mortality of approximately 80%. Visualization of an intimal flap (**Figure 72.4**) by ultrasound has a sensitivity as high as 80% and specificity of 100% for dissection.

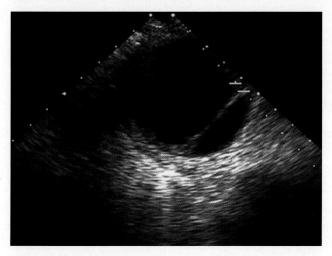

**Figure 72.4** Aortic dissection showing an intimal flap, visualized in the descending aorta by transesophageal echocardiography.

Selected References

1. Fojtik JP, Costantino TG, Dean AJ. The diagnosis of aortic dissection by emergency medicine ultrasound. *J Emerg Med.* 2007;32:191-196.
2. Khan IA, Nair CK. Clinical, diagnostic, and management perspectives of aortic dissection. *Chest.* 2002;122:311-328.
3. Taylor RA, Moore CL. Echocardiography. In: Cosby KS, Kendall JL, eds. *Practical Guide to Emergency Ultrasound.* 2nd ed. Wolters Kluwer; 2014:55-74.

# 73 | AORTIC DISSECTION

Lev Deriy, Brian Starr, Carlos E. Vazquez, Pamela Y.F. Hsu, Eli L. Torgeson, and Neal S. Gerstein

1. A 68-year-old man with a 50 pack-year smoking history, hypertension, and peripheral vascular disease is admitted to the hospital with pain in the chest and abdomen, hypotension, and diaphoresis. **Figure 73.1** and ▶ **Video 73.1** were obtained on point-of-care transesophageal echocardiography (TEE).

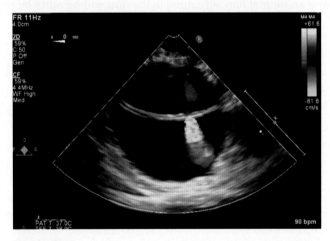

**Figure 73.1**

Which of the following answers is *most* correct?
A. This is a type A dissection and surgical management is indicated
B. This is a type B dissection and medical management is indicated
C. This is a type B dissection and surgical management is indicated
D. Unable to determine the type of dissection without additional imaging of ascending aorta

2. A 62-year-old man presents to the Emergency Department complaining of 2 hours of chest pain. An electrocardiogram (ECG) showed 2 mm of ST-elevation in the inferior leads (II, III, aVF). His vital signs show HR 105 bpm, BP 182/103 mm Hg, $SpO_2$ 97% on room air, and RR 18/min. Which of the following findings on point-of-care ultrasound (POCUS) would be *most likely* to change the management of this patient?

   A. Significant regional wall motion abnormalities
   B. Severely dilated right ventricle with tricuspid annular plane systolic excursion (TAPSE) <16 mm
   C. Dilated ascending aorta with severe aortic regurgitation
   D. Dilated left ventricle with global hypokinesis and moderate mitral regurgitation

3. A 45-year-old man with a history of aortic aneurysm and hypertension presents with chest and back pain and is discovered to have a dissecting aortic aneurysm. He is taken for emergent surgical repair. **Figure 73.2** shows the TEE obtained.

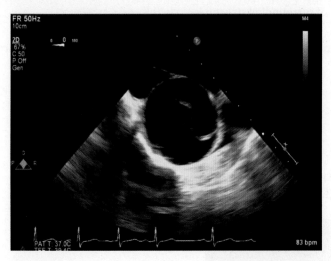

**Figure 73.2**

Which of the following echocardiographic findings is *most* consistent with identification of the false lumen (FL) in a patient being evaluated for acute aortic dissection?
   A. The false lumen expands in systole.
   B. The false lumen has high-velocity color Doppler flow without spontaneous echo contrast or clot present.
   C. The false lumen demonstrates diastolic collapse.
   D. The false lumen has lower velocity color Doppler flow with spontaneous echo contrast and clot present.

4. Which of the following TEE views is the *most* useful for the diagnosis of a type A aortic dissection?

   A. Midesophageal four-chamber view
   B. Upper esophageal aortic arch short-axis view
   C. Midesophageal aortic valve short-axis view
   D. Midesophageal aortic valve long-axis view

5. Which of the following statements comparing TEE and transthoracic echocardiography (TTE) examination of the aorta is *most* accurate?

    A. Although TEE has better resolution for the proximal aorta, TTE has higher sensitivity for aortic dissection than TEE in the descending aorta.
    B. The lower-frequency transducer used during TEE examinations provides deeper tissue penetration.
    C. There is a shorter distance between the transducer and the area of interest in TTE examination.
    D. TEE allows for examination of nearly the entire descending thoracic aorta in both short- and long-axis planes.

6. Which of the following is *most* helpful in differentiating an artifact from an aortic dissection flap?

    A. An artifact should be seen in multiple views.
    B. An artifact moves synchronously with the heart.
    C. A dissection flap has color Doppler flow in the same direction on both sides.
    D. An artifact moves independently of surrounding structures.

7. Which of the following echocardiographic findings is the *most* likely to be associated with acute aortic dissection?

    A. Tricuspid regurgitation
    B. Aortic stenosis
    C. Mitral regurgitation
    D. Aortic regurgitation

8. A 71-year-old woman presents for repair of a type A thoracic aortic dissection. Intraoperative TEE image is obtained as shown in **Figure 73.3** and ▶ **Video 73.2**.

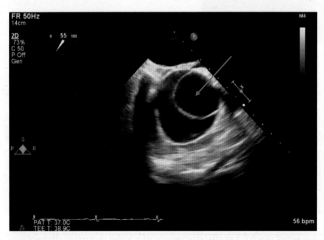

**Figure 73.3**

In this image during systole, what structure does the *arrow* point to?
A. Descending aorta, false lumen
B. Ascending aorta, false lumen
C. Ascending aorta, true lumen (TL)
D. Descending aorta, true lumen

9. In **Figure 73.4**, what is the name of the structure indicated by the *white asterisk* in this suprasternal notch view that can be mistaken for a dissection flap?

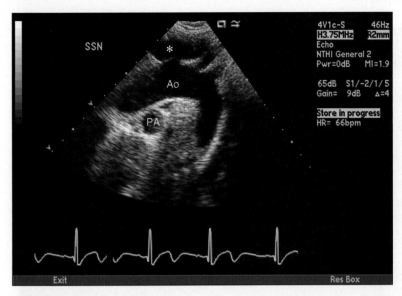

**Figure 73.4**

A. Trachea
B. Brachiocephalic artery
C. Brachiocephalic vein
D. Azygos vein

10. A 75-year-old woman is undergoing an aortic root repair for a type A dissection. The white arrows in **Figure 73.5** are pointing to what structure?

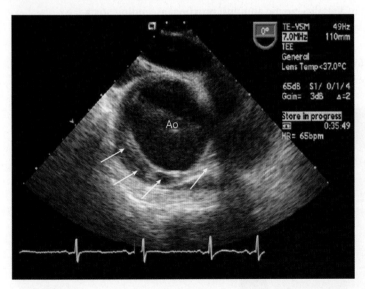

**Figure 73.5**

A. Calcifications in the descending aorta
B. Intramural hematoma in the ascending aorta
C. Normal wall thickening in the descending aorta
D. Take-off of the brachiocephalic artery in the ascending aorta

**11.** A 70-year-old man presents to the Emergency Department with angina and pain radiating to his back. In the TTE image shown in **Figure 73.6**, what are the names of *each* of the structures identified by the blue, red, green, and white arrows?

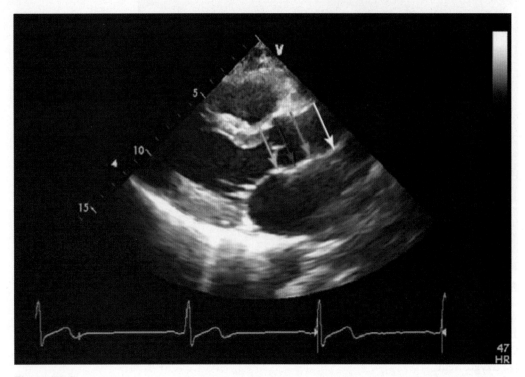

**Figure 73.6**

    **A.** Aortic annulus; sinus of Valsalva; sinotubular junction; proximal ascending aorta
    **B.** Aortic annulus; sinotubular junction; sinus of Valsalva; proximal ascending aorta
    **C.** Sinotubular junction; sinus of Valsalva; aortic annulus; proximal ascending aorta
    **D.** Sinus of Valsalva; sinotubular junction; aortic annulus; proximal ascending aorta

**12.** An 83-year-old man presents for emergency type A aortic dissection repair. Intraoperative TEE is performed revealing the image in **Figure 73.7**. What does this M-mode image demonstrate?

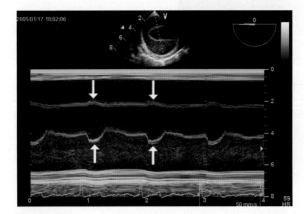

**Figure 73.7**

    **A.** False lumen expansion during systole
    **B.** True lumen expansion during systole
    **C.** False lumen expansion during diastole
    **D.** True lumen expansion during diastole

**13.** **Figure 73.8** shows a type A aortic dissection. Which of the following is the site of the intimal tear?

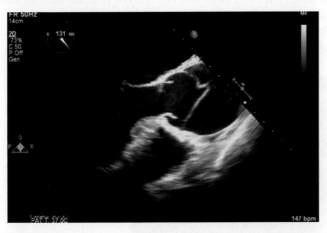

**Figure 73.8**

   **A.** Aortic valve annulus
   **B.** Sinus of Valsalva
   **C.** Sinotubular junction
   **D.** Proximal ascending aorta

**14.** A 69-year-old man with a history of hypertension arrives in the Emergency Department with a 3-day history of anterior chest pain. A bedside TTE is performed (see **Figure 73.9**).

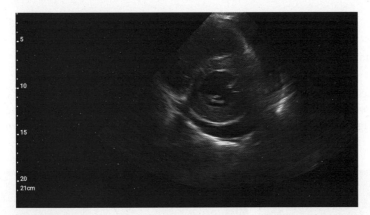

**Figure 73.9**

Which of the complications of aortic dissection is represented?
   **A.** Aortic regurgitation
   **B.** Intramural hematoma
   **C.** Pleural effusion
   **D.** Pericardial effusion

15. A 22-year-old man with an unknown past medical history is brought to the Emergency Department following a head-on motor vehicle collision. His BP is 85/55 mm Hg, HR 120 bpm, RR 22/min, and SpO$_2$ 90% on non-rebreather face mask. Chest radiography shows a widened mediastinum, and a POCUS examination is performed. Based on **Figure 73.10**, which letter corresponds to the *most likely* site of aortic pathology in this scenario?

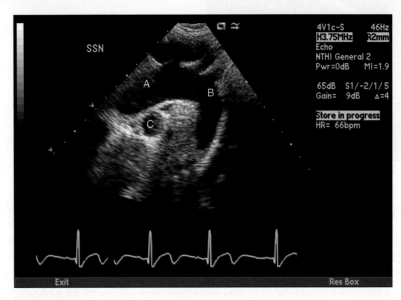

**Figure 73.10**

A. A
B. B
C. C
D. The most common site is not in Figure 73.10

16. A 25-year-old weightlifter is being evaluated in the Emergency Department after a sudden onset of chest and abdominal pain during a weightlifting competition. An abdominal ultrasound is performed and is shown in **Figure 73.11A**. In **Figure 73.11B**, the color flow Doppler image frozen in systole shows which of the following?

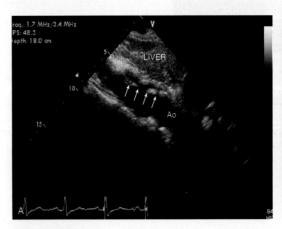
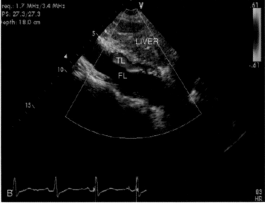

**Figure 73.11**

A. An aortic dissection with flow toward the probe in the true lumen
B. An aortic dissection with flow toward the probe in the false lumen
C. An aortic dissection with flow away from the probe in the true lumen
D. An aortic dissection with flow away from the probe in the false lumen

**17.** For the patient in **Question 73.16**, what is the *most appropriate* next step in his management?

    **A.** Admit the patient to the intensive care unit for medical management
    **B.** Call vascular surgery to proceed with open abdominal aorta repair
    **C.** Obtain additional imaging of the aorta
    **D.** Proceed with endovascular abdominal aorta repair

**18.** Which of the following is true regarding the use of TTE in the assessment of a patient with suspected acute aortic dissections?

    **A.** Transthoracic echo has been shown to be more sensitive than TEE for the identification of aortic dissections.
    **B.** The suprasternal view with transthoracic echo is able to visualize portions of the ascending aorta not visible on TEE.
    **C.** Transthoracic echo provides suboptimal views of the aortic valve and left ventricular outflow tract (LVOT).
    **D.** Transthoracic echo cannot be used to identify the complications of dissection.

**19.** A 75-year-old man is being evaluated for a possible aortic dissection in the Emergency Department after sudden onset of sharp chest, back, and abdominal pain. Physical examination reveals BP in his right arm 178/99 mm Hg and 90/51 mm Hg in his left. Additionally, his left femoral pulse is diminished. Abdominal ultrasound reveals a dissection into his left common iliac artery. Based on **Figure 73.12**, where would you expect the site of pathology to be?

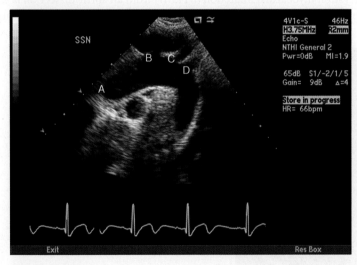

**Figure 73.12**

    **A.** A
    **B.** B
    **C.** C
    **D.** D

**20.** For the patient in question 19, what additional ultrasound finding is *most* likely associated with his diagnosis?

    **A.** More than three B-lines per sonographic lung field
    **B.** Absence of lung sliding in the left lung
    **C.** Bowing of the interventricular septum toward the left ventricle
    **D.** Presence of a left pleural effusion

# Chapter 73 ▪ Answers

**1.** Correct Answer: D. Unable to determine the type of dissection without additional imaging of ascending aorta.

*Rationale:* The right pulmonary artery (PA) is typically seen between the probe and the proximal portion of the ascending aorta in a short-axis view. Since there is no PA in Figure 73.1, it likely represents a dissection in descending aorta. Aortic dissection involving any portion of the ascending aorta (Stanford A) is a surgical emergency with a mortality rate up to 1% to 2% *per hour* in the first 48 hours if untreated. In comparison, dissections of the descending aorta are managed primarily with medical therapy, including aggressive HR and BP control, with surgical and/or endovascular repair only for cases causing end-organ damage or rapid expansion. Because the management differs so greatly, identification of the correct type of dissection is extremely important and cannot be made without evaluation of the ascending portion of the aorta.

### Selected Reference

1. Baron T, Flachskampf FA. Echocardiography in acute aortic dissection. In: Flachskampf FA, Neskovic AN, Picard MH, eds. *Emergency Echocardiography* Taylor & Francis Group.

**2.** Correct Answer: C. Dilated ascending aorta with severe aortic regurgitation

*Rationale:* Aortic dissection infrequently presents as acute myocardial ischemia/infarction if the dissection flap extends into the ostium of the coronary artery, causing acute occlusion and ST-segment changes. Distinguishing a primary ST-elevation myocardial infarction (STEMI) from an aortic dissection is essential because the treatment for myocardial infarction and delay of dissection repair can be fatal for patients with aortic dissection.

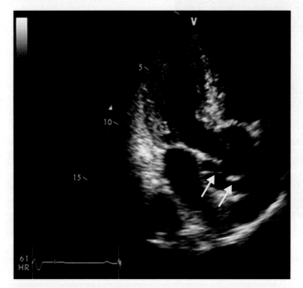

**Figure 73.13** Apical three-chamber (long-axis) view demonstrating a Type A aortic dissection with a dissection flap in the ascending aorta.

Visualization of an intimal flap, most commonly seen in the parasternal long-axis, apical three-chamber (see **Figure 73.13**), and/or apical five-chamber view, directly supports the diagnosis of aortic dissection. Indirect evidence of dissection includes a dilated ascending aorta, aortic regurgitation, and pericardial effusion. POCUS has been shown to be a valuable tool with high specificity for the diagnosis of aortic dissection.

### Selected References

1. Chenkin J. Diagnosis of aortic dissection presenting as ST-elevation myocardial infarction using point-of-care ultrasound. *J Emerg Med.* 2017;53(6):880-884.
2. Jayasuriya S. Statistics for the echo boards. In: Sorrell VL, Jayasuriya S, eds. *Questions, Tricks, and Tips for the Echocardiography Boards.* 2nd ed. Wolters Kluwer; 2019:7-9.

3. Correct Answer: D. The false lumen has lower velocity color Doppler flow with spontaneous echo contrast and clot present

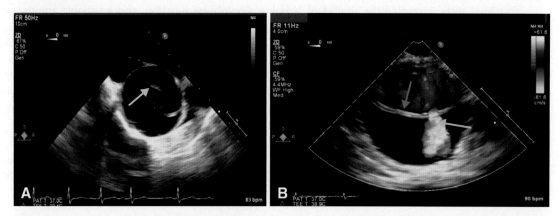

**Figure 73.14** A. A midesophageal ascending aorta short-axis view of a dissecting aneurysm. The yellow arrow is pointing toward the false lumen expansion during diastole. B. A descending aorta short-axis view. The blue arrow is pointing toward the true lumen expansion during systole. The green arrow is pointing toward a jet from the true lumen to the false lumen during systole.

*Rationale:* Identification and differentiation between the true lumen and the false lumen in aortic dissection can be challenging. Size, vessel origination, and presence of flow can be misleading. Some features that can be helpful in making this determination (as shown in **Figure 73.14**) include:
- There is a systolic expansion (*blue arrow*) and diastolic collapse of the true lumen.
- The false lumen expands in diastole (*yellow arrow*).
- The true lumen has high-velocity flow without spontaneous echo contrast.
- The false lumen has lower-velocity flow with spontaneous echo contrast and/or thrombus.
- Flow occurs between the true lumen and the false lumen during systole (*green arrow*).

### Selected References

1. Goldstein SA, Evangelista A, Abbara S, et al. Multimodality imaging of diseases of the thoracic aorta in adults: from the American Society of Echocardiography and the European Association of Cardiovascular Imaging Endorsed by the Society of Cardiovascular Computed Tomography and Society for Cardiovascular Magnetic Resonance. *J Am Soc Echocardiogr.* 2015;28:119-118.
2. Rasalingam R. *The Washington Manual of Echocardiography.* Wolters Kluwer; 2013.

4. Correct Answer: D. Midesophageal aortic valve long-axis view

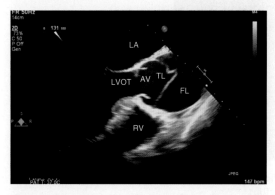

**Figure 73.15** Midesophageal aortic valve long-axis view.

*Rationale:* The midesophageal aortic valve long-axis view in **Figure 73.15** is obtained by slight withdrawal of the probe from the midesophageal long-axis view while maintaining a transducer omniplane angle of 120° to 140°. Reducing the depth of field allows concentrated imaging of the LVOT, aortic valve, and proximal aorta, including the sinuses of Valsalva, sinotubular junction, and a variable amount of the tubular ascending aorta. This view is useful in evaluating the aortic valve, aortic root dimensions, and proximal ascending aorta, as it allows for visualization of the entire aortic root and proximal ascending aorta. Color flow Doppler can help in identifying aortic regurgitation, flow in the true lumen and/or false lumen, and flow through the intimal tear. The midesophageal four-chamber view does not provide visualization of the ascending aorta, the upper esophageal aortic arch view does not provide optimal visualization of the aortic valve, and the midesophageal short-axis aortic valve view does not provide adequate visualization of the ascending aorta.

## Selected Reference

1. Hahn R, Abraham T, Adams MS, et al. Guidelines for performing a comprehensive transesophageal echocardiographic examination: recommendations from the American Society of Echocardiography and the Society of Cardiovascular Anesthesiologists. *J Am Soc Echocardiogr.* 2013;26:921-964.

**5.** Correct Answer: **D. TEE allows for examination of nearly the entire descending thoracic aorta in both short- and long-axis planes**

*Rationale:* TEE examination of the aorta is superior to TTE because of the shorter distance in general between the transducer and the area of interest. The use of a higher-frequency transducer also provides a better resolution at shallow depth. TEE allows examination of almost the entire descending thoracic aorta from the diaphragm to the arch in both long- and short-axis planes.

The sensitivity and specificity of TEE for the diagnosis of aortic dissection are both very high. The specificity is less than 100% because of misinterpretation of ultrasound artifacts. Careful examination of multiple views helps avoid these false-positive diagnoses.

## Selected Reference

1. Otto CM. *Echocardiography Review Guide: Companion to the Textbook of Clinical Echocardiography.* 4th ed. Elsevier; 2019.

**6.** Correct Answer: **B. An artifact moves synchronously with the heart**

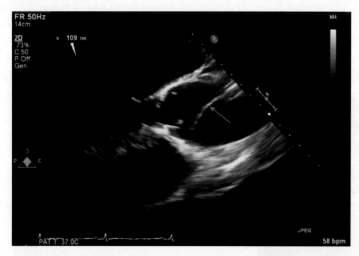

**Figure 73.16** Midesophageal aortic valve long-axis view. The *blue arrow* is pointing toward the dissection flap.

*Rationale:* It is very important to distinguish a dissection flap from an echocardiographic artifact (e.g., mirror or reverberation artifact) to avoid unnecessary intervention. The real flap (**Figure 73.16**, *arrow*) usually has a discrete sharp edge, is visualized in multiple views, moves independently of the surrounding structures, and has oppositely directed blood flow on color flow Doppler (**Figure 73.17**). An artifact is usually longitudinal, moves with the movement of the heart, and may interrupt color flow Doppler, but the direction of flow is the same on both sides.

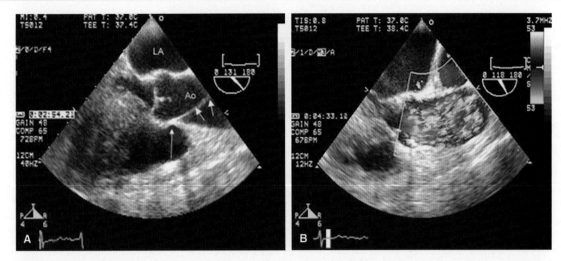

**Figure 73.17** Midesophageal aortic valve long-axis view. **A:** This image shows a common artifact that could be confused with a dissection. This is a classic side lobe artifact arising (*small arrows*) from a rather bright echo at the sinotubular junction (*vertical arrow*) resulting in an unnatural curvilinear echo extending along the direction of the scan plane within the lumen of the aorta. **B:** With color flow imaging there is no margination of flow by the linear echo, helping to confirm that this is artifact rather than a true dissection flap.

### Selected References

1. Diseases of the aorta. In: Armstrong WF, Ryan T, eds. *Feigenbaum's Echocardiography.* 8th ed. Wolters Kluwer; 2019:611-650.
2. Vegas A. *Perioperative Two-Dimensional Transesophageal Echocardiography: A Practical Handbook.* 2nd ed. Springer; 2012.

## 7. Correct Answer: D. Aortic regurgitation

*Rationale:* Propagation of the dissection proximally can involve the aortic valve causing acute aortic regurgitation due to the aortic annulus dilation and/or prolapse of the dissection flap. Aortic stenosis may predispose to aortic aneurysm, which may increase the likelihood of aortic dissection, but it is not the most likely association. Other valvular complications related to connective tissue disease may be present in rare cases, but tricuspid and mitral valvulopathies are not typically associated with aortic dissection.

### Selected References

1. Goldstein SA, Evangelista A, Abbara S, et al. Multimodality imaging of diseases of the thoracic aorta in adults: from the American Society of Echocardiography and the European Association of Cardiovascular Imaging Endorsed by the Society of Cardiovascular Computed Tomography and Society for Cardiovascular Magnetic Resonance. *J Am Soc Echocardiogr.* 2015;28:119-118.
2. Otto C. *Echocardiography Review Guide.* 4th ed. Elsevier; 2020.

## 8. Correct Answer: C. Ascending aorta, true lumen

*Rationale:* The goals of perioperative TEE in the evaluation of aortic dissection include the following: (a) establishing the diagnosis, (b) localizing primary and secondary entry sites, (c) differentiating true lumen from false lumen, (d) evaluating the aortic valve for insufficiency, (e) establishing involvement of the coronary arteries, and (f) ruling out associated conditions such as pericardial effusions and tamponade. The TEE image (Figure 73.3) shows the ascending thoracic aorta in short axis. The right pulmonary artery (PA) is typically seen between the transducer and the proximal portion of the ascending aorta in a short-axis view. The superior vena cava (SVC) or a portion of the right atrium (RA) can be seen on the left side of the screen and the main PA on the right side of the screen. The indicated lumen is bulging toward the other lumen during systole, as indicated by the ECG tracing on the lower left portion of Figure 73.3. Bulging of the true lumen toward the false lumen is expected during systole (immediately after the R-wave on the ECG tracing). The TEE image (**Figure 73.18** and ▶ **Video 73.2**) from the same patient shows a collapsed TL during diastole.

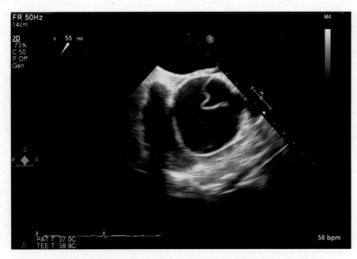

**Figure 73.18** Ascending aorta short-axis transesophageal echocardiography (TEE) view during diastole

Selected Reference

1. Perrino AC Jr, Reeves ST. Chapter 17: *Transesophageal echocardiography in the intensive care unit*. In: *A Practical Approach to Echocardiography*. 2nd ed. Philadelphia: Lippincott Williams & Wilkins; 2008.

**9.** Correct Answer: **C. Brachiocephalic vein**

*Rationale:* The brachiocephalic (innominate) vein can be mistaken for a dissection flap in the suprasternal notch view. Obtaining other views of the ascending aorta with and without color Doppler may help to distinguish the vein from a dissection flap.

Selected Reference

1. Rao PK, Quader N. Diseases of the great vessels. In: Quader N, Makan M, Perez P, eds. *The Washington Manual of Echocardiography*. 2nd ed. Wolters Kluwer; 2017:220-241.

**10.** Correct Answer: **B. Intramural hematoma**

*Rationale:* The goals of perioperative TEE in the evaluation of aortic dissection include the following: (a) establishing the diagnosis, (b) localizing primary and secondary entry sites, (c) differentiating true lumen from false lumen, (d) evaluating the aortic valve for insufficiency, (e) establishing involvement of the coronary arteries, and (f) ruling out associated conditions such as pericardial effusions and tamponade.

Figure 73.5 shows the ascending aorta in the short axis along with the classic crescentic shape of an intramural hematoma (*white arrows*). When the vasa vasorum ruptures into the media, blood and the ensuing thrombus create an intramural hematoma. About one-third of intramural hematomas progress to overt aortic dissection or rupture and hence are clinically treated similarly to dissection.

Selected Reference

1. Rao PK, Quader N. Diseases of the great vessels. In: Quader N, Makan M, Perez P, eds. *The Washington Manual of Echocardiography*. 2nd ed. Wolters Kluwer; 2017:220-241.

**11.** Correct Answer: A. Aortic annulus; sinus of Valsalva; sinotubular junction; proximal ascending aorta

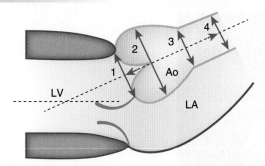

**Figure 73.19** The four sites in the parasternal long-axis view (PSAX) where the proximal aorta should be measured: (1) the aortic annulus, (2) the sinus of Valsalva, (3) the sinotubular junction, (4) the proximal ascending aorta. Ao, aorta; LA, left atrium; LV, left ventricle.

*Rationale:* TTE is an invaluable tool in evaluating the aortic valve and the aortic root for pathology. **Figure 73.19** shows the aortic root including the aortic valve in the long axis. This view provides great detail into the pathology of these structures (regurgitation, dissection, abscess, etc.). Knowing the names of the above structures can greatly assist in delineating the exact location of pathology, especially in type A aortic dissections. In order, arrow 1 = aortic annulus; arrow 2 = sinus of Valsalva; arrow 3 = sinotubular junction; arrow 4 = proximal ascending aorta. Dissections in these areas can also help predict immediate cardiac complications (coronary involvement, valve involvement).

### Selected References

1. Lang RM, Badano LP, Mor-Avi V, et al. Recommendations for cardiac chamber quantification by echocardiography in adults: an update from the American Society of Echocadiography and the Europeans Association of Cardiovascular Imaging. *J Am Soc Echocardiogr.* 2015;28:1-39.
2. Rao PK, Quader N. Diseases of the great vessels. In: Quader N, Makan M, Perez P, eds. *The Washington Manual of Echocardiography.* 2nd ed. Wolters Kluwer; 2017:220-241.

**12.** Correct Answer: B. True lumen expansion during systole

*Rationale:* The TEE image (Figure 73.7) is taken in motion mode (or M-mode), which reveals expansion of the true lumen during early systole with the intimal flaps moving toward the false lumen. Spontaneous echo contrast can also be visualized in the lower false lumen from stagnant flow. The false lumen is often larger than the TL, especially in chronic dissections. The true lumen is identified by forward systolic flow, whereas flow in the false lumen is complicated and variable.

### Selected Reference

1. Payne KJ, Ikonomidis JS, Reeves ST. Transesophageal echocardiography of the thoracic aorta. In: Perrino AC, Reeves ST, eds. *Practical Approach to Transesophageal Echocardiography.* 2nd ed. Wolters Kluwer; 2008:321-347.

**13.** Correct Answer: **C. Sinotubular junction**

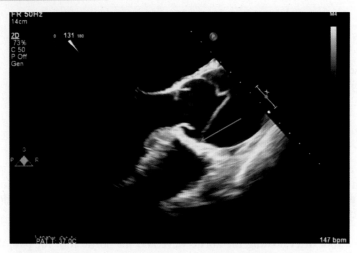

**Figure 73.20** Midesophageal aortic valve long-axis view demonstrating the dissection entry site (*arrow*).

*Rationale:* The intimal tear in a type A dissection most commonly occurs just above the sinotubular junction (**Figure 73.20**). The best view to evaluate the entry site is midesophageal aortic valve long-axis view. This view is useful in evaluating the aortic valve, aortic root dimensions, and proximal ascending aorta. Color flow Doppler can help to identify aortic regurgitation, flow in the true lumen and/or false lumen, and flow across the intimal tear.

### Selected References

1. David S, Merry AF. *Practical Perioperative Transesophageal Echocardiography*. Saunders/Elsevier; 2003.
2. Hahn R, Abraham T, Adams MS, et al. Guidelines for performing a comprehensive transesophageal echocardiographic examination: recommendations from the American Society of Echocardiography and the Society of Cardiovascular Anesthesiologists. *J Am Soc Echocardiogr*. 2013;26:921-964.

**14.** Correct Answer: **D. Pericardial effusion**

*Rationale:* In this parasternal short-axis view, an echolucent area deep to the left ventricle is visible and is consistent with a pericardial effusion. A pericardial effusion can result from either transudative accumulation across the thin wall of the FL or from a rupture of the dissection into the pericardium (hemopericardium). Aortic regurgitation can occur when the dissection flap involves the aortic root, but is not evident in Figure 73.9. Intramural thrombosis is common within the false lumen from nonlaminar blood flow, but is not apparent in Figure 73.9 of the right and left ventricles. A transudative pericardial effusion is also common with chronic aortic dissection; however, this effusion tracks anterior to the descending aorta, differentiating it from a pleural effusion, which would track distal to the descending aorta. Additionally, the right ventricle appears dilated in this view.

### Selected References

1. Black JH, III, Manning WJ. *Clinical Features and Diagnosis of Acute Aortic Dissection in UptoDate*; August 2019.
2. Rao PK, Quader N. Diseases of the great vessels. In: Quader N, Makan M, Perez P, eds. *The Washington Manual of Echocardiography*. 2nd ed. Wolters Kluwer; 2017:220-241.

**15.** Correct Answer: B. B

*Rationale/Critique:* Traumatic aortic injuries are often associated with deceleration injuries as well as blunt trauma to the chest. While many patients with a significant traumatic aortic injury die before they arrive at the hospital, an aortic injury should be suspected in patients who have a widened mediastinum on their initial chest x-ray. The thoracic aorta is usually not well-visualized with traditional transthoracic views, but the suprasternal view is capable of showing portions of the aortic arch. The most common site of traumatic aortic injury is at the isthmus, distal to the left subclavian take-off, represented by *arrow B* in Figure 73.10. The most common site for an *ascending* aortic dissection is within a few centimeters of the aortic valve, represented by *arrow A. Arrow C* shows the right pulmonary artery.

Selected References
1. Mirvis SE, Bidwell JK, Buddemeyer EU, et al. Value of chest radiography in excluding traumatic aortic rupture. *Radiology*. 1987;163:487-493.
2. Rao PK, Quader N. Diseases of the great vessels. In: Quader N, Makan M, Perez P, eds. *The Washington Manual of Echocardiography*. 2nd ed. Wolters Kluwer; 2017:220-241.
3. Sidebotham D, Merry A, Legget M. *Practical Perioperative Transoesophageal Echocardiography*. Elsevier Limited; 2003.

**16.** Correct Answer: A. An aortic dissection with flow toward the probe in the true lumen

*Rationale:* Aortic dissection can occur following intense physical exertion, and abdominal ultrasound is capable of identifying a dissection in the abdominal aorta, although its sensitivity is low enough that it should not be relied upon as a sole imaging modality if clinical suspicion is high. This longitudinal view shows the true lumen as smaller than the false lumen and demonstrates blood flow toward the probe during systole. In contrast, flow is absent in the larger false lumen. One would expect to see expansion of the TL during systole as well.

Selected References
1. Rao PK, Quader N. Diseases of the great vessels. In: Quader N, Makan M, Perez P, eds. *The Washington Manual of Echocardiography*. 2nd ed. Wolters Kluwer; 2017:220-241.
2. Sidebotham D, Merry A, Legget M. *Practical Perioperative Transoesophageal Echocardiography*. Elsevier Limited; 2003.

**17.** Correct Answer: C. Obtain additional imaging of the aorta

*Rationale:* Although the abdominal aorta is involved, it is not clear as to whether the ascending aorta or aortic root may be involved. Aortic dissection involving the ascending aorta is considered a surgical emergency. Mortality may increase by 1% to 2% *per hour* after symptom onset and until surgical treatment. In contrast, Type B dissections are most commonly treated medically, with a goal of decreasing aortic pressure over time (dP/dt) via anti-impulse therapy. Beta-blockade is the mainstay, with vasodilators added if BP cannot be brought down to a systolic BP of 100 to 120 mm Hg, once the HR has consistently been brought to <60 bpm. Abdominal aortic dissections complicated by signs of malperfusion are candidates for endovascular procedures. Hemodynamically stable patients without a high suspicion of an ascending aortic dissection may be imaged with computed tomography (CT) angiography or magnetic resonance imaging (MRI) angiography. Hemodynamically unstable patients with a high suspicion for type A dissection should be immediately transferred to the operating room where the diagnosis can be confirmed with TEE prior to incision.

Selected References
1. Goldstein SA, Evangelista A, Abbara S, et al. Multimodality imaging of diseases of the thoracic aorta in adults: from the American Society of Echocardiography and the European Association of Cardiovascular Imaging Endorsed by the Society of Cardiovascular Computed Tomography and Society for Cardiovascular Magnetic Resonance. *J Am Soc Echocardiogr*. 2015;28:119-118.
2. Svensson LG, Adams DH, Bonow RO, et al. Aortic valve and ascending aorta guidelines for management and quality. *Ann Thorac Surg*. 2013;95:1-66.
3. Tsai TT, Nienaber CA, Eagle KA. Acute aortic syndromes. *Circulation*. 2005;112:3802-3813.

**18.** Correct Answer: B. The suprasternal view with TTE is able to visualize portions of the ascending aorta not visible on TEE.

*Rationale:* Echocardiography, CT, MRI, and aortography have all been used to diagnose aortic dissection. There has been increasing interest in the use of TTE in the assessment of the patient at risk, particularly in cases of suspected ascending aortic dissections. TTE does not involve ionizing radiation, can be performed at the bedside, requires no sedation, and provides good visualization of the LVOT, aortic root, and initial portions of the ascending aorta. In some individuals, TTE is capable of visualizing the distal ascending aorta, proximal aortic arch, and great vessel branching pattern/involvement. Part of this area is considered the "blind spot" of TEE, where the air from the trachea prevents visualization from the esophagus. Additionally, TTE allows for assessment of aortic regurgitation, regional wall motion abnormalities, LV dysfunction, and pericardial effusions, all important factors when preparing for surgical repair.

Selected References
1. Meredith EL, Masani ND. Echocardiography in the emergency assessment of acute aortic syndromes. *Eur J Echocardiogr.* 2009 Jan;10(1):i31-i39. doi:10.1093/ejechocard/jen251.
2. Sobczyk D, Nycz K. Feasibility and accuracy of bedside transthoracic echocardiography in diagnosis of acute proximal aortic dissection. *Cardiovasc Ultrasound.* 2015;13:15. Published 2015 Mar 25. doi:10.1186/s12947-015-0008-5.

**19.** Correct Answer: D. D

*Rationale:* The patient has an aortic dissection that has compromised perfusion to the left upper and lower extremity as noted by the physical examination findings of BP/pulse differences. In this suprasternal view (Figure 73.12) *A* represents the ascending aorta, *B* the brachiocephalic trunk, *C* the left carotid artery, and *D* the left subclavian artery (LSCA). Since the BP in the right arm is not affected, the dissection is likely originating distal from the brachiocephalic trunk (*B*). Moreover, dissection involving brachiocephalic trunk (*B*) and the left carotid artery (*C*) would likely have a profound neurologic manifestation not mentioned in the question. The diminished perfusion to the left upper and lower extremities points toward LSCA (*D*) as an originating site for the aortic dissection. Alternatively, the LSCA could be involved by the retrograde dissection originating more distally, in the descending thoracic and abdominal aorta, but since the descending thoracic and abdominal aorta are not included in the answers, the most likely site for this pathology is LSCA (D).

Selected References
1. Black JH, III, Manning WJ. *Clinical Features and Diagnosis of Acute Aortic Dissection in UptoDate*; August 2019.
2. Rao PK, Quader N. Diseases of the great vessels. In: Quader N, Makan M, Perez P, eds. *The Washington Manual of Echocardiography*. 2nd ed. Wolters Kluwer; 2017:220-241.

**20.** Correct Answer: D. Presence of a left pleural effusion

*Rationale:* All of the answer choices represent abnormalities found on a POCUS examination. More than three B-lines per sonographic field suggest an interstitial disease process (e.g., pulmonary edema), and fewer than three B-lines is a normal finding. Absence of lung sliding in the nondependent portions of the left lung field suggests either pneumothorax or adhesion of the parietal and visceral pleura, which would not be expected with an aortic dissection. Bowing of the interventricular septum toward the left ventricle would be expected in pathologies that cause overload of the right ventricle (e.g., pulmonary embolism). Transudative pleural effusions occur in 19% of aortic dissections, much more commonly when they are chronic. Other extra-aortic complications of aortic dissection that can be evaluated by ultrasound include aortic regurgitation, pericardial effusion, cardiac wall motion abnormalities, hemoperitoneum, and hypovolemia.

Selected References
1. Black JH, III, Manning WJ. *Clinical Features and Diagnosis of Acute Aortic Dissection in UptoDate*; August 2019.
2. Lee FC. Lung ultrasound-a primary survey of the acutely dyspneic patient. *J Intensive Care.* 2016;4(1):57. doi:10.1186/s40560-016-0180-1.
3. Sidebotham D, Merry A, Legget M. *Practical Perioperative Transoesophageal Echocardiography*. Philadelphia: Elsevier Limited; 2003.

# 74 | INVASIVE LINE PLACEMENT: CENTRAL LINE, ARTERIAL LINE, AND PERIPHERAL IV PLACEMENT

John P. Gaillard, Casey D. Bryant, and Jonathan T. Jaffe

1. An 83-year-old man with chronic obstructive pulmonary disease (COPD) (FEV$_1$ 50% of predicted) presents to the Emergency Department with progressive dyspnea and wheezing. His vital signs are temperature 37.1°C, BP 132/74 mm Hg, HR 94 bpm, respirations 22/min, and SpO$_2$ 92% on 4 L/min O$_2$ via nasal cannula. Due to the inability to place a peripheral IV, you place a central line in the patient's left subclavian vein. A postprocedure chest x-ray shows a pattern consistent with COPD and a small right-sided pleural effusion. The following ultrasound image (**Figure 74.1**) is obtained from the left chest.

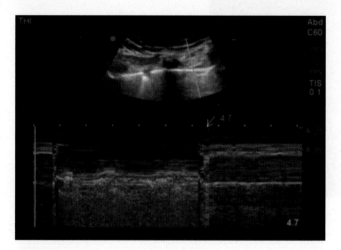

**Figure 74.1**

Based on Figure 74.1, which of the following is indicated?
A. Immediate needle decompression of the left chest
B. Bronchodilators and steroids
C. Left-sided tube thoracostomy
D. Right-sided tube thoracostomy

2. Based on the ultrasound images shown in **Figure 74.2**, which of the following locations is the preferred puncture site for a right femoral arterial line?

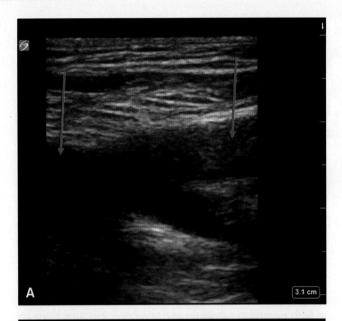

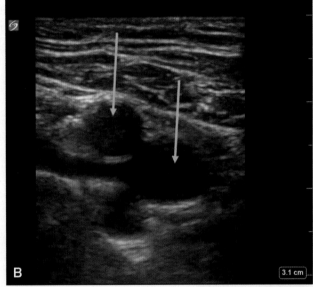

**Figure 74.2**

A. **RED** arrow
B. **PURPLE** arrow
C. **GREEN** arrow
D. **BLUE** arrow

3. Which of the ultrasounds shown in **Figure 74.3** best identifies the internal jugular vein?

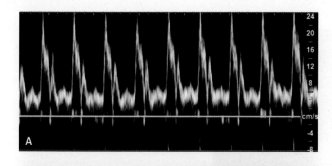

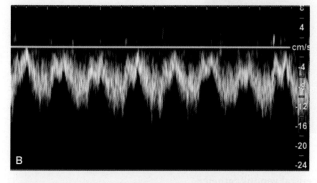

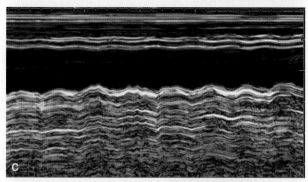

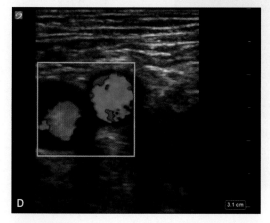

**Figure 74.3**

A. Figure 74.3A
B. Figure 74.3B
C. Figure 74.3C
D. Figure 74.3D

4. Based on **Figure 74.4**, which of the following is the best course of action regarding central venous catheter placement?

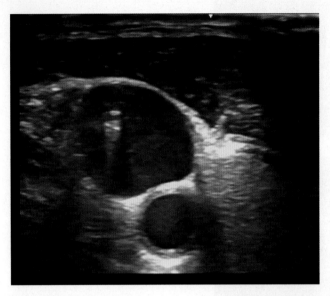

**Figure 74.4**

A. This is an acceptable site to place a central venous catheter.
B. Going proximal to this site is recommended.
C. Going distal to this site is recommended.
D. Finding an alternative vessel is recommended.

5. A nurse asks you for assistance with obtaining peripheral IV access on a patient in the intensive care unit who was admitted with endocarditis associated with intravenous drug abuse. During the course of the procedure, you obtain the ultrasound shown in **Figure 74.5** without getting blood return into the catheter.

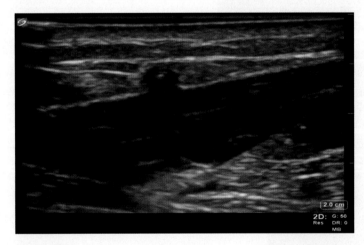

**Figure 74.5**

Which of the following is the next best step?
A. Advance the needle further because it most likely is against the anterior wall of the vein.
B. Advance the catheter off the needle into the vein because the image confirms correct placement.
C. Apply color to the vessel to check for lack of flow because there was no flash despite being in the vein.
D. Obtain a long access view of the needle to identify the tip because you may have gone through the back wall of the vein.

6. You are caring for a 32-year-old woman in septic shock from a urinary source. Despite adequate fluid resuscitation, she remains on vasopressor medications, and you are planning to place an arterial line using ultrasound guidance for hemodynamic monitoring. You obtain **Figure 74.6** during cannulation and have blood return in the catheter device.

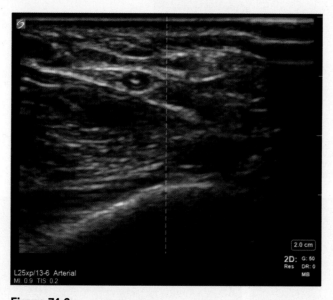

**Figure 74.6**

Which of the following is the *most* correct statement regarding ultrasound guidance for radial artery cannulation versus the palpation technique in adults?
A. Ultrasound guidance requires **more attempts** and takes a **longer amount of time** to achieve successful cannulation.
B. Ultrasound guidance requires **more attempts** but takes a **shorter amount of time** to achieve successful cannulation.
C. Ultrasound guidance requires **fewer attempts** but takes a **longer amount of time** to achieve successful cannulation.
D. Ultrasound guidance requires **fewer attempts** and takes a **shorter amount of time** to achieve successful cannulation.

7. You are preparing to place a radial arterial line and are assessing the vessel for patency and appropriateness. The patient is on venoarterial extracorporeal membrane oxygenation (ECMO) with vasopressor and inotrope support. On vessel assessment, pulsatility is not evident given the patient's current low-flow state. You employ alternative methods for vessel evaluation and you are concerned that the vessel may not be patent due to lack of flow noted on color and pulsed-wave Doppler imaging. **Figure 74.7** shows your current approach and findings.

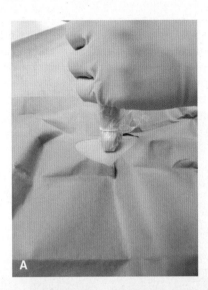

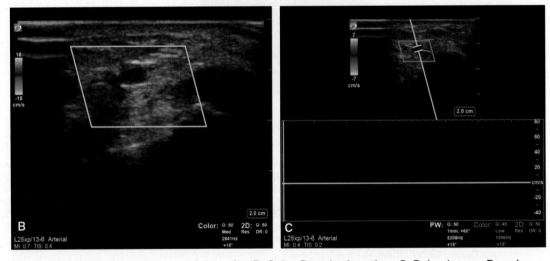

**Figure 74.7** A. Probe position on right wrist. B. Color Doppler imaging. C. Pulsed-wave Doppler imaging.

Which property or principle is contributing the most to the lack of flow noted on ultrasound?
**A.** Doppler shift
**B.** Bernoulli's principle
**C.** Acoustic impedance
**D.** Nyquist limit

# Chapter 74 ▪ Answers

**1.** Correct Answer: **B. Bronchodilators and steroids**

*Rationale:* Figure 74.1 shows a lung point sign: the point at which the lung (visceral pleura) begins to separate from the chest wall (parietal pleura). Initially thought to be pathognomonic for pneumothorax, a lung point sign can also be seen in patients with blebs from COPD or other disease processes in which the lung is adherent to the chest wall (e.g., asbestosis). This is confirmed by the presence of a lung pulse, that is, movement of the heart transmitted to and sensed at the pleural space, which can be seen on the right side of the image. The patient in this question is having a COPD exacerbation, so choice B is correct. Based on the vital signs, the patient is not in extremis, so choice A is incorrect. In a stable patient with COPD, you should obtain further imaging (computed tomography [CT] scan) before placing a chest tube, so choice C is incorrect. A small pleural effusion is not likely to cause significant dyspnea, so choice D is incorrect.

### Selected Reference

1. Aziz SG, Patel BB, Ie SR, Rubio ER. The lung point sign, not pathognomonic of a pneumothorax. *Ultrasound Q*. 2016; 32(3):277-279.

**2.** Correct Answer: **A. RED arrow**

*Rationale:* **Figure 74.8A** shows a longitudinal view of the common femoral artery and its bifurcation into the superficial femoral artery and the deep femoral artery. **Figure 74.8B** shows a transverse view of the superficial femoral artery, the deep femoral artery, and the common femoral vein at the junction with the greater saphenous vein. The ideal location for femoral artery puncture is in the common femoral artery proximal to the bifurcation (choice A). This area is usually above the middle third of the femoral head (not pictured here). Puncture into the superficial femoral artery (choices B and C) increases the likelihood of unsuccessful cannula placement and increases the incidence of retroperitoneal bleeding and pseudoaneurysms. Choice D is the femoral vein. See **Figure 74.8** for additional details.

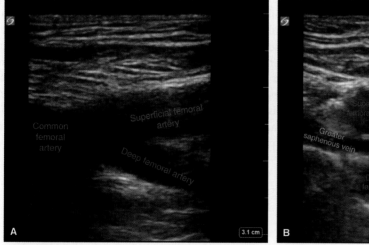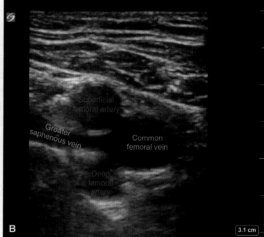

**Figure 74.8**

### Selected Reference

1. Turi ZG. Ending "poke until you get a gusher": part II-the evidence based approach to vascular access revisited. *Catheter Cardiovasc Interv*. 2017;89(7):1185-1192.

**3.** Correct Answer: B. Figure 74.3B

*Rationale:* Figure 74.3B shows pulsed-wave Doppler tracing of a vein, evidenced by the flow away from the probe during systole and diastole at a relatively slow velocity. Figure 74.3A shows pulsed-wave Doppler of an artery, evidenced by flow only during systole at a relatively faster velocity. Figure 74.3C shows M-mode without a corresponding B-mode image. M-mode alone is not used to identify a specific vessel. Since there is no B-mode image with the M-mode tracing, it would be difficult to differentiate an artery from a vein. Figure 74.3D shows color Doppler with flow going away and coming toward the probe. Based on this limited information, it would be difficult to differentiate the artery from the vein, although real-time visualization may help identify the appropriate vessel.

### Selected Reference

1. Troianos CA, Hartman GS, Glas KE, et al. Guidelines for performing ultrasound guided vascular cannulation: recommendations of the American Society of Echocardiography and the Society of Cardiovascular Anesthesiologists. *J Am Soc Echocardiogr.* 2011;24:1291-1318.

**4.** Correct Answer: D. Finding an alternative vessel is recommended.

*Rationale:* Figure 74.4 shows a thrombus within the internal jugular vein. Whenever a thrombus is visualized on ultrasound, it is recommended to find an alternative vessel for central line placement, so choice D is correct. Central line placement in this vessel would increase the risk of dislodging part or all of the thrombus, leading to a pulmonary embolism.

### Selected References

1. Saugel B, Scheeren TWL, Teboul JL. Ultrasound-guided central venous catheter placement: a structured review and recommendations for clinical practice. *Crit Care.* 2017;21(1):225.
2. Silverberg MJ, Kory P. Intensive care ultrasound: II. Central vascular access and venous diagnostic ultrasound. *Ann Am Thorac Soc.* 2013;10(5):549-556.

**5.** Correct Answer: D. Obtain a long access view of the needle to identify the tip because you may have gone through the back wall of the vein.

*Rationale:* The next step in this scenario is to verify the needle tip. There are several ways to confirm whether you are in the vessel with your needle or catheter. This can be accomplished by scanning in a proximal to distal motion while remaining in transverse orientation or by switching to a longitudinal view (choice D is correct). Ideally, the tip should be followed throughout the procedure, although it is not uncommon to lose or misidentify it, often resulting in overly deep placement of the needle. This tends to occur more frequently when using the transverse approach; however, this method is performed more rapidly and with more success than the long-axis technique. It is important to remember that the image on the screen is simply a cross section and can represent any location along the length of the needle. Clearly, a portion of the needle is within the vessel in this image, but it is impossible to know from Figure 74.5 alone where the tip is located (choices A and B are incorrect, see **Figure 74.9**). Although color Doppler can help look for flow, it will not help confirm correct placement of the needle (choice C is incorrect).

Longitudinal view
of needle and vein

Transverse view of
needle and vein

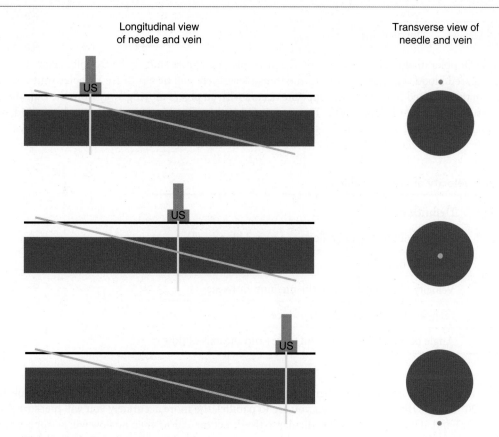

**Figure 74.9** Comparison of short-axis and long-axis views.

Selected References
1. Joing S, Strote S, Caroon L, et al. Videos in clinical medicine. Ultrasound-guided peripheral i.v. placement. *N Engl J Med.* 2012;366(25):e38.
2. Mahler SA, Wang H, Lester C, Skinner J, Arnold TC, Conrad SA. Short- vs long-axis approach to ultrasound-guided peripheral intravenous access: a prospective randomized study. *Am J Emerg Med.* 2011;29(9):1194-1197.

**6.** Correct Answer: D. Ultrasound guidance requires **fewer attempts** and takes a **shorter amount** of time to achieve successful cannulation.

*Rationale:* The ability to obtain radial artery access for hemodynamic or blood gas monitoring is a critical skill when caring for sick patients. Factors increasing difficulty of access include obesity, edema, vessel scarring, atherosclerosis, hypotension, and vasopressor use. Each attempt increases the chance of hematoma formation and vessel spasm, which increases the difficulty of subsequent attempts. In their systematic review and meta-analysis of randomized controlled trials (RCTs), Shiloh, et al. showed a 71% improvement in the likelihood of first-pass success rates when ultrasound guidance was utilized in comparison to the palpation technique. Another high-quality systematic review by White, et al. showed improved first-pass success rates, reduction in overall time to cannulation, and reduction in the number of attempts when ultrasound guidance is used for cannulation of the radial artery in both adults and pediatric patients.

Selected References
1. Shiloh AL, Savel RH, Paulin LM, Eisen LA. Ultrasound-guided catheterization of the radial artery: a systematic review and *meta-analysis* of randomized controlled trials. *Chest.* 2011;139(3):524-529.
2. Shiver S, Blaivas M, Lyon M. A prospective comparison of ultrasound-guided and blindly placed radial arterial catheters. *Acad Emerg Med.* 2006;13(12):1275-1279.
3. White L, Halpin A, Turner M, Wallace L. Ultrasound-guided radial artery cannulation in adult and paediatric populations: a systematic review and meta-analysis. *Br J Anaesth.* 2016;116(5):610-617.

**7.** Correct Answer: A. Doppler shift

*Rationale:* Doppler imaging is dependent on the principle of Doppler shift or the Doppler effect. For any object (e.g., red blood cell) moving toward the transducer, there will be a positive Doppler shift with an increase in the reflected frequency. The opposite occurs with an object moving away from the transducer, with a resultant negative Doppler shift. The magnitude of the effect is relative to the angle of incidence $[f_d = (f_t \times 2u \times \cos\theta)/c]$. In order to determine the velocity of flow of a particular area, it can be rewritten as $[u = (f_d \times c)/(f_t \times 2\cos\theta)]$. The variables are defined in **Table 74.1**:

**Table 74.1 Velocity of Flow Variables**

| Variable | Definition |
| --- | --- |
| $u$ | Velocity of the moving reflector (e.g., red blood cell) |
| $f_d$ | Received frequency |
| $c$ | Velocity of sound waves in the medium or tissue |
| $f_t$ | Frequency emitted by the transducer |
| $\theta$ | Angle between the ultrasound waves and the axis of flow |

The angle of insonation is important when assessing flow with Doppler as the cosine of 0° is one, while the cosine of 90° is zero. Therefore, the closer you are to parallel, the more accurately you will measure flow. On the other hand, if you insonate perpendicular to the direction of flow, then no flow will be appreciated. In this example, the initial images were obtained using a perpendicular orientation to the radial artery in a critically ill patient with a low-flow state. The ultrasound probe was then angled a slight amount to bring the ultrasound waves more in line with the direction of flow.

The Bernoulli principle is built upon the principle of conservation of energy and refers to the inverse relationship of pressure and flow velocities.

Acoustic impedance in human ultrasound is a physical property relating to the resistance of the medium (tissue, fluid, etc.) through which the sound waves are traveling.

The Nyquist limit represents the minimal sampling rate that must be used to prevent aliasing and is equal to one-half of the pulse repetition frequency.

Knowing the principles of the Doppler effect, you make the following adjustment and obtain **Figure 74.10**.

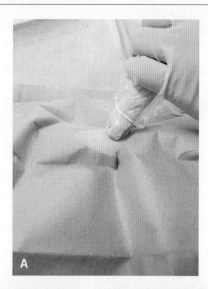

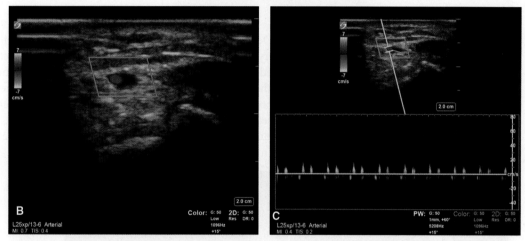

**Figure 74.10** A. Adjusted probe position relative to radial artery flow. B. Color wave Doppler imaging with flow demonstrated. C. Color and pulsed-wave Doppler imaging demonstrating pulsatile flow.

### Selected References

1. Kremkau FW. Physics and instrumentation. In: Lang R, Goldstein S, Kronzon I, Khandheria B, Mor-Avi V, eds. *ASE's Comprehensive Echocardiography*. Elsevier, Inc.; 2016:1-18.
2. Kremkau FW, Badano LP, Muraru D. Physics and instrumentation. In: Lang R, Goldstein S, Kronzon I, Khandheria B, Mor-Avi V, eds. *ASE's Comprehensive Echocardiography*. Elsevier, Inc.; 2016:1-18.
3. Merritt CRB. Physics of ultrasound. In: Rumack C, Levine D, eds. *Diagnostic ultrasound*. 5th ed. Elsevier, Inc.; 2018:1-33.

### Acknowledgment

The authors gratefully acknowledge Drs. Braghadheeswar Thyagarajan and Shelby Harris for their assistance with acquiring photos for Question 74.7.

# 75 | THORACENTESIS AND CHEST TUBE PLACEMENT

Casey D. Bryant, John P. Gaillard, and Jonathan T. Jaffe

1. A 45-year-old man presents to the Emergency Department with shortness of breath and chest pain. His past medical history includes coronary artery disease with stenting 3 years ago, ongoing tobacco smoking, and type 2 diabetes mellitus, controlled with oral medications. The shortness of breath and chest pain began 2 hours prior to arrival while the patient was coughing. The patient arrives dyspneic, tachypneic, and is using accessory muscles for breathing. Lung auscultation is diminished on the left without wheezes or rhonchi. Vital signs on presentation include temperature 37.2°C, HR 135 bpm, BP 100/60 mm Hg, RR 32/min, and SpO$_2$ 93% on a non-rebreather mask at 15 L/min. You evaluate the patient with point-of-care ultrasound and obtain **Figure 75.1.**

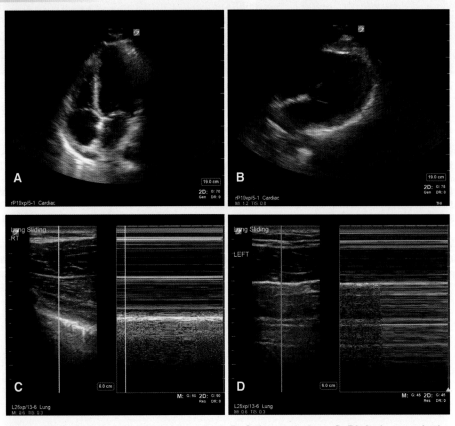

**Figure 75.1** A. Apical four-chamber view. B. Subcostal view. C. Right lung apical. D. Left lung apical.

What would be the *most* appropriate next step?
A. Pericardiocentesis
B. Chest tube placement
C. Fluid resuscitation, cultures, and antibiotics
D. Endotracheal intubation

2. On postoperative day 4 after coronary artery bypass grafting (CABG) surgery, a 54-year-old man is noted to have a new left-sided pleural effusion without evidence of interstitial or alveolar edema on chest x-ray obtained for an increased oxygen requirement. The chest drain placed in surgery was removed the day prior for minimal serosanguinous output, and there is no evidence of pleural effusion on the most recent chest x-ray 8 hours earlier. You are planning for drainage of the effusion via thoracentesis using point-of-care ultrasound (POCUS) guidance and obtain **Figure 75.2**.

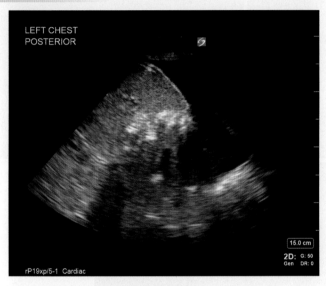

**Figure 75.2** Left posterior thorax.

What would be the most appropriate next step?
A. Perform drainage at this site
B. Obtain a computed tomography (CT) scan to evaluate further
C. Evaluate the effusion at other intercostal spaces
D. Defer drainage in favor of diuresis

3. You are caring for a 72-year-old woman in the intensive care unit (ICU) after a surgical mitral valve replacement, two-vessel coronary arterial bypass graft (CABG), maze procedure, and left atrial appendage excision. Her postoperative course has been complicated by copious respiratory secretions, renal failure, and sepsis. She remains intubated. On chest x-ray obtained this morning, her right thorax has a large opacification. Lung markings are difficult to discern in the lower thorax, and the mediastinum appears appropriately positioned. You decide to investigate her right thorax further with point-of-care ultrasound (**Figure 75.3**).

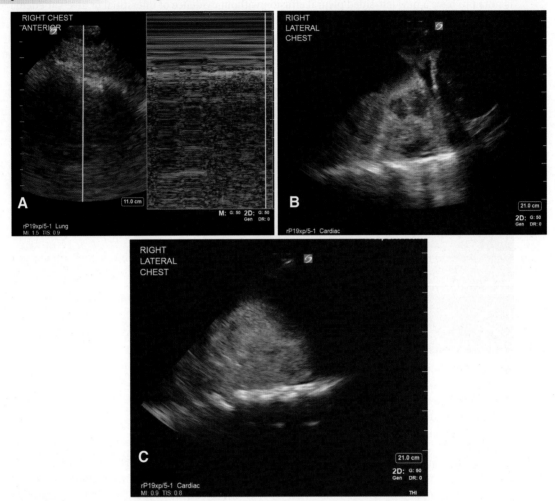

**Figure 75.3** A. Right thorax anterior chest wall. B. Right thorax at the level of the diaphragm. C. Right thorax above the diaphragm.

What would be the most appropriate next step?
A. Send the patient for a CT chest with intravenous contrast to obtain more information
B. Aggressive chest physiotherapy followed by bronchoscopy if no improvement
C. Start inhaled bronchodilators and steroids
D. Perform tube thoracostomy

# Chapter 75 ▪ Answers

**1.** Correct Answer: B. Chest tube placement

*Rationale:* The ultrasound images (Figure 75.1) of the left chest demonstrate a finding known as the lung point sign. The lung point sign is the location where the visceral and parietal pleura separate due to a pneumothorax. This finding is dynamic during the respiratory cycle, as demonstrated by **Figure 75.4** and ▶ **Video 75.1.**

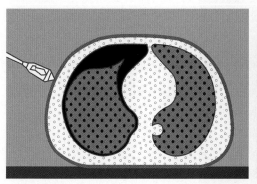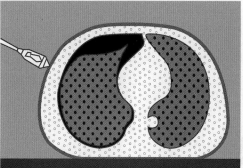

**Figure 75.4** Theoretical explanation of the lung point. Left, at expiration, the pneumothorax has a defined volume. A probe placed at a point slightly anterior to the lung level will display a pneumothorax pattern. Right, at inspiration, we must imagine that the lung volume slightly increases, therefore increasing the surface of the lung in contact with the wall. The probe remaining at the same location will immediately display fleeting lung patterns.

Although it is not found in all patients with pneumothorax, the lung point sign has a specificity approaching 100% when it is identified. Sensitivity has been reported to range from 66% to 92%. Another lung ultrasound finding that is less specific for pneumothorax includes a lack of lung sliding, which can be shown in a number of pathologies including atelectasis, pulmonary contusions, acute respiratory distress syndrome (ARDS), and pleural adhesions. This patient is presenting with a clinical syndrome consistent with pneumothorax, and rapidly deployed POCUS can be used to further confirm the diagnosis. In a stable patient, in whom there remains diagnostic uncertainty, additional imaging studies (e.g., chest x-ray or CT) may be considered.

With a clear diagnosis and a patient in extremis, proceeding directly to placement of a chest tube to relieve the pneumothorax would be appropriate. The images of the heart do not demonstrate any evidence of a pericardial effusion. There was no clear evidence presented in the question stem to suggest this is an infectious process. Intubation can likely be avoided with definitive management of the pneumothorax. Additionally, intubation and positive pressure ventilation will likely worsen the pneumothorax, leading to worsening tension physiology.

Selected References
1. Aziz SG, Patel BB, Ie SR, Rubio ER. The lung point sign, not pathognomonic of a pneumothorax. *Ultrasound Q.* 2016 Sep;32(3):277-279.
2. Lichtenstein D, Mezière G, Biderman P, Gepner, A. The "lung point": an ultrasound sign specific to pneumothorax. *Intensive Care Med.* 2000;26:1434-1440.
3. Lichtenstein DA, Mezière G, Lascols N, et al. Ultrasound diagnosis of occult pneumothorax. *Crit Care Med.* 2005;33:1231-1238.
4. Soldati G, Testa A, Sher S, Pignataro G, La Sala M, Silveri NG. Occult traumatic pneumothorax: diagnostic accuracy of lung ultrasonography in the emergency department. *Chest.* 2008;133:204-211.
5. Volpicelli G. Sonographic diagnosis of pneumothorax. *Intensive Care Med.* 2011;37:224-232.

**2.** Correct Answer: C. Evaluate the effusion at other intercostal spaces

*Rationale:* The pleural effusion shown is simple in appearance (hypoechoic) and appropriate for bedside drainage, with or without leaving a chest tube in place, but the intercostal space shown in Figure 75.2 would put the patient at risk for diaphragm and/or spleen puncture. The proceduralist should continue evaluating the effusion in different intercostal spaces to identify a more appropriate drainage site. Upon further investigation with the ultrasound, successful drainage was performed at the site shown in **Figure 75.5**.

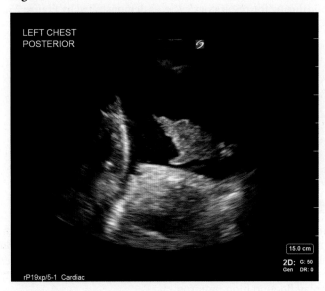

**Figure 75.5** Left posterior thorax.

A CT scan is not necessary in this situation, as the diagnosis is clear. Given the large appearance of the effusion, drainage is preferred over diuresis. Thoracentesis with ultrasound guidance (either dynamic or static performed immediately beforehand) has been shown to be a safer procedure with less complications in comparison to marking of the spot with drainage at a later time and drainage based on physical examination.

The American College of Emergency Physicians, the British Thoracic Society, the Society of Critical Care Medicine, the Society of Hospital Medicine, and the American College of Chest Physicians all recommend using ultrasound guidance for thoracentesis.

Selected References
1. Feller-Kopman D. Ultrasound-guided thoracentesis. *Chest.* 2006 Jun;129(6):1709-1714.
2. Dancel R, Schnobrich D, Puri N, et al.; Society of Hospital Medicine Point of Care Ultrasound Task Force, Soni NJ. Recommendations on the use of ultrasound guidance for adult thoracentesis: a position statement of the Society of Hospital Medicine. *J Hosp Med.* 2018 Feb;13(2):126-135.
3. Havelock T, Teoh R, Laws D, Gleeson F. BTS Pleural Disease Guideline Group. Pleural procedures and thoracic ultrasound: British Thoracic Society pleural disease guideline 2010. *Thorax.* 2010;65(suppl 2):ii61-ii76.

**3.** Correct Answer: D. Perform tube thoracostomy

*Rationale:* Anterior thorax imaging demonstrates normal-appearing M-mode confirming the presence of lung sliding, which argues against large volume atelectasis. Figure 75.3 obtained in the right lower thorax at the level of the diaphragm demonstrates a finding known as the "thoracic spine sign." This finding has been shown in a prospective trial to be highly specific (92.9%, 95% confidence interval [CI] 81.9%-97.7%) for clinically significant pleural effusions that were concomitantly noted on CT imaging. The sensitivity was 73.7% (95% CI 48.6%-89.9%), but this improved to 92.9% (95% CI 64.2%-99.6%) once trace effusions were excluded from the data set.

The heterogeneous appearance of the effusion in this clinical scenario presented suggests hemothorax, and additional imaging with CT is not necessary. It is appropriate to proceed directly to tube thoracostomy for drainage of suspected hemothorax. Upon placement, 1400 mL of dark venous-appearing blood was removed from the pleural space with an improvement in the patient's $FiO_2$ requirement. Chest physiotherapy and bronchoscopy may be appropriate if there is evidence of mucus plugging, but the normal lung sliding observed argues against that. There are no clinical indicators of bronchospasm to suggest that bronchodilators or steroids would be useful in this situation.

## Selected Reference

1. Dickman E, Terentiev V, Likourezos A, Derman A, Haines L. Extension of the thoracic spine sign: a new sonographic marker of pleural effusion. *J Ultrasound Med.* 2015 Sep;34(9):1555-1561.

Jonathan T. Jaffe, Casey D. Bryant, and John P. Gaillard

1. A 56-year-old man with a history of peptic ulcer disease and cirrhosis is admitted to the Emergency Department for abdominal pain. His vital signs are temperature 38.2°C, HR 114 bpm, BP 97/54 mm Hg, RR 22/min, and SpO$_2$ 93% on 2 L nasal cannula. He is in mild distress with clear lungs and a distended abdomen that is diffusely tender to palpation. He is given a 30 mL/kg bolus of lactated Ringer's solution and started on broad-spectrum antibiotics, with a plan to perform a diagnostic paracentesis. During the preparation for the procedure, **Figure 76.1** is obtained from the left lower quadrant.

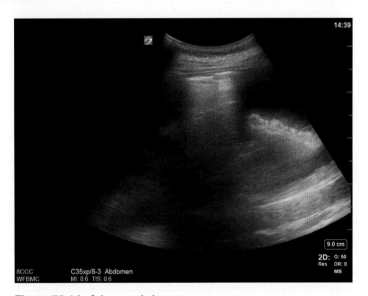

**Figure 76.1** Left lower abdomen.

What is the *most appropriate* next step in his management?
A. Proceed with paracentesis
B. Surgical consultation
C. Evaluate other sites for paracentesis
D. Computed tomography (CT) abdomen/pelvis

2. A 62-year-old woman with a history of alcoholic cirrhosis presents to the Emergency Department with abdominal distension and fever. Her vital signs show a temperature of 38.5°C, HR 110 bpm, BP 97/54 mm Hg, RR 20/min, and SpO$_2$ 95% on 2 L nasal cannula. Her abdomen is tense and diffusely tender, prompting a clinical concern for spontaneous bacterial peritonitis. During preparation for a diagnostic paracentesis, **Figure 76.2** is obtained.

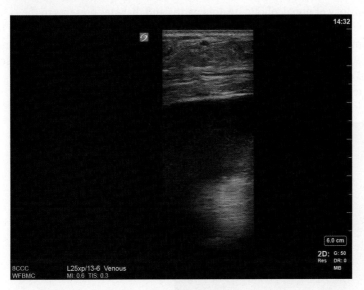

**Figure 76.2** Right lower abdomen.

What is the next best step in her management?
A. Evaluate different sites for paracentesis.
B. Proceed with paracentesis at this location.
C. Evaluate with color flow Doppler.
D. Refer procedure to Interventional Radiology.

3. A 55-year-old man with a history of hepatitis C is admitted to the hospital for shortness of breath and abdominal distension. His is nontoxic appearing and states that his symptoms are similar to the symptoms he had 2 weeks ago when a paracentesis was performed to remove 5 L of ascites. Prior to the procedure, **Figure 76.3** is obtained.

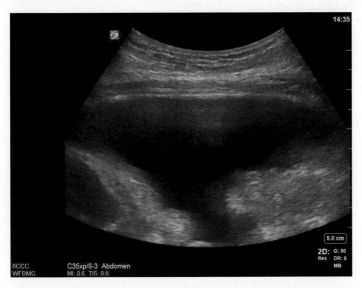

**Figure 76.3** Lower middle abdomen.

What is the *most appropriate* next course of action?
A. Switch to high-frequency linear probe and apply color Doppler.
B. Mark site and perform paracentesis as planned.
C. Use sterile probe cover and perform procedure under real-time guidance.
D. Increase depth to see entirety of pocket.

4. A 44-year-old woman with a history of nonalcoholic steatohepatitis and diabetes presents to the Emergency Department with fever, abdominal pain, and vomiting. She is writhing on the stretcher in pain. Her vital signs show a temperature of 37.9°C, HR 127 bpm, BP 110/62 mm Hg, RR 20/min, and SpO$_2$ 96% on room air. She has mild jaundice and her abdomen has a positive fluid wave. An ultrasound image is obtained (**Figure 76.4**), the site is marked, and she is prepped and draped for a diagnostic paracentesis while she continues to writhe in pain.

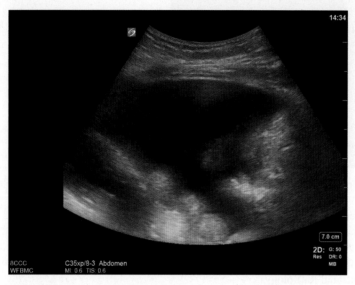

**Figure 76.4** Left lower abdomen.

What is the best course of action?
A. Provide local anesthetic and proceed with paracentesis.
B. Refer procedure to Interventional Radiology.
C. Provide adequate analgesia and perform the procedure under real-time ultrasound guidance.
D. Find a different pocket of fluid to minimize complication risk.

# Chapter 76 ▪ Answers

---

**1.** Correct Answer: B. Surgical consultation

*Rationale:* Figure 76.1 shows an abdomen with free air and ascites. Although the patient is at risk for spontaneous bacterial peritonitis, this presentation is much more concerning for perforated viscus and emergent surgical consultation is most appropriate (Choice B is correct). Although the diagnosis of perforated viscus is not commonly made with ultrasound, it is important to recognize air when it is seen. It most often appears as an echogenic stripe representing the peritoneum associated with deep artifactual reverberation echoes with a comet tail appearance. Detection can be operator-dependent and certain patient maneuvers and positions, such as deep breathing and left lateral decubitus position, can be helpful. One study found the sensitivity of ultrasound for free air in acute abdominal pain patients to be 85% and the specificity to be 100%, making it a valuable diagnostic tool. With this finding, paracentesis should not be performed (Choices A and C are incorrect). Although a CT scan would be helpful in confirming the presence of intraperitoneal air and may be able to identify the source of the injury, the decision to perform more diagnostic testing should occur after surgical consultation in an acutely ill patient with generalized peritonitis, as delays in surgery may be associated with worse survival (Choice D is incorrect).

### Selected References
1. Bohnen J, Boulanger M, Meakins JL, McLean APH. Prognosis in generalized peritonitis: relation to cause and risk factors. *Arch Surg.* 1983;118(3):285-290. doi:10.1001/archsurg.1983.01390030017003.
2. Hefny AF, Abu-Zidan FM. Sonographic diagnosis of intraperitoneal free air. *J Emerg Trauma Shock.* 2011;4:511-513. doi:10.4103/0974-2700.86649.
3. Moriwaki Y, Sugiyama M, Toyoda H, et al. Ultrasonography for the diagnosis of intraperitoneal free air in chest-abdominal-pelvic blunt trauma and critical acute abdominal pain. *Arch Surg.* 2009;144(2):137-141. doi:10.1001/archsurg.2008.553.

---

**2.** Correct Answer: A. Evaluate different sites for paracentesis

*Rationale:* Figure 76.2 shows a vessel above the large pocket of ascites. Although placing color on Figure 76.2 could confirm this, it is not necessary (Choice C is incorrect). It is likely that moving your probe a few centimeters would avoid the vessel and the procedure could be performed safely at the bedside (Choice A is correct; Choice D is incorrect). Generally, paracentesis is performed with a low-frequency curvilinear probe, but it is reasonable to use a high-frequency linear probe to help identify superficial vasculature, which could contribute to additional bleeding from the procedure. Blind techniques for paracentesis utilize either the infraumbilical midline or the lower quadrants superior and medial to the anterior superior iliac spine to avoid the inferior epigastric vessels. Ultrasound allows entry sites at other parts of the abdominal wall, provided that vessels are actively avoided. This vessel could easily be punctured with a paracentesis attempt, inadvertently leading to the creation of an abdominal wall hematoma (Choice B is incorrect).

### Selected References
1. Ennis J, Schultz G, Perera P, Williams S, Gharahbaghian L, Mandavia D. Ultrasound for detection of ascites and for guidance of the paracentesis procedure: technique and review of the literature. *Int J Clin Med.* 2014;05(20):1277-1293. doi:10.4236/ijcm.2014.520163.
2. Nicolaou S, Talsky A, Khashoggi K, Venu V. Ultrasound-guided interventional radiology in critical care. *Crit Care Med.* 2007;35(5 suppl.). doi:10.1097/01.CCM.0000260630.68855.DF.
3. Runyon MS, Marx JA. Peritoneal procedures. In: Roberts JR, Custalow CB, Thomsen TW, Hedges JR, eds. *Roberts & Hedges' Clinical Procedures in Emergency Medicine.* 6th ed. Elsevier/Saunders; 2014:852-872.

---

**3.** Correct Answer: D. Increase depth to see entirety of pocket

*Rationale:* Although Figure 76.3 appears to show an adequate pocket for performing paracentesis, it is important to optimize the image prior to performing the procedure. With a depth of only 5 cm, it is impossible to fully characterize the deeper structures. The depth should be increased at the minimum to see the bottom of the pocket and identify what is immediately deep to the fluid. Ideally, the entire abdominal contents should be visualized with a starting depth ranging from 12 to 25 cm depending on the patient (Choice D is correct). Looking for blood vessels with the high-frequency linear probe is a good consideration and a reasonable decision, but should be performed after optimizing the image (Choice A is incorrect). The pocket appears large, but this is misleading by the shallow depth. One study showed that 1 cm of fluid between the most superficial bowel loop and the peritoneum correlates with 1 L of ascitic fluid; however, the average depth in that study was 5 cm with no measurements <1.5 cm. Figure 76.3 may represent an adequate location to perform the procedure, but the image should be improved, and other sites scanned prior to deciding on inserting the needle here (Choice B is incorrect). It is often provider preference whether to perform the procedure using ultrasound guidance. It would be a reasonable choice in this case if this shallow pocket is the best available entry site, but this decision should be made after obtaining the best possible images (Choice C is incorrect).

### Selected References

1. Ennis J, Schultz G, Perera P, Williams S, Gharahbaghian L, Mandavia D. Ultrasound for detection of ascites and for guidance of the paracentesis procedure: technique and review of the literature. *Int J Clin Med.* 2014;05(20):1277-1293. doi:10.4236/ijcm.2014.520163.
2. Irshad A, Ackerman SJ, Anis M, Campbell AS, Hashmi A, Baker NL. Can the smallest depth of ascitic fluid on sonograms predict the amount of drainable fluid? *J Clin Ultrasound.* 2009;37(8):440-444. doi:10.1002/jcu.20616.
3. Millington SJ, Koenig S. Better with ultrasound: paracentesis. *Chest.* 2018;154(1):177-184. doi:10.1016/j.chest.2018.03.034.
4. Nicolaou S, Talsky A, Khashoggi K, Venu V. Ultrasound-guided interventional radiology in critical care. *Crit Care Med.* 2007;35(5 suppl.). doi:10.1097/01.CCM.0000260630.68855.DF.
5. Runyon MS, Marx JA. Peritoneal procedures. In: Roberts JR, Custalow CB, Thomsen TW, Hedges JR, eds. *Roberts & Hedges' Clinical Procedures in Emergency Medicine.* 6th ed. Elsevier/Saunders; 2014:852-872.

**4.** Correct Answer: C. Provide adequate analgesia and perform the procedure under real-time ultrasound guidance

*Rationale:* Figure 76.4 obtained shows an adequate pocket of fluid that could be used to perform a paracentesis (Choice D is incorrect). However, it is important that the patient remain still after a site is located with ultrasound and marked. In this scenario, in which the patient is writhing in the bed, it is possible that the fluid pocket could have shifted and the previously marked location is no longer the ideal site of entry (Choice A is incorrect). Options are to recheck with a sterile probe cover and mark the site again or to use a sterile probe cover and perform the procedure under real-time ultrasound guidance (Choice C is correct). Since an adequate pocket was seen before the patient was moving, it is reasonable to assume that one will still be present for subsequent attempts at the bedside without having to send her to Interventional Radiology (Choice B is incorrect).

### Selected References

1. Ennis J, Schultz G, Perera P, Williams S, Gharahbaghian L, Mandavia D. Ultrasound for detection of ascites and for guidance of the paracentesis procedure: technique and review of the literature. Int J Clin Med. 2014;05(20):1277-1293. doi:10.4236/ijcm.2014.520163.
2. Millington SJ, Koenig S. Better with ultrasound: paracentesis. *Chest.* 2018;154(1):177-184. doi:10.1016/j.chest.2018.03.034.
3. Runyon MS, Marx JA. Peritoneal procedures. In: Roberts JR, Custalow CB, Thomsen TW, Hedges JR, eds. *Roberts & Hedges' Clinical Procedures in Emergency Medicine.* 6th ed. Elsevier/Saunders; 2014:852-872.

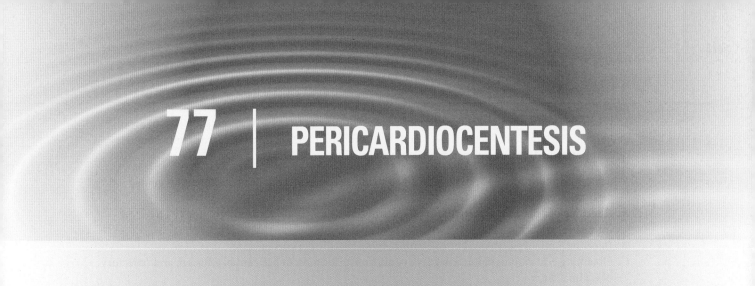

# 77 | PERICARDIOCENTESIS

Rachel C. Frank and Dusan Hanidziar

1. A 39-year-old woman presents to the Emergency Department 12 hours after the onset of rhinorrhea, nasal congestion, and cough. She reports pleuritic chest pain, shortness of breath, and light-headedness. Her electrocardiogram (ECG) reveals sinus tachycardia with low voltage and electrical alternans. Her HR is 124 bpm, and BP is 88/66 mm Hg, with pulsus paradoxus of 15 mm Hg.

A still image from her echocardiogram is shown in **Figure 77.1.**

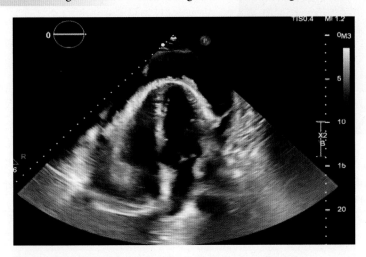

**Figure 77.1** Apical four-chamber view during diastole.

Which of the following pericardial effusions can be *most* safely drained via pericardiocentesis?
**A.** Effusion due to pericarditis measuring 22 mm in diastole adjacent to the right ventricular free wall
**B.** Effusion due to aortic dissection or myocardial rupture
**C.** Effusion in a patient with severe pulmonary hypertension
**D.** Organized pericardial hematoma

2. A 74-year-old man is admitted to the post-anesthesia care unit (PACU) following placement of a permanent pacemaker. His medical history includes sinus node dysfunction, hypertension, diabetes, and chronic kidney disease requiring hemodialysis. Four hours later, he develops shortness of breath, and his vital signs are notable for a HR of 125 bpm and a BP of 82/68 mm Hg. Cardiac ultrasound is quickly performed, and a large pericardial effusion is visualized.

Which of the following steps can be performed to increase the safety of echocardiography-guided pericardiocentesis?
A. Checking platelet count, partial thromboplastin time (PTT) and prothrombin time (PT)/ international normalized ratio (INR)
B. Injecting 5 mL of agitated saline to confirm entry into the pericardial space
C. Obtaining echocardiographic images to confirm size, location of pericardial effusion, and trajectory of optimal entry
D. All of the above

3. A 62-year-old man is admitted to the intensive care unit (ICU) with shock. His ECG reveals sinus tachycardia with low voltage and electrical alternans. His vital signs are significant for HR 101 bpm, BP 84/66 mm Hg, with pulsus paradoxus of 14 mm Hg, respiratory rate 25/min. His echocardiogram is shown in **Figure 77.2**.

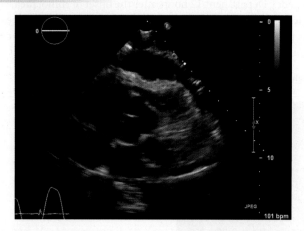

**Figure 77.2** Right ventricular outflow tract collapse during diastole.

The patient is diagnosed with cardiac tamponade. The decision is made to perform emergent pericardiocentesis. What is the optimal position to enter the pericardial space?
A. Subcostal
B. Parasternal
C. Apical
D. Echocardiography-guided to find the area of the largest effusion with no vital organs in the anticipated path of entry

# Chapter 77 ▪ Answers

1. Correct Answer: A. Effusion due to pericarditis measuring 22 mm in diastole adjacent to the right ventricular free wall

*Rationale:* An effusion measuring 22 mm in diastole is large, and it would be safe to perform echocardiography-guided pericardiocentesis. Effusions that are the result of aortic dissection or myocardial rupture are a surgical emergency. In these cases, pericardiocentesis may delay definitive surgical intervention or exacerbate bleeding. In severe pulmonary hypertension (right ventricular systolic pressure > 70 mm Hg), the right ventricular free wall may be splinted by the effusion and rapid draining of the effusion may result in worsening tricuspid regurgitation and right ventricular failure. However, the benefits of pericardiocentesis for a patient with tamponade (even when concomitant pulmonary hypertension is present) outweigh the risks of worsening right ventricular function. Nevertheless, caution should be taken to ensure that the effusion is not drained completely. Organized pericardial hematomas (particularly those following cardiac surgery) may not be easily drained by pericardiocentesis. These effusions are optimally managed with surgical intervention.

### Selected Reference

1. De Carlini CC, Maggiolini S. Pericardiocentesis in cardiac tamponade: indications and practical aspects. *E-Journal Cardiol Pract.* 2017;15(19). Available online https://www.escardio.org/Journals/E-Journal-of-Cardiology-Practice/Volume-15/ Pericardiocentesis-in-cardiac-tamponade-indications-and-practical-aspects.

---

**2.** Correct Answer: **D. All of the above**

*Rationale:* Echocardiography-guided pericardiocentesis can increase the safety of emergency pericardiocentesis. This includes obtaining images in different planes to identify the largest effusion diameter in a location amenable to drainage. Additional steps can be taken by the medical team to increase the safety of the procedure. Optimally, in patients undergoing this procedure, identification and reversal of coagulopathy would take place prior to intervention, provided that the patient is stable enough to wait for laboratory data to return. In nonemergent procedures, cross-matched packed red blood cells should also be available in case of a bleeding complication. Once the pericardial fluid has been aspirated and the needle removed, injecting 5 mL of agitated saline through the sheath into the pericardial space confirms entry into the pericardial space. This is an important safety check prior to dilation. Bubbles should be seen in the pericardial space and not in the ventricles or atria of the heart.

### Selected References

1. Adler Y, Charron P, Imazio M, et al. 2015 ESC Guidelines for the diagnosis and management of pericardial diseases: The Task Force for the Diagnosis and Management of Pericardial Diseases of the European Society of Cardiology (ESC) Endorsed by: The European Association for Cardio-Thoracic Surgery (EACTS). *Eur Heart J.* 2015;36(42):2921-2964.
2. De Carlini CC, Maggiolini S. Pericardiocentesis in cardiac tamponade: indications and practical aspects. *E-Journal Cardiol Pract.* 2017;15(19). Available online https://www.escardio.org/Journals/E-Journal-of-Cardiology-Practice/Volume-15/ Pericardiocentesis-in-cardiac-tamponade-indications-and-practical-aspects.

---

**3.** Correct Answer: **D. Echocardiography-guided to find the area of the largest effusion with no vital organs in the anticipated path of entry**

*Rationale:* Although the subxiphoid approach has been utilized historically, complication rates may be lower if the site is selected based on echocardiography to identify the area with the largest amount of pericardial fluid and reduce the potential for organ injury. The apical approach utilizes a trajectory in the fifth to seventh intercostal space, approximately 1 to 2 cm lateral to the apical impulse. This approach risks accidental left ventricular puncture; however, the thicker left ventricle is more likely to seal following iatrogenic puncture compared to the thin-walled right ventricle. The left lung is at risk for pneumothorax due to the trajectory of the approach.

The subxiphoid approach is between the xiphoid process and the left costal margin at a 15° to 30° angle cpehlad. This approach can risk injury to the right atrium, liver, and peritoneal cavity if the angle is incorrectly directed. This distance is often longer to reach the pericardial space than with other approaches. However, the risk of pneumothorax is lower. The parasternal approach utilizes the fifth intercostal space close to the sternal border. If insertion is more than 1 cm laterally, there is an increased risk of pneumothorax and damage to vasculature. All puncture sites occurring in intercostal spaces should be done directly above the rib, to avoid the subcostal neurovascular bundle. Active continuous echocardiography during the procedure improves safety as well, improves safety compared to methods in which a static image is obtained at the beginning of the procedure and pericardial space is entered based on the operator's memorized trajectory. Real-time echocardiography allows for the identification of organs moving into the anticipated trajectory that may not have been appreciated on the initial images.

### Selected References

1. Adler Y, Charron P, Imazio M, et al. 2015 ESC Guidelines for the diagnosis and management of pericardial diseases: The Task Force for the Diagnosis and Management of Pericardial Diseases of the European Society of Cardiology (ESC) Endorsed by: The European Association for Cardio-Thoracic Surgery (EACTS). *Eur Heart J.* 2015;36(42):2921-2964.
2. De Carlini CC, Maggiolini S. Pericardiocentesis in cardiac tamponade: indications and practical aspects. *E-Journal Cardiol Pract.* 2017;15(19). Available online https://www.escardio.org/Journals/E-Journal-of-Cardiology-Practice/Volume-15/ Pericardiocentesis-in-cardiac-tamponade-indications-and-practical-aspects.

# 78 | ENDOTRACHEAL INTUBATION

Jan Kasal and Chakradhar Venkata

**1.** A 46-year-old man is admitted to the Emergency Department after a high-speed motor vehicle collision. He has suspected bilateral rib fractures and develops respiratory distress and hypoxemia. The decision is made to intubate. After intubation, his SpO$_2$ remains 82% on 100% FiO$_2$, and there is resistance to delivering breaths. His BP is 130/60 mm Hg, and HR is 110 bpm. An ultrasound image of the right chest during ventilation is performed and shown in **Figure 78.1**.

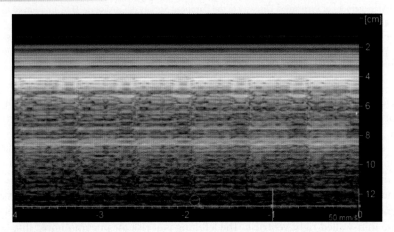

**Figure 78.1**

Which of the following statements is *most* likely to be correct?
A. There is a right-sided pneumothorax
B. There is a left mainstem intubation
C. There is no esophageal intubation
D. There is no issue related to intubation

2. A 47-year-old woman with acute respiratory distress syndrome (ARDS) from COVID-19 infection is in the intensive care unit (ICU) on venovenous extracorporeal membrane oxygenation (VV ECMO). She becomes agitated and pulls at her endotracheal tube (ETT) and nasogastric (NG) tube. Because she is oxygenated and ventilated with ECMO, the team decides to perform a neck ultrasound to evaluate tube positioning (▶ Video 78.1 and Figure 78.2).

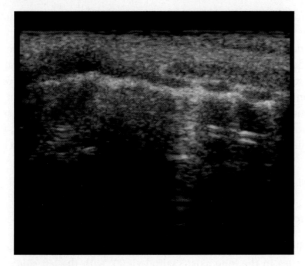

Figure 78.2

These findings are *most* consistent with which of the following?
A. The ETT is in the esophagus.
B. The ETT is in the trachea.
C. The venous ECMO cannula is in the internal jugular vein.
D. The NG tube has been displaced.

3. A 50-year-old woman with *Legionella* pneumonia complicated by ARDS is scheduled for percutaneous tracheostomy. Ultrasound of the neck done just prior to cannulation is displayed in ▶ Videos 78.2A and B and Figure 78.3A and B.

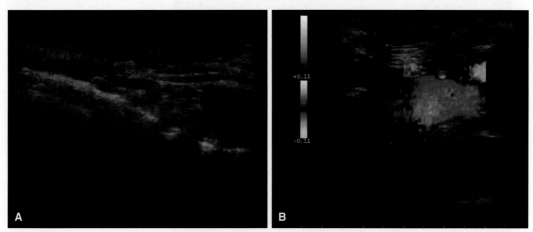

Figure 78.3

Which is the most likely structure seen in ▶ Videos 78.2A and B and Figure 78.3A and B?
A. Pulmonary artery
B. Brachiocephalic artery (BA)
C. Superior vena cava
D. Left subclavian artery

# Chapter 78 ▪ Answers

**1.** Correct Answer: B. There is a left mainstem intubation

*Rationale:* The M-mode ultrasound in Figure 78.1 shows vertical movement extending from the pleura to the bottom of the screen at regular intervals, representing brief movements of lung tissue. These movements correlate with heartbeats, and this ultrasound pattern is called the lung pulse. The lung pulse confirms the presence of both layers of pleura and excludes pneumothorax at that location. Air between the pleural layers (pneumothorax) would reflect the ultrasound waves, and no cardiac movement could be seen. Normal ventilation should produce a "beach sign" on M-mode. Since this pattern is not seen during ventilation, one should consider the possibility of pneumothorax, or lack of lung movement for other reasons. Because the presence of lung pulse rules out pneumothorax, a lack of ventilation to the right lung is most likely, from esophageal intubation, left-mainstem intubation, or another process obstructing ventilation to the right lung.

Selected Reference
1. Lichtenstein D. *Lung Ultrasound in the Critically Ill.* Springer; 2016, Chapter 31 and 34.

**2.** Correct Answer: B. The ETT is in the trachea

*Rationale:* Ultrasound can be a useful adjunct for examination of the upper airway. The ultrasound shown demonstrates a 2D view of the trachea in the long axis (sagittal view), with the left side of the image cephalad, and the right caudad, using a linear transducer. In **Figure 78.4**, the cricoid cartilage (CC, on the left side) and tracheal cartilages (TC, on the right side of the screen) are visible. Cartilage has an oval hypoechoic appearance. The bright line just below the cartilages represents the air-mucosa (A-M) interface. Reverberations (R, below A-M) represent comet tail artifacts. The ETT is seen as a double line structure, better seen on the right of the screen. Because air does not conduct ultrasound waves well, to make the ETT visible, the cuff was filled here with normal saline. This examination is consistent with endotracheal intubation (choice B is correct). The esophagus and internal jugular veins are not visible in the image (choices A, C are incorrect).

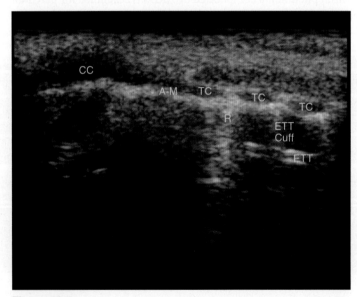

**Figure 78.4**

An esophageal intubation will appear lateral to the anterior trachea on a transverse image taken approximately 1 inch above the suprasternal notch (the "double-tract" sign, *white arrows*, **Figure 78.5**). The tube diameter visible on the ultrasound is too large for a misplaced NG tube (choice D is incorrect). Also, the well-visible tube segment is due to the cuff filled with saline surrounding the tube, something that would not be possible with an NG tube. In a study by Arya et al., ultrasound identified 100% of tracheal intubations and 83% of esophageal intubations.

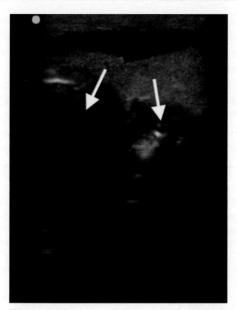

**Figure 78.5**

## Selected References

1. Arya R, Schrift D, Choe C, Al-Jaghbeer M. (2019). Real-time tracheal ultrasound for the confirmation of endotracheal intubations in the intensive care unit: an observational study. *J Ultrasound Med.* 2019 Feb;38(2):491-497.
2. Chou HC, Chong KM, Sim SS, et al. (2013). Real-time tracheal ultrasonography for confirmation of endotracheal tube placement during cardiopulmonary resuscitation. *Resuscitation.* 2013;84(12):1708-1712.
3. Kundra P, Mishra SK, Ramesh A. Ultrasound of the airway. *Indian J Anaesth.* 2011;55(5):456-462.
4. Raphael DT, Conard FU, 3rd. Ultrasound confirmation of endotracheal tube placement. *J Clin Ultrasound.* 1987;15(7):459-462.

**3.** Correct Answer: B. Brachiocephalic artery (BA)

*Rationale:* Ultrasound may be beneficial during percutaneous dilatational tracheostomy (PDT). It may identify aberrant vessels, help in selecting the optimal location for tracheal puncture, and guide the needle insertion into the trachea, similar to ultrasound-guided vascular access.

Figure 78.3A is a 2D view of the trachea in the long (sagittal) axis. There is a sizable pulsatile structure localized caudally (at the right side of the screen), consistent with an aberrant blood vessel. Figure 78.3B shows color Doppler of the same view and demonstrates pulsatile arterial flow.

In this case, the percutaneous tracheostomy was canceled based on the ultrasound findings and concerns about the increased risk of vascular injury. Computed tomography (CT) demonstrated the BA (*yellow arrow*) anteriorly to the trachea (**Figure 78.6**). The patient underwent open surgical tracheostomy at a later date.

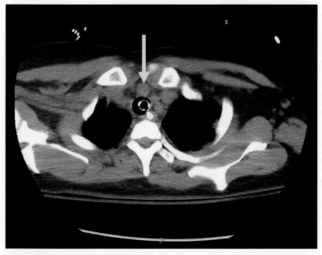

**Figure 78.6**

BA injury during PDT is an infrequent, but potentially life-threatening complication. Recognizing the vessel located in the tract of planned percutaneous cannulation should alert physicians to the possibility of an aberrant BA course, and safer options should be considered, such as obtaining further preprocedural imaging first or planning for an open tracheostomy.

Ultrasound can be incorporated into the standard procedure of PDT, which typically also includes bronchoscopy guidance. The advantage of ultrasound is the ability to identify vascular structure; the benefit of bronchoscopy is the ability to directly visualize the needle in the airway and reduce the risk of posterior tracheal wall injury. The ultrasound and bronchoscopy may complement each other, but may not necessarily be interchangeable. Few studies so far have examined solely ultrasound-guided PDT versus solely bronchoscopy-guided PDT. In one study, the ultrasound for PDT was noninferior to bronchoscopy.

## Selected References

1. Aggarwal R, Soni KD, Goyal K, Singh GP, Sokhal N, Trikha A. Does real time ultrasonography confer any benefit during bronchoscopy guided percutaneous tracheostomy: a preliminary, randomized controlled trial. *Indian J Crit Care Med.* 2019;23(5):236-238.
2. Gobatto ALN, Besen BAMP, Tierno PFGMM, et al. Ultrasound-guided percutaneous dilational tracheostomy versus bronchoscopy-guided percutaneous dilational tracheostomy in critically ill patients (TRACHUS): a randomized noninferiority controlled trial. *Intensive Care Med.* 2016;42(3):342-351.
3. Hulde N, Köppen M, Gratzke M, Kisch-Wedel H, Brenner P, Huge V. Hemorrhage of the innominate artery during percutaneous dilatation tracheotomy. *Anaesthesist.* 2018;67(6):448-451.
4. Lopes-Pimentel P, Villamizar MA, Romero N, Koo M. Innominate artery dolichoectasia identified during ultrasound assessment prior to percutaneous tracheostomy. *Rev Esp Anestesiol Reanim.* 2016;63(2):125-126.
5. Sharma SD, Kumar G, Hill CS, Kaddour H. Brachiocephalic artery haemorrhage during percutaneous tracheostomy. *Ann R Coll Surg Engl.* 2015;97(2):e15-e17.

Chuan-Jay Jeffrey Chen and Jarone Lee

1. A 24-year-old man with a history of intravenous heroin use presents with erythema and swelling of the left second finger over the proximal interphalangeal (PIP) joint. His finger is held in flexion due to the swelling, limiting the images able to be obtained using ultrasound gel and the linear probe. What is the next best step to assess the swelling?

   A. Order a computed tomography (CT) scan of the hand
   B. Consult the hand surgery service
   C. Submerge the hand in a water bath
   D. Use warmed ultrasound gel

2. Which of the following features of **Figure 79.1** best suggests the diagnosis of abscess?

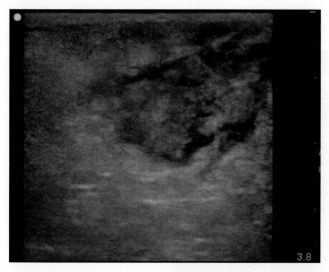

**Figure 79.1**

   A. "Dirty" shadowing
   B. "Clean" shadowing
   C. Cobblestoning
   D. Posterior acoustic enhancement

3. A 3-year-old girl presents with significant redness and swelling over her forearm. On physical examination, you perceive a 2 cm area of fluctuance. You obtain the point-of-care ultrasound image shown in **Figure 79.2** over the area of fluctuance.

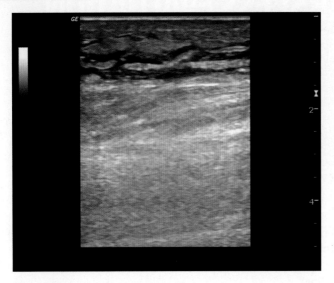

**Figure 79.2**

How deep should you make your incision?
A. No incision
B. 0.5 cm
C. 1.2 cm
D. >2 cm

4. A 28-year-old woman presents with a painful, swollen lump in her right groin. You obtain the ultrasound image shown in **Figure 79.3**.

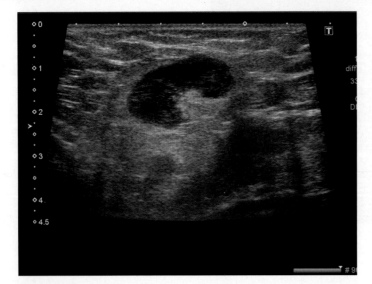

**Figure 79.3**

What is the next best step?
A. Needle aspiration
B. Incision and drainage
C. Decreased depth of image
D. Color Doppler evaluation

5. A 59-year-old woman presents with swelling over her left axilla worsening over the last 4 days. She appears uncomfortable. You perform ultrasound over the area of swelling (**Figure 79.4**).

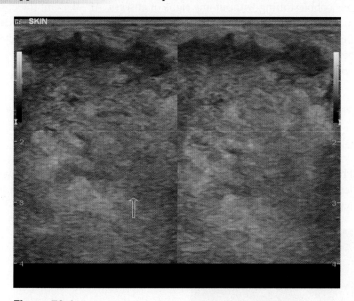

**Figure 79.4**

Which of the following should be performed next?
A. M-mode measurement
B. Downward probe pressure
C. Increasing image gain
D. Decreasing image gain

# Chapter 79 ▪ Answers

**1.** Correct Answer: C. Submerge the hand in a water bath

*Rationale:* Using ultrasound to assess abscesses, lacerations, or other pathology within the hand or foot can be difficult due to significant pain, anatomic restrictions, or other factors that limit the ability of the probe to make contact with the skin. Water baths can significantly decrease discomfort without compromising imaging quality. Warmed ultrasound gel would increase contact with the skin. While CT imaging or a hand surgery consult may also reveal an abscess, they take significantly more time and resources than using a simple water bath.

Selected References
1. Blaivas M, Lyon M, Brannam L, Duggal S, Sierzenski P. Water bath evaluation technique for emergency ultrasound of painful superficial structures. *Am J Emerg Med*. 2004;22(7):589-593.
2. LeDonne S, Sengupta D. US probe: Ultrasound water bath for distal extremity evaluation. http://www.emdocs.net/us-probe-ultrasound-water-bath-for-distal-extremity-evaluation/
3. Shih J. Ultrasound for the win! 53M with right index finger swelling. https://www.aliem.com/2017/07/ultrasound-win-53m-right-index-finger-swelling/

**2.** Correct Answer: D. Posterior acoustic enhancement

*Rationale:* Because abscesses are fluid-filled spaces, ultrasound waves are less attenuated and hence tissues deep to the abscess appear hyperechogenic (posterior acoustic enhancement). "Dirty" shadowing suggests air or gas, which scatters ultrasound waves. "Clean" shadowing suggests a solid object that does not permit ultrasound waves to pass through, such as bone or gallstones. Cobblestoning suggests cellulitis without abscess.

Selected Reference
1. O'Rourke K, Kibbee N, Stubbs A. Ultrasound for the evaluation of skin and soft tissue infections. *Mo Med*. 2015;112(3):202-205.

**3.** Correct Answer: A. No incision

*Rationale:* The image demonstrates cobblestoning without any signs of abscess. At ~0.5 cm, the epidermis/dermis layer gives way to subcutaneous tissue, which in this case is filled with subcutaneous edema. Beyond 1.2 cm lies muscle. While Figure 79.2 is a single still image, there are no clear fluid collections, areas with septae or sediment, defined areas with significant posterior acoustic enhancement, or other signs of abscess. Therefore, no incision is indicated.

Selected Reference
1. O'Rourke K, Kibbee N, Stubbs A. Ultrasound for the evaluation of skin and soft tissue infections. *Mo Med.* 2015;112(3):202-205.

**4.** Correct Answer: D. Color Doppler evaluation

*Rationale:* Color Doppler should be applied to distinguish an abscess from a reactive lymph node, which can mimic an abscess, with tenderness and fluctuance. In this case, applying color Doppler would show clear features of a lymph node, that is, hilar blood flow (see **Figure 79.5**).

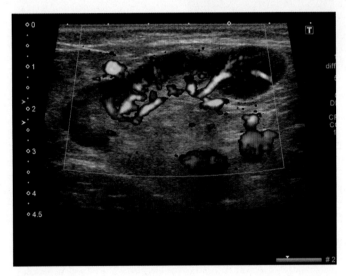

**Figure 79.5**

Selected References
1. Ultrasound assessment of abscess and cellulitis. In: Baston CM, Moore C, Krebs EA, Dean AJ, Panebianco N. eds. *Pocket Guide to POCUS: Point-of-Care Tips for Point-of-Care Ultrasound.* McGraw-Hill; Accessed May 05, 2021. https://accessmedicine-mhmedical-com.ezp-prod1.hul.harvard.edu/content.aspx?bookid=2544&sectionid=210344732 https://accessmedicine.mhmedical.com/content.aspx?bookid=2544&sectionid=210344732
2. Grimm LJ, Carmody KA. Abscess evaluation with bedside ultrasonography. https://emedicine.medscape.com/article/1379916-overview#a8

**5.** Correct Answer: B. Downward probe pressure

*Rationale:* In Figure 79.4, the abscess lies deep to the superficial stripe of hypoechogenicity at 0.5 cm deep. Applying downward pressure with the probe would cause the fluid within the abscess to create an image of swirling echogenicity on the screen, helping the operator identify where the actual abscess is.

Selected References
1. Chen KC, Lin AC, Chong CF, Wang TL. An overview of point-of-care ultrasound for soft tissue and musculoskeletal applications in the emergency department. *J Intensive Care.* 2016;4:55. doi:10.1186/s40560-016-0173-0.
2. Ultrasound assessment of abscess and cellulitis. In: Baston CM, Moore C, Krebs EA, Dean AJ, Panebianco N. eds. *Pocket Guide to POCUS: Point-of-Care Tips for Point-of-Care Ultrasound.* McGraw-Hill; Accessed May 05, 2021. https://accessmedicine-mhmedical-com.ezp-prod1.hul.harvard.edu/content.aspx?bookid=2544&sectionid=210344732

# 80 | LUMBAR PUNCTURE

Andrew N. Chalupka and Emily E. Naoum

1. What is the level most anatomically amenable to spinal puncture in the elderly?

   A. L2-L3
   B. L3-L4
   C. L4-L5
   D. L5-S1

2. When using static ultrasound guidance to perform a lumbar puncture, what are the most common view(s) to obtain?

   A. Paramedian sagittal and transverse
   B. Paramedian sagittal and midline sagittal
   C. Paramedian sagittal alone
   D. Transverse alone

3. What are the advantages of using ultrasound guidance for lumbar neuraxial procedures?

   A. More accurate identification of a specific lumbar intervertebral space
   B. Increased success rate
   C. Improved safety profile
   D. All of the above

4. **Figure 80.1** depicts a lumbar neuraxial ultrasound obtained in the paramedian sagittal view.

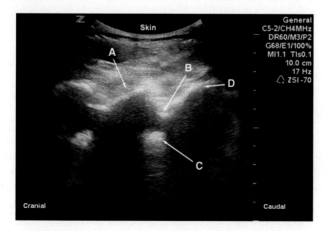

**Figure 80.1**

Select the correctly paired label.
A. Transverse process
B. Ligamentum flavum
C. Anterior longitudinal complex
D. L5 vertebral body

5. **Figure 80.2** depicts a lumbar neuraxial ultrasound obtained in the transverse view.

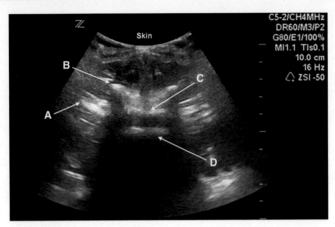

**Figure 80.2**

Select the correctly paired label.
A. Articular process
B. Transverse process
C. Vertebral body
D. Posterior longitudinal ligament complex

# Chapter 80 ▪ Answers

1. **Correct Answer: D. L5-S1**

*Rationale:* In the elderly, degenerative changes and difficulties in positioning the patient may contribute to difficulty in accessing the intrathecal space. The paramedian approach offers an alternative to the midline approach that can overcome inadequate flexion or a calcified interspinous ligament. The size of the inter-laminar space can influence the success of lumbar puncture. Ultrasound analysis of the influence of age on spinal anatomy has demonstrated that younger patients have larger interlaminar spaces than elderly patients, and that in all patients the L5-S1 interspace has the largest interlaminar height.

Selected Reference
1. Bae J, Park SK, Yoo S, Lim YJ, Kim JT. Influence of age, laterality, patient position, and spinal level on the interlamina space for spinal puncture. *Reg Anesth Pain Med.* 2020;45:27-31.

2. **Correct Answer: A. Paramedian sagittal and transverse**

*Rationale:* The combination of paramedian sagittal and transverse sonographic views yields useful information in determining a patient's lumbar spine anatomy. The paramedian sagittal view allows identification of the lumbosacral junction and the determination of the precise levels of laminae and transverse processes. The transverse view allows identification of the spinous and articular processes, as well as the angle of rotation in the case of scoliosis. Both views can be used to identify the anterior and posterior complexes, yielding information about the depth at which the epidural space will be reached.

Selected Reference
1. Chin A, van Zundert A. Chapter 23: Spinal anesthesia. In: Hadzic A, eds. *Hadzic's Textbook of Regional Anesthesia and Acute Pain Management,* 2nd ed. McGraw-Hill; 2017.

3. **Correct Answer: D. All of the above**

*Rationale:* A systematic review and meta-analysis of 31 clinical trials demonstrated that when used for placement of spinal and epidural anesthetics and performance of lumbar punctures, lumbar neuraxial ultrasound provided several advantages: improved identification of specific vertebral levels, increased procedural success rate, and improved safety.

In one study, compared with gold standard computed tomography (CT), ultrasound was able to correctly identify a given intervertebral space in up to 90% of cases. Conversely, other studies have shown palpation to be notoriously unreliable, with accurate identification of spaces as infrequent as 29% of the time. The increased success rate of ultrasound-guided procedures was attributable to the correlation between ultrasound-measured depth and actual needle depth. Evidence for safety outcomes varied, with strong evidence for a decrease in the number of attempts and a nonsignificant trend toward a lower incidence of headache. No difference was found in the rate of spinal/epidural hematoma, although being such a rare event, no study was sufficiently powered to detect a difference (and indeed, no hematomas were observed in any study included in the analysis). Nevertheless, the authors of the meta-analysis note that it can be reasonably concluded that decreasing the number of procedural attempts, as ultrasound guidance does, would decrease the risk of spinal/epidural hematoma.

### Selected References

1. Broadbent CR, Maxwell WB, Ferrie R, Wilson DJ, Gawne-Cain M, Russell R. Ability of anaesthetists to identify a marked lumbar interspace. *Anaesthesia*. 2000 Nov;55(11):1122-1126.
2. Perlas A, Chaparro LE, Chin KJ. Lumbar neuraxial ultrasound for spinal and epidural anesthesia: a systematic review and meta-analysis. *Reg Anesth Pain Med*. 2016 Mar-Apr;41(2):251-260.

4. **Correct Answer: B. Ligamentum flavum**

*Rationale:* **Figure 80.3** demonstrates the appropriate location of the ultrasound transducer anatomically demonstrated on a patient and the relative positioning against a model spine. Ideal imaging allows identification of the sacrum caudally and characterization of lumbar levels to increase the accuracy when identifying the ideal site for neuraxial block or lumbar puncture. The anterior and posterior complexes can be seen and ligamentum flavum may be utilized to estimate an appropriate depth of insertion for epidural placement and/or anticipated distance to the dural sac.

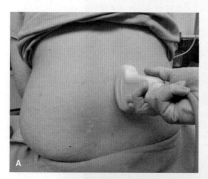
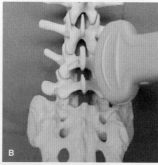
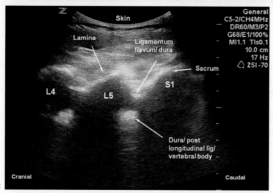

**Figure 80.3**

Selected References

1. Balki M. Locating the epidural space in obstetric patients—ultrasound a useful tool: continuing professional development. *Can J Anesth*. 2010;57:1111-1126.
2. Norris MC. Chapter 35: Neuraxial anesthesia. In: Barash PG, Cullen BF, Stoelting RK, eds. *Clinical Anesthesia*, 8th ed. Wolters Kluwer Health/Lippincott Williams; 2017.
3. Perlas A, Chaparro LE, Chin KJ. Lumbar neuraxial ultrasound for spinal and epidural anesthesia: a systematic review and meta-analysis. *Reg Anesth Pain Med*. 2016 Mar-Apr;41(2):251-260.

**5.** Correct Answer: **D. Posterior longitudinal ligament complex**

*Rationale:* **Figure 80.4** demonstrates the appropriate location of the ultrasound transducer anatomically demonstrated on a patient and the relative positioning against a model spine. Ideal imaging allows identification of the spinous and articular processes, as well as the angle of rotation in the case of scoliosis. The anterior and posterior complexes can also be identified and utilized to estimate an appropriate depth of insertion for epidural placement and/or anticipated distance to the dural sac.

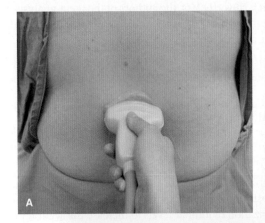
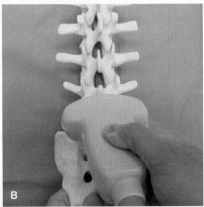
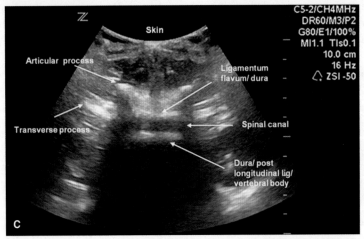

**Figure 80.4**

Selected References

1. Balki M. Locating the epidural space in obstetric patients—ultrasound a useful tool: continuing professional development. *Can J Anesth*. 2010;57:1111-1126.
2. Norris MC. Chapter 35: Neuraxial anesthesia. In: Barash PG, Cullen BF, Stoelting RK, eds. *Clinical Anesthesia*, 8th ed. Wolters Kluwer Health/Lippincott Williams; 2017.
3. Perlas A, Chaparro LE, Chin KJ. Lumbar neuraxial ultrasound for spinal and epidural anesthesia: a systematic review and meta-analysis. *Reg Anesth Pain Med*. 2016 Mar-Apr;41(2):251-260.

# 81 | TRANSCRANIAL DOPPLER

Etienne J. Couture and Andre Y. Denault

1. What is the correct association of signal depth and direction when assessing the middle cerebral artery through the temporal window?

   A. Depth 20 to 25 mm, positive velocities
   B. Depth 20 to 25 mm, negative velocities
   C. Depth 45 to 55 mm, positive velocities
   D. Depth 45 to 55 mm, negative velocities

2. What is the sequence of Doppler flow pattern of the middle cerebral artery in a situation where normal intracranial pressure progresses to intracranial hypertension leading to cerebral circulatory arrest?

   A. Normal tracing, biphasic flow, normal systolic flow and reduced diastolic flow, systolic spikes, no flow
   B. Normal tracing, systolic spikes, biphasic flow, normal systolic flow and reduced diastolic flow, no flow
   C. Normal tracing, normal systolic flow and reduced diastolic flow, biphasic flow, systolic spikes, no flow
   D. Normal tracing, normal systolic flow and reduced diastolic flow, systolic spikes, biphasic flow, no flow

3. How is the Lindegaard index (LI) calculated?

   A. Mean flow velocity in the middle cerebral artery/Mean flow velocity in the extracranial portion of the ipsilateral internal carotid artery
   B. (Systolic flow velocity − Diastolic flow velocity) × 3 + Diastolic flow velocity
   C. (Systolic flow velocity − Diastolic flow velocity)/Mean flow velocity
   D. (Systolic flow velocity − Diastolic flow velocity)/Systolic flow velocity

# Chapter 81 ▪ Answers

**1.** Correct Answer: C. Depth 45 to 55 mm, positive velocities

*Rationale:* The majority of the transcranial Doppler examination in the intensive care unit is done through the temporal acoustic window using a lower frequency probe (1-2 MHz) like that used for echocardiography. The depth, direction of blood flow, and cerebral blood flow velocity range are used to identify the insonated vessel through the temporal acoustic window (**Table 81.1**).

**Table 81.1 Normal Blood Flow Velocity Using Transcranial Doppler**

| Artery | Depth (mm) | Direction of Flow | Peak Velocity (cm/s) | Mean Velocity (cm/s) | End-Diastolic Velocity (cm/s) | Pulsatility Index | Resistance Index | Diameter (mm) |
|---|---|---|---|---|---|---|---|---|
| MCA | M1: 40-65 | Toward | 90-110 | 55-75 | 35-55 | 0.81-0.97 | 0.54-0.62 | 2.0-4.0 |
|  | M2: 30-40 |  |  |  |  |  |  |  |
| ACA | 60-80 | Away | 80-90 | 50-60 | 30-40 | 0.76-0.92 | 0.53-0.59 | 1.6-2.1 |
| PCA | P1: 55-80 | Toward | 66-81 | 42-53 | 26-33 | 0.78-0.97 | 0.53-0.60 | 2.0-3.0 |
|  | P2: 60-70 | Away |  |  |  |  |  |  |

ACA, anterior cerebral artery; M1, middle cerebral artery, sphenoidal or horizontal segment; M2, middle cerebral artery, insular segment; MCA, middle cerebral artery; P1, precommunicating posterior cerebral artery; P2, postcommunicating posterior cerebral artery; PCA, posterior cerebral artery. Toward stands for positive velocities, Away stands for negative velocities.

## Selected References

1. Alexandrov AV, Sloan MA, Wong LK, et al. Practice standards for transcranial Doppler ultrasound: part I—test performance. *J Neuroimaging.* 2007;17(1):11-18.
2. Couture EJ, Desjardins G, Denault AY. Transcranial Doppler monitoring guided by cranial two-dimensional ultrasonography. *Can J Anaesth.* 2017;64(8):885-887.
3. Rigamonti A, Ackery A, Baker AJ. Transcranial Doppler monitoring in subarachnoid hemorrhage: a critical tool in critical care. *Can J Anaesth.* 2008;55(2):112-123.

**2.** Correct Answer: C. Normal tracing, normal systolic flow and reduced diastolic flow, biphasic flow, systolic spikes, no flow

*Rationale:* A normal transcranial Doppler tracing of the middle cerebral artery, found from a temporal acoustic window at a depth around 4 to 6 cm with a flow direction toward the probe, is characterized by a positive Doppler signal of approximately 100 cm/s in systole and 50 cm/s at end diastole. Increases in intracranial pressure will first show a reduction of diastolic flow velocity, followed by a slightly decreased duration of systolic flow, and then the absence of diastolic flow. If the intracranial pressure is above the diastolic blood pressure, it will preclude diastolic cerebral blood flow.

The progression of intracranial pressure will then lead to the three stages of intracranial circulatory arrest, characterized by distinct flow velocity patterns that succeed one another in the following order: oscillating flow, systolic spike flow, and absence of flow. Oscillating flow is characterized by an antegrade systolic flow with a retrograde diastolic flow in one cardiac cycle. As intracranial hypertension progresses, the ratio of the area under the curve of the antegrade systolic and the retrograde diastolic flow will decrease from highly positive to 1 (equal flow forward in systole and backward in diastole). Further progression of intracranial hypertension will produce only brief systolic spikes of less than 200 ms, without any other flow during the rest of the cardiac cycle. When intracranial pressure reaches mean arterial blood pressure, there will be no blood flow in the major intracranial arteries (**Figure 81.1**).

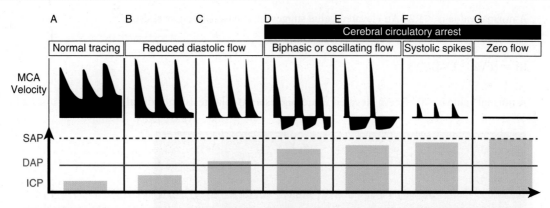

**Figure 81.1** Intracranial hypertension and circulatory arrest. Transcranial Doppler changes in the MCA flow with a progressive increase in ICP are shown compared with a normal MCA flow pattern and normal ICP (*panel A*). The initial stages of increased ICP typically show patterns of systolic peaks with a progressive reduction in diastolic velocities and decreased systolic flow duration (*panels B and C*). The three patterns that correspond to intracranial circulatory arrest are shown: biphasic oscillating flow (*panels D and E*), systolic spike flow (*panel F*), and zero flow (*panel G*). ICP, intracranial pressure; DAP, diastolic arterial pressure; MCA, middle cerebral artery; SAP, systolic arterial pressure.

### Selected References

1. Denault AY, Vegas A, Lamarche Y, Tradif J-C, Couture P. *Basic Transesophageal and Critical Care Ultrasound.* 1st ed. CRC Press, Taylor & Francis Group; 2018.
2. Hassler W, Steinmetz H, Pirschel J. Transcranial Doppler study of intracranial circulatory arrest. *J Neurosurg.* 1989;71(2):195-201.

---

**3.** Correct Answer: A. Mean flow velocity in the middle cerebral artery/Mean flow velocity in the extracranial portion of the ipsilateral internal carotid artery

*Rationale:* Cerebral vasospasm following aneurysmal subarachnoid hemorrhage may lead to delayed cerebral ischemia and infarction with devastating consequences. Cerebral vasospasm peaks at 3 to 7 days after aneurysmal subarachnoid hemorrhage and can last for up to 14 days. Angiography and computed tomography (CT) angiogram are useful tools in the diagnosis of cerebral vasospasm. Transcranial Doppler serves as a simple, noninvasive, bedside tool that can also monitor cerebral blood flow velocities without transport, ionizing radiation, invasive vascular access, or intravenous contrast use. Proximal vasospasm reduces the diameter of the vessel lumen, increasing its mean blood flow velocity, whereas distal vasospasm will tend to increase the pulsatility index (PI) rather than increasing mean blood flow velocity.

LI can be used to differentiate increased cerebral flow velocity caused by vasospasm from hyperemia by comparing intra- to extracranial blood flow velocities. LI is the mean flow velocity (FVm) in the middle cerebral artery divided by the FVm in the extracranial portion of the ipsilateral internal carotid artery. Hyperemia will correspond to an LI < 3 and cerebral vasospasm to an LI > 3, with severe vasospasm graded as an LI > 6.

Transcranial Doppler monitoring (**Figure 81.2**) allows measurement of peak systolic flow velocity (FVs) and end-diastolic flow velocity (FVd), whereas FVm, PI, and resistance index (RI) are calculated from FVs and FVd. Automated modules of analysis in ultrasound machines can calculate FVm as an area under a traced Doppler profile.

FVm can be calculated from the following formula:

$$FVm = [FVs + (2 \times FVd)]/3$$

or

$$FVm = (FVs - FVd)/3 + FVd$$

PI can be calculated from the following formula:

$$PI = (FVs - FVd)/FVm$$

A normal value is <1.2. An elevated value suggests increased vascular resistance. RI can be calculated from the following formula:

$$RI = (FVs - FVd)/FVs$$

A normal value is <0.75. An elevated value suggests vascular resistance distal to the site of insonation.

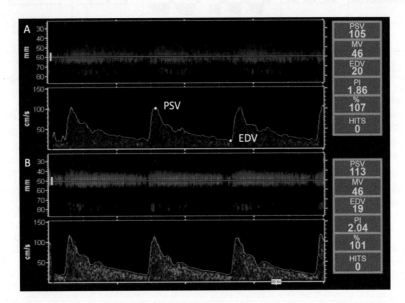

**Figure 81.2** Transcranial Doppler of left (A) and right (B) middle cerebral artery. Transcranial Doppler–derived blood velocity before and aortic valve repair in a 69-year-old man with severe chronic aortic regurgitation. Note the reduced end-diastolic velocities (EDV) and the elevated pulsatility index (PI) from 1.86 and 2.04 (normal: 0.8-1.2) in the left and right middle cerebral artery. %, percentage mean velocity (MV) values compared with baseline; HITS, high-intensity transient signals; PSV, peak systolic velocity.

Selected Reference

1. Rasulo FA, De Peri E, Lavinio A. Transcranial Doppler ultrasonography in intensive care. *Eur J Anaesthesiol.* 2008;25:167-173.

# APPENDIX

# ATTRIBUTION LIST: FIGURES, TABLES, AND VIDEOS

## CHAPTER 3

### Figure 3.2

Reprinted with permission from Abbas S, Peng P. Basic principles and physics of ultrasound. In: Peng P, Finlayson R, Lee S. Bhatia A, eds. *Ultrasound for Interventional Pain Management.* Springer; 2020. Figure 1.15.

### Table 3.1

Derived from Azhari H. *Basics of Biomedical Ultrasound for Engineers.* John Wiley & Sons, Inc.; 2010.

## CHAPTER 4

### Figure 4.1

From Physics and instrumentation. In: Armstrong WF, Ryan T, eds. *Feigenbaum's Echocardiography.* 8th ed. Wolters Kluwer; 2019:9-37. Figure 2.16.

## CHAPTER 5

### Figure 5.1

From Oh JK, Park S, Pisralu SV, Nkomo VT. Native valvular heart disease. In: Oh JK, Kane GC, eds. *The Echo Manual.* 4th ed. Wolters Kluwer; 2019:307-362. Figure 13.33g.

### Figure 5.2

From Physics and instrumentation. In: Armstrong WF, Ryan T, eds. *Feigenbaum's Echocardiography.* 8th ed. Wolters Kluwer; 2019:9-37. Figure 2.39.

### Figure 5.3

Reprinted with permission from Central venous access. In: Marino PL, eds. *Marino's The ICU Book.* 4th ed. Wolters Kluwer; 2014:17-39. Figure 2.6.

Garcia-Cortes RS, Rao PK, Quader N. Transesophageal echocardiography In: Quader N, Makan M, Perez J, eds. *The Washington Manual of Echocardiography.* 2nd ed. Wolters Kluwer; 2017:294-324.

## CHAPTER 10

### eFigure 10.1

Zimmerman JM, Coker BJ. The nuts and bolts of performing focused cardiovascular ultrasound (FoCUS). Anesth Analg. 2017 Mar;124(3):753-760. doi: 10.1213/ANE.0000000000001861. PMID: 28207445.

## CHAPTER 12

### Figure 12.1

From Left and right atrium, and right ventricle. In: Armstrong WF, Ryan T, eds. *Feigenbaum's Echocardiography.* 8th ed. Wolters Kluwer; 2019:158-193. Figure 7.14.

### Figure 12.2

Reprinted with permission from Garcia-Cortes RS, Rao PK, Quader N. Transesophageal echocardiography. In: Quader N, Makan M, Perez J, eds. *The Washington Manual of Echocardiography.* 2nd ed. Wolters Kluwer; 2017:294-324. Figure 21.22.

### Figure 12.3

Reprinted with permission from Mitral valve disease. In: Feigenbaum H, Armstrong WF, Ryan T, eds. *Feigenbaum's Echocardiography.* 6th ed. Wolters Kluwer; 2004:306-340. Figure 11.32.

## CHAPTER 15

### Figure 15.19

From Bertrand PB, Levine RA, Isselbacher EM, Vandervoort PM. Fact or artifact in two-dimensional echocardiography: avoiding misdiagnosis and missed diagnosis. *J Am Soc Echocardiogr.* 2016;29:381-391.

### Table 15.1

Adapted from Bertrand PB, Levine RA, Isselbacher EM, Vandervoort PM. Fact or artifact in two-dimensional echocardiography: avoiding misdiagnosis and missed diagnosis. *J Am Soc Echocardiogr.* 2016;29:381-391.

### Figure 15.20

From Bertrand PB, Levine RA, Isselbacher EM, Vandervoort PM. Fact or artifact in two-dimensional echocardiography: avoiding misdiagnosis and missed diagnosis. *J Am Soc Echocardiogr.* 2016;29:381-391. doi:10.1016/j.echo.2016.01.009.

### Figures 15.21, 15.22, and 15.26

From Bertrand PB, Levine RA, Isselbacher EM, Vandervoort PM. Fact or artifact in two-dimensional echocardiography: avoiding misdiagnosis and missed diagnosis. *J Am Soc Echocardiogr.* 2016;29:381-391. doi:10.1016/j.echo.2016.01.009.

### Figure 15.27

Adapted from Bertrand PB, Levine RA, Isselbacher EM, Vandervoort PM. Fact or artifact in two-dimensional echocardiography: avoiding misdiagnosis and missed diagnosis. *J Am Soc Echocardiogr.* 2016;29:381-391. doi:10.1016/j.echo.2016.01.009 and Bertrand PB, Grieten L, De Meester P, et al. Etiology and relevance of the figure-of-eight artifact on echocardiography after percutaneous left atrial appendage closure with the Amplatzer Cardiac Plug. *J Am Soc Echocardiogr.* 2014;27:323-8 e1. doi:10.1016/j.echo.2013.11.001.

## CHAPTER 20

### Figure 20.5

From Geleijnse ML, Di Martino LF, Vletter WB, et al. Limitations and difficulties of echocardiographic short-axis assessment of paravalvular leakage after 8 transcatheter aortic valve implantation. *Cardiovasc Ultrasound.* 2016 Sep;14(1):37. https://creativecommons.org/licenses/by/4.0/; https://creativecommons.org/publicdomain/zero/1.0/. Figure 2.

## CHAPTER 21

### Figure 21.3

Reprinted from Nagueh SF, Smiseth OA, Appleton CP, et al. Recommendations for the evaluation of left ventricular diastolic function by echocardiography: an update from the American Society of Echocardiography and the European Association of Cardiovascular Imaging. *J Am Soc Echocardiogr.* 2016 Apr;29(4):277-314. Copyright © 2016 American Society of Echocardiography. With permission.

## CHAPTER 22

### Figure 22.4

Derived from Evaluation of systolic function of the left ventricle. In: Armstrong WF, Ryan T. *Feigenbaum's Echocardiography.* 8th ed. Philadelphia, PA: Wolters Kluwer; 2019:100-127. Figure 5.36.

### Figure 22.5

Reprinted with permission from Evaluation of systolic function of the left ventricle. In: Armstrong WF, Ryan T. *Feigenbaum's Echocardiography.* 8th ed. Philadelphia, PA: Wolters Kluwer; 2019:100-127. Figure 5.8.

### Figure 22.6

Reprinted with permission from Evaluation of systolic function of the left ventricle. In: Armstrong WF, Ryan T. *Feigenbaum's Echocardiography.* 8th ed. Philadelphia, PA: Wolters Kluwer; 2019:100-127. Figure 5.53.

### Figure 22.7

Reprinted with permission from The echocardiographic examination. In: Feigenbaum H, Armstrong WF, Ryan T. *Feigenbaum's Echocardiography.* 6th ed. Philadelphia, PA: Lippincott, Williams & Wilkins; 2005:105-137. Figure 5.27.

### Figure 22.9

Reprinted from Ahmadpour H, Shah AA, Allen JW, Edmiston WA, Kim SJ, Haywood LJ. Mitral E point septal separation: a reliable index of left ventricular performance in coronary artery disease. *Am Heart J.* 1983;106(1 Pt 1):21-28. Copyright © 1983 Elsevier. With permission.

### Figure 22.10

Reprinted with permission from Evaluation of systolic function of the left ventricle. In: Armstrong WF, Ryan T. *Feigenbaum's Echocardiography.* 8th ed. Philadelphia, PA: Wolters Kluwer; 2019:100-127. Figure 5.9.

### Figure 22.11

Reprinted with permission from Evaluation of systolic function of the left ventricle. In: Armstrong WF, Ryan T. *Feigenbaum's Echocardiography.* 8th ed. Philadelphia, PA: Wolters Kluwer; 2019:100-127. Figure 5.2.

### Figures 22.12 and 22.13

Reprinted from Lang RM, Badano LP, Mor-Avi V, et al. Recommendations for cardiac chamber quantification by echocardiography in adults: an update from the American Society of Echocardiography and the European Association of Cardiovascular Imaging. *J Am Soc Echocardiogr.* 2015;28(1):1-39.e14. Copyright © 2015 Elsevier. With permission. Figures 5 and 4.

### Figure 22.14

Reprinted with permission from Hemodynamics. In: Armstrong WF, Ryan T. *Feigenbaum's Echocardiography.* 8th ed. Philadelphia, PA: Wolters Kluwer; 2019:194-216. Figures 8.5 and 8.6.

### Figure 22.15

Reprinted with permission from Evaluation of systolic function of the left ventricle. In: Armstrong WF, Ryan T. *Feigenbaum's Echocardiography.* 8th ed. Philadelphia, PA: Wolters Kluwer; 2019:100-127. Figure 5.1.

## CHAPTER 23

### Figure 23.1

Reproduced from Denault A, Vegas A, Lamarche Y, Tardif J-C, Couture P. *Basic Transesophageal and Critical Care Ultrasound.* Taylor and Francis, CRC Press; 2018; with permission of Taylor and Francis Group, LLC, a division of Informa plc.

### Figure 23.2

Adapted from Lang RM, Badano LP, Mor-Avi V, et al. Recommendations for cardiac chamber quantification by echocardiography in adults: an update from the American Society of Echocardiography and the European Association of Cardiovascular Imaging. *J Am Soc Echocardiogr.* 2015;28(1):1-39.e14; Denault A, Vegas A, Lamarche Y, Tardif J-C, Couture P. *Basic Transesophageal and Critical Care Ultrasound.* Taylor and Francis, CRC Press; 2018.

### Figure 23.4

Reproduced from Denault A, Vegas A, Lamarche Y, Tardif J-C, Couture P. *Basic Transesophageal and Critical Care Ultrasound.* Taylor and Francis, CRC Press; 2018; with permission of Taylor and Francis Group, LLC, a division of Informa plc.

## CHAPTER 25

### Figures 25.1, 25.3, 25.6, 25.18, and 25.44

Courtesy of Jina Bai, PA-C, New York Hospital—Weill-Cornell Medical Center.

### Figure 25.37

Reprinted from Matsumura Y, Fukuda S, Tran H, et al. Geometry of the proximal isovelocity surface area in mitral regurgitation by 3-dimensional color Doppler echocardiography: difference between functional mitral regurgitation and prolapse regurgitation. *Am Heart J.* 2008 Feb;155(2): 231-238. Copyright © 2008 Elsevier. With permission. Figure 3.

### Figure 25.38

Used with permission from https://www.cardioserv.net/wp-content/uploads/2017/06/Angles-768x573.jpeg at https://www.cardioserv.net/echo-mitral-valve/. Copyright © CardioServ.

### Figure 25.39

From Lancellotti P, Tribouilloy C, Hagendorff A, et al. Recommendations for the echocardiographic assessment of native valvular regurgitation: an executive summary from the European Association of Cardiovascular Imaging. *Eur Heart J Cardiovasc Imaging.* 2013 Jul;14(7):611-644. By permission of Oxford University Press. Copyright © 2021 European Society of Cardiology. Figure 23.

### Video 25.16

From Thomas B, Durant E, Barbant S, Nagdev A. Repeat point-of-care echocardiographic evaluation of traumatic cardiac arrest: a new paradigm for the emergency physician. *Clin Pract Cases Emerg Med.* 2017 May 23;1(3):194-196. Copyright: © 2017 Thomas. https://creativecommons.org/licenses/by/4.0/

### Figure 25.48B

Reproduced with permission of Medtronic, Inc.

### Figure 25.48C

Stented pericardial bioprosthesis courtesy of Carpentier-Edwards Magna.

### Figure 25.50

Reprinted from Tsang W., Freed BH, Lang RM. Quantification of mitral regurgitation. In: Lang RM, Goldstein SA, Kronzon I, Khandheria B, Mor-Avi V, eds. *ASE's Comprehensive Echocardiography.* 2nd ed. Elsevier; 2016:Chapter 116. Copyright © 2016 Elsevier. With permission. Figure 116.7.

### Figure 25.56

Reprinted from Sidebotham DA, Allen SJ, Gerber IL, Fayers T. Intraoperative transesophageal echocardiography for surgical repair of mitral regurgitation. *J Am Soc Echocardiogr.* 2014 Apr;27(4):345-366. Copyright © 2014 American Society of Echocardiography. With permission. Figure 7B.

## CHAPTER 28

### Figure 28.1

Reprinted with permission from Cabell CH, Abrutyn E, Karchmer AW. Cardiology patient page. Bacterial endocarditis: the disease, treatment, and prevention. *Circulation.* 2003;107(20):e185-e187. Figure 1.

### Figures 28.2, 28.3, and 28.4

Reprinted with permission from Sordelli C, Severino S, Ascione L, Coppolino P, Caso P. Echocardiographic assessment of heart valve prostheses. *J Cardiovasc Echogr.* 2014;24(4):103-113. Figures 5, 8, and 10.

### Figure 28.6

Reprinted with permission from Lerakis S, Hayek SS, Douglas PS. Paravalvular aortic leak after transcatheter aortic valve replacement: current knowledge. *Circulation.* 2013;127:397-407. Figure 2A.

### Figure 28.7

Reprinted from Merritt-Genore H, Siddique A, Um J, Moulton M, Markin NW. Rare but real: tension pneumopericardium in a patient with a left ventricular assist device. *CASE.* 2017;1(6):230-232. Copyright © 2017 by the American Society of Echocardiography. Figure 3.

## CHAPTER 29

### Figure 29.2

Reprinted with permission from Left and right atrium, and right ventricle. In: Armstrong WF, Ryan T. *Feigenbaum's Echocardiography.* 8th ed. Philadelphia, PA: Wolters Kluwer; 2019:158-193. Figure 7.37.

### Figure 29.3

Reprinted with permission from Aortic valve disease. In: Armstrong WF, Ryan T. *Feigenbaum's Echocardiography.* 8th ed. Philadelphia, PA: Wolters Kluwer; 2019:240-281. Figure 10.67B.

### Figure 29.4

Reprinted with permission from Left and right atrium, and right ventricle. In: Armstrong WF, Ryan T. *Feigenbaum's Echocardiography.* 7th ed. Philadelphia, PA: Wolters Kluwer; 2010:185-216. Figure 8.11.

### Figure 29.5

Reprinted with permission from Cheung AT. Prosthetic valves. In: Perrino AC, Reeves ST, eds. *A Practical Approach to Transesophageal Echocardiography.* 2nd ed. Wolters Kluwer; 2008:257-280. Figure 13.14.

### Figure 29.6

Reprinted with permission from Saghir MS, Banerjee S, Cooper DH. Infective endocarditis. In: Rasalingam R, Makan M, Pérez JE, eds. *The Washington Manual of Echocardiography.* Philadelphia, PA: Wolters Kluwer; 2013:180-191. Figure 14.5a.

### Figure 29.7

Reprinted with permission from Cresci S. Hypertrophic cardiomyopathy. In: Quader N, Makan M, Pérez JE, eds. *The Washington Manual of Echocardiography.* 2nd ed. Philadelphia, PA: Wolters Kluwer; 2017:103-117. Figure 9.2a.

### Figure 29.9

Reprinted with permission from The echocardiographic examination. In: Armstrong WF, Ryan T. *Feigenbaum's Echocardiography.* 7th ed. Philadelphia, PA: Wolters Kluwer; 2010:91-122. Figure 5.25.

### Figures 29.10 and 29.11

Reprinted with permission from Cresci S. Hypertrophic cardiomyopathy. In: Quader N, Makan M, Pérez JE, eds. *The Washington Manual of Echocardiography.* 2nd ed. Philadelphia, PA: Wolters Kluwer; 2017:103-117. Figure 9.4bc.

### Figure 29.15

Reprinted with permission from Jadbabaie F. Right ventricle, right atrium, tricuspid and pulmonic valves. In: Perrino AC, Reeves ST, eds. *A Practical Approach to Transesophageal Echocardiography.* 3rd ed. Philadelphia, PA: Wolters Kluwer; 2014:424-436. Figure 20.10.

### Tables 29.1 and 29.2

Adapted from Infective endocarditis. In: Armstrong W, Ryan T, eds. *Feigenbaum's Echocardiography.* 8th ed. Wolters Kluwer; 2019:347-376.

## CHAPTER 30

### Figure 30.2

From Fernandes FH, Amaral LV, Borges PA, França VE, Silva JB, Gardenghi G. Patent foramen ovale closure with prosthesis for occlusion of atrial septal defect in lipomatous hypertrophy of atrial septum. Report of two cases. *J Transcat Intervent.* 2020;28:eA20200003. Figure 1.

### Video 30.3

From Masses, tumors, and source of embolus. In: Armstrong WF, Ryan T, eds. *Feigenbaum's Echocardiography.* 8th ed. Wolters Kluwer; 2019:651-691. Figure 21.18b (Video).

## CHAPTER 31

### Figures 31.1 and 31.2

From Foster E. Echocardiographic evaluation of the pericardium. *UpToDate.* Wolters Kluwer; 2019. Retrieved June 26, 2019, from https://www.uptodate.com/contents/echocardiographic-evaluation-of-the-pericardium#H27.

### Figure 31.3

Reprinted from Klein AL, Abbara S, Agler DA, et al. American Society of Echocardiography clinical recommendations for multimodality cardiovascular imaging of patients with pericardial disease: endorsed by the Society for Cardiovascular Magnetic Resonance and Society of Cardiovascular Computed Tomography. *J Am Soc Echocardiogr.* 2013 Sep;26(9):965-1012. e15. Copyright © 2013 Elsevier. With permission.

## CHAPTER 32

### Figure 32.3

Reprinted with permission from Echocardiography in systemic disease and clinical problem solving. In: Armstrong WF, Ryan T, eds. *Feigenbaum's Echocardiography.* 7th ed. Wolters Kluwer; 2010:741-755. Figure 24.52.

**Figure 32.4**

From Kim J, Kim SM, Lee SY, et al. A case of severe aortic valve regurgitation caused by an ascending aortic aneurysm in a young patient with autosomal dominant polycystic kidney disease and normal renal function. *Korean Circ J.* 2012 Feb;42(2):136-139. Figure 2.

**Figures 32.5 and 32.7**

Reprinted with permission from Diseases of the aorta. In: Armstrong WF, Ryan T, eds. *Feigenbaum's Echocardiography.* 7th ed. Wolters Kluwer; 2010:633-665. Figures 21.18 and 21.56.

**Figures 32.6 and 32.10**

Reprinted with permission from The echocardiographic examination. In: Armstrong WF, Ryan T, eds. *Feigenbaum's Echocardiography.* 7th ed. Wolters Kluwer; 2010:91-120. Figure 5.43.

**Figure 32.8**

Reprinted with permission from Infective endocarditis. In: Armstrong WF, Ryan T, eds. *Feigenbaum's Echocardiography.* 7th ed. Wolters Kluwer; 2010:361-383. Figure 14.18.

**Figure 32.9**

From The comprehensive echocardiographic examination. In: Armstrong WF, Ryan T, eds. *Feigenbaum's Echocardiography.* 8th ed. Wolters Kluwer; 2019:61-99. Figure 4.17.

**Figure 32.11**

Reprinted with permission from Conrad CF, Cambria RP. Open thoracoabdominal aortic aneurysm repair. In: Fischer JE, ed. *Fischer's Mastery of Surgery.* 7th ed. Wolters Kluwer; 2019:2279-2327. Figure 198.1.

**CHAPTER 33**

**Figures 33.1, 33.2, 33.6, and 33.10**

Reprinted with permission from Congenital heart disease. In: Armstrong WF, Ryan T, eds. *Feigenbaum's Echocardiography.* 8th ed. Wolters Kluwer; 2019:544-607. Figures 19.41, 19.32, 19.122, and 19.39.

**Figure 33.3**

Reprinted with permission from Contrast echocardiography. In: Armstrong WF, Ryan T, eds. *Feigenbaum's Echocardiography.* 8th ed. Wolters Kluwer; 2019:38-60. Figure 3.19.

**Figures 33.5 and 33.9**

Reprinted with permission from Hypertrophic and other cardiomyopathies. In: Armstrong WF, Ryan T, eds. *Feigenbaum's Echocardiography.* 8th ed. Wolters Kluwer; 2019:539-560. Figures 18.19 and 18.58.

**Figure 33.7**

Reprinted with permission from Dilated cardiomyopathy. In: Armstrong WF, Ryan T, eds. *Feigenbaum's Echocardiography.* 8th ed. Wolters Kluwer; 2019:507-537. Figure 17.7.

**Figure 33.8**

Reprinted with permission from Echocardiography in systemic disease and specific clinical presentations. In: Armstrong WF, Ryan T, eds. *Feigenbaum's Echocardiography.* 8th ed. Wolters Kluwer; 2019:692-726. Figure 22.75.

**CHAPTER 34**

**Table 34.1**

From Brady WJ, Aufderheide TP, Chan T, et al. Electrocardiographic diagnosis of acute myocardial infarction. Emerg Med Clin North Am 2001;19:295-320.

**Figure 34.3**

Reprinted with permission from Lamabert AS. Mitral regurgitation. In: Perrino AC, Reeves ST, eds. *A Practical Approach to Transesophageal Echocardiography.* 2nd ed. Wolters Kluwer; 2008:171-188. Figure 8.6.

**Figure 34.5A**

Reproduced from Dominguez F, González-López E, Padron-Barthe L, Cavero MA, Garcia-Pavia P. Role of echocardiography in the diagnosis and management of hypertrophic cardiomyopathy. *Heart.* 2018;104(3):261-273; with permission from BMJ Publishing Group Ltd. Figure 3D.

**Figures 34.7 and 34.14**

Reprinted with permission from Olusesi O, Yeung M. Ischemic heart disease and complications of myocardial infarction. In: Quader N, Makan M, Perez P, eds. *The Washington Manual of Echocardiography.* 2nd ed. Wolters Kluwer; 2017:81-92. Figure 7.8A.

**Figure 34.10**

Reprinted with permission from Culp WC Jr, Knight WL. Echo rounds: three-dimensional transesophageal echocardiography of papillary muscle rupture. *Anesth Analg.* 2010 Aug;111(2):358-360. Figure 1.

**CHAPTER 35**

**Figure 35.15**

From Nagueh SF, Smiseth OA, Appleton CP, et al. Recommendations for the evaluation of left ventricular diastolic function by echocardiography: an update from the American Society of Echocardiography and the European Association of Cardiovascular Imaging. *J Am Soc Echocardiogr.* 2016;29:277-314. Figure 8.

**CHAPTER 37**

**Figures 37.1, 37.2BD, 37.4ABC, 37.7A, and 37.8**

Reprinted with permission from Congenital heart diseases. In: Armstrong WF, Ryan T, eds. *Feigenbaum's Echocardiography.* 7th ed. Wolters Kluwer; 2010:561-632. Figures 20.44, 20.88A, 20.78A, 20.72A, 20.74, 20.66, 20.45, and 20.78BC.

**Figures 37.2A, 37.4D, 37.5, 37.6, 37.7BD, 37.9, and 37.10A, B-F**

Reprinted with permission from Congenital heart diseases. In: Armstrong WF, Ryan T, eds. *Feigenbaum's Echocardiography.* 8th ed. Wolters Kluwer; 2019:544-610. Figures 19.98, 19.67AC, 19.95A, 19.78AB, 19.54, 19.57AC, 19.39, 19.63, and 19.64.

**Figure 37.2C**

Reprinted with permission from The echocardiographic examination. In: Armstrong WF, Ryan T, eds. *Feigenbaum's Echocardiography.* 7th ed. Wolters Kluwer; 2010:91-121. Figure 5.24.

**Figure 37.3**

From Smer A, Nanda NC, Akdogan RE, Elmarzouky ZM, Dulal S. Echocardiographic evaluation of mitral valve regurgitation. *Mini-invasive Surg.* 2020;4:52. Figure 1.

**CHAPTER 38**

**Figures 38.1 and 38.2**

Reprinted with permission from Brenes JC, Asher CR. Cardiac ultrasound artifacts. In: Klein AL, ed. *Clinical Echocardiography Review.* 2nd ed. Wolters Kluwer; 2018:15-29. Figures 2.2 and 2.20AB.

**Figure 38.3**

Reprinted with permission from Echocardiography and coronary artery disease. In: Armstrong WF, Ryan T, eds. *Feigenbaum's Echocardiography.* 8th ed. Wolters Kluwer; 2019:427-459. Figure 15.65.

**Figure 38.4**

Reprinted from Eddicks S, Kivelitz D, Breitwieser C, et al. Right ventricular metastasis caused by a renal cell carcinoma (Grawitz tumor): case report. *J Am Soc Echocardiogr.* 2006 Aug;19(8):1073.e11-15. Copyright © 2006 American Society of Echocardiography. With permission. Figure 2.

**Figure 38.5**

Reprinted from Weems WB, Aronson S, Yang X, Jayakar D, Jeevanandam V, Lang RM. Papillary fibroelastoma of the aortic valve. *J Am Soc Echocardiogr.* 2002 Apr;15(4):382-384. Copyright © 2002 American Society of Echocardiography. With permission. Figure 1.

**Figure 38.7**

Reprinted with permission from Weiner SD, Tumors HS. Masses, and source of emboli. In: Klein AL, ed. *Clinical Echocardiography Review.* 2nd ed. Wolters Kluwer; 2018:519-533. Figure 29.3.

**Figure 38.8**

Reprinted with permission from Left and right atrium, and right ventricle. In: Armstrong WF, Ryan T, eds. *Feigenbaum's Echocardiography.* 8th ed. Wolters Kluwer; 2019:158-193. Figure 7.40.

## CHAPTER 41

**Figure 41.13**

Reprinted by permission from Monnet X, Teboul JL. Passive leg raising. *Intensive Care Med.* 2008;34:659-663. Figure 1.

**Figure 41.15**

Courtesy of Mark Hamlin, MD and from Marik PE, Monnet X, Teboul JL. Hemodynamic parameters to guide fluid therapy. *Ann Intensive Care.* 2011 Mar 21;1(1):1. Copyright © 2011 Marik et al; licensee Springer. https://creativecommons.org/licenses/by/2.0/. Figure 4.

## CHAPTER 42

**Figure 42.14CD**

Reprinted from Mitter SS, Shah SJ, Thomas JD. A test in context: E/A and E/e' to assess diastolic dysfunction and LV filling pressure. *J Am Coll Cardiol.* 2017 Mar 21;69(11):1451-1464. Copyright © 2017 by the American College of Cardiology Foundation. With permission. Figures 1 and 2.

## CHAPTER 45

**Figure 45.24**

Reprinted from Ono R, Falcão LM. Takotsubo cardiomyopathy systematic review: pathophysiologic process, clinical presentation and diagnostic approach to Takotsubo cardiomyopathy. *Int J Cardiol.* 2016 Apr 15;209:196-205. Copyright © 2016 Elsevier. With permission. Figure 2.

## CHAPTER 46

**Figure 46.1**

From Laselle BT, Kendall JL. Trauma. In: Cosby KS, Kendall JL, eds. *Practical Guide to Emergency Ultrasound.* 2nd ed. Wolters Kluwer; 2014:21-54. Figure 3.11c.

**Figure 46.2**

Reprinted with permission from Vachha BA, Tsai LL, Lee KS, Camacho MA. Diagnostic imaging in acute surgical care. In: Britt LD, Peitzman A, Barie P, Jurkovich G, eds. *Acute Care Surgery.* Wolters Kluwer; 2013:104-126. Figure 9.5.

**Video 46.1**

Courtesy of Dr. Justin Bowra and *The Pocus Atlas.* From Bowra J. Trauma. *The POCUS Atlas.* Accessed December 4, 2020. https://www.thepocusatlas.com/trauma/g6302hr5hk6l2cu7vgvwu4yf57y9jn.

**Figure 46.5**

From Laselle BT, Kendall JL. Trauma. In: Cosby KS, Kendall JL, eds. *Practical Guide to Emergency Ultrasound.* 2nd ed. Wolters Kluwer; 2014:21-54. Figure 3.53.

**Figure 46.6**

From Huang C, Liteplo AS, Noble VE. Lung and thorax. In: Cosby KS, Kendall JL, eds. *Practical Guide to Emergency Ultrasound.* Wolters Kluwer; 2014:75-83. Figure 5.6.

**Figure 46.7**

From Huang C, Liteplo AS, Noble VE. Lung and thorax. In: Cosby KS, Kendall JL, eds. *Practical Guide to Emergency Ultrasound.* 2nd ed. Wolters Kluwer; 2014:75-83. Figure 5.9.

**Video 46.2**

Courtesy of Dr. Dr Justin Bowra and *The Pocus Atlas.* From Bowra J. Pulmonary/Lung. *The POCUS Atlas website.* Accessed December 4, 2020. https://www.thepocusatlas.com/lung/9kalmbf8y6j0nrspwvv876nyem83t5.

**Figure 46.9**

From Huang C, Liteplo AS, Noble VE. Lung and thorax. In: Cosby KS, Kendall JL, eds. *Practical Guide to Emergency Ultrasound.* 2nd ed. Wolters Kluwer; 2014:75-83. Figure 5.16.

**Video 46.3**

Courtesy of E. Liang Liu, MD.

**Figure 46.10**

From Pericardial diseases. In: Armstrong WF, Ryan T, eds. *Feigenbaum's Echocardiography.* 8th ed. Wolters Kluwer; 2019:217-239. Figure 9.26.

**Figure 46.11**

From Pericardial diseases. In: Armstrong WF, Ryan T, eds. *Feigenbaum's Echocardiography.* 8th ed. Wolters Kluwer; 2019:217-239. Figure 9.25.

**Video 46.4**

Courtesy of Dr. Shahad Al Chalaby and *The Pocus Atlas.* From Alerhand S. Pericardial tamponade. *The POCUS Atlas* website. Accessed December 4, 2020. https://www.thepocusatlas.com/echocardiography/pericardial-tamponade.

**Video 46.5**

Courtesy of Dr. Stephen Alerhand and *The Pocus Atlas.* From Alerhand S. Cardiac tamponade. *The POCUS Atlas* website. November 15, 2017. Accessed December 4, 2020. https://www.thepocusatlas.com/echocardiography/2017/11/15/cardiac-tamponade.

## CHAPTER 47

**Video 47.1**

Reprinted from Cavayas YA, Sampson C, Yusuff H. A 17-year-old male adolescent with shortness of breath, fever, and right pleuritic chest pain. *Chest.* 2017 Oct;152(4):e85-e87. Copyright © 2017 American College of Chest Physicians. With permission. Video 1.

**Figures 47.1, 47.2, 47.3, and 47.6**

Courtesy of Dr. Allison C. Ferreira.

**Figure 47.4**

Courtesy of Andrew T. Young.

**Figure 47.7**

Reprinted with permission from Boretsky KR. Images in anesthesiology: point-of-care ultrasound to diagnose esophageal intubation: "The Double Trachea." *Anesthesiology.* 2018;129(1):190. Figure 1.

## CHAPTER 49

**Figure 49.2**

From Blanco P, Aguiar FM, Blaivas M. Rapid Ultrasound in Shock (RUSH) velocity-time integral: a proposal to expand the RUSH protocol. *J Ultrasound Med.* 2015 Sep;34(9):1691-700. Copyright © 2016 by the American Institute of Ultrasound in Medicine. Reprinted by permission of John Wiley & Sons, Inc. Figure 4.

**Figure 49.8**

Reprinted with permission from Jozwiak M, Depret F, Teboul JL, et al. Predicting fluid responsiveness in critically ill patients by using combined end-expiratory and end-inspiratory occlusions with echocardiography. *Crit Care Med. 2017*;45:e1131-e1138. Figure 1.

**Figure 49.9**

Reprinted from Beaubien-Souligny W, Bouchard J, Desjardins G, et al. Extracardiac signs of fluid overload in the critically ill cardiac patient: a focused evaluation using bedside ultrasound. *Can J Cardiol. 2017*;33(1):88-100. Copyright © 2016 Canadian Cardiovascular Society. With permission. Figure 5.

**Figure 49.10**

Reprinted with permission from Barjaktarevic I, Toppen WE, Hu S, et al. Ultrasound assessment of the change in carotid corrected flow time in fluid responsiveness in undifferentiated shock. *Crit Care Med.* 2018;46:e1040-e1046. Figure 1.

## CHAPTER 50

**Figure 50.3D**

Reprinted from Nagueh SF, Smiseth OA, Appleton CP, et al. Recommendations for the evaluation of left ventricular diastolic function by echocardiography: an update from the American Society of Echocardiography and the European Association of Cardiovascular Imaging. *J Am Soc Echocardiogr.* 2016 Apr;29(4):277-314. Figure 14. Copyright © 2016 American Society of Echocardiography. Published by Mosby, Inc. All rights reserved.

**Figure 50.39**

From Oh JK. Assessment of diastolic function. In: Oh JK, Kane GC, Seward JB, Tajik AJ, eds. *The Echo Manual.* 4th ed. Wolters Kluwer; 2019. Figure 8.8B.

**Figure 50.40**

From Giannakopoulos G, Rey F, Müller H. Pathophysiology of the aortic regurgitation Doppler signal end-diastolic notching: "A-dip insight." *Echocardiography.* 2020 Jul;37(7):1116-1119. Copyright © 2020 Wiley Periodicals LLC. Reprinted by permission of John Wiley & Sons, Inc. Figure 1.

**Figure 50.41**

Reprinted from Silbiger JJ. Pathophysiology and echocardiographic diagnosis of left ventricular diastolic dysfunction. *J Am Soc Echocardiogr.* 2019 Feb;32(2):216-232.e2. Copyright © 2018 by the American Society of Echocardiography. With permission. Figure 14.

**Figure 50.47**

Reprinted from Nagueh SF, Smiseth OA, Appleton CP, et al. Recommendations for the evaluation of left ventricular diastolic function by echocardiography: an update from the American Society of Echocardiography and the European Association of Cardiovascular Imaging. *J Am Soc Echocardiogr.* 2016 Apr;29(4):277-314. Copyright © 2016 American Society of Echocardiography. With permission. Figure 8.

**Figure 50.59**

Adapted from Abudiab MM, Chebrolu LH, Schutt RC, Nagueh SF, Zoghbi WA. Doppler echocardiography for the estimation of LV filling pressure in patients with mitral annular calcification. *JACC Cardiovasc Imaging.* 2017 Dec;10(12):1411-1420. Copyright © 2017 by the American College of Cardiology Foundation. With permission.

## CHAPTER 52

**Figure 52.5**

Reprinted by permission from Springer Nature: Springer Nature. Goffi A, Kruisselbrink R, Volpicelli G. The sound of air: point-of-care lung ultrasound in perioperative medicine. *Can J Anaesth.* Figure 3.

**Figure 52.8**

Images adapted from http://pie.med.utoronto.ca/POCUS.

## CHAPTER 53

**Figure 53.6**

Reprinted with permission from Mongodi S, Stella A, Orlando A, Mojoli F. B-lines visualization and lung aeration assessment: mind the ultrasound machine setting. *Anesthesiology.* 2019;130(3):444. Figure 1.

**Video 53.8, Figure 53.8, and Video 53.11**

Courtesy of Dr. Gregory Mints, MD.

**Table 53.1**

Data from Copetti, R, Soldati G, Copetti P. Chest sonography: a useful tool to differentiate acute cardiogenic pulmonary edema from acute respiratory distress syndrome. *Cardiovasc Ultrasound.* 2008 Apr 29;6:16.

## CHAPTER 54

**Figure 54.16**

Image provided courtesy of Dr. James Rippey.

## CHAPTER 57

**Video 57.1**

From Arya R, Schrift D, Choe C, Al-Jaghbeer M. Real-time tracheal ultrasound for the confirmation of endotracheal intubations in the intensive care unit: an observational study. *J Ultrasound Med.* 2019;38(2):491-497. Copyright © 2018 by the American Institute of Ultrasound in Medicine. Reprinted by permission of John Wiley & Sons, Inc. Video 1.

**Figure 57.2**

Reproduced with permission from John Wiley & Sons: Arya R, Schrift D, Choe C, Al-Jaghbeer M. Real-time tracheal ultrasound for the confirmation of endotracheal intubations in the intensive care unit: an observational study. J Ultrasound Med. 2019;38(2):491-497.

**Figures 57.3 and 57.4**

With permission from The Scandinavian Airway Management course www.airwaymanagement.dk.

## CHAPTER 59

**Figure 59.1**

Reprinted with permission from Laya BF, Amini B, Zucker EJ, Kilborn T, Vargas SO, Lee EY. In: Lee EY, ed. *Pediatric Radiology: Practical Imaging Evaluation of Infants and Children.* Wolters Kluwer; 2018:358-458. Figure 6.3.

**Figure 59.2**

Reprinted with permission from Left and right atrium, and right ventricle. In: Armstrong WF, Ryan T, eds. *Feigenbaum's Echocardiography.* 8th ed. Wolters Kluwer; 2019:158-193. Figure 7.73.

**Figure 59.3**

Reprinted with permission from Davis A, Boone LT. Ischemic heart disease and complications of myocardial infarctions. In: Anderson B, Park MM, eds. *Basic to Advanced Clinical Echocardiography.* Wolters Kluwer; 2021:265-281. Figure 16.16.

**Figure 59.4**

Reprinted with permission from Moradi A, Sud K, Danik J. Mitral valve disease in the cardiac care unit. In: Herzog E, ed. *Herzog's CCU Book.* Wolters Kluwer; 2018:397-406. Figure 36.3.

**Figure 59.5**

Reprinted with permission from Infective endocarditis. In: Armstrong WF, Ryan T, eds. *Feigenbaum's Echocardiography.* 8th ed. Wolters Kluwer; 2019:347-376. Figure 13.45.

## Figure 59.6

Reprinted with permission from Echocardiography in systemic disease and clinical problem solving. In: Armstrong WF, Ryan T, eds. *Feigenbaum's Echocardiography*. 7th ed. Wolters Kluwer; 2010:741-774. Figure 24.30.

## Figures 59.7 and 59.10

Reprinted with permission from Barron KR, Wagner M. Does the patient have a pneumothorax? In: Bornemann P, ed. *Ultrasound for Primary Care*. Wolters Kluwer; 2021:97-103. Figures 14.6 and 14.9.

## Figure 59.8

Reprinted with permission from Obstructive disease and ventilatory failure. In: Marini JJ, Dries DJ. *Critical Care Medicine*. 5th ed. Wolters Kluwer; 2019:525-546. Figure 25.5.

## Figure 59.9

Reprinted with permission from Taylor RA, Moore CL. Echocardiography. In: Cosby KS, Kendall JL, eds. *Practical Guide to Emergency Ultrasound*. 2nd ed. Wolters Kluwer; 2014:55-74. Figure 4.33.

## CHAPTER 60

### Figure 60.2A

Reprinted with permission from Lichtenstein DA, Meziere G, Lascols N, et al. Ultrasound diagnosis of occult pneumothorax. *Crit Care Med*. 2005;33(6):1231-1238.

### Figure 60.2BD

From Huang C, Liteplo AS, Noble VE. Lung and thorax. In: Cosby KS, Kendall JL, eds. *Practical Guide to Emergency Ultrasound*. 2nd ed. Wolters Kluwer; 2014:75-83. Figure 5.8.

### Figure 60.2C

From Roch A, Bojan M, Michelet P, et al. Usefulness of ultrasonography in predicting pleural effusions >500 mL in patients receiving mechanical ventilation. *Chest*. 2005;127(1):224-232.

### Figure 60.3AB

From Laselle BT, Kendall JL. Trauma. In: Cosby KS, Kendall JL, eds. *Practical Guide to Emergency Ultrasound*. 2nd ed. Wolters Kluwer; 2014:21-54. Figures 3.79 and 3.78.

### Figure 60.6

From French AJ, English J, Stone MB, Frazee BW. Soft tissue and musculoskeletal procedures. In: Cosby KS, Kendall JL, eds. *Practical Guide to Emergency Ultrasound*. 2nd ed. Wolters Kluwer; 2014:319-349. Figure 22.26a.

## CHAPTER 61

### Figure 61.1

Reprinted with permission from Fentress M. Does the patient have cholelithiasis or cholecystitis?. In: Bornemann P, ed. *Ultrasound for Primary Care*. Wolters Kluwer; 2021:151-157. Figure 22.4C.

### Figures 61.3, 61.14, and 61.29

Reprinted from Oppenheimer DC, Rubens DJ. Sonography of acute cholecystitis and its mimics. *Radiol Clin North Am*. 2019 May;57(3):535-548. Copyright © 2019 Elsevier. With permission. Figures 1B and 10CD.

### Figures 61.8 and 61.25AB

Reprinted from Connor-Schuler R, Binz S, Clark C. Portal venous gas on point-of-care ultrasound in a case of cecal ischemia. *J Emerg Med*. 2020 Mar;58(3):e117-e120. Copyright © 2019 Elsevier. With permission. Figures 1-3.

### Figures 61.11 and 61.26

Reprinted from Irshad A, Anis M, Ackerman SJ. Current role of ultrasound in chronic liver disease: surveillance, diagnosis and management of hepatic neoplasms. *Curr Probl Diagn Radiol*. 2012 Mar-Apr;41(2):43-51. Copyright © 2012 Elsevier. With permission. Figures 1 and 3.

### Figure 61.12B

Reprinted with permission from Siegel MJ, Masand PM. Liver. In: Siegel MJ, ed. *Pediatric Sonography*. 5th ed. Wolters Kluwer; 2019:211-272. Figure 7.62C.

### Figure 61.16

Reprinted by permission from Pace J, Arntfield R. Focused assessment with sonography in trauma: a review of concepts and considerations for anesthesiology. *Can J Anaesth*. 2018 Apr;65(4):360-370. Figure 9.

### Figure 61.17

Reprinted from Copelan A, Bahoura L, Tardy F, Kirsch M, Sokhandon F, Kapoor B. Etiology, diagnosis, and management of bilomas: a current update. *Tech Vasc Interv Radiol*. 2015 Dec;18(4):236-243. Copyright © 2015 Elsevier. With permission. Figure 1.

### Figure 61.22

From Xiang H, Han J, Ridley WE, Ridley LJ. Mickey mouse signs. *J Med Imaging Radiat Oncol*. 2018 Oct;62 Suppl 1:92. Copyright © 2018 The Royal Australian and New Zealand College of Radiologists. Reprinted by permission of John Wiley & Sons, Inc. Figure 1A.

### Figure 61.24

Reprinted by permission from Minault Q, Gaiddon C, Veillon F, Venkatasamy A. The champagne sign. *Abdom Radiol (NY)*. 2018 Oct;43(10):2888-2889. Figure 1A.

## CHAPTER 62

### Figure 62.4

Adapted from Denault AY, Couture EJ, Sia YT, et al. Right ventricle, right atrium, tricuspid and pulmonic valves. In: Perrino AC, Reeves ST, eds. *A Practical Approach to Transesophageal Echocardiography*. 4th ed. Philadelphia, PA: Wolters Kluwer; 2020:345-380. Figure 14.11; Amsallem M, Kuznetsova T, Hanneman K, et al. Right heart imaging in patients with heart failure: a tale of two ventricles. *Curr Opin Cardiol*. 2016;31(5):469-482; and Tang WH, Kitai T. Intrarenal venous flow: a window into the congestive kidney failure phenotype of heart failure? *JACC Heart Fail*. 2016;4(8):683-686.

### Table 62.1

Adapted from Amsallem M, Kuznetsova T, Hanneman K, et al. Right heart imaging in patients with heart failure: a tale of two ventricles. *Curr Opin Cardiol*. 2016;31(5):469-482; Tang WH, Kitai T. Intrarenal venous flow: a window into the congestive kidney failure phenotype of heart failure? *JACC Heart Fail*. 2016;4(8):683-686; Perrino AC, Reeves ST, eds. *A Practical Approach to Transesophageal Echocardiography*. 4th ed. Wolters Kluwer; 2020.

## CHAPTER 63

### Figure 63.1

Reprinted with permission from Branney SW, Wolfe RE, Moore EE, et al. Quantitative sensitivity of ultrasound in detecting free intraperitoneal fluid. *J Trauma Acute Care Surg*. 1995;39(2):375-380. Figure 1.

### Figure 63.2

Reprinted with permission from Auckland AK. Unexplained hematocrit drop. In: Sanders RC, ed. *Clinical Sonography: A Practical Guide*. 5th ed. Wolters Kluwer; 2016:588-595. Figure 45.7.

### Figure 63.3

Courtesy of Dr. Rohan Panchamia, Weill Cornell Medical Center.

### Figure 63.5

Reprinted with permission from Indiran V, Vinoth Kumar R, Jefferson B. Enhanced peritoneal stripe sign. *Abdom Radiol (NY)*. 2018 Dec;43(12):3518-3519. Figure 1.

**Figures 63.4 and 63.12**

From Goudie A. Detection of intraperitoneal free gas by ultrasound. *Australas J Ultrasound Med.* 2013 May;16(2):56-61. Copyright © 2013 Australasian Society for Ultrasound in Medicine. Reprinted by permission of John Wiley & Sons, Inc. Figures 1 and 4.

**Figures 63.6A-D and 63.13**

Reprinted by permission from Asrani A. Sonographic diagnosis of pneumoperitoneum using the "enhancement of the peritoneal stripe sign." A prospective study. *Emerg Radiol.* 2007 Apr;14(1):29-39. Figures 1ab, 2b, and 3b.

**Figures 63.7AC and 63.9**

Reprinted with permission from Laselle BT, Kendall JL. Trauma. In: Cosby KS, Kendall JL, eds. *Practical Guide to Emergency Ultrasound.* 2nd ed. Wolters Kluwer; 2014:21-53. Figures 3.62, 3.43, and 3.37.

**Figure 63.7B**

Reprinted with permission from Kelley K, Rose JS, Bair AE. Fundamentals of ultrasound. In: Cosby KS, Kendall JL, eds. *Practical Guide to Emergency Ultrasound.* 2nd ed. Wolters Kluwer; 2014:10-20. Figure 2.11a.

**Figure 63.8**

Reprinted with permission from Focused assessment with sonography for trauma (FAST). In: Loukas M, Burns D, eds. *Essential Ultrasound Anatomy.* 1st ed. Wolters Kluwer; 2020:246-258. Figure 12.3.

**Figure 63.10**

Reprinted with permission from Stratta E, Johnson K. Does the patient have ascites? In: Bornemann P, ed. *Ultrasound for Primary Care.* Wolters Kluwer; 2021:143-150. Figure 21.4.

**Figure 63.11**

Reprinted with permission from Rao VV, Haddad R. Ultrasound basics: physics, transducers, conventions, terminology, and artifacts. In: Bornemann P, ed. *Ultrasound for Primary Care.* Wolters Kluwer; 2021:3-12. Figure 1.24.

## CHAPTER 66

**Figure 66.10**

From Wang RC, Knight RS. First trimester pregnancy. In: Cosby KS, Kendall JL, eds. *Practical Guide to Emergency Ultrasound.* 2nd ed. Wolters Kluwer; 2014:218-235. Figure 15.1ab.

**Figure 66.11**

Reproduced with permission from Auckland A. Sonographic assessment of the ectopic pregnancy. In: Stephenson SR, Dmitrieva J, eds. *Diagnostic Medical Sonography: Obstetrics and Gynecology.* Wolters Kluwer; 2018:371-390. Figure 17.12.

**Figure 66.12**

Reprinted with permission from Ward VL, Estroff JA. Radiologic imaging. In: Emans SJ, Laufer MR, DiVasta A, eds. *Emans, Laufer, Goldstein's Pediatric and Adolescent Gynecology.* 7th ed. Wolters Kluwer; 2020:575-609. Figure 37.42.

**Figure 66.13**

Reprinted with permission from Ovaries and adnexa. In: Doubilet PM, Benson CB, Benacerraf BR, eds. *Atlas of Ultrasound in Obstetrics and Gynecology.* 3rd ed. Wolters Kluwer; 2019:436-459. Figure 31.2.1ab.

**Figure 66.14**

Reprinted with permission from Iyer RS, Chapman T. *Pediatric Radiology: The Essentials.* Wolters Kluwer; 2015. Figure 45.3.

**Figure 66.15**

Reprinted with permission from Ovaries and adnexa. In: Doubilet PM, Benson CB, Benacerraf BR, eds. *Atlas of Ultrasound in Obstetrics and Gynecology.* 3rd ed. Wolters Kluwer; 2019:436-459. Figure 31.9.3ab.

## CHAPTER 67

**Figures 67.8, 67.9, 67.11, 67.12, 67.13AB, 67.14, 67.15, Videos 67.7, 67.8, 67.10, 67.11, 67.12AB, 67.13AB, and 67.15**

Reprinted with permission from Dean AJ. Abdominal aorta. In: Cosby KS, Kendall JL, eds. *Practical Guide to Emergency Ultrasound.* 2nd ed. Wolters Kluwer Health; 2014:156-171. Video 10.21AB, Figure 10.21, Video 10.17, Figure 10.26, Video 10.8AB, Video 10.1, Figure 10.4B, Video 10.2, Video 10.8DE, Video 10.20AB, Video 10.3.

**Figure 67.22**

Reprinted with permission from Hannon KM. Vascular structures. In: Kawamura D, Lunsford B, eds. *Abdomen and Superficial Structures.* 3rd ed. Wolters Kluwer; 2013:57-100. Figure 4.13.

## CHAPTER 68

**Figure 68.2**

Reprinted with permission from El-Boghdadly K, Kruisselbrink R, Chan VWS, Perlas A. Images in anesthesiology: gastric ultrasound. *Anesthesiology.* 2016;125(3):595.

## CHAPTER 69

**Figure 69.1**

Reprinted with permission from Cosby KS, Kendall JL. Right upper quadrant: liver, gallbladder, and biliary tree. In: Cosby KS, Kendall JL, eds. *Practical Guide to Emergency Ultrasound.* 2nd ed. Wolters Kluwer; 2014:133-155. Figure 9.34a.

**Figure 69.2**

Reprinted with permission from Dean AJ. Abdominal aorta. In: Cosby KS, Kendall JL, eds. *Practical Guide to Emergency Ultrasound.* 2nd ed. Wolters Kluwer; 2014:156-171. Figure 10.33.

**Figures 69.3 and 69.18**

Reprinted with permission from Bailitz J. A problem-based approach to resuscitation of acute illness or injury. In: Cosby KS, Kendall JL, eds. *Practical Guide to Emergency Ultrasound.* 2nd ed. Wolters Kluwer; 2014:96-107. Figure 7.12.

**Figure 69.4**

Reprinted with permission from Smith EA, Smith WL. Pediatric imaging. In: Farrell TA, ed. *Radiology 101.* Wolters Kluwer; 2020:144-174. Figure 5.47.

**Figure 69.5**

Reprinted with permission from Cosby KS, Kendall JL. Right upper quadrant: liver, gallbladder, and biliary tree. In: Cosby KS, Kendall JL, eds. *Practical Guide to Emergency Ultrasound.* 2nd ed. Wolters Kluwer; 2014:133-155. Figure 9.41.

**Figure 69.6**

Reprinted with permission from Laselle BT, Kendall JL. Trauma. In: Cosby KS, Kendall JL, eds. *Practical Guide to Emergency Ultrasound.* 2nd ed. Wolters Kluwer; 2014:21-54. Figure 3.22.

**Figure 69.7**

Reprinted with permission from Tayal VS, Lewis MR. Does the patient have a bowel obstruction? In: Bornemann P, ed. *Ultrasound for Primary Care.* Wolters Kluwer; 2021:158-162. Figure 23.4.

**Figure 69.8**

Reprinted with permission from Bogler DM. Possible renal mass. In: Sanders RC, ed. *Clinical Sonography: A Practical Guide.* 5th ed. Wolters Kluwer; 575-587. Figure 44.7.

**Figures 69.9 and 69.10**

Reprinted with permission from Bieker TM. The gallbladder and biliary system. In: Kawamura D, Nolan T, eds. *Abdomen and Superficial Structures.* 4th ed. Wolters Kluwer; 2018:171-211. Figures 6.30 and 6.33.

**Figure 69.11**

Reprinted with permission from Daffner RH, Hartman M. Abdominal radiographs. In: Daffner RH, Hartman M, eds. *Clinical Radiology*. 4th ed. Wolters Kluwer; 2014:215-251. Figure 7.3a.

**Figure 69.12**

Reprinted with permission from Murakami ME, Cernigliaro JG. Imaging in gynecologic emergencies. In: Benrubi GI, ed. *Handbook of Obstetric and Gynecologic Emergencies*. 4th ed. Wolters Kluwer; 2011:354-378. Figure 28.15.

**Figure 69.13**

Reprinted with permission from Fentress M. Does the patient have cholelithiasis or cholecystitis?. In: Bornemann P, ed. *Ultrasound for Primary Care*. Wolters Kluwer; 2021:151-157. Figure 22.4.

**Figure 69.14**

Reprinted with permission from Brant W. Abdomen ultrasound. In: Klein J, Vinson EN, Brant WE, Helms CA, eds. *Brant and Helms' Fundamentals of Diagnostic Radiology*. 5th ed. Wolters Kluwer; 2019:1156-1191. Figure 50.44.

**Figure 69.15**

From Llewellyn ME, Jeffrey RB, DiMaio MA, Olcott EW. The sonographic "bright band sign" of splenic infarction. *J Ultrasound Med*. 2014 Jun;33(6):929-938. Copyright © 2016 by the American Institute of Ultrasound in Medicine. Reprinted by permission of John Wiley & Sons, Inc. Figure 2.

**Figure 69.16**

Reprinted with permission from Invasive procedures and surgical asepsis. In: Penny SM, ed. *Introduction to Sonography and Patient Care*. 2nd ed. Wolters Kluwer; 2021:387-409. Figure 13.2.

**Figure 69.17**

Reprinted with permission from Laselle BT, Kendall JL. Trauma. In: Cosby KS, Kendall JL, eds. *Practical Guide to Emergency Ultrasound*. 2nd ed. Wolters Kluwer; 2014:21-54. Figure 3.11D.

**Figure 69.19**

Reprinted with permission from Milicevic MN. Echinococcal cyst—open and laparoscopic approach. In: Fischer J, ed. *Fischer's Mastery of Surgery*. 7th ed. Wolters Kluwer; 2019:1294-1314. Figure 106.5.

**Figure 69.20**

Reprinted with permission from Rybyinski A. Sonography-guided interventional procedures. In: Kawamura D, Nolan T, eds. *Abdomen and Superficial Structures*. 4th ed. Wolters Kluwer; 2018:795-811. Figure 27.11.

**Figure 69.21**

Reprinted with permission from Smith EA, Trout AT. Abdomen. In: Klein J, Vinson EN, Brant WE, Helms CA, eds. *Brant and Helms' Fundamentals of Diagnostic Radiology*. 5th ed. Wolters Kluwer; 2019:1495-1530. Figure 69.49.

**Table 69.1**

From Shekarchi B, Rafsanjani SZH, Fomani NSR, Chahardoli M. Emergency department bedside ultrasonography for diagnosis of acute cholecystitis; a diagnostic accuracy study. *Emerg (Tehran)*. 2018;6(1):e11. http://creativecommons.org/licenses/by/3.0/. Table 2.

## CHAPTER 70

**Figure 70.1AB**

Courtesy of John L. Kendall. From Fox JC, Vandordaklou N. Lower extremity venous studies. In: Cosby KS, Kendall JL, eds. *Practical Guide to Emergency Ultrasound*. 2nd ed. Wolters Kluwer; 2014:254-263. Figures 17.6a, 17.7, 17.13D, and 17.11ab.

**Figure 70.1C,D,E**

Reprinted with permission from Brant WE, Dougherty RS. Vascular ultrasound. In: Brant WE, Helms C, eds. *Fundamentals of Diagnostic Radiology*. 4th ed. Wolters Kluwer; 2013:954-978. Figure 39.32.

**Figure 70.2A,B**

Reprinted with permission from Talbot SR, Oliver M. Duplex imaging of the lower extremity venous system In: Kupinski AM, ed. *LWW Sonography: The Vascular System*. Wolters Kluwer; 2013:209-229. Figure 14.23.

**Figure 70.2C**

Courtesy of John L. Kendall. Reprinted with permission from Fox JC, Vandordaklou N. Lower extremity venous studies. In: Cosby KS, Kendall JL, eds. *Practical Guide to Emergency Ultrasound*. 2nd ed. Philadelphia, PA: Wolters Kluwer; 2014: 254-263. Figure 17.13D.

**Figure 70.3**

From Masses, tumors, and source of embolus. In: Armstrong WF, Ryan T, eds. *Feigenbaum's Echocardiography*. 8th ed. Wolters Kluwer; 2019:651-691. Figure 21.47.

**Figure 70.4**

Reprinted with permission from Moneta GL, Zaccardi MJ. Duplex evaluation of lower extremity arterial occlusive disease. In: Zierler R, Dawson D, eds. *Strandness's Duplex Scanning In Vascular Disorders*. 5th ed. Wolters Kluwer; 2016:151-163. Figure 12.1ab.

**Figure 70.5**

Reprinted with permission from Caps MT, Mraz BA. Upper extremity venous thrombosis. In: Zierler R, Dawson D, eds. *Strandness's Duplex Scanning in Vascular Disorders*. 5th ed. Wolters Kluwer; 2016:250-273. Figure 20.12b.

**Figure 70.6**

Reprinted with permission from Peripheral venous systems. In: Arger PH, Iyoob SD, eds. *Complete Guide to Vascular Ultrasound*. Wolters Kluwer; 2005:55-74. Figure 5.23a.

**Figure 70.7**

Reprinted with permission from Peripheral venous systems. In: Arger PH, Iyoob SD, eds. *Complete Guide to Vascular Ultrasound*. Wolters Kluwer; 2005:55-74. Figure 5.24.

**Figure 70.8**

Reprinted with permission from Bailitz J. A problem-based approach to resuscitation of acute illness or injury. In: Cosby KS, Kendall JL, eds. *Practical Guide to Emergency Ultrasound*. 2nd ed. Wolters Kluwer; 2014:96-107. Figure 7.8.

**Figure 70.9**

Images courtesy of Karen Cosby. From Fox JC, Vandordaklou N. Lower extremity venous studies. In: Cosby KS, Kendall JL, eds. Practical Guide to Emergency Ultrasound. 2nd ed. Philadelphia, PA: Wolters Kluwer; 2014:254-263. Figure 17.11ab.

**Table 70.2**

Adapted from Needleman L. Update on the lower extremity venous ultrasonography examination. *Radiol Clin North Am*. 2014;52:1359-1374.

**Figure 70.12**

Reprinted with permission from Eidem BW, O'Leary PW. Quantitative methods in echocardiography—basic techniques. In: Eidem BW, Cetta F, Johnson J, Lopez L, eds. *Echocardiography in Pediatric and Adult Congenital Heart Disease*. 3rd ed. Wolters Kluwer; 2021:42-66. Figure 3.18.

## CHAPTER 71

**Figure 71.3**

Reprinted with permission from Haystead C, Bowie JD, Kliewer MA, et al. Ultrasound. In: Provenzale JM, Nelson RC, Vinson EN, eds. *Duke Radiology Case Review*. 2nd ed. Wolters Kluwer; 2012:487-537. Figure 9.15A.

**Figure 71.4**

Reprinted with permission from Rybyinski A. Sonography-guided interventional procedures. In: Kawamura D, Nolan T, eds. *Abdomen and Superficial Structures*. 4th ed. Wolters Kluwer; 2018:795-811. Figure 27.20.

**Figure 71.5**

Reprinted with permission from Helms WE. Vascular ultrasound. In: Klein J, Vinson EN, Brant WE, Helms CA, eds. *Brant and Helms' Fundamentals of Diagnostic Radiology*. 5th ed. Wolters Kluwer; 2019:1252-1276. Figure 54.29.

## CHAPTER 72

**Figure 72.2**

Reprinted with permission from Dean AJ. Abdominal aorta. In: Cosby KS, Kendall JL, eds. *Practical Guide to Emergency Ultrasound*. 2nd ed. Wolters Kluwer; 2014:156-171. Figure 10.27b.

**Figure 72.4**

Reprinted with permission from Taylor RA, Moore CL. Echocardiography. In: Cosby KS, Kendall JL, eds. *Practical Guide to Emergency Ultrasound*. 2nd ed. Wolters Kluwer; 2014:55-74. Figure 4.45.

## CHAPTER 73

**Figures 73.4, 73.10, and 73.12**

Reprinted with permission from Rao PK, Quader N. Diseases of the great vessels. In: Quader N, Makan M, Perez P, eds. *The Washington Manual of Echocardiography*. 2nd ed. Wolters Kluwer; 2017:220-241. Figure 17.8.

**Figure 73.5**

Reprinted with permission from Rao PK, Quader N. Diseases of the great vessels. In: Quader N, Makan M, Perez P, eds. *The Washington Manual of Echocardiography*. 2nd ed. Wolters Kluwer; 2017:220-241. Figure 17.6.

**Figure 73.7**

Reprinted with permission from Payne KJ, Ikonomidis JS, Reeves ST. Transesophageal echocardiography of the thoracic aorta. In: Perrino AC, Reeves ST, eds. *Practical Approach to Transesophageal Echocardiography*. 2nd ed. Wolters Kluwer; 2008:321-347. Figure 16.11.

**Figure 73.11**

Reprinted with permission from Rao PK, Quader N. Diseases of the great vessels. In: Quader N, Makan M, Perez P, eds. *The Washington Manual of Echocardiography*. 2nd ed. Wolters Kluwer; 2017:220-241. Figure 17.11.

**Figure 73.13**

Reprinted with permission from Jayasuriya S. Statistics for the echo boards. In: Sorrell VL, Jayasuriya S, eds. Questions, Tricks, and Tips for the Echocardiography Boards. 2nd ed. Wolters Kluwer; 2019:7-9. Figure 2.1a.

**Figure 73.17**

From Diseases of the aorta. In: Armstrong WF, Ryan T, eds. *Feigenbaum's Echocardiography*. 8th ed. Wolters Kluwer; 2019:611-650. Figure 20.50.

**Figure 73.19**

From Lang RM, Badano LP, Mor-Avi V, et al. Recommendations for cardiac chamber quantification by echocardiography in adults: an update from the American Society of Echocardiography and the European Association of Cardiovascular Imaging. *J Am Soc Echocardiogr*. 2015;28:1-39.

## CHAPTER 74

**Figure 74.1**

Reprinted with permission from Aziz SG, Patel BB, Ie SR, Rubio ER. The lung point sign, not pathognomonic of a pneumothorax. *Ultrasound Q*. 2016;32:277-279.

## CHAPTER 75

**Figure 75.4**

From Lichtenstein DA, Mezière G, Lascols N, et al. Ultrasound diagnosis of occult pneumothorax. *Crit Care Med*. 2005 Jun;33(6):1231-1238. Figure 9.

## CHAPTER 79

**Figure 79.1**

Courtesy of Meghan Herbst under the Creative Commons License: https://wikem.org/wiki/File:Isoechoic_abscess.png (https://creativecommons.org/licenses/by-sa/3.0/).

**Figure 79.3**

Courtesy of Dr Dinesh Brand under the Creative Commons License.

**Figure 79.4**

Image courtesy of Dr. Maulik S Patel under the Creative Commons License.

## CHAPTER 80

**Figures 80.3 and 80.4**

Reprinted with permission from Balki M. Locating the epidural space in obstetric patients—ultrasound a useful tool: continuing professional development. *Can J Anesth*. 2010;57:1111-1126.

## CHAPTER 81

**Figure 81.1**

Reproduced from Denault A, Vegas A, Lamarche Y, Tardif J-C, Couture P. *Basic Transesophageal and Critical Care Ultrasound*. 1st ed. Taylor and Francis, CRC Press; 2018; with permission of Taylor and Francis Group, LLC, a division of Informa plc.

**Figure 81.2**

Adapted from Azzam MA, Couture EJ, Beaubien-Souligny W, Brassard P, Gebhard CE, Denault AY. A proposed algorithm for combining transcranial Doppler ultrasound monitoring with cerebral and somatic oximetry: a case report. *Can J Anaesth*. 2021;68:130-136.

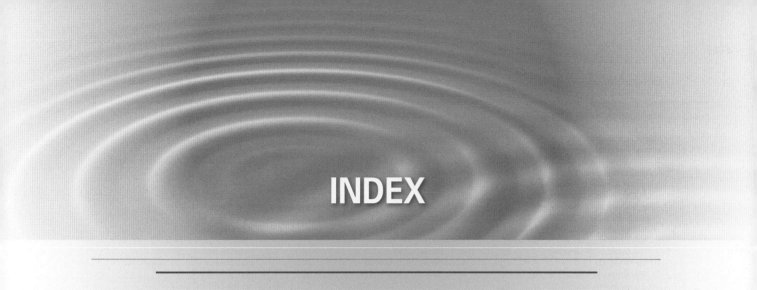

# INDEX

**Note:** Page numbers followed by *f* and *t* indicate figures and tables respectively.